YO-ART-740

Clinical Pharmacology

Basic Principles in Therapeutics

EDITED BY

Kenneth L. Melmon, M.D.

Associate Professor of Medicine and Pharmacology,
and Chief, Division of Clinical Pharmacology,
University of California School of Medicine, San Francisco, California

AND

Howard F. Morrelli, M.D.

Associate Professor of Medicine and Pharmacology,
and Vice Chairman (House Staff Affairs), Department of Medicine,
University of California School of Medicine, San Francisco, California

THE MACMILLAN COMPANY
New York

COLLIER-MACMILLAN LIMITED *London*
COLLIER-MACMILLAN CANADA LIMITED *Toronto*

Copyright © 1972, The Macmillan Company

PRINTED IN THE UNITED STATES OF AMERICA

All rights reserved. No part of this book may be reproduced or transmitted in any form or by any means, electronic or mechanical, including photocopying, recording, or any information storage and retrieval system, without permission in writing from the Publisher.

THE MACMILLAN COMPANY
866 Third Avenue, New York, New York 10022
COLLIER-MACMILLAN CANADA, LTD., Toronto, Ontario

Library of Congress catalog card number: 76–152818

PRINTING   23456789   YEAR   23456789

DEDICATION

*This book is dedicated
to the
proposition
that the quality of therapeutics
can be improved;
and to the
patients, investigators, teachers, students,
and their families
who have made this proposition
tenable.*

PREFACE

> Even in medicine, though it is easy to know what honey, wine and hellebore,
> cautery and surgery are, to know how and to whom and when to apply them
> so as to effect a cure is no less an undertaking than to be a physician.
> ARISTOTLE, Nicomachean Ethics, Vol. IX

DETAILED pharmacologic knowledge stands alone as a basic science, but successful therapeutics requires application of this information to disease-induced abnormalities in individual patients. Aristotle did not claim that physicians were successful, only that they attempted to be. There is abundant information that physicians generally are poor therapists, despite their detailed knowledge of the pathogenesis of disease and the pharmacology of specific drugs that can alter a disease. The consequences of poor therapy include both toxic reactions to drugs and unchecked or even exacerbated disease. No longer can it be said, "The diagnosis is always more important than the treatment." Therapeutics must not continue to lag so far behind pharmacology, physiology, biochemistry, and pathophysiology, which serve as its base. Much information must be applied to clinical settings to allow major improvements in the management of disease and decreases in the incidence, morbidity, and mortality of drug toxicity.

This textbook was written (1) to help medical students understand how to approach the problems of administration of drugs to man, and (2) to show house staff and practicing physicians who learned therapeutics in a "hand-me-down" fashion that this instructional approach at best fosters mediocrity in therapeutics and should be replaced by a more efficacious and satisfying method. A consistent approach to therapeutic settings is possible, and the organization of the book generally describes the rationale for therapeutic decisions. An underlying principle herein is that the pathophysiology of disease and basic facts of pharmacology must be interdigitated in order to select drugs and establish therapeutic objectives. Once a category of drug is considered, the therapist must recall and use the basic principles of drug administration (Unit I); then the specific factors of disease and drug that justify bringing them together must be contemplated, so that the dynamics of pharmacology and pathophysiology can be put into perspective in the therapeutic plan (Unit II). Once the therapeutic objectives have been set, a plan must be made and implemented to observe, recognize, and evaluate the effects of drug administration (Unit III). The student may then evaluate his ability to recognize and apply principles in programmed problem-solving situations, taken from actual cases of the clinical pharmacology consultation service, University of California Medical Center, San Francisco (Unit IV).

Successful use of this book requires knowledge of both pharmacology and medicine. It does not replace the basic textbook in either discipline; rather, it is a supplement to both. Unit II does not include all, or even most, of the important diseases or drugs that might be discussed. The approach described in each chapter—physiology, pathophysiology, pharmacology, and, finally, the integration of these subjects—is consistent, can be applied at the bedside, and constitutes what the editors consider to be active clinical pharmacology. Such an approach can be subdivided into guidelines (principles), and some clinical states lend themselves more readily than others to illustration of principles that can be applied broadly. We hope the reader will find that principles applicable to one disease also apply to other disorders, for that is what makes them principles. They should help to stimulate thought rather than to propagate dogma or provide further recipes for therapeutics.

The contributors have demonstrated extraordinary diligence and patience in writing this innovative textbook. The editors thank their colleagues, fellows, house staff, and students for encouragement, criticism, and help during the long gestation period. They are greatly indebted for the thoughtful criticism and suggestions made by Arthur P. Grollman, Jr., M.D., associate professor of pharmacology and medicine, Albert Einstein College of Medicine, Bronx, New York. They are also indebted to Peggy Langston for editorial assistance in preparing the final manuscript.

KENNETH L. MELMON
HOWARD F. MORRELLI

CONTRIBUTORS

Becker, Charles E., M.D. Director, Acute Detoxification Study Unit, San Francisco General Hospital, San Francisco, California

Bertino, Joseph R., M.A., M.D. Professor of Medicine and Pharmacology, Yale University School of Medicine, New Haven, Connecticut

Bourne, Henry R., M.D. Instructor of Medicine and Pharmacology, University of California School of Medicine, San Francisco, California

Cohen, Allen B., M.D. Research Fellow, Cardiovascular Research Institute, University of California School of Medicine, San Francisco, California

Fenster, L. Frederick, M.D. Clinical Associate Professor of Medicine, University of Washington School of Medicine; Department of Medicine, Mason Clinic, Seattle, Washington

Hollister, Leo E., M.D. Associate Professor of Medicine, Stanford University School of Medicine, Stanford, California; Medical Investigator, Veterans Administration Hospital, Palo Alto, California

Hryniuk, William M., M.D. Assistant Professor of Medicine, University of Manitoba School of Medicine, Winnipeg, Manitoba, Canada

Marsh, John C., M.D. Associate Professor of Medicine and Pharmacology, Yale University School of Medicine, New Haven, Connecticut

Melmon, Kenneth L., M.D. Associate Professor of Medicine and Pharmacology, and Chief, Division of Clinical Pharmacology, University of California School of Medicine, San Francisco, California

Miller, Russell L., M.D. Trainee, Clinical Pharmacology, University of California School of Medicine, San Francisco, California

Morrelli, Howard F., M.D. Associate Professor of Medicine and Pharmacology, and Vice Chairman (House Staff Affairs), Department of Medicine, University of California School of Medicine, San Francisco, California

Nies, Alan S., M.D. Assistant Professor of Medicine and Pharmacology, Vanderbilt University School of Medicine, Nashville, Tennessee

Rowland, Malcolm, Ph.D. Associate Professor of Pharmacy and Pharmaceutical Chemistry, University of California School of Pharmacy, San Francisco, California

Sharp, Geoffrey W. G., Ph.D. Associate Professor of Physiology, Harvard Medical School; Chief, Biochemical Pharmacology Unit, Massachusetts General Hospital, Boston, Massachusetts

Smith, William M., M.D., M.P.H. Associate Clinical Professor of Medicine, University of California School of Medicine; Director, U.S.P.H.S. Cooperative Drug Study; Director, United States Public Health Service Hospital, San Francisco, California

Thier, Samuel O., M.D. Associate Professor of Medicine, University of Pennsylvania School of Medicine; Associate Director, Medical Services, University of Pennsylvania Hospital, Philadelphia, Pennsylvania

Thomson, Pate D., M.D. Assistant Clinical Professor of Medicine, University of California School of Medicine, San Francisco, California

Weser, Elliot, M.D. Professor and Head, Section of Gastroenterology, and Deputy Chairman, Department of Physiology and Medicine, University of Texas Medical School, San Antonio, Texas

Williams, Hibbard E., M.D. Associate Professor of Medicine, University of California School of Medicine; Chief, Medical Services, San Francisco General Hospital, San Francisco, California

CONTENTS

Unit I
Basic Principles of Drug Administration

Unit II
Pathophysiologic and Pharmacologic Considerations in Drug Administration

Unit III
Recognition and Evaluation of Effects of Drug Administration

xi

Unit IV
Clinical Examples of the Use of Drugs

UNIT I
BASIC PRINCIPLES OF DRUG ADMINISTRATION

Chapter 1

DRUG CHOICE IN DISEASE

William M. Smith and *Kenneth L. Melmon*

THERAPY AS A SCIENCE

Contemporary Therapeutics

Each act of treatment is a complex experiment worthy of the rigorous logic customarily applied to diagnostic or laboratory activities. In any clinical situation, the proper choice and use of drugs constitute an experiment and demand a scientific approach for maximum effectiveness and safety. As with any experiment, a well-conceived plan, careful execution, and an objective appraisal are required.

The physician's job only begins when he establishes an accurate diagnosis; the ultimate test of his skills is reflected in the outcome of his therapy. Maximum satisfaction accrues to the patient and the doctor when successful treatment is predictable and if it results from application of the scientific method. Then intellectual as well as humanitarian goals are fulfilled. Furthermore, when therapeutics is approached methodically, the skilled clinician will be respected as a scientist and can take justifiable pride in having achieved this recognition with complex man as his object of study.

The scientific method is as applicable to daily clinical treatment as it is to experimental therapeutics. In the former instance, the goal in an individual patient is to equal or surpass the best results of similar earlier "experiments," whereas in experimental therapeutics the intent is to inquire or innovate. Feinstein has emphasized that good clinical judgment involves the scientific application of human capabilities. An important aspect of clinical judgment is the selection and appraisal of therapeutic agents. "The therapeutic decisions of clinical judgment require valid evidence, logical analysis, and demonstrable proof. Their scientific quality can be discerned, assessed, and improved by the same rational procedures used for any other act of experimental science" (Feinstein, 1967).

The rational choice of therapeutic agents involves these prerequisites: (1) an accurate diagnosis; (2) a thorough knowledge of the data related to the pathophysiology of the disease; (3) a knowledge of the basic pharmacology and biochemistry of the drug and its metabolites, and the kinetics of the compound in normal and diseased man; (4) the ability to transfer such knowledge to effective bedside action; (5) reasonable expectations of the relation of pathophysiology and pharmacology so that the drug's effect can be anticipated; and (6) a plan to make specific measurements that will reveal efficacy and toxicity and will set the course for continued therapy.

Major purposes of this book are to develop awareness of therapeutic principles, to help promote transference of pharmacologic knowledge to bedside situations, and to convince the physician that therapy may be more effective and rewarding if objectivity is used to assess the results of a decision.

It is ironic that diagnostics has attained a sophisticated scientific state at a time when therapeutic decisions rest largely on impression, sentiment, and uncritical, perhaps misleading, advertising. The enormity of the problem and the consequences of this paradox are readily appreciated when the underlying forces are considered.

A pharmacologic revolution began during World War II, has advanced rapidly over the past 25 years, and is responsible for what Modell has called "the drug explosion" (Modell, 1961). The practicing physician must choose among thousands of new drugs. The number of medicaments available in the early 1960s approached 200,000; 90% of those most commonly prescribed did not exist prior to World War II (Brown, 1955). Over 7000 new prescription products were introduced between 1948 and 1963; the current therapeutic arsenal includes over 7200 drugs and drug combinations (American Medical Association, 1971). The turnover is so rapid that approximately 70% of these were unknown or unavailable 15 years ago, when over half of all physicians received their pharmacotherapeutic training in medical school. This pace has slowed only moderately as a result of the Kefauver-Harris legislation of 1962. Further slowing may occur due to new FDA regulations, recent government-sponsored reviews of drug prescriptions (Task Force, 1968), and the *Final Report* of the Task Force on Prescription Drugs (1969). Nonetheless, physicians are overwhelmed by the sheer volume of new drugs, particularly when so much "investigation" related to drugs is inadequate (Editorial, 1969). Much of this "investigation" is conducted by clinicians, but since a first-rate clinician is not necessarily a good investigator the resultant poor data may lead to erroneous marketing decisions and advertising claims. Consequently, teachers of medicine often turn first to literature on drug research for examples of poor investigation and invalid conclusions.

Another aspect of the problem, which has important economic consequences, is the tendency for physicians to prescribe by brand name rather than by generic name. Generic prescribing is the use of chemically equivalent products that, whenever available, cost considerably less than brand-name products, often as little as one-third. The physician is responding to his most immediate source of drug information, the manufacturers' advertising, but he adds another dimension to the problem of modern therapeutics. He must be reassured that *chemical* equivalence equals *clinical* equivalence, and it has been demonstrated that this is not necessarily so. On the basis of available evidence, however, the Task Force on Prescription Drugs

(1969) concluded that lack of clinical equivalence among chemical equivalents has been grossly exaggerated, and that the use of low-cost chemical equivalents can yield important savings to patients.

Even if all the new drugs were necessary, effective, and safe, the therapists' problem would still be alarming. However, many drugs are duplicates, single preparations of prefabricated mixtures of many drugs, or so poorly tested that they cannot be seriously considered. The uncritical clinical use of these agents by physicians, as well as irrational polypharmacy, has predisposed the public to an alarming increase of iatrogenesis in disease (Modell, 1963; Lasagna, 1965; Moser, 1969; Melmon, 1971). Fortunately, this has been accompanied by a slow but definite awareness of major areas of therapeutic hazards: drug interaction and adverse drug effects (Smith *et al.*, 1966; Morrelli and Melmon, 1968). The credulity of physicians should have been taxed (but often was not) by claims that each of a plethora of nearly identical agents could be "best" for a given medical indication. It is time to use the scientific techniques that allow us to choose and use available preparations wisely. Logical branch points analogous to those of a computer can be set in our own minds, eliminating the need for rote memorization of the myriad facts about each drug.

Unfortunately, despite the conscientious efforts of pharmacology and medicine departments, and of ethical pharmaceutical houses, the physician's education has rarely equipped him with a critical approach to therapy; nor in his busy practice has he felt it necessary or possible to apply rigorous thought to therapeutic decisions. There can be no doubt, however, that inadequate thinking about drug choice has caused many therapeutic deficiencies and serious drug reactions, some of which we are not even equipped to recognize. A conservative estimate of the number of prescriptions filled each year in the United States exceeds one billion, or over four for every man, woman, and child in the country (Gosselin, 1968). In addition, approximately 25 to 30 million patients are admitted yearly to the hospital, each receiving an average of 14 drugs during his stay (Cluff *et al.*, 1964). No wonder the number of untoward reactions is increasing at an alarming rate!

Acute drug toxicity is a common medical emergency. If intended as self-mutilation, we easily recognize it; drug overdosage has become the most rapidly increasing means of suicide. However, we must also appreciate some more subtle but equally alarming facts. More than a decade ago it was reported that 5% of 1000 consecutive admissions to a major medical center were a direct consequence of well-intentioned and conscientiously prescribed drugs (Barr, 1955). This does not mean that physicians are basically careless, irrational, or ignorant. Rather, the uncritical and wide use of drugs seems related to a gap that exists between the teaching of pharmacology as a basic science and as a clinical science. As a result, there have developed (1) a lack of appreciation of the risk involved in using drugs, namely, that no drug is devoid of toxicity and that useful, potent drugs can cause serious morbidity and mortality; (2) a lack of awareness that potential drug reactions and interactions increase proportionally to the number of drugs administered; (3) little familiarity with the principles of controlled drug evaluation; (4) no effective professional program for continuing education in pharmacotherapy; (5) no objective, well-organized, and concise source of drug information; and (6) a dependence on the pharmaceutical industry to fill the gap.

Drug advertisements frequently are misleading and reflect economic realities such as the cost of drug research, the pharmaceutical firms' desire to share in the market for a particular class of drug, and the brief duration of the potential market (often because therapeutic claims are not upheld or untoward effects are eventually recognized). Such advertisements can place unreasonable pressure on the therapist, leading to irrational therapeutics. Similar claims may have encouraged Osler's observation that one should treat as many patients as possible with a new drug while it still has the power to heal.

Medicine has made great strides since Voltaire's satiric description of physicians as "men who prescribe medicine of which they know little, to cure diseases of which they know less, in human beings of which they know nothing." And yet, if the profession has ever been in danger of irrational and irresponsible therapeutic practices, it is now. Physicians are characteristically rational and responsible, but it is nearly impossible for them to appear so if they respond to the pressures of time, uncritical reading, industrial advertising, and the persuasion of "detail men" and patients to use the flood of new drugs without proper education in therapeutics and without sufficient knowledge about or rational expectations of each drug.

The yield from the drug explosion has been excessive, actually going beyond the availability of competent clinical investigators to assess the efficacy and safety of new drugs. However, the ability of practicing physicians to assimilate the essential knowledge of therapeutics and to develop competence in prescribing drugs rationally has not been exceeded and should not be replaced by decisions based on conditioned behavior.

This book constitutes another acceptance of the challenge implied by Lasagna in 1964 when he cited the tragedy of declining education in pharmacology at a time when it is most needed. We make an effort to demonstrate the feasibility of teaching rational therapeutics. We recognize that the education of physicians in this matter cannot be left to chance or commercial enterprises. The authors agree with Lasagna that "our society's handling of the problems created by the pharmacological revolution of the last quarter of the century leaves much to be desired" (Lasagna, 1964). But we add that we have within our grasp the means to begin correcting our therapeutic ways, by virtue of the intelligence and drive of the physician, the effective techniques of education, and the sincere desire of the teacher and student to correct their deficiencies.

This chapter reviews historically and conceptually the evolution of the discipline of clinical pharmacology, including the methods of therapeutic investigation and the proper evaluation of sources of information on the choice of drugs.

Historical Perspective

Our focus on the state of contemporary therapeutics may be sharpened if it is placed in historical perspective (Garrison, 1929). As medicine emerged from its medieval eclipse, discarding the bonds of Galenism (Galen, A.D. 131–201) with its elaborate system of polypharmacy, teleology, pragmatism, and dogmatism, it enjoyed a rebirth of the scientific spirit in the tradition of Hippocrates (460–370 B.C.) and Aristotle (384–322 B.C.). Paracelsus (1493–1541) was perhaps the most notable early leader who rejected Galenical tradition and witchcraft and advocated experimentation. Although alchemy, philosophy, and astronomy remained his pillars of faith, among his contributions can be found the precursors of chemical pharmacology and experimental therapeutics.

His successors in the seventeenth century included outstanding scientists such as Harvey (1578–1657), Malpighi (1628–94), Descartes (1596–1650), and Sydenham (1624–89). Sydenham, more than anyone since Hippocrates, emphasized the importance of clinical inspection and observation in the nosology of disease. However, except for the introduction of mineral baths and chemicals, therapeutics remained largely a mixture of quackery and faith healing. Botanicals, ground bones, powdered excrement of animals, and insects were the favored medicaments.

The eighteenth century brought further accent on observation and classification in the sciences. This was accompanied by the rise of surgeons and physiologists such as Hunter (1718–83), Cruikshank (1745–1800), Hales (1677–1761), Priestley (1733–

1804), and Lavoisier (1743–94). Clinical medicine's major thrust was in improved bedside diagnostic technique and initial efforts at correlation with post-mortem findings. Noteworthy contributors were Withering (1741–99), Morgagni (1682–1771), Heberden (1710–1801), Jenner (1749–1823), and Rush (1745–1813). However, progress in therapeutics was limited; and, with the exception of inoculation for prevention of smallpox, therapeutics remained principally apothecary medicine. Three editions of the London *Pharmacopoeia* detailed the extracts, powders, syrups, spirits, oils, inorganics, and pro-prietaries available at that time. Bloodletting, emetics, and cathartics were the most popular modalities and at best were indiscriminate in their usual failure to help and in their occasional harmful consequences.

Many of the errors of logic that occurred during this period have persisted into the modern era. The placebo effect was unknown at that time, and undoubtedly many of the harmless medicaments were associated with improvement and received the stamp of efficacy. Such uncritical labels have been retained from generation to generation and are accepted primarily on faith or authority. Ignorance of the natural history of disease also led to erroneous conclusions about therapies. These conclusions, too, became cemented into the "traditional wisdom" of practice. Such *post-hoc* reasoning was the architect of most premodern and, some would say, current-day therapeutics.

The nineteenth century witnessed an organized advancement of science on most frontiers. Although medicine is said to have entered the modern era of clinical science with Claude Bernard (1813–78), diagnosis remained imprecise and therapy largely ineffective, so that the practice of medicine yielded very little to scientific inquiry. Furthermore, the ethical and moral standards of the day largely interdicted significant "experimentation" in humans. The investigators did not recognize that every treatment in medicine is an experiment (although most are faulty when not so designed).

Physicians who were motivated toward scientific experimentation rejected patients as objects of research and turned to the laboratory and various models of disease in animals. This approach has both assets and limitations. Among the limitations are species variation, which can be critical in the pharmacologic effect of a drug, and the fact that models of disease in animals may not duplicate the disease in man. The pharmacokinetics and pharmacologic effects in the animal model may have little relevance for therapeutics in man. We were yet to learn that only man can serve as the final model to establish the efficacy and toxicity of any new drug (witness thalidomide).

The early development of pathology as a basic medical science offered pathologist-physicians the opportunity to apply emerging laboratory technology to diagnosis. Precision in diagnostics improved much faster than in therapeutics. The influence of outstanding pathologists and clinicians such as Virchow (1821–1902), Rokitansky (1804–78), Graves (1796–1853), Bright (1789–1858), and Addison (1793–1860) sharpened the thrust of critical and accurate diagnostics. The classification of disease by morbid anatomy became paramount, and the major challenge for clinicians was the correlation of their observations with postmortem findings—witness the continued and effective use of the clinical and pathologic correlations as teaching tools.

Progress in the basic medical sciences revealed the abysmal ignorance, folly, and superstition that surrounded the "healing arts" and led to the therapeutic nihilism of the early twentieth century. Sir William Osler (1849–1919), an exemplar of this philosophy, was a major contributor to the pre-eminent status of the science of diagnostics.

Clinicians of that era, which persisted well into the middle third of this century, had the burdensome heritage of earlier errors of logic, the tyranny of authority, and an accumulation of subjective interpretations and axioms regarding therapy that were based on personal experience, anecdotal descriptions, and testimonials. Therapy was not approached as an experimental science, and most medical treatment was based on the biases of both the healed and the healers. Progress in therapeutics was limited principally to the important but undramatic deletion of ineffective and toxic substances. With this background, it is not surprising that we entered the postwar pharmaceutical boom with a number of conceptual barriers to the development of a science of therapeutics.

Conceptual Barriers

Foremost among these barriers is the notion that the scientific method is not applicable to the treatment of patients, owing to uncontrollable and multiple variables in the human or to weaknesses in clinical testing techniques. This conceptual obstacle applies to all aspects of clinical science and is not unique to therapeutics.

Feinstein's insights into this problem are artfully presented in his book *Clinical Judgment*, which is highly recommended to all who are interested in the "science of therapeutics" (Feinstein, 1967). We have begun to appreciate that clinical phenomena can be discussed and described with predictable precision, meaningful classification, and logical analysis of measurements. We can construct experiments yielding valid conclusions concerning pharmacology and the treatment of patients. Measurements of discrete rather than continuous variables often consist of enumerated attributes that have been critically observed and given precise verbal descriptions. Such measurements can be quantitated as readily as numerical dimensions. That such attributes are useful in predicting the course of a disease state or the response to a drug should not seem surprising. We have entered an age when seemingly random and unrelated observations may be analyzed to predict activities almost as complex as the physiology and pathology of the human. If a cybernetic approach can make accurate predictions of changes in the world's economy, similar use of simultaneous equations relating multiple factors in man could be applied to therapeutics.

Digital computers, employing the mathematical concepts of set theory, symbolic logic, and Boolean algebra, have already indicated the validity of such clinical observations and reasoning in the quantitative evaluation of therapy (Irvington House, 1964; Feinstein, 1964, 1967, 1968).

Another barrier embedded in our thinking is the idea that phenomena or changes in morbid anatomy observed in sick people can be meaningfully classified in terms of traditional disease entities. A diagnostic label attached to a patient's disease narrows subsequent thought processes related to etiology, pathogenesis, prognosis, and therapy of the disease. Although the taxonomy of disease is the central component of clinical communication, the taxonomy in use today is unfortunately based on the morbid anatomy described by pathologists over the past two centuries. Such description encourages the physician to think of diseases as static entities abstract from the sick human being, incapable of change and not requiring dynamic readjustment of therapeutic agents. If the disease in a patient is not considered dynamic, major changes in the pharmacokinetics of drugs critical for control of the disease will be ignored. Thus, the contracted volume of distribution (V_d) or altered rates of clearance (see Chapters 2 and 5) of intravenously administered lidocaine in a patient with heart failure results in a higher-than-expected concentration of lidocaine in plasma after standard doses are administered. If the heart failure is reversed but the arrhythmia persists and lidocaine is still needed, a greater dose would be necessary to achieve efficacy. *Principle: Realization that a disease state is dynamic is a key to rational and effective therapeutics. A disease course represents a sequence, not a single event.*

A disease label should usually indicate a spectrum of possible courses. Therapeutic literature that refers to subjects with a given disease, but which is not precise as to its stage, yields uninterpretable data. It may be virtually impossible to tell if patients in different series had the same disease, let alone the same stage of it.

The problem of evaluating response to therapy is great, but not overwhelming. The morbid anatomy, as well as the altered function (as documented by laboratory tests or bedside observations) and the natural course of the disease, must be considered. Such information is generally available, allowing a physician to think of a disease as a process with discrete or continuous variables, all subject to potential analysis and all required for appraisal of the state of the disease, therapeutics, and prognosis.

What is myocardial infarction? It has a specific morbid anatomy, but what of the multiplicity of clinical and therapeutic inferences contained in the label? Various hemodynamic, autonomic, and blood-clotting changes must be considered before therapy (see Chapter 5). The failure to establish comprehensive but consistent criteria for this diagnosis, as a basis for correlating prognosis and response to therapy, is partially responsible for the unresolved conflict over the value of anticoagulants in the management of myocardial infarction. Similarly *pulmonary emphysema, chronic bronchitis, nephritis,* and *cerebral arteriosclerosis* are terms surrounded by ambiguous inferences of both diagnostic and therapeutic significance.

Ambiguity also arises in diseases classified subjectively by functional state, for example, hyperkinetic children. Upon observing that not all such children improved with amphetamine therapy, Lasagna demonstrated in his sample that only those with underlying brain damage improved (Lasagna, 1969). Failure to emphasize nosology in clinical trials undoubtedly accounts for some of the apparent discrepancies between studies.

Another barrier to be dispelled is the concept that empiricism should be condemned a priori. Practical therapeutics is greatly extended by the therapeutic scientist who makes valid, systematic, and controlled empiric observations on ways to change the outcome of clinical events, even though the causes and mechanisms of such change are not understood. Clinicians have come to accept the idea that the principal motive for research is the discovery of *causes*. The legitimacy of seeking answers to the *how* questions—for example, the hows of treatment—in addition to the *whys* of etiology and pathogenesis, must be accepted as potentially worthy endeavors for medical scientists and must be valued among the methods used in providing rational therapeutics with ammunition.

There are many instances in which medical knowledge of "why" is not necessary for effective therapy (at least on an interim basis) and additional instances in which the knowledge of "why" does not lead promptly to better therapy. The former is illustrated by the efficacy of red-blood-cell transfusion to a patient with an undiagnosed anemia and angina secondary to the lowered oxygen-carrying capacity of the blood. The latter is illustrated by the frustration created by therapeutic failures in diseases such as the porphyrias in which diagnosis is chemically elegant, and pathogenesis at the molecular level is known to some extent (Meyer and Marver, 1971a, 1971b).

In addition, there are examples of recognition of appropriate treatment for an abnormal condition long before its "causes" or the pharmacology of the drugs for its therapy are fully understood. Relevant examples are the successful treatment of essential hypertension by rauwolfia alkaloids and the amelioration of a specific psychosis with monoamine oxidase inhibitors. In each case the pathophysiology of the disease is still unclear and the pharmacology of the drugs was not well known when they were found to be efficacious.

Many important discoveries have been made empirically. Withering's use of foxglove in "dropsy" and the Indians' use of cinchona bark for "fevers" are among the more notable. Serendipity was equally involved in the discovery of the clinical relevance of the oxygen electrode and the discovery of insulin and its proper use. *Principle: Empiricism per se should not be a barrier to therapeutic progress.*

Evolution of Therapeutic Investigation

Prior to Claude Bernard, investigations in medicine were based on observation. Clinical manifestations were classified empirically or inferentially, and, on the basis of the subsequent course of events, conclusions were drawn regarding both causes and cures. This approach, in vogue since Hippocrates, was subject to many pitfalls and logical fallacies. The medical scientists of the seventeenth, eighteenth, and nineteenth centuries revived and refined the observational approach, but applied it principally to diagnostics.

The active experimental approach introduced by Bernard was intended primarily to facilitate the discovery of mechanisms of disease, but his definition of an "experimenter" clearly fits the physician's role in therapeutics.* A similar approach was introduced into pharmacology by Bernard's predecessor, Magendie (1783–1855). However, little of the basic knowledge gained in pharmacology was applied to clinical therapeutics. Scientists generally pursued their interests in the laboratory, where precision and reproducibility were possible and prestige and academic advancement more certain. There, the study of body tissue and fluids and animal models of disease (whether or not relevant to man) led to dramatic expansion of our knowledge in the basic medical sciences of physiology, biochemistry, and pharmacology. Still, the clinical application of these facts was primarily toward the understanding of etiology and pathogenesis of disease in man. There was little transference of basic pharmacologic knowledge to establishing the diagnosis, altering the course of disease, or anticipating the effects of drug-induced alteration of the *milieu intérieur*. Little attempt was made to distinguish pharmacology from therapeutics, or to determine whether or by what means a disease state could alter the pharmacology of a drug. Neither was an attempt made to distinguish between observation of a drug effect in an animal model and application of the drug to diseased man, where multiple organ systems might be affected, polypharmacy necessary, and assets and liabilities of drug interaction encountered. No attention was paid to the adverse effects of drugs. Although homeopathy (which might be considered a systematic approach to drug therapy of disease) was never accepted by the medical community, neither were the principles of rational therapeutics. Drugs were considered neither potent nor potentially dangerous tools.

Progress in therapeutic investigation was further restrained by the drift of scientists away from the clinical setting toward the laboratory. Moral considerations concerning experimentation in man encouraged such drift. However, the validity of the experimental method for medical and therapeutic investigation was established. The clinicians' training for such investigative careers included academic work in the basic sciences, mathematics, philosophy, and formal logic. The result, "medical progress," was associated with an ever-widening intellectual gap between the bedside physician and the academic clinician (who became barely distinguishable from the basic scientist). Nonetheless, a foundation was being laid for the science of diagnostics and the emergence of the discipline of clinical pharmacology and experimental therapeutics. The application of science has revolutionized diagnostics and will unquestionably increase the efficacy of therapeutics.

Just as earlier medical scientists found a clinical orientation to be somewhat of a handicap in the laboratory, where their attention was more and more directed away from disease in man and toward molecular biology, inevitably a restitution occurred, with the recognition that in

---

* "We give the name experimenter to the man who applies methods of investigation, whether simple or complex so as to make natural phenomena vary, or so as to alter them with some purpose or other" (Bernard, 1865).

the final analysis, "the best subject for the study of man is man himself." *Principle: The ultimate test of the efficacy and risk-to-benefit ratio of a drug occurs in patients exhibiting the disease in question.*

Modern clinical investigators are emerging who are competent and comfortable both in the laboratory and at the bedside. They function in both areas and can serve as liaison between the practitioner of medicine and the basic medical scientist. Many have been called clinical physiologists. Some are clinical pharmacologists. In the future, others may function in similar capacities linking other basic sciences with clinical application, by uniting the philosophy and logic of both disciplines and making transference from one subject to the other simple and highly rewarding.

Clinical Pharmacology: A Discipline for Rational Therapeutics

Clinical pharmacologists try to overcome the barriers that inhibit application of the scientific method to therapeutics. Recognition and concern for this problem emerged along with the pharmaceutical revolution and resultant "drug explosion" of the past quarter century. New antibiotics and chemotherapeutic agents appeared, necessitating the development of clinical trials for their evaluation (Medical Research Council, 1948, 1950a, 1950b, 1952, 1954). Results had been clear in the case of penicillin treatment of acute infection, where success was dramatic and untoward effects were few. However, with subsequent new therapeutic agents, inadequacies of testing were evident. Therapeutic trials of the sulfonamides, for example, did not prevent extensive use of compounds that ultimately proved dangerously toxic, and early trials of streptomycin in pulmonary tuberculosis were encouraging but inconclusive.

Thus, a new discipline appeared, its growth fostered in England (Daniels, 1951; Hill, 1951, 1952) and its title, "clinical pharmacology," suggested in America (Gold, 1952). Numerous clinical pharmacology "units" have been established in the past decade, with primary emphasis on either clinical investigation or pharmacology. Initially, at least, most eschewed the "testing" of drugs.

Clinical pharmacology as an independent academic discipline is concerned with the effectiveness of drugs in man. This concern includes three principal approaches to medical investigation and teaching (Chalmers, 1964). The first of these is the study of the pharmacology of drugs in man, that is, the disposition of the drug (absorption, distribution, metabolism, and elimination) (see Chapter 2) and its

mechanism of action. The second involves the study of drug actions to investigate the pathophysiology of diseases of a particular organ system. These two approaches involve pharmacologists and clinical investigators, neither of whom may have a primary interest in evaluating the efficacy of a drug in a patient with a given disease. The third and unifying approach deals specifically with the documentation of the safety and efficacy of drugs in man.

The clinical pharmacologist is concerned with the interdigitation of therapeutics with basic pharmacologic principles, research methodology, biostatistics, and clinical acumen. An essential product of these relationships is the clinical trial, a prerequisite to rational therapeutics.

The Clinical Trial: The Instrument of Rational Therapy

The word "drug" has many definitions. The noun comes from the Middle English word *drogge*, meaning dry, which combined as *drogge vate* meant dry cask or barrel and referred to "dry" rather than liquid contents. The barrel is hardly dry or empty in the twentieth century! *Webster's Unabridged Dictionary* defines *drug* as a substance used as medicine (in turn a substance or preparation used in treating disease) or in making medicines for internal or external uses. According to the Food, Drug, and Cosmetic Act of 1938, a drug is a substance recognized in an official pharmacopoeia or formulary; a substance intended for use in the diagnosis, cure, mitigation, treatment, or prevention of disease in men or other animals; a substance other than food (although we now know that at least some foods should be included) intended to affect the structure or function of the body of man or other animals; and a substance intended for use as a component of a medicine, but not a component, part, or accessory of a device. There are additional definitions of drugs that may reflect on therapeutics; the noun is also used to describe a commodity that lies on hand or is not salable (pharmaceutical houses seem to have laid that definition to rest). When used as a verb, *drug* often refers to an act in which poisoning is intended!

In the broadest sense, clinical trials are not new. Whenever a clinician treats a patient, he conducts a "clinical trial." The results of the trial may be dramatic, as when a disease associated with a uniformly fatal outcome is reversed or cured by a new therapeutic maneuver. Then a single result may be sufficient to establish that a drug is effective. Such observations, carefully described and recorded in only a few patients by astute clinicians, have accounted for notable therapeutic progress. All observations are in a sense comparisons either with the natural history of the disease or with alternate modes of therapy representing the "control." Retrospective analysis may suggest or sometimes establish the value of dramatically effective drugs, such as penicillin to cure pneumococcal infections, insulin to prevent diabetic keto-acidosis, glucose to reverse hypoglycemia, potassium to reverse hypokalemia, or citrus fruits to cure scurvy. However, most drug trials must be more carefully designed if real but subtle benefits are to be discovered. Prospective comparisons are also essential to eliminate fallaciously accepted therapies.

The evaluation of new drugs in man begins only after extensive developmental activities by the biologic and chemical research divisions of a pharmaceutical corporation, accompanied by quality control, product development, and legal action. All are conducted in accordance with federal regulations established in the Food, Drug, and Cosmetic Act of 1938 and the Kefauver-Harris Amendments of 1962. The original act provided only for clearance of drugs for safety; the amendments required that efficacy also be demonstrated prior to approval by the government for routine use in man. After review of the accumulated experimental data in animals (usually a year or more after the initial decision to begin exploratory research), a decision may be made to undertake studies in man.

An FDA Form 1571, a Notice of Claimed Investigational Exemption for a New Drug (IND), is filed, which informs the FDA that the evaluation of the drug's efficacy and safety in man is to begin. The FDA is responsible for promptly reviewing the IND to ensure that its data adequately support the manufacturer's claim that the drug is safe for clinical trial in man.

The IND contains the following information: (1) a description of the chemistry and biologic activity of the drug; (2) the specific dosage forms to be given to man; (3) specifications of the quality control measures employed in the manufacture of the drug, and identification of all ingredients; (4) a description of equipment, procedures, and facilities used in the drug's manufacture; (5) the names and qualifications of the individuals to conduct the initial studies; (6) a signed statement of each investigator acknowledging his understanding of the nature of the drug, his responsibilities to personally supervise the studies, and his agreement to observe the requirements regarding use of volunteers and informed written consent; (7) a description of the facilities available for the studies; (8) protocols concerning dose, route, and duration of administration of the drug, as well as the clinical and laboratory examinations to be made; (9) data sheets provided to each investigator before he begins studies, detailing all that is known about the drug, its indications, and possible side effects; and (10) specified observations that should be reported at once.

Drug trials are conducted in three phases (Figure 1–1). Phase 1 is the first administration to humans and usually involves only a small number of normal volunteers. This phase is principally concerned with establishing dosage range and biologic activity of the drug in man.

Phase 2 is usually divided into early (a) and late (b) portions and involves administration of the drug to a few selected patients with the disease against which the drug may be useful. There is often a delay after phase 2a to conduct a review of possible toxicity in animals and to carry out special animal studies on reproductive processes before proceeding further in man. Phase 2b is a resumption or continuation of 2a studies, but therapy lasts longer and final decisions regarding dosage form are made prior to launching into the broad clinical trials of phase 3.

Phases 1, 2a, and 2b are usually conducted or supervised by a clinical pharmacologist who is responsible for selecting the investigators who will participate in the phase 3 trials. These clinical investigators are provided with data sheets updated by phase 2 studies, and with FDA Form 1573, on which they agree to study the drug under the conditions specified in the IND for evaluation of the drug's efficacy in the clinical conditions for which it is intended.

Phase 3 studies must include controlled clinical trials by a sufficient number of qualified investigators on a patient population large enough to provide data permitting evaluation of the drug's efficacy and safety.

A scientific methodology has developed for clinical trials. The methods ensure critical and unbiased data-gathering, subject to statistical analysis, and eliminate psychic and other environmental influences on results (Waife and Shapiro, 1959; Mainland, 1960; Hill, 1962). Studies in humans must be controlled. The controlled clinical trial is designed to compare treatments in patients; by controlling or equalizing all variables except the drug, such comparisons are rendered convincing. *Principle: A controlled clinical trial ensures that "the comparisons we make are as precise, as informative, and as convincing as possible" (Hill, 1960).*

The prospectively planned, controlled clinical trial substitutes a scientific experiment for the inevitably biased observational approach. This substitution incorporates the skills of a careful and objective investigator. Claude Bernard pointed out that the scientist differs from the metaphysician and the philosopher in that the scientist fails to be satisfied with his a priori idea and the consequences of his deductive logic alone, but additionally requires the experimental test (Bernard, 1865).

Important prerequisites to the conduct of valid and effective clinical trials (as well as to the treatment of a given patient) must be satisfied before the appropriate experimental and statistical design are considered.

The therapeutic objective must be clearly

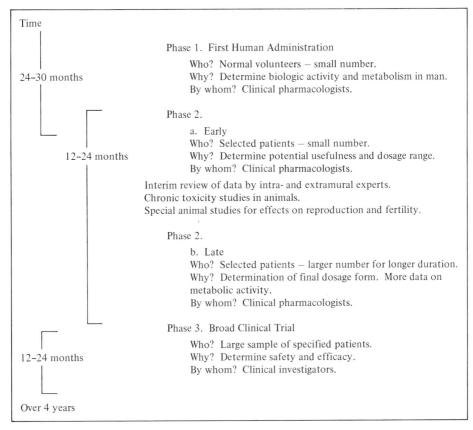

Time

Phase 1. First Human Administration

Who? Normal volunteers — small number.

24–30 months

Why? Determine biologic activity and metabolism in man.

By whom? Clinical pharmacologists.

Phase 2.

a. Early

Who? Selected patients — small number.

12–24 months

Why? Determine potential usefulness and dosage range.

By whom? Clinical pharmacologists.

Interim review of data by intra- and extramural experts.

Chronic toxicity studies in animals.

Special animal studies for effects on reproduction and fertility.

Phase 2.

b. Late

Who? Selected patients — larger number for longer duration.

Why? Determination of final dosage form. More data on metabolic activity.

By whom? Clinical pharmacologists.

Phase 3. Broad Clinical Trial

Who? Large sample of specified patients.

12–24 months

Why? Determine safety and efficacy.

By whom? Clinical investigators.

Over 4 years

Figure 1–1. Drug trials.

identified. A proper and well-stated objective is the key to the logic of the experimental and statistical design, as it forms the basis for choosing the index of accomplishment and for stratifying patients into groups with comparable natural prognosis. Whether the objective can be achieved ethically must also be considered and will influence the type of controls to be employed. If orthodox therapy cannot ethically be withheld, the design will be limited to the use of standard therapy, rather than a placebo, as the control.

The index of accomplishment must be preset and relevant to the therapeutic objective. If, for example, the objective were control of bacteriuria, an appropriate index would be a reduction of the quantitative bacterial count in serial urine cultures. Changes in the formed elements in the urinary sediment would be a less satisfactory and perhaps misleading index, since the drug specific for the organism may also be nephrotoxic. The index of accomplishment must also be discriminating and sensitive. If two organisms were responsible for the urinary tract infection and one was known to be, or likely to be,

resistant to the antibiotic to be tested, colony counts of the resistant organism alone would be invalid, insensitive, and indiscriminating. If clinical cure were related to a limited reduction in the bacterial count, an index dependent on sterility of the urine would place an inappropriate demand on the therapy and would be insensitive to the objective. Similarly, life or death would be grossly insensitive as indices of the effectiveness of short-term therapy in a patient with urinary tract infection. Such an index was appropriately chosen by Ponce de Leon in his quest for eternal youth, and by Pasteur in his more modest search for a cure for rabies. A life-or-death index, however, would be insensitive (although perhaps valid) if applied to the efficacy of a uricosuric agent in a patient with gout and hyperuricemia.

Once the preferred measurement is selected, criteria must be established to determine how much change in the indices will be necessary before the therapy can be considered a success. A scale of accomplishment must be considered. These predetermined criteria may be changes in a specific measurement, for example, mg/100 ml changes in serum cholesterol in a patient with hypercholesterolemia. In some conditions such as cancer, simple categories, such as *cured, improved, no change,* or *worse,* may be appropriate if they are well defined and reproducible.

The final prerequisite for a useful study is detailed understanding of the natural history of the disease to be treated; its clinical behavior can then be classified and appropriate groups for comparison can be established. Composition of such groups is a clinical (not a statistical) consideration requiring precise observation of clinical events.

Subject Selection. The importance of selecting a proper sample, that is, one qualitatively appropriate or representative of the population for which therapy is intended, cannot be overemphasized. The goal of the clinical trial, in fact, is to be able to generalize the findings to future patients.

The objective of subject selection is to set up truly comparable groups, in which each patient or group is equally likely to respond. Therefore, the groups must be homogeneous for all characteristics affecting prognosis. Feinstein has referred to this process as "correlated prognostic stratification" and considers it the crux of clinical logic in experimental therapeutics (Feinstein, 1968).

Sample Size. If results of experimental trials are to be convincing, quantitative or statistical considerations must be included. Sample size is influenced by numerous factors, including patient availability, known results of no treatment or of the standard regimen, expected performance of the test drug (usually best based on a pilot study), expected drop-out rate, and the clinicians' judgment as to what constitutes a meaningful result.

In addition to the traditional fixed-sample-size schemes, sequential analysis designs are frequently utilized (Armitage, 1960; Cornfield, 1966). Using these designs, "success or failure" decisions (as between matched pairs of subjects) can be made while the study is in progress. Such serial analysis permits the earliest possible recognition of a clear outcome, more effective safety monitoring, and termination of a study earlier than with fixed sample sizes. This may result in earlier availability of a good drug or preferred regimen.

On the average, sequential design employs fewer subjects than do fixed-sample-size studies. The sequential design is not applicable to all problems, however, and its end point is a conclusion that treatment A is, or is not, better than treatment B. If A is not as good as B, further information is not necessary. However, if A is better than B, the study does not estimate how much better. Then a much longer time, or even an additional study, may be required to give magnitude to the difference observed.

Drug Dosage. The dosage of a drug in a clinical trial must be carefully chosen. The optimal dose, that is, one that works well in most patients and produces a minimum of side effects, is seldom known before a clinical trial begins. If the dose chosen is too low, a real difference between the experimental and control groups may be too slight to be appreciated. False conclusions of "no efficacy" may result, leading to rejection of a potent drug. If the dose is too high, toxic reactions may obscure any therapeutic merit. *Principle: Inflexibility or mischoice of a dosage regimen is detrimental in both experimental and clinical settings.*

Phase 1 and phase 2 studies (see page 10 and Figure 1–1) usually identify the useful portion of the dose-response curve, but such studies do not impose absolute limits on the dosage chosen for an individual. In most experimental and therapeutic attempts, graded doses should be employed, based on knowledge of the disease state and pharmacokinetics of the drug. Such planning often allows quantification of results and identification of the occasional instance where a threshold effect is operative, for example, the studies on the use of levodopa for Parkinson's disease (see Chapter 11).

Placebo Effect. A placebo has been defined as "any therapeutic procedure (or component thereof) which is given (1) deliberately to have an effect, or (2) unknowingly and has an effect on a symptom, syndrome, disease, or patient; but which is objectively without specific activity for the condition being treated" (Shapiro, 1964) (see Chapter 14). The placebo effect is the change produced by a placebo. Such subjective responses may occur in any therapeutic procedure and are difficult to control.

Approximately 35% of patients studied are "placebo reactors" (Beecher, 1955) (see Chapter 14). If not eliminated by preliminary testing, these patients present special methodologic problems during design of drug evaluations. In a drug trial in which subjective responses to therapy are measured, it is difficult to control for placebo effect. For this reason, studies using sedatives, hypnotics, analgesics, relaxants, tranquilizers, antipruritics, and antiemetics are especially difficult. They demand the most sophisticated experimental design and statistical analysis. The "preference technique" that incorporates controls for placebo effect into a sequential design has proved to be an effective and easily performed method for evaluating relative drug efficacy of symptomatic drugs (Jick *et al.,* 1966).

The more suggestible the patient, the more likely he is to obtain relief from either a placebo or an active drug. A positive history of many symptoms commonly thought to be drug side effects can be obtained from healthy people not taking any medication (Reidenberg and Lowenthal, 1968). The "placebo reactor" must be recognized as a functional type and "controlled for" in all studies (Lasagna *et al.*, 1958; Beecher, 1959; Wolf, 1959; Shapiro, 1964).

Control of Bias. The *sine qua non* of the clinical trial is its controls. "Clinical trial" and "controlled clinical trial" should be synonymous. However, as emphasized by Hill (1951, 1952), even those not so designed do in fact have controls. Control may only be a recollection of past personal experience; however inappropriate this may be, it may nonetheless serve as a basis for comparison. Past personal experience and previously recorded observations are referred to as historical controls. Properly, controls should be concurrent. Only in the case of a uniformly fatal disease, for example, tuberculous meningitis in the preantibiotic era, would the historical control be justified. Historical controls can afford no protection against bias or placebo effects and are therefore most often too treacherous for use. *Principle: The selection of the control is as critical as the selection of the experimental group.*

Basically, control is achieved by either of two methods: the use of separate groups for control and treatment, or alternation of test drug and placebo in the same subjects. The former requires either random selection of large homogeneous groups or careful matching of a series of pairs, a difficult endeavor.

Assignment of patients to experimental or control groups by the use of random-number tables is the preferred method. Assignment of alternate cases to control or experimental groups is notoriously subject to conscious or subconscious manipulation. The use of serially numbered, sealed envelopes containing the regimen assignment in random order has been effective. Separate sets of envelopes may be provided for specific subgroups, if it is essential to stratify for sex, age category, or separate treatment centers. If the sample size is large enough, such stratification is seldom necessary; random distribution usually results in equality in large groups. When the subject serves as his own control, the comparison is likely valid and fewer subjects are required. One must be certain, however, that the disease has not undergone spontaneous progression or remission during the course of the study.

Double-Blind Technique. This technique has as its primary purpose the control of personal bias while the investigator is observing and measuring the response to therapy. Conscious and unconscious preferences, desires, fears, and other psychic forces in the investigator *and* the subject must be effectively dealt with if the true pharmacologic or therapeutic effect of a drug is to be recognized. Extratherapeutic factors are particularly important when subjectivity plays any role in the comparisons (see Chapter 14). These factors may have either positive or negative influences on the subject, depending upon the investigator's or subject's attitudes toward the illness. Most subjects want to please the investigator and to get well, but exceptions are too numerous and variable to disregard. In addition to a desire to benefit the patient, physicians may have preconceived biases for or against the treatment or the experiment.

The double-blind technique as originally conceived (Gold *et al.*, 1937) effectively reduces the influence of extratherapeutic factors. The investigator and the subject are "blind" as to whether a placebo or an active drug is being taken. However, "blinding" per se does not eliminate bias; it merely distributes it equally so that bias alone cannot account for a result. The method thereby prevents false-positive results, but may reduce the sensitivity of the observations and lead to false-negative results (Modell and Houde, 1958).

Double-blind procedures also alleviate the need to make decisions on allocation of an active agent or a placebo to subjects with a serious disease not responsive to known agents.

Extraneous Influences. Randomization has already been mentioned in regard to the selection of subjects where it serves to eliminate bias in the assignment of regimen. This technique is also used to distribute equally among the treatment and control groups the many extraneous forces of the environment that impinge on study subjects. Randomization does not eliminate the forces and, like the double-blind technique, may therefore reduce sensitivity. The preservation of sensitivity of the method is much more dependent on control of the circumstances of the study and upon selection of homogeneous subjects than it is on random (hopefully equal) distribution of their differences (Figure 1–2).

SOURCES OF DRUG INFORMATION

In the present setting of burgeoning pharmaceutical productivity and inadequate pharmacotherapeutic education, the physician's need for objective, concise, and well-organized information on drugs is obvious. Among the available sources are medical journals; drug compendia; textbooks and manuals of pharmacology and

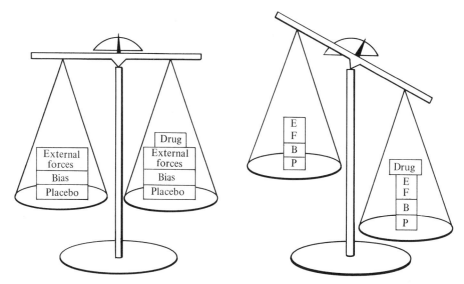

Figure 1–2. Diagrammatic representation of experimental designs for clinical evaluation. *Left*: Excessive dead-weighting to prevent chance occurrence from swinging the balance reduces sensitivity to the extent that drug effects do not swing balance and hence cannot be measured. *Right*: Reduction of dead-weighting through appropriate design makes it possible to measure pharmacodynamic effects of same intensity with same balance. (From Modell, W., and Houde, R. W.: Factors influencing clinical evaluation of drugs, with special reference to the double-blind technique. *J.A.M.A.*, **167**:2190–99, 1958.)

therapeutics; professional seminars, conventions, and society meetings; direct-mail advertising and unsolicited throwaway journals; detail men; and pharmacy newsletters. Despite this cornucopia of drug information, responsible medical spokesmen insist that most practicing physicians are unable to extract the objective and unbiased data required for the practice of rational therapeutics (Task Force, 1968).

The most popular source of information, described as most useful in a recent industry survey, is the *Physicians' Desk Reference* (PDR). The brand-name manufacturers, whose products (2600 in the 1970 edition) are cross-indexed by brand name, manufacturer, indication, generic name, and pharmacologic action, support it. No comparative data on efficacy, safety, or cost are included; the information is largely identical to the package inserts. The compendium on drugs written by the Council on Drugs of the AMA circumvents some of these objections (American Medical Association, 1971).

All textbooks of medicine and pharmacology consider therapeutics to some extent, but none has succeeded in fully bridging the gap between pharmacology as a basic science and as a clinical science.

Drug formularies, particularly in view of the growing importance of hospital-based medical practice, have considerable potential for the promotion of rational prescribing. "The formulary system is a method used by the medical staff of a hospital, working through a Pharmacy and Therapeutics Committee, to evaluate and to select, from among numerous medicinal agents available, those that are considered most useful therapeutically and to list dosage forms in which they may be administered most effectively" (*American Hospital Formulary Service*, 1967).

Industry advertising, whether it be by direct mailing, journals, displays, professional courtesies, or the detail man, is intended to be persuasive rather than educational. The pharmaceutical industry cannot, should not, and indeed does not purport to be responsible for educating physicians in the use of drugs. Nonetheless, by default, it has become a most significant influence.

Over 1500 journals are published regularly in the United States. These vary from controlled-circulation publications sent free to prescriber populations and aimed specifically at physicians reputed to be prolific prescribers, to the journal *Clinical Pharmacology and Therapeutics*, which is devoted primarily to the objective evaluation of the actions and effects of drugs in man. In between are numerous journals of general medical interest, such as *New England Journal of*

Medicine, Annals of Internal Medicine, Archives of Internal Medicine, and *Postgraduate Medicine*, paid for by individual subscription, and usually offering timely, objective therapeutic reports. Specialty journals are concerned with understanding and treating diseases of specific organ systems.

At the present time, the preferred source for information on the rational use of drugs in man is the current scientific medical literature. Although reliable information on drug use usually may be found in any of these journals, each article should be subjected to the critical appraisal discussed below and judged according to the principles presented.

As educational institutions address themselves more directly to the problems of modern therapeutics, lectures and seminars become more widely available. The spoken word, no more sanctified than the written, is more given to flirting with speculation on unsubstantiated early data or personal experience. Thus, lectures too must be judged against the following principles.

PRINCIPLES FOR EVALUATING CURRENT LITERATURE

The most reliable basis for interpreting the current literature on drug efficacy and toxicity in man is a thorough understanding of the philosophy and salient features of the clinical trial. To summarize briefly:

1. The purpose of the controlled clinical trial is the evaluation of efficacy and toxicity of drugs in man.

2. The guiding philosophy is the experimental rather than the observational approach.

3. The essence of such clinical trials is comparison.

4. The validity of the comparison depends on the accuracy and appropriateness of the measurements and on the elimination of bias.

5. The goal is to be able to generalize the findings to future patients, that is, to make inferences.

6. The strength of the inference depends on the validity of the comparison.

Approaching the Paper

Based on the above principles, every drug evaluation report should be confronted by four general questions:

1. What is the objective of the investigator?
2. Are his methods appropriate and sensitive enough for the distinction he wishes to make?
3. Is the statistical design sound?
4. Do his data justify his conclusions?

Many other questions attend these, and it may be of value for the reader of drug evaluations to construct a full set that he routinely applies to each report.

We should not accept data and conclusions based upon the status of the authors. However, the reliability of drug evaluations is favorably influenced by an academic milieu, where the experimental rather than the observational approach is cultivated. The experimental approach certainly can be applied elsewhere, but does not thrive to the same extent as in institutions of medical education. Therefore, be aware of the source of the report.

More has been said about the art of "getting published" than the art of "getting read." "Catchy" titles abound and do not guarantee a meaningful report. Often titles are not as informative as they might be, and one should always look beyond them. Titles quoted during scholarly sessions may only serve to identify a glib or uncritical reader.

The qualified clinical investigator rarely includes a "claim" in a title. A student would be wise to use a cautious, skeptical approach to any report whose title has the flavor of hucksterism. Furthermore, the mere inclusion of "double-blind" in the title should not be assumed to guarantee the reliability and validity of the data and conclusions. The use of the double-blind technique is no assurance of valid results in an otherwise poorly designed study. *Principle: Never permit the technique to sanctify the results.*

A helpful title may do no more than inform the reader whether the report is a pilot study or a definitive study, and whether it employed human or animal subjects. This information may permit an immediate decision as to the usefulness of the report or provide an appropriate frame of reference through which it can be approached. *Principle: Preliminary or pilot studies are of interest to other investigators, but rarely provide a basis for reaching decisions on drug choices in disease.*

Animal studies, which are usually concerned with basic pharmacology or with the screening of new drugs, likewise seldom have immediate relevance in choosing drugs for patients. The general problem of species differences, or of differences between diseases in man and models of disease in animals, places further limitation on the value of animal studies to the therapist. The presence of a desired effect and the absence of undesired effects in animals does not guarantee that either is true in humans (Koppani, 1960).

Clinical trials may have two fundamentally different purposes, each legitimate. One or the other, however, may not pertain to selection of a drug for patients. In one type of investigation, the pharmacologic action of a drug is at issue, whereas the other is concerned with drug efficacy in a particular disease. Do not assume that the results in one necessarily apply to the other. It is therefore important to determine if the study was conducted using subjects having the disease for which the drug is advocated. *Principle: For a report to have maximum relevance to patient care, its subjects should have had the same condition as the patient in question.*

Objectives of the Evaluation

A good investigator strives to identify and control all factors that may interfere with or aid in evaluation of his data. As we evaluate his report, we must seek answers to specific questions before we can conclude that he was successful.

1. Is there a well-defined (simple) objective? Has a question or hypothesis been stated clearly (succinctly)?

2. Has the author defined the response indicative of efficacy or safety?

3. Do you understand what he considers to be clinically important or meaningful? Do you agree?

Bear in mind that efficacy and toxicity are variables rather than fixed quantities. A narrow therapeutic margin is acceptable if the treatment is for a serious or fatal disease. Indeed, meager clinical benefit and nearly certain adverse reactions may be acceptable in the treatment of cancer. However, to justify use of a drug in a self-limited, nonfatal illness, therapy must be effective in most subjects and must not produce adverse reactions.

These decisions of clinical importance are often more fundamental than the specific statistical design permitting the investigator to judge the "significance" of the findings. They are based on the investigator's knowledge of the disease for which the drug is being evaluated. A few illustrative examples of such decisions are:

1. Should a new drug for lowering serum cholesterol be used in the management of heart disease?

   a. What decrease in cholesterol levels would you demand in subjects considered to be at increased risk (levels over 280 mg/100 ml) in order to consider a test drug effective?

   b. What proportion of patients with coronary heart disease must be protected from further clinical events before a drug under evaluation for lowering cholesterol is considered effective?

   c. What incidence of adverse reactions would be acceptable in such studies, particularly reactions as disabling as cataracts?

2. Should a new drug be used in the management of postoperative pain?

   a. What difference between the proportion of patients with postoperative pain relieved by a test drug, as compared with a placebo, would you accept as showing efficacy?

   b. What difference would you require if the new drug were being compared to an established analgesic?

A paper should present a concise statement of the question or hypothesis, and it should have clinical importance. Appropriate examples based on the questions posed might be:

1. The annual mortality rate from recurrent myocardial infarction will be reduced by 50% in males aged 45 to 55 whose mean cholesterol level is lowered more than 20% by drug A.

2. Will the dose of new analgesic agent A, by young males following inguinal herniorraphy under spinal anesthesia, be 25% less than the standard drug (indicating 25% greater effectiveness)?

3. Will the use of new analgesic A (known to be effective) be associated with a 50% reduction in postoperative nausea, vomiting, ileus, or urinary retention, as compared with the standard agent?

Methods and Statistical Design

Does the author indicate the possibility for an error in inference? This question approaches the problem of whether the subjects were representative of the patient population for which the therapy is intended. It also involves consideration of the following:

1. How sensitive were his methods?

2. Were patient and observer bias controlled?

3. What extraneous influences, presumably uncontrollable, were at play, and how were they dealt with?

Two types of errors may be made. A type 1 error is made when a "false hypothesis" is accepted. Rejection of a "true hypothesis" is a type 2 error.

Customarily under the null hypothesis (no real difference), the investigator decides in advance what "level of significance" he will accept as indicating a significant difference. Translated, this means that the author is indicating the probability of making a type 1 error, that is, of accepting a false hypothesis. This probability usually is 5% (0.05) or 1% (0.01). Stated another way, if a hypothesis is false, the author's samples should not indicate otherwise more than 5%, or 1%, of the time. The probability of making this type of error is commonly designated alpha (α).

Avoidance of type 1 errors depends on the

magnitude of the drug's pharmacodynamic action, selection of the proper dosage, the accuracy of the measurements, and the sensitivity of the methods. Sensitivity is increased by selection of subjects who are homogeneous and appropriate for the measurements to be made. "Homogeneous" means that all the subjects in a group are equally likely, before treatment, to respond to the agent under study. Sensitivity is further enhanced by maintenance of constant conditions for the control and experimental groups by eliminating all possible extraneous forces (Modell, 1960).

Type 2 errors may be avoided by the proper use of controls and by the elimination or neutralization of bias. This aspect of statistical design has received considerable attention and includes the techniques of randomization, double-blinding, control groups, crossover controls, and recognition of the placebo effect. These techniques tend to reduce sensitivity and thereby increase the likelihood of a type 1 error (Barron and Bukantz, 1967).

Modell has called attention to the consequence of efforts to eliminate bias, and his papers should be consulted for a lucid presentation of the implications of balancing (Modell and Houde, 1958; Modell, 1960). The equal distribution or "dead-weighting" of bias, placebo effect, and extraneous forces, which interfere with recognition of the pharmacodynamic force being evaluated, is illustrated in Figure 1–2.

The "sensitivity of the methods" embraces the specific measurement techniques themselves, as well as the more general sensitivity of the methods of clinical investigation. Their combination must be appropriate for the distinction the investigator is trying to make. For example, the fraction of air expired in the first second of expiration is a more sensitive method to detect airway obstruction than physical examination of the chest.

Has the author included an internal control, such as a standard therapy? The capability of recognizing a drug reaction is vital to the interpretation of a negative result.

Do the data permit construction of a dose-response curve? That is, are the methods sensitive enough to detect increments of drug action? Such sensitivity is essential to provide quantitative significance to a positive result.

Are the criteria for response appropriate? The specificity of the criterion must be examined. The clinical response in rheumatic fever may be dramatic, without corresponding changes in sedimentation rate or antistreptolysin antibody titers.

Subjects must also be representative of the population about which the investigator plans to make a therapeutic inference. Therefore, the use of a random or purposive selection will depend on the objectives of the investigation. In any event, the reader must be aware that this decision will greatly influence not only the validity of the data but also their relevance to his patient's problem.

The reader might ask the following questions before proceeding to the author's results and conclusions: Were the subjects selected at random, or by purposive sampling? What bias was introduced or avoided? Is the population chosen from diseased patients, ambulatory normals, hospitalized patients, or institutionalized volunteers? These and many other factors in selection may influence the response to the drug under investigation. Who was rejected? Who dropped out of the study? What bias did this introduce? Criteria for selection of subjects may either increase the sensitivity or obscure important drug effects.

Interpretations and Conclusions

Assuming that the answers to the questions addressed by the paper have been satisfactory (we believe that reliable data have been obtained and one or more of the standard methods for statistical analysis were applied), the only remaining concern of the reader should be the logical construction of the author's conclusions. Remember that proper statistical analysis in itself does not assure that the original data were valid or worth collecting. *Principle: The statistical answer may mislead one to assume that the data were both valuable and valid.*

In most papers by good clinical investigators, the conclusions are self-evident. One area of frequent confusion, however, concerns the interpretation of the "not significant" verdict (Hill, 1953; Mainland, 1963). Does this mean that the trial was inadequate, or that the methods lacked sensitivity, or should "not significant" be understood to mean "not real," "nonexistent," "unimportant," or merely "not proved"?

"Significantly different" was originally defined as a rare occurrence among random samples of the same population. "Rare" meant that the occurrence was likely in less than 5% of the total distribution (outside ±2 standard deviations in a normally distributed variable). "Not significant" meant not rare in the same sense. A statistical test of significance is merely a statement of the likelihood or probability that whatever differences are seen in the data are due to chance. To equate "no significant differences" with "no real differences" is a fallacy. Fisher explicitly stated that the "null hypothesis (no difference) is never proved," and that "not significant" meant simply "not proved" (Fisher,

1935). This discussion represents more than a semantic problem since many investigators who know the meaning of "not significant" may act in some situations as if "not significant" means "nonexistent" or "unimportant." The key word is *act*. What use are we going to make of the verdict? Our use of the verdict will depend on the risk we are willing to take. If we decide to pool the A and B treatment groups because they were "not significantly different" and to compare them with the control C, we are acting as if A and B treatments are not really different in their effects. If our assumption is untrue, we are assuming a risk we have not quantitated. The use an author makes of a "not significant" verdict depends on the purpose of his investigation and upon his fund of additional and not necessarily related knowledge. The most valuable use of "not significant" may be to avoid pursuit of false leads consisting of apparently strong incidental associations. If we can show that such associations frequently occur by chance, we should not pursue them even at the risk of rare type 1 errors.

In summary, when seeking information from the current literature on the choice, use, and evaluation of drugs in man, have a clear idea of what you are looking for. Select articles that present results from controlled clinical trials in humans with the disease in question. Immediately read the summary to confirm that the title was not misleading and that the report will be of value to you. This is a checkpoint (Figure 1–3)!

Next, read the introduction. Is the therapeutic objective well defined? Has the author chosen a relevant and sensitive index of accomplishment? Does this have clinical importance? Checkpoint! If the answers are not "yes," it is unlikely that it will be fruitful to proceed.

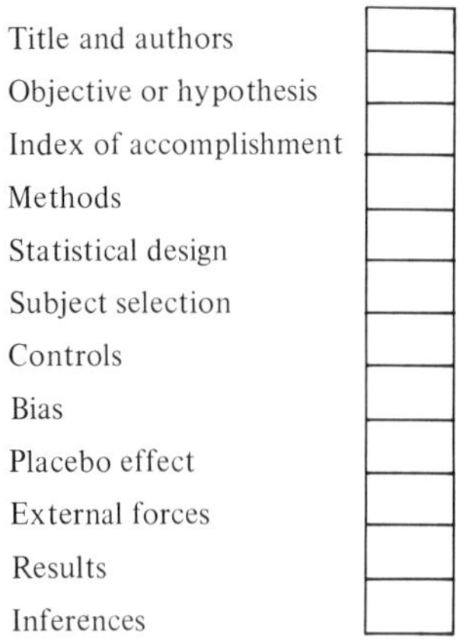

If still "on target" at this point, examine the "methods" carefully:

Were subjects chosen appropriately?
Are the measurement techniques sensitive?
Was the drug dose appropriate?
Was the statistical design sound?

Be prepared to stop at any of these checkpoints, or at least to make careful note of your reservations.

Do the data justify the conclusions? *If the paper is bad, disregard it and do not quote it.*

The literature on the use of drugs in man will be stimulating, useful, and rewarding if approached in this way.

THE PATHWAY TO RATIONAL THERAPEUTICS

Role of the University

Improved medical education is essential to achieve the objective of rational prescribing; it must occur at both undergraduate and postgraduate levels. The teaching of therapeutics, the training and support of clinical pharmacologists, and the supervision and conduct of clinical drug trials are key features of the universities' role. Furthermore, academicians have an obligation to cooperate and collaborate with both industry and government in achieving shared objectives.

Role of Industry

The interest of the pharmaceutical industry is clear; its resources and potential are great. While not responsible for rational therapeutics, industry must be responsive to societal needs. It has a moral obligation to the community to control its own practices, particularly as they may contribute to irrational prescribing. Drug manufacturers must accept the obligation to market only the best of their products: those that fill an unmet need and do not result in needless duplication. Industry could increase its already significant support of research and educational programs in collaboration with the academic community. Industry can and should play an important role in ensuring the success of governmental efforts to establish reliable, objective, well-organized, and concise sources of drug information.

Role of Government

Federal agencies, notably the Food and Drug Administration and the United States Public Health Service, have both regulatory and supportive responsibilities in the production, testing, marketing, and use of drugs in man. These functions derive from the basic responsibility to protect the public's health. In so doing, government must walk a difficult tightrope because it is

Title and authors
Objective or hypothesis
Index of accomplishment
Methods
Statistical design
Subject selection
Controls
Bias
Placebo effect
External forces
Results
Inferences

Figure 1–3. Drug report checkpoints.

also in the public's interest to support and protect an atmosphere of free inquiry, avoiding unnecessary restrictions that impede the development of useful new drugs. Among the specific contributions government can make toward rational prescribing are expanded support for educational programs in clinical pharmacology and creation of reliable, useful sources of drug information. Federal agencies could also enhance both scientific and public communication, the latter directed toward a better understanding of the need for, and benefits derived from, clinical investigation.

Role of Practitioners

If rational therapeutics consists of selection of the right drug for the right patient in the right amounts at the right times (Task Force, 1968), the prescribers play the most strategic role. Rational prescribing is dependent on the physicians' exercise of good clinical judgment on many points. In addition to the safety and efficacy of the drug in the immediate clinical situation, these include the advantages or disadvantages of alternative choices, the most appropriate dosage form, duration of therapy, potential side effects or adverse reactions, and the possibility of drug interactions. If university, industry, and government each fulfill their role, and if each adopts an understanding, communicative, and collaborative stance toward the others, the pharmaceutical revolution will proceed rationally and practicing physicians will respond with performance of rational therapeutics.

REFERENCES

AMA Drug Evaluations, 1st ed. American Medical Association, Chicago, 1971.

Armitage, P.: *Sequential Medical Trials.* Blackwell Scientific Publications, Oxford, 1960.

American Hospital Formulary Service: A Collection of Drug Monographs and Other Information. American Society of Hospital Pharmacists, Washington, D.C., 1967.

Barr, D. P.: Hazards of modern diagnosis and therapy: the price we pay. *J.A.M.A.*, 159:1452–56, 1955.

Barron, B. A., and Bukantz, S. C.: The evaluation of new drugs: current Food and Drug Administration regulations and statistical aspects of clinical trials. *Arch. Intern. Med. (Chicago)*, 119:547–56, 1967.

Beecher, H. K.: The powerful placebo. *J.A.M.A.*, 159: 1602–1606, 1955.

———: *Measurement of Subjective Response.* Oxford University Press, New York, 1959.

Bernard, C.: *An Introduction to the Study of Experimental Medicine.* Paris, 1865. Translation by H. C. Greene. Dover Publications, New York, 1957.

Brown, E. A.: Problems of drug allergy. *J.A.M.A.*, 157: 814–19, 1955.

Chalmers, T. C.: Clinical pharmacology as an academic discipline. *New Eng. J. Med.*, 270:140–41, 1964.

Clapp, R. F.: *Study of Purchase Problems and Policies.*

Dept. of Health, Education, and Welfare—Welfare Administration, Research Report #2. U.S. Government Printing Office, Washington, D.C., 1966.

Cluff, L. E.; Thornton, G. F.; and Seidl, L. G.: Studies on the epidemiology of adverse drug reactions. I. Methods of surveillance. *J.A.M.A.*, 188:976–83, 1964.

Cornfield, J.: Sequential trials, sequential analysis and the likelihood principle. *Amer. Statist.*, 20:18–23, 1966.

Daniels, M.: Clinical evaluation of chemotherapy in tuberculosis. *Brit. Med. Bull.*, 7:320–26, 1951.

Editorial: The drug efficacy study. *New Eng. J. Med.*, 280:1177–79, 1969.

Feinstein, A. R.: Symptomatic patterns, biologic behavior, and prognosis in cancer of the lung: practical applications of Boolean algebra and clinical taxonomy. *Ann. Intern. Med.*, 61:27–43, 1964.

———: *Clinical Judgment.* Williams & Wilkins Co., Baltimore, 1967.

———: Clinical epidemiology. I–III. The clinical design of statistics in therapy. *Ann. Intern. Med.*, 69:1287–312, 1968.

Fisher, R. A.: *The Design of Experiments.* Oliver & Boyd, Ltd., London, 1935.

Garrison, F. H.: *An Introduction to the History of Medicine.* W. B. Saunders Co., Philadelphia, 1929.

Gold, H.: "The proper study of mankind is man." *Amer. J. Med.*, 12:619–20, 1952.

Gold, H.; Kwit, N. T.; and Otto, H.: The xanthines (theobromine and aminophylline) in the treatment of cardiac pain. *J.A.M.A.*, 108:2173–79, 1937.

Gosselin, R. D., & Co.: *National Prescription Audit.* Dedham, Mass., 1968.

Hill, A. B.: The clinical trial. *Brit. Med. Bull.*, 7:278–82, 1951.

———: The clinical trial. *New Eng. J. Med.*, 247:113–19, 1952.

———: The philosophy of the clinical trial. National Institutes of Health Annual Lectures, Washington, D.C., 1953.

———: *Controlled Clinical Trials.* Conference of Council for International Organizations of Medical Sciences. Blackwell Scientific Publications, Oxford, 1960.

Hill, Sir A.: *Statistical Methods in Clinical and Preventive Medicine.* Oxford University Press, New York, 1962.

Irvington House: Rheumatic fever in children and adolescents: a long-term epidemiologic study of subsequent prophylaxis, streptococcal infection, and clinical sequelae. *Ann. Intern. Med.*, 60(suppl. 5):1–129, 1964.

Jick, H.; Slone, D.; Dinan, B.; and Muench, H.: Evaluation of drug efficacy by a preference technique. *New Eng. J. Med.*, 275:1399–1403, 1966.

Koppani, T.: Symposium on the study of drugs in man. I. From animal to human: some basic principles of comparative pharmacology. *Clin. Pharmacol. Ther.*, 1:7–15, 1960.

Lasagna, L.: Problems of drug development. *Science*, 145:362–67, 1964.

———: Drug toxicity in man: the problem and the challenge. *Ann. N.Y. Acad. Sci.*, 123:312–15, 1965.

———: Presented at the International Symposium on amphetamines and related compounds in Milan, Italy. Reported in *Med. World News*, May 9, 1969.

Lasagna, L.; Laties, V. G.; and Dohan, L. J.: Further studies on "pharmacology" of placebo administration. *J. Clin. Invest.*, 37:533–37, 1958.

Mainland, D.: The clinical trial: some difficulties and suggestions. *J. Chron. Dis.*, 11:484–96, 1960.

———: The significance of "nonsignificance." *Clin. Pharmacol. Ther.*, 4:580–86, 1963.

Medical Research Council: Streptomycin treatment of pulmonary tuberculosis. *Brit. Med. J.*, 2:769–82, 1948.

Medical Research Council: Clinical trials of antihistaminic drugs in the prevention and treatment of the common cold. *Ibid.*, **2**:425–29, 1950a.

———: Treatment of pulmonary tuberculosis with streptomycin and para-aminosalicylic acid. *Ibid.*, **2**:1073–85, 1950b.

———: The prevention of streptomycin resistance by combined chemotherapy. *Ibid.*, **1**:1157–62, 1952.

———: A comparison of cortisone and aspirin in the treatment of early cases of rheumatoid arthritis. *Ibid.*, **1**:1223–27, 1954.

Melmon, K. L.: Preventable drug reactions: causes and cures. *New Eng. J. Med.*, **284**: 1361–68, 1971.

Meyer, U., and Marver, H.: Chemically induced porphyria: Increased microsomal heme turnover after treatment with allylisopropylacetamide. *Science*, **171**: 64–66, 1971a.

———: Intermittent acute porphyria (IAP): Clinical demonstration of a genetic defect in porphobilinogen (PBG) metabolism. *Clin. Res.*, **14**:398, 1971b.

Modell, W.: The sensitivity and validity of drug evaluations in man. *Clin. Pharmacol. Ther.*, **1**:769–76, 1960.

———: The drug explosion. *Clin. Pharmacol. Ther.*, **2**:1–7, 1961.

———: Hazards of new drugs: the scientific approach is necessary for the safest and most effective use of new drugs. *Science*, **139**:1180–85, 1963.

Modell, W., and Houde, R. W.: Factors influencing clinical evaluation of drugs, with special reference to the double-blind technique. *J.A.M.A.*, **167**:2190–99, 1958.

Morrelli, H. F., and Melmon, K. L.: The clinician's approach to drug interactions. *Calif. Med.*, **109**:380–89, 1968.

Moser, R. H.: *Diseases of Medical Progress: A Study of Iatrogenic Disease*, 3rd ed. Charles C Thomas, Publisher, Springfield, Ill., 1969.

Reidenberg, M. M., and Lowenthal, D. T.: Adverse non-drug reactions. *New Eng. J. Med.*, **279**:678–79, 1968.

Shapiro, A. K.: Etiological factors in placebo effect. *J.A.M.A.*, **187**:712–14, 1964.

Smith, J. W.; Seidl, L. G.; and Cluff, L. E.: Studies on the epidemiology of adverse drug reactions. V. Clinical factors influencing susceptibility. *Ann. Intern. Med.*, **65**:629–40, 1966.

Task Force on Prescription Drugs, Dept. of Health, Education, and Welfare: *Background Papers*. U.S. Government Printing Office, Washington, D.C., 1968.

———: *Final Report*. U.S. Government Printing Office, Washington, D.C., 1969.

Waife, S. O., and Shapiro, A. P. (eds.): *The Clinical Evaluation of New Drugs*. Paul B. Hoeber, Inc., New York, 1959.

Wolf, S.: The pharmacology of placebos. *Pharmacol. Rev.*, **11**:689–704, 1959.

Chapter 2

DRUG ADMINISTRATION AND REGIMENS

Malcolm Rowland

Recommended dosage regimens are found in textbooks of pharmacology, formularies, and the pharmaceutical manufacturers' package inserts. These schedules have proved satisfactory in limited but carefully supervised clinical studies. Until the last few decades, the fate of drugs in man was virtually unknown, and a reasonable dosage regimen was established empirically by carefully titrating the patient with the drug until a desired response with minimum side effects was achieved. Clinical trials are now more extensive and sophisticated and are preceded by pharmacologic, toxicologic, metabolic, and kinetic investigations in animals (see Chapter 1). Data derived from studies in animals are the basis for prediction of the therapeutic dose and suitable dosage regimens in man. However, the fate of the drug in man must be studied (phase 1 testing) to test the predictions or to suggest suitable modifications in dosage schedules.

A drug in man is subject to physical and chemical processes that may markedly alter its effectiveness or toxicity. Many of these processes are well known, so that accurate predictions can be made about the fate of a given drug in a given patient. The clinician should be familiar with available information on the absorption, distribution, metabolism, and excretion of the drugs he uses. This knowledge allows him to predict likely pharmacokinetic changes, and to plan his course accordingly. If the physician fails to understand these processes, he runs the risk of giving ineffective treatment or causing dangerous toxicity.

After entering the circulation, drugs simultaneously distribute into various parts of the body and are eliminated. Distribution generally occurs much more rapidly than elimination. The major organs responsible for the elimination of drugs are the liver, which transforms the drug into one or more metabolites, and the kidneys, which excrete variable amounts of the drug and its metabolites. Many drugs are eliminated via the feces after biliary excretion. The qualitative nature of these processes and the rates at which they occur must be considered in choosing the best agent to be administered to a patient for a specific phase of a disease. A long-acting antibiotic that requires infrequent administration may be advantageous in the treatment of an infection, but a long-acting soporific might be undesirable for treatment of insomnia.

Drugs are sometimes given once. Usually they are repetitively administered to maintain a constant concentration of drug in the blood or tissues, thereby achieving a uniform response. Optimum control is attained by adjustment of the dose and of the interval between doses. If a dose interval is too frequent or if the dose is too large, drug levels rise and lead to toxic effects (see Chapter 15). If the drug is given too infrequently or in too small a dose, drug therapy may be ineffective. The patient's age, weight, degree of adiposity, and hepatic and renal function, as well as his individual responsiveness to the drug and the simultaneous effects of other drugs, must be considered when planning a therapeutic regimen (see Chapter 14). *Principle: Correct assessment of a drug regimen requires knowledge of the therapeutic dose and of the speed of drug elimination in that patient.*

In clinical practice, situations frequently arise in which multiple drug therapy is indicated. A wide variety of therapeutic agents stimulate enzymes that are responsible for the metabolism of drugs. It may be necessary to increase the dose or frequency of administraton of a drug when it is used in combination with enzyme-stimulating agents. Conversely, other drugs may inhibit enzyme systems; this may necessitate a decrease in the frequency or size of the dose (see Chapter 16). A drug may displace another either from its site of action (receptor) or from a plasma or tissue protein. If displacement occurs at the site of action, the effect of the first drug is decreased, whereas displacement from proteins can increase the drug's effect by increasing the concentration of drug at its receptor (see Chapters 16 and 17). A drug may also influence the renal excretion or the intestinal absorption of another drug (see Chapters 16 and 17).

Patients with renal disease slowly eliminate drugs predominantly cleared by the kidneys and require a decreased frequency of drug administration (see Chapter 3). If a choice exists between two agents, one of which is primarily eliminated by the kidneys while the other is primarily eliminated by hepatic metabolism, the latter drug should be used in patients with renal impairment; otherwise, drug accumulation and toxicity may result. Patients with liver disease may metabolize drugs more slowly and may require less frequent administration of drugs (see Chapter 4). Drugs may distribute more slowly in certain cases of altered hemodynamics, for example, congestive heart failure. Initially, more drug than usual remains in the vascular system, reaching the brain and heart. A normal dose may cause toxicity, and a readjustment of the dosage schedule for these patients may be necessary. *Principle: The state of a patient's health can drastically alter his dose requirements.*

In preliminary drug testing, the chemical is administered to test subjects, usually in capsules. In this form the chemical may be efficacious. When the same drug is clinically given as a drug formulation, that is, a tablet, emulsion, suspension, or suppository, different results may be seen. A formulation contains a variety of materials that may stabilize the drug, hasten the disintegration and dissolution of the agent, or simply improve acceptance by the patient.

Many of these excipients can modify the rate and amount of absorption of drug. Sometimes a change in the dosage form of a drug makes the difference between success or failure in drug therapy. *Principle: The fact that a particular formulation contains a specified amount of active chemical does not guarantee that this drug will be liberated upon administration.*

Summary Principle: The decision to use any particular drug is dependent not only upon its pharmacologic properties but also upon the health of the patient, the rate at which the drug is eliminated, the simultaneous use of other drugs, and the route and dosage form of the agent to be administered. Only after considering each of these factors can a rational judgment be made regarding the "drug of choice."

FACTORS INFLUENCING DRUG ABSORPTION AND DISPOSITION

Most drugs are reversibly bound to receptors, and the effect of the drug is directly related to its concentration in the fluid surrounding the receptor. The concentration of drug in tissue may depend on its concentration in plasma, because in most instances drug is conveyed to tissues via the blood. Accordingly, the onset, duration, and intensity of the pharmacologic effect should be reflected by the concentration of the drug in plasma. Figure 2–1 lists some of the factors that influence the amount and persistence of drug in the body, and consequently its pharmacologic effect. This scheme is complex, but some general quantitative principles regarding drug administration can be advanced.

A minimum tissue concentration of drug is required for a desired response. This concentration is related to a particular concentration of drug in plasma (the minimum effective concentration, MEC). As long as the concentration of drug is maintained above the MEC, an effect is observed, and the intensity of the effect increases as the concentration increases, until a maximum response or toxicity is produced. The greater the rate of drug absorption, the more rapidly drug levels in plasma and tissues rise, resulting in an earlier onset and a greater intensity of pharmacologic effect. If drug absorption is very slow, plasma concentrations of drug may never reach the MEC, and no effect will be observed (Figure 2–2).

Passage of Drugs Across Membranes

A drug must often cross several membranes to reach its receptor. This transfer is usually accomplished by passive diffusion. In addition, special drug transport mechanisms, that is, facilitated diffusion and active transport, allow substances to pass across cell membranes at a faster rate than does simple

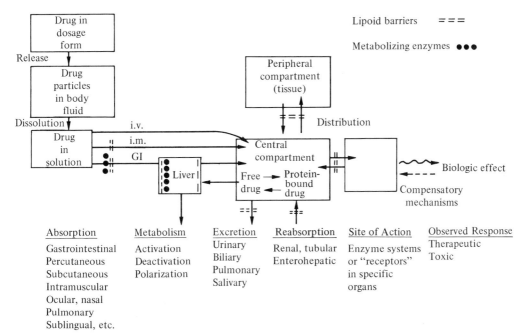

Figure 2–1. Diagram illustrating the factors that influence the onset, duration, and intensity of drug effects. Note that the drug must dissolve before being absorbed, and that it passes across many lipoid barriers and some metabolizing systems before reaching the site of action. (From Barr, W. H.: Principles of biopharmaceutics. *Amer. J. Pharm. Educ.*, **52**:958–81, 1968.)

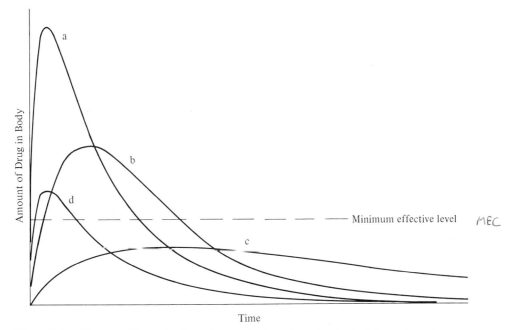

Figure 2–2. Diagram illustrating how changes in the rate and extent of drug absorption can influence both the duration of action and the efficacy of drug therapy. The same dose is given on different occasions:

Case a: Drug absorbed rapidly and completely. This produces a prompt response.

Case b: Drug absorbed completely but more slowly. This produces a delayed, but sometimes more prolonged response.

Case c: Drug absorbed completely but so slowly that drug levels never reach the minimum effective level and, therefore, therapy is ineffective.

Case d: Drug absorbed rapidly but incompletely. This produces a prompt but transient response.

diffusion (Ariens, 1964; Binns, 1964; Shanker, 1964; Korn, 1966; Stein, 1967).

Passive Diffusion. Passive diffusion is characterized by the movement of drug molecules down a concentration or electrochemical gradient without cellular expenditure of energy. The transfer is neither saturable nor inhibited by other materials and is only slightly sensitive to temperature changes.

Most cells are in very close proximity to a capillary. Passage of drug across short distances is usually rapid, but diffusion may be hindered by the intervening cell membranes. The membranes may be single (e.g., erythrocyte and capillary walls) or complex (e.g., the multicellular intestinal epithelium and structures associated with the passage of drug into the brain). Although the membrane's complexity may determine the time necessary for passage of a molecule, any membrane may be considered a barrier through which the diffusion of a molecule is slower than it would be through a similar layer of water.

The driving force for drug transfer is the difference between the concentrations of the diffusing species on either side of the membrane ($C_{out} - C_{in}$). The rate of penetration of the drug through this barrier is related to the concentration gradient by Fick's law of diffusion:

$$\text{Rate of penetration} = \frac{-DAK(C_{out} - C_{in})}{\Delta x} \quad (1)$$

where D is the diffusion coefficient of the drug molecule within the membrane, K is the partition coefficient of the molecule between the membrane and the aqueous phase on either side of the membrane, and A and Δx are the area and thickness of the membrane, respectively. The minus sign denotes loss of drug from the outside when the concentration outside is greater than that on the inside. The more lipid soluble the molecule, the higher its partition coefficient; the greater the surface area of the membrane, the more rapid is molecular transfer through a lipoidal membrane. Smaller molecules, by possessing a higher diffusion coefficient, diffuse through the membrane more rapidly than do larger molecules. The fraction $DKA/\Delta x$ is frequently called the permeability constant (P) of the system. The distribution of drugs between plasma and tissue (uptake into or release from tissue) continues until the concentrations of drug in plasma and tissue water are equal and net transfer is nil.

The time required to reach equilibrium depends on the permeability constant; the higher the value, the more rapidly the drug diffuses across the membrane to establish equilibrium. The most important determinant of the permeability constant is the partition coefficient, K. When highly lipid-soluble drugs are used, penetration is sufficiently rapid that only a single passage of blood through an organ is necessary to establish equilibrium between tissue and plasma. Rate of drug uptake into tissues is then limited by the flow rate of blood.

Many drugs are organic acids or bases. It is usually assumed that only nonionized lipid-soluble drugs pass through lipid-rich membranes. The ionized molecule is thought to be too polar to penetrate the lipoidal barrier. This concept is known as the "pH partition hypothesis," or the theory of nonionic diffusion. The rate of passage of a drug through a membrane is therefore dependent upon the pH of the environment and the dissociation constant (pK_a) of the drug (i.e., the pH at which the nonionized and ionized drug concentrations are equal), since according to the Henderson-Hasselbalch equation:

$$pH = pK_a + \log\frac{(\text{nonionized})}{(\text{ionized})} \quad \text{(for a base)} \quad (2a)$$

$$pH = pK_a + \log\frac{(\text{ionized})}{(\text{nonionized})} \quad \text{(for an acid)} \quad (2b)$$

with the sign ( ) denoting concentration. For example, the local anesthetic lidocaine is a base with a pK_a of 7.89. Therefore, at pH 7.89, equal concentrations of the nonionized base and positively charged ionized lidocaine (formed by the amine accepting a hydrogen ion) are present in solution. Alkalinizing the solution (raising the pH) increases the fraction of nonionized drug thereby increasing drug transfer. Conversely, the more acidic the medium (the lower the pH), the greater the concentration of ionized drug; transfer of lidocaine is therefore decreased. If a drug is a strong acid or base, it is more highly ionized at physiologic pH and crosses membranes more slowly.

Equilibrium is achieved when the nonionized concentrations of drug are equal on both sides of the membrane. When a pH differential exists across the membrane, the concentrations (nonionized plus ionized) of drug on either side of the membrane are unequal. Basic drugs (amphetamine, mecamylamine, antihistamines, etc.) accumulate in the more acidic fluids (including intracellular). Acidic molecules (salicylates, phenobarbital, etc.) are found in higher concentrations in the more alkaline extracellular fluids. Recent work suggests that ionized molecules are also transported through membranes; this process may account for some drug transfer (Kakemi *et al.*, 1969).

In many instances, equilibrium is not achieved, either because drug diffuses from a small volume into a much larger volume (e.g., absorption of drugs from the gastrointestinal tract into body fluids) or because drug is rapidly removed by elimination so that the concentration of drug on the inner side of the membrane (C_{in}) is virtually negligible compared to that on the outside (C_{out}); the drug then diffuses unidirectionally. In most biologic systems the volume (V) of the system from which the drug diffuses remains reasonably constant. Under these circumstances the Fick equation simplifies to:

$$\frac{dC_{out}}{dt} = -kC_{out} \quad (3)$$

where k (equal to $DAK/V\Delta x$) is a proportionality constant with units of time $^{-1}$. Since the term $dC_{out}/C_{out}\,dt$ is the fractional rate of change in the concentration, k can be regarded as the fraction of drug removed from the site per unit time. Such processes, where *the rate of transfer of drug is proportional to the amount remaining*, are said to follow *first-order kinetics.* Data describing first-order kinetics may be represented by the above differential equation, but the integral form is more common:

$$C = C_0 e^{-kt} \tag{4}$$

where C_0 is the initial drug concentration and e is the base of the natural logarithm. According to this equation, the concentration falls exponentially and the fraction remaining (C/C_0) at a given time is independent of the initial concentration. While first-order processes are prevalent, occasionally *the rate of drug transfer or loss is constant and independent of the concentration of drugs*; such processes are said to obey *zero-order kinetics* (see page 33). Under such circumstances the concentration falls at a constant rate, so that the fractional rate of decline, rather than being constant as seen in the case of first-order processes, is lower with larger initial drug concentrations.

To ascertain whether drug transfer proceeds by first-order kinetics, a semilogarithmic plot of the declining concentration (or amount) against time may be constructed. This yields a straight line:

$$\log C = \log C_0 - \frac{k}{2.3} t \tag{5a}$$

or if both sides of equation 4 had been multiplied by the volume, V:

$$\log A = \log A_0 - \frac{k}{2.3} t \tag{5b}$$

where A_0 is the amount initially present, and A the amount remaining after time t. Semilogarithmic plots are usually derived from logarithms to the base 10. The value 2.3 is the relation between the natural logarithm and logarithms to the base 10. In either case, the value of k can be determined from the slope of the plotted line (Figure 2–3). It is clinically more useful to calculate the half-life ($t_{1/2}$) that is, the time required for the concentration (or amount) to decrease to one-half its initial value. If the half-life is known, k is readily found, because at the half-life $C = 1/2\, C_0$ and $\log_e 2$ is 0.693. Therefore:

$$k = \frac{0.693}{t_{1/2}} \tag{6}$$

Principle: For a first-order process, the half-life, given by the time required for the concentration to decline by one-half, is independent of concentration. As a first approximation, absorption of drugs from gastric, intestinal, intramuscular, subcutaneous, and rectal sites, drug distribution throughout the body, and the renal excretion and metabolism of many drugs obey first-order kinetics.

Facilitated Diffusion. Glucose is too large and too polar a molecule to pass through the aqueous pores of cell membranes. Nonetheless, it rapidly diffuses into red blood cells. To explain the ability of glucose and other molecules to be transferred rapidly across membranes, facilitated diffusion has been proposed. In facilitated diffusion, a postulated carrier complexes with the drug molecule in the membrane. The complex is then translocated across the membrane at a much faster rate than that associated with the diffusion of drug alone. Transport of drug occurs down a concentration gradient. Unlike simple

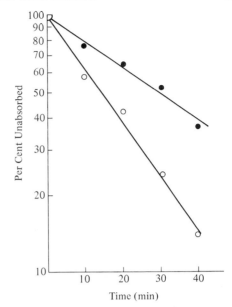

Figure 2–3. Absorption of salicylic acid (○) and aspirin (●) from the stomach of man. The drugs were given in solution. The absorption of both drugs is satisfactorily described by first-order kinetics, with the half-life for absorption being 15 minutes and 30 minutes, respectively. (From Levy, G.; Gumtow, R. H.; and Rutowski, J. M.: The effect of dosage form upon the gastrointestinal absorption rate of salicylates. *Canad. Med. Ass. J.*, **85**:414–19, 1961.)

diffusion, the postulated carrier can be saturated at high drug concentrations, and other materials can inhibit or compete for the same carrier system. This system requires no cellular energy and is only slightly sensitive to temperature changes. Facilitated diffusion is responsible for the rapid transport of other sugars and amino acids into the human erythrocyte.

Active Transport. Endogenous compounds and drugs may be transported across membranes against a concentration gradient. This "uphill" or active transport requires metabolic energy and can be readily inhibited by metabolic inhibitors or by alterations in temperature. Relative selectivity, saturability, and competitive inhibition are also characteristic of active transport processes. Transport of sodium out of cells, renal tubular reabsorption of glucose, secretion of acids and bases by the renal tubular cell into the tubular lumen, removal of many endogenous acids from the brain, and intestinal absorption of 5-fluorouracil are achieved by active transport.

Passage of Drugs into the Central Nervous System (CNS) and Across the Placenta. Although some acids are actively secreted from the CNS, most drugs enter or leave the brain and cerebrospinal fluid (CSF) by passive diffusion. Entry of drug into the brain is principally via cerebral capillaries, although some polar drugs first appear in the CSF apparently via the choroid plexus. The apparent exclusion of some drugs from the CNS is attributed to a "blood-brain barrier." This barrier may be due to the sheath of lipoidal glial cells that surrounds capillaries of the brain, which could reduce the rate of entry of some compounds. The drug's rate of entry can be correlated with its oil-to-water partition coefficient, degree of ionization at plasma pH, and its binding to plasma proteins. An increase in lipid solubility and a decrease in ionization or binding enhances entry. For example, thiopental is a very lipid-soluble, weak acid (pK_a 7.6). It enters the brain so rapidly that the membranes no longer appear to prevent drug transfer, and the initial rate of uptake becomes directly related to blood flow. In contrast, Evans blue dye is a water-soluble, ionized, highly protein-bound substance that cannot enter brain tissue or CSF. Most drugs lie between these extremes. *Principle: To produce a central effect, a drug must be somewhat lipid soluble.* A notable exception is alpha-methyldopa, an amino acid, which is actively transported into the brain and subsequently metabolized to alpha-methylnorepinephrine. A basic drug that acts on the nervous system may be altered to produce a selective peripheral effect by quaternization of the drug, which decreases its lipid solubility and makes it virtually unavailable for transfer to the central nervous system.

The time required to produce equilibrium of drug concentration between plasma and tissue is a function of the permeability of the membrane for that drug (see page 24). For drugs that enter freely into the CNS, equilibrium is attained in a short time, and the concentration of drug in brain rapidly reflects changes in its plasma concentration. For drugs that enter the CNS very slowly, days or weeks on a constant drug regimen may be required before peak concentrations are found in brain. Chronic accrual of such drugs may lead to adverse central effects which may persist for a considerable time after reduction of the concentration of drug in plasma. *Principle: Response or toxicity to a drug may not appear simultaneously with drug administration or cease promptly when the drug is discontinued.*

Many drugs, including barbiturates, local anesthetics, volatile anesthetics, and sulfonamides, have been detected in fetal blood. The characteristic withdrawal syndrome (from narcotics) and occasional hypoglycemic episodes seen in newborns whose mothers take narcotics or oral hypoglycemic agents indicate that these drugs also pass across the placenta. Passage may actually be encouraged by the large surface area available for diffusion and the rich vascular supply to the placenta. Transfer is by passive diffusion; the higher the oil-to-water partition coefficient of a drug and the lower the degree of ionization and protein binding in the blood, the more rapidly it passes into the fetus. *Principle: Placental membranes are lipoidal in character and differ little from other membranes of the body in respect to the passage of drugs.*

The placenta contains enzymes capable of metabolizing drugs. The degree of protection this confers on the fetus is still unknown. However, a rule of thumb useful in any clinical setting is particularly applicable in this instance: *Do not use drugs unless there is a clear indication for their administration* (Goldstein *et al.*, 1968; Moya, 1970; Ginsberg, 1971).

Routes of Administration

Drugs are given topically, enterally, by inhalation, or parenterally. The enteral route includes oral and rectal administration. Parenteral routes include intravenous, intramuscular, and subcutaneous injections when a systemic effect is desired, and tissue infiltration, spinal injections, and epidural injections when a localized action is sought. Drugs injected into the cerebrospinal fluid may exit and cause systemic effects. Inhalation and topical application usually produce intensive local effects, but occasionally systemic effects are also produced.

Intravenous Injection. When the clinical setting requires immediate response, drugs are most often given intravenously. This mode of administration can result in a predictable concentration of drug in blood and in an extremely rapid response. For example, when thiopental is administered for seizures, control often ensues within seconds of injection. However, the rate of injection should be slow enough to prevent excessively high drug concentrations in plasma, which may produce local pain and perhaps undesirable cardiovascular and central effects. One or two minutes for injection is generally sufficient, but if problems arise in the first few seconds, drug administration should be stopped. This route also provides a method for precise and continual drug therapy using an infusion via an intravenous drip. The concentration of drug in the fluid and the fluid's flow rate into the patient determine the rate of drug delivery. If even more precise drug delivery is required, an infusion pump can be used. For example, labor can be induced and controlled with an intravenous infusion of oxytocin. This drug is very rapidly destroyed in the body, and the necessary control could not be attained if other methods or routes of administration were used. Intravenous infusion might also be considered when a drug's therapeutic index is narrow.

Despite the many advantages of the intravenous route, it is not without its liabilities. Insoluble materials cannot be given in this manner, as they may cause embolism. The intravenous route is used with difficulty for chronic drug administration, owing to the hazards of thrombophlebitis, infection, and infiltration of drug into subcutaneous tissues. Once injected, the drug reaches high concentrations rapidly and cannot be withdrawn; extraordinary care must be taken to ensure that the correct dose is given.

Intra-arterial Injection. This route is reserved for situations requiring localization of drug in a particular organ. It is especially useful when toxic materials must be injected, since, by concentrating the drug locally, it reduces the risk of producing toxic concentrations in the systemic circulation. For example, an antineoplastic nitrogen mustard can be injected intra-arterially at a tumor site. Combinations of this drug with radiopaque materials may ensure proper placement of drug in very high concentrations in the organ being visualized by roentgenography. All precautions taken during intravenous administration of drugs are applicable when drugs are given by the intra-arterial route.

Intramuscular and Subcutaneous Injection. Quantitative drug administration is guaranteed by use of intramuscular or subcutaneous injections, but the rate of drug absorption may be variable. An injection is usually made into the muscles of the buttock, thigh, or arm, or the subcutaneous tissue of the arm or thigh. Greater volumes of drug solution can usually be given by the intramuscular route than by the subcutaneous route. Both routes are generally reserved for patients in whom a fairly rapid response is desired, but in whom intravenous administration is either too dangerous or unnecessary, or suitable veins cannot be found. In addition, these routes are chosen for administration of drugs that are poorly absorbed from or destroyed within the gastrointestinal tract. Drug absorption from intramuscular and subcutaneous sites is usually rapid (especially from an aqueous solution). However, uptake from these sites may be delayed and erratic, particularly when solutions of salts of sparingly soluble acids and bases are injected. For example, quinidine hydrochloride is acidic. The buffer capacity of tissues at the injection site is sufficiently high that it raises the pH of the injection solution. This pH shift causes the sparingly soluble quinidine base to precipitate at the site; absorption is prolonged as drug slowly dissolves into the tissue fluids. The initial pH of a solution of the sodium salt of diphenylhydantoin is around 12. The extreme alkalinity of the solution may cause severe pain following its intramuscular injection. As the pH of the injected solution decreases, the drug precipitates and is absorbed slowly (Ditlefsen, 1957; Ballard, 1968; Wallis *et al.*, 1968).

In some disease states, such as accelerating hypertension, shock, or congestive heart failure, changes in blood flow around the site of injection may become the limiting factor in drug absorption from muscle. Rubbing or heating the skin around the injection site may increase local blood flow and aid in drug absorption. Coadministration of epinephrine with the local anesthetics extends their duration of action by producing vasoconstriction. The intramuscular and subcutaneous routes may be contraindicated when shock or malignant hypertension limits blood flow through muscle. Furthermore, as the patient recovers from either state, blood flow to the site, and consequently drug absorption, will increase at a time when the agent may no longer be necessary, and adverse effects may occur.

Neutral, sparingly soluble drugs are dissolved in nonaqueous solvents (vehicles) that are either miscible or immiscible with water (e.g., polyethylene 300 and peanut oil, respectively). The water-miscible solvents are removed more rapidly, and the drug precipitates at the injection site. Because the drug then has limited solubility, it dissolves slowly and low concentrations of drug are obtained in the blood for prolonged periods (see Prolonged-Release Dosage Forms, page 46).

Oral Administration. The alimentary canal is the most popular route of drug administration. Oral preparations account for more than 80% of all drugs prescribed; rectal suppositories are occasionally employed. Ingested drug is available to absorption sites (gastric and intestinal epithelium) for a finite period, sometimes as long as 1 or 2 days. For certain drugs (including griseofulvin and bishydroxycoumarin) this time is insufficient for complete absorption. The efficacy of the oral route for medication is judged by both the rate and the extent of absorption. Either incomplete or slow absorption can account for ineffective therapy (Figure 2–2, page 23).

Large *intra*patient variations exist in the absorption rates of drugs, even when the drugs are taken in solution (Shanker, 1964). Many of the differences in absorption may be explained by the "pH partition hypothesis." Numerous physiologic factors add to the variation, for example, rate of production, nature and composition of the gastric and intestinal juices, rate of gastric emptying, gastrointestinal motility, presence or absence of food, pathologic state of the gastrointestinal tract, and position of the patient (see Chapter 4). Even larger *inter*patient variations may occur when drugs are used clinically, because the agents are ingested in solid dosage form (Wagner, 1961). Absorption of a drug from tablet or capsule is influenced by many of the physiologic factors mentioned above, but also depends upon solubility, particle-size distribution, chemical form, and crystalline structure of the drug, as well as several manufacturing variables (e.g., the compression force used to make the tablets, and the "inert" materials that can either hasten or retard disintegration and dissolution of the tablet). Consequently, dosage forms might be described as "drug delivery systems" from which a drug is designed to be made completely available to the absorption sites in a predictable and reproducible manner. *Principle: Comparisons between drug preparations containing the same active compound should take into account the rate and extent of drug absorption.*

Gastrointestinal Absorption of Drugs from Solution. Drugs in simple solution are usually absorbed rapidly and completely unless they form insoluble complexes with the intestinal juices or unless they are unstable in the intestinal tract. Absorption is still rapid from hydroalcoholic solutions (elixirs), even if the drug precipitates when the solution is diluted by the gastric juice. Liquid suspensions contain materials that are only sparingly soluble in water. Some suspensions, such as the antacids, are not intended for absorption. Others are given in the hope that in a well-dispersed system, dissolution is hastened and absorption is enhanced. The absorption of such suspensions largely depends upon the size of the particles since this determines the surface area available for dissolution of drug. The smaller the particles, the larger the surface area. For example, the sparingly soluble sulfonamide sulfadiazine is absorbed more rapidly when the particles in suspension are reduced from 20μ to less than 2μ in diameter. Absorption from a suspension is almost always more rapid than from a tablet of the same drug.

The "pH partition hypothesis" states that the absorption of drugs from the alimentary canal can be explained by the passive diffusion of the nonionized, lipid-soluble molecules across a lipid membrane. Very weakly acidic or basic lipid-soluble drugs that are essentially nonionized at all physiologic pHs are absorbed from the stomach and intestine, whereas very strong acids, which remain largely ionized except at pH 1 to 2, are poorly absorbed. Polar molecules, whether neutral (mannitol) or ionized (neomycin), are either absorbed poorly or not at all, unless they are sufficiently small to pass through the pores of the membrane (e.g., urea). Moderately strong bases (e.g., ephedrine, pK_a 9.3; amphetamine, pK_a 9.9) are negligibly absorbed from the acidic gastric contents, but rapidly from the intestinal fluids, which have a much lower hydrogen ion concentration (pH 5 to 8). Moderately strong acids (e.g., salicylic acid, pK_a 3) are absorbed from the stomach, but more rapidly from the duodenum. The enormous increase in the available surface area in the duodenum (as opposed to the stomach) created by the intestinal villi more than compensates for the decrease in the concentration of nonionized acid. This observation emphasizes the critical importance of gastric emptying time to absorption of drug.

Drugs are absorbed less rapidly as they proceed down the intestine, primarily because the surface area for absorption is decreased. Nonetheless, absorption from the rectum is sufficient to make it an effective route for drug administration. Absorption can occur via the lymphatic system, presumably by passive diffusion, but lymph flow at the absorption site is negligible compared to blood flow, and this route has minor quantitative importance in the intestinal absorption of drugs (DeMarco and Levine, 1969).

If the pH partition hypothesis were the sole determinant of drug absorption, highly ionized molecules would not be absorbed. Nonetheless, quaternary ammonium compounds, which are always ionized, are absorbed after oral ingestion, although absorption is slow, erratic, and incomplete. Because toxicity is associated with accidental ingestion of quaternary ammonium herbicides, and orally administered hexamethonium is effective in man, exceptions to the hypothesis may be important. Presumably, these compounds are absorbed by specialized transport processes, but whether the processes are active or facilitated is unknown. Excluding certain vitamins (riboflavin, thiamine, and nicotinamide), only drugs such as 5-fluorouracil and 5-bromouracil, which are structurally related analogs of a naturally occurring compound, have conclusively been shown to be absorbed by active transport processes. In rats, the ionized species of acidic and basic drugs penetrate through the intestinal wall. Even if the observation in rats can be extrapolated to man, the quantitative significance of these findings in the overall absorption of drugs is unknown (Levine and Pelikan, 1964; Ther and Winne, 1971).

Absorption of Drugs in Different Dosage Forms. Tablets and capsules are the most prevalent and convenient forms of medication. Reliable and predictable medication depends on several factors, as illustrated in Figure 2–4. Factors that influence the gastrointestinal absorption of drugs in different dosage forms have been reviewed (Levy, 1963). Examples are presented here to illustrate the importance of some of these variables. In most cases, disintegration of a tablet into small particles in the gastrointestinal fluid hastens dissolution by providing a larger surface area of drug. Consequently, absorption is more rapid and perhaps more complete. The importance of disintegration is emphasized by the required pharmacopeial tests of disintegration that form an integral part of the quality control of solid dosage forms. Deaggregation of the particles must follow disintegraton if rapid dissolution is to occur. However, rapid disintegration does not ensure rapid dissolution. Consider the extreme case of the tablet of glass beads that could be made to disintegrate rapidly; dissolution does not follow. Not so extreme, but more relevant, is the case of the patient who was stabilized on one brand of prednisone. Upon switching to another brand, his condition deteriorated and reverted to normal only when the original product was used. A difference in the rate of dissolution of prednisone from these

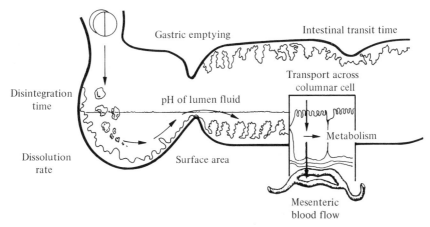

Figure 2–4.   Factors influencing the rate and extent of drug absorption after ingestion of a tablet. The tablet must disintegrate, and drug must dissolve before absorption occurs. The rate and extent of absorption can be influenced by the stomach-emptying time and the presence of drug-metabolizing enzymes in the intestinal wall. (From Barr, W. H.: Principles of biopharmaceutics. *Amer. J. Pharm. Educ.*, **52**:958–81, 1968.)

two preparations was responsible for the change in the patient's condition, even though both the active and inactive preparations disintegrated within minutes when tested in an *in vitro* apparatus (Levy *et al.*, 1964). *Principle: A drug must dissolve in the fluids of the gut before absorption can take place.*

A very water-soluble drug such as neomycin dissolves rapidly, but it crosses the intestinal wall slowly. Neomycin is principally used to suppress the growth of intestinal bacteria. With most drugs, the rate of dissolution is slower than the intrinsic absorption of the drug, and dissolution is the rate-limiting step in the overall removal of drug from the gastrointestinal tract. Dissolution rates cannot be directly measured clinically; evidence that dissolution is the rate-controlling step in drug absorption is derived from studies showing that a drug is absorbed more slowly from a solid dosage form than from solution. Occasionally the dissolution rate of sparingly soluble drugs is so protracted that dissolution controls not only the absorption process but also the overall rate of elimination of the drug from the body; the drug is present in blood for a prolonged period after a single dose. Information about the absorption of a given preparation should be sought if a patient's response to that preparation is inadequate. *Principle: Dissolution or absorption of a drug can be rate limiting in the overall absorption process.*

The manner in which a dosage form is prepared can substantially affect the therapeutic efficacy of the pharmacologic agent (Nelson, 1962). Differences in activity between dosage forms occasionally arise from variations in the nature and amount of the materials used in the manufacturing process, for example, stabilizing materials, binders that maintain tablet integrity prior to ingestion, lubricants that aid in the manufacturing process, and ingredients that promote disintegration of the solid dosage form upon ingestion. Because of these potential variations, absorption of many drugs is most rapid and reliable from a simple powder-filled capsule. However, some drugs (especially those that are poorly soluble) are best administered in another dosage form; hydrochlorothiazide has lower diuretic activity in capsule form than in a well-formulated tablet (Tannenbaum *et al.*, 1968).

Iron must be in the reduced state to be absorbed, but it is oxidized in the gastric fluid. Salicylates irritate the stomach and cause bleeding; penicillin G and erythromycin are unstable in the acidic contents of the stomach. To avoid the adverse effects of drug contact with gastric contents, the agents are often enteric coated with a material resistant to gastric fluid but not to alkaline intestinal fluids. Theoretically, drug release is prevented in the stomach, but these products have not been as reliable as uncoated tablets. Breakdown may occur in the stomach, or absorption may be incomplete (Levy and Hollister, 1964; Hollister and Kanter, 1965; Leonards and Levy, 1965). Absorption of drug may be delayed for as long as 20 hours after ingestion owing either to delayed gastric emptying or to delayed breakdown of the protective coating of the tablet in the intestine. *Principle: Enteric-coated tablets should not be given when an immediate effect is desired.*

The rate of solution of a drug in the gastrointestinal fluids, an important aspect in drug absorption, depends primarily upon the surface area of the particle exposed to these fluids and the concentration of drug at the dissolving surface. The drug is usually present in saturated solution around the particle. Numerous factors can alter either of these variables.

A decrease in particle size hastens dissolution because the surface area of the drug is increased. With many drugs, such changes increase the rate but not the extent of absorption, as absorption of the original dosage form would have been complete before the contents of the intestine reached the rectum. Nonetheless, even though absorption may be complete, therapy may be ineffective if the drug is too slowly absorbed (Figure 2–2, Case c, page 23). The critical effects of slow but complete absorption may be less apparent in multiple dosing. In contrast, when sparingly soluble drugs are administered, the concentration of drug at the dissolving surface is so very low that dissolution is slowed to the extent that absorption is incomplete and the drug appears in the feces. If drug is not absorbed in the upper gastrointestinal tract, it probably will not be absorbed at all, because dissolution of drug particles and access of drug to absorption sites is reduced with increasing condensation of the gastrointestinal contents. Griseofulvin, bishydroxycoumarin, and spironolactone are poorly soluble drugs that are incompletely absorbed. The problems created by insolubility were not fully appreciated when spironolactone was first used. Since its introduction, the therapeutic dose has been reduced by twentyfold (500 mg to 25 mg) by micronization of the drug into smaller particles. Evidently, only 5% or less of the drug was absorbed in early preparations. A similar, but not so drastic, difference is seen with various preparations of griseofulvin. This drug is a lipid-soluble molecule with aqueous solubility of 10 mg per liter, and is given in daily doses of 0.5 to 1.0 g. Numerous clinical studies have verified the incomplete absorption of this drug in man and have shown that decreasing the particle size of the drug leads to greater physiologic availability. The 500-mg tablet previously used has been replaced by a tablet containing 250 mg of micronized drug. However, absorption of this drug is still incomplete (Rowland et al., 1968).

The potassium salt of penicillin V yields higher peak concentrations of antibiotic in plasma than does the free acid form. Similar results are obtained with the salts of other acidic and basic drugs. More rapid absorption of the salt form is not due only to its increased solubility, since the buffer capacity of the gastric and intestinal juices is adequate to neutralize rapidly any liberated salt without producing major changes in pH. The absorption difference between the salt and the free acid is explained by a difference in concentration of the saturated solution of antibiotic around the dissolving particle. For penicillin V, this concentration corresponds to the low aqueous solubility of the acid; hence dissolution is slow. In contrast, the solution immediately in contact with potassium penicillin is a saturated solution of this salt; the solubility of the

salt is much greater than that of the free acid and dissolution increases accordingly. Even if the penicillin V precipitates when the dissolving salt enters the acidic gastric contents, a saturated solution is produced in the gastric juices and the absorption rate is increased, although one should not disregard the vast surface area presented by the precipitating acid. In this special case, destruction of penicillin V in the gastric contents is reduced by hastening drug absorption, and more antibiotic reaches the systemic circulation (Lee et al., 1958). The sodium or potassium salt of many acids (e.g., barbiturates, sulfonamides, and penicillin) and the hydrochloride or sulfate salt of many basic drugs are used in tablets to enhance absorption. In addition, many bases and some acids are liquids, rendering them unsuitable for incorporation into solid dosage forms; this disadvantage is overcome by formation of their salts. In rare instances a salt may be more slowly absorbed than the free drug. Warfarin is such an apparent anomaly, in that a tablet of the sodium salt is more slowly absorbed than the free acid (O'Reilly et al., 1966). As the salt begins to dissolve into the acidic gastric contents, the sparingly soluble free acid may precipitate onto the outside of the particles of the tablet. The precipitation may further delay disintegration and retard absorption. Tablets containing free acid disintegrate and deaggregate, thereby creating a greater surface area for dissolution. In contrast, the larger conglomerates of the tablet containing the salt are surrounded by precipitated insoluble material. Hence, salts of sparingly soluble acids and bases may not always be absorbed more readily than preparations containing the free drug. In some instances the choice between the preparations may be based on the undesirable effects of the cation. Thus, in patients with infection, congestive heart failure, or renal disease, it may be safer to give the acid rather than its sodium or potassium salt.

It is common practice to increase the rate of dissolution of a drug by using the salt form of the agent or by decreasing the particle size, thereby making absorption rapid and complete. In some drugs these manipulations are unwise and can be hazardous. The oral hypoglycemic agent, tolbutamide, is weakly acidic and could be easily formulated as a rapidly dissolving salt, yielding high concentrations of drug in blood. A sudden marked depression of the concentration of blood sugar would ensue, with obvious detrimental effects. Accordingly, tolbutamide is formulated with a particle size that dissolves slowly, and the gradual release from the product results in therapeutic concentrations of drug in blood that are maintained for extended periods (Figure 2–2, Case b, page 23). There are additional reasons for seeking slow absorption of a drug. The most common side effect associated with nitrofurantoin is gastrointestinal irritation and occasional emesis due to a central action of the drug, probably dependent on high concentrations of nitrofurantoin in blood. This drug was originally prepared in tablets containing small particles. The tablet preparation was replaced by capsules containing larger crystals that decreased the rate but not the extent of absorption; the side effects were reduced without compromising the therapeutic effect of the drug (Paul *et al.*, 1967).

The crystalline form of a drug can influence its absorption. Crystalline novobiocin yields insignificant blood levels of drug; only the amorphous material (a calcium salt) has a large enough surface area to allow effective dissolution. When a drug exhibits polymorphism, differences in its availability for absorption may be related to a particular crystalline form. Only one of the polymorphic forms of chloramphenicol palmitate can be absorbed well enough to be of clinical value (Aguiar *et al.*, 1967).

Complexation of a drug in gastrointestinal fluids may alter the rate and perhaps the extent of its absorption. The complexing agent may be mucin, proteinaceous materials, electrolytes, or other substances. Sometimes the resulting complex is insoluble, as in the case of tetracycline and divalent calcium ions. In this instance, absorption of the antibiotic is significantly reduced if the drug is taken with milk, food, or other sources of calcium ions (Sweeney *et al.*, 1957). Complexes that are larger and more polar than the drug alone, even when they are soluble, frequently diffuse less readily than the drug across cell membranes.

Gastric Emptying and Gut Motility. The stomach acts as a reservoir, regulating the delivery of materials to the small intestine. Because the absorptive capacity of the intestine is greater than that of the stomach, gastric emptying time is a critical determinant of the absorption rate of drugs, particularly when the drugs are in solution (i.e., liquid preparations and drugs that rapidly disperse and dissolve) (Hunt and Knox, 1968). When basic drugs are retained in the acidic environment of the stomach, their absorption is slowed. In contrast, acidic drugs like salicylic acid and penicillin G can be absorbed from the stomach but are far more rapidly absorbed from the intestine. The dissolution of drugs, which frequently is a limiting factor in drug absorption, is hastened by peristalsis in the intestine. An increase in the rate of stomach emptying might therefore minimize differences in the absorption rates of different formulations of a drug. *Principle: Any factor that shortens gastric emptying increases the overall absorption rate of acidic and basic compounds.*

Gastric emptying appears to be an exponential function. The half-life of gastric emptying normally is 20 to 60 minutes, although many factors influence the rate of this process. Gastric emptying is slowed by emotion, vigorous exercise, pain, hot meals, and high concentrations of electrolytes or hydrogen ions; it is speeded by hunger, mild exercise, cold meals, dilute solutions, and lying on the right side. Meals of normal content leave the stomach within 4 hours. Frequently, drug absorption is more rapid when the patient has been fasting. Absorption of drugs may be hampered when the drugs are trapped in food particles. Disease states may affect gastric emptying. Emptying rates are significantly lower in patients with gastric ulcers than in normal subjects or those with duodenal ulcers (George, 1968), whereas some surgical procedures hasten gastric emptying.

Although the stomach contents are emptied exponentially, the removal of a single undisintegrated tablet, for example, an enteric-coated product, is a random process and can vary from 15 minutes to 7 hours (Blythe *et al.*, 1959). Such variability leads to erratic and unpredictable delivery of whole tablets (especially enteric-coated tablets) into the intestine. Consequently, control of concentration of drug in blood can be difficult with such dosage forms.

The pharmacologic effect or the dosage form of drugs can modify gastric emptying. Amphetamine (Northrup and van Liere, 1963), anticholinergic drugs, and morphine (Sacchetti *et al.*, 1964) slow stomach emptying. Nitrofurantoin absorption is slowed if the drug is suspended in a methylcellulose thickening agent (Seager, 1968), perhaps because the methylcellulose decreases the rate of gastric emptying (Levy and Jusko, 1965). *Principle: Gastric emptying can be an important determinant of a patient's response to a drug.*

The motility of the gut also plays a role in the absorption of drugs. As peristalsis increases, disintegration and deaggregation of the product are hastened; dissolution and absorption are enhanced. The effects of peristalsis on enhanced absorption may be countered by the decreased transit time of materials in the gastrointestinal tract. For poorly soluble substances, the overall effect of increased peristalsis could be diminution of the amount of drug absorbed.

Alternate Routes for Drug Administration. *Rectal Absorption.* Drugs given rectally, usually in the form of suppositories, are used for local therapy or for systemic effects. Drugs cross the rectal mucosa by the same mechanism operative in other parts of the alimentary canal. Although the rectum receives a rich vascular and lymphatic supply, it is devoid of villi and has a relatively small surface area. Since drug absorption from the rectum is usually slow, rectal medication is most often reserved for situations in which the oral route is unsatisfactory. It is employed in children and in patients with severe gastrointestinal disturbances. The rectal route has decided advantages over the oral route when the drugs are destroyed in the intestinal fluids or cause gastric irritation. In the past, it was assumed that drugs that are rapidly destroyed by the liver could be given via the rectal route to bypass the portal circulation. This is true only for the parts of the rectum drained by the inferior and middle hemorrhoidal veins, as the superior hemorrhoidal vein enters the hepatic portal circulation via the inferior mesenteric vein. Dose requirements are either the same or slightly more than those for orally administered drugs. Aminophylline, aspirin, and the anti-emetic prochlorperazine are available as rectal suppositories. Similar preparations may be inserted into the vagina to achieve a primarily localized effect. Typically, vaginal suppositories contain either anti-infectives, antiprotozoal agents, or hormones (Schwarz, 1966).

Suppository bases contain materials that either dissolve, soften, or melt in the rectum. Vehicles that melt, such as cocoa butter, do so within minutes of insertion, whereas water-soluble vehicles, such as polyethylene glycol, dissolve slowly because the rectum contains only a few milliliters of fluid. (More water can be withdrawn from the mucosal cells, resulting in cellular dehydration and local irritation. This process is probably the mechanism whereby a gelatin suppository acts as a laxative.)

Dissolution of drug from a suppository may be the rate-limiting step for the overall absorption process. The salt form and particle size of the drug consequently become significant factors affecting its absorption rate. Drug availability depends largely upon retention of the material. Retention can be variable, especially when the suppositories are prepared with water-miscible bases and are expelled before dissolution of the base is complete.

Percutaneous Absorption. Dermatologic preparations include ointments, creams, and pastes. Bases include soft paraffin wax, wool fat, emulsions, and water-soluble polyethylene glycol. The preparation is usually intended to act locally to treat itching and eczema, to increase the thickness of the keratin layer, to soften or protect the skin, to provide antisepsis, or to bring antiparasitic and anti-inflammatory agents to affected skin. Drugs penetrate the skin layers, but only a small percentage of the applied drug is usually absorbed. Application of drugs to the skin is an ineffective means of producing high concentrations of drug in the lower dermal layers. Therefore, when treating conditions associated with these tissues, it is preferable to give the drug systemically, for example, oral griseofulvin to treat dermatophytoses. In contrast, volatile, lipid-soluble liquids, such as chloroform, can be absorbed in substantial amounts through the skin, because the drug is exposed to a large surface area. Many substances, including corticosteroids, boric acid, and quaternary ammonium compounds, can be significantly absorbed when applied to burns or

other lesions that denude extensive areas of skin. Some materials may conceivably enhance the percutaneous absorption of drugs. Dimethyl-sulfoxide (DMSO) has enthusiastic advocates, but its place in clinical practice is unestablished.

Absorption from the Oral Cavity. The oral mucosa is richly vascular; drugs can be rapidly absorbed from this surface. Drugs may be given sublingually or simply placed in the mouth. These routes have three main advantages over absorption of drugs from the gastrointestinal fluids. The drug is not exposed to the gastric and intestinal contents where it might be destroyed, and the venous drainage of the oral cavity bypasses the liver. Excess drug can easily be removed from the mouth if the desired effect occurs sooner or more intensely than expected. These routes cannot be used if large doses of drug are required or if the drug irritates the oral mucosa. Drugs that are effectively administered by the oral cavity include nitroglycerin (sublingual) for rapid relief of angina and certain testosterone formulations (Gibaldi and Kanig, 1965).

Summary Principle: When a drug is in solution, the critical determinants of its absorption include (1) the chemical composition of the membrane it must cross; (2) the vascularity at and blood flow to the site; (3) the surface area exposed to the solution; (4) the contact time of the drug at the site of absorption; and (5) physicochemical properties of the drug, that is, lipid solubility, pK_a, and molecular size. When dissolution becomes the rate-limiting step in drug absorption, the solubility of the drug, its salt form, the surface area available for dissolution, the nature and volume of the vehicle, and other pharmaceutical factors become additional determinants. Rational application of this knowledge can reduce uncertainty in drug administration.

Routes of Elimination

The concentration of drug in blood and tissues rises when the rate of absorption exceeds the rate of elimination. Eventually these rates equalize, and thereafter elimination exceeds absorption. Hepatic metabolism and renal excretion are the major mechanisms of elimination. Less important mechanisms include loss via the biliary tract, excretion via the lungs, or elimination in sweat and other secretions.

Elimination is dependent on the distribution of drugs, which is determined in part by binding of drugs to macromolecules, especially proteins. Extensive binding of a drug with tissue components reduces the fraction of the dose in blood and delays excretion and metabolism. Similarly, the uptake of very lipid-soluble materials into fat reduces their rate of elimination.

Metabolism. Most therapeutic agents are soluble in lipids, allowing them to cross the gastrointestinal lumen and other membranes. This same property allows almost quantitative reabsorption from the nephron, and some drugs would remain in the body indefinitely but for their enzymatic conversion into more polar compounds. Drug-metabolizing enzymes oxidize, reduce, hydrolyze, or conjugate compounds (with acetate, glycine, sulfate, or glucuronic acid), often making them more soluble in water. They generally differ from enzymes involved in intermediary metabolism by their lack of specificity, although succinylcholine and procaine are hydrolyzed by pseudocholinesterase. The enzymes usually are located in the endoplasmic reticulum of hepatic cells, but the gastrointestinal mucosa, placenta, kidney, and plasma are also capable of drug metabolism.

The location of drug-metabolizing enzymes may determine the dose requirement for a drug. When hepatic enzymes clear a drug rapidly, larger oral doses may be required than one would have predicted from dose response studies obtained from intravenous administration (Shand *et al.*, 1970).

Sometimes chemicals must be metabolized before they are active (e.g., Prontosil to sulfanilamide, phenacetin to acetaminophen, alpha-methyldopa to alpha-methylnorepinephrine); sometimes both parent molecule and metabolite are active (e.g., both acetohexamide and its reduced form, hydroxyhexamide, possess hypoglycemic activity).

Metabolism of drugs is described by Michaelis-Menten enzyme kinetics. According to this model, the rate of metabolism (dA_m/dt) is defined by:

$$\frac{dA_m}{dt} = \frac{V_{\max} \cdot C}{K_m + C} \tag{7a}$$

where C is a concentration of a drug in blood or plasma, $V_{\max}$ is the maximum velocity, and K_m is the Michaelis-Menten constant. The constant, $V_{\max}$, is the maximum production rate of metabolite, and it is a function of the total amount of metabolizing enzyme, whereas $1/K_m$ indicates the affinity between substrate and enzyme. By definition, K_m is the concentration at which the rate of metabolism is one-half the maximum. Strictly speaking, the concentration of drug should be that in solution around the metabolic site. In practice, this concentration cannot be measured. However, when metabolism takes place in a highly perfused organ, such as the liver, diffusion equilibrium of many drugs between blood and this organ is rapidly established. Then concentrations of drug in blood are proportional to those at the metabolic site, and substitution of the latter by the former is reasonable.

Within the dose range of many therapeutic agents, only a small fraction of the total available metabolic sites are occupied ($K_m > C$). Consequently, the above equation reduces to:

$$\text{Rate of metabolism} = kC \tag{7b}$$

where k is the proportionality constant equal to $V_{\max}/K_m$, with units of volume per unit time. Under these circumstances, metabolism is a first-order process; that is, the rate of metabolism is directly proportional to the concentration of the drug. In many therapeutic settings, therefore, the fraction cleared per unit time is independent of the dose.

With some drugs, all of the enzyme becomes occupied ($C > K_m$) as doses are increased, and the rate of metabolism becomes maximal ($V_{\max}$), constant (zero order), and independent of the concentration and dose of drug. The fraction of the dose eliminated in a given time decreases, and the pharmacologic effect is disproportionately prolonged with increasing dose. As drug concentration falls, a point is reached when the kinetics of metabolism gradually change from a zero-order process back to a first-order process. (See Dose-Dependent Drug Kinetics, page 49.)

Phenobarbital, 3,4-benzpyrene, and DDT are a few of the several hundred compounds that induce drug-metabolizing enzymes (Conney, 1967) (see Chapter 16). Studies have usually been conducted in animals, and stimulation is reflected in acceleration in the overall rate of metabolism. Both enhancement of the rate of enzyme synthesis (induction) and stabilization of the existing enzyme account for the increase in the total mass of the enzyme, which hastens metabolism. Changes in binding between drug and enzyme, which can be interpreted as a change in the nature of the enzyme, occur infrequently.

The converse of stimulation is inhibition, either competitive or noncompetitive. In competitive inhibition, the inhibitor reversibly binds to and competes for the metabolic site on an enzyme, thereby reducing the rate of metabolism of the drug. An increasing concentration of drug displaces and eventually overrides the competitive inhibitor, so that the maximum rate of drug metabolism does not change. Noncompetitive inhibition involves the irreversible interaction of the inhibitor with the enzyme, so that the total number of available metabolic sites and the maximum metabolic rate are decreased. The clinical significance of enzyme induction and inhibition is discussed in Chapters 3, 4, 5, 7, 15, and 16 (Williams, 1959; Goldstein *et al.*, 1968; Parke, 1968; Conney, 1969; Anders, 1971).

Urinary Excretion. The kidneys receive 20% of the cardiac output and maintain the composition of body fluids. Although 125 ml/min of protein-free filtrate pass through the glomeruli, only 1 to 2 ml of the filtrate appear in the urine. The enormous capacity of the nephron to reabsorb water often results in high urinary concentration of solutes, including drugs. Many polar drugs or polar metabolites are excreted predominantly by the kidneys (see Chapter 3).

The renal clearance of a substance can be regarded as the volume of plasma that is completely cleared of that substance by the kidney per unit time. This concept of clearance also applies to any organ that metabolizes (e.g., liver) or secretes a drug from the plasma (e.g., stomach or intestine). The renal clearance cannot exceed renal plasma flow, and the ratio of the clearance/renal plasma flow is the extraction ratio for that compound. When the ratio is 1, renal clearance equals renal plasma flow. The excretion rate of the compound is related to the renal clearance by

$$\text{Excretion rate} = \text{Renal clearance} \times \text{Plasma concentration} \qquad (8)$$

In a therapeutic range, some drugs have a constant clearance equal to the glomerular filtration rate (GFR = 125 ml/min); others have a constant value far exceeding the GFR (e.g., penicillin's clearance is 500 ml/min); and in a few drugs, clearance fluctuates. *Principle: If the renal clearance of a compound remains constant,* *its excretion rate is directly proportional to its plasma concentration.*

Urinary excretion is complex and depends on glomerular filtration, active secretion in the proximal convoluted tubules, and passive diffusion in the distal portion of the nephron (Figure 2–5).

The glomerular filtrate has the same concentration and pH as plasma, with the exception of proteins, which are too large to filter through this membrane. Therefore, when the glomerular filtration of a drug is assessed, the fraction bound to protein must be considered. Glomerular filtration alone would slowly eliminate most drugs, especially those that are highly protein bound. Fortunately, a major contribution to urinary excretion of drug is active secretion at the proximal portion of the nephron. Two types of transport systems are present: organic acid transport (e.g., penicillin, probenecid, hippurates, esters and ether glucuronides, phenols and sulfates) and organic base transport (e.g., procaine, mecamylamine, and N-methylnicotinamide). In each, the structural requirements for the drugs are minimal. The excretion of penicillin G (500 ml/min) far exceeds the expected 50 ml/min based solely on the GFR and the fraction bound to plasma protein (0.6). Evidently, displacement of this antibiotic from protein is not rate limiting in the secretory process.

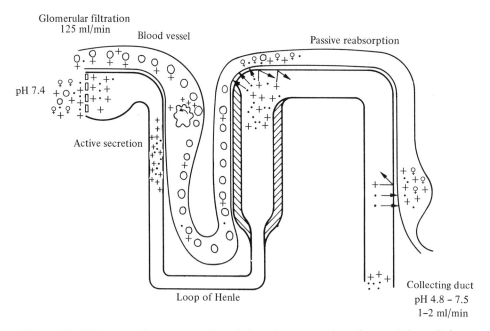

Figure 2–5. Diagrammatic representation of the urinary excretion of a weak base. It is assumed that the kidney is a large nephron, that only the ionized drug (+) is bound to plasma proteins (○) and is actively secreted into the proximal tubules, and that only the nonionized drug (·) is passively reabsorbed.

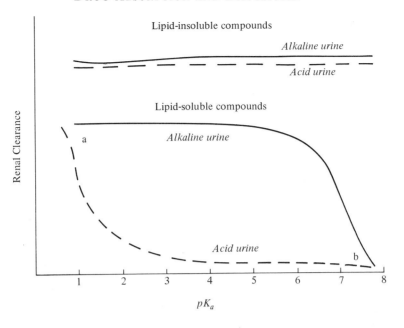

Figure 2–6. Schematic representation of the influence of pK_a on the renal clearance of organic acids under conditions of acidic and alkaline urine. It is assumed that only the undissociated molecule is reabsorbed and that all the undissociated lipid-soluble acids have the same permeability characteristics. Note that changes in permeability will change the position of the curves and that for an impermeable acid the renal clearance is high and insensitive to changes in urinary pH. Points *a* and *b* denote regions at which clearance of lipid-soluble acids is pH insensitive. (From Weiner, I. M., and Mudge, G. H.: Renal tubular mechanisms for excretion of organic acids and bases. *Amer. J. Med.*, **36**:743–62, 1964.)

Active tubular secretion can be saturated, and the maximum secretion is defined as the tubular secretory maximum (T_m) for the drug. In therapeutic practice, the secretion rate of a drug rarely approaches its T_m. Like all active processes, secretion of a drug into the nephron can be competitively inhibited. For example, probenecid, which is slowly eliminated, reduces tubular secretion of penicillin.

Despite glomerular filtration and active secretion, the renal clearance of many drugs is low because they are substantially reabsorbed from the distal portion of the nephron. The mechanism may involve passive diffusion of lipid-soluble materials across the renal cell into the peritubular capillaries, where equilibrium between drug in the luminal fluid and that in the peritubular blood vessels is probably never achieved. Therefore, the extent of reabsorption becomes a function of the rate of reabsorption of a drug, which is described by the modified Fick equation.

Continual reabsorption of water, which increases the concentration of drug in the lumen, and the low concentration of drug in the peritubular blood (especially if the drug is extensively bound to plasma proteins) favor reabsorption of drug. For some neutral nonpolar drugs, such as the antifungal agent griseofulvin, reabsorption can be so extensive that the renal clearance is almost zero. Conversely, mannitol, xylose, and other neutral polar substances are too water soluble and lack suitable partition charac-

teristics for reabsorption; therefore, large amounts of these drugs are found in the urine.

The renal clearance of many acidic and basic drugs varies over the normal urinary pH range (4.8 to 7.5). These observations are explained by the same pH partition hypothesis employed to describe the effect of pH on the absorption of drugs from the gastrointestinal tract. An alkaline urine leads to lowering of the concentration of nonionized acid, a commensurate decrease in reabsorption, and elevation in the net renal clearance (Figure 2–6). *Principle: With basic drugs, the more acidic the urine, the higher the clearance; the opposite is found with acidic drugs.*

The extent to which urinary pH influences renal clearance of a compound depends to a large degree on the compound's pK_a. At any pH, the pK_a determines the ratio of nonionized to ionized drug (see Henderson-Hasselbalch equation, page 24). At one extreme, strong acids (pK_a less than 2), regardless of the plasma or urinary pH (compatible with life), are still many units away from the pK_a. Therefore, the concentration of nonionized drug is extremely low, and its rate and extent of reabsorption is small; its urinary clearance is high and insensitive to changes in urinary pH. Although reabsorption of these compounds may be changed by changes in pH (e.g., a unit change in urinary pH produces a tenfold change in the concentration of non-ionized drug), the change in net clearance is minor. At the other extreme, weak acids (pK_a greater than 7.5), e.g., barbital (pK_a 7.7), are so sufficiently nonionized, over the entire physiologic urinary pH range, that a high concentration gradient for reabsorption always exists. Therefore, the resultant relatively low renal clearance is insensitive to changes in urinary pH. *Principle: Only when acids have a pK_a of 3 to 7.5 is reabsorption sensitive (responsive) enough to changes in pH that renal clearance can be greatly influenced.*

The renal clearance of salicylic acid (pK_a 3.0) is extremely sensitive to small changes in urinary pH. The same concepts apply to bases. Those that are moderately weak (pK_a less than 8) are reabsorbed at all urinary pHs, whereas excretion of stronger bases is very sensitive to urinary pH. Frequently, the excretion of drugs with an intermediate pK_a is further increased by diuretics, because dilution of urinary constituents also reduces reabsorption of drug.

Independent of acid or base strength, the nonionized moiety must partition favorably into the membrane before reabsorption occurs. For example, both penicillin G and salicylic acid have similar pK_a values ($pK_a = 3.0$), but only salicylic acid is sufficiently lipid soluble to be reabsorbed. The urinary excretion of electrolytes exhibits a diurnal variation, simultaneously influencing urinary pH, which is low at night and higher during the day (Elliot *et al.*, 1959). If the excretion of a drug is susceptible to changes in urinary pH, the excretion rate fluctuates even throughout the day. Such fluctuation should not be confused with enterohepatic recycling of the drug.

When the urinary pH is maintained near 7.5, 0.5% of the antihistamine chlorpheniramine is excreted in the urine. The rise to 20% excretion when the urine is acidified to pH 4.8 is unlikely to be of great consequence (Beckett and Wilkinson, 1965). In contrast, amphetamine is largely dependent upon renal excretion; with analogous changes in urinary pH, the percentage of the dose excreted increases from 2% to 70% (Beckett and Rowland, 1965). The excretion of both amines is sensitive to changes in pH, but the increase is consequential only for amphetamine. *Principle: The extent to which urinary pH changes alter the rate of drug elimination depends upon the contribution of renal clearance to overall drug loss.*

Alkaline or acidic adjustments in urinary pH are frequently employed to enhance the elimination of acidic and basic substances during a drug overdose (see Chapter 17). Sometimes renal clearance of a drug assumes greater importance at higher doses. For example, only 2 to 5% of salicylic acid is usually excreted unchanged following normal doses, and the drug is rapidly eliminated. Most of the drug appears in the urine as the glycine conjugate, salicyluric acid, a polar metabolite that is rapidly cleared and insensitive to changes in urinary pH. Despite the fact that urinary clearance of salicylic acid is exquisitely sensitive to urinary pH, alkalinization of urine would appear to be ineffective in altering the duration of the drug in a patient with salicylate overdose. However, alkalinization *is* efficacious because the glycine conjugation mechanism becomes saturated at high doses. The drug's half-life becomes markedly prolonged, and urinary excretion of salicylic acid becomes a major factor in elimination (see Dose-Dependent Drug Kinetics, page 49, and Chapter 17). Saturation of the metabolic processes for other drugs may occur during drug overdose; efforts to increase elimination of the drug by alkalinizing or acidifying the urine may be more successful than one would initially suspect on the basis of normal-dose pharmacokinetic data (Weiner and Mudge, 1964). *Principle: Knowledge of the physicochemical properties of the drug molecule, that is, pK_a, lipid solubility, and the overall importance of renal clearance for drug elimination, may allow manipulation of renal function to enhance or slow elimination of the drug.*

Biliary Excretion. Many drugs and their metabolites are actively transported by hepatic cells from blood to bile. Some of the metabolites are formed within the hepatic cells, where transport systems for both acids and bases have been found. Some actively transported substances, for example, bromsulfophthalein (BSP), are used to assess hepatic function. BSP excretion can be compromised when patients take drugs that compete for the same transport system. Rifamycin is readily taken up and secreted into the bile; it presumably competes for the same transport system as BSP and inhibits transport of the latter agent (Dettli and Spring, 1968). *Principle: Tests of physiologic function employing pharmacologic agents must be clearly understood before they can be properly applied or interpreted.*

Drugs or their metabolites (particularly glucuronides) are prone to biliary excretion if they are polar and if their molecular weight exceeds 300, for example, erythromycin, chloramphenicol, many hormones, dyes, and antidepressants. Advantage is taken of the predictable biliary excretion of certain tetracyclines and some penicillins to treat infections of the biliary tract.

The drugs or metabolites secreted into the gastrointestinal tract via biliary excretion may be reabsorbed (establishing enterohepatic cycling). Conjugated metabolites may be hydrolyzed by enzymes in the gut before reabsorption. The pharmacologic significance of recycling depends on the fraction of the dose excreted by the bile. When the quantity is substantial, the effects of a single dose may be prolonged, for example, the laxative effect of phenolphthalein or the sedative effect of glutethimide. If the gallbladder is emptied intermittently (as in man), quanta of drug are presented periodically to the intestinal epithelium. When these quanta are absorbed, a transient rise in the plasma concentration of drug may occur.

Most of the data on biliary excretion of a drug in man are determined from studies in patients with bile duct fistulas. These patients are abnormal, and care should be exercised in extrapolating these results to normal subjects (Smith, 1966; Stowe and Plaa, 1968). *Principle: When a drug appears in the feces after oral administration, parenteral administration may determine the contribution of the biliary system to the amount of drug in the feces.*

Alternate Routes of Excretion. Drugs can be excreted into the intestinal fluids, saliva, sweat, tears, expired gases, and milk. Except for the elimination of general anesthetics by the lungs, excretion via these routes is unimportant. However, the secretion of drugs into milk is a major concern for the developing infant or for the consumer of dairy products who may ingest pesticides and antibiotics in milk. The consequences of this subtle method of exposure to drugs are discussed in Chapters 14, 15, and 16.

Protein Binding

Proteins can complex with drugs, resulting in a wide variety of effects. Some drugs, such as actinomycin, complex with nuclear proteins and interfere with protein synthesis; some bind with a protein receptor and elicit a pharmacologic response; some interact with an enzyme and may inhibit the enzyme and/or be metabolized; some reversibly complex with circulating and tissue proteins, effectively reducing the total amount of unbound or "free" drug in solution.

Ionic, van der Waals, hydrogen, and hydrophobic binding forces contribute in varying degrees to protein binding. Ionic interactions occur between amino acids of the protein, which possess a charge at plasma pH, and the ionized portion of many acidic and basic drugs. Hydrophobic bonds are formed between the more lipophilic regions of the drug and the protein molecule. Lipophilic molecules often have affinity for plasma proteins. Thiopental

is more lipid soluble and more avidly bound to albumin than is its oxygen analog, pentobarbital. Conversely, if a molecule is small, neutral, and water soluble (e.g., alcohol, urea, or caffeine), it is negligibly bound by proteins and distributes fairly evenly throughout the body-water spaces. Most studies of protein binding have focused upon the interaction between drugs and plasma proteins. Tissue proteins are also important but are difficult to isolate and study. Albumin is the most important and abundant plasma protein (4 g/100 ml) and possesses about 200 ionizable groups per molecule with a net negative charge on 18 groups at pH 7.4. Albumin has a high affinity for many drugs, but binds anions (e.g., penicillins, sulfonamides, warfarin, bishydroxycoumarin, and salicylic acid) much more strongly and in more significant amounts than cations.

The binding of a drug to plasma and tissue proteins can influence the distribution of the drug, the rate at which it passes through membranes, the intensity of its pharmacologic effect, and the drug's elimination rate.

Protein binding alters drug distribution. Only free drug diffuses into tissues because the protein-drug complex is unable to cross cell membranes. As protein binding lowers the concentration of free drug in solution, the gradient responsible for diffusion and passage of drug into tissues decreases and transfer slows. Bishydroxycoumarin is avidly bound to albumin and tissue proteins; it leaves plasma slowly, whereas antipyrine, which is poorly bound, distributes very rapidly (Nagashima *et al.*, 1968). Equilibrium is established for protein-bound drugs when the concentration of the free portion is equal in the water of all tissues. Although the total concentration of sulfonamide in plasma is high at equilibrium, the concentration of the free drug is equal in plasma and cerebrospinal fluid (which has a very low concentration of protein).

Protein binding pharmacologically inactivates a drug. Unless protein is removed from plasma, chemical assays of the drug determine total concentration, whereas many biologic assays (e.g., the plate assay for antibiotics) measure only the activity of free drug. (Broth dilution, by promoting dissociation of the drug-protein complex, tends to minimize the effect of protein binding.) When a comparison of similar antibiotics is based only on total concentrations of drug in plasma, *caveat emptor*! High concentrations of one drug may be due to its high binding affinity to albumin and of another to high concentration of free drug. The clinical efficacy of the two drugs may be quite different despite equivalent total concentrations. Protein binding may also influence the doses of drugs given to patients with hypoalbuminemia. If the drug is ordinarily bound in significant amounts to albumin, the patient's response to therapy must be assessed and appropriate adjustments in the dose must be made. *Principle: Interpretation of drug concentrations recorded in studies using various assays for the drug must be made with knowledge of the assay techniques.*

Protein binding is reversible. Removal of drug by metabolism or excretion allows dissociation of the drug-protein complex. Addition of drug promotes further formation of complex. *Principle: Protein binding acts as a temporary store of drug and tends to prevent large fluctuations in the concentration of free drug in the body fluids.*

The formation of a drug-protein complex is described by the law of mass action:

$$\text{Drug} + \text{Protein} \underset{k_2}{\overset{k_1}{\rightleftharpoons}} \text{Drug-protein complex} \qquad (9)$$
$$(D) \qquad (P) \qquad\qquad (DP)$$

Equilibrium association constant (K)

$$= \frac{\text{Association rate constant } (k_1)}{\text{Dissociation rate constant } (k_2)}$$

$$= \frac{(DP)}{(D_{\text{free}})(P_{\text{free}})} \qquad (10)$$

where (D_{free}) and (P_{free}) are the free concentrations of drug and protein, respectively. The concentration of drug-protein complex at equilibrium is denoted by (DP). The association and dissociation rate constants, k_1 and k_2, are extremely high, and for practical purposes equilibrium is established instantaneously. The magnitude of the equilibrium association constant (K) varies from almost zero, when there is no protein binding of a drug, to 10^6 liters per mole when almost all the drug is bound to protein. The warfarin-albumin complex has a K of 1.25×10^5 liters per mole, and very low concentrations of free warfarin exist in solution at therapeutic doses (O'Reilly, 1967). This anticoagulant possesses a much higher inherent activity than would have been surmised on the basis of total concentrations in plasma. This kinetic description considers a drug-protein complex in which a mole of albumin binds a mole of drug, but often there are a number of binding sites on a protein. When binding sites differ, each is characterized by a distinct association constant, and there may be several identical sites (with the same K) on each protein molecule.

The total capacity of a protein to bind with a drug is the product of the number of binding sites per protein molecule and the total amount of protein. As the drug concentration in plasma increases, there is a concomitant decrease in the number of available binding sites, and the percentage of free drug rises. If all the protein binding sites are occupied, any addition of drug increases the concentration of unbound drug. Conversely, either lowering the dose or raising the protein concentration decreases the per-centage of free drug. Although drugs may bind to albumin, the fraction of unbound drug in plasma for many drugs is reasonably constant over a wide therapeutic range, because there are enormous amounts of protein in the plasma and tissues relative to the amount of drug. The concentration of albumin in plasma is 5.8×10^{-4} M (total amount, 120 g; molecular weight, 69,000). Therefore, if we assume only 1 to 1 binding, 1.74 millimoles (120/69,000) of drug are required to occupy all the available sites on the albumin in plasma. If the molecular weight of a drug is 200, 0.34 g is needed to saturate binding sites. In practice, this estimate is low, as an equal amount of albumin is present in accessible tissues. Often the therapeutic dose is much less than the saturation dose, and the number of available binding sites on albumin (P_{free}) remains substantially unchanged. Therefore, the ratio of the bound drug to the free drug remains relatively constant (see equation 10). When the concentration of drug becomes exceedingly high, the percentage of free drug significantly increases as the dose increases. This is seen clinically when drugs with high association constants are given in gram doses (e.g., sulfonamides, phenylbutazone).

When determining albumin's role in drug distribution, other factors must be considered, for example, the body-water spaces and other binding sites. Even the simplest model, in which plasma albumin is the only site for binding and the drug distributes into total body-water spaces (42 liters), demonstrates that if a drug has an association constant (K) of 10^4 liters per mole, 73% of a 1-millimole dose (300 mg if molecular weight is 300) is unbound, and the percentage of free drug does not rise significantly upon increasing the dose (Martin, 1965). Usually a K of 10^4 represents a strongly bound drug, corresponding to a situation in which approximately 83% of the drug in plasma is bound to albumin. Only if the association constant is much higher (10^5 to 10^6 liters per mole) would changes in free-drug concentration over the therapeutic dose range be substantial. In practice, even then the changes in unbound drug are not as dramatic as would be expected. Usually a portion of drug is also bound to tissue components, leaving more sites available on the plasma albumin for each millimole of drug ingested. Accordingly, the amount of free albumin does not decrease as rapidly as predicted from the above model, nor after large doses does the amount of unbound drug increase as rapidly.

Semisynthetic penicillins that have a high association constant are given in doses of 500 to 1000 mg, but after they are discontinued the percentage of drug bound to serum albumin remains constant. Oxacillin has a K of about 10^5 liters per mole, and after 500 mg are given intramuscularly, 95% of the drug in plasma is bound to proteins over a concentration range of 4 to 20 μg of antibiotic per milliliter of plasma. Further analysis shows that a significant fraction of the dose is bound to tissue, indicating that the total number of available binding sites in the body is greater than those provided by albumin. Therefore, even moderate doses of antibiotic cannot occupy a substantial fraction of the available protein-binding sites (Kunin, 1966).

The percentage of drug bound to albumin is often derived from *in vitro* measurements. If 80% binding is found *in vitro*, dangerous inferences might be made as to its *in vivo* effects on drug distribution and pharmacologic effects. If possible, the equilibrium concentration of free drug should be known, since the percentage bound can vary with total concentration of drug. More importantly, for some drugs (especially bases) which have a large volume of distribution (page 42), only a small percentage of the total dose is present in the plasma (the rest being in the tissues). Consequently, 80% binding to albumin *in vitro* may correspond to only a small fraction of the total dose *in vivo*. In such a setting, abnormalities of albumin concentration or complete displacement of the drug from albumin would have little effect on the concentration of free drug or the effects of a standard dose of drug. *Principle: The relevance of* in vitro *tests can be established only after the drug is used* in vivo.

Only free drug is filtered through the glomerulus. If glomerular filtration is the principal route of drug elimination (e.g., suramin [Ott and Seeger, 1955] and chlortetracycline [Sirota and Saltzman, 1950]), protein binding decreases the rate of drug elimination. The converse is true during hypoalbuminemia (Wyers and Van Munster, 1961). Unfortunately, analogous predictions are far more difficult to make for drugs that are metabolized by the liver or actively secreted by the renal tubule or bile duct. In these circumstances, binding to albumin does not necessarily imply a slow rate of removal. After standard doses, approximately 60% of penicillin G in plasma is bound to albumin, and yet practically all the penicillin presented to the kidney is cleared. The same applies to the hepatic extraction of the highly bound bromsulfophthalein. In either case dissociation of the drug-protein complex is sufficiently rapid that it is not the rate-limiting step in elimination.

One might assume that the speed of elimination of a protein-bound drug decreases with time after drug administration, since the percentage of free drug decreases as the total amount in the body diminishes. The assumption holds for some sulfonamides (Kruger-Thiemer *et al.*, 1965), but these particular drugs (1) are given in gram doses, (2) are highly protein bound ($K = 10^5$ liters per mole), and (3) are primarily removed by glomerular filtration. Lacking this therapeutically uncommon combination of circumstances, protein binding alone does not affect the disappearance rate of drug over time (overall shape of the plasma concentration-time curve).

The drug-binding capacity of albumin is large but finite. Drugs with a high association constant, when given in large doses, compete for sites occupied by other drugs. The displacement elevates the free concentration of displaced drug and may result in its producing a more intense and often unwanted pharmacologic response. *Principle: When the association constant (K) of a drug is high, any factor producing a small displacement of the drug may markedly enhance the pharmacologic effects of the drug.* There are many examples of this important type of drug interaction (see Chapter 16). The elevation in concentration of free drug depends upon the amounts of each drug and their respective association constants. *Principle: A clinically noticeable drug interaction based on displacement of one drug by another from common plasma and perhaps tissue protein-binding sites is most often seen when the second drug has a high association constant and is given in large doses.*

If a drug is displaced from protein, the increased concentration of free drug in body water may result in an increased extravascular concentration of drug. The glomerular filtration rate of drug increases, but metabolism and active renal or hepatic secretion (dependent upon the total plasma concentration) decrease. Whether displacement from proteins hastens or retards elimination depends on the balance of these processes (Figure 2–7).

Both a drug-drug displacement interaction and stimulation of drug-metabolizing enzymes can lower the concentration of a drug in plasma. Time factors can be used to distinguish between these mechanisms. In drug-drug displacement there may be an initial sudden increase in the plasma concentration of the first drug, followed by a rapid redistribution of the new unbound species and diminution in the plasma concentration of drug. Evidence of enzyme stimulation is usually not seen for days (Goldstein, 1949; Meyer and Guttman, 1968).

ABSORPTION AND DISPOSITION KINETICS FOLLOWING DRUG ADMINISTRATION

Intravenous Bolus

After injection, drugs mix with a small volume of plasma, forming a bolus which is promptly diluted by the circulating blood. The

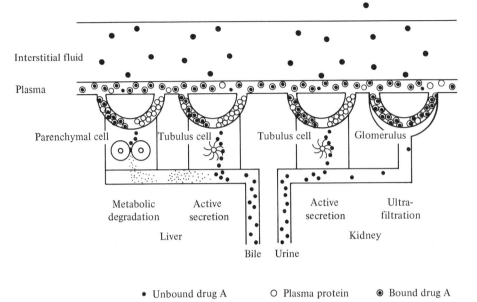

Intracellular fluid

Interstitial fluid

Plasma

Parenchymal cell   Tubulus cell   Tubulus cell   Glomerulus

Metabolic   Active   Active   Ultra-
degradation   secretion   secretion   filtration

Liver   Kidney

Bile   Urine

• Unbound drug A   ○ Plasma protein   ◉ Bound drug A

a

Intracellular fluid

Interstitial fluid

Plasma

Parenchymal cell   Tubulus cell   Tubulus cell   Glomerulus

Metabolic   Active   Active   Ultrafiltration
degradation   secretion   secretion

Liver   Kidney

Bile   Urine

○ Unbound drug B   ◎ Bound drug B

b

40

cardiac output per minute equals the total blood volume, extensive dilution occurs within 2 minutes of injection, and mixing is essentially complete within 10 minutes. Large macromolecules (such as albumin) or molecules that are very tightly bound to plasma proteins (such as Evans blue dye and bishydroxycoumarin) do not leave the vascular system readily and can be used to determine the plasma volume. However, most drugs rapidly diffuse into the surrounding tissues as they pass through capillary beds. Even during the first few moments after injection, while the drug physically mixes with plasma, it distributes into a much larger volume. Nonetheless, a very high concentration of most drugs in plasma can be produced if the injection is too rapid. The incidence of lidocaine's central nervous system toxicity is proportional to its rate of administration. Most often, an arrhythmia can be readily controlled without producing toxicity if the rate of infusion of the initial bolus is approximately 1 mg/kg of body weight/min, in the absence of heart failure (see Chapter 5). *Principle: The rate of injection of a drug must be commensurate with the clinical need and should be as slow as possible.*

As drug passes from highly perfused to less-well-perfused tissues, and drug redistribution occurs, the patterns of distribution become complex. Important factors that influence distribution include (1) the extent of binding of drug to circulating and tissue proteins and other components of cells, (2) regional differences in pH, (3) the permeability characteristics of specific membranes to the drug, and (4) the lipid content of the cells. Tissue uptake of a drug is dependent upon the mass of tissue and the rate of blood flow to it, as well as the partition coefficient of the drug between blood and tissue. The volume of various tissues does not correlate with the flow rate of blood through them. For example, the adrenals constitute 0.03% of body weight but receive 500 ml of blood/100 ml of tissue/min. In contrast, adipose tissue accounts for 15 to 20% of body weight but receives only 2 ml of blood/100 ml of tissue/min (Mapleson, 1963).

These figures vary in a normal individual and change even more drastically in some diseases (e.g., congestive heart failure, hypovolemic shock, and gram-negative sepsis) (see Chapter 5). Differences in perfusion may account for differences in the time required to bring tissue concentrations of drug into equilibrium with concentrations in plasma. In the kidney, liver, heart, and brain, which are richly perfused, equilibrium is established rapidly if the drug readily crosses membranes. Thereafter, concentrations of drug in tissues reflect changes in concentrations in plasma.

Other factors affect uptake of drugs by tissues. If drugs do not freely cross membranes, uptake may be slow despite adequate perfusion. Drugs enter muscle and viscera more slowly than they enter the very highly perfused organs; however, because these tissues have considerable mass, they can significantly affect overall distribution of drug. Fat-soluble compounds partition slowly into the poorly perfused adipose tissue. In time, however, substantial amounts of drug, like DDT or other pesticides, can accumulate in the fat, which then acts as a reservoir for drug and maintains concentrations of the drug in plasma after the administration of drug is discontinued. Special properties of tissues may also affect distribution of drug. Bones accumulate most drugs poorly, but certain antibacterial agents and ions (tetracycline, calcium, and strontium) are incorporated into bone and persist for long periods. The thyroid, salivary glands, and kidneys are capable of actively transporting iodides against a concentration gradient (see Chapter 7); some pigmented tissues like the retina and skin may concentrate phenothiazines, tricyclic antidepressants (see Chapter 11), and "antimalarial" agents (see Chapter 9).

Distribution accounts for much of the early decline in concentration of drug in plasma, but clearance of drug by metabolism and excretion occurs simultaneously, and eventually clearance becomes a predominant factor in decreasing plasma levels of drug. Consider the kinetics

Figure 2–7. *a.* Schematic representation of the excretion in kidney and liver of a drug (*A*) with a strong protein binding but a high rate of dissociation of the drug-protein complex. Note the glomerular filtration is restricted to the unbound drug. Active excretion and metabolic degradation extend themselves to the total plasma concentration of the drug. The concentration in interstitial fluid and the unbound concentration in plasma are both low.

b. Schematic representation similar to that depicted in *a* but now in the presence of a second drug (*B*), displacing the original one from the plasma proteins. Note that the excretion by glomerular filtration is increased because of the increase in the concentration of unbound drug. The active excretion and metabolic degradation are decreased because of the decrease in plasma concentration of the drug, which is the result of the redistribution, leading to increased interstitial and possibly intracellular concentrations after displacement.

(*a* and *b* from Ariens, E. J.: Modulation of pharmacokinetics by modification of the various factors involved. *Farmaco* [*Sci.*], **24**:3–102, 1969.)

following injection of a dose of thiopental, a lipid-soluble anesthetic (Mark and Brand, 1964). Anesthesia is induced within seconds as concentrations in plasma rise and rapidly equilibrate with brain. However, even though the drug is slowly metabolized, the concentration in brain rapidly declines and the patient regains consciousness within 20 minutes. The rapid fall in plasma concentrations of drug is related to redistribution of drug from brain and other well-perfused organs to other tissues (Figure 2–8). Despite the high lipid-partition characteristics of this drug, uptake into adipose tissues, which are poorly perfused, is too slow to account for this early rapid redistribution. Redistribution primarily results from movement of the drug into lean tissues. The latter do not have a high affinity for thiopental, but their perfusion and mass are sufficient to make a substantial contribution to uptake of drug. In addition, although the liver slowly metabolizes thiopental, the percentage of the dose presented to it is so high that a significant fraction of a dose is eliminated by this route during the first 20 minutes after injection (Saidman and Eger, 1966). Adipose tissue, which plays only a modest role in early redistribution, acts as a reservoir for the drug and becomes increasingly important with time.

If drugs were not eliminated, their concentrations in blood would ultimately equilibrate with all organs and a state of distribution equilibrium would be achieved. This state is approached but very rarely reached, since elimination is always operating. With thiopental, many hours elapse before concentrations of drug in blood and tissues decline at the same rate of 15% per hour, which represents the rate constant for metabolism. *Principle: For practical purposes, distribution equilibrium is achieved when the rate of loss of drug from the blood corresponds to the rate of loss of drug from the body.*

Apparent Volume of Distribution. Each drug distributes throughout the body in a characteristic manner. The apparent volume of distribution (V_d) is given by:

$$V_d = \frac{\text{Amount of drug in the body}}{\text{Concentration of drug in the blood}} \qquad (11)$$

The V_d is defined as that volume of fluid into which the drug *appears* to distribute with a concentration equal to that in blood. It assumes that the body acts as a *single homogeneous container* or *compartment* with respect to the drug.

Plasma or plasma water can also serve as the basis for analysis, but each results in a different value for V_d. Consider, for example, a drug almost entirely bound to albumin. If plasma or whole blood is analyzed, the resulting value of V_d is the plasma volume or the blood volume, respectively. If plasma water is assayed, an enormous value for V_d is calculated because most of the drug is elsewhere. In order to understand the significance of V_d, the physician must know the basis for its calculation. In fact, V_d is a contrived but useful term. The most common method used to determine V_d is intravenous injection of a known amount of drug and determination of the concentration of drug in plasma or blood over time. The concentration of drug is often plotted

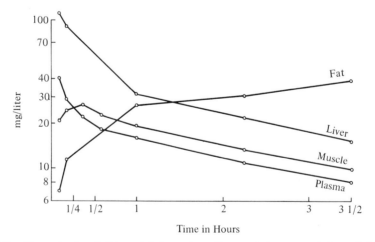

Figure 2–8. Tissue levels of thiopental in a dog after an intravenous bolus of thiopental (25 mg/kg). Note the early rapid fall in plasma levels, the rapid equilibration of thiopental between that in plasma and liver, the moderately rapid uptake of thiopental by muscle, and the slow accumulation of this lipid-soluble drug in fat. (From Brodie, B. B.; Bernstein, E.; and Mark, L. C.: Role of body fat in limiting the duration of action of thiopental. *J. Pharmacol. Exp. Ther.*, **105**:421–26, 1952.)

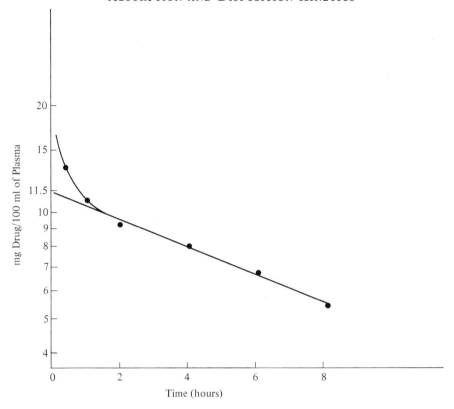

Figure 2–9. Plasma levels of sulfaethylthiadiazole after intravenous administration of 2 g of drug. Note the early distribution phase followed by the elimination phase. (From Swintosky, J. V.; Robinson, M. J.; and Foltz, E. L.: Sulfaethylthiadiazole. II. Distribution and disappearance from the tissues following intravenous injection. *J. Amer. Pharm. Ass.* [*Sci. Ed.*], **46**:403–11, 1957. Reproduced with permission of the copyright owner.)

against time on semilogarithmic paper (Figure 2–9). Graphed in this manner, the initial or distribution phase can readily be distinguished from the slower elimination phase. The monoexponential character of the elimination phase is typical for many drugs whose metabolism and/or renal excretion obey first-order kinetics. Consequently, during the elimination phase the body can be considered as one homogeneous container or compartment of volume, V_d, in which irreversible first-order rate constants account for drug elimination. Extrapolation of the straight line in Figure 2–9 to zero time gives the concentration of drug in plasma (C_o), assuming instantaneous distribution of the dose injected, and V_d is simply computed by dose/C_o. In the example in Figure 2–9, following injection of 2 g of sulfaethylthiadiazole intravenously, $C_o = 11.4$ mg/100 ml of plasma, and therefore V_d is 17.4 liters. The time required for distribution equilibration is usually 1 to 5 hours. The above calculation assumes that little or no drug is lost during the distribution phase. Although this is true for most drugs, some are extensively metabolized and excreted during the "distribution phase," when a high fraction of the dose is in the vascular system. Extrapolation of the elimination phase to zero time on the semilogarithmic plot

does not adequately compensate for early loss of drug; C_o is lower than it would be if all the drug were present. Since the numerator (i.e., dose) is fixed, the value of V_d can be influenced by drug elimination. Therefore, caution is indicated in ascribing any *physiologic* meaning to a variance in V_d of a drug between subjects or between animals and man, as an associated variance in the rate of elimination can contribute to variance in V_d calculated in the above manner.

The volume of distribution of iodinated-131 albumin, thiosulfate, and deuterated water corresponds to the plasma volume, extracellular volume, and total body-water spaces, respectively. Normally, these values are around 4%, 20%, and 60% of body weight. However, each value is lower in obese subjects. Drugs usually distribute in a far more complex and specific manner, and their calculated V_d is a fictitious volume, bearing little if any resemblance to the actual volume occupied by the drug. The V_d is useful in calculating the amount of drug in the body when the concentration of drug in plasma is known, or in predicting the concentration in plasma following a given dose. Often, the value of V_d is characteristic of a drug and constant over a wide dose range and might better be called a volume constant. The constant for a drug may vary under special and unusual circumstances. For example, with drugs that are highly protein bound, the V_d may be greater at higher doses. This could arise if the available sites on the plasma proteins became occupied and the free fraction of drug increased, causing a larger quantity of drug to leave the vascular space.

Many acids, including salicylates, sulfonamides, penicillins, and anticoagulants, are either highly protein bound or too water soluble to enter cellular water and adipose tissues in significant amounts. Therefore, their V_d is low (approximately 0.15 to 0.3 liters/kg). In contrast, bases are avidly taken up by many tissues. Concentrations in plasma are low, and V_d exceeds the volume of the total body fluids; for example, the V_d for amphetamine is around 3 liters/kg.

Elimination Half-Life. Once the distribution phase is complete, the plasma concentration of drug (C), and therefore the amount of drug in the body (A_b, equal to $V_d C$), decline exponentially. *Principle: Drug elimination usually proceeds by first-order kinetics.* Therefore, the amount of drug eliminated in a unit of time is proportional to the amount of drug in the body at that time:

$$A_b = D_o e^{-K_d t} \tag{12}$$

where K_d is the elimination rate constant for the drug (units of reciprocal time) and D_o is the dose of drug injected (see First-Order Absorption, page 47). If the dose and K_d are known, the amount of drug in the body at any time can be calculated. The value of K_d is determined from the slope of a semilogarithmic plot of the declining plasma concentration of the drug against time. For sulfaethylthiadiazole, 9.3% of the drug present at any time is eliminated each hour (Figure 2–9).

More commonly, the rate of drug removal is expressed by its chemical or elimination half-life ($t_{1/2}$), that is, the time required for the amount of drug in the body to decrease by one-half. The elimination half-life is related to K_d by:

$$t_{1/2} = \frac{0.693}{K_d} \tag{13}$$

The $t_{1/2}$ of sulfaethylthiadiazole is 0.693/0.093, or 7.5 hours, and the time required to reach 50% of any amount of drug is always 7.5 hours. When the renal clearance of a drug is constant, with the rate of excretion being proportional to the concentration of drug in plasma, the half-life

of a drug can also be calculated from urinary excretion data. This method is particularly useful when the concentration of drug in plasma is low but large amounts of drug are present in urine (Wagner *et al.*, 1965; Nitowsky *et al.*, 1966).

In practice, the disposition kinetics of any drug are assessed over its accepted useful dose range. When V_d and K_d do not vary as the dose increases, the system is "linear" and predictions of concentrations in the body after repeated dosing can be made, provided the expected concentrations are within the dose range studied. Occasionally the system is nonlinear (either V_d, K_d, or both change with dose), making predictions far more difficult (see Dose-Dependent Drug Kinetics, page 49).

Elimination Half-Life and Total Body Clearance. The clearance of a drug is defined as the volume of blood cleared of drug by metabolism and excretion per unit time. By definition, this is also the number of milliliters of V_d cleared per unit time and therefore equal to $K_d V_d$. Appropriately, $K_d V_d$ is termed the total body clearance and is the sum of the drug's metabolic (eq. 7b) and renal clearance (eq. 8):

Total body clearance ($K_d V_d$)
= Metabolic clearance ($k_m V_d$)
   + renal clearance ($k_e V_d$)   (14)

where k_m and k_e are the first order metabolic and excretion rate constants, respectively. For sulfaethylthiadiazole, the total body clearance is 1.62 liters/hr. For a given clearance, the larger the V_d, the smaller the K_d; hence the $t_{1/2}$ increases. If the clearance and V_d of a drug are known, the $t_{1/2}$ can be readily ascertained. Furthermore, a change in $t_{1/2}$ can be computed following a change in either of these two determinants. *Principle: The $t_{1/2}$ depends on the clearance of drug and on the manner in which the drug distributes.*

The $t_{1/2}$ of a drug depends on the events following its administration. If compounds undergo hepatic metabolism and renal excretion, elimination is affected by the ability of these organs to remove the drug, blood flow to the organs, and the fraction of the total dose remaining in the vascular system.

The maximal total body clearance usually is the sum of blood flow to the liver and kidneys (approximately 3 liters/min). If a drug were cleared to this extent and only distributed into the vascular system (5 liters), its $t_{1/2}$ would be extremely short, that is, 1.2 minutes. If the drug distributed into total body-water spaces, that is, $V_d = 42$ liters, the $t_{1/2}$ would be 10 minutes. Creatinine distributes in this manner, but it is cleared only by glomerular filtration. If the total body clearance equals 125 ml/min (the GFR), $t_{1/2} = 4$ hours, which agrees with experimental data. Although it is cleared similarly, inulin has a $t_{1/2}$ of 1.3 hours, because it distributes only extracellularly. The V_d of many bases is greater than 200 liters/70 kg in man, and even if the drug were effectively cleared (e.g., the total body clearance is 0.25 liters/min), the $t_{1/2}$ of the drug would be in excess of 10 hours.

The clearance of a drug can be used to quantitatively assess renal function (creatinine or para-aminohippuric acid clearance) and hepatic function (bromsulfophthalein clearance). These measurements can be used to calculate dosage regimens. If V_d and K_d are known, the total body clearance of a drug can be determined. However, a more direct and accurate method requires determination of the *total* area under the blood drug concentration-time curve $\left(\int_0^\infty C \, dt \right)$. Division of the dose by this area gives the total body clearance, since the rate of drug elimination is $K_d V_d C$. The amount of drug eventually eliminated is equal to the dose administered and is the sum of all the amounts eliminated in each time interval, that is, the integral of the amount of drug eliminated in each time interval between infinite time and zero.

$$\text{Dose} = \int_0^\infty dA_b = K_d V_d \int_0^\infty C \, dt \tag{15a}$$

or

$$K_d V_d = \frac{\text{Dose}}{\int_0^\infty C \, dt} \tag{15b}$$

Provided clearance is constant, even if the concentration-time curve is multiphasic, the correct clearance can be obtained by the above formula. In other words, clearance is model independent. This is not surprising, since clearance is the product of the blood flow through and the extraction ratio of an organ removing the drug. For example, if the liver were the only organ responsible for drug elimination, it would make no difference whether clearance was measured directly across this organ or estimated from drug concentrations in blood. If k_e and K_d are known, the rate constant for metabolism (k_m) can be calculated and the renal and metabolic clearance can be derived from the total body clearance. (In determining the volume of distribution from the total body clearance, the use of area measurements and K_d gives a slightly different value than that derived from $V_d - \text{Dose}/C_o$, because the area during the distribution phase is included in the total area measurement. For present purposes, the difference can be disregarded.)

Intravenous Infusion

Some clinical conditions are best managed by constant prolonged concentrations of drug. A known infusion rate is achieved simply by fixing the flow rate and the concentration of the drug in the intravenous fluid. Lidocaine is administered in this manner to control ventricular arrhythmias; antibiotics are similarly administered to treat severe infections. *Principle: A constant concentration of drug in tissues depends on a constant (zero-order) rate of infusion.*

As drug enters the body, some is removed, and the concentration continues to rise until the rate of drug elimination equals the infusion rate (Figure 2–10). Thereafter, if input is constant, it is continually balanced by elimination, and a plateau concentration of drug is maintained. The rate of change of drug concentration in the body is the difference between the rate of infusion (R_o) and the rate of elimination ($K_d V_d C$). The concentration, given by:

$$C = \frac{R_o}{V_d K_d} (1 - e^{-K_d t}) \tag{16}$$

continues to rise throughout the infusion until a plateau is reached, when the rate of change in the concentration of drug is zero, and $R_o = K_d V_d C^*$. The magnitude of the plateau concentration (C^*) depends upon the rate of infusion (R_o), the elimination-rate constant of that drug (K_d), and its volume of distribution (V_d). K_d and V_d are fixed; therefore, *the plateau concentration of drug is directly related to the infusion rate.* Doubling the infusion rate may immediately produce a rapid increase in the concentration of drug in blood, but eventually only leads to a doubling of the plateau concentration. *Principle: The time required to reach the plateau concentration is determined solely by the drug's elimination rate constant (K_d) and is completely independent of the rate of drug infusion.* When a drug has been infused for a time equal to its elimination half-life, the value of the term $(1 - e^{-K_d t})$ is 0.5, since $K_d t_{1/2} = 0.693$ and $e^{-0.693} = 0.5$; one-half of the plateau concentration is reached at this time. Similarly, at twice the half-life, the concentration is 75%, at 3 half-lives 87.6%, and at 3.3 half-lives 90% of the plateau concentration. The half-life of penicillin G is 0.5 hours; consequently, a plateau concentration in blood is seen within 1.5 to 2 hours. Tetracycline, with a half-life of 8 hours, requires up to 27 hours to reach 90% of the plateau concentration. *Principle: For a given infusion rate, if the elimination half-life of a drug is in minutes, the plateau concentration is reached in minutes; if the half-life is in hours, many hours are required.*

The infusion rate (R_o) is calculated to produce the desired therapeutic concentration of drug. If the V_d of the drug is unknown, the rate of infusion can be calculated from the observed therapeutic dose. For example, the therapeutic dose of tetracycline is 250 mg, which has a $t_{1/2}$ of 8 hours; that is, $K_d = 0.086$ hours^{-1}. Therefore, R_o is 250 × 0.086, or 21.5 mg/hr; after 26 hours (3.3 × 8 hours), 225 mg of drug (90% of 250 mg) will be present in the body. When the infusion is terminated, drug levels will decline

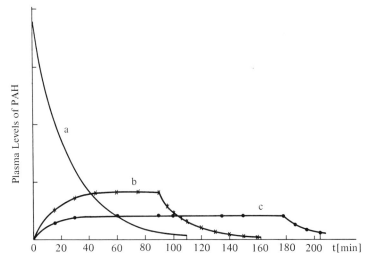

Figure 2–10. Plasma levels of para-aminohippuric acid following an intravenous bolus and infusion. The subject (31.8 kg) received 720 mg of para-aminohippuric acid (PAH) on one occasion as a single bolus (*a*), on another occasion as an infusion over a period of 90 minutes (*b*), and on another occasion as an infusion over a period of 180 minutes (*c*). Note that the half-life of PAH is approximately 20 minutes, and that, as expected, it takes 60 minutes to approach plateau levels of this drug. Also, doubling the infusion rate yields twice the plasma levels of PAH. (From Gladtke, E.: Pharmakokinetische Prüfung der Vollständigkeit der Absorption nach Dost. *Antibiot. Chemother.* [*Basel*], **12**:159–69, 1964, S. Karger, Basel/New York, 1970.)

in an exponential fashion. If the infusion rate is reduced by one-half, the new plateau concentration will be one-half the initial value. The rate at which drug concentration falls from the initial to this new value is dependent solely upon the elimination constant for the drug. A concentration halfway between the initial and final concentrations (i.e., 3/4 of the initial value) is reached when the drug has been infused at half the initial rate for a time equal to the half-life of the drug.

When high concentrations of drug are needed immediately, an intravenous bolus must be given, followed by an infusion. By adjusting the relationship between the size of the bolus and the infusion rate, any concentration of drug in blood can be rapidly obtained and maintained. The size of the bolus is generally based on the drug's average therapeutic dose (D_o). The infusion rate is $K_d D_o$ (D_o $0.693/t_{1/2}$); and, if the infusion is continued for a number of hours (h), the total dose administered will be $D_o + D_o \times 0.693h/t_{1/2}$. Returning to the example of tetracycline, for an infusion period of 24 hours the total dose given would be 250 mg + (250 × 0.693 × 24/8) mg, or 770 mg.

Prolonged-Release Dosage Forms

Prolonged-release dosage forms are intended to attain rapidly and maintain a steady concentration of drug in blood or tissues, without resorting to an intravenous infusion. One intention in using these preparations is to reduce the dosing frequency, to make therapy convenient, and to improve compliance by the patient. In addition, by maintaining a reasonably constant plasma concentration of drug, excessive peaking is avoided and side effects, which may be associated with peak concentrations of drug, might be lessened. Perhaps a more uniform concentration of drug in blood and tissues might be paralleled by a more uniform pharmacologic effect and response. Although oral and parenteral prolonged-release dosage forms exist, the former are far more frequently used. In either case, with dissolution being the rate-limiting step in drug absorption, the rate of solution of the drug from the dosage form into the surrounding fluids at the absorption site is controlled and slowed, by either chemical or physical techniques. If a uniform rate of release of drug from these preparations is possible, analogous to a constant intravenous infusion, steady concentrations of drug can be achieved in tissues.

Oral prolonged-release dosage forms are generally designed so that the desired concentration of drug in blood is maintained for 8 to 12 hours. The preparations contain a rapidly dissolving portion that initially releases drug equal to the normal therapeutic dose, and a more slowly dissolving portion that releases a maintenance or sustaining dose, the size of which depends upon the initial dose and the elimination half-life of the drug. (Sustaining dose = $D_o \times 0.693 \times h/t_{1/2}$, where D_o is the normal therapeutic dose and h is the number of hours desired to extend the duration of action; see discussion of constant infusion regimen, page 52.) Reduction in the rate of absorption is achieved in different ways. A drug may be coated with water-insoluble materials such as waxes, ethyl cellulose, and related materials, or embedded in a matrix that slowly erodes upon transit through the gastrointestinal tract. Release of drug may depend upon the hydrolysis or digestion rate of the waxes or upon the pH or the enzymatic activity of the intestinal fluids. A number of drugs, especially amines, have been complexed with ion-exchange resins; release of amine from resin is mainly a function of the ionic strength of the gastrointestinal fluids. In addition, solubility of some drugs has been decreased by the formation of insoluble tannates. Occasionally, prolongation of concentrations of drug in blood is pharmacologically achieved by using a drug interaction (see Chapter 16). An example is probenecid, which reduces the renal secretion of penicillin.

Not every drug is a suitable candidate for incorporation into prolonged-release dosage forms. These dosage forms should normally be restricted to drugs with small therapeutic doses and relatively short half-lives (less than 10 hours), which otherwise would need to be taken frequently during the day and night. The total dose in a single prolonged-release dosage form is always greater than that in the ordinary unit dose. Accordingly, the potential hazard is greater (if all the drug is rapidly absorbed), and, therefore, drugs having small therapeutic indexes (e.g., anticoagulants, digitalis) should not be used in these dosage forms.

Although the elimination half-life of many drugs varies over a wide range, both the size of the dose and the release characteristics of the dosage form are constant, being based on average clinical data. Furthermore, unlike plain tablets, many drugs in this form cannot be broken by the patient when less than a unit dose is required. In some regimens, an intermittent rather than a continuous schedule may be more efficacious (e.g., aminosalicylic acid is used intermittently in treating patients with tuberculosis). Although the peaks and nadirs of concentration of drug in blood are reduced, they still occur when the patient takes a dosage regimen of a drug in a prolonged-release form.

Unlike oral prolonged-release dosage forms, parenteral therapy is not restricted in frequency of administration by the transit time of materials along the gastrointestinal tract. Thus, these dosage forms can be given daily, weekly, or monthly. Intramuscular implants can last for months, but their use has been restricted to hormones, including desoxycorticosterone acetate, estradiol, and testosterone. These drugs are extremely insoluble, and solution from the pellet form limits the rate of absorption. Because dissolution is very slow, the surface area of the implant remains essentially the same for the duration of drug release; in this way a constant pattern of release is obtained. These preparations were originally designed to imitate the assumed steady continuous activity of endocrine glands and would theoretically avoid the fluctuations between deficiency and excess of the hormone. Most glands are now known to secrete intermittently, and diurnal variation in concentration of some hormones may

be critical to their physiologic effects (see Chapter 7).

A variety of parenteral depot forms exist in which the drug is injected either as a suspension or as a solution. In selected diabetics, insulin may be given at infrequent (daily) intervals, because advantage is taken of the crystalline form of this hormone. These large crystals dissolve slowly; hence prolonged absorption from the injection site is made possible. To achieve the desirable prompt action, the crystals are mixed with the high-surface-area amorphous insulin. In this manner a prompt and prolonged (12- to 18-hour) response to insulin is achieved. In penicillin therapy, the advent of an intramuscular suspension of the sparingly soluble benzathine salt provided a way to obtain extended and persistent (but low) antibiotic concentrations in tissues. Prolonged levels are also achieved by the intramuscular injection of procaine penicillin suspended in an oil containing aluminum stearate. The oil retards absorption by preventing contact dissolution of this salt by the aqueous medium. The addition of aluminum stearate further retards dissolution by increasing the viscosity of this preparation at the injection site. The liberated procaine penicillin is hydrolyzed to penicillin G on absorption into the blood stream. These dosage forms are very convenient for prophylaxis in children with rheumatic fever in whom compliance is important (Ballard and Nelson, 1970).

First-Order Absorption

Absorption of drugs usually proceeds by first-order kinetics. Exceptions include sparingly soluble drugs and those absorbed by active or facilitated absorption. All the drug is initially present at the absorption site, and the absorption rate is maximal; thereafter it declines exponentially. The decline in absorption is accompanied by a rise in the body levels of the drug and an increased rate of drug elimination. A maximum level is reached when the rate of drug absorption equals the rate of drug removal; thereafter body levels of drug decline (Figure 2–11). The faster the absorption, the earlier peak levels are reached. If absorption is too slow, the concentration of drug in blood and tissues may never reach therapeutic levels (Figure 2–2, page 23). Differences in absorption may occur when the same dose is administered via different routes or when various dosage forms are given.

The amount of drug in the body (A_b) at any time is then described by:

$$A_b = \frac{D_o k_a}{k_a - K_d} (e^{-K_d t} - e^{-k_a t}) \tag{17}$$

where D_o is the dose administered (or FD_o, if only a fraction, F, is absorbed) and k_a is the absorption rate constant of the drug. Absorption normally is faster than elimination ($k_a > K_d$). Following absorption, the fall in concentration depends on elimination; the elimination half-life

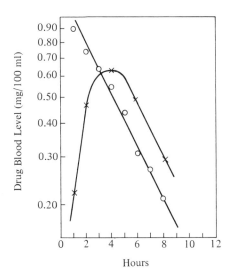

Figure 2–11. Average blood levels of theophylline in 11 subjects receiving 0.5 g of aminophylline by rapid intravenous injection (○) and one subject receiving 0.5 g of aminophylline orally (×). Note that after absorption is complete, blood levels of theophylline after oral administration decline parallel to those following intravenous administration. (From Swintosky, J. V.: Illustrations and pharmaceutical interpretations of first-order drug elimination rate from the bloodstream. *J. Amer. Pharm. Ass.*, **45**:395-400, 1956.)

of the drug can be estimated from a semilogarithmic plot of the decline phase (Figure 2–11). On occasion, absorption is slower than elimination ($k_a < K_d$) and continues well after peak levels are reached. Then the half-life for the decline phase is equal to the absorption half-life of the drug. Correct designation of the decline phase is ensured by intravenous administration of the drug.

The rate and extent of drug absorption are important in therapeutics. Direct measurements of absorption of drug from the stomach are occasionally made (Figure 2–3, page 25). More often, the rate of drug absorption is deduced from the shape of the plasma level-time curve of the drug. The absorption data are expressed as the cumulative percentage of the dose absorbed plotted against time, or analyzed further to derive information as to the kinetics of the absorption process (Wagner and Nelson, 1964; Levy, 1965).

Usually the total body clearance of a drug is constant. Then the total area under the plasma concentration-time curve is proportional to the dose absorbed and independent of the rate of absorption. Area analysis forms the basis for estimation and comparison of the extent of absorption when the same dose is given in different dosage forms or by different routes of administration.

More Complicated Kinetic Systems

The concept of the body as a single space or compartment into which drug instantaneously distributes and from which elimination proceeds by a first-order process is both simple and useful; simple because this model is the most rudimentary one acceptable and yet can be used to satisfy most of the available data; useful because it provides a concise method of describing the data and for defining terms such as clearance, elimination half-life, and volume of distribution. These terms can be used in calculating suitable dosage regimens and in establishing the possible effects of disease states on the kinetics of drug absorption and disposition. However, the one-compartment model does not describe the initial rapid distribution phase. This requires at least two compartments: an initial dilution space and another space into which the drug distributes more slowly. Even a two-compartment model may be inadequate. For example, when thiopental concentrations in blood are plotted on semilogarithmic paper, a triphasic or triexponential curve is observed, perhaps indicating the need for a three-compartment model (Price *et al.*, 1960). Study of ferrokinetics, which includes slowly equilibrating pools, homeostatic regulatory mechanisms, erythrocyte production, and hemolysis, requires even more complex models (Wasserman *et al.*, 1965). The degree of complexity of data analysis is determined by the intended use of that data. Three approaches are taken: curve fitting, compartmental analysis, and physiologic modeling. In all cases, the digital computer is used for rapid analysis of the data.

Curve fitting is pragmatic and requires adequate description of the observed data by a mathematical equation. No physiologic interpretation is given to the equation, but it can be useful when the model predicts the results of variable therapeutic maneuvers (e.g., the shape of the curve following an infusion or multiple dosing can be forecast). Therefore, an optimum infusion rate and dosage regimen can be established for any desired drug concentration.

Compartmental analysis consists of formulating a model that contains the minimum number of compartments that adequately fits the observed data. Between any pair of compartments are two rate constants denoting reversible transfer of drug, while elimination is represented by an irreversible rate constant out of a compartment. If three compartments are used to describe a triexponential curve, there is no way of knowing the relationship of any one compartment to any other. The arrangement of compartments is usually based on pertinent physiologic or biochemical data. From the data and a given model, the individual rate constants can be calculated and the amount of drug in each compartment at any time can be defined. The main virtue of this approach is that it examines the data in a more discriminatory way than merely describing the shape of the curve, and it has the possibility of associating a given rate constant or volume term of the model with a physiologic counterpart. Compartmental analysis has been successful in shedding light on the qualitative aspects of drug distribution and elimination. This approach has also proved useful in quantitatively describing certain diseases of the liver (using bilirubin kinetics) and disorders of calcium and protein metabolism (Berlin *et al.*, 1968).

Physiologic modeling takes into account the various parts of the body, such as liver, brain, kidney, muscle, fat, and skin. The blood flow to each organ, membrane permeability to the drug, protein binding, partition of drug between plasma and tissue, and mass of tissue are considered. When these parameters for each tissue are known, the kinetics of drug disposition can be predicted. The model is proved or fails when its predictions are matched with observed data. Although physiologic modeling is the best way to gain insight into the kinetics of drug distribution and elimination, the approach is rarely used because a large amount of data is required to design the model, and reasons for discrepancies between the model and the data are hard to pinpoint (Bischoff and Dedrick, 1968; Wagner, 1968b; Bischoff *et al.*, 1970).

Dose-Dependent Drug Kinetics

Active and facilitated transport, metabolism, renal and biliary secretion, and protein binding of drugs are saturable processes. In most clinical settings the concentration of drug at the appropriate site is assumed to be below the capacity of the particular system, therefore following first-order kinetics. Although this approximation is often useful, deviations from linearity occur frequently enough after therapeutic doses to warrant some discussion.

One example of dose-dependent elimination kinetics is illustrated by salicylic acid (SA). When the amount of SA or aspirin (which is rapidly hydrolyzed to SA) is raised from 300 mg to 10 g, the time required for the first 50% of the dose to be removed from the body (half-life) increases from 3 hours to 20 hours (Table 2–1). In man, elimination of SA is dependent on glycine conjugation to form salicyluric acid (SAU), glucuronidation of SA, and excretion of unchanged drug in the urine (Levy, 1965). When the dose is 300 mg (equivalent to a single aspirin tablet), elimination follows first-order kinetics and the percentages of loss contributed by each process are 80%, 17%, and 3%, respectively. When doses are above 300 mg of SA, glycine conjugation in man becomes limiting and the rate of formation of SAU eventually reaches a maximal and constant value, regardless of further increases in the dose of salicylate. Consequently, with increasing dose the frac-

Table 2–1. MEAN HALF-LIFE OF SALICYLATE ELIMINATION IN ADULT HUMANS AS REPORTED IN THE LITERATURE*†

DRUG	Dose grams	Dose mmoles	ROUTE	Half-Life (HOURS)
Sodium salicylate	0.25	1.6	i.v.	2.4
Aspirin	1.0	5.6	Oral	5.0
Aspirin	1.3	7.2	Oral	6.1
Salicylic acid	1.3	9.4	i.v.	6.1
Sodium salicylate	10–20	62.5–125	i.v.	19.0

* Independent of route of administration, as the dose of salicylate is increased, the time taken to eliminate one-half of the drug from the body progressively increases due to a limited capacity to glycine conjugate salicylic acid at high doses of the drug.
† From Levy, G.: Pharmacokinetics of salicylate elimination in man. *J. Pharm. Sci.*, **54**:959–67, 1965. Reproduced with permission of the copyright owner.

tional rate of loss of SA from the body diminishes, SA concentrations in blood are prolonged, and glucuronidation and renal excretion of SA become increasingly important in elimination of the drug. The data suggest that SA elimination may be accelerated by co-administration of glycine, thereby raising the saturable point in glycine conjugation. Unfortunately, such a change has not been demonstrated (Nelson *et al.*, 1966). The data also suggest that increasing the dosage regimen from 300 mg to 2 g of SA three times daily, by producing a higher initial level of salicylate that saturates the glycine conjugation mechanism, results in a more prolonged half-life and a disproportionately greater accumulation of drug in the body.

Man has a limited capacity to sulfate and glucuronidate some drugs (see Chapter 15). The mild oral sedative salicylamide (SAM) is metabolized rapidly and exclusively to these conjugates, primarily in the liver and gut wall. Critical factors in the efficacy of this drug are the dose and the rate of absorption. As the dose increases, the sulfate and then the glucuronide conjugation mechanisms become saturated, a greater percentage of SAM appears in the systemic circulation unchanged, and more pronounced effects are seen (Figure 2–12). Decreasing the rate of absorption of SAM slows the rate of presentation of the drug to the metabolic sites, and more drug is metabolized as it passes through the gut wall and liver (Barr, 1969). Dose-dependent kinetics are also important when bishydroxycoumarin (Nagashima *et al.*, 1968), phenylbutazone (Burns *et al.*, 1953), methotrexate, and diphenylhydantoin

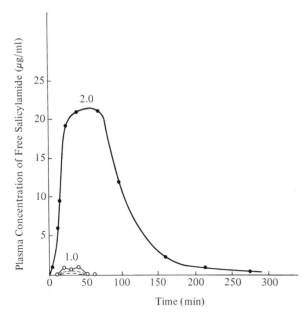

Figure 2–12. Plasma levels of salicylamide after various doses of the drug. The subject received 0.3 g (dotted lines), 1 g (○), and 2 g (●) in solution on separate occasions. At low doses the drug is extensively metabolized as it passes through the gut wall and through the liver. Only at very high doses are the enzymes saturated, and plasma levels of salicylamide then rise disproportionately. (From Barr, W. H.: Factors involved in the assessment of systemic or biological availability of drug products. *Drug Inform. Bull.*, 1969, pp. 27–44.)

(Arnold and Gerber, 1970) are given to man. Suitable dosage regimens for drugs exhibiting dose-dependent kinetics in the therapeutic dose range defy easy calculation and are established by careful titration of the patient with the drug (Dayton *et al.*, 1967; Levy, 1968). *Principle: If a choice exists between two drugs and one exhibits dose-dependent kinetics whereas the other does not, the latter drug should be chosen.*

Relationship Between Pharmacologic Effect and Time

It is reasonable to expect a relationship (sometimes complex) between the pharmacologic effect of a reversibly bound drug and its concentration in plasma. When there is a physiologic, homeostatic control mechanism to reverse the pharmacologic effect of a drug (e.g., the sympathomimetic response to hypotensive agents such as nitroglycerin), when the drug distributes slowly into the tissues where it acts, or when the drug must be metabolized before it is active, the relationship of pharmacologic effect to drug concentrations in blood may be difficult to recognize. However, examination of simple relationships may demonstrate the value of looking for these relationships in clinical settings.

Imagine that a drug is removed from a receptor by a first-order process (rate constant, k). As the amount of drug (A) declines, there is some minimal value ($A_{\min}$) below which a response is no longer observed. The duration of effect (t_D) is related to the logarithm of the dose administered (D_o), since:

$$A_{\min} = D_o e^{-k t_D} \tag{18a}$$

or

$$t_D = \frac{2.3}{k} \log \frac{D_o}{A_{\min}} \tag{18b}$$

For example, if k is 2.3 hr^{-1} and D_o is twice $A_{\min}$, $t_d = \log 2$ or 0.3 hour. Raising the dose by tenfold only increases the duration of effect to 1.3 hours (log 20). A semilogarithmic plot of dose against duration of action should yield a straight line with slope $2.3/k$ and intercept $A_{\min}$ (Figure 2–13). Estimation of k is then possible even when tissues in which the response is generated cannot be sampled, or when assays of the drug in plasma are inadequate.

A smaller second dose of local anesthetic appears to be as effective as the first injection. A single 5-mg amphetamine tablet ($t_{1/2} = 12$ hours) taken at 8:00 A.M. may be effective for 4 hours, but after a second dose at noon the stimulant effects may last until late evening. The response is increased because the total amount of drug in the body is equal to $A_{\min} + D_o$. The greater the amount of drug remaining at the termination of effect of the first dose, the greater the intensity and duration of effect of the second dose. No further increase in magnitude and duration of effect is anticipated after the third and fourth doses, because when the effect subsides, the $A_{\min}$ does not change. The effects of many drugs are closely related to their chemical concentrations in tissues. Dosage intervals chosen in relation to the duration of action of a second dose of drug can prevent accumulation of drug in tissues. *Principle: For many drugs, administration of an equal dose just after termination of the effect of the first dose can produce a*

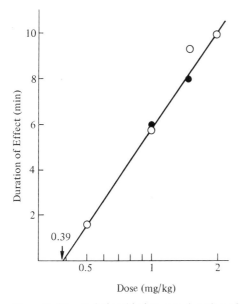

Figure 2–13. Relationship between duration of effect and dose administered. Human subjects were given an intravenous dose of an anesthetic CI-581. Note the linear relationship between duration of coma and the logarithm of the dose and that the value for the minimum effective dose is 0.39 mg/kg of body weight. (From Levy, G.: Kinetics of pharmacologic effects. *Clin. Pharmacol. Ther.*, **7**:362–72, 1966; based on the data from Domino, E. F.; Chodoff, P.; and Corssen, G.: Pharmacologic effects of CI-581, a new dissociative anesthetic, in man. *Clin. Pharmacol. Ther.*, **6**:279–91, 1965.)

more intense and prolonged response than that seen with the first dose.

If the duration of effect of a third and subsequent dose surpasses that of the second dose, the pharmacologic effect terminates during the distribution phase of the drug. Thiopental and lidocaine fall into this category. The first injection produces a rapid effect but a prompt termination as the drug concentration in plasma, brain, heart, and other well-perfused organs rapidly declines owing to redistribution of drug into muscle, skin, and fat. After the second equal dose, the duration of action is more prolonged because of the pre-existing drug in these less well-perfused tissues, which slows further distribution of drug from blood. A third dose, given at the same pharmacologic end point, should produce an even longer response as the amount of the drug in the body continues to rise; and, if the minimum effective concentration of drug at the site of action remains constant (i.e., no tolerance to the pharmacologic effects of the drug occurs), the duration of effect will extend until the amount of drug lost due to metabolism and excretion during this interval equals the amount of drug injected. When a patient is given such a drug, successive doses should be reduced to avoid accumulation of drug in tissues and attendant toxicity (Levy, 1966). *Principle: A drug's short duration of action should not necessarily be attributed to rapid elimination.*

DOSAGE REGIMENS

Some drugs (e.g., aspirin, hypnotics, antinausea agents, succinylcholine, and *d*-tubocurarine) are given as a single dose. More frequently, drugs are given on a continuous basis. The first dose or the first few doses of digitalis are larger than maintenance doses and are given to rapidly produce therapeutic concentrations of the drug in blood or tissue. Later, supplementary doses are given at intervals that allow maintenance of this therapeutic concentration. Inappropriate choice of the maintenance dose or the dosing interval leads to ineffective therapy or to accumulation of drug.

Most drugs are given six times, three times, twice, or once daily. The decision to use a particular dosage frequency is dependent on several factors, but the drug's half-life ($t_{1/2}$) is the most important. *One suitable and frequently adopted plan is to give the initial therapeutic dose (D^*) followed by half that dose at intervals equal to the half-life of the drug.* For example, 250 mg of oxytetracycline provides effective antimicrobial concentrations in blood. Its elimination half-life in man is 8 hours. Therefore, a reasonable schedule (which has proved acceptable) is 500 mg initially, followed by 250 mg every 8 hours.

This regimen is clinically unsuitable for drugs with very short or long half-lives, such as penicillin and digitoxin, which have $t_{1/2}$ values of 30 minutes and 9 days, respectively. Penicillin would have to be given too frequently, whereas if digitoxin were given every 9 days the fluctuation in concentration of drug in tissues would produce ineffective levels of drug or toxicity. The compliance of the patient taking digitoxin would probably be poor (he would likely forget to take the drug every ninth day) (see Chapter 14). Accordingly, it is useful to derive a general formula that can be used for all drugs. The supplemental dose replaces the drug lost during the dosing interval (T). Repeating this dose at the dosing interval ensures adequate drug levels. This maintenance dose is given by the difference between the initial dose (D^*) and the amount of drug remaining ($D^*e^{-K_dT}$, for an intravenous dose) at the end of the dosing interval. One can either choose the dosing interval and calculate the maintenance dose or specify the minimum acceptable concentration of drug in the body and determine the appropriate dosing interval. If the dosing interval is much longer than $t_{1/2}$, the initial dose must be increased so that an effective dose still exists at the end of the dosing interval. Only 0.3% of a dose of penicillin G remains at the end of the usual dosing interval of 4 hours (8 half-lives); therefore, initial and maintenance doses are equal. This dosage regimen is feasible because penicillin is not toxic at the high initial concentrations produced in blood and tissues. For many drugs, the therapeutic/toxic ratio is large, and wide fluctuations in concentrations in blood and tissues are tolerable. If the therapeutic index or ratio is small and the $t_{1/2}$ is short (e.g., norepinephrine, oxytocin), the drug must be administered by infusion. At the other extreme, drugs with very long half-lives are usually administered daily, although less frequent dosing is theoretically justified. If the daily dosing interval is a small fraction of the $t_{1/2}$, the effect is similar to that produced by a continuous infusion. The maintenance dose is then equal to D^*K_dT. This maintenance dose equation may be used as a guideline in calculating digitoxin regimens. An initial dose of 1.0 to 1.5 mg of digitoxin is given. With a $t_{1/2}$ of 9 days, the daily maintenance dose is calculated to be between 0.075 and 0.12 mg (e.g., $1.0 \times 0.693/9 \times 1$), which is within the range found empirically. Moreover, this drug has a low therapeutic ratio and index, and this regimen ensures that digitoxin concentrations do not fluctuate by more than 10% throughout the day.

The above considerations are based on information derived from intravenous administration of drug. The data also apply to drugs given by other routes, provided absorption is complete and more rapid than elimination (e.g., digitoxin). When absorption is slow, the ratio of the initial dose to the maintenance dose may require correction for the amount of drug eliminated during attainment of peak concentrations in blood. In rare instances, absorption is slower than elimination; under these circumstances the dosing frequency is determined by the half-life of drug absorption and not of elimination. When absorption is incomplete, larger oral doses are necessary than those indicated by intravenous studies. This difference between the oral and intravenous dose may also arise if the drug is extensively cleared in the first passage through the liver (page 44).

Although dosage regimens can be calculated by the above methods, a fixed dose is often given at fixed intervals for convenience. Because drugs are eliminated exponentially (by first-order processes), residual drug from the first dose always exists at the time of the next dose. Consequently, drug progressively accumulates until, within the dosing interval, the amount lost equals the amount administered. The concentration of drug then fluctuates around a mean or plateau concentration. There are three determinants of drug concentration: How rapidly is the plateau reached? What is the degree of fluctuation around the plateau concentration? What is the degree of accumulation?

Figure 2–14 depicts the amount of drug in the body plotted against time after repetitive dosing at a fixed interval, given intravenously and orally. Whether maximum, minimum, or average concentrations are considered during accumulation of drug, the similarity to the rise in body concentrations of drug following a constant intravenous infusion is apparent. With an infusion, 1 half-life and 3.3 half-lives were required to reach 50% and 90% of the plateau concentration, respectively. Similar results were obtained with chronic administration of drug. For example, penicillin ($t_{1/2} = 0.5$ hour) reaches plateau concentrations in 2 hours; between 1 and 3 weeks must elapse before plateau concentrations are reached with phenobarbital ($t_{1/2} = 2$ to 6 days) (Butler et al., 1954). If the time required to reach half the plateau concentration of drug is known, the biologic half-life can be determined, even when this value is difficult to calculate from a single-dose study (e.g., those hampered by technical difficulties in analysis of small concentrations of drug in blood). *Principle: The shorter the half-life of a drug, the more rapidly its concentration in blood approaches the plateau value.*

Theoretically, an initial large dose of drug can

Figure 2–14. *a.* Body levels of a drug given intravenously on a fixed-dose, fixed-time interval regimen. One gram of the drug is given every 8 hours, and the drug has an elimination half-life of 12 hours. Note that 90% of the peak level is reached within 40 hours, that the area under the plasma curve during a dosing interval at the steady state is equal to the total area under the plasma curve for a single dose, and that at the steady state, the difference in the amount of drug in the body between the maximum and minimum levels is equal to the dose, that is, 1 g.

b. Body levels of a drug given orally on a fixed-dose, fixed-time interval regimen. This is the same drug as in *a*, except given orally with the half-life for absorption of 1.4 hours (k = 0.5 hr^{-1}). Comments made about the intravenous route are equally applicable to the oral route, except that the difference between the amount of drug in the body between maximum and minimum levels at the steady state no longer equals the dose.

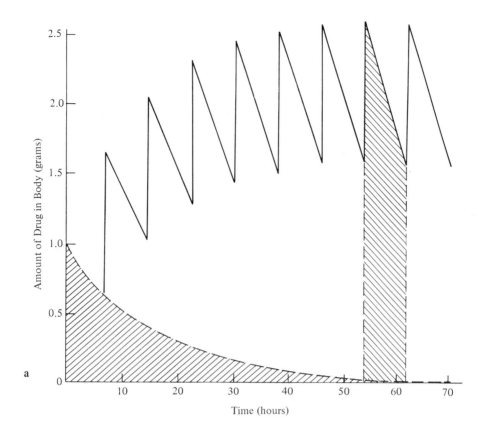

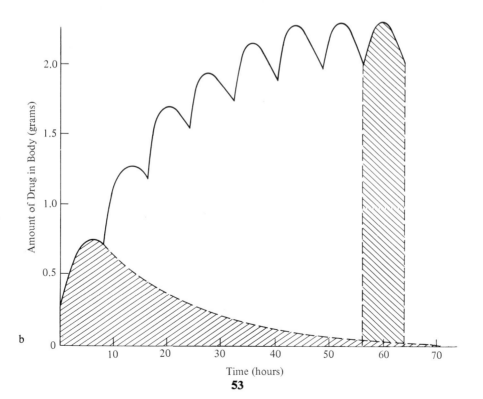

be given to achieve therapeutic concentrations, followed by smaller maintenance doses. However, the patient sometimes responds unfavorably to the loading dose. Gradual accumulation of drug is a safer and more convenient means of drug delivery. Fixed-dose regimens have become popular, but a therapeutic effect may not be seen until several doses of drug have been given. In addition, the maximum effects (therapeutic and toxic) of a drug do not occur until drug accrual is maximal. *Principle: The physician and pharmacist must be able to calculate the time at which maximal accrual of drug will occur on a fixed-dose schedule and must carefully observe the patient until this time passes.*

When intravenous doses are given at regular intervals (T), the amount of drug in the body at the end of the first interval (Ab_{T_1}) is defined by:

$$Ab_{T_1} = D_o e^{-K_d T} \tag{19}$$

following a dose (D_o). When this dose is repeated, drug accumulates in a geometric fashion (Figure 2–14). The corresponding amounts of drug in the body immediately following (Ab_{o_n}), during (Ab_{t_n}), and at the end (Ab_{T_n}) of the dosing interval after the nth dose are:

$$Ab_{o_n} = D_o \frac{1 - e^{-nK_d T}}{1 - e^{-K_d T}} \tag{20a}$$

$$Ab_{t_n} = Ab_{o_n} e^{-K_d t} \tag{20b}$$

$$Ab_{T_n} = Ab_{o_n} e^{-K_d T} \tag{20c}$$

As the number of doses increases, $e^{-nK_d T}$ approaches zero, and the corresponding asymptotic values $Ab_{o\infty}$, $Ab_{t\infty}$, and $Ab_{T\infty}$ are:

$$Ab_{o\infty} = D_o/1 - e^{-K_d T} \tag{21a}$$

$$Ab_{t\infty} = Ab_{o\infty} e^{-K_d t} \tag{21b}$$

$$Ab_{T\infty} = Ab_{o\infty} e^{-K_d T} \tag{21c}$$

The difference between the asymptotic maximum and the minimum amount of drug in the body is equal to the dose (D_o). The amount of drug in the body at any time is related to its corresponding asymptotic value by $1 - e^{-nK_d T}$, and the shape of the curve drawn through these values, be they maxima, minima, or intermediate, is identical to the constant infusion curve. If the dosing interval T is much longer than the $t_{1/2}$ of the drug, the asymptotic value may be reached after only a few doses.

Many aspects of dosage regimens can be derived by considering the average amount of drug in the body at the plateau level rather than by calculating the amount of drug present over time (Wagner *et al.*, 1965). Provided total body clearance ($K_d V_d$) is independent of dose and the drug is completely absorbed, then the administered dose (D_o) is given by:

$$D_o = K_d V_d \int_0^\infty C \, dt \tag{22}$$

Upon a fixed dose–fixed time schedule, at the steady state, this dose is eventually lost during the dosing interval so that:

$$D_o = K_d V_d \int_{t_1}^{t_2} C_\infty \, dt \tag{23}$$

Where $T = t_2 - t_1$, C_∞ denotes the concentration of drug at times during the dosing interval at the steady state, and the integral $\int_{t_1}^{t_2} C_\infty \, dt$ is the area over the time T at this steady-state level, which must then equal the total area under the plasma concentration curve following a single dose (Figure 2–14). In addition, the average concentration at this asymptotic level (C_{av}) is readily determined, since:

$$C_{av} = \frac{\text{Area over the dosing interval at the steady-state level}}{\text{Dosing interval } (T)} \tag{24a}$$

or

$$C_{av} = D_o/K_d V_d T \tag{24b}$$

If the drug is ingested rather than injected, and only a fraction (F) is absorbed, then FD_o must be substituted for D_o.

Considerations based on this concept hold true for more complex models, and C_{av} is also independent of the rate of absorption. However, the more rapid the absorption, the greater the variation of the plasma concentrations of drug about C_{av} during a dose interval. Even so, the differences observed following a single dose by various routes are less apparent after multiple doses if the amount of drug in the body at the steady state is large compared to this single dose. Alternatively, assuming that all the drug is absorbed, equation 24b can be rearranged to give:

$$V_d C_{av} = D_o/K_d T \quad \text{or} \quad 1.44 \, D_o t_{1/2}/T \tag{25}$$

If T and $t_{1/2}$ are known, the average amount of drug in the body at steady state ($V_c C_{av}$) can be computed. Thus, when $T = t_{1/2}$, $V_d C_{av} = 1.44 \, D_o$. For example, the $t_{1/2}$ of desipramine in one patient was 33 hours, and he received 75 mg of drug every 8 hours (Van Rossum, 1968). Therefore, the average amount of drug in the body at the steady state was six times the dose, or 150 mg. *Principle: Given quantitative information following a single dose of drug, one can estimate the average amount of drug in the body at the plateau concentration under a variety of dosage schedules.*

In determining dosage regimens, it is also necessary to know the extent of drug accumulation. The definition for the degree of drug accumulation depends on the reference point. Drug accumulation may be defined by the relationship between the cumulative maxima or minima and the dose (D_o), but a simple and meaningful index is the drug-amount ratio (R_A) (Wagner, 1967):

$$R_A = \frac{\begin{array}{c}\text{Average amount of drug in the body during}\\ \text{a dosage interval at the equilibrium state}\end{array}}{\begin{array}{c}\text{Average amount of drug absorbed following}\\ \text{a single dose}\end{array}} \tag{26a}$$

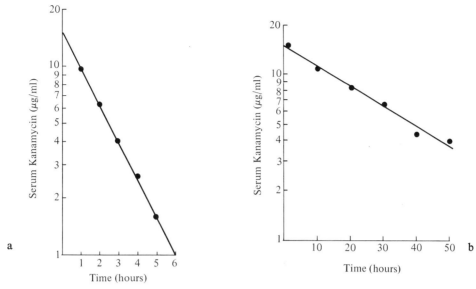

Figure 2–15. Serum levels of kanamycin in patients with normal (*a*) and low (*b*) creatinine clearance. Each subject received 7 mg/kg of body weight intramuscularly. In the subject with the creatinine clearance approaching normal values (83 ml per minute), kanamycin is eliminated rapidly ($t_{1/2}$ = 1.5 hours), whereas the subject with severe renal failure (Cl_{cr} = 8 ml per minute) eliminates the drug very slowly ($t_{1/2}$ = 25 hours), necessitating a different dosage regimen in the two cases. Note also the very rapid absorption of kanamycin from the intramuscular site. (From Orme, B. M., and Cutler, R. E.: The relationship between kanamycin pharmacokinetics: distribution and renal function. *Clin. Pharmacol. Ther.*, **10**:543–50, 1969.)

Assuming all the drug is absorbed, the denominator is the dose (D_o), while the numerator ($V_d C_{av}$) is given by $D_o/K_d T$; therefore:

$$R_A = 1/K_d T \quad \text{(or } 1.44\, t_{1/2}/T) \tag{26b}$$

In the particular example with desipramine, $R_A = 6$. According to this definition, there is no accumulation of drug when the dosing interval is greater than 1.44 $t_{1/2}$. For example, if the elimination half-life of a drug is 16 hours, drug accumulation is prevented if the therapeutic dose is given once daily. The amount of drug in the body fluctuates about this average value, $V_d C_{av}$; however, if the range is tolerable (in terms of therapeutic effect and toxicity), the daily single-dose regimen is satisfactory.

A daily dose of 0.1 mg of digitoxin could be used instead of a single large digitalizing dose. The half-life of digitoxin is 9 days; therefore, the R_A is 1.44 × 9/1, or 13 (i.e., the average amount of drug present at equilibrium is 1.3 mg). This concentration may not be reached for approximately 1 month, and beneficial results may not be seen for the first 1 or 2 weeks. However, since congestive heart failure may be mild and chronic, digitoxin therapy may be needed for years. Therefore, a therapeutic approach that produces a gradual rise to the desired level of drug may be superior in some circumstances to administration of a large loading dose that could produce serious toxicity. Conversely, if gradual accumulation produces toxicity, days may pass before drug levels fall. Such situations are all too common in clinical settings and are usually related to failure to carefully observe the patient until a desirable effect of the drug is obtained. If the patient is sent home or asked to visit the office at infrequent intervals, toxicity may appear subtly; and, when toxicity becomes overt, countermeasures may be required for some time.

On the positive side, an interesting example is given by phenobarbital. A regimen of 30 mg three times daily is common, and an effect is seen within the first few doses. However, the half-life is between 2 and 6 days, 1.44 $t_{1/2}/T$ is 9.6 to 26, and at equilibrium between 260 and 780 mg are present in the body. Few toxicities are experienced with this dosage schedule, although administration of an equivalent amount of drug in a single large dose could prove disastrous. Perhaps tolerance to barbiturate develops during the 1- to 3-week period of drug accrual. The same tolerance would not be likely for digitalis.

Cumulative and noncumulative drugs do not exist; rather, the degree of accumulation is dependent upon the relationship between the dosing interval and the elimination half-life of the drug. If the half-life is known, the degree of accumulation can be defined for any dosing interval. In this way, toxicity following chronic drug administration can be avoided (see Chapter 15). *Principle: With reversibly bound drugs, accumulation is a function of dosing, not an intrinsic property of the drug.*

Dosage Regimens and Age

The renal, hepatic, and perhaps biliary clearance and the body distribution of a drug change throughout life. Individual responsiveness and tolerance to a drug may also be a function of age, but there have been few well-designed clinical studies in this area. The most profound changes are seen in the neonate and the infant. Some metabolic enzymes are virtually absent in the fetus and appear only after days or weeks have elapsed. Renal function is incompletely developed at birth. Also, only the delivery date and not the biochemical age of the neonate is known. Furthermore, the electrolyte and fluid balance of a child can change dramatically during illness. These facts make extrapolation of adult dosage regimens to pediatric situations tenuous. Body surface area may be used as a basis for translation of an adult initial dose, but cannot be used to determine the maintenance dose and dosing interval. There is no substitute for a cautious and prudent approach to the treatment of children, especially premature and newborn infants. If possible, at the earliest stages of therapy, concentrations of the drug in blood should be monitored and, when necessary, corrections made in the dosage regimen, so that a minimum effective concentration derived from studies in adults is maintained (Done, 1964; Yaffe, 1966; Sereni and Principii, 1968).

Dosage Regimens in Disease States

Accepted dosage schedules may require drastic modification in patients with renal failure, liver disease, or altered hemodynamics. The initial therapeutic dose is rarely adjusted, except on the basis of kilograms of body weight, unless the drug has a very narrow therapeutic range and there is reason to suspect altered drug distribution (e.g., in edematous or obese patients). The most profound adjustments in dose involve the size and frequency of the supplementary doses. This is especially true for those drugs that are primarily eliminated via the kidneys in a patient with severely impaired renal function. The same considerations probably apply to drugs that require hepatic metabolism in a patient with liver disease. Much less is known about the quantitative aspects of liver disease and drug dosage. Unlike renal function, which can be fairly well evaluated with clearance

of creatinine, inulin, or PAH, hepatic drug metabolic function cannot be easily measured.

Most studies pertaining to the effects of disease on dose requirements have been related to modified antibiotic regimens in patients with renal failure (Kunin, 1967). Antibiotics are readily analyzed in biologic fluids, and the concentration of drug in plasma correlates with efficacy. The elimination kinetics of chloramphenicol and erythromycin, which are more or less completely metabolized, undergo only small changes when patients have renal impairment. Major readjustments in dosage schedules are necessary with gentamicin, streptomycin, and kanamycin when patients are anuric, because these drugs are almost totally excreted unchanged in the urine.

Kanamycin appears unmetabolized in the urine, is not bound to plasma proteins, and has an apparent volume of distribution similar to the extracellular volume (19% of the total body weight). The antibiotic is poorly absorbed from the gastrointestinal tract and, therefore, is given intramuscularly or intravenously. It possesses a low therapeutic index, and nephrotoxicity and ototoxicity are associated with high doses. Dosage regimens must be carefully considered in patients with renal failure. For varying degrees of renal function, the urinary clearance of kanamycin is always about 76% of the inulin clearance (Cl_{in}) and 60% of the creatinine clearance (Cl_{cr}) and is therefore directly proportional to the glomerular filtration rate (Orme and Cutler, 1969). It is therefore possible to calculate the half-life of kanamycin under any circumstances, since:

$$t_{1/2} = \frac{0.693 V_d}{\text{Renal clearance of kanamycin}} \qquad (27a)$$

For kanamycin, this equation further reduces to:

$$t_{1/2} \text{ (hr)} = \frac{0.693 \times 0.19 \times \text{body weight in grams}}{60 \times 0.6 \times \text{creatinine clearance}} \\ \text{(ml/min)} \qquad (27b)$$

$$= 3.7 \times \frac{\text{Body weight in kg}}{\text{Creatinine clearance (ml/min)}} \qquad (27c)$$

In patients with normal renal function, Cl_{cr} is 125 ml/min/1.73 m² of body surface area, which corresponds to a 70-kg man of average height. Accordingly, the expected half-life of kanamycin is 2.1 hours, which agrees with the observed data. This formula also predicts a half-life of 21.7 hours in a patient with severe renal impairment ($Cl_{cr} = 8$ ml/min). This value is in close accord with the observed value of 25 hours (Figure 2–15). Therefore, suitable dosage regimens of kanamycin consist of 7 mg/kg of body weight initially, followed by 3.5 mg/kg every half-life (corresponding to 2 hours and 25 hours in the examples discussed above). In practice, 7 mg/kg can be administered every three half-lives; and, although the concentration of drug in plasma falls to low levels, the regimen is clinically efficacious. In an anuric patient, a single 7-mg/kg dose should suffice unless the patient is hemodialyzed; in this instance, approximately 50% of the drug is removed and must be replaced. Thus, if the patient's weight and creatinine clearance are known, an adequate, safe regimen for this antibiotic can be designed. If the V_d of kanamycin per kilogram of body weight is the same in two subjects, the half-life of the drug is inversely proportional to the creatinine clearance per kilogram of body weight. Thus, if the creatinine clearance, corrected for body weight, is one-fourth normal, the expected kanamycin half-life is approximately 8 hours. It should also be possible to correlate kanamycin half-life with serum creatinine concentrations, thereby further simplifying the measurements, since:

$$\text{Serum creatinine} = \frac{\text{Creatinine production rate}}{\text{Creatinine clearance}} \quad (28)$$

While the production rate of creatinine is fairly constant for an individual, it is dependent on muscle mass and, therefore, decreases in the elderly. Thus, it is possible for two patients to have the same concentrations of creatinine in serum but different Cl_{cr}. Nevertheless, dosage regimens for kanamycin based on serum creatinine levels may be sufficiently accurate for clinical purposes (Cutler and Orme, 1969) (see Chapter 3).

Digoxin is primarily excreted by the kidney. In patients with normal renal function, its half-life is 1.6 days, and 63% appears in the urine unchanged. In anuric patients this glycoside is not excreted; therefore, the 4.6-day half-life represents only metabolism. Like kanamycin, the renal clearance of this drug is proportional to the Cl_{cr}; assuming a relatively constant metabolic clearance, it is possible to predict the half-life of digoxin from Cl_{cr} data.

Digoxin has a narrow therapeutic index, and, when the amount of drug in the body exceeds 1.7 mg, toxicity may be imminent. Therefore, accumulation is defined in respect to peak concentrations in blood rather than to average body content. An initial or digitalizing dose of between 0.7 and 1.5 mg is usually taken in three divided doses over a period of 10 hours to avoid toxicity. Once digitalization is accomplished, a daily maintenance dose replaces drug losses. After the first day, the amount of drug remaining is equal to $e^{-K_d t}$, which corresponds to 65% of the loading dose in the patient without renal disease and 86% in anuric patients; the respective maintenance doses are 35% and 14% of the digitalizing dose. Sometimes the loading dose is omitted and control of heart failure is achieved by gradual accrual of drug. The daily dose is constant but is chosen on the basis of the desired eventual plateau concentrations, which must be equal to the omitted digitalizing dose (approximately 1.1 mg). The daily digoxin dose is thus 0.4 and 0.16 mg, respectively. Although 2 weeks ($3.3 t_{1/2}$) are required to reach 90% of 1.1 mg in the anuric patient, this concentration is achieved within 5 days in the patient with normal renal function. Also, should the renal function of the patient change, the new digoxin half-life can be calculated from the new creatinine clearance, and the daily dose can be corrected to ensure an optimal drug concentration (Jelliffe, 1968). These calculations are not a substitute for careful patient monitoring, but serve to indicate the kinetic basis of digoxin therapy. Adjustments for thyroid function, electrolyte balance, and gastrointestinal function of the patient are necessary (see Chapters 3 and 5), but some of the empiricism in digitalis therapy can be avoided by using this quantitative approach.

The argument can be made that kanamycin and digoxin are exceptions and that most drug regimens defy accurate quantitation in patients with renal or hepatic malfunction. However, a sound understanding of the kinetics of these two drugs can foster rational choice of dosage schedules (Dettli et al., 1970; Jelliffe et al., 1970; Koch-Weser and Klein, 1971; McHenry et al., 1971).

In summary, the appropriateness of the usual recommended regimen for a given patient depends upon his resemblance to patients examined in small but carefully supervised clinical trials. Ideally, drug disposition should be studied in the individual patient. When disease-induced changes in kinetics of drug absorption or disposition or drug interactions occur, they should be carefully documented. Final drug concentrations in blood are independent of the initial dose, which only serves to rapidly establish a therapeutic effect; accordingly, there is some margin for error in the size of the initial dose. Although the initial therapeutic dose might be selected on the basis of body weight, this is rarely done for adults because the V_d per kilogram of body weight of a drug is reasonably constant and the range in body weight is no greater than the acceptable two- to fivefold therapeutic plasma concentration range obtained with most drugs. However, such corrections should be made when the drug is to be given to obese or emaciated patients and to children.

Principle: Both the size and the frequency of the maintenance dose are dependent on the half-life of the drug. This half-life can vary as a result of physiologically, pharmacologically, or pathologically induced changes in the total body clearance and perhaps in the volume of distribution of the drug. Such variations should be anticipated by the physician and the pharmacist, and proper adjustments should be made in dose and dose interval.

If the glomerular filtration rate (inulin or creatinine clearance), the renal plasma flow (PAH clearance), and the urinary pH are known, it should be possible to predict variations in the renal clearance of drug. Unfortunately, at present there are no indices of the metabolic clearance of drugs. Consequently, it is not possible to predict either the actual $t_{1/2}$ of a drug that is eliminated primarily by metabolism or the expected changes in $t_{1/2}$ of such a drug in a patient with a diseased liver. In general, there is a narrow range in the half-life of a therapeutic agent eliminated primarily by sulfate or glucuronide conjugation, and the $t_{1/2}$ for the agent listed in the literature may be valuable in designing an adequate dosage regimen for such a drug. However, when oxidation or reduction is the major metabolic route, wide variance in the $t_{1/2}$ may necessitate different dosage schedules in different patients. Ideally, the concentration of drug in blood and/or the excretion rate of the drug in urine should be measured; these values would be excellent adjuncts to observations of therapeutic effects in the patient. Using both quantitative measurements of drug and observations of its pharmacologic effect, the physician and the pharmacist should be able to make suitable adjustments in the dosage schedule. Although at present the measurement of concentrations of drug in blood appears impractical, as the specificity of new drugs increases, as physicians use fewer drugs at one time in a patient (see Chapter 15), and as chemical analytic techniques improve, we may be in a position to analyze drugs and to use the data wisely. Perhaps inert compounds will be found that can be used to assess the clearance of the major metabolic pathways. The information so derived would aid in predicting an adequate dosage schedule for any drug, thereby reducing much of the present uncertainty in drug therapy.

REFERENCES

Aguiar, A. J.; Krc, J., Jr.; Kinkel, A. W.; and Samyn, J. C.: Effect of polymorphism on the absorption from chloramphenicol palmitate. *J. Pharm. Sci.,* **56**: 847–53, 1967.

Anders, M. W.: Enhancement and inhibition of drug metabolism. *Ann. Rev. Pharmacol.,* **11**:37–56, 1971.

Ariens, E. J. (ed.): *Molecular Pharmacology: The Mode of Action of Biologically Active Compounds,* Vol. I. Academic Press, Inc., New York, 1964.

————: Modulation of pharmacokinetics by modification of the various factors involved. *Farmaco* [*Sci.*], **24**:3–102, 1969.

Arnold, K., and Gerber, N.: The rate of decline of diphenylhydantoin in human plasma. *Clin. Pharmacol. Ther.,* **11**:121–34, 1970.

Ballard, B. E.: Biopharmaceutical considerations in subcutaneous and intramuscular drug administration. *J. Pharm. Sci.,* **57**:357–78, 1968.

Ballard, B. E., and Nelson, E.: Prolonged-action pharmaceuticals. In Martin, E. W. (ed.): *Pharmaceutical Sciences,* 13th ed. Mack Publishing Co., Easton, Pa., 1970, pp. 1699–1728.

Barr, W. H.: Principles of biopharmaceutics. *Amer. J. Pharm. Educ.,* **52**:958–81, 1968.

————: Factors involved in the assessment of systemic or biological availability of drug products. *Drug Inform. Bull.,* 1969, pp. 27–44.

Beckett, A. H., and Rowland, M.: Urinary excretion kinetics of amphetamine in man. *J. Pharm. Pharmacol.,* **17**:628–39, 1965.

Beckett, A. H., and Wilkinson, G. R.: Influence of urine pH and flow rate on the renal excretion of chlorpheniramine in man. *J. Pharm. Pharmacol.,* **17**: 256–57, 1965.

Berlin, N. I.; Berman, M.; Berk, P. D.; Phang, J. M.; and Waldman, T. A.: The application of multicompartment analysis to problems of clinical medicine. *Ann. Intern. Med.,* **68**:423–48, 1968.

Binns, T. B. (ed.): *Symposium: Absorption and Distribution of Drugs.* Williams & Wilkins Co., Baltimore, 1964.

Bischoff, K. B., and Dedrick, R. L.: Thiopental pharmacokinetics. *J. Pharm. Sci.,* **57**:1346–51, 1968.

Bischoff, K. B.; Dedrick, R. L.; and Zaharko, D. S.: Preliminary model for methotrexate pharmacokinetics. *J. Pharm. Sci.,* **59**:149–54, 1970

Blythe, R. H.; Grass, G. M.; and Macdonnell, D. R.: The formulation and evaluation of enteric coated aspirin tablets. *Amer. J. Pharm.,* **131**:206–16, 1959.

Brodie, B. B.; Bernstein, E.; and Mark, L. C.: Role of body fat in limiting the duration of action of thiopental. *J. Pharmacol. Exp. Ther.,* **105**:421–26, 1952.

Burns, J. J.; Rose, R. K.; Chenkin, T.; Goldman, A.; Schulert, A.; and Brodie, B. B.: The physiological disposition of phenylbutazone (Butazolidin) in man, and a method for its estimation in biological material. *J. Pharmacol. Exp. Ther.,* **109**:346–57, 1953.

Butler, T. C.; Mahaffee, C.; and Waddell, W. J.: Phenobarbital: studies of elimination, accumulation, tolerance and dosage schedules. *J. Pharmacol. Exp. Ther.,* **111**:425–35, 1954.

Conney, A. H.: Pharmacological implications of microsomal enzyme induction. *Pharmacol. Rev.,* **19**:317–66, 1967.

————: Drug metabolism and therapeutics. *New Engl. J. Med.,* **280**:653–60, 1969.

Cutler, R. E., and Orme, B. M.: Correlation of serum creatinine concentration and kanamycin half-life. *J.A.M.A.,* **209**:539–42, 1969.

Dayton, P. G.; Cucinell, S. A.; Weiss, M.; and Perel, J. M.: Dose dependence of drug plasma level decline in dogs. *J. Pharmacol. Exp. Ther.,* **158**:305–16, 1967.

DeMarco, T. J., and Levine, R. R.: Role of the lymphatics in the intestinal absorption and distribution of drugs. *J. Pharmacol. Exp. Ther.,* **169**:142–51, 1969.

Dettli, L., and Spring, P.: Factors influencing drug elimination in man. *Farmaco* [*Sci.*], **23**:757–812, 1968.

Dettli, L.; Spring, P.; and Habersang, R.: Drug dosage in patients with impaired renal function. *Postgrad. Med. J. Suppl.,* **46**:32–35, 1970.

Ditlefsen, E. M.: Quinidine concentration in blood and excretion in urine following parenteral administration as related to congestive heart failure. *Acta Med. Scand.*, **159**:105–109, 1957.

Done, A. K.: Developmental pharmacology. *Clin. Pharmacol. Ther.*, **5**:432–79, 1964.

Elliot, J. S.; Sharp, R. F.; and Lewis, L.: Urinary pH. *J. Urol.*, **81**:339–43, 1959.

George, J. D.: Gastric acidity and mobility. *Amer. J. Dig. Dis.*, **13**:376–83, 1968.

Gibaldi, M., and Kanig, J.: Absorption of drugs through the oral mucosa. *J. Oral Ther.*, **1**:440–50, 1965.

Ginsberg, J.: Placental drug transfer. *Ann. Rev. Pharmacol.*, **11**:387–408, 1971.

Gladtke, E.: Pharmakokinetische Prüfung der Vollständigkeit der Absorption nach Dost. *Antibiot. Chemother. (Basel)*, **12**:159–69, 1964.

Goldstein, A.: The interaction of drugs and plasma proteins. *Pharmacol. Rev.*, **1**:102–65, 1949.

Goldstein, A.; Aronow, L.; and Kalman, S. M.: *Principles of Drug Action: The Basis of Pharmacology.* Harper & Row, New York, 1968, pp. 160–94, 206–79.

Hollister, L. E., and Kanter, S. L.: Studies of delayed-action medication. IV. Salicylates. *Clin. Pharmacol. Ther.*, **6**:5–11, 1965.

Hunt, J. N., and Knox, M. T.: Control of gastric emptying. *Amer. J. Dig. Dis.*, **13**:372–75, 1968.

Jelliffe, R. W.: An improved method of digoxin therapy. *Ann. Intern. Med.*, **69**:703–17, 1968.

Jelliffe, R. W.; Buell, J.; Kalaba, R.; Sridhar, R.; Rockwell, R.; and Wagner, J. G.: An improved method of digitoxin therapy. *Ann. Intern. Med.*, **72**:453–64, 1970.

Kakemi, K.; Arita, T.; Hori, R.; Konishi, K.; Nishimura, M.; Matsui, H.; and Nishimura, T.: Absorption and excretion of drugs. XXXIV. An aspect of the mechanism of drug absorption from the intestinal tract in rats. *Chem. Pharm. Bull. (Tokyo)*, **17**:255–61, 1969.

Koch-Weser, J., and Klein, S. W.: Procainamide dosage schedules, plasma concentrations and clinical effects. *J.A.M.A.*, **215**:1454–60, 1971.

Korn, E. D.: Structure of biological membranes. *Science*, **153**:1491–98, 1966.

Kruger-Thiemer, E.; Diller, W.; and Bunger, P.: Pharmakokinetic models regarding protein binding of drugs. *Antimicrob. Agents Chemother.*, 1965, pp. 183–91.

Kunin, C. M.: Clinical pharmacology of the new penicillins. II. Effect of drugs which interfere with binding to serum proteins. *Clin. Pharmacol. Ther.*, **7**:180–88, 1966.

———: A guide to the use of antibiotics in patients with renal failure. *Ann. Intern. Med.*, **67**:151–58, 1967.

Lee, C.; Froman, R. O.; Anderson, R. C.; and Chen, K. K.: Gastric and intestinal absorption of potassium penicillin V and the free acid. *Antibiot. Chemother. (Basel)*, **8**:354–60, 1958.

Leonards, J. R., and Levy, G.: Absorption and metabolism of aspirin administered in enteric-coated tablets. *J.A.M.A.*, **193**:99–104, 1965.

Levine, R. R., and Pelikan, E. W.: Mechanisms of drug absorption and excretion. Passage of drugs out of and into the gastrointestinal tract. *Ann. Rev. Pharmacol.*, **4**:69–84, 1964.

Levy, G.: Biopharmaceutical consideration in dosage form design and evaluation. In Sprowls, J. B. (ed.): *Prescription Pharmacy.* J. P. Lippincott Co., Philadelphia, 1963, pp. 31–94.

———: Pharmacokinetics of salicylate elimination in man. *J. Pharm. Sci.*, **54**:959–67, 1965.

———: Kinetics of pharmacologic effects. *Clin. Pharmacol. Ther.*, **7**:362–72, 1966.

———: Dose dependent effects of pharmacokinetics.

In Tedeschi, D. H., and Tedeschi, R. E. (eds.): *Importance of Fundamental Principles in Drug Evaluation.* Raven Press, New York, 1968, pp. 141–72.

Levy, G.; Gumtow, R. H.; and Rutowski, J. M.: The effect of dosage form upon the gastrointestinal absorption rate of salicylates. *Canad. Med. Ass. J.*, **85**:414–19, 1961.

Levy, G.; Hall, N. A.; and Nelson, E.: Studies on inactive prednisone tablets. *Amer. J. Hosp. Pharm.*, **21**:402, 1964.

Levy, G., and Hollister, L. E.: Failure of the U.S.P. disintegration test to assess physiological availability of enteric coated tablets. *New York J. Med.*, **64**:3002–3005, 1964.

Levy, G., and Jusko, W. J.: Effect of viscosity on drug absorption. *J. Pharm. Sci.*, **54**:219–25, 1965.

McHenry, M. C.; Gavan, T. L.; Gifford, R. W.; Guerkink, N. A.; Van Ommen, R. A.; Town, M. A.; and Wagner, J. G.: Gentamicin dosages for renal insufficiency. *Ann. Intern. Med.*, **74**:192–97, 1971.

Mapleson, W. W.: An electric analogue for uptake and exchange of inert gases and other agents. *J. Appl. Physiol.*, **18**:197–204, 1963.

Mark, L. C., and Brand, L.: Where does the Pentothal go? *Bull. N.Y. Acad. Med.*, **40**:476–82, 1964.

Martin, B. K.: Potential effect of the plasma proteins on drug distribution. *Nature (London)*, **207**:274–76, 1965.

Meyer, M. C., and Guttman, D. E.: The binding of drugs to plasma proteins. *J. Pharm. Sci.*, **57**:895–918, 1968.

Moya, F.: Uptake, distribution and placental transfer of drugs in obstetrical anesthesia. In Shnider, S. (ed.): *Obstetrical Anesthesia: Current Concepts and Practice.* Williams & Wilkins Co., Baltimore, 1970, pp. 13–28.

Nagashima, R.; Levy, G.; and O'Reilly, R. A.: Comparative pharmacokinetics of coumarin anticoagulants I.V. *J. Pharm. Sci.*, **57**:1888–95, 1968.

Nelson, E.: Physicochemical and pharmaceutic properties of drugs that influence the results of clinical trials. *Clin. Pharmacol. Ther.*, **3**:673–81, 1962.

Nelson, E.; Hanan, M.; and Levy, G.: Comparative pharmacokinetics of salicylate elimination in man and rats. *J. Pharmacol. Exp. Ther.*, **153**:159–96, 1966.

Nitowsky, H. M.; Matz, L.; and Berzofsky, J. A.: Studies on oxidative drug metabolism in the full-term newborn infant. *J. Pediat.*, **69**:1139–49, 1966.

Northup, D. W., and Van Liere, E. J.: Effect of the isomers of amphetamine and desoxyphedrine on gastric emptying in man. *J. Pharmacol. Exp. Ther.*, **109**:358–60, 1963.

O'Reilly, R. A.: Studies on the coumarin anticoagulant drugs: interaction of human plasma albumin and warfarin sodium. *J. Clin. Invest.*, **46**:829–37, 1967.

O'Reilly, R. A.; Nelson, E.; and Levy, G.: Physicochemical and physiologic factors affecting the absorption of warfarin in man. *J. Pharm. Sci.*, **55**:435–37, 1966.

Orme, B. M., and Cutler, R. E.: The relationship between kanamycin pharmacokinetics, distribution and renal function. *Clin. Pharmacol. Ther.*, **10**:543–50, 1969.

Ott, H., and Seeger, C.: Untersuchungen zur Frage Germaninbindung an die Serumproteine. *Z. Ges. Exp. Med.*, **125**:455–68, 1955.

Parke, D. V.: *The Biochemistry of Foreign Compounds.* Pergamon Press, New York, 1968.

Paul, H. E.; Hayes, K. J.; Paul, M. F.; and Borgmann, A. R.: Laboratory studies with nitrofurantoin. *J. Pharm. Sci.*, **56**:882–85, 1967.

Price, H. L.; Kovnat, P. J.; Safer, J. N.; Conner, E. H.; and Price, M. L.: The uptake of thiopental by body tissues and its relation to the duration of narcosis. *Clin. Pharmacol. Ther.*, **1**:16–22, 1960.

Rowland, M.; Riegelman, S.; and Epstein, W. L.: Absorption kinetics of griseofulvin in man. *J. Pharm. Sci.*, **57**:984–89, 1968.

Sacchetti, G.; Nicolis, F. B.; and Roncoroni, L.: Evaluation in man of the effects of an anticholinergic agent on the gastric emptying by a quantitative x-ray method. *J. Pharmacol. Exp. Ther.*, **145**:393–98, 1964.

Saidman, L. J., and Eger, E. I.: The effect of thiopental metabolism on the duration of anesthesia. *Anesthesiology*, **27**:118–26, 1966.

Schwarz, T. W.: Molded solid dosage forms: suppositories. In Sprowls, J. B., and Beal, H. M. (eds.): *American Pharmacy*. J. P. Lippincott Co., Philadelphia, 1966, pp. 311–31.

Seager, H.: The effect of methyl cellulose on the absorption of nitrofurantoin from the gastrointestinal tract. *J. Pharm. Pharmacol.*, **20**:968–69, 1968.

Sereni, F., and Principii, N.: Developmental pharmacology. *Ann. Rev. Pharmacol.*, **8**:453–66, 1968.

Shand, D. G.; Nuckolls, E. M.; and Oates, J. A.: Plasma propranolol levels in adults. *Clin. Pharmacol. Ther.*, **11**:112–20, 1970.

Shanker, L. W.: Physiological transport of drugs. In Harper, N. J., and Simmonds, A. B. (eds.): *Advances in Drug Research*, Vol. I. Academic Press, Inc., New York, 1964, pp. 72–106.

Sirota, J. H., and Saltzman, A.: The renal clearance and plasma protein binding of Aureomycin in man. *J. Pharmacol. Exp. Ther.*, **100**:210–18, 1950.

Smith, R. L.: The biliary excretion and enterohepatic circulation of drugs and other organic compounds. *Progr. Drug Res.*, **9**:299–360, 1966.

Stein, W. D.: *The Movement of Molecules across Cell Membranes*. Academic Press, Inc., New York, 1967.

Stowe, C. M., and Plaa, G. L.: Extrarenal excretion of drugs and chemicals. *Ann. Rev. Pharmacol.*, **8**:337–56, 1968.

Sweeney, W. M.; Hardy, S. M.; Bornbush, A. C.; and Ruegsegger, J. M.: Absorption of tetracycline in human beings as affected by certain excipients. *Antibiot. Med. Clin. Ther.*, **4**:642–56, 1957.

Swintosky, J. V.: Illustrations and pharmaceutical interpretations of first order drug elimination rate from the bloodstream. *J. Amer. Pharm. Ass.*, **45**:395–398, 1956.

Tannenbaum, P. J.; Rosen, E.; Flanagan, T.; and Crosley, A. P.: The influence of dosage form on the activity of a diuretic agent. *Clin. Pharmacol. Ther.*, **9**:598–604, 1968.

Ther, L., and Winne, D.: Drug absorption. *Ann. Rev. Pharmacol.*, **11**:56–70, 1971.

Van Rossum, J. M.: Pharmacokinetics of accumulation. *J. Pharm. Sci.*, **57**:2162–64, 1968.

Wagner, J. G.: Biopharmaceutics: absorption aspects. *J. Pharm. Sci.*, **50**:359–87, 1961.

———: Biopharmaceutics: gastrointestinal absorption aspects. *Antibiot. Chemother.* (*Basel*), **12**:53–84, 1964.

———: Drug accumulation. *J. Clin. Pharmacol.*, **7**: 84–88, 1967.

———: Biopharmaceutics. *Drug Intelligence*, **2**:30–34, 1968a.

———: Pharmacokinetics. *Ann. Rev. Pharmacol.*, **8**:67–94, 1968b.

Wagner, J. G., and Nelson, E.: Kinetic analysis of blood levels and urinary excretion in the absorptive phase after single doses of drug. *J. Pharm. Sci.*, **53**: 1392–1403, 1964.

Wagner, J. G.; Northam, J. I.; Alway, C. D.; and Carpenter, O. S.: Blood levels of drug of the equilibrium state after multiple dosing. *Nature* (*London*), **207**:1301–1302, 1965.

Wallis, W.; Kutt, H.; and McDowell, F.: Intravenous diphenylhydantoin in treatment of acute repetitive seizures. *Neurology* (*Minneap.*), **18**:513–16, 1968.

Wasserman, L. R.; Sharney, L.; Gevirtz, N. R.; Schwartz, L.; Weintraub, L. R.; Tendler, P.; Dumont, A.; Dreilling, D.; and Witte, M.: Study of iron kinetics. I. Interpretation of ferrokinetic data in man. *J. Mount Sinai Hosp. N.Y.*, **32**:262–304, 1965.

Weiner, I. M., and Mudge, G. H.: Renal tubular mechanisms for excretion of organic acids and bases. *Amer. J. Med.*, **36**:743–62, 1964.

Williams, R. T.: *Detoxication Mechanisms: The Mechanisms and Detoxication of Drugs, Toxic Substances and other Organic Compounds*, 2nd ed. John Wiley & Sons, New York, 1959.

Wyers, P. J. H., and Van Munster, P. J. J.: The disappearance of Evans blue dye from the blood in normal and nephrotic subjects. *J. Lab. Clin. Med.*, **58**: 375–85, 1961.

Yaffe, S. J: Some aspects of perinatal pharmacology. *Ann. Rev. Med.*, **17**:213–34, 1966.

UNIT II
PATHOPHYSIOLOGIC AND PHARMACOLOGIC CONSIDERATIONS IN DRUG ADMINISTRATION

Chapter 3

RENAL DISORDERS

Samuel O. Thier and *Geoffrey W. G. Sharp*

This chapter illustrates aspects of renal function involved in the use of pharmacologic agents. An exhaustive review of such agents is not undertaken since an enormous number of drugs depend upon the kidney as a site of action and/or a determinant of pharmacokinetics (see Chapter 2). The authors consider *selected* aspects of renal physiology and pathophysiology that affect drug use. When principles are illustrated, the reader is to understand that only selected examples are presented and that the principles also apply to other drugs.

Diuretics are discussed in detail since they are the most important class of drugs acting directly on the kidney and since they illustrate best how knowledge of drug mechanism and site of action is used to develop a therapeutic strategy. Selected renal diseases are discussed to illustrate specific problems in therapy and general problems in the evaluation of widely accepted but poorly substantiated modes of therapy. Finally, the pathophysiology of advanced renal failure is reviewed and special considerations in the treatment of this state are presented.

As principles of therapeutics are developed for specific and general circumstances, one overriding principle must be kept in mind: *Principle: An understanding of the basic concepts of renal physiology and the chemical nature of drugs is mandatory in order to master the principles of therapeutics that pertain not only to renal disease but also to any disease whose treatment may be affected by renal function.*

ASPECTS OF RENAL PHYSIOLOGY IMPORTANT TO THERAPEUTIC CONSIDERATIONS

Excretory Function

The important function of the kidneys is to regulate the volume and composition of body fluids, and consequently, drug distribution and excretion. The renal mechanisms for handling drugs are no different from those described for endogenous substances. The renal clearance of many drugs may be altered by changes in filtration, reabsorption, secretion, or metabolism. Renal mechanisms may be the means for excretion of pharmacologic agents or may themselves be targets of these agents.

The concept of glomerular filtration has been introduced in Chapter 2. Substances are filtered at the glomerulus if they are not protein bound and if they are small enough to pass the selective barrier of the glomerular apparatus. The greater its binding to proteins, the less readily a substance is filtered. If a substance is freely filtered and neither reabsorbed nor secreted by the tubule, clearance of that substance is a measure of the glomerular filtration rate. If net tubular reabsorption occurs, the rate of excretion is less than the filtration rate, whereas net tubular secretion accelerates the rate of excretion.

Kidney function may affect the duration of action of some drugs, the doses required for therapeutic effects, and the chemical form of drug to be given. The effects of some drugs on the kidney may directly alter kinetics of other drugs or may indirectly alter kinetics by changing volume and chemical composition of body fluids. In addition, cumulative and perhaps toxic effects of drugs at renal and extrarenal sites must be anticipated when there are drug- or disease-induced changes in renal function.

Renal mass is lost in most forms of renal failure, resulting in decreased excretory function via compromised glomerular filtration and tubular secretion. Reduction in tubular reabsorptive capacity may enhance excretion of certain substances, but such an enhancement usually is quantitatively less important than the reduction in filtered load. Thus, drug retention and drug toxicity are usually the clinical problems.

The excretion of substances cleared by filtration is markedly reduced during uremia. If standard doses are given at standard time intervals, the drugs accumulate and toxicity results. Recognition of the altered kinetics permits rescheduling of doses to provide appropriate therapeutic levels while avoiding toxicity. Similar alterations in dosage may be necessary for secreted drugs such as ampicillin, whereas penicillin has an alternate hepatic clearance mechanism. Still other agents, although not toxic themselves, may produce toxic metabolites that accumulate during renal failure (e.g., the ototoxic metabolite of ethacrynic acid).

As a rule, renal failure reduces requirements for drugs that are directly excreted or whose active or toxic metabolites are excreted by the kidney. However, the accumulation of some metabolites ordinarily cleared by the kidney (e.g., the metabolites of chloramphenicol) may have no pharmacologic effect (Kunin et al., 1959). *As* *long as the active or toxic form of the drug does not accumulate, dose schedules need not be altered.*

During renal failure, substances metabolized by the kidney may accumulate or be dissipated slowly. Insulin requirements in diabetic patients with renal failure may diminish in part because insulin is no longer effectively metabolized by the kidney (Rabkin et al., 1970). Although there are few data documenting a significant role for the kidney in drug metabolism, the theoretic possibility for such a role must be considered. The logic of such a consideration should be clear, and the question should be raised as new drugs are introduced.

Renal Toxicity of Primary Drug

When drugs are retained in the body, drug toxicity should be anticipated. Regardless of the mechanism responsible for the retention, the toxicity may further damage kidneys and create a cycle of accelerating toxicity and renal damage. Such a cycle could best be avoided by careful selection of drugs and their dose intervals, but once started it usually must be broken by withdrawing the agent.

Sodium colistimethate, an antibiotic of the polymyxin group, produces renal tubular damage ranging from mild dysfunction to acute tubular necrosis (Elwood et al., 1966). Administration of sodium colistimethate in the presence of renal insufficiency may result in toxic concentrations within the kidneys. The greater the toxicity, the more likely additional antibiotic therapy is to enhance and to prolong it. During renal failure, sodium colistimethate or similar agents should be used only if other antibiotics less dependent on renal excretion are unsuitable, and then only with the knowledge that "new" kinetics of excretion are operative and must be utilized in determining the dosage.

A number of other drugs produce dose-related toxic damage to the kidney. Sensitivity reactions resulting in vasculitis, glomerulitis, glomerulonephritis, and perhaps tubular damage may also occur. These lesions should be considered, particularly if extrarenal manifestations of hypersensitivity are present (e.g., skin eruption, arthralgia, or eosinophilia). In either toxic or hypersensitivity reactions, withdrawal of the offending drug is indicated (Schreiner and Maher, 1965).

Extrarenal Toxicity of Drugs

Extrarenal toxicity in renal failure occurs when a compound largely dependent on the kidney for excretion, but having little direct effect on the kidneys, is used to treat disease. Digoxin is primarily excreted in an unchanged form by the kidney (Doherty *et al.*, 1964). Retention of digoxin produces cardiac toxicity, and if cardiac output is reduced, renal perfusion decreases and both the cardiac and renal systems suffer further. Kanamycin can damage the eighth cranial nerve and is capable of producing both renal and extrarenal toxicity.

Renal and extrarenal toxicity of the metabolic products of drugs must also be anticipated and recognized. The possible renal toxicity of phenacetin metabolites (Bluemle and Goldberg, 1968) and the ototoxicity of ethacrynic acid metabolites (Schneider and Becker, 1966) are examples. Although there are few other documented examples, anticipation of such possibilities facilitates their recognition.

Redefinition of Drug Form with Renal Failure

The route of administration and the form of the drug must be kept in mind when treating a patient with renal failure. Penicillin provides an example of the need to change from a potentially toxic to a nontoxic form of the same drug during renal failure. Penicillin G is usually given as the potassium salt, which contains 1.7 mEq of potassium per million units of penicillin. During renal failure, there is a tendency to retain potassium, and it may be preferable to use sodium penicillin.

Resistance to vitamin D develops during renal failure. Vitamin D is ordinarily converted to the active metabolite 25-hydroxychole-calciferol, which facilitates calcium absorption from the intestinal lumen. In patients with renal failure, formation of this active metabolite is impaired and calcium is poorly absorbed from the gut. There is usually no need for vitamin D therapy in uremia, but for the few patients who do require such treatment specific principles must be considered. Theoretically, administration of the active form of vitamin D is preferred, but large doses of vitamin D provide adequate active metabolite (Avioli *et al.*, 1969). Vitamin D resistance can be treated by (1) altering the form of the vitamin, (2) altering the route of calcium administration, or (3) giving large enough quantities of vitamin D to provide adequate amounts of active metabolite despite inefficient production.

Drugs That Depend on Renal Excretion for Their Action

Drugs that depend upon renal excretion for their action, such as nitrofurantoin, are ineffective in sterilizing urine of patients with renal failure. During renal failure nitrofurantoin does not appear in the urine in significant concentration (Sachs *et al.*, 1968). *Principle: Sensitivity of an organism to an antibiotic is not the only deter-minant of the drug's efficacy. If a drug does not reach the site of its intended effect, there can be no benefit.*

Relatively specific tubular transport systems for reabsorption and secretion exist. Glucose and amino acids are freely filtered and almost completely reabsorbed in the proximal tubule by stereospecific, saturable, energy-dependent mechanisms. Specific genetic defects in the transport of these molecules have been described. In addition, reabsorption of these substances is reduced in disorders that depress all proximal tubular function (e.g., Fanconi syndrome). Organic acids and bases are both reabsorbed and secreted in the proximal tubule (Weiner and Mudge, 1964). Substances may affect these secretory or reabsorptive mechanisms, thereby dramatically altering excretory rates. Selective interference with reabsorption or secretion may provide flexibility in the use of drugs that are organic acids. Since renal mechanisms are few, a drug acting upon any aspect of renal function or utilizing a specific mechanism may interfere with a second drug's action or excretion. Thus, the action of a second drug may be enhanced or reduced, although the pharmacologic action of the second drug may be totally unrelated to that of the first.

Probenecid, which utilizes the tubular organic acid transport system, inhibits reabsorption of uric acid, producing uricosuria (Goodman and Gilman, 1970). When probenecid was found to compete for organic acid transport in the tubular secretory system, a role for probenecid in inhibiting secretion of the organic acid penicillin was defined. Probenecid can enhance penicillin activity or reduce the dose of penicillin required to produce a desired blood level (although the availability of penicillin makes this no longer clinically necessary). Other agents utilizing the organic acid transport pathways may have clinically significant biphasic effects, inhibiting secretion at low doses and reabsorption at high doses (Yü and Gutman, 1959). In low doses, salicylates inhibit uric acid secretion, elevating serum uric acid concentrations and antagonizing uricosuric agents such as probenecid (an example of two organic acids interfering with each other). At higher doses salicylates inhibit the quantitatively more significant reabsorptive mechanism and produce uricosuria.

Less obvious interactions of drugs related to renal function may occur when one drug interacts with a metabolite of a second drug. If the metabolite is pharmacologically active, the interaction assumes therapeutic importance. For example, allopurinol inhibits the enzyme xanthine oxidase, reducing uric acid production (Goodman and Gilman, 1970). Allopurinol is metabolized to alloxanthine, which also inhibits xanthine oxidase and has a longer duration of action than does its parent drug. Alloxanthine, but not allopurinol, is reabsorbed by the same mechanism as uric acid. The addition of a uricosuric agent to a regimen of allopurinol may be intended to facilitate the lowering of serum uric acid by increasing urinary uric acid at a time when uric acid production is reduced. In fact, the combination may reduce the effectiveness of allopurinol when the uricosuric agent increases the loss of alloxanthine and reduces the inhibition of xanthine oxidase (Elion et al., 1968).

An organic acid such as sulfinpyrazone may be used to inhibit secretion of another drug, thus raising the plasma level of the second drug. Organic acids frequently are protein bound. This binding limits their availability for filtration at the glomerulus. If sulfinpyrazone displaces the second drug from proteins, making it available for increased glomerular filtration, the plasma concentration of the second drug may be lowered (Anton, 1961). *Principle: The principles of anticipation of drug interaction hold for all pharmacologic agents. Knowledge of drug structure and of the rate and mechanism of action should permit a prediction of the interaction and effect. An apparent failure to achieve the anticipated drug response should suggest unsuspected renal dysfunction or the unsuspected administration of a second drug.*

Summary Principles: (1) Pharmacokinetics of drugs are altered by change in their rate of excretion. This process usually requires a reduction in drug dosage and frequency of administration. (2) When drugs and their metabolites are excreted in reduced amounts by the kidney, toxicity of these agents at both renal and extrarenal sites must be anticipated. (3) Modification of drug form or route of administration may be required during renal failure. (4) Drugs dependent on renal excretion for their action become less effective when excretory function is reduced. (5) Drugs utilizing the same excretory mechanism (e.g., organic acids) interact, either directly or indirectly. These interactions may have therapeutic usefulness, but may also interfere with therapeutic intent.

Acid-Base Regulation

The body's extracellular fluid environment is maintained relatively constant at approximately pH 7.4; intracellular fluid is generally more acidic. The pH of body fluids is regulated by three interrelated systems:

1. The chemical buffers—solutions of weak acids and their salts in extracellular fluid, cells, and bone, including carbonic acid–bicarbonate, phosphates, and proteins.

2. The respiratory system, which compensates for changes in systemic pH by altering pCO_2, and thereby regulates the carbonic acid concentration of body fluids.

3. The kidneys, which regulate normal buffer concentrations by excreting excess bicarbonate or excess hydrogen ion as titratable acid and/or ammonium ion.

An acid is defined as a proton (H^+) donor (e.g., carbonic acid, H_2CO_3). A base is a proton acceptor (e.g., bicarbonate ion, HCO_3^-) that combines with hydrogen ion to form an acid. Ordinarily the kidney maintains whole-blood bicarbonate at 26 to 28 mM and the respiratory system regulates carbonic acid at 1.3 to 1.4 mM. This balance determines the pH of plasma and interstitial fluid and influences the pH of cells.

The numerical pH is the negative logarithm of hydrogen ion concentration; hence, minor changes in pH units reflect large changes in hydrogen ion concentration.

Henderson-Hasselbalch Equation. The law of mass action states that for the reaction:

$$HA \rightleftharpoons H^+ + A^- \tag{1}$$

the concentration of the three components involved will have the relationship:

$$\frac{[H^+][A^-]}{[HA]} = K \tag{2}$$

The more H^+ and A^- required to satisfy this equation, the stronger the acid. Weak acids are only partially dissociated; strong acids are almost completely ionized.

If we rearrange the second equation:

$$[H^+] = K\frac{[HA]}{[A^-]} \tag{3}$$

and then apply logarithms:

$$\log [H^+] = \log K + \log \frac{[HA]}{[A^-]} \tag{4}$$

Multiply throughout by -1:

$$-\log [H^+] = -\log K + \log \frac{[A^-]}{[HA]}$$

But $-\log [H^+] = pH$, and by analogy we can define $-\log K$ in the same term (i.e., pK). If we do this, we have:

$$pH = pK + \log \frac{[A^-]}{[HA]} \tag{5}$$

so that $pH = pK$ when the acid is 50% dissociated. The Henderson-Hasselbalch equation (Henderson, 1908; Hasselbalch, 1917) is used in discussion of acid-base regulation.

pK_a expresses the degree of dissociation of a chemical (acid or base) into its component ions in solutions of various pH (see Chapter 2). The pK_a of a chemical is characteristic for that substance and is inversely proportional to its acidity. When the pK_a is known, one can predict the change in ionization of the substance that occurs with the addition of acid or base to the system. Knowledge of the pK_a of a chemical is important in predicting its degree of ionization and distribution in the body and its excretion rate. Many drugs are weak acids or weak bases and therefore exist in ionized or nonionized forms, depending upon their pK_a and the local pH. Ionized drugs penetrate cell membranes less readily than do nonionized drugs; differences in pH across the membrane may significantly affect the distribution of the drug between intracellular and extracellular spaces. Weak acids, for example, have a relatively low intracellular concentration, as the more alkaline plasma "traps" ions in extracellular fluid. Changes in systemic pH may alter the intracellular/extracellular ratio of a drug and, depending on the location of the drug's receptor, may alter its pharmacologic effect. For example, the weak acid phenobarbital becomes ionized to a greater extent as hydrogen ion concentration falls. Since phenobarbital crosses membranes easily in the nonionized form but with difficulty in the ionized form, the drug accumulates on whichever side of the cell membrane has a lower hydrogen ion concentration. In extracellular acidosis phenobarbital moves intracellularly, where it exerts its pharmacologic action, and coma deepens. Raising the pH of extracellular fluid reverses this phenomenon. Weak bases behave in the opposite fashion, exiting from cells as extracellular pH falls. This shift from cells may enhance drug action if the site of action is extracellular. Thus, the weak base mecamylamine, an antihypertensive agent, leaves cells during extracellular acidosis and accumulates at an extracellular site, where it exerts its pharmacologic effect, producing more severe hypotension than would be expected of the same dose at normal pH (Payne and Rowe, 1957).

Buffers. Carbonic acid dissociates into hydrogen ion and bicarbonate ion and has a pK_a of 6.1:

$$pH = pK_a + \log \frac{[HCO_3^-]}{[H_2CO_3]}$$

In a closed system, if the amount of carbonic acid is increased, the pH is decreased by the resultant dissociation of carbonic acid to provide more H^+. Similarly, if the bicarbonate (HCO_3^-) is increased, the pH increases as the added base takes up hydrogen ion. From the equation

$$H^+ = K \frac{[H_2CO_3]}{[HCO_3^-]}$$

we see that increasing the bicarbonate decreases the $[H^+]$. The bicarbonate/carbonic acid buffer system therefore donates H^+ when the $[H^+]$ is lowered and accepts H^+ when the $[H^+]$ is raised. Buffer systems operate most efficiently near their pK_a (relatively large amounts of acid or base are needed to change pH). In the body, the carbonic acid buffer system ($pK = 6.1$) must function at pH 7.4. The bicarbonate buffer system is effective at pH 7.4 because the carbonic acid concentration is controlled independently by the respiratory system and the bicarbonate ion concentration is controlled by the kidneys. Ideally, the pK_a of carbonic acid would be 7.4, for variations in $[H^+]$ or $[HCO_3^-]$ would then result in a smaller change in pH than in the true circumstance.

Phosphate provides another buffer system. If phosphoric acid is titrated with sodium hydroxide, three reactions occur:
1. At approximately pH 2, H_3PO_4 is 50% dissociated to $H^+ + H_2PO_4^-$.
2. At pH 6.8, $H_2PO_4^-$ is 50% dissociated to $H^+ + HPO_4^{--}$.
3. At pH 11.8, HPO_4^{--} is 50% dissociated to $H^+ + PO_4^{---}$.
Thus, by our previous definition, the pK_a of H_3PO_4 is 2; of $H_2PO_4^-$, 6.8; and of HPO_4^{--}, 11.8.

Knowing the pK_a allows calculation of the amounts of each of the phosphate ions present at any pH. For example, $H_2PO_4^-$ has a pK_a of 6.8. At pH 7.4 one could calculate that $7.4 = 6.8 + \log \frac{[HPO_4^{--}]}{[H_2PO_4^-]}$. The $\log \frac{[HPO_4^{--}]}{[H_2PO_4^-]}$ must be 0.6, which is the log of 4/1. Thus, at pH 7.4 each mole of phosphate exists as 0.8 M of HPO_4^{--} and 0.2 M of $H_2PO_4^-$. HPO_4^{--} is either an acid or a base, depending upon whether it donates or accepts a hydrogen ion. In biologic fluids there are many different buffer systems, each with a different pK_a that reacts to a change of pH. The titration curve of a biologic fluid is therefore complex. Furthermore, many important biologic substances, particularly proteins, have several dissociating groups on the same molecule. Dissociation of such groups occurs as the pH is raised. Those groups with low pK_a values dissociate before groups with high pK_a values.

Acid Production. The complexity of acid-base equilibrium becomes clear when one considers a single (though major) source of H^+: the interaction of CO_2 and water to form carbonic acid:

$$CO_2 + H_2O \underset{\text{carbonic anhydrase}}{\rightleftharpoons} H_2CO_3 \qquad (6)$$

and the equilibration of carbonic acid with its ions:

$$H_2CO_3 \rightleftharpoons H^+ + HCO_3^- \qquad (7)$$

Each CO_2 molecule introduced into the blood stream liberates one hydrogen ion. The amount of CO_2 carried in the blood is governed by the rate of hydration of CO_2, the rate of hydrogen ion removal, and the partial pressure of CO_2. The rate of equation 6 is influenced by the enzyme carbonic anhydrase, while the extent of equation 7 depends upon the availability and capacity of buffer system bases. When all else is stable, the pCO_2 regulates breathing by its effect on midbrain respiratory centers (Lambertson, 1968). Such regulation is critical for the stability of body pH. Therefore, drugs affecting the respiratory center and impairing this regulatory mechanism may alter acid-base status (e.g., morphine sulfate).

Cell metabolism releases large quantities of CO_2 and hydrogen ion. The hydrogen ion is fixed by combination with bases and eliminated, so that release and fixation are constant. For instance:

$$CO_2 + H_2O \longrightarrow H_2CO_3 \longrightarrow H^+ + HCO_3^-$$

and elimination of CO_2 in the lungs requires that:

$$H^+ + HCO_3^- \longrightarrow H_2CO_3 \longrightarrow CO_2 + H_2O$$

so the total contribution of the hydrogen ion formed when CO_2 is released is zero. If bicarbonate were inappropriately lost by excretion into the urine, hydrogen ion retention and acidosis would result. Conversely, administration of bicarbonate reduces the concentration of hydrogen ion and results in alkalosis.

Whenever an uncharged organic compound is converted to a charged anion, a hydrogen ion is formed; whenever a charged anion is converted to an uncharged form, a hydrogen ion is fixed. For example, lactate accumulation during severe exercise leads to temporary acidosis, but this is corrected during subsequent metabolism of the excess lactate. Alkalosis occurs when sodium lactate or citrate is administered. During the metabolism of lactate or citrate, hydrogen ion is removed from solution. Advantage is taken of these latter reactions in the treatment of metabolic acidosis.

Acidosis and alkalosis are likely to occur only when exogenous administration or endogenous production of acid or alkali exceeds removal by metabolism and/or excretion. The metabolic acidosis of uncontrolled diabetes mellitus provides a good example. In this condition, fat breakdown occurs so rapidly that acetoacetic acid and betahydroxybutyric acid accumulate. This accumulation of keto acids exceeds the normal buffer and excretory mechanisms responsible for acid-base regulation, and diabetic acidosis ensues. If insulin is administered, keto acid production is reduced and acid-base balance is restored.

A source of net hydrogen ion production requiring buffering is the catabolism of sulfur-containing amino acids, including methionine and cysteine (Lemann and Relman, 1959). Protein foods and catabolic conditions are therefore acidifying. The

reactions mentioned so far can acidify only temporarily, when the hydrogen ion is produced faster than it can be removed by metabolic processes.

All acidifying and alkalinizing processes are influenced by buffer systems that mitigate but *do not prevent* a change in pH. The respiratory center responds to changes in pH to initiate compensation.

Regulation of Acid-Base Balance by the Respiratory System. The major buffer system guarding against severe metabolic acidosis is the bicarbonate–carbonic acid system. Administration of acid results in the following reaction:

$$H^+ + HCO_3^- \longrightarrow H_2CO_3 \longrightarrow H_2O + CO_2$$
$$\longrightarrow \text{Eliminated by the lungs}$$

Respiratory function is required to remove CO_2 and lower the H_2CO_3 concentration in blood.

Metabolic acidosis normally results in increased ventilation, which corrects the pH by lowering pCO_2. Metabolic alkalosis can be partially corrected by hypoventilation, with attendant elevation of pCO_2.

Respiratory influences on acid-base balance can be predicted by using the two equations:

$$CO_2 + H_2O \to H_2CO_3 \to HCO_3^- + H^+ \qquad (8)$$
$$\text{(}CO_2 \text{ accumulation during hypoventilation)}$$

$$H^+ + HCO_3^- \to H_2CO_3 \to H_2O + CO_2 \qquad (9)$$
$$\text{(}CO_2 \text{ loss during hyperventilation)}$$

If equation 8 is predominant, respiratory acidosis occurs. If equation 9 is predominant, the result is respiratory alkalosis. The rise in total CO_2 characteristic of respiratory *acidosis* is also seen in metabolic *alkalosis*, and the fall in total CO_2 seen in respiratory *alkalosis* is also characteristic of metabolic *acidosis* (see Figure 3–1 for alterations in respiratory and metabolic acidosis and alkalosis).

Isolated measurements of total CO_2 in blood therefore do not allow distinction of metabolic acidosis from respiratory alkalosis nor of metabolic alkalosis from respiratory acidosis. The clinical condition of the patient and arterial pH measurements readily distinguish these conditions.

Regulation of Acid-Base Balance by the Kidney. In the final stage of correction of metabolic acidosis, bicarbonate is restored to normal; respiratory accommodation is incapable of this step, extraction of hydrogen ion from the body fluids by the kidneys being required. If excess hydrogen ion is introduced and a metabolic acidosis results, H^+ reacts with $HCO_3^- \to H_2CO_3 \to CO_2 + H_2O$ (buffer protection), and pCO_2 is lowered by hyperventilation (respiratory compensation).

Removal of excess hydrogen ion and restoration of normal bicarbonate concentration are accomplished by the secretion of hydrogen ion into the urine. To acidify the urine, three processes must operate effectively: (1) bicarbonate reabsorption; (2) formation of titratable acid; and (3) ammonium production (Figure 3–2).

The tubular secretion of hydrogen ion results in removal of luminal bicarbonate so that (1) bicarbonate is not inappropriately lost in the urine, and (2) further hydrogen ion secretion may acidify

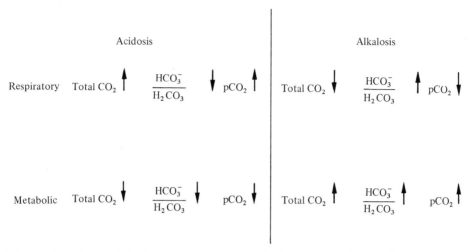

Figure 3–1. Abnormalities in respiratory and metabolic acidosis and alkalosis. The arrows indicate the direction of change from normal.

the urine. Maximum free hydrogen ion secretion is gradient limited at urine pH 4.5. A low concentration of free hydrogen ion (less than 1 mEq per liter) produces a pH of 4.5 and limits further secretion. The secretion of 50 to 100 mEq of hydrogen ion per day required for acid-base balance can be achieved only if hydrogen ion can be excreted into the urine without lowering pH to less than 4.5. One means of accepting large amounts of hydrogen ion without precipitously lowering pH is a buffer system. Buffer systems (e.g., phosphate buffer) accounting for the titratable acidity of the urine are utilized. Formation of titratable acid by titration of phosphate buffer with hydrogen ion allows quantitatively significant amounts of acid to be excreted without lowering urine pH to below 4.5. Phosphate excretion may increase in acidosis, as phosphate is removed from bone to provide increased buffer. The production of ammonia by deamination of glutamine and other amino acids reduces hydrogen ion concentration by forming ammonium ion (Pitts, 1964; Stone and Pitts, 1967).

The slow adaptive increase of ammonia production and its excretion as ammonium ion are the major chronic adaptations to acidosis.

Acidosis. Failure of bicarbonate reabsorption results in acidosis with inappropriately alkaline urine and may be the result of a primary defect in bicarbonate reabsorption in the proximal tubule or of a defect in the ability to secrete hydrogen ion against a gradient in the distal tubule. Ineffective acid secretion may also occur in chronic nephritis when ammonia production falls as a function of reduced tubular mass. In the latter case, the urine may have a pH of 4.5 but may contain quantitatively insufficient hydrogen ion to maintain acid-base balance. Failure to excrete titratable acid is rarely a problem.

Metabolic acidosis may result either from production or administration of acid at a rate faster than the normal kidney can excrete it, or from an inability of the diseased kidney to excrete normal amounts of acid. In either situation, administration of acidifying drugs (e.g., ammonium chloride, calcium chloride) or drugs that impair acid excretion (e.g., carbonic anhydrase inhibitors) aggravates the acidosis. When renal function is normal, the acidosis produced by acidifying salts or carbonic anhydrase inhibitors limits the diuretic effect of these drugs (see Diuretics, page 76).

During acidosis, the change in hydrogen ion concentration may alter protein-bound/free ratios of drugs, shift drugs intracellularly or extracellularly, increase or decrease sensitivity to drugs, and produce pathologic states requiring treatment. In acidosis, weakly acidic drugs bound to plasma protein may be dissociated from the proteins, producing an increase in the free or active form of the drug.

Acidosis may also reduce sensitivity to drugs. Part of the resistance to insulin in the diabetic patient with acidosis results from the acidosis per se. This resistance to insulin is in part due to the reduction in glycolysis produced by the acidosis. Sensitivity to catecholamines is also reduced during acidosis, which frequently complicates states of poor tissue perfusion. The acidosis increases the requirements of drug for a standard pressor effect to greater-than-ordinary doses. Whether the decreased pharmacologic effect of the drug is related to decreased receptor sensitivity or to alteration of metabolism or renal handling of the drug is not yet known.

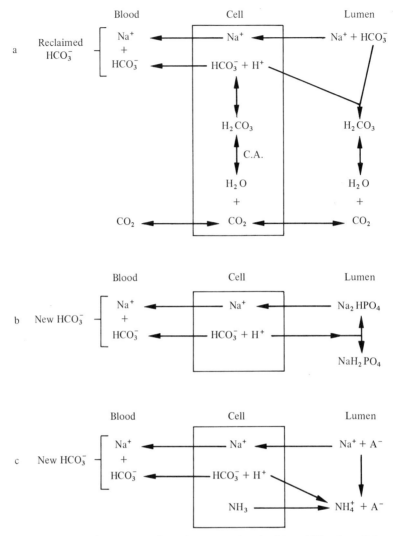

Figure 3–2. Diagrammatic representation of processes involved in acidification of the urine.
   a. Mechanism for bicarbonate reclamation. (C.A. = carbonic anhydrase.) One possible
   action of carbonic anhydrase is shown. It is possible that carbonic anhydrase may catalyze
   the reaction $OH^- + CO_2 \leftrightarrow HCO_3^-$.
   b. A mechanism for the formation of titratable acid.
   c. Mechanism for ammonium ion production.

Treatment of metabolic acidosis requires treatment of the underlying disease (i.e., treatment of diabetes mellitus, correction of poor tissue perfusion, removal of acidifying drugs, etc.). In addition, approximately one-half of the acid load is buffered intracellularly and one-half extracellularly, allowing calculation of bicarbonate deficit (Swan and Pitts, 1955). This calculation provides only an estimate of the bicarbonate requirement, since the rates of acid production, metabolism, and excretion vary with therapy. The objective of bicarbonate therapy is to restore buffering capacity, but replacement should be accomplished slowly and cautiously. Therapy proceeds under changing conditions; that is, as acidosis is corrected circulatory function may improve, which itself corrects acidosis. A calculated replacement may prove excessive, resulting in alkalosis.

Alkalosis, hypokalemia, or hypocalcemia may develop with bicarbonate therapy and complicate the disease state. As metabolic acidosis develops, potassium leaves cells and is excreted by the kidney. Depletion of total exchangeable potassium may be masked by an apparently normal or even mildly elevated serum potassium concentration, and the physiologic effect of potassium (expressed on the electrocardiogram) should be monitored. If acidosis is abruptly corrected, the potassium may move back into cells, resulting in hypokalemia with its attendant effects on muscular, neuromuscular, and cardiac functions. If uremia develops slowly, hypocalcemia may be present and become evident during sudden reduction of hydrogen ion concentration, resulting in tetany.

Careful thought should precede the choice of an "alkalinizing" solution (Schwartz and Waters, 1962). The use of lactate rather than bicarbonate has been advocated, with shaky foundation. Because lactate must be metabolized to bicarbonate to produce buffering effects, there is no advantage to its use. In fact, lactate administration is associated with some risk in the patient with hypoxemia or hypoperfusion because the lactate may not be metabolized. The sodium lactate will not add to the acidosis, but the physician may assume he has provided adequate therapy when he has not, in the absence of lactate metabolism. The organic buffer trishydroxymethylaminomethane (THAM) has been advocated in patients who are hypervolemic and edematous. Although often chosen to avoid further unnecessary and detrimental sodium administration, THAM in its commercially available form must be given in fluid volumes greater than those required for comparable buffering from bicarbonate and may in fact be a less effective buffer at intracellular sites. *Principle: Before choosing alternative agents for a desired effect, the physician should define his objectives and note whether the alternative therapy will be as good as the standard therapy. An alternative agent should not be selected if it will aggravate one aspect of a disease while ameliorating another. This principle is particularly applicable when the standard agent has only minor disadvantages associated with its use.*

Alkalosis. The reabsorption of bicarbonate by the renal tubule is a linear function of the filtered load. Most bicarbonate is reabsorbed in the proximal tubule by a mechanism that is limited by the concentration of filtered bicarbonate that can be reabsorbed. This maximum concentration or T_m HCO_3^- is usually in the range of 2.6 mEq/100 ml and is a protection against alkalosis. For example, all filtered bicarbonate above 2.6 mEq/100 ml is excreted. The T_m HCO_3^- may be elevated by increased pCO_2, increased adrenal steroids, decreased chloride, decreased potassium, and decreased extracellular volume. Elevation of the T_m

HCO_3^- permits the maintenance of an elevated serum bicarbonate level (metabolic alkalosis).

The principles related to altered drug availability, sensitivity, and movement across membranes during acidosis also apply to alkalosis. Alkalosis rarely occurs spontaneously during renal failure, but may result from drug action on the kidney (diuretics or steroids) or from vigorous and poorly controlled treatment of acidosis. The critical role of chloride ion in alkalosis has recently been recognized (Schwartz et al., 1968). Chloride, a permeable anion, is readily reabsorbed with sodium. Chloride depletion may occur in a number of circumstances (e.g., diuresis, vomiting, or compensation for respiratory acidosis). Whenever chloride is unavailable for reabsorption with sodium, potassium and hydrogen ion are secreted to accompany the relatively impermeable anions (bicarbonate, phosphate, and sulfate) in the urine. In a hypochloremic state, perpetuation of alkalosis and hypokalemia should be anticipated; alkalosis can be corrected only after replacement of chloride. Administration of chloride without potassium may correct the alkalosis but does not reverse the potassium depletion. Administration of potassium without chloride not only fails to correct the alkalosis but may not result in positive potassium balance. Potassium chloride is the logical treatment for hypokalemic, hypochloremic alkalosis. Better tasting, better appearing, or less caustic potassium salts are more readily accepted by patients but are ineffective. Potassium chloride, a caustic salt, was produced in an enteric-coated form because of its unpalatability; however, the tablets delivered the salt in high concentration to the lower small bowel, where it produced ulcerations. This problem has been obviated by administering potassium chloride in a flavored liquid form and by explaining to the patient that the drug *must* be taken. *Principle: The drug form may be of critical therapeutic importance. The role of the physician cannot be delegated to a pharmaceutical firm that provides an esthetically pleasing, nontoxic, but ineffective preparation.*

Alkalosis has the opposite effect of acidosis on drug action. One area of therapeutic difficulty is encountered during the administration of catecholamines. Although acidosis reduces vascular sensitivity to catecholamines and administration of alkali should restore responsiveness, if the catecholamines are administered in an alkaline solution, they are oxidized to inactive compounds. Therefore, during acidosis with hypotension, catecholamines should not be administered through the same intravenous tubing used for bicarbonate. *Principle: Availability* of drugs may be affected by the mode of their administration. Ineffective mixtures are best anticipated and avoided by a knowledge of the chemistry of the drugs, in addition to their pharmacologic effects.

Therapeutic Implications of the Urinary pH.
The pH of the urine is an important determinant of drug excretion, drug action, and the solubility of chemicals in the urine.

Nonionic diffusion, which effects the movement of weak acids into and out of cells, affects acidic or basic drugs. For example, the excretion of the weak acids phenobarbital and salicylate may be markedly enhanced by alkalinizing the urine. Weak bases such as quinidine or amphetamine are ionized in acid urine, poorly reabsorbed by the tubular cell, and therefore more rapidly excreted. Although this principle may be used to facilitate excretion of toxic amounts of drugs, rapid excretion of other agents may cancel their therapeutic effectiveness. Probenecid, which is nearly completely reabsorbed from acid urine, is effective as a uricosuric agent because it inhibits uric acid reabsorption, but it may be rendered less effective if the urine is alkalinized (Weiner et al., 1960). In alkaline urine, probenecid is ionized and its reabsorption is markedly reduced. Thus, it is less available to inhibit uric acid reabsorption. The frequently employed combination of probenecid and alkalinization of the urine in patients with gout has theoretic and practical drawbacks. Similar rapid excretion of a drug dependent on urinary pH applies to many weak acids, including such antibacterial agents as nitrofurantoin (Woodruff et al., 1961). Streptomycin is considerably more effective in alkaline urine, whereas mandelamine is effective only in acid urine. Some sulfa drugs are relatively insoluble in acid urine and may precipitate; alkalinization of the urine in patients receiving certain sulfas may protect against precipitation.

Summary Principles: (1) Changes in extracellular pH alter drug binding to protein, raising or lowering the concentration of the free, active form of the drug and requiring modification of dosage schedules. (2) Changes in extracellular and intracellular pH alter drug distribution across cell membranes. Movement of drug to higher or lower concentration at the site of action modifies drug activity. (3) Responsiveness to drugs is altered by changes in free-drug concentration or distribution. Failure of a drug to act in the face of major changes in pH should suggest such a possibility. (4) The excretion of weak acids and weak bases may be affected by changes in urinary pH. Toxic drugs may be removed and the action of therapeutic agents prolonged by altering urine pH.

Effectiveness of therapeutic agents may be reduced by inattention to these mechanisms. (5) Treatment of acid-base abnormalities is always directed at the underlying disorder. Correction of buffer component concentration should proceed slowly with frequent re-evaluation of the extent of correction. The untoward physiologic effects of correction of acid-base abnormalities must be borne in mind.

Regulation of Volume and Tonicity

The major reabsorptive sites of the nephron are the proximal convoluted portion of the tubule, the loop of Henle, and the distal convoluted portion of the tubule (Figure 3-3). Knowledge of the functional divisions permits identification of the site of action of diuretics and allows the logical development of therapeutic programs.

In the proximal tubule:

1. Isosmotic reabsorption of 60 to 70% of ions and water is accomplished by active reabsorption of sodium.

2. High permeability to water allows the passive reabsorption of water with sodium. The osmotic activity of the tubular fluid is equal to that of the interstitial fluid and plasma (Frazier, 1968; Earley and Daugharty, 1969).

In the loop of Henle:

1. Both diluting and concentrating mechanisms are affected by the sodium reabsorptive capacity.

2. Reabsorption of 20 to 30% of the filtered sodium occurs via active transport systems that are "physiologically nonsaturable"; that is, saturation of the sodium transport system cannot be demonstrated under physiologic conditions.

3. The ascending limb is impermeable to water. The active transport of sodium out of a segment of the nephron that is impermeable to water ultimately leaves fluid in the tubule that is hypotonic to plasma. This hypotonic fluid may be conceived to consist of two separate volumes, one isosmotic with plasma and the other free of osmotic activity (solute free water or "free water"). Free-water production then occurs in the ascending limb of the loop of Henle, depending upon the volume of sodium-containing filtrate delivered to that site, the active transport of sodium, and the tubule's impermeability to water.

4. The tubular fluid in the early distal region remains hypotonic regardless of load, and the medullary interstitium is made hypertonic by the active extrusion of sodium from the segment of the tubule impermeable to water (Jamison et al., 1967; Jamison, 1968).

5. Two segments of the ascending limb are

Proximal Convolution   Distal Convolution

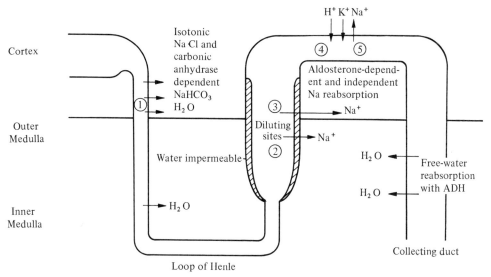

Figure 3–3. Diagram of the nephron indicating functional areas involved in salt and water regulation.

active in dilution of the urine: the medullary portion and the cortical portion. The medullary portion is also responsible for concentration of the interstitium and is necessary for the reabsorption of free water from the distal nephron. The cortical diluting segment of the ascending limb has no effect on medullary interstitium or on free-water reabsorption.

In the distal tubule (including the collecting duct):

1. Reabsorption of the remaining 5% of filtrate occurs.

2. Urine is not hypertonic under any conditions in the convoluted portion.

3. In the collecting duct, high concentration gradients can be found between blood and urine; in water diuresis the osmotic activity may be only one-fourth that of blood, whereas in water-deprivation states the osmotic activity may be four times that of blood.

4. The tubule's permeability to water in the collecting duct is increased by antidiuretic hormone (ADH), the concentration of ADH being high in states of water deprivation and low in normal states. A hypertonic medullary interstitium is necessary for maximal concentration of urine in response to ADH (Berliner and Bennett, 1967).

5. Sodium reabsorption enhances potassium and hydrogen secretion and is in part dependent upon the action of aldosterone (Morgan and Berliner, 1968). *The presence of aldosterone-dependent and -independent sodium reabsorptive mechanisms suggests the possibility of two specific pharmacologic interventions at this site.*

Two interdependent regulatory systems are responsible for the normalization of body fluid volume and electrolyte composition: (1) extracellular fluid volume, regulated primarily by the retention or excretion of sodium; and (2) total solute concentration, regulated by the renal excretion of water and by varying water intake.

In general, extracellular fluid volume is maintained by the balanced intake and excretion of sodium. Increased sodium intake results in increased sodium loss, because the expansion of extracellular fluid and vascular volume leads to increased glomerular filtration, decreased aldosterone secretion, and operation of physical and perhaps humoral factors. Sodium loss is self-limited by a reversal of these processes. Hormonal control of the rate of sodium excretion is achieved by aldosterone, secreted in response to a decrease in the "effective renal perfusion." Aldosterone stimulates the sodium reabsorptive mechanisms in the kidney, large intestine, sweat glands, and salivary glands until sodium balance is achieved (Laragh and Kelly, 1964). Simultaneously, it stimulates both potassium and hydrogen ion excretion from the distal tubule. The excretion of potassium and hydrogen ions is facilitated by the electrochemical gradient produced when sodium is actively transported out of the distal tubule, leaving behind relatively impermeable anions. Other factors, both physical (i.e., alterations of renal tubular geometry, changes in renal interstitial pressure, changes in capillary oncotic pressure, etc.) and humoral, may play a role in the regulation of sodium balance. One feature of considerable interest and controversy is the possibility of a "sodium-excreting factor" or "third factor," stemming from the observation that expansion of extracellular fluid volume causes a decrease in sodium reabsorption in the proximal tubule independent of glomerular filtration rate and aldosterone effect (de Wardener et al., 1961; Bricker, 1967).

Renal Perfusion. Renal blood flow is approximately 4 ml/g of tissue per minute, a flow rate higher than that of any other organ, representing about 25% of the cardiac output. This rate of flow is crucial to the kidney's regulation of body fluid composition by filtering and processing a large volume of blood. Renal blood flow is normally regulated by the resistance of the afferent and efferent arterioles and by the blood pressure in cases of extreme pressure variation. Vascular autoregulation is highly developed in the kidney; a constant glomerular filtration rate is maintained over a wide range of blood pressures. Stimulation of sympathetic nerves produces vasoconstrictor activity and rapidly reduces blood flow and filtration rate. There is no evidence of vasodilator nerve function in the kidney. Epinephrine, norepinephrine, and serotonin reduce blood flow and filtration; angiotensin reduces renal blood flow without impairment of filtration.

A single measurement of blood flow provides information about the adequacy of renal perfusion but reflects little about blood flow in different parts of the kidney. Distribution of renal blood flow has been defined by studying the washout of radioactive krypton from the kidney after its injection into the renal artery. The blood flow to the cortex is 80% of the total; to the outer medulla, 10 to 15%; and to the inner medulla, only 3 to 5%. The distribution of blood flow may be altered, correlating with salt retention when inner cortical and outer medullary flow increases or with sodium loss when outer cortical flow increases. Inner cortical flow correlates with perfusion of nephrons with long loops of Henle. These nephrons are relative "salt retainers," whereas the short-loop nephrons of the outer cortex are relative "salt wasters." Some diuretics may act by altering renal distribution of blood flow (Thorburn et al., 1963; Barger, 1966).

Pharmacologic modification of glomerular filtration rate, sodium reabsorption, and aldo-

sterone activity has been accomplished. The elucidation of further humoral and physical factors controlling sodium reabsorption may lead to the development of more effective therapeutic agents.

Two mechanisms appear capable of regulating tonicity of body fluids. Under conditions of water loss with increased serum sodium concentration, thirst stimulates increased water intake. At the same time, increased secretion of ADH leads to concentration of urine and to water retention. When thirst and water reabsorption have returned serum tonicity to normal, the need to drink is reduced, ADH secretion falls, and the permeability of the collecting duct to water is decreased.

Consequences of Loss of Volume Regulation. When sodium regulatory function is impaired during renal failure, regulation of extracellular fluid volume is compromised. Normally the kidneys excrete from less than 1 mEq to greater than 300 mEq of sodium per day, but the patient with renal failure often has a greater obligatory loss of sodium and a smaller excretory capacity. In renal failure, sodium restriction may result in sodium deficiency with hypovolemia; too large a sodium intake leads to sodium retention and hypervolemia. A steady state must be established in which the patient maximally perfuses his kidneys and has neither congestive heart failure nor hypovolemia. Either hypovolemia or hypervolemia may result in reduced renal perfusion and in accelerated deterioration of renal function. In the steady state any change in the patient's program should be examined for its potential to produce salt deficits or excesses. Potent diuretics such as furosemide or ethacrynic acid may be effective even when renal function is significantly reduced and may induce severe hypovolemia. Some cathartics produce salt loss from the gastrointestinal tract and may precipitate hypovolemia, whereas others contain large amounts of sodium and induce hypervolemia. Sodium may be present in unexpected sources. Antacids, for example, may contain sufficient sodium to upset the delicate balance in a patient with renal failure. Exchange resins such as Kayexalate can effectively reduce serum potassium levels (removing approximately 1 mEq of K^+/g of resin), but the exchange returns to the patient 2 to 3 mEq of Na^+/g of resin (Evans et al., 1953).

In addition to effects on renal function, alteration in extracellular volume alters the effectiveness of vasoactive drugs. Blood pressure is a function of intravascular volume, dependent in part on the cardiac output and peripheral resistance (see Chapter 5). Response to a standard dose of a pressor substance is less than expected if the patient is hypovolemic, whereas antihypertensive agents produce exaggerated effects during hypovolemia.

Summary Principles: (1) Renal failure blunts physiologic responses to increased or decreased extracellular fluid volume. Drugs that expand or contract volume must be used with great care. (2) Changes in extracellular fluid volume may exaggerate or depress the action of drugs that alter vasomotor responses. (3) The therapeutic strategy of volume regulation is to avoid hypovolemia or hypervolemia, either of which further impairs renal function.

Regulation of Potassium

The kidney largely controls the rate of potassium excretion. Intake greater than need requires an increase in potassium excretion and vice versa. Potassium is subject to reabsorption after glomerular filtration; more than 90% is removed from the lumen of the nephron before reaching the distal tubule. At the distal tubule both reabsorption and secretion of potassium can occur. High rates of distal sodium reabsorption generate high transepithelial potentials and aid the passive movement of potassium into the urine. Potassium secretion is stimulated by nonreabsorbable anions (which raise electrical potentials), increased delivery of sodium to the distal tubule, and adrenal hormones (which stimulate distal sodium reabsorption). Potassium retention may occur if delivery of sodium to the distal tubule is reduced by sodium chloride depletion or by diminished renal perfusion. Reduction in sodium-retaining adrenal secretions also enhances potassium retention. In normal subjects excessive potassium retention by increased dietary potassium is difficult to achieve. In patients with renal failure, however, potassium content of the diet assumes greater importance and may produce excess or deficiency of this cation. In primary or secondary adrenocortical overactivity or following diuretic administration, potassium depletion commonly occurs and either may have serious direct consequences or may modify other forms of therapy (e.g., digitalis) (Giebisch and Windhager, 1964; Malnic et al., 1966).

During renal failure, maximum excretion and reabsorption of potassium are reduced. Although hypokalemia or hyperkalemia may occur, depending upon potassium intake, in practice potassium retention is more common. Acidosis shifts potassium from an intracellular to an extracellular location, decreasing the ratio of potassium (intracellular/extracellular) across cell membranes and increasing excitability of conduction and pacemaking tissue. Even small changes in extracellular fluid potassium can have dramatic effects.

Potassium excess may result from ingestion, decreased excretion, or increased tissue release (hemolysis or tissue necrosis). In addition, commercially available premixed electrolyte solutions, potassium penicillin G, salt substitutes, and low-sodium products prepared with potassium-exchange resins are sources of excess potassium that should be avoided in renal failure.

Potassium depletion is not common in typical chronic renal failure, but does occur during both acidosis and alkalosis of renal or extrarenal origin. Hypokalemia is characterized by skeletal muscle weakness, leading to paralysis, cardiac arrhythmias, ileus, tetany, respiratory arrest, and increased sensitivity to drugs whose mechanism of action is dependent on alteration of the sodium-potassium pump (e.g., digitalis). The therapeutic steps used to correct hypokalemia depend on the presence of attendant acidosis or alkalosis. Since potassium shifts to extracellular sites during acidosis, hypokalemia during acidosis represents more severe total body potassium depletion than does hypokalemia associated with alkalosis. Potassium depletion generally occurs in acquired renal acidifying defects, which are usually accompanied by sodium wasting. As hypovolemia develops, potassium is secreted by the distal tubule as maximum sodium retention is attempted. In most circumstances re-expansion of blood volume by administration of sodium and correction of the acidosis reduces the potassium loss. Potassium concentration in serum should be determined frequently during correction of acidosis. Correction of acidosis with hypokalemia requires large potassium supplements and careful monitoring. In renal tubular acidosis with reduced bicarbonate reabsorption in the proximal tubule, persistent potassium loss may be particularly frustrating. In this disorder, $NaHCO_3$ therapy may only partially correct the acidosis and leads to inordinate sodium delivery to the distal tubule. The result is exaggerated potassium loss and a continuing need for potassium supplementation even after correction of acidosis.

Several attempts have been made to estimate potassium requirements from measurements of serum potassium. The serum potassium is the result of a complex set of factors, but serum pH is one of the most important. At normal pH (~ 7.4) reduction of serum potassium to less than 3 mEq per liter reflects a deficit of 200 mEq or more of total body potassium (Scribner and Burnell, 1959). As serum potassium falls further, total-body-potassium deficits rise exponentially.

A correction factor has been calculated for serum potassium during acidosis of about 0.5 to 1.0 mEq per liter rise in potassium for each 0.1 pH unit fall in extracellular pH (Scribner and Burnell, 1959). Such estimates of potassium requirements represent averages and are applicable to individual cases only as guidelines. Potassium replacement requires administration of less than the estimated requirement and careful monitoring of the effects of therapy.

Since it is the physiologic effect of potassium that is important, the efficacy and safety of progressive replacement may be estimated by observations of changes in the electrocardiogram. Electrocardiographic changes monitor the electrophysiologic events occurring as a result of changing potassium concentrations. These changes may be a more sensitive measure of potassium effect than is the serum potassium concentration.

Summary Principles: (1) Potassium excess and potassium depletion produce alterations in cell membrane function that may produce fatal electrophysiologic events. Drugs that also affect electrophysiologic events must be used with knowledge of potassium concentration and effect. (2) Potassium salts of many drugs and unexpected sources of potassium must be guarded against in renal failure. (3) Replacement of potassium deficit must take into account measured deficits relative to serum potassium levels, alterations in serum potassium levels with variations in pH, and physiologic effects of potassium. Replacement should be gradual with re-evaluation of therapy at frequent intervals.

Endocrine Function of the Kidney

The kidney is a site of both hormone action and hormone production. The effects of hormones that act on the kidney have been modified pharmacologically. Similar modifications of the action of renal hormones, which produce striking physiological effects, have not been accomplished.

Erythropoietin. The secretion rate of erythropoietin is primarily determined by the pO_2 of the blood. Renal damage or disease diminishes erythropoietin production, contributing to the anemia of chronic renal failure (Stohlman, 1968).

Renin. Renin is secreted from the juxtaglomerular apparatus in response to a decrease in perfusion pressure of afferent glomerular arterioles and occurs when the intravascular volume or renal perfusion is decreased. As renin secretion may be controlled by changes in the luminal sodium concentration at the region of the macula densa, pharmacologic regulation of renin secretion may be possible. Renin generates an inactive decapeptide (angiotensin I) from a specific plasma alpha-globulin substrate. Converting enzyme then hydrolyzes the decapeptide to the octapeptide, angiotensin II. Angiotensin II is a potent pressor agent and stimulates the secretion of aldosterone, resulting in increased blood pressure, sodium retention, and expansion of the extracellular fluid volume (Haber, 1969).

Prostaglandins. The physiologic role of these fatty-acid derivatives is not known. Natriuresis has been demonstrated following infusion of 0.1 to 2 μg/min of prostaglandin E into the renal artery. Prostaglandins have been isolated from the renal medulla; a mixture of them was named medullin. Experiments *in vitro* have shown that these hormones stimulate transepithelial sodium transport, increase the water permeability of the collecting duct, and inhibit the action of ADH. The importance of these substances lies not in our present knowledge but in a definition of their position in the normal physiologic regulation of vasomotor activity and sodium balance (Bergstrom, 1967).

DIURETICS

The diuretics are by far the most important group of pharmacologic agents acting directly on the kidney. Although designed to produce negative sodium balance, they affect tonicity control, acid-base regulation, potassium balance, renal perfusion, and the effect of hormones on the kidney. Examination of the diuretics illustrates how knowledge of chemical structure, mechanisms of action, site of action and toxicity is useful in the design of effective therapeutic programs.

Diuretic therapy used to correct edema or hypertension depends upon the pathophysiology of the disease, the pharmacology and kinetics of diuretics, and the physiologic changes that diuretics can induce. A variety of potent, orally effective diuretics is currently available for the treatment of hypertension, as well as for edema, and commonly is used in patients with congestive heart failure, cirrhosis, nephrosis, and protein-losing enteropathy.

Studies on the mechanisms of edema formation have shown that whatever the primary disturbance, the result is an increased renal retention of sodium, which in turn leads to expansion of total exchangeable sodium. Decreased renal excretion of sodium may in some instances be primarily due to reduced perfusion of the kidneys, with consequent reduction in total filtration rate. In other instances, altered distribution of blood flow may be at fault, leading to selective perfusion of juxtamedullary nephrons that reabsorb sodium more efficiently owing to their longer loops of Henle. Most commonly, however, the renal disturbance seems to reside in the regulation of tubular function.

Diuresis is an increase in the rate of formation of urine and may be either physiologic or pharmacologic. For practical reasons, this discussion is restricted to the diuresis associated with an increase in the excretion of sodium, promoting a negative sodium balance. The net loss of sodium from body fluids contracts the overexpanded extracellular fluid space. The maneuvers necessary to produce diuresis are sometimes simple. In the early stages of congestive heart failure, reduction of sodium in the diet often effects a negative sodium balance and weight loss in the patient. However, as the disease progresses and the magnitude of renal sodium retention increases, diuretics are required. The effectiveness of diuretics depends on sodium ingestion; restriction of sodium intake may be an essential part of diuretic therapy. Palatability of the diet may become a limiting factor in effective therapy. Although the main effect of diuretics is to remove sodium, they may influence other ions as well. Diuretics constitute a threat to electrolyte homeostasis (Goldberg, 1967).

Diuresis may be induced by:

1. Osmotically active diuretics.
2. Acid-forming salts.
3. Inhibition of sodium reabsorption in the renal tubule.
4. Inhibition of the enzyme carbonic anhydrase.
5. Antagonism of aldosterone.
6. Diuretics with less precisely defined mechanisms of action.
   a. Thiazide derivatives
   b. Furosemide
   c. Ethacrynic acid
7. Agents that affect the distribution of blood flow in the kidney (possibly a mechanism of action of ethacrynic acid or furosemide).
8. Agents that block the entry of sodium into the tubule. Each class of drug may produce toxicity, either by interference with electrolyte balance or by mechanisms independent of its diuretic action. Since diuretics act by modifying the normal or abnormal excretory process, a clear understanding of renal function is essential before proper use of diuretic agents can be considered.

Mechanism of Action

Osmotic Diuretics. Any substance that passes the glomerular membrane and is not completely reabsorbed from the renal tubule has some osmotic diuretic effect, which retains water in the tubule. The retained water in the proximal tubule produces an increased concentration gradient (from lumen to cell) for sodium ion and thereby limits sodium reabsorption. Consequently, urine flow increases. Examples of osmotic diuretics are mannitol, urea, and glucose; the latter is responsible for the diuresis seen in diabetes mellitus. Osmotic diuretics have minimal efficacy unless large quantities are administered. However, in an edematous patient, the sodium reabsorptive mechanisms may be working maximally and even high doses may be ineffective. Osmotic diuretics might theoretically be useful when further depression of renal function produced by other classes of diuretics is contraindicated.

Since the osmotically active materials also effect overexpansion of the extracellular fluid compartment, pulmonary edema may be precipitated by their use.

Acid-Forming Salts. Salts having a labile cation and a fixed (nonmetabolizable) anion may have both an acidifying and a diuretic effect. By definition, fixed ions cannot be changed, whereas labile ions can be converted to uncharged forms. An example of such a salt is ammonium chloride. Chloride is a fixed anion, whereas the ammonium ion is a labile cation. The ammonium ion can be converted to urea with the production of a hydrogen ion, which is dissipated with bicarbonate as CO_2 and H_2O. The result is acidosis and replacement of bicarbonate by chloride derived from the salt. Thus, chloride is presented to the tubule in excess, and both sodium and potassium are excreted as chlorides along with water. To a lesser extent, the excretion of calcium is also increased. The extent of diuresis and the mobilization of sodium, potassium, and water depend upon the size of the acid load, the capacity of the kidney to secrete acid, and the state of the mechanisms regulating renal excretion of cations.

The duration of diuretic action of acid-forming salts is determined by the rate of adaptation of the kidney to the acidosis. When the amount of ammonia produced by the kidney is equal to the amount of chloride administered, ability to excrete acid equals the acid load, and diuresis of sodium, potassium, and water ceases. Ordinarily significant natriuresis and kaliuresis ceases after 3 or 4 days of continuous administration of ammonium chloride, but calcium loss persists.

Mercurial Diuretics. Mercurial diuretics were introduced into medical practice at the beginning of this century. Many of the organic mercurials are derivatives of mercuripropanol; they have a chain of not less than three carbon atoms and a mercury atom at the end of the chain. Perhaps

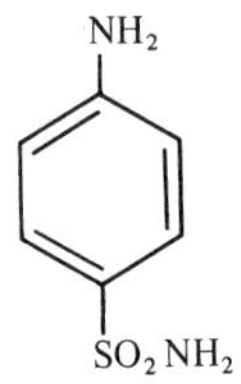

Sulfanilamide

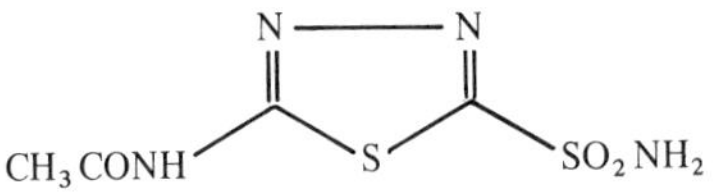

Acetazolamide

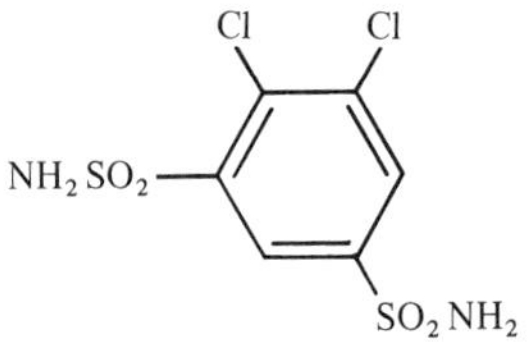

Dichlorophenamide

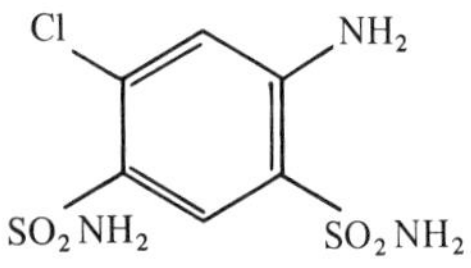

Chlorodisulfamyl-
aniline

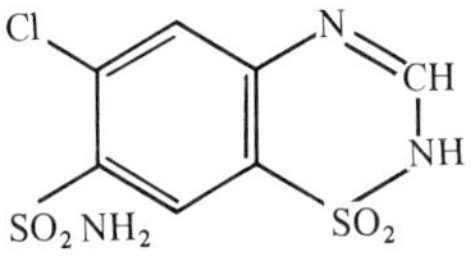

Chlorothiazide

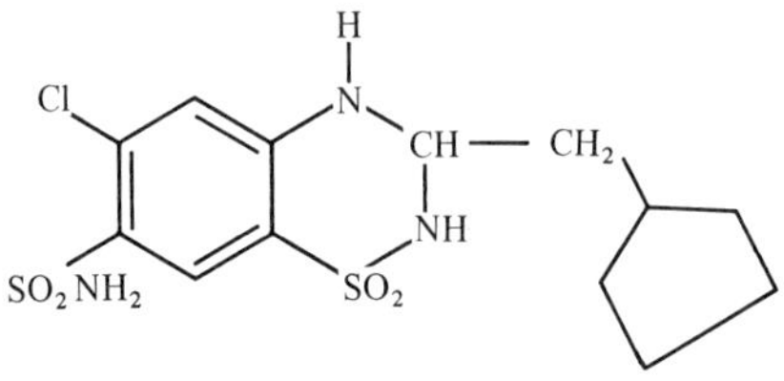

Cyclopenthiazide

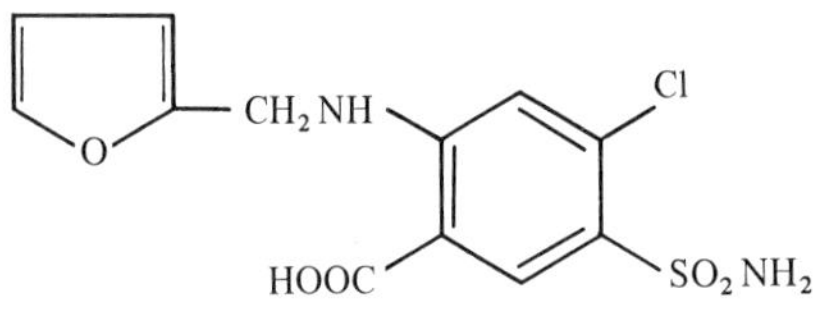

Furosemide

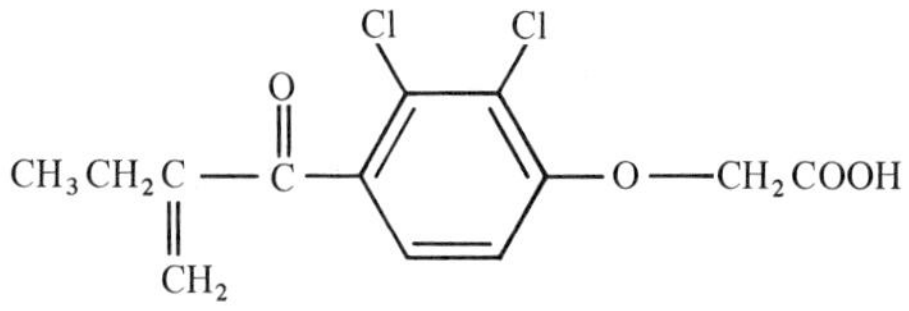

Ethacrynic Acid

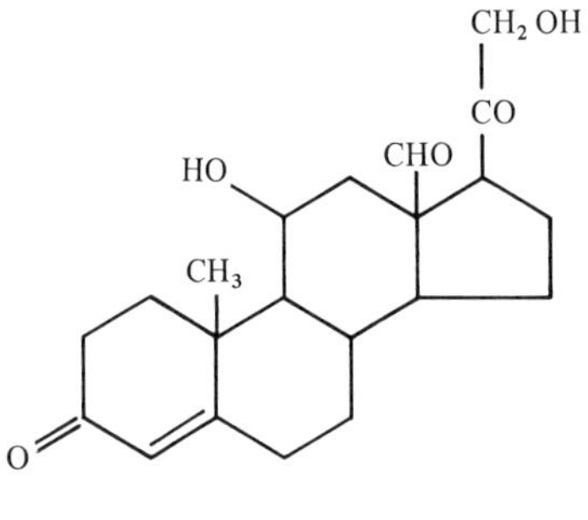

Aldosterone

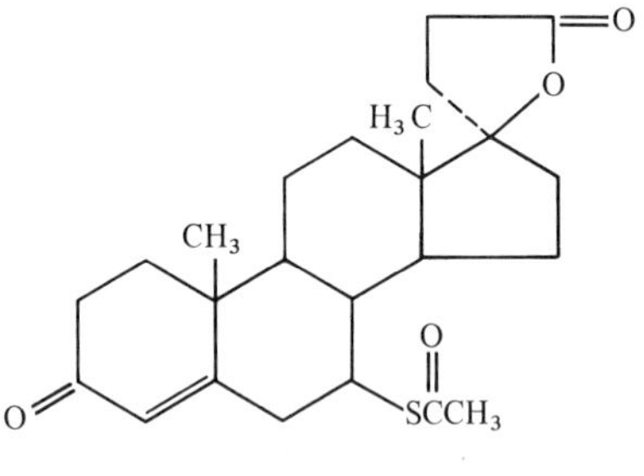

Spironolactone

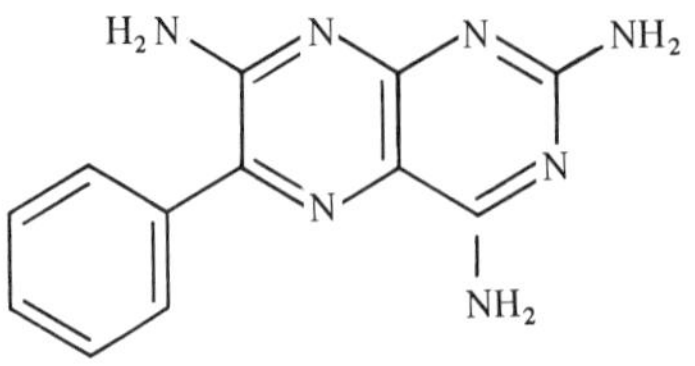

Triamterene

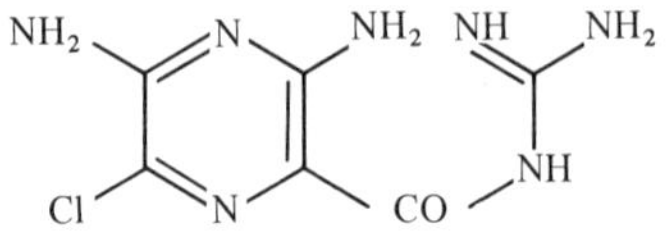

Amiloride

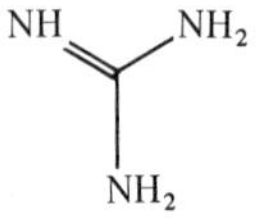

Guanidine

this configuration fulfills the spatial requirements for combination of the mercurial with an enzyme essential for active transport processes. However, merbaphen, the first mercurial agent to be used as a diuretic, does not have this configuration, and inorganic mercurial salts also have diuretic activity. The possibility that the renal intracellular release of mercury as mercuric ion is responsible for the diuretic action is supported by the fact that all known organomercurial diuretics are acid labile and release the mercuric ion after rupture of the carbon chain. Perhaps this process can help to explain the potentiation of the pharmacologic actions of mercurial diuretics by acidifying salts. The liberation of mercuric ion may account for nephrotoxicity when excessive quantities of these diuretics are given to patients with uremia or congestive heart failure.

Organomercurials are administered parenterally because they are poorly absorbed by the oral route. The desirability of oral administration of any drug has led to the development of compounds such as chlormerodrin, which are effective when given by mouth, but nausea, vomiting, and diarrhea are likely to occur. The development of potent nonmercurial diuretics has eliminated the need for oral mercurial diuretics.

The organomercurials have a gradual onset of action, reaching a peak activity within about 2 hours. The effect is probably due to inhibition of sodium-transport processes with subsequent block of chloride and water movement. More sodium and chloride reaches the distal tubule under such conditions, and secretion of potassium and hydrogen ions may be stimulated by the increased sodium load and secondary aldosteronism. One consequence of this process is the development of alkalosis, which inhibits the diuretic action of mercurials. Acidification by ammonium chloride restores diuretic responsiveness. *Principle: Understanding the mechanism of action of a drug often suggests proper combined therapy.*

Refractoriness to organomercurials may also be due to an extremely low glomerular filtration rate. If given in repeated doses to patients with renal insufficiency or congestive heart failure, mercurials may produce acute tubular necrosis. If such an effect is feared, theophylline or caffeine may be useful because they increase glomerular filtration rate. However, it is advisable to avoid the use of mercurials in renal failure and to choose an equally potent, less toxic diuretic (e.g., furosemide).

Carbonic Anhydrase Inhibitors. Modern developments in our understanding of the pharmacology of diuretics stem from data regarding: (1) the role of carbonic anhydrase in renal electrolyte transport, (2) the observation that sulfanilamide produces an alkaline urine and metabolic acidosis, and (3) the development of the theory of hydrogen and sodium exchange in urinary acidification.

Sulfanilamide was the first drug used to test the possibility that interfering with the supply of hydrogen ions could inhibit sodium reabsorption. In three edematous patients, sulfanilamide inhibition of carbonic anhydrase resulted in sodium, bicarbonate, and water diuresis (Schwartz, 1949). Within a year of this report, acetazolamide, a carbonic anhydrase inhibitor, was introduced. This was the first effective oral nonmercurial diuretic. Its diuretic potency is not so great as that of the mercurials

---

Figure 3–4. Formulas for selected diuretic compounds. The sulfonamides, carbonic anhydrase inhibitors, chlorothiazides, and furosemide all contain a sulfamyl group despite marked differences in their modes and sites of action. Sulfanilamide is shown because it is used in the first demonstration of diuresis due to inhibition of carbonic anhydrase activity. Acetazolamide, the first nonmercurial orally active diuretic, is a potent inhibitor of carbonic anhydrase. It causes a diuresis with increased amounts of sodium and potassium bicarbonate in the urine. Dichlorphenamide is also a carbonic anhydrase inhibitor, but this compound elicits a modest increase of chloride excretion that is not characteristic of the inhibitors of carbonic anhydrase. Chlorodisulfamylaniline, despite the presence of two sulfamyl groups, causes the excretion of relatively more chloride than bicarbonate, so that it is not included in the class of diuretics that act by inhibition of carbonic anhydrase. This compound is similar in structure to chlorothiazide, the prime member of a series of orally administered diuretics that have considerable ability to cause the excretion of sodium and chloride. Cyclopenthiazide is almost 1000 times more potent than chlorothiazide.

Furosemide, which contains a sulfamyl group, and ethacrynic acid are the most effective diuretics currently available and are capable of producing massive diuresis. The structural similarities of aldosterone and spironolactone are apparent. However, a competition ratio of at least 1000:1 (spironolactone:aldosterone) is required for inhibition of aldosterone-induced sodium retention. Triamterene amd amiloride are examples of diuretics that block the entry of sodium into the renal cells at the tubular membrane. Their formulas are drawn to emphasize the similarity of one portion of each molecule to guanidine. Tetrodotoxin, which blocks the movement of sodium across cell membranes, also contains the guanidinium moiety.

and it has a slower onset of action. However, the action of acetazolamide is self-limited, because after chronic use the carbonic anhydrase inhibition results in an acidosis of sufficient magnitude to provide enough hydrogen ions to drive the reaction without enzymatic assistance. An intermittent course of treatment is therefore desirable. Under these conditions sodium, potassium, and bicarbonate excretion are all increased; the effect on chloride is minimal but the loss of potassium may be great. The use of the compound, however, led to the development of more effective and less toxic diuretics.

Thiazides. Studies of structure-activity relationships in carbonic anhydrase inhibitors led to the development of other classes of diuretics, which, while retaining the sulfamyl group necessary for carbonic anhydrase inhibitory activity, do not act by virtue of this property (e.g., chlorothiazide). The thiazide diuretics, which may be administered orally, have high potency, a considerable effect on chloride excretion, and little effect on bicarbonate.

Thiazides do not mimic diuretics that act by inhibition of carbonic anhydrase but, rather, resemble the mercurials in their ability to enhance excretion of equivalent amounts of sodium and chloride. *Perhaps in no other class of drugs is the fallacy of assuming a common mechanism of action by chemically similar drugs illustrated so well* (Figure 3–4). Unlike the mercurials, however, the diuretic response is not inhibited by alkalosis (nor is it affected by acidosis). Thiazides do increase potassium excretion. In very high dosage their inherent carbonic anhydrase inhibitory activity may cause excretion of bicarbonate.

The maximal diuretic effects of the thiazides appear to be equivalent. Whereas potency and potency changes may be estimated by comparing the amounts by weight of each agent required to produce a certain submaximal response, the expression of submaximal activity in dosage terms is not a measure of the true (or required) efficacy of diuretic agents. The dose-response curves of these compounds are parallel, suggesting similar modes of action. However, the dosage (aside from toxicity and side effects) is irrelevant in one respect—if a diuretic is less active than another member of the group, its dosage should simply be increased. A major concern during diuretic therapy is the *maximal* ability to remove sodium, chloride, and water from the body. Essentially, therefore, if all thiazides have the same maximal activity, their therapeutic activities are equal.

Aldosterone Antagonists. In the distal tubule, sodium and chloride are reabsorbed and potassium and hydrogen ion are secreted. During metabolic acidosis, potassium secretion is low relative to hydrogen ion secretion; in alkalosis, the opposite occurs. To extend the logic, potassium depletion increases hydrogen ion secretion and may cause metabolic alkalosis. Potassium chloride "loading" produces acidosis. Aldosterone and other adrenocortical steroids stimulate sodium reabsorption and, when given in excess, produce potassium depletion and metabolic alkalosis. However, in edematous states, when aldosterone secretion rates are high, potassium depletion and alkalosis may not occur. If proximal sodium reabsorption is high, little sodium is presented to the distal tubule for reabsorption in exchange for potassium and hydrogen ion. Thus, despite an increased hormonal drive for potassium exchange, little occurs. However, aldosterone-secretion rates modify the response to diuretics. If aldosterone secretion is high and a diuretic such as chlorothiazide is administered, sodium reabsorption is inhibited at a point proximal to the distal tubular convolution, and excretion of potassium and hydrogen ion may increase owing to the increased load of sodium presented to and reabsorbed by the distal tubule in exchange for potassium and hydrogen ion.

Two possibilities for aldosterone antagonism, and hence sodium diuresis, are apparent: (1) inhibition of the synthesis of aldosterone in the adrenal cortex and (2) inhibition of the action of aldosterone in the renal tubule. The former approach has not as yet been successful because of lack of selectivity among the inhibitors tested, because of toxicity of the drugs tested, and, in the case of heparinoids, because of the necessity of administration by injection.

Effective antagonists of the peripheral effects of aldosterone, the spironolactones, have been developed. These compounds induce sodium excretion and potassium retention in salt-loaded, adrenalectomized rats treated with aldosterone, but are inactive if no aldosterone is present. The spironolactones compete with aldosterone for receptor sites in the tubules and, therefore, act only when mineralocorticoid is present. Aldosterone antagonists are poorly absorbed, have a delayed onset of action, are not very potent, and must be used in high dosage (see Chapter 2). They are useful as supplementary therapy because they can reduce the potassium depletion caused by other diuretics.

Ethacrynic Acid and Furosemide. These compounds are the most potent diuretics developed. They cause striking diuretic effects even in patients already responding maximally to other compounds (e.g., thiazides). Although furosemide contains a sulfamyl group, its action is unlike that of the carbonic anhydrase inhibitors or thiazides. The effects of furosemide and ethacrynic acid are similar. These agents have a rapid onset and short duration of action and inhibit sodium transport in most of the ascending limb of the loop of Henle. Potassium and hydrogen ion excretion increases during diuresis with both agents, suggesting that there is little direct effect at the distal tubule. These potent compounds can cause hypovolemia, potassium depletion, and alkalosis. Their activity is unaffected by alkalosis or acidosis.

Triamterene and Amiloride. The action of these compounds is unique. The inhibition of sodium transport results from interaction of the agent with the luminal surface of the tubule, thus preventing the passage of sodium across the membrane. Triamterene and amiloride appear to have their main effects distally; by blocking sodium reabsorption, they reduce potassium loss at this site. The effects of triamterene and amiloride therapy are similar to those of aldo-sterone antagonists, but are not dependent on the presence of aldosterone.

Intrarenal Distribution of Blood Flow and Diuretic Action

Redistribution of flow within the kidney correlates with remarkable changes in renal function. The outer cortical nephrons with short loops are "relative salt losers," whereas the juxtamedullary nephrons, with long loops of Henle, are "relative salt retainers." An increase in medullary flow therefore produces sodium retention, but an increase in cortical flow results in sodium loss. During congestive heart failure cortical blood flow is decreased and the outer medullary blood flow rises. Increased activity of the sympathetic nervous system results in this blood flow pattern and is probably responsible for the changes seen during congestive heart failure. Although alpha-adrenergic blocking agents can reverse the pattern of blood flow

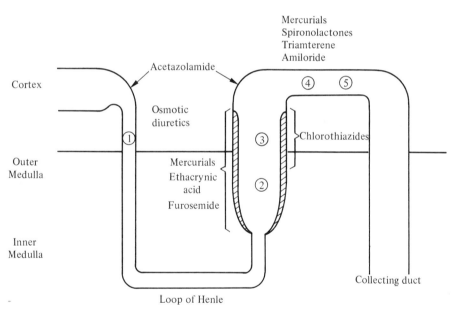

Figure 3–5. Sites of diuretic action.

Site 1. Proximal tubule. A diuretic acting at this site produces *increased* free-water production or reabsorption and *increased* potassium loss.

Site 2. Medullary diluting segment of ascending limb. A diuretic acting at this site produces *decreased* free-water production or reabsorption and *increased* potassium loss.

Site 3. Cortical diluting segment of ascending limb. A diuretic acting at this site produces *decreased* free-water production, does not affect free-water reabsorption, and *increases* potassium loss.

Site 4. Aldosterone-sensitive portion of distal tubule. A diuretic acting at this site produces *decreased* potassium loss, but acts only in the presence of aldosterone.

Site 5. Aldosterone-insensitive portion of distal tubule. A diuretic acting at this site produces *decreased* potassium loss.

Table 3–1. METHODS USED IN THE DETERMINATION OF SITE OF ACTION

PROXIMAL TUBULE	LOOP OF HENLE	DISTAL TUBULE

Micropuncture:
  Free flow
  Split oil droplet
  Stopped flow
  Microperfusion
Excretion patterns of water and
  electrolytes
	Effects on free-water clearance
	  during diuresis
	Effects on free-water reabsorp-
	  tion during dehydration
	Micropuncture
		Excretion patterns, particularly
		  K^+ and H^+

produced by sympathetic activity, this effect has not been used therapeutically. Furosemide and ethacrynic acid produce increased cortical flow and decreased medullary flow.

Sites of Action of Diuretics (Table 3–1)

Consideration of the effects of diuretics on electrolyte excretion provides several clues to their sites of action. Spironolactones, triamterene, and amiloride decrease potassium excretion, suggesting an action on the distal tubule (Figure 3–5, sites ④ and ⑤). The low maximal fractional excretion of sodium suggests that inhibition at this site could account for the total effect of these agents. The mercurial-induced fall in free-water clearance during an osmotic diuresis indicates an action on the ascending limb of the loop of Henle (Figure 3–5, sites ② and ③).

Thiazides affect free-water clearance but not solute/free-water reabsorption. Ethacrynic acid and furosemide affect both. Therefore, etha-

crynic acid and furosemide affect most of the ascending limb and both diluting sites (Figure 3–5, sites ② and ③). Thiazides affect the second (cortical) diluting site (Figure 3–5, site ③).

Acetazolamide produces a urinary electrolyte pattern different from that of the other weak diuretics. Proximal inhibition of carbonic anhydrase raises bicarbonate and decreases chloride excretion. Distal inhibition of carbonic anhydrase increases potassium excretion because of the hydrogen ion deficit. A urine with high sodium, potassium, and bicarbonate concentrations suggests both proximal and distal inhibition of carbonic anhydrase (Figure 3–5, site ① and less defined distal site).

Accepted explanations exist for the modes of action of only four types of diuretics: (1) osmotic diuretics, (2) carbonic anhydrase inhibitors, (3) aldosterone antagonists, and (4) compounds that block sodium transport.

The consequence of carbonic anhydrase inhibition is clear, although the chemical nature

Table 3–2. EFFECTS OF DIURETICS ON ELECTROLYTE EXCRETION*

AGENT	CHANGES IN URINARY ELECTROLYTES				MAXIMAL FRACTIONAL EXCRETION OF SODIUM	INHIBITORY FACTORS		SITE OF ACTION (see Figure 3–5 for site numbers)
	Na^+	K^+	Cl^-	HCO_3^-	%	Acidosis	Alkalosis	
Weak diuretics								
Acetazolamide	↑	↑	↑	↑	~4	+		1
Spironolactone	↑	↓	↑	↑	~2			4
Triamterene	↑	↓	↑	↑	~2			5
Amiloride	↑	↓	↑	↑	~2			5
Moderately effective diuretics								
Thiazide compounds	↑	↑	↑	↑	~8			3
Potent diuretics								
Organomercurials	↑	↑	↑		~20		+	2,3 ?4–5
Furosemide	↑	↑	↑		~23			2,3
Ethacrynic acid	↑	↑	↑		~23			2,3

* Modified from Goldberg, M.: The physiology and pathophysiology of diuretic agents. In Fulton, W. F. M. (ed.): *Modern Trends in Pharmacology and Therapeutics.* Butterworth & Co., Ltd., London, 1967, pp. 41–75.

Table 3–3. COMPLICATIONS

DIURETIC	HYPER-URICEMIA	HYPO K$^+$	HYPER K$^+$	ACIDOSIS	ALKALOSIS	OTHER
Osmotic	—	+	—	—	+ contraction	Hyper- or hypo-osmolality
Acid-forming salts	—	+	—	+	—	
Organomercurials	—	+	+ (rare, acute)	—	+	Tubular necrosis, hypersensitivity reactions
Acetazolamide	?	+	—	+	—	Urinary tract calculi, hepatic coma
Thiazides	+	+	—	—	+	Cutaneous vasculitis, agranulocytosis, thrombocytopenia, anemia, pancreatitis, glucose intolerance, hepatic coma
Ethacrynic acid	+	+	—	—	+	Hyper- and hypoglycemia, gastrointestinal bleeding, deafness, hepatic coma
Furosemide	+	+	—	—	+	Glucose intolerance, deafness, hepatic coma
Spironolactone	—	—	+	—	—	Gynecomastia
Triamterene	—	—	+	+	—	Azotemia
Amiloride	—	—	+	+	—	Azotemia

of the enzyme-inhibitor interaction is not. Aldosterone antagonists are competitive, displacing the hormone from its nuclear receptor sites to inhibit sodium-retaining activity. Triamterene and amiloride act at the luminal cell surface of the distal tubule and prevent sodium transport. This action occurs mainly in the distal tubule and is effective even in the absence of aldosterone.

Summary Principles: (1) Knowledge of the sites and mechanisms of diuretic action permits rational selection of individual agents and rational combinations of these agents (Table 3–2, Figure 3–5).

a. Resistance to diuretics, which occurs with diminishing glomerular filtration rate, can be explained in part by the increased reabsorption of sodium from the proximal tubule. Diuretics acting on the more distal nephron become progressively less effective as the glomerular filtration rate falls. Knowledge of the site of action of diuretics allows the physician to select agents affecting the more proximal portion of the nephron, which logically should be preferred as the total filtered sodium decreases and as progressively less sodium reaches the distal tubule.

b. Drugs that act at different sites, such as furosemide and thiazides, have additive natriuretic effects.

c. Drugs that act at the same site through different mechanisms, such as spironolactone and triamterene, may also be additive in effect.

d. The action of one drug may negate an undesirable effect of a second agent. For example, the potassium loss of thiazide therapy may be reduced by adding spironolactone or triamterene.

(2) There is a logical pharmacologic basis for utilizing more than one agent in a diuretic program. Drug companies have marketed combinations of diuretics in a single tablet. Such combinations fix the relative doses of the diuretics and make the therapeutic program less flexible.

(3) In addition to the site and mechanism of drug action, potency and side effects of diuretics must be considered in designing a therapeutic program (Tables 3–2 and 3–3). *Treatment should utilize the least potent, least toxic agent that will accomplish the desired diuresis.* (The relative potencies of diuretics are listed in Table 3–2, and the toxic complications in Table 3–3.)

TREATMENT OF RENAL DISEASE

Glomerular Disease

A discussion of the pathogenesis of glomerular diseases, particularly the acute glomerulonephritides and the nephrotic syndrome, is beyond the scope of this chapter, but both groups of disorders have been ascribed to immunologic mechanisms. With the possible exception of "Goodpasture's" syndrome (a necrotizing glomerulitis with pulmonary hemorrhage), the cause-and-effect relationship between immunologic processes and clinical states is unproved

(Lerner *et al.*, 1967). Nevertheless, it is common practice to give drugs directed at the suspected immune process in idiopathic nephrotic syndrome and selected glomerulonephritides. Corticosteroids and antimetabolites are widely used, and favorable responses to their administration have been reported. A favorable clinical response may not prove that an immunologic etiology is present, as the "immunosuppressive" drugs have anti-inflammatory effects. Few controlled studies of these drugs have been performed, and unsuccessful treatment programs are less likely to be reported than are apparently successful ones. Since glomerulonephritis and the nephrotic syndrome may have numerous etiologies, the physician should be skeptical of dogmatic statements about efficacy or lack of efficacy of programs in these broad clinical states. Adequately controlled studies of clearly defined pathologic and clinical entities are necessary. It is as important to recognize an inadequately supported program of therapy as it is to see the logic of a carefully proved effective regimen. At present, treatment of glomerulonephritis and nephrotic syndrome is largely symptomatic; attention is focused on controlling edema with diet and diuretics, and on treating other complications such as hypertension. Diets providing large quantities of protein for patients with nephrotic syndrome may be effective in the absence of azotemia. The use of steroids and/or immunosuppressive agents should be utilized for nephrotic syndrome only with a knowledge of their risks and with an understanding that their place in the therapeutic program is theoretic.

Interstitial Nephritis

A group of disorders, now classed as interstitial nephritis, was for a long time considered to represent bacterial pyelonephritis. Evidence now indicates that interstitial nephritis may result from bacterial infection, genetic factors, toxins, or other undetermined etiologies (Heptinstall, 1966). Careful definition of etiology is critical to any discussion of drug effectiveness. Antibiotic therapy is ineffective in toxic interstitial nephritis, and antibiotics could conceivably produce such a lesion. To treat toxic nephritis, the toxin must be removed. In the genetically determined disorders little effective therapy has been developed. In true bacterial interstitial nephritis, antibiotic therapy may be useful. The treatment of infection in the urinary tract is based on principles that are broadly applicable. *Obstruction must be corrected, adequate urine flow assured, and foreign bodies removed when possible. Antibacterial therapy should be specific for the organism identified, that is, chosen according to bacterial sensitivity to antibiotics. A bactericidal drug of low toxicity unlikely to allow development of bacterial resistance is preferred.*

Antibiotics should be chosen with knowledge of their bacteriostatic or bactericidal properties. Knowledge of the drug's excretion is required (e.g., filtration of sodium colistimethate and secretion of penicillin). Alterations of excretion rates with modification of chemical structure must be borne in mind (e.g., oxacillin is excreted more slowly than penicillin G). Likewise, alteration of toxicity with chemical modification of the parent compound must be considered (e.g., cephaloridine is far more nephrotoxic than cephalothin, although their antibacterial spectra are similar). The pH of the urine must be considered in selection of an antibacterial program (e.g., alkalinization facilitates the pharmacologic effect of streptomycin, obviates the effectiveness of mandelamine, and increases the solubility of sulfa compounds).

If interstitial infection is to be treated, it should be diagnosed beyond doubt, and the antibiotic chosen should achieve adequate tissue concentrations. Nitrofurantoin may adequately sterilize urine but may fail to eradicate tissue infection. The subject of asymptomatic bacteriuria and its relationship to interstitial nephritis remains to be clarified. Some investigators feel that bacteriuria can be correlated with a host of renal and vascular complications; others consider asymptomatic bacteriuria to be benign (Petersdorf, 1966; Kass and Zinner, 1969). In general, most authors agree that asymptomatic bacteriuria of more than 10^5 colonies per milliliter of urine should be treated. If the same organism sensitive to the same drugs recurs after therapy has been discontinued, inadequate dose or duration of therapy is likely. A more prolonged course of therapy and/or a higher dose may result in sterilization of the urine. If a second organism accounts for the recurrence, a series of changes in antibiotic therapy is unlikely to effect urine sterilization (Turck *et al.*, 1966). Continuous long-term therapy, however, may suppress infection or prevent recurrences. The pattern of recurrent infections with changing organisms is common in elderly women and need not cause alarm in this group. A similar pattern in males and in younger or pregnant females should be pursued much more vigorously, as it may indicate significant anatomic or functional abnormality of the urinary tract.

Alterations in antibiotic programs during renal failure have been based on (1) altered kinetics of antibiotic excretion, (2) toxicity of the antibiotics, and (3) action of metabolic products of the antibiotic. In general, reduced dose and frequency of administration are indicated for drugs excreted by the kidney. A change from a drug primarily excreted by the kidney (e.g., tetracyline) to one alternatively secreted in the bile (e.g., erythromycin) may be useful. Metabolism of an antibiotic to an inactive though retained metabolite (e.g., chloramphenicol) allows the same dosage schedule used in the absence of renal insufficiency.

Urinary Tract Calculi

Prevention of crystal precipitation is the goal of treatment in urinary tract calculus disease. Calcium phosphate and magnesium ammonium phosphate are relatively insoluble in alkaline urine and become increasingly soluble as urine pH falls. Calcium oxalate is also insoluble at alkaline pH but does not become very soluble even if the pH falls below 6.0. Uric acid and cystine, on the other hand, are soluble in alkaline urine but not in acid urine. *Principles: Treatment of renal stone disease optimally includes (1) reduction of the excretion of the precipitating substance* (i.e., treatment of the cause of hypercalcemia, interference with oxalate production, inhibition of uric acid production, etc.); *(2) increase of urine volume so that any given quantity of precipitable substance exists at the lowest possible concentrations; and (3) adjustment of urine pH to permit increased solubility.*

A few specific therapeutic approaches have been attempted. Inhibitors of crystal formation in urine such as magnesium (Neuman and Newman, 1968) and pyrophosphate (given as neutral phosphate) (Fleisch et al., 1964) have been employed with some success in the treatment of patients with calcium stones.

In uric acid stone disease, reduction in uric acid production with the xanthine oxidase inhibitor allopurinol has been successful. Although allopurinol reduces uric acid excretion, it increases the excretion of xanthine and hypoxanthine, which have finite solubilities. Reports of xanthine stones are now appearing, indicating that one form of stone disease may be converted to another by therapy (Greene et al., 1969).

Diets deficient in methionine have been relatively unsuccessful in preventing cystine production and stone formation (Zinneman and Jones, 1966). Alkalinization of the urine is helpful, but cystine solubility does not change markedly until urine pH rises above 7.5. Since the kidney cannot elevate urine pH much above 8.0, there is little leeway in this approach. *Principle: The effect of altering urine pH depends on the pK$_a$ of the compounds in question.*

Advantage has been taken of the phenomenon of disulfide exchange. In this reaction, a sulfhydryl-containing compound exchanges with one-half of a disulfide compound, producing a mixed disulfide (R'SH + RS–SR $\rightleftharpoons$ R'S–SR + RSH) (Crawhall and Watts, 1968). D-Penicillamine has been used to produce a mixed disulfide when reacted with cystine. The mixed disulfide is approximately 50 times more soluble than cystine. Although the basic disorder of amino acid transport in cystinuria is unaffected, clinical manifestations of stone formation can be treated effectively. The numerous allergic reactions to D-penicillamine stress the importance of attempting a simpler program of administration of fluid and alkali before proceeding to the more effective but potentially more dangerous form of therapy.

ALTERED RENAL PHYSIOLOGY AS A CONSEQUENCE OF RENAL FAILURE (PATHOPHYSIOLOGY AND CLINICAL MANIFESTATIONS OF UREMIA)

Advanced renal failure resulting from a variety of disorders leads to a clinical and chemical picture known as uremia. Uremia as a clinical state can be recreated on the basis of the pathophysiology of renal function. In simplest terms, renal failure is a state in which waste products are retained, volume and tonicity regulation of body fluids are impaired, potassium homeostasis is compromised, acid-base regulation is inadequate, calcium and phosphorus metabolism are abnormal, red-blood-cell production and survival are decreased, blood clotting is defective, and regulation of blood pressure is difficult.

During renal failure nitrogenous waste products are retained. Elevation of either blood urea or creatinine is useful as an index of nitrogen retention. Serial determinations of both urea and creatinine concentrations in blood may aid evaluation of renal function (Dossetor, 1966). Urea is cleared by filtration and reabsorption (largely diffusion), whereas creatinine is cleared almost entirely by filtration. There may be some secretion of creatinine, particularly at high serum concentrations. Thus, changes in urine flow rate allowing greater reabsorption affect urea more than creatinine. When urine flow is reduced owing to decreased renal perfusion or to postrenal obstruction, blood urea concentration rises out of proportion to creatinine concentration in blood. Similarly, urea concentrations may be affected by extrarenal events, including exogenous protein intake (diet), endogenous protein load (gastrointestinal bleeding), catabolic drugs (glucocorticosteroids), and antianabolic drugs (tetracycline), all raising concentrations of urea in blood while having little effect on the serum creatinine. *The extrarenal factors that alter serum urea must be recognized, since they do not necessarily reflect changes in renal function, but may result in increasing azotemia in patients with renal failure.*

Whether urea itself contributes to the clinical picture of uremia has been debated, but nitrogenous waste products, in general, may account for the headache, malaise, nausea, and vomiting seen during uremia. Urea may contribute to these symptoms, and in addition precipitates in sweat ducts contribute to the pruritus of uremia. Visible precipitation, particularly about the mouth, produces the classic "uremic frost." Other retained waste products may play a role in blood-clotting abnormalities, platelet dysfunction (Stewart and Castaldi, 1967), peripheral neuropathy (Tyler, 1968), and insulin insensitivity of uremia (Hampers *et al.*, 1966). The retention of normally filtered and excreted waste products should alert the physician to the possibility that pharmacologic agents or metabolites may be similarly retained.

Acid-base abnormalities during renal failure are largely confined to problems of acid retention, which reduces buffer levels and leads to a fall in serum bicarbonate concentration. The depletion of bone buffers may lead to demineralization. Acidosis may contribute to the headache, nausea, and vomiting of renal failure and may alter drug activity and distribution.

Loss of fine control of volume of body fluids predisposes to congestive heart failure or hypovolemia. Either state further reduces renal perfusion and produces deterioration of renal function. Loss of tonicity regulation is less likely to produce difficulties, if the thirst mechanism is intact, unless the patient does not have access to water or receives inappropriate intravenous fluids. A relatively fixed intake independent of demand may lead to hypernatremia or hyponatremia.

In addition to the inability to handle extremes of volume or tonicity, the patient with renal failure is unable to regulate potassium balance. Potassium retention readily occurs in renal failure and may cause fatal arrhythmias. While hyperkalemia may be more common in uremia, hypokalemia may occur during strict potassium restriction or as a consequence of diuretic therapy and may also occur in certain forms of renal disease (e.g., renal tubular acidosis, pyelonephritis).

Phosphate retention occurs in patients with uremia, lowering the serum calcium. Vitamin D resistance also occurs, associated with reduced intestinal absorption of calcium. Calcium concentrations in serum fall, stimulating parathormone release, which results in bone resorption and calcium mobilization. Although the relative roles of these factors have not been defined clearly, the end results—hypocalcemia, hyperphosphatemia, bone disease, and persistently elevated parathormone levels—are consistently observed in uremia. Occasionally the parathormone production becomes autonomous and persistent, necessitating parathyroid surgery.

Magnesium retention may occur in uremia, leading to somnolence and coma, but usually does not occur without magnesium ingestion (antacids, cathartics, etc.). Hypomagnesemia is uncommon in advanced renal failure.

In renal disease, erythropoietin production is reduced and renin production is increased. The reduced erythropoietin production and shortened red-cell survival time result in anemia. The shortened red-cell survival in uremia correlates with retention of nitrogenous waste products. Normal red blood cells introduced into uremic patients have shortened survival times, whereas cells from uremic patients transfused into normal volunteers survive for nearly normal periods. Platelet dysfunction in uremia may be associated with bleeding. Excess of renin may contribute to hypertension, leading to nosebleeds, headaches, encephalopathy, cardiac hypertrophy, and acceleration of peripheral vascular disease.

The patient with advanced chronic renal failure is a sallow, anemic, fatigued individual with headache, nausea, and vomiting. His skin may show excoriation, bruises, and uremic frost. He may complain of paresthesias, muscle cramps or twitching, or even generalized seizures. His blood pressure probably is elevated, and a pericardial friction rub resulting from a characteristic but unexplained fibrinous pericarditis may be heard. His state of hydration and his serum sodium concentration depend on his previous intake of water and electrolytes. His respiration may be deep and sighing as he compensates for metabolic acidosis.

Laboratory studies show a normochromic, normocytic anemia with normal numbers of platelets. Urinalysis reveals reduced concentrating and diluting ability, probably with proteinuria resulting from glomerular damage, and/or reduced tubular reabsorption of protein. Changes in urinary sediment are variable. Waste product retention is reflected by elevated blood urea and creatinine levels. Serum calcium is usually low, phosphorus and potassium high. *The constellation of clinical and laboratory abnormalities in the uremic patient can be predicted as the consequence of reduced renal function. Just as there is a logical physiologic basis for the development of uremia, there is a logical physiologic basis for principles of therapeutics that are instituted to ameliorate uremia or depend on renal function.*

Unusual requirements for or altered responses

to pharmacologic agents accompany uremia, whether these agents are intended to affect renal or extrarenal function. The failing kidney may be less responsive to drugs that act directly on it. Diuretics become progressively less effective as intrinsic renal disease progresses.

Uricosuric agents reduce tubular reabsorption of filtered uric acid. During renal failure, filtration of uric acid is diminished and the tubules become insensitive to drugs altering reabsorption; uric acid is retained, and uric acid plasma concentrations must be lowered by another method. Allopurinol provides alternative therapy by reducing synthesis of the uric acid. *Principle: During renal failure, pharmacologic approaches aimed at correcting kidney-induced abnormalities may employ drugs with extrarenal sites of action.*

SPECIAL CONSIDERATIONS IN THE TREATMENT OF RENAL FAILURE

When the kidney is unable to function, volume and composition of body fluids must be regulated by therapeutic programs. In addition to alterations in drug dosage, the route of administration, potential toxicity and interactions, and alterations in diet may be considered. Sodium and potassium intake must be controlled, along with intake of calcium, phosphate and magnesium.

Calcium

Phosphate retention, parathyroid activity, and vitamin D metabolism are important determinants in the development of the bone disease and calcium abnormalities associated with renal failure. The treatment of symptomatic hypocalcemia, which occurs in few uremic patients, must take into account each contributory factor. Thus, phosphates should be reduced by limiting dietary intake (dairy products) and by promoting gastrointestinal loss with magnesium-free antacids, which bind phosphorus in the intestinal lumen. Because oral calcium salts are unlikely to be absorbed, treatment of significant hypocalcemia may require parenteral calcium. Vitamin D "resistance" can be overcome with large doses of vitamin D. Parathyroid secretion is reduced as serum calcium concentrations rise. *These modes of therapy are directed at reversing the results, not the cause, of renal insufficiency.* If the renal insufficiency is corrected by dialysis or by successful transplantation, calcium abnormalities will be less important (except in rare instances of autonomous parathormone secretion).

Hypocalcemia may complicate clinical situations other than renal failure. Neuromuscular irritability can be enhanced by low serum concentrations of calcium, high serum concentrations of potassium, or low hydrogen ion concentration. The extent of irritability depends on the relationship between these ions. If acidosis is too rapidly corrected in a patient with hypocalcemia, tetany may occur. Similarly, tetany may not occur at low calcium concentrations if potassium is depleted, but may appear if potassium is too rapidly replaced. *When hypocalcemia is present, the treatment of acidosis or hypokalemia must proceed slowly and hypocalcemia should be simultaneously corrected.*

Magnesium

Antacids bind phosphates in the gastrointestinal lumen and are thereby useful in the treatment of hypocalcemia. However, since some antacids contain high concentrations of sodium and/or magnesium, the choice of these gels may be critical. Ordinarily, magnesium is excreted by the kidney; if excess magnesium is administered in the form of gels, hypermagnesemia may cause somnolence or coma and cardiac arrhythmias.

Hypomagnesemia may occur in renal disorders when tubular function is abnormal, especially in patients who are being given diets deficient in magnesium. If neuromuscular irritability or a state resembling delirium tremens develops in an individual with renal failure, hypomagnesemia should be considered and, if proved by laboratory studies, treated with magnesium replacement (Randall, 1969).

Protein

Regulation of protein intake also is employed; when most dietary protein is in the form of essential amino acids and the total intake is restricted, azotemia can be controlled and acidosis limited. Such dietary therapy reduces the clinical symptoms of uremia and may mask the usual evidence of deterioration, but probably does not alter the total life expectancy of the patient (Lewis and Magill, 1968).

Dietary management of renal failure also reduces the required frequency of dialysis (making the patient's life more bearable and opening more positions in dialysis programs). The main disadvantages have been the reduction of the usual warning signs of impending uremic death and the requirement for additional therapy in the form of alkali and exchange resin for removal of potassium. Furthermore, life is not prolonged, and the discomfort of the program for the patient frequently results in hostility toward the therapeutic program and the physician who prescribed it.

When all conservative medical and dietary

forms of treatment have failed, dialysis and transplantation are available to the patient. Either peritoneal dialysis or extracorporeal hemodialysis may be used to remove waste products, excess fluids, and toxins, as well as to alter the chemical composition of body fluids.

Dialysis

Volume. Dialysis may abruptly alter volume, producing either hypovolemia or hypervolemia. Such changes in volume may be made to correct fluid overload and/or to restore responsiveness to drugs, such as hypotensive agents. Another therapeutic problem accompanying volume shifts affects the central nervous system. During dialysis, when urea is rapidly removed from extracellular fluid, a disequilibrium is established between intracellular (high) and extracellular (low) urea concentrations. Urea does not exit as quickly from cells as from the extracellular space. The osmolality of brain may increase and water may enter brain cells, producing cerebral edema with headache and seizures. This complication may be avoided either by lowering urea concentration in plasma slowly enough to provide time for equilibration between the compartments or by providing osmotically active material that remains extracellular (e.g., mannitol) to increase the osmolality of the extracellular fluid.

Electrolytes and Acid-Base Correction. Dialysis is particularly well suited to correction of electrolyte and acid-base abnormalities. However, the same principles applicable to the rate of correction of acidosis or alkalosis apply to dialysis. Since potassium is readily dialyzed, hypokalemia is a danger. Rapid potassium reduction in a patient who is adequately digitalized produces arrhythmias, as digoxin is cleared slowly by dialysis procedures (Doherty *et al.*, 1967).

Drug Removal. Dialysis can be used both to eliminate and to administer drugs, altering the pharmacokinetics of the drug and the kinetics of drug action. Knowledge of the rates of dialysis of pharmacologic agents is required to redefine dosage regimens. Because dialysis can remove drugs, it may be used to treat selected drug toxicities when the drugs are dialyzable. Centers with large dialysis units have compiled lists of toxins that may be effectively treated by dialysis (Maher and Schreiner, 1968). *Principles: (1) A toxin may be bound in tissues and be unavailable for effective dialysis (e.g., glutethimide). In this case dialysis may not be beneficial. (2) Administration of a second drug capable of preferentially binding the toxin and removing it from tissue may allow dialysis of the complex (e.g., mercurials*

bound by BAL may then be dialyzed). (3) The use of substances in the dialyzing fluid that bind toxins or in which toxins have a higher solubility is not theoretically sound. The theory contends that toxins enter these dialyzing fluids or bind to them and may then be removed at higher-than-usual rates. In fact, the rate of removal of a toxin is a function of the concentration gradient across the dialyzing membrane and of the characteristics of the membrane. If the dialysis fluid contains no toxin, the gradient across the membrane will be infinite and the rate of removal maximal. Thus, if the volume of dialysis fluid is such that a significant concentration of toxin never accumulates, a maximum rate of toxin removal is achieved that is not affected by substances in the dialysate. *Recognition of the goal of a therapeutic maneuver and assessment of its theoretic and practical achievement are mandatory.*

Numerous complications of dialysis result from differential rates of movement of solute and solvent (e.g., hypernatremia), from absorption of substances from the dialysate (e.g., hyperglycemia), and from blind entrance into a body cavity (peritoneal dialysis) (e.g., infection, bleeding, and perforation of the bowel). Unexpected complications, such as hypercalcemia, may result from variation in calcium ion content of tap water used for dialysis. Dialysis is an effective form of therapy to aid or substitute for the failing kidney and to provide the patient with a longer life expectancy. A patient maintained on dialysis may be considered for renal transplantation.

Transplantation

A discussion of renal transplantation is beyond the scope of this chapter, but a few therapeutic principles may be considered. The main problem of transplantation has been allograft rejection. Rejection is lessened by (1) careful selection of compatible donors, (2) corticosteroid therapy, (3) immunosuppressive therapy, (4) antilymphocyte therapy (radiation and antilymphocyte antiserum), and (5) anticoagulant therapy. These programs are aimed at reducing the likelihood of rejection, suppressing the rejection reaction, and preventing damage from responses to rejection such as intravascular coagulation. A great risk attends these approaches. A means of detecting the key antigens responsible for rejection and specifically blocking them without interfering with the remainder of the host's defense mechanisms would be more desirable.

The second problem of transplantation is that compensatory mechanisms operative in the patient with renal failure may become suddenly unopposed. One such mechanism, hyperparathyroidism, may result in hypercalcemia, which is itself nephrotoxic (McIntosh et al., 1966). Recognition that compensatory mechanisms may persist unopposed allows steps to be taken to blunt these mechanisms. For example, after transplantation, serum phosphorus may fall owing to renal and gastrointestinal losses. The renal losses result from the action of parathormone on the proximal tubule of the normal transplanted kidney; the gastrointestinal losses occur via antacid gels given to the transplant recipient when he is taking high doses of glucocorticoids. The fall in serum phosphorus permits a rise in serum calcium, which may be blunted by an adequate phosphate intake.

Summary Principle: The kidney is a major organ that determines drug kinetics and is a major site of drug action. Renal function must be considered in the development of most therapeutic strategies. The principles of therapeutics illustrated by examples utilizing the kidney apply to all organ systems.

REFERENCES

Anton, A. H.: A drug-induced change in the distribution and renal excretion of sulfonamides. *J. Pharmacol. Exp. Ther.*, **134**:291–303, 1961.

Avioli, L. V.; Sook, W. L.; Birge, S. J.; Slatopolsky, E.; and DeLuca, H. F.: The nature of the defect in intestinal calcium absorption in chronic renal disease. *J. Clin. Invest.*, **48**:4a, 1969.

Barger, A. C.: Renal hemodynamic factors in congestive heart failure. *Ann. N.Y. Acad. Sci.*, **139**:276–84, 1966.

Bergstrom, S.: Prostaglandins: members of a new hormonal system. *Science*, **157**:382–91, 1967.

Berliner, R. W., and Bennett, C. M.: Concentration of urine in the mammalian kidney. *Amer. J. Med.*, **42**:777–89, 1967.

Bluemle, L. W., and Goldberg, M.: Renal accumulation of salicylate and phenacetin—possible mechanisms in the nephropathy of analgesic abuse. *J. Clin. Invest.*, **47**:2507–14, 1968.

Bricker, N. S.: The control of sodium excretion with normal and reduced nephron populations: the preeminence of third factor. *Amer. J. Med.*, **43**:313–21, 1967.

Crawhall, J. C., and Watts, R. W. E.: Cystinuria. *Amer. J. Med.*, **45**:736–55, 1968.

de Wardener, H. E.; Mills, I. H.; Clapham, W. F.; and Hayter, C. J.: Studies on the efferent mechanism of the sodium diuresis which follows the administration of intravenous saline in the dog. *Clin. Sci.*, **21**:249–58, 1961.

Doherty, J. E.; Flanigan, W. J.; Perkins, W. H.; and Ackerman, G. L.: Studies with tritiated digoxin in anephric human subjects. *Circulation*, **35**:298–303, 1967.

Doherty, J. E.; Perkins, W. H.; and Wilson, M. C.: Studies with tritiated digoxin in renal failure. *Amer. J. Med.*, **37**:536–44, 1964.

Dossetor, J. B.: Creatinemia versus uremia: the relative significance of blood urea nitrogen and serum creatinine

concentration in azotemia. *Ann. Intern. Med.*, **65**:1287–99, 1966.

Earley, L. E., and Daugharty, T. M.: Sodium metabolism. *New Eng. J. Med.*, **281**:72–86, 1969.

Elion, G. B.; Yu, T. F.; Gutman, A. B.; and Hitchings, G. H.: Renal clearance of oxipurinol, the chief metabolite of allopurinol. *Amer. J. Med.*, **45**:69–77, 1968.

Elwood, C. M.; Lucas, G. D.; and Muehrcke, R. C.: Acute renal failure associated with sodium colistimethate treatment. *Arch. Intern. Med. (Chicago)*, **118**:326–34, 1966.

Evans, B. M.; Hughes Jones, N. C.; Milne, M. D.; and Yellowlees, H.: Ion-exchange resins in the treatment of anuria. *Lancet*, **2**:791–95, 1953.

Fleisch, H.; Bisaz, S.; and Care, A. D.: Effect of orthophosphate on urinary pyrophosphate excretion and prevention of urolithiasis. *Lancet*, **1**:1065–67, 1964.

Frazier, H. S.: Renal regulation of sodium balance. *New Eng. J. Med.*, **279**:868–75, 1968.

Giebisch, G., and Windhager, E. E.: Renal tubular transfer of sodium, chloride, and potassium. *Amer. J. Med.*, **36**:643–69, 1964.

Goldberg, M.: The physiology and pathophysiology of diuretic agents. In Fulton, W. F. M. (ed.): *Modern Trends in Pharmacology and Therapeutics*. Butterworth & Co., Ltd., London, 1967, pp. 41–75.

Goodman, L. S., and Gilman, A. (eds.): *The Pharmacological Basis of Therapeutics*, 4th ed. The Macmillan Co., New York, 1970.

Greene, M. L.; Fujimoto, W. Y.; and Seegmiller, T. E.: Urinary xanthine stones—a rare complication of allopurinol therapy. *New Eng. J. Med.*, **280**:426–27, 1969.

Haber, E.: Pathophysiologic studies of the renin-angiotensin system. *New Eng. J. Med.*, **280**:148–55, 1969.

Hampers, C. L.; Soeldner, J. S.; Doak, P. B.; and Merrill, J. P.: Effect of chronic renal failure and hemodialysis on carbohydrate metabolism. *J. Clin. Invest.*, **45**:1719–31, 1966.

Hasselbalch, K. A.: Die Berechnung der Wassertoffzahl des Blutes aus der freien und gebundenen Kohlensaure derselben und die Sauerstoffbindung des Blutes als Funktion der Wassetstoffzahl. *Biochem. Z.*, **78**:112–44, 1917.

Henderson, L. J.: The theory of neutrality regulation in the animal organism. *Amer. J. Physiol.*, **21**:427–48, 1908.

Heptinstall, R. H.: *Pathology of the Kidney*. Little, Brown & Co., Boston, 1966.

Jamison, R. L.: Micropuncture study of segments of thin loop of Henle in the rat. *Amer. J. Physiol.*, **215**:236–42, 1968.

Jamison, R. L.; Bennett, C. M.; and Berliner, R. W.: Countercurrent multiplication by the thin loops of Henle. *Amer. J. Physiol.*, **212**:357–66, 1967.

Kass, E. H., and Zinner, S. H.: Bacteriuria and renal disease. *J. Infect. Dis.*, **120**:27–46, 1969.

Kunin, C. M.; Glazko, A. J.; and Finland, M.: Persistence of antibiotics in blood of patients with acute renal failure. II. Chloramphenicol and its metabolic products in the blood of patients with severe renal disease or hepatic cirrhosis. *J. Clin. Invest.*, **38**:1498–1508, 1959.

Lambertson, C. J.: Chemical control of respiration at rest. In Mountcastle, V. B. (ed.): *Medical Physiology*, 12th ed. C. V. Mosby Co., St. Louis, 1968.

Laragh, J. H., and Kelly, W. G.: Aldosterone: its biochemistry and physiology. *Advances Metab. Dis.*, **1**:217–62, 1964.

Lemann, J., Jr., and Relman, A. S.: The relation of sulfur metabolism to acid-base balance and electrolyte excretion: the effects of DL-methionine in normal man. *J. Clin. Invest.*, **38**:2215–23, 1959.

Lerner, R. A.; Glassock, R. J.; and Dixon, F. J.: The role of antiglomerular basement membrane antibody in the pathogenesis of human glomerulonephritis. *J. Exp. Med.*, 126:99–104, 1967.

Lewis, E. J., and Magill, J. W.: Symposium: Proceedings of the Conference on the Nutritional Aspects of Uremia. *Amer. J. Clin. Nutr.*, 21:346–643, 1968.

McIntosh, D. A.; Peterson, E. W.; and McPhaul, J. J.: Autonomy of parathyroid function after renal homotransplantation. *Ann. Intern. Med.*, 65:900–907, 1966.

Maher, J. F., and Schreiner, G. E.: The dialysis of poisons and drugs. *Trans. Amer. Soc. Artif. Intern. Organs*, 14:440–53, 1968.

Malnic, G.; Klose, R. M.; and Giebisch, G.: Micropuncture study of distal tubular potassium and sodium transport in rat nephron. *Amer. J. Physiol.*, 211:529–47, 1966.

Morgan, T., and Berliner, R. W.: Permeability of the loop of Henle, vasa recta and collecting duct to water, urea and sodium. *Amer. J. Physiol.*, 215:108–15, 1968.

Neuman, W. F., and Newman, M. W.: *The Chemical Dynamics of Bone Mineral.* University of Chicago Press, Chicago, 1968.

Payne, J. P., and Rowe, G. G.: The effects of mecamylamine in the cat as modified by the administration of carbon dioxide. *Brit. J. Pharmacol.*, 12:457–60, 1957.

Petersdorf, R. G.: Asymptomatic bacteriuria: a therapeutic enigma. In Ingelfinger, F. J.; Relman, A. S.; and Finland, M. (eds.): *Controversy in Internal Medicine.* W. B. Saunders Co., Philadelphia, 1966, pp. 302–12.

Pitts, R. F.: Renal production and excretion of ammonia. *Amer. J. Med.*, 36:720–42, 1964.

Rabkin, R.; Simon, N. M.; Steiner, S.; and Colwell, J. A.: Effect of renal disease on renal uptake and excretion of insulin in man. *New Eng. J. Med.*, 282:182–86, 1970.

Randall, R. E.: Magnesium metabolism in chronic renal disease. *Ann. N.Y. Acad. Sci.*, 162:831–46, 1969.

Sachs, J.; Taggert, G.; Noell, P.; and Kunin, C. M.: Renal function and urinary recovery of nitrofurantoin. *New Engl. J. Med.*, 278:1032–35, 1968.

Schneider, W. J., and Becker, E. L.: Acute transient hearing loss after ethacrynic acid therapy. *Arch. Intern. Med. (Chicago)*, 117:715–17, 1966.

Schreiner, G. E., and Maher, J. F.: Drugs and the kidney. *Ann. N.Y. Acad. Sci.*, 123:326–32, 1965.

Schwartz, W. B.: Effect of sulfanilamide on salt and water excretion in congestive heart failure. *New Eng. J. Med.*, 240:173–77, 1949.

Schwartz, W. B.; Van Ypersele de Strihou, C. V.; and Kassirer, J. P.: Role of anions in metabolic alkalosis and potassium deficiency. *New Eng. J. Med.*, 279:630–39, 1968.

Schwartz, W. B., and Waters, W. C., III: Lactate versus bicarbonate. *Amer. J. Med.*, 32:831–33, 1962.

Scribner, B. H., and Burnell, J. M.: Interpretation of serum potassium concentration. *Metabolism*, 5:468–79, 1959.

Stewart, J. H., and Castaldi, P. A.: Uremic bleeding: reversible platelet defect corrected by dialysis. *Quart. J. Med.*, 36:409–23, 1967.

Stohlman, F., Jr.: The kidney and erythropoiesis. *New Eng. J. Med.*, 279:1437–40, 1968.

Stone, W. J., and Pitts, R. F.: Pathways of ammonia metabolism in the intact functioning kidney of the dog. *J. Clin. Invest.*, 46:1141–50, 1967.

Swan, R. C., and Pitts, R. F.: Neutralization of infused acid by nephrectomized dogs. *J. Clin. Invest.*, 34:205–12, 1955.

Thorburn, G. D.; Kopald, H. H.; Herd, J. A.; Hollenberg, M.; O'Morchoe, C. C.; and Barger, A. C.: Intrarenal distribution of nutrient blood flow determined with krypton[85] in unanesthetized dog. *Circ. Res.*, 13:290–307, 1963.

Turck, M.; Anderson, K. N.; and Petersdorf, R. G.: Relapse and reinfection in chronic bacteremia. *New Eng. J. Med.*, 275:70–73, 1966.

Tyler, R. H.: Neurologic disorders in renal failure. *Amer. J. Med.*, 44:734–48, 1968.

Weiner, I. M., and Mudge, G. H.: Renal tubular mechanisms for excretion of organic acids and bases. *Amer. J. Med.*, 36:743–62, 1964.

Weiner, I. M.; Washington, J. A., II; and Mudge, G. H.: On the mechanism of action of probenecid on renal tubular secretion. *Bull. Johns Hopkins Hosp.*, 106:333–46, 1960.

Woodruff, M. W.; Malvin, R. L.; and Thompson, I. M.: The renal transport of nitrofurantoin: effect of acid-base balance upon its excretion. *J.A.M.A.*, 175:98–101, 1961.

Yü, T. F., and Gutman, A. B.: Study of the paradoxical effects of salicylate in low, intermediate, and high dosage on the renal mechanism for excretion of urate in man. *J. Clin. Invest.*, 38:1298–1315, 1959.

Zinneman, H. H., and Jones, J. E.: Dietary methionine and its influence on cystine excretion in cystinuric patients. *Metabolism*, 15:915–21, 1966.

Chapter 4

HEPATIC AND GASTROINTESTINAL DISORDERS

I. HEPATIC DISORDERS

L. Frederick Fenster

UNIQUE CHARACTERISTICS OF THE LIVER AND ITS DISEASES: THERAPEUTIC IMPLICATIONS

The physician is rarely able to provide more than supportive and symptomatic treatment for primary disorders of the liver. Proven curative therapy is largely restricted to focal disorders, such as hepatic abscess or localized hepatic tumors (benign or malignant), surgical techniques being crucial in each case. Common hepatic disorders, such as hepatitis (viral, drug, or toxic) and cirrhosis, affect the liver diffusely. Therapy must support the patient long enough for natural reparative and regenerative processes to take place. Although this goal is not as dramatic and exciting as the application of surgical remedies, it is nevertheless complex and demanding with significant rewards for both patient and physician. Since the liver is the metabolic "engine room" of the body, the results of its functional deterioration are diverse and far-reaching. An enlightened therapeutic program for a patient with life-threatening liver disease, for example, must take into consideration such major factors as (1) nutritional needs

and proper dietary therapy; (2) changes in central nervous system function, especially those related to protein intake and drugs; (3) altered renal function; (4) fluid and electrolyte imbalance; (5) serum protein abnormalities; (6) blood-clotting aberrations; (7) abnormal glucose metabolism; and (8) alterations in circulatory dynamics. As a result of this multiplicity of deranged functions, the physician attempting to provide optimal supportive therapy for a patient with advanced liver disease must understand fluid and electrolyte balance, renal function, the proper use of diuretics, ammonium metabolism, and many other aspects of internal medicine. In addition, he must keep the main goals and priorities of treatment in mind and, above all, avoid creating new disorders with his therapy. In many diseases, the internist's pen is mightier than the surgeon's sword.

Because most therapeutic measures in primary liver disorders are necessarily supportive or symptomatic, being largely directed at the complications of the disease, the principal goal is often to "buy time" (Davidson, 1966). For example, most cases of viral hepatitis are benign, and the patients eventually regain normal liver structure and function. Therapy in such instances is dictated by the patient's symptoms; the physician must act as the patient's liver *pro tempore*. In fulminant hepatitis with coma, therapy is directed at keeping the patient alive long enough to permit liver regeneration. In decompensated alcoholic cirrhosis, abstinence from alcohol is by far the most important long-term therapeutic maneuver. Although reduction of ascites may be indicated in some patients to improve comfort, appetite, and respiratory dynamics, it is not often crucial in treatment. More often, the primary goal is to assure physical and psychologic comfort, adequate food intake, and rest for the patient while the liver recovers from the toxic effects of alcohol. All too often the patient and physician regard ascites as a challenge, much like Mount Everest, the conquest of which becomes the misdirected objective of treatment. This approach often results in ill-advised therapeutic paracenteses or in overzealous use of potent diuretics, either of which may precipitate hepatic encephalopathy or progressive oliguric renal failure (the "hepatorenal syndrome").

"Playing for time" in the treatment of liver disease is based on two important characteristics of mammalian liver: its metabolic "reserve" and its great capacity for regeneration (Simpson, 1963). Only a small percentage of the normal complement of liver cells must function well for adequate metabolic performance. This "liver reserve" is illustrated by the remarkably good hepatic function of patients with massive replacement of the liver by carcinoma or cysts, and by the fact that the normal liver is able to conjugate and excrete many times more than the usual daily bilirubin load. After severe diffuse injury to liver cells, even limited regeneration may significantly improve liver function. If the causative factor in the disease process can be removed or suppressed, regeneration usually occurs, with resultant clinical improvement. For example, the removal of extrahepatic obstruction in patients with secondary biliary cirrhosis may result in remarkable clinical and histologic improvement (Bunton and Cameron, 1963). In liver disease associated with alcoholism, withdrawal of the toxin and improved nutrition often lead to marked improvement in liver function and structure, although certain consequences of the disruption of liver architecture (i.e., scarring and alterations in vasculature) may be permanent. In active postnecrotic cirrhosis, the destructive process may subside and allow regeneration to dominate over continuing inflammation and necrosis, tipping the scales in favor of clinical improvement or remission. However,

for unknown reasons (whether persistent infection, "autoimmunity," or self-perpetuating vascular aberrations) many cases continue to progress inexorably, and regenerative forces never adequately compensate. To use a rather macabre illustration, one might prefer to have alcoholic cirrhosis, not only because of the presumed greater pleasure in the early stages but also because a known etiologic factor can be withdrawn to allow regeneration to become dominant.

CATEGORIES AND EXAMPLES OF THERAPEUTIC APPROACHES TO LIVER DISORDERS

Withdrawal, Depletion, or Antagonism of a "Toxic" or Offending Substance

Alcoholic Liver Disease and the Withdrawal of Alcohol. The therapeutic value of withdrawing a toxic substance is most obvious in alcoholic liver disease. Ethanol is a hepatic toxin, causing biochemical and structural hepatic abnormalities in virtually all subjects who consume large quantities, irrespective of the associated dietary intake (Rubin and Lieber, 1968c). The relative importance of alcohol and dietary deficiencies in the pathogenesis of Laennec's cirrhosis is still controversial and will not be discussed here (Erenoglu et al., 1964; Reynolds et al., 1965; Rubin and Lieber, 1968b). Furthermore, in nearly all stages of alcoholic liver disease, abstinence from alcohol results in improved liver function and a more favorable prognosis, whether because of withdrawal of alcohol, better nutrition, or both. Most chronic alcoholic patients admitted to the hospital do not have fully developed Laennec's cirrhosis but, rather, alcoholic fatty liver, a completely reversible condition when alcohol is withdrawn. Once cirrhosis is established, irreversible scarring with its secondary effects takes place, but liver function still may improve considerably when alcohol is withdrawn and liver parenchymal cell regeneration occurs.

A critical retrospective study of survival in Laennec's cirrhosis (Powell and Klatskin, 1968) demonstrated that more patients who abstained from alcohol after initial diagnosis survived after 5 years (63%) than those who continued to imbibe (40.5%). Because of the refractoriness of alcoholism as a social and psychiatric disorder, most patients with alcoholic liver disease do not abstain (only 33% in the above series). We must deal with patients who continue to drink and to consume marginal diets. Although the ultimate prognosis is poor in such patients, effective palliative and symptomatic treatment is still possible in many; they should not be rejected as "hopeless" cases.

Withdrawal of Offending Drugs. Because many drugs have been implicated in the production of hepatic abnormalities, withdrawal of a drug that either causes a liver disorder or adversely affects its management has assumed increasing importance. Extensive review of the subject is beyond the scope of this discussion (Popper *et al.*, 1965b; Sherlock, 1965, 1966; Klatskin, 1969). Almost any drug, given the right circumstances and patient, can cause hepatic functional and/or structural abnormalities. All too often, such reactions are called simply "drug hepatitis" or "toxic reaction" without consideration of the many possible pathogenetic mechanisms which include (1) direct toxicity, a dose-related liver injury that results in patients given high enough doses; (2) interference with hepatic secretion or excretion via competitive inhibition or other mechanisms; and (3) hypersensitivity reactions. Certain hepatic drug reactions attributed to hypersensitivity may actually result from genetically determined biochemical alterations that are silent physiologically or biochemically until a drug is administered (Motulsky, 1965, 1969). Unless other clinical evidence of hypersensitivity (e.g., fever, rash, and eosinophilia) is present, this type of reaction should probably be termed "idiosyncratic" rather than "allergic" or "hypersensitive."

Drugs utilized in the management of patients with known liver disease may often lead to complications, again making drug withdrawal crucial in treatment. Examples include the role of diuretics or narcotics in precipitating hepatic encephalopathy and the progressive azotemia caused by high doses of neomycin in some patients with renal functional impairment. *Principle: The physician must be alert to the potential role of drugs in the production of both primary liver disorders and their complications. The possibilities of such adverse effects are numerous. Whenever a patient develops new evidence of liver dysfunction or new problems in management, drug effects may be involved.*

Treatment Directed at Reducing Blood Ammonium Concentration.* Hepatic encephalopathy is a complex syndrome resulting from many interacting factors (Webster, 1965; Sherlock, 1968; Conn, 1969). Whatever the ultimate causes, most patients with hepatic precoma or coma have increased levels of arterial blood ammonium, and attention has been focused on the role of ammonium as a major "toxic" factor in the pathogenesis of this disorder. A direct cause-and-effect relationship between encephalopathy and blood ammonium concentration has not been demonstrated conclusively. It is possible that ammonium serves merely as an excellent "marker" or indicator of other undefined factors that are more directly involved in the production of the central nervous system aberrations, as does porphobilinogen excess in porphyria. Whatever the precise mechanisms, the correlation of clinical status with blood ammonium levels has been consistent enough to lead to the widespread use of the term "ammonia intoxication" and has directed attention to pharmacologic means of lowering the blood ammonium concentration in the treatment of hepatic encephalopathy.

The ammonium content of the blood may be influenced by several factors, including (1) the action of bacteria to produce ammonia in the distal small intestine and colon from protein and urea (which diffuses across the intestinal wall into the lumen) (Walser and Bodenlos, 1959; Webster and Gabuzda, 1959), and (2) production of ammonium by the renal tubules (the major source of circulating ammonium in normal man at rest) (Owen *et al.*, 1960). These factors rarely lead to significant elevations of blood ammonium in the absence of severe liver disease and/or extensive shunting of portal blood into the systemic circulation, whether spontaneous or surgically induced.

Published evidence indicates that measures that lower blood ammonium concentration can often reverse the course of hepatic encephalopathy, although no strictly controlled studies have been reported. Therapy is most effective in patients with "exogenous" hepatic precoma, in which an obvious precipitating event such as intestinal bleeding or excessive protein intake has occurred (Chalmers, 1960). When coma supervenes in the course of progressive liver-cell failure without an obvious precipitating cause ("endogenous coma"), therapy is far less rewarding.

The first step in the treatment of hepatic encephalopathy is the withdrawal or control of any precipitating factors, which may include (1) drugs known to have potentiating effects (e.g., sedatives, tranquilizers, narcotics, and diuretics); (2) hypovolemia, which may occur after overvigorous diuresis or paracentesis; (3) electrolyte abnormalities, especially hypokalemia (Read *et al.*, 1959; Baertl *et al.*, 1963; Artz *et al.*, 1966; Sherlock *et al.*, 1966); (4) intercurrent infection; and (5) gastrointestinal bleeding. There is evidence that more ammonia is released from the protein of red blood cells than from equivalent

---

* Ammonia is released in the gut and may diffuse from blood into the brain, but at physiologic pH more than 99% of ammonia exists as the ammonium ion (Warren *et al.*, 1960; Brown *et al.*, 1967).

amounts of casein (Bessman et al., 1958) or plasma protein (Bessman and Hawkins, 1963); thus very little bleeding may initiate precoma.

Because the gut contributes most to the elevated ammonium levels in most instances of "ammonia intoxication," it is the primary target of therapy. Elimination of protein from the diet is the first step in the early phases of encephalopathy and should be automatic in patients with precoma or coma. This subject is discussed later in regard to dietary treatment of liver disease. Vigorous purging of the colon with laxatives and enemas in an attempt to reduce the substrates for ammonia production is the next logical step. In patients with intermittent or chronic encephalopathy, a state of "controlled" diarrhea is sometimes useful. Some patients are so labile that a single day of relative constipation may induce coma (perhaps an example of the "auto-intoxication" referred to in older literature). When antacids are utilized in the treatment of upper intestinal bleeding associated with actual or potential hepatic coma, those agents with laxative effects should be chosen. *Principle: Aim for as many desirable pharmacologic effects as possible from a single agent.*

Alteration of the Intestinal Flora. The bacterial content of the lower intestine cannot be eliminated or even reduced for more than a few days, but its species can be altered. The aim of such therapy is to change the flora, qualitatively and/or quantitatively, so that less ammonia is formed. Gram-negative organisms (particularly *Proteus*, coliforms, and *Bacteroides*) appear to be the principal ammonia producers (Phear and Ruebner, 1956).

For acute alteration of the colonic flora, antibiotics must be used. To minimize the potential dangers of systemic superinfection and to achieve prompt high concentrations in the bowel lumen, poorly absorbed antibacterial agents are used. Neomycin has become the prototypic drug for this purpose, for it is effective, has an appropriate spectrum of activity, and is poorly absorbed, and (of no small import) there is now extensive experience with it. Kanamycin also seems highly suitable.

When neomycin is given orally in doses of 4 to 12 g per day, there is prompt and marked suppression of stool bacterial counts, particularly of coliforms (Dawson et al., 1957; Fisher and Faloon, 1957; Fast et al., 1958). With continued administration in high doses, resistant strains of *Escherichia coli, Streptococcus faecalis*, micrococci, and yeasts may become prominent. Neomycin often induces some degree of diarrhea, which may be helpful in itself. In comatose patients, neomycin may be given through a nasogastric tube or by enema (Najarian et al.,

1959), although the latter is less reliable in its effect. Dosage must be individualized. In order to achieve a prompt effect, high doses (6 to 12 g) are usually given for the first 1 to 2 days or until the patient improves. (Coma in this setting *is*, after all, a life-threatening situation.) The dose may then be reduced to 1 to 4 g per day or discontinued altogether, according to the clinical response.

Although neomycin is poorly absorbed, ototoxicity and nephrotoxicity have been reported in patients with impaired renal function (Kunin et al., 1960; Last and Sherlock, 1960; Berk and Chalmers, 1970). If the drug is used in such patients, its dose should be reduced and the serum creatinine concentration monitored. Tetracyclines may be useful substitutes in the acute management of "ammonia intoxication" in uremic patients, because these drugs may not be so dependent on renal excretion as are other alternatives (Lieber and Davidson, 1960; Jones and Davidson, 1962; Davidson, 1964). However, recent data make the use of tetracyclines untenable in uremic patients at standard doses (see Chapter 10).

Other potential complications of neomycin therapy include (1) severe diarrhea, with consequent potassium depletion, which may aggravate encephalopathy (Artz et al., 1966); and (2) enteric superinfection with resistant *Staphylococcus aureus*, leading to fulminant staphylococcal enterocolitis (Tisdale et al., 1960).

When neomycin is used continuously for more than a week, periodic gram stains of the stool are indicated. When staphylococcal colonization occurs, simple omission of the drug for a few days will usually suffice. If clinical evidence of an enteritis is present, the condition should be actively treated with a suitable antibiotic (e.g., oral vancomycin).

Long-term neomycin therapy is sometimes necessary in patients with chronic or episodic hepatic encephalopathy. When low doses (0.5 to 2 g per day) are utilized, complications are rare. This program may allow patients with protein sensitivity (the "one-meatball syndrome") to consume adequate protein without ill effects, promoting improved nutrition and liver function. Malabsorption may result when large doses of neomycin are ingested for a week or more, but this phenomenon is clinically mild, readily reversible, and rarely seen with the use of clinically recommended dose schedules (Jacobson et al., 1960; Faloon et al., 1966; Dobbins, 1968). A neomycin-induced intestinal lactase deficiency could theoretically lead to milk intolerance (Cain et al., 1968).

Neomycin is now widely accepted as a valuable agent in the treatment of "ammonia intoxication," but because of the life-threatening nature of coma and the impressive clinical evidence that neomycin is an effective adjunct in treatment, strictly controlled studies have not been performed (Chalmers, 1968). The use of neomycin has a logical basis; it produces the desired effect on the colonic flora and leads to a reduction in blood ammonium concentrations, which is associated with clinical improvement in most instances. Whether the apparent beneficial effect is due to suppression of ammonium accumulation or of some other product is not known (Zieve, 1966). *Principle: Successful therapy, based on logical premises, does not prove the accuracy of the premises. The therapy may work for other reasons.*

Other means of reducing ammonia production in the gut include (1) the feeding of *Lactobacillus acidophilus* (Macbeth *et al.*, 1965; Read *et al.*, 1966); (2) the use of a synthetic disaccharide, lactulose, which is not hydrolyzed and reaches the colon, where its bacterial fermentation leads to changes in fecal pH and bacterial flora (Bircher *et al.*, 1966; Elkington *et al.*, 1969; Ma *et al.*, 1969; Brown *et al.*, 1971); (3) attempts to reduce bacterial urease activity by the induction of jack bean urease immunity (Thompson and Holmes, 1967); and (4) the oral administration of a highly potent and specific inhibitor of bacterial urease acetohydroxamic acid (Fishbein *et al.*, 1965; Summerskill *et al.*, 1968). The ultimate usefulness of these measures requires further study.

Methods to Lower Blood Ammonium Directly. Based on the theory that high blood concentrations of ammonium are directly toxic to the brain, attempts have been made to lower the ammonium concentration by intravenous infusions of L-arginine and glutamic acid to increase urea synthesis. Enthusiastic reports of efficacy (Walshe, 1953; Najarian and Harper, 1956) are countered by controlled studies that failed to show a beneficial effect (Alexander *et al.*, 1955; Reynolds *et al.*, 1958). Since patients with decompensated cirrhosis usually have normal or elevated plasma levels of amino acids, including arginine and glutamic acid (Wu *et al.*, 1955; Zinneman *et al.*, 1969), it seems unlikely that lack of substrate for ammonium "detoxification," rather than hepatic enzyme deficiency, is a limiting factor. This form of therapy has not been altogether successful; undesirable side effects (e.g., systemic acidosis) have been noted (Baertl and Gabuzda, 1959).

More heroic approaches to "detoxify" the blood of patients in hepatic coma have been tried. Hemodialysis or peritoneal dialysis, by correcting fluid and electrolyte disturbances and lowering urea levels, may be at least transiently beneficial. In addition, blood ammonium levels can be acutely lowered by these methods (Kiley *et al.*, 1958; Nienhuis *et al.*, 1963; Keynes, 1968). Exchange transfusions of blood or plasmapheresis recently have become popular in treating the coma of fulminant hepatitis (Trey *et al.*, 1966; Berger *et al.*, 1967; Jones *et al.*, 1967), but there is no convincing evidence that this approach results in improved survival (Reynolds, 1969). Cross-circulation with another human, a very formidable undertaking with major ethical, technical, and logistic problems, has resulted in dramatic, prompt alleviation of coma in a few patients (Burnell *et al.*, 1967). This approach is obviously not suitable for patients with presumed viral hepatitis, but an experience utilizing a baboon in cross-circulation has been reported (Bosman *et al.*, 1968). The use of isolated perfused pig or cadaver livers in extracorporeal circulation is another experimental approach (Sen *et al.*, 1966; Eiseman, 1967; Abouna *et al.*, 1969). The ultimate answer to the problem of hepatic failure may be cadaveric liver homotransplantation, but many major problems remain to be solved.

Depletion of Circulating Bile Acids: Use of Cholestyramine in Pruritus. Pruritus is a common and often disabling symptom of many hepatobiliary diseases, particularly those involving chronic cholestasis (McPhedran and Henderson, 1965). Although it has been suggested for years that increased serum and tissue concentrations of bile acids are the cause of the itching, correlations have not always been convincing (Carey, 1958; Osborn *et al.*, 1959). The availability of cholestyramine has stimulated renewed interest in this problem. Cholestyramine is an insoluble chloride salt of a basic anion-exchange resin, with a strong affinity for bile salts (cholates) in the intestine. It exchanges chlorides for cholates, forming an insoluble complex that is excreted in the feces. It complexes to varying extents with other substances, including bilirubin, steroid hormones, and drugs (Lester *et al.*, 1962; Gallo *et al.*, 1965; Sjövall and Sjövall, 1966). In adequate dosage, cholestyramine prevents the reabsorption of bile salts via the enterohepatic circulation, depletes the bile salt pool, and reduces the serum bile salt concentration. Other events might logically follow: (1) increased bile salt synthesis from cholesterol by the liver, with subsequent reduction in serum cholesterol concentration; (2) deficient micelle formation in the gut with steatorrhea; (3) decreased absorption of fat-soluble vitamins; (4) interference with the absorption of other drugs; and (5) binding of bilirubin, possibly leading to a reduction in serum bilirubin levels in some forms of jaundice

(Lottsfeldt *et al.*, 1963; Spiegel *et al.*, 1965; Datta and Sherlock, 1966; Fallon and Woods, 1968; Northcutt *et al.*, 1969).

The principal role of cholestyramine is in the management of severe pruritus, particularly that associated with primary biliary cirrhosis (Van Itallie *et al.*, 1961; Schaffner *et al.*, 1965; Datta and Sherlock, 1966). The advent of this drug was a major advance in symptomatic therapy. In most patients, refractory itching can be controlled. Dramatic resolution of skin xanthomata has occurred in some patients, presumably owing to interference with intestinal absorption of lipids and to mobilization of tissue cholesterol for accelerated bile salt synthesis (Keczkes *et al.*, 1964). Pruritus associated with other forms of chronic cholestasis can be controlled with this agent, but it is ineffective if complete biliary obstruction is present, since there is no enterohepatic circulation to interrupt. The same patterns of bile salt elevations seen in obstructive jaundice are observed in patients with pruritus of pregnancy; these patients also respond to cholestyramine, even if they do not manifest gross hyperbilirubinemia (Sjövall and Sjövall, 1966; Lutz and Margolis, 1969).

Cholestyramine has a pungent odor and is unpleasant to take; patients who are not severely distressed by their itching often refuse it. Mild intestinal symptoms, such as nausea, diarrhea, or constipation, occur often in the early stages of treatment but usually subside with continued administration. Steatorrhea has not been a significant problem, but the possibility of fat-soluble vitamin deficiency must be anticipated and prevented (Schaffner *et al.*, 1965; Datta and Sherlock, 1966; Gross and Brotman, 1970). Intestinal impaction has been attributed to the drug (Cohen *et al.*, 1969). As cholestyramine may bind other drugs given simultaneously, the interval between the administration of this drug and that of other medication should be as long as possible (Northcutt *et al.*, 1969) (see Chapter 16).

The striking relief of pruritus, associated with a sharp drop in bile acid blood concentrations, suggests a role for bile acids in pruritus. This is not convincing proof of a cause-and-effect relationship. Cholestyramine has many actions, including that of binding conjugates of steroid hormones, and the depletion of substances other than bile salts may be responsible for its remarkable antipruritic effect. *Principle: Knowledge of the mechanism of a drug action may allow greater understanding of the pathogenesis of a disease state.*

Recently another potential use for cholestyramine has been suggested (Hofmann, 1967). Patients with a diseased or surgically absent terminal ileum frequently develop significant diarrhea and steatorrhea, presumably owing to deficient reabsorption of bile salts (Hardison and Rosenberg, 1967). This troublesome diarrhea may be due mainly to a cathartic action of the unabsorbed bile salts, and treatment with cholestyramine has been suggested (Hofmann and Poley, 1969). Steatorrhea is worsened by this therapy, an undesirable response in some patients; if steatorrhea is the major abnormality, treatment with bile salts is more logical.

The development and use of cholestyramine llustrate how the application of a new drug may (1) lead to a significant new mode of therapy for a refractory clinical symptom (i.e., pruritus of cholestasis), (2) add new insight into the pathogenesis of the symptom (i.e., the role of bile acids in the production of pruritus), and (3) provide new evidence in related areas (i.e., cholesterol metabolism and the diarrhea of distal small-bowel disease).

Depletion of Excessive Tissue Iron in the Treatment of Hemochromatosis. At least four varieties of hemochromatosis may be distinguished: (1) primary or idiopathic; (2) that associated with chronic anemia, particularly when erythroid hyperplasia is present; (3) that following cirrhosis; and (4) that produced by excessive iron intake, as in the Bantus (Kent and Popper, 1968). In most forms of hemochromatosis, iron accumulation in the liver and other tissues precedes the development of significant tissue damage (i.e., cirrhosis), but the exact relationship between parenchymal iron overload and tissue damage is unclear. While cirrhosis has not been induced in experimental animals by iron overloading per se, iron loading potentiates liver damage when another toxic factor, such as carbon tetrachloride or ethionine, is added, or when a deficient diet coexists (Goldberg and Smith, 1960; MacDonald, 1960; Kent *et al.*, 1964). It has not been disproved that iron per se is toxic, since the long-term animal experiments that would mimic the situation in patients are virtually impossible to perform. An attempt to remove the excessive iron is considered essential in the therapy of this syndrome. Patients with fully developed hemochromatosis have a total body iron in excess of normals by 15 to 40 g. An effort to remove this surplus iron from the tissues must be vigorous enough to reduce iron by 0.5 g per week. Phlebotomy is the only practical method currently available to accomplish this goal. Since a pint of whole blood contains approximately 250 mg of iron, one to three phlebotomies per week deplete iron by 10 to 30 g in a year. A program of serial phlebotomies, carried out for months or years, has resulted in apparent clinical and biochemical improvement in many patients (Grosberg, 1961; Brody and McKenzie, 1962; Duffy and Meister, 1963; Block *et al.*, 1965; Knauer *et al.*, 1965; Weintraub *et al.*, 1966). Patients so treated must be followed closely, with monitoring of hemoglobin and serum albumin concentrations. After a suitable interval, serial liver biopsies are probably the best indicator of response to therapy. Despite many enthusiastic reports of improved liver structure and function, better diabetic control, and a happier patient, no critical evaluation of therapy with appropriate controls has been reported. A program of serial phlebotomies leads to a close patient-physician relationship and requires patients with good motivation and willingness to cooperate in a dramatic, painful, time-consuming form of therapy. These factors might lead to a more effective treatment regimen in such matters as diet, diabetic control, and abstinence from alcohol and may result in clinical improvement (MacDonald, 1964). *Principle: Selection of patients for an intensive form of therapy often leads to differences in ancillary measures that must be considered in evaluating the result* (see Chapter 1).

Some patients with hemochromatosis cannot tolerate a program of repeated phlebotomies. Patients with advanced cirrhosis and hypoalbuminemia may not tolerate the loss of protein; patients with chronic anemia are not amenable to this approach. Efforts have been made to develop an effective means of treating such patients with iron-chelating agents, such as desferrioxamine B and diethylenetriaminepentaacetic acid (Moeschlin and Schnider, 1963; Hwang and Brown, 1964). Although significant mobilization and excretion of parenchymal iron can be achieved with these drugs, the quantities of iron removed are considerably less than those achieved by frequent phlebotomies: the equivalent of 1 to 2 pt of blood per month. In addition, these agents must be given parenterally and daily. The acute increase in urinary iron excretion produced by these drugs has also been utilized as a diagnostic test of parenchymal iron overload (Lloyd *et al.*, 1964; Walsh *et al.*, 1964; Harker *et al.*, 1968; Smith *et al.*, 1969). *Principle: A therapeutic effect can have diagnostic implications.*

In summary, patients with hemochromatosis have both excessive tissue iron deposits and tissue damage (in liver, pancreas, heart, etc.), and the iron may, in some unknown way, contribute to or potentiate the tissue damage. Therapeutic attempts to remove the excessive iron deposits are logical. This goal of therapy can be achieved quickly with phlebotomies, more slowly with iron-chelating drugs. The effect of the depletion of excess tissue iron on the clinical status and longevity of the patient remains to be critically appraised.

Depletion of Excessive Tissue Copper in the Treatment of Wilson's Disease. Wilson's disease (hepatolenticular degeneration) is a rare disorder characterized by accumulation of copper in various tissues and by variable clinical manifestations, which usually reflect degeneration of the central nervous system and the liver. It is an autosomal, recessively inherited disease, and about 1 in 200 of the general population is heterozygous for the abnormal gene (Sternlieb and Scheinberg, 1968). A deficiency in ceruloplasmin, an alpha-2-globulin that normally binds serum copper and probably plays a crucial role in the regulation of copper metabolism, is found in 95% of cases. The exact pathophysiology of Wilson's disease is unknown, but presumably the disorder in copper metabolism is primary and induces tissue damage by interference with tissue enzymes (Bearn, 1966). The histopathology of the liver is characteristic, especially in the early stages, but not specific (Scheinberg and Sternlieb, 1959; Anderson and Popper, 1960; Silverberg and Gellis, 1962; Levi *et al.*, 1967). The central nervous system manifestations and histopathology closely mimic other types of chronic liver disease with encephalopathy (with or without portal systemic shunts) (Victor *et al.*, 1964; Popoff *et al.*, 1965), thus raising questions about the presumed toxic action of copper.

The use of penicillamine (beta,beta-dimethylcysteine) has generated great interest in the therapy and etiology of Wilson's disease. Penicillamine is a chelating agent that can bind tissue copper and induce significant urinary copper excretion. When it is combined with a low-copper diet, a prolonged negative copper balance can be achieved. Administered over long periods, with the dosage adjusted to ensure continued urinary copper excretion of at least 1 mg per day, this agent leads to improvement in most patients (Sternlieb and Scheinberg, 1964). The neurologic manifestations are more likely than the hepatic to respond dramatically, but improvement is sometimes noted in the latter as well (Denny-Brown, 1964). As penicillamine is toxic, producing a variety of undesirable side effects, close observation during treatment is required. Periodic assays of urinary copper excretion are also necessary to ensure that the drug is accomplishing its desired effect, since some patients become refractory with time. The benefit of this therapy is still questionable because no controlled studies have been reported. The apparent effectiveness of copper depletion therapy in some patients with this disease and the poor prognosis of the untreated patient make it unlikely that a critical controlled study will be done. This quandary has been discussed in relation to the prophylactic use of penicillamine in asymptomatic patients (Editorial, 1968; Sternlieb and Scheinberg, 1968). The theory that excessive copper is "toxic" in this disease is only a working hypothesis, but is supported by considerable evidence, particularly the clinical experience with penicillamine. *Principle: Carefully gleaned clinical experience may justify the use of a drug despite incomplete information regarding its pharmacologic effects and the pathogenesis of the disorder being treated* (see Chapter 1).

Replacement of a Deficient Substance

Bile Salt Therapy. Bile salts normally play a major role in fat digestion by creating a micellar suspension of the products of pancreatic enzymatic lipolysis (Hofmann, 1965). The liver forms the primary bile acids, cholic acid and chenodeoxycholic acid, from cholesterol and secretes them into the bile as glycine and taurine conjugates. Deoxycholic acid, a secondary bile acid, is a bacterial metabolite of cholic acid that is reabsorbed and then re-excreted by the liver. Similarly, chenodeoxycholic acid may be converted to lithocholic acid by intestinal bacteria and recirculated via the enterohepatic circulation (Van Itallie and Hashim, 1963). The maintenance of a bile salt pool sufficient for normal fat absorption depends upon an efficient enterohepatic circulation, for 90 to 95% of bile salts excreted in the bile each day are reabsorbed, predominantly in the terminal ileum (Heaton et al., 1968). Bile salts are also major determinants of the rate and volume of bile flow (Wheeler, 1961; Javitt, 1969).

Intraluminal bile salts may be deficient in any disorder associated with (1) decreased hepatic production, (2) obstruction (intrahepatic or extrahepatic) of the flow of bile, (3) diversion of the bile (as in biliary fistula or T-tube drainage of bile duct), or (4) interference with reabsorption via the enterohepatic circulation. Theoretically, oral administration of bile salts may overcome any intraluminal deficiency present in patients with chronic liver disease (particularly of the cholestatic type) (Atkinson et al., 1956), or with diversion of the bile to the outside (DePalma et al., 1967), thus promoting better fat absorption and nutrition. Unfortunately, there are no critical studies of this form of therapy. Studies of the steatorrhea that follows resection of the terminal ileum have demonstrated a bile salt deficiency (secondary to interruption of the enterohepatic circulation), and administration of taurocholate has decreased fat malabsorption (Hardison and Rosen-

berg, 1967). The total bile salt pool is about 4 g, and it "turns over" as often as twice during a single meal! Therefore, if replacement therapy is to be effective, large doses of bile salts must be ingested, often resulting in distressing diarrhea. There is little justification for the small doses of bile salts, often combined with similarly inadequate quantities of pancreatic enzymes, contained in many commercial preparations.

Although not strictly replacement therapy, bile salts have also been used to promote increased bile flow in patients with infection of the biliary tree or with multiple small common-duct stones without jaundice (Harvey, 1965). The theoretic aim of therapy is to "wash out" the small stones or infectious exudate by the choleretic effect of bile salts. In some cases bile salts exert a bacteriostatic effect and may lyse pneumococci (Goodman and Gilman, 1970). Bile salts may be utilized to alter favorably the phospholipid/cholesterol ratio in bile of patients with gallstones (Swell and Bell, 1968). The goal in this instance is to increase cholesterol solubility and to prevent or dissolve the stones. There is good evidence both in dogs (Schmidt et al., 1938) and in man (Swell and Bell, 1968; Thistle and Schoenfield, 1971) that oral administration of conjugated bile salts increases bile concentration of bile acids, phospholipids, and cholesterol, especially the former two. In contrast, administration of dehydrocholic acid (the oxidized, unconjugated bile acid) leads to hydrocholeresis and produces a relatively large quantity of bile low in total solids and viscosity. Secretin and other choleretics have been utilized, with similar effects (Grossman et al., 1949; Schwartz, 1962; Waitman et al., 1969). Theoretically, one might use one of the hydrocholeretics to achieve increased flows of more dilute bile when treating common bile duct "gravel." The administration of conjugated bile salts in this setting might increase bile flow, but the viscosity of the bile would also increase, for the effect on bile flow is due to the absorption and biliary excretion of the administered bile salts (Ivy, 1944). However, if the goal were to increase the solubility of cholesterol in bile, administration of the conjugated bile salts would be preferable. These considerations of bile salt therapy in biliary tract disorders are highly theoretic. Despite a surfeit of commercially available bile salt–containing drugs, no critical studies assessing their clinical application have been published. *Principle: Theoretically sound applications of drug therapy require scientifically controlled observations for documentation of a therapeutic effect.* Because certain secondary bile acids can produce liver damage in experimental animals (Palmer and Hruban, 1966), and as most commercial bile salt preparations contain animal bile salts about which little is known, these drugs should not be used freely.

Albumin Infusions. Patients with cirrhosis and ascites usually have low serum albumin concentrations, owing to decreased synthesis by the liver and to the dilutional effect of peripheral edema and ascites. Although other factors may be involved in some cases, portal hypertension and plasma colloid osmotic pressure are the major determinants of ascites formation in cirrhosis (Atkinson and Losowsky, 1961). The higher the portal pressure and the lower the serum albumin concentration (the major determinant of colloid osmotic pressure), the more persistent and refractory ascites tends to be. Although subsidence of liver inflammation and/ or infiltration may lead to a decrease in portal hypertension in some cases, the elevated pressure in advanced cirrhosis is difficult to alter except by surgical means. Most efforts have been directed at correcting the serum albumin deficit as a means of treating ascites (Faloon et al., 1949; Post et al., 1951). When large amounts of salt-poor albumin are given intravenously for a few weeks, serum albumin concentration can be effectively increased and maintained with continued periodic infusions (Wilkinson and Sherlock, 1962). Ascitic fluid albumin also increases, for it is in equilibrium with the serum albumin. In some patients, especially those with relatively mild degrees of portal hypertension, drug-induced diuresis may be potentiated by this approach (Losowsky and Atkinson, 1961; Vlahcevic et al., 1967). The treatment has dangers, however, especially the frequent precipitation of bleeding from esophageal varices (Faloon et al., 1949; Havens and Bluemle, 1950; Post et al., 1951). In addition, some patients develop even more ascites. This very expensive form of therapy has produced no significant long-term benefit, and the development of more potent diuretics has largely obviated its usefulness. The same may be said for utilization of intravenous infusions of autologous ascitic fluid, an attempt to accomplish the same end by less expensive means (Britton and Nakamoto, 1960; Yamahiro and Reynolds, 1961; Kaisei, 1962).

The use of albumin or ascitic fluid infusions has been studied in the management of the "hepatorenal syndrome." In its pure form, this syndrome consists of progressive (and usually fatal) renal failure due to severe hepatic decompensation, usually with jaundice and ascites. Renal failure is not the result of obstruction, infection, acute tubular necrosis, or other detectable causes (Eisner and Levitt, 1961); the basic defect appears to be functional rather than structural (Koppel et al., 1969). Such patients usually have a normal or high cardiac output, normal or supernormal blood volume, decreasing renal plasma flow and glomerular filtration rate, and good tubular function with preservation of urinary concentrating ability (Baldus et al., 1964a, 1964b; Shear et al., 1965). The progressive azotemia is related to decreased "effective" renal perfusion, and because these patients exhibit altered hemodynamics with decreased peripheral resistance (Lancestremere et al., 1962) but increased renal vascular resistance, expansion of the plasma volume may improve renal perfusion. The results of this approach have been discouraging. Although rare patients respond with a rise in urine output and a decrease in azotemia, the effect is generally transient and the almost uniformly fatal outcome is only delayed (Reynolds et al., 1967; Tristani and Cohn, 1967). Patients with low or normal blood volumes are more likely to respond. If, indeed, there is a decrease in "effective plasma volume" in patients with normal or high blood volumes, this defect is not readily correctable simply by further volume expansion. Other more important pathogenetic factors (particularly alterations in intrarenal hemodynamics) will probably be defined before this syndrome is understood and hence amenable to therapy (Papper and Vaamonde, 1968). *Principle: Effective therapy must often await elucidation of the pathophysiology of the disorder.*

Miscellaneous Replacement Therapy. Most patients with alcoholic liver disease are not underweight (as 1 oz of ethanol contains 150 kcal), but their protein intake is usually inadequate and B-complex vitamins are often depleted (Leevy et al., 1965). Routine administration of these vitamins seems appropriate in these patients, although in the absence of overt clinical evidence of specific deficiencies such therapy is probably not of major importance. Because of the experimental evidence in rats that alcohol increases choline requirements (Klatskin et al., 1954), administration of lipotropic agents, such as choline and methionine, has been advocated in the treatment of alcoholic cirrhosis (Cayer, 1947; Cayer and Cornatzer, 1950). There is no evidence, however, that deficiency of these substances is important in the pathogenesis of clinical liver disease or that their administration is beneficial (Gabuzda et al., 1950). Some degree of steatorrhea is often present in many forms of biliary tract disease (Barona et al., 1962; Linscheer et al., 1966; Losowsky and Walker, 1969), resulting in depleted body stores of fat-soluble vitamins, particularly vitamins D and K. Parenteral vitamin D therapy may be especially important in patients with prolonged cholestasis, such as that due to primary biliary cirrhosis. However, this approach does not forestall the bone abnormalities that complicate that disease, although calcium absorption is improved (Kehayoglou *et al.*, 1968). Parenteral administration of vitamin K is designed to correct deficiencies in factors VII, IX, and X and in prothrombin, which may result from (1) inadequate bacterial production of vitamin K in the intestinal lumen (as during administration of antibiotics, including neomycin), (2) steatorrhea (as that stemming from deficiency in bile salt excretion), or (3) impaired liver function. Parenteral vitamin K corrects the deficiency so long as liver function remains relatively intact. The response to vitamin K is usually rapid, occurring within 12 hours. In advanced parenchymal liver disease, the liver is unable to utilize the supplemental vitamin to produce the deficient clotting factors. The prothrombin time may actually worsen in severe liver disease, for reasons yet unclear (Unger and Shapiro, 1948; Finkel, 1961; Douvres, 1965). The paradoxical depression of prothrombin time sometimes seen in patients with advanced liver disease prohibits continued administration of vitamin K to such patients (Steigmann *et al.*, 1959). *Principle: Observe the effect of a drug on specific objectives; too much of a good thing may be detrimental.*

Prophylactic Measures in Liver Disease

Gamma Globulin in the "Prevention" of Viral Hepatitis. Immune gamma globulin, when given soon after exposure to infected material, greatly reduces the incidence of subsequent *clinically apparent* infectious hepatitis (Krugman *et al.*, 1960). Because the antibody content of gamma globulin varies according to the immune status of the donor, it is not possible to recommend an ideal or standard prophylactic dose. In general, the larger the dose, the longer the protection lasts. For short-term exposures, administration of 0.01 to 0.02 ml/lb, preferably within a few days of exposure, is recommended (Krugman, 1963; Grady, 1968). A larger dose of 0.06 ml/lb is recommended for pregnant or postmenopausal females, individuals subjected to prolonged or continuous exposure in highly endemic areas, and patients with pre-existing hepatic disease. *Principles: (1) Both stool and blood of patients with infectious hepatitis are maximally infectious during the prodromal or preicteric phase, and most patients are no longer infectious 2 to 3 weeks after the onset of jaundice. (2) The earlier the prophylaxis after exposure, the more likely solid prophylaxis will ensue. (3) Gamma globulin does not prevent but, rather, attenuates, the illness in exposed persons.* The

evidence that gamma globulin in large doses reduces the incidence of post-transfusion viral hepatitis is still conflicting and inconclusive (Mirick *et al.*, 1965; Holland *et al.*, 1966; Grady and Bennett, 1970). Rapidly developing research regarding the "Australia antigen" may lead to early revision of these concepts.

Use of Mannitol in Surgical Patients with Obstructive Jaundice. Severe degrees of jaundice in the surgical patient may predispose in some way to hypotension and/or postoperative renal failure. (This observation probably led to an erroneous concept of a hepatorenal syndrome due to a "toxic" effect of the bile pigment on the renal tubules.) Additional evidence in experimental animals and man has elucidated this association. Patients undergoing surgery for obstructive jaundice have an unusually high incidence of postoperative renal failure (Williams *et al.*, 1960; Dawson, 1968). The renal defect resembles that of acute tubular necrosis, and its pathogenesis may be due to a relative hypovolemia, perhaps due to the action of some retained bile constituent on tubular function, leading to an inappropriate natriuresis and to increased renal salt and water losses (Topuzlu and Stahl, 1966). Whatever the mechanism, preliminary evidence indicates that mannitol has a protective effect (Dawson, 1968). Interest in mannitol therapy should not lead the physician to ignore the patient's hydration status and blood volume. Although the value of mannitol in the routine management of icteric patients undergoing surgery is not proved, it may be advisable to start intensely jaundiced patients on mannitol infusions before surgery and to continue therapy for at least 48 hours afterward (Editorial, 1968).

Miscellaneous Therapy in Liver Disease

Use of Anabolic Steroids in the Treatment of Chronic Liver Disease. Testosterone and some of its synthetic analogs have been used as anabolic agents in the management of several chronic wasting diseases to improve appetite, promote positive nitrogen balance, and increase protein synthesis. Alcoholic liver disease is often associated with severe nutritional deficiencies, and anabolic steroids have been advocated in its treatment for over 2 decades. Prolonged use of these agents promotes positive nitrogen balance in such patients (Gabuzda *et al.*, 1950; Grossman and Yalow, 1965). However, this form of treatment has not been proved to lead to more rapid clinical and histologic improvement than do alcohol withdrawal and diet alone. Alcoholic patients with extensive noncirrhotic fatty metamorphosis (and only mild functional abnormalities) can be "defatted" more rapidly when treated with anabolic steroids (Jabbari and Leevy, 1967; Mendenhall, 1968). This effect may result from increased lipoprotein synthesis, allowing more rapid removal of hepatic fat. The only well-controlled study of the effects of short-term anabolic steroid therapy in patients with advanced decompensated Laennec's cirrhosis failed to show a beneficial effect on either liver function or histology (Fenster, 1966). On the basis of the evidence at hand, it may be reasonable to administer anabolic steroids to malnourished alcoholics with fatty livers to speed reconstitution of normal liver architecture. Whether long-term treatment of patients with alcoholic cirrhosis is clinically beneficial remains to be demonstrated. C-17-substituted analogs of testosterone frequently impair biliary secretion, leading to bromsulfophthalein (BSP) retention in many cases and occasionally to frank jaundice. To avoid confusion in the management of such patients, testosterone propionate is the agent of choice, even though it must be administered parenterally.

Adrenocortical Steroids in the Management of Liver Disease. Corticosteroids are widely used in the treatment of liver disorders. Unfortunately, almost no adequately controlled studies of their effects have been conducted (Goldgraber and Kirsner, 1959). Rationales for their use include (1) many active parenchymal liver diseases are inflammatory disorders, and adrenal steroids are "anti-inflammatory"; and (2) patients with active liver disease usually have elevated serum immune globulin levels and increased hepatic gamma globulin production (Cohen et al., 1960). These observations, plus certain clinical features of "autoimmune" disorders, suggest that immune factors may play a role in the perpetuation and progression of certain types of chronic liver disease (MacKay and Wood, 1961; Gelzayd and Kirsner, 1967; Doniach and Walker, 1969). Hepatic conjugation of hydrocortisone may be impaired in liver disease, but serum levels are generally normal (Brown and Englert, 1961). Pituitary suppression may occur in some patients, owing to slow conjugation that leads to high free-cortisol levels (Tucci and Martin, 1966).

Although steroid therapy may lead to a more rapid clinical and biochemical recovery in acute benign viral hepatitis, the incidence of relapse is increased (Evans et al., 1953). Treatment is not justified in routine cases. Although steroids have been strongly advocated in fulminant viral hepatitis with precoma or coma (Katz et al., 1962), their administration has not been proved

to save lives in this highly lethal condition. Occasionally, patients have shown such dramatic improvement that many physicians are convinced of the beneficial effect of these drugs. *Principle: It is difficult to decide on the basis of present evidence whether some severely ill patients do respond to steroids, or whether they "respond" because the disease is in fact not so severe. The use of steroids in this setting may be justified on the basis of "games theory"; that is, what is the outcome if the physician fails to give a potentially therapeutic agent in an otherwise potentially fatal disease? This decision-making process is much less rational, but sometimes operationally justifiable in therapeutics.*

Patients with viral hepatitis-induced subacute hepatic necrosis (Tisdale, 1966) have a severe histologic lesion and tend to have a prolonged clinical course, with the eventual development of cirrhosis in a significant percentage of cases (Boyer and Klatskin, 1970). The term "chronic active hepatitis" is used loosely, but generally refers to patients with continuing clinical and histologic evidence of "smoldering" hepatitis lasting many months or years, with the eventual development of postnecrotic cirrhosis. Many of these patients are young females with "rheumatic" clinical features and very high serum gamma globulin concentrations. In subacute necrosis and "chronic active hepatitis," steroid therapy has been widely considered (Page and Good, 1960; Kern et al., 1963; Mistilis and Schiff, 1964; Cook et al., 1968). Most hepatologists feel that corticosteroids are of definite value, since clinical and functional improvement usually results. However, there is no convincing evidence that the underlying lesion is influenced favorably, or that the eventual outcome is altered (Vakil et al., 1965). Corticosteroids, when used, should be started in large doses (e.g., 30 to 60 mg of prednisone per day) and tapered in a stepwise manner with careful monitoring of liver function tests. The aim is to taper to the lowest dosage compatible with continued improvement or control, hopefully in the range of 10 to 20 mg of prednisone per day. As in other steroid-treated chronic disorders, the complications of therapy may become more distressing than the primary disease (Jacobs, 1963).

There is less theoretic justification for corticosteroid therapy in alcoholic liver disease. Two recent controlled studies of alcoholic hepatitis suggested possible benefits in the most critically ill patients (Helman et al., 1971; Porter et al., 1971). Some patients with primary biliary cirrhosis appear to respond temporarily to steroid therapy (Carman and Giansiracusa, 1955). Two studies of chronic steroid treatment in cirrhosis of mixed etiology showed conflicting results (Wells, 1960; Copenhagen Study Group, 1969). Sarcoidosis with clinically significant liver involvement (sometimes progressing to granulomatous cirrhosis) is an accepted indication for steroid therapy. Drug-induced hepatitis, especially that due to hypersensitivity, may respond well to steroid therapy, but results have been variable.

Corticosteroids are widely used in the treatment of active liver disease, particularly subacute hepatic necrosis and chronic active hepatitis. In the latter disorders, such treatment effectively suppresses the clinical and laboratory manifestations of active disease, but it has not been proved to have a beneficial effect on the underlying histopathology. Controlled studies adequate for a definitive evaluation are still lacking.

Use of Corticosteroids as a Diagnostic Test. A few patients with presumed viral hepatitis have laboratory and histologic features that are not diagnostic of acute parenchymal disease but suggest extrahepatic biliary obstruction. This "cholangiolitic" or "cholestatic" hepatitis may be difficult to manage since laparotomy is the only definitive way of reaching a diagnosis, a step best avoided if hepatitis is present. Because most patients with acute viral hepatitis respond to adrenal steroid therapy with a fairly sharp decline in jaundice, a steroid trial of 5 to 8 days may be a useful diagnostic test in problem cases (Summerskill et al., 1961; Pruzanski, 1966; Wruble et al., 1966). The following principles apply to this approach to differential diagnosis: (1) a dose equivalent to 30 to 60 mg of prednisone should be used; (2) patients with complete extrahepatic obstructive jaundice often show some decline in jaundice (Katz et al., 1957); (3) a fall in bilirubin concentration of at least 40% is required for the presumptive diagnosis of hepatitis; (4) this test is intended only to distinguish viral (not drug) hepatitis from extrahepatic obstruction; (5) this approach is probably useful only when moderate-to-marked degrees of jaundice are present; and (6) the test is most helpful when a positive response occurs, for lack of response does not exclude hepatitis. The mechanism of the reduction of serum bilirubin in response to steroid administration is obscure, for reduction may occur without associated changes in fecal or urinary urobilinogen, urinary bilirubin, or rate of red-cell breakdown (Williams and Billing, 1961; Aach, 1969). A steroid trial is an empiric test of limited diagnostic value. If the patient responds, the steroids may be tapered slowly. If the test is negative, the steroids may be stopped. Pituitary-adrenal suppression is not expected after such short-term therapy;

however, if the patient requires surgery, the remote possibility of transient adrenal insufficiency should be kept in mind. *Principle: A single drug may have many effects; thus, steroids used as a diagnostic test could suppress adrenal function critical to survival during a surgical procedure prompted by the result of the original test.*

Use of "Immunosuppressive" Therapy in Liver Disease. Immune mechanisms may play a role in the initiation and/or perpetuation of certain types of chronic liver injury (MacKay and Wood, 1961). The evidence for this role is largely indirect. For example, circulating antibodies or cell-mediated immune mechanisms have not been shown conclusively to initiate human hepatic injury (Gelzayd and Kirsner, 1967). A better case can be made for the possible role of antigen-antibody complexes in the perpetuation of liver injury (Popper et al., 1965a). The clinical and serologic features of "chronic active" hepatitis suggest that "autoimmune" factors are involved. This concept has led to the use of the purine analog 6-mercaptopurine and its derivative azathioprine (Imuran) in therapy. The original rationale for the use of these agents in liver disease was that of "immunosuppression." Uncontrolled experiences with moderate doses indicated an apparent beneficial effect in many patients (MacKay et al., 1964; Page et al., 1964; Geenen et al., 1966; MacKay, 1968). However, immune responses and immune globulin levels were usually unaffected, even in those patients who seemed to benefit. When doses of 1.0 to 2.0 mg/kg of body weight were utilized, there was a high incidence of bone marrow suppression and initial worsening of jaundice, with occasional fatal results (Krawitt et al., 1967). Recent evidence indicates that smaller doses of these agents (0.5 to 1.0 mg/kg) may be effective, while avoiding the toxic reactions complicating higher doses (Mistilis and Blackburn, 1967; Sjöberg and Welin, 1967). As patients with severe active liver disease may be very sensitive even to these low doses, it is wise to begin therapy with very small amounts, gradually increasing the dose until a desired effect is achieved. Frequent blood counts and liver function tests must be obtained during therapy.

At present, 6-mercaptopurine and azathioprine appear to be useful in the treatment of certain types of chronic active liver disease, although no controlled experiences prove this contention. A trial of one of these drugs seems indicated in patients who are refractory to corticosteroids, or in whom the complications of steroid therapy are disabling. If such therapy is truly effective, the reasons are obscure. In addition to possible effects on immune mechanisms, these agents may have important anti-inflammatory properties or inhibitory effects on virus replication. *Principle: The "name" or "type" of a drug does not necessarily reflect its in vivo pharmacologic effect at all doses, its mode of action or toxicity in a given disease state, or its desirability in the treatment of a disorder with a poorly defined pathogenesis.*

Use of Vasopressin in the Treatment of Bleeding Esophageal Varices. Massive upper intestinal bleeding in a patient with cirrhosis may be due to a variety of lesions, including peptic ulcer, esophagogastritis, esophageal laceration, and esophageal varices. When esophageal varices are the cause of hemorrhage, the mortality is at least 50% in patients with alcoholic cirrhosis and is formidable in those with other types as well. In addition to transfusions and supportive care, the Sengstaken-Blakemore tube has traditionally been used in such patients to tamponade the bleeding veins. However, the excessive mortality associated with its use has led to its abandonment in many centers and to reliance on the use of vasopressin (Conn and Simpson, 1967). Vasopressin (Pitressin) is a purified preparation of antidiuretic hormone separated from oxytocic hormone, one vial containing 20 pressor units. When 20 units are diluted in 20 to 100 ml of saline or dextrose/water and injected intravenously over 10 to 30 minutes, the portal pressure decreases by an average of 39 to 46% (Shaldon and Sherlock, 1960; Shaldon et al., 1961). This effect is due largely to preportal splanchnic arteriolar constriction, with an associated decrease in blood flow to the abdominal organs and a fall in portal venous return. The effect is not specific for the splanchnic circulation, and generalized vasoconstriction occurs (including the coronary bed). Stimulation of smooth muscle by vasopressin leads to intestinal colic, bowel evacuation, and pallor in most patients. This therapy is dangerous, and coronary thrombosis or mesenteric infarction has been precipitated in some patients. In addition, the decrease in hepatic blood flow is undesirable. However, the life-threatening nature of bleeding varices, particularly in alcoholic cirrhotics, appears to justify the risks if such therapy is effective. *Principle: A toxic drug may be justified in a life-threatening clinical setting, if the potential benefit is sufficiently great.*

The use of vasopressin is based on the premise that prolonged reduction of pressure in the bleeding varices will lead to clotting and hemostasis. This goal can be accomplished in a high proportion of cases, as demonstrated by a double-blind, controlled study (Merigan et al., 1962). The major therapeutic problem has been the high frequency of recurrent bleeding after the effect of the drug has dissipated in 30 to 60 minutes. This relapse rate has led to recommendations that serial courses be given, even when the bleeding has apparently stopped (Conn and Dalessio, 1962; Conn and Simpson, 1968). *Principles: (1) Electrocardiographic monitoring is mandatory during the use of vasopressin. (2) Pharmacologic activity may be absent in some instances, and unless the patient shows some evidence of a drug effect (pallor, abdominal colic, defecation, etc.) it is wise to try a different supply of drug (one must have evidence of drug action before evaluating its clinical effect)* (Sherlock, 1964). *(3) Vasopressin should never be injected directly into the vein without prior dilution, and its infusion should never take less than 10 minutes. (4) If bleeding continues after one course, a second course using a maximum of 40 units is indicated; tachyphylaxis is said not to occur* (Heimburger et al., 1960). *(5) Cessation of bleeding after vasopressin therapy does not prove that varices were the source.* Some authors have suggested the use of this agent in other types of upper intestinal bleeding or to provide a more bloodless operative field, because of the decrease in blood flow to all abdominal organs (Shaldon et al., 1961; Delaney et al., 1966). However, the drug's pressor effect may aggravate bleeding from an artery at the base of a peptic ulcer.

Vasopressin appears to be a simple and useful mode of therapy in the management of a difficult and often lethal condition. Its use is based on the pathophysiologic principle that bleeding from varices is related in part to high portal pressure. Vasopressin accomplishes the desired pharmacologic effect; that is, it lowers portal pressure acutely and significantly. Still more important, it is effective in stopping the massive bleeding from esophageal varices. Survival rate in these patients is limited by the high rate of recurrent bleeding and the nature of the underlying liver disease.

Enzyme Induction and the Treatment of Hepatic Disorders. The phenomenon of enzyme induction in the liver and its pharmacologic implications have attracted increasing interest in recent years. The activities of drug-metabolizing enzymes in liver microsomes can be markedly enhanced when animals are treated with various drugs, hormones, insecticides, and carcinogens (Conney, 1967; Kappas and Song, 1968). More than 200 such agents, including many commonly used drugs, have this effect. This is a relatively new and exciting area of study, with tremendous implications for clinical pharmacology. Enzyme induction was first applied therapeutically in the treatment of congenital unconjugated hyperbilirubinemia. Serum unconjugated bilirubin is normally converted to bilirubin diglucuronide in liver microsomes by the enzyme glucuronyl transferase, an essential step prior to its excretion in bile. Theoretically, the induction of increased transferase activity could promote more rapid conjugation and excretion of bilirubin, thus lowering serum bilirubin levels. Phenobarbital, when administered chronically in low doses, does indeed cause a lowering of serum bilirubin concentration in several types of chronic unconjugated hyperbilirubinemia (Yaffee et al., 1966; Crigler et al., 1967; Kreek and Sleisenger, 1968; Whelton et al., 1968b). Treatment of pregnant women in the last few weeks of pregnancy decreases the concentration of bilirubin in the neonate, a potentially useful form of therapy in the prevention of kernicterus (Maurer et al., 1968; Trolle, 1968; Ramboer et al., 1969). Phenobarbital administration also decreases serum bilirubin concentrations in chronic intrahepatic cholestasis (Thompson and Williams, 1967).

Although phenobarbital therapy lowers the serum bilirubin level in patients with several different hepatic disorders, the evidence that it does so by enzyme induction in man is still indirect, and different mechanisms may be equally important (Klaassen and Plaa, 1968). For example, phenobarbital may accelerate the production of enzymes responsible for bilirubin catabolism or it may affect the hepatic uptake of bilirubin. In rats, phenobarbital enhances the biliary excretion of indocyanin green, which is not biotransformed prior to excretion (Klaassen and Plaa, 1968). Reliable determinations of glucuronyl transferase activity, which are needed to demonstrate enzyme induction, are difficult to perform on liver specimens obtained by needle biopsy. Whatever the mechanisms involved, the study of drug-enzyme interactions promises to lead to important, perhaps innovative, developments in clinical pharmacology (Thompson et al., 1969). *Principle: Consistent questioning of a concept in drug therapy does not alter the therapeutic usefulness of a proved drug but may allow development of more specific drugs as well as elucidation of both basic mechanisms of disease and new concepts in therapeutics.*

ADDITIONAL TOPICS THAT ILLUSTRATE PRINCIPLES OF THERAPY

Antibiotics and Cholangitis

Suppurative infections of the biliary system (cholangitis) are usually surgical problems, for mechanical obstruction is present in most cases. However, antibiotic therapy may be vital in preventing bacteremia, in controlling the progression of infection while planning surgical intervention, or in instances when surgery is impossible or inadvisable. What should dictate the choice of an antibiotic for the treatment of such a patient? As always, the first consideration is the nature of the organism proved or suspected to be present. This dictates the use of an antibiotic with a suitable spectrum of activity. Given the fact that several antibiotics are appropriate, excretion of the active drug in bile may be critical. In theory, higher concentrations of antibiotic can be achieved at the site of infection by this route than can be delivered via the blood (with secondary diffusion into the bile duct or gallbladder). There are few studies of biliary excretion of antibiotics in man (Pulaski and Fusillo, 1955; Twiss et al., 1956; Kunin and Finland, 1959; Preston et al., 1959, 1960; Hammond and Griffiths, 1961; Ayliffe and Davies, 1965; Khan and Scott, 1967; Acocella et al., 1968; Mortimer et al., 1969), but three tentative principles may be stated. *Tentative Principles: (1) Drugs that are normally concentrated in the liver may be absent, or present in greatly reduced concentrations in the bile, when severe liver functional impairment is present* (Brette et al., 1965; Weinstein and Dalton, 1968). *(2) The concentration of antibiotics in bile is low in patients with obstructive jaundice* (Mortimer et al., 1969). *(3) The selective excretion and concentration of an antibiotic in bile probably result in relatively lower serum and tissue levels.* Antibiotics that are excreted in man in potentially effective concentrations in bile include the tetracyclines, the synthetic penicillins (especially alpha-amino-benzylpenicillin [ampicillin]), and the rifamycins. Thus, it is reasonable to consider one of these drugs in the treatment of selected patients with cholangitis if the antimicrobial spectrum is appropriate for the suspected pathogen. This consideration is paramount. *Principle: Drug availability at the desired site of action may be altered, that is, increased or decreased, by the primary disease state; this must be considered before selection of a therapeutic agent.*

Dietary Therapy

The importance of dietary manipulations in the treatment of various liver diseases has generally been overemphasized. In most instances, only a well-balanced, nutritionally adequate diet is required. In a few circumstances, however, specific diets are important. Patients with fluid retention require sodium restriction. In such cases, salt substitutes are sometimes valuable to ensure a palatable diet. A high-protein diet may shorten the duration of illness in infectious hepatitis (Chalmers et al., 1955). In the treatment of hepatic failure with coma, the infusion of 20% glucose into the vena cava has been recommended, but there is no proof of its efficacy. Patients with encephalopathy should be treated with protein withdrawal, at least initially, with the following considerations: (1) as prolonged complete protein deprivation is incompatible with histologic improvement in patients with alcoholic liver disease, the period of radical protein restriction should be as brief as possible; (2) the addition of small doses of neomycin often permits increased protein intake without precipitating encephalopathy; (3) some patients demonstrate a "liver flap" or asterixis for weeks at a time without other evidence of progressive hepatic encephalopathy, and they should not be arbitrarily subjected to severe protein restriction; and (4) treatment of a new patient with liver failure should begin with a moderately reduced protein intake (such as 30 or 40 g), and the intake should be increased as the patient's tolerance is determined. Great differences in protein tolerance exist among patients with the same degree of hepatic failure, and therapy in each case must be individualized.

In the treatment of severe alcoholic cirrhosis in which malnutrition is often present, certain principles apply. *Principles: (1) Clinical, but not histologic, improvement may occur when alcohol abstinence is combined with severe protein restriction and negative nitrogen balance* (Eckhardt et al., 1950). *(2) Clinical (and sometimes histologic) improvement usually ensues with the use of a high-calorie, high-protein intake, even when large amounts of alcohol are consumed* (Erenoglu et al., 1964; Reynolds et al., 1965). *(3) A low-protein intake, plus continued alcohol, regularly leads to clinical and histologic deterioration* (Erenoglu et al., 1964). *(4) Adequate dietary protein is necessary to achieve a positive nitrogen balance* (Gabuzda et al., 1950). *(5) Clinical and histologic improvement (including mobilization of hepatic fat) regularly occurs when diets adequate in calories and protein and high in fat are used* (Mindrum and Schiff, 1955). Patients with decompensated alcoholic liver disease should receive a palatable, well-balanced diet containing adequate (70 to 100 g) dietary protein. Increasing the dietary protein to higher levels may increase the positive nitrogen balance and hasten a return to a more "normal" nutritional state, but it may not promote more rapid clinical improvement (Chalmers, 1958). Unless the patient actively drinks alcohol, there is no scientific basis for a low-fat diet, which not only sacrifices the caloric value of fat but also makes a palatable diet more difficult to devise (Crews and Faloon, 1962). This conclusion applies to other forms of liver disease as well.

Patients with chronic cholestasis (such as primary biliary cirrhosis) may develop significant steatorrhea, in which case a low-fat diet may provide partial symptomatic relief. The administration of medium-chain triglycerides (MCT) has been suggested in a variety of malabsorptive conditions, including subacute and chronic liver disease (Burke and Danks, 1966; Linscheer et al., 1966). The therapeutic rationale for their use is discussed in Chapter 4, Part II.

Fluid and Electrolyte Disturbances and the Use of Diuretics in Cirrhosis

Patients with cirrhosis frequently have dramatic alterations in fluid and electrolyte balance (e.g., hypokalemia) (Artman and Wise, 1953; Heinemann and Emirgil, 1960; Shear et al., 1969); impaired ability to excrete a water load, possibly the result of greatly decreased delivery of fluid to the distal tubule with consequent hyponatremia despite a supernormal total body sodium (Schedl and Bartter, 1960); and ascites and edema, associated with marked secondary hyperaldosteronism and sodium retention (Henley et al., 1960).

Fluid retention does not necessarily indicate a need for vigorous diuretic therapy. With the array of very potent diuretic drugs available, it is increasingly important for the physician to use good judgment in deciding when and how to use them (Laragh, 1967). The overall goals of therapy *at the particular stage of liver disease present* must be kept in mind. Patients with parenchymal liver failure require good nutrition, rest, and *time* for recovery. Since tense ascites may contribute to anorexia, produce respiratory embarrassment, and potentiate variceal bleeding, a controlled diuresis is desirable in such patients. In other cases, ascites is a secondary problem that becomes easier to manage as liver function improves.

The vigorous use of diuretics in patients with advanced and decompensated cirrhosis may induce hyponatremia, hypokalemia, alkalosis, and hypovolemia, any of which may precipitate hepatic encephalopathy (Read et al., 1959; Baertl et al., 1963; Sherlock et al., 1966). Careful monitoring of the patient's mentation, the presence or absence of a "liver flap," and fluid and electrolyte balance is imperative.

It is advisable to begin diuretic therapy with relatively small doses and observe the effect, for responses to diuretics vary widely and are not always predictable. Truly refractory ascites is rare if diuretics are used intelligently and are given in high enough doses to achieve the desired effect. *Principles: (1) Spironolactone, by blocking the action of aldosterone at the distal tubule (and thereby promoting increased sodium excretion and potassium conservation), is a very useful adjunct, but is not often effective alone in patients with avid sodium reabsorption. (2) The use of spironolactone or triamterene in combination with other diuretics may prevent the development of hypokalemia and alkalosis. (3) If hypokalemia develops, potassium should be given as the chloride* (Kassirer and Schwartz, 1966) *unless acidosis exists* (Shear *et al.*, 1969). *(4) The development of hypovolemia may prevent further diuresis, which may be remedied by the cautious use of salt-poor albumin or plasma infusions. (5) Mild hyponatremia is common in such patients and should not cause alarm if it is asymptomatic. (6) Marked hyponatremia and refractory ascites may respond to mannitol infusions* (Sherlock, 1963b) *or moderate doses of corticosteroids when combined with water restriction* (Carbone and Matthews, 1960; Redeker *et al.*, 1960; Gantt *et al.*, 1962).

EFFECT OF LIVER DISEASE IN PLANNING DRUG THERAPY OF OTHER DISORDERS

Role of the Liver in Drug Metabolism and Excretion (see also Chapter 2)

Drug detoxification takes place primarily in the smooth endoplasmic reticulum of the liver. Drug molecules are converted to a more polar form, thus rendering lipid-soluble materials more water soluble for urinary or biliary excretion. This conversion is accomplished by oxidation and other reactions, usually followed by conjugation (Marver and Schmid, 1968). The duration of highly nonpolar drug action is generally limited by the rate of conversion to inactive metabolites, and dysfunction of these hepatic microsomal systems allows many therapeutic agents to evoke their responses for a prolonged time (Hargreaves, 1968). The administration of drugs often leads to an increase in the smooth endoplasmic reticulum and in microsomal drug-metabolizing enzymes. Induction is a nonspecific adaptation, without specificity for the drug administered and without apparent relation to drug action or structure. Enzyme induction leads to accelerated biotransformation of many drugs and thus potentially alters the duration and intensity of drug action (see Chapter 16).

A secondary role of the liver in drug metabolism is that of biliary excretion. This action is more important in the metabolism of endogenous substances such as bilirubin, steroid hormones, bile salts, and cholesterol (Wheeler, 1965). Drugs excreted primarily in the bile, such as cholecystographic media, bromsulfophthalein (BSP), indocyanin green, and rose bengal, are utilized in the diagnosis of hepatobiliary disorders. Many drugs compete for biliary excretion with other drugs and with endogenous substances, resulting in clinically important effects. For example, BSP, indocyanin green, rose bengal, and certain cholecystographic media may cause transient hyperbilirubinemia by competing with bilirubin for biliary excretion (Bolt *et al.*, 1961; Billing, 1965). As the hyperbilirubinemia is largely unconjugated, the site of competition is apparently within the liver cell and not at the excretory surface. In the case of oral contraceptives and androgenic 17-alkylated steroids, inhibition of bilirubin excretion seems to take place at the canalicular level, resulting in conjugated hyperbilirubinemia (Kory *et al.*, 1959). Biliary excretion of a drug may permit its metabolism or deconjugation from glucuronide by intestinal bacteria and/or recirculation via the enterohepatic circulation. These processes may affect the drug's metabolic fate and activity. Unfortunately, little is known about this aspect of drug metabolism (Williams *et al.*, 1965).

Altered Drug Metabolism in Patients with Liver Disease

Drug metabolism may be significantly impaired by liver disease (see Chapter 2). Special precautions are generally recommended in the administration of drugs to such patients. Despite the theoretic logic of this assumption there are few objective data to support it. Several early studies of the rate of metabolism and/or duration of effect of drugs metabolized in the liver did not show significant differences between normal controls and patients with advanced cirrhosis (Sessions *et al.*, 1954; Weiner *et al.*, 1954; Brodie *et al.*, 1959; Marcus and Kapadia, 1964; Nelson, 1964). At least two explanations are possible: (1) the liver's reserve capacity for the metabolism of drugs is great; and (2) in the studies quoted, no allowance was made for the possible role of other drugs in stimulating metabolism of the test drug by enzyme induction. A recent study of patients with hepatic cirrhosis demonstrated significant elevation and prolongation of blood levels of phenylbutazone only in those patients who were not pretreated with other drugs (Levi *et al.*, 1968). *Principle: Drug metabolism is affected by many diverse factors, including the administration of other drugs* (see Chapter 16).

In some instances, altered drug metabolism in patients with liver disease is clinically important. The rate of conversion of active chloramphenicol to its inactive metabolites is markedly decreased in some patients with cirrhosis (Kunin *et al.*, 1959; Suhrland and Weisberger, 1963), a phenomenon that may lead to a high incidence of bone marrow depression. When azotemia is *not all exhaled via lung?*

also present, choice of this drug would appear to be particularly unwise. Paraldehyde is often used to treat the agitation of alcoholics with liver disease, with the assumption that its pulmonary excretion ensures safety. Most of this drug is metabolized in the liver, and prolonged depression of the central nervous system is occasionally seen after standard doses in cirrhotic patients (Levine *et al.*, 1940; Sherlock, 1963a). Ergot poisoning appears to be common in the presence of liver disease, presumably because of decreased detoxification (Whelton *et al.*, 1968a). Tolbutamide has produced prolonged hypoglycemic reactions in patients with cirrhosis (Cohn *et al.*, 1964), but hypoglycemia occurs spontaneously in patients with liver disease and in patients taking tolbutamide in the absence of liver disease. In summary, alterations in the biotransformation of drugs by the diseased liver may lead to undesirable drug effects, but proven examples of this phenomenon are few and clinical concern may have been overemphasized. *Principle: Observe the patient's response to therapy; do not rely on preconceptions.*

Liver disease may affect drug metabolism in other ways. Portal hypertension may impair absorption of nutrients and drugs as a result of venous stasis and edema of the intestinal mucosa (Enquist *et al.*, 1965). The presence of ascites or edema may alter the distribution of drugs. The urinary excretion of D-xylose after *oral* administration, a screening test for intestinal malabsorption, is inaccurate in cirrhotics. Ascites leads to falsely low values because xylose enters the ascitic fluid and is unavailable for renal excretion (Marin *et al.*, 1968). Other theoretic hazards in the interpretation of this test are extensive portal systemic shunting and decreased D-xylose metabolism, which may increase D-xylose urinary excretion (Price *et al.*, 1967).

Altered Sensitivity to Drugs

Patients with liver disease may react unpredictably to a drug without any known alterations in the metabolism of the agent. Patients at the threshold of hepatic encephalopathy are often very sensitive to the administration of sedatives, particularly morphine (Laidlaw *et al.*, 1961). These effects are presumably due to drug action upon an already "sensitive" brain, rather than to impaired metabolism with a prolonged drug effect (Levi, 1965). Sensitivity to bishydroxycoumarin (Dicumarol) in patients with abnormal liver function may reflect changes in the biochemical mechanisms involved in the synthesis of prothrombin or in protein binding, rather than an impaired rate of metabolism of the drug (Reisner *et al.*, 1949; Brodie *et al.*, 1959). An abnormal drug response does not necessarily

establish altered drug metabolism, even in patients with severe liver disease.

Alcohol and Drug Effects

Because of the frequent association between alcoholism and liver disease, the relationship between alcohol and drugs deserves comment. Alcohol often potentiates the action of sedatives; this may simply reflect alcohol's central nervous system depressant effects. Alcoholics, when not intoxicated, are often resistant to the action of sedatives and anesthetics. In this regard, ethanol, like other drugs, may induce microsomal enzymes in both rats and man (Rubin and Lieber, 1968c). Chronic alcohol administration leads to hypertrophy of the smooth endoplasmic reticulum with increased activity of drug-metabolizing enzymes. Clearance of several drugs is significantly increased in nonintoxicated chronic alcoholics (Kater *et al.*, 1969). Ethanol, in concentrations commonly found in intoxicated persons, may inhibit the *in vitro* activity of a variety of microsomal enzymes and may account for some of the clinical observations noted above (Rubin and Lieber, 1968c; Rubin *et al.*, 1970).

Considering the widespread use of alcohol in our society, it is surprising that so few investigations have been concerned with alcohol-drug interactions, which might have great social and medical significance (Soehring and Schuppel, 1966; Becker, 1970).

Hepatic "Drug Reactions" in Patients with Pre-existent Liver Disease

Is it logical and ethical to treat a patient with liver disease with a drug implicated in the production of hepatic damage in other patients? The answer may appear obvious, but many modifying factors must be taken into account. A physician may have excellent reasons for giving chlorpromazine to a patient with viral hepatitis. An anesthesiologist may feel that halothane is the anesthetic of choice in a cirrhotic patient. A glass of wine may improve the morale and appetite of a patient with cirrhosis or hepatitis. What are the important principles in dealing with this question?

The indications for drug selection and the likelihood of accomplishing the desired therapeutic result must be established. No other drug should be available that could produce the same therapeutic effect with less risk. The physician should then consider the probability that the drug in question will cause liver damage and the effect of this damage on the patient. For example, chlorpromazine-induced cholestatic jaundice occurs in 0.5 to 1% of patients receiving the drug for 2 or more weeks. If the patient has no history of a previous hepatic reaction to phenothiazines (in which case the drug is obviously contraindicated), chlorpromazine may be used with the knowledge that prolonged administration has 1 chance in 200 of inducing cholestatic jaundice. Although hepatic reactions are usually benign, they may run a long course and greatly complicate management (Zimmerman, 1963). Liver damage due to hypersensitivity does not occur with greater frequency in patients with antecedent liver disease. If a patient develops hepatic damage, the superimposition of two different disease processes can lead to diagnostic problems. The acceptability of the risk depends on the urgency for the use of the drug and on the clinical setting. If an energetic medical student with infectious hepatitis complained of "being constrained" by hospitalization, one would offer a consoling phrase or find out *why* he felt constrained, not drug him with antipsychotic medications. If a schizophrenic were "climbing the walls," the risk might be worth the therapeutic effect.

"Halothane hepatitis" is probably due to individual hypersensitivity and is relatively rare, occurring about once in 1000 to 10,000 exposures (more often after repeated exposures). Unlike the relatively innocuous cholestatic type of hepatic reaction associated with chlorpromazine, halothane causes a severe lesion with high mortality. Often the patient develops unexplained fever or mild hepatic functional abnormalities after an initial exposure, only to develop a fatal and fulminant hepatitis following reexposure (Trey et al., 1968). These clues must be considered before halothane is used in any patient! A hepatic reaction to halothane is no more likely to occur in a patient with cirrhosis than in others. However, such a reaction, superimposed on an already severely diseased liver, greatly increases the risk of mortality. Halothane may be safely administered to a patient with cirrhosis, provided the patient has shown no evidence of sensitivity to the drug in a prior administration (Jones et al., 1965; Klatskin, 1968). Repeated exposures to halothane probably should be avoided (Chadwick and Jennings, 1964).

The advisability of alcohol administration in a patient with active liver disease is debatable. Large amounts of alcohol are hepatotoxic, including dose-related metabolic and histologic changes seen in every person. Dietary factors and the initial status of the liver, however, may be important determinants of clinically significant effects of alcohol on the liver. Patients with alcoholic cirrhosis usually improve clinically and histologically as long as they consume a nutritious diet, even when given large amounts of alcohol. Since such patients have a refractory psychosocial disorder that can be controlled only by complete avoidance of alcohol, "therapeutic" use is contraindicated in most instances. In other types of liver disease (e.g., postnecrotic cirrhosis), modest amounts of alcohol probably will not produce deleterious effects on the course of the liver disorder if nutrition is adequate.

In some situations, the existence of previous or current liver dysfunction makes a hepatic reaction to drugs more likely. Liver functional reserve is reduced during pregnancy, as manifested by decreased capacity for bilirubin and BSP excretion (Thorling, 1955; Combes et al., 1963). Large parenteral doses of tetracycline have been implicated in the production of acute severe fatty liver of pregnancy, a highly lethal condition that may take place spontaneously (Schultz et al., 1963; Kunelis et al., 1965). Tetracycline-associated disorders may also occur in nonpregnant patients, but pregnancy and/or pyelonephritis seem to be predisposing factors (Peters et al., 1967). The increased metabolic demands and diminished hepatic reserve in pregnancy make the pregnant patient especially likely to react to large doses of tetracycline. It appears reasonable to avoid the use of this drug in doses higher than 1 g per day (Whalley et al., 1964).

Oral contraceptives frequently lead to BSP retention and, less commonly, to elevated serum alkaline phosphatase and serum glutamate-pyruvate transaminase activity. Jaundice rarely occurs and is usually associated with relatively "pure" cholestasis on liver biopsy (Ockner and Davidson, 1967). Most evidence assigns responsibility to the estrogenic component of these drugs (Urban et al., 1968). Women with prior episodes of cholestasis and/or severe pruritus of pregnancy are much more likely to develop cholestasis (Kreek et al., 1967b). The hepatic reaction is reversible and nonprogressive. Patients with primary biliary cirrhosis, postnecrotic cirrhosis, constitutional hyperbilirubinemia (Gilbert's syndrome), benign familial recurrent cholestasis, and Dubin-Johnson syndrome may develop increased jaundice when exposed to oral contraceptives (Kleiner et al., 1965; Schaffner, 1966; Gartner and Arias, 1969; Mowat and Arias, 1969). Exacerbations of hepatic porphyria may follow the use of contraceptives and other drugs (Zimmerman et al., 1966; DeMatteis, 1967).

II. GASTROINTESTINAL DISORDERS

L. Frederick Fenster and Elliot Weser

CHARACTERISTICS OF GASTROINTESTINAL DISEASE PERTINENT TO THERAPEUTICS

One has only to observe the consumer dollars spent in the United States for drugs designed to cure real and imagined gastrointestinal disorders (a stroll through any drugstore is enlightening in this respect), the widespread attention given to special diets, and the prevalence of gastrointestinal complaints in any clinic or hospital sample to realize that the care and feeding of the gut is an important topic. Gastrointestinal symptoms are so common that any practitioner of medicine must become involved in their diagnosis and management. In fact, gastrointestinal disorders are the greatest cause of disability and loss of work in the United States.

Certain characteristics are typical of gastrointestinal disorders and have pertinence to therapeutics. First, emotional disturbances play major roles in pathogenesis and symptomatology. From one half to two thirds of patients seen in everyday medical practice suffer mainly from disorders of psychic origin, and of these at least half complain predominantly of intestinal symptoms (Lewis, 1953). In addition, patients with a proven structural ("organic") abnormality of the intestinal tract often have their difficulties precipitated, exacerbated, or intensified by emotional factors. Indeed, the fact that the patient clearly relates symptoms to emotional upsets may lead the unwary physician to discount important symptoms of structural disease. The gut is a common "target organ" for emotional stress, a fact that must be kept in mind in designing rational therapy. A closely related factor is the prevalence of numerous myths and fantasies about the interrelationships between food, drink, bowel habits, and health. Failure to consider these factors may nullify an otherwise sound therapeutic program. Second, the intestinal tract is highly exposed, being the first line of defense against innumerable natural and unnatural substances, including nutrients, toxins, irritants, and drugs. Accordingly, a consideration of possible adverse effects of ingested substances is important in the study, diagnosis, and management of gastrointestinal disorders. Third, most intestinal problems are chronic and/or recurrent. Unless surgical therapy is appropriate and successful, the management of peptic ulcer disease, inflammatory bowel diseases, and reflux esophagitis (not to mention the irritable colon syndrome) involves a long-term program emphasizing symptomatic, supportive, and empiric treatment. Dramatic cures with medical treatment are not common, and useful therapeutic approaches often require considerable persistence on the part of both patient and physician. Because of these features, controlled studies of therapeutic methods are essential (Truelove and Wright, 1964). *Principle: The more chronic and fluctuating the natural history of a disease, the more difficult it is to determine the value of a treatment program, and the more crucial are carefully controlled trials.*

109

CATEGORIES AND EXAMPLES OF THERAPEUTIC APPROACHES TO GASTROINTESTINAL DISORDERS

Withdrawal, Depletion, or Antagonism of a "Toxic" or Offending Substance

Withdrawal of Offending Drugs. Adverse effects of drugs on the gastrointestinal tract range from simple irritative symptoms to life-threatening hemorrhage. Most antibiotics given orally produce a variety of intestinal symptoms such as anorexia, nausea, abdominal pain, and diarrhea (Fekety, 1968). These effects are usually dose related and are probably due to direct irritation of the gut and/or alteration of the bacterial flora. Overgrowth of resistant bacteria or fungi may lead to more serious complications, such as enterocolitis due to *Staphylococcus aureus*. Several drugs (e.g., neomycin) adversely affect intestinal absorption (Dobbins, 1968). Small-bowel ulcerations may be caused by enteric-coated potassium chloride (Boley *et al.*, 1965; Buchan and Houston, 1965). Several agents, including salicylates, corticosteroids, reserpine, phenylbutazone, and indomethacin, have been implicated (often with insufficient evidence *in man*) in upper gastrointestinal bleeding due to gastritis or peptic ulcer. The adverse effects of chronic laxative abuse are well known. In some patients, corticosteroids and possibly thiazide diuretics predispose to pancreatitis (Schrier and Bulger, 1965). In evaluating gastrointestinal symptoms thought to be secondary to drug ingestion, the "toxic effects" of placebos must be kept in mind (Beecher, 1955) (see Chapter 14); controlled studies in this area of investigation are essential (Kerr and Davidson, 1958).

Cathartics. Because of the conviction that a daily and bountiful bowel movement is a prerequisite for good health, misuse of laxatives is widespread. The mechanism of action of many cathartics, often assumed to be one of simple bowel irritation, is not well understood (Phillips *et al.*, 1965). Whatever the mechanism, chronic use of many over-the-counter laxatives has resulted in a variety of syndromes, some difficult to recognize and, in part because of patient refractoriness, still more difficult to reverse. These include the surreptitious use of cathartics to cause a factitious diarrhea (rarely associated with protein-losing enteropathy); chronic hypokalemia; and "cathartic colon," which may be confused with inflammatory bowel disease (Litchfield, 1959; Kramer and Pope, 1964; Rawson, 1966; Ziter, 1967; Heizer *et al.*, 1968; Fleischer *et al.*, 1969). Withdrawal of the cathartic usually results in partial or complete reversal of the physiologic abnormality. A successful therapeutic program entails a multi-faceted approach, including patient education, management of emotional problems, and the use of diet and relatively innocuous cathartics and enemas in progressively decreasing amounts. Convincing the patient (and his relatives) that the *character* of his stools is more important than their *frequency* is probably the most important aspect of therapy.

Salicylates. A majority of patients ingesting moderate doses of salicylates over a few days develop increased fecal blood loss (Grossman *et al.*, 1961; Scott *et al.*, 1961; Beeken, 1968). The magnitude of blood loss is not great (usually two to four times control values), but is potentially important in the pathogenesis of iron-deficiency anemia in menstruating females or in patients with inadequate bone marrow reserve. The relationship between salicylate ingestion and major upper gastrointestinal hemorrhage is less clear, with only circumstantial evidence implicating the drug as a precipitating factor (Parry and Wood, 1967). The more common occult bleeding is associated with endoscopically visible gastric mucosal lesions (Thorsen *et al.*, 1968). Given these facts, salicylates should be withdrawn from patients who show evidence of iron-deficiency anemia or who have potential bleeding sites in the upper gut, especially peptic ulcers. However, assuming compelling reasons for utilizing this valuable analgesic, can the gastric mucosal damage be prevented or minimized? We know that (1) acetylsalicylic acid is an organic acid with a pK_a of 3.5; 50% is ionized at pH 3.5 and 99% at pH 5.5; (2) in the undissociated, lipid-soluble form, acetylsalicylic acid is rapidly absorbed through the gastric mucosa; (3) mucosal damage with bleeding is thought to be intimately associated with drug absorption, perhaps owing to disruption of the lipid-protein layer on the surface of the mucosal cell, allowing gastric hydrochloric acid to act on the unprotected mucosa (Davenport, 1967, 1969); and (4) the mucosal damage can be prevented by neutralization of the gastric contents (Thorsen *et al.*, 1968; Davenport, 1969; Leonards and Levy, 1969) (see Chapter 2).

Some degree of mucosal injury and bleeding may be a necessary concomitant of rapid gastric absorption of salicylates. Neutralization of gastric acidity, although protective to the mucosa, may also reduce gastric absorption and lead to lower peak blood levels (Cooke and Hunt, 1970). If neutralization is deemed advisable, potent antacids should be utilized. The small amount of antacids present in most "buffered-aspirin" preparations is probably insufficient to affect the pH of gastric contents, and taking the drug with meals has no protective effect (Stephens *et al.*, 1968). An unresolved question is the effect of particle size and rate of solution on the degree of mucosal damage (Levy and Hayes, 1960; Györy and Stiel, 1968) (see Chapter 2).

Corticosteroids. Peptic ulcer is one of many potential complications of corticosteroid therapy (Spiro and Milles, 1960). Patients with rheumatoid arthritis treated with large doses of steroids have an increased incidence of peptic ulcer, but the same does not hold true when steroids are utilized in the treatment of non-rheumatic disorders such as skin disease, inflammatory bowel disease, and asthma (Cooke, 1967). Because arthritic patients almost invariably receive salicylates and other anti-rheumatic drugs along with steroids, it is likely that these agents are in some way responsible for the difference. Unfortunately, there are no good prospective trials in which not only steroids but also other antirheumatic drugs are taken into account in the evaluation of complicating ulcers. How do steroids contribute to the development of peptic ulcers in patients with rheumatoid arthritis? Corticosteroids may have at least a permissive role in the pathogenesis of ulcers (Engel, 1955), and chronic prednisone treatment leads to augmentation of stimulated gastric acid secretion (Strickland *et al.*, 1969). Corticosteroids may affect gastric mucus secretion, perhaps interfering with normal protective mechanisms (Sun, 1969). Whatever the mechanism, the physician should follow certain principles while awaiting further information. *Principles: (1) A baseline upper gastrointestinal x-ray should be obtained prior to initiation of long-term steroid therapy. (2) Concomitant salicylates, phenylbutazone, indomethacin, and related drugs should be avoided in the patient on chronic steroid therapy. (3) Steroids should be reduced to the minimum effective dose (complications are much less frequent when doses are less than the equivalent of 20 mg of prednisone per day (Spiro and Milles, 1960)). (4) A high index of suspicion for the development of an ulcer is advisable, remembering that these ulcers are often atypical and relatively asymptomatic.* An hourly antacid program has not been shown to prevent the development of "steroid ulcers," but such a routine would seem theoretically wise in the patient with rheumatoid arthritis. If a patient on steroid therapy develops an ulcer, the drug should be withdrawn if possible. In most instances, these ulcers *do* heal despite continued steroid treatment, but healing may be unusually slow.

Withdrawal of Dietary Factors. *Gluten-Free*

Diet in Celiac Disease. The role of dietary gluten in celiac disease illustrates how a food may cause intestinal disorders. A gluten-free diet is efficacious in the treatment of celiac disease in both children and adults (Dicke *et al.*, 1953; French *et al.*, 1957; Benson *et al.*, 1964; McDonald *et al.*, 1964). With strict adherence to this diet, intestinal absorptive function usually improves within several weeks. On the other hand, the striking morphologic alterations of the small intestine associated with untreated celiac disease revert more slowly and may require many months for restoration of normal histology. Strict adherence to the gluten-free diet is necessary for a significant, if not complete, remission. Once a biochemical and histologic remission is achieved, reingestion of gluten produces a recurrence of clinical, absorptive, and morphologic abnormalities (Benson *et al.*, 1964). Instillation of gluten or toxic fractions into the ileum of patients with celiac disease results in dramatic changes in function and histology at the site of instillation (Rubin *et al.*, 1962). Although the toxicity of dietary gluten in celiac disease is well established, the precise nature of the toxic factor and its mechanism of action is unknown.

Lactose Withdrawal in Lactase Deficiency. Many people are deficient in intestinal lactase and are unable to hydrolyze ingested lactose. Failure to hydrolyze lactose prevents its normal absorption, and increased quantities of the sugar remain in the intestinal lumen, inducing an osmotic diarrhea. Bacterial metabolism of the sugar in the colon produces organic acids (such as lactic and acetic acids) that lower the pH of the stool and further contribute to the diarrhea (Bayless and Huang, 1969). Lactase deficiency may be secondary to diseases affecting the small intestine or may be primary, on a congenital or genetic basis. An unusually high incidence of lactase deficiency has been reported in Negroes and Asian adults (Bayless and Rosensweig, 1966; Cook and Kajubi, 1966; Davis and Bolin, 1967; Huang and Bayless, 1968), indicating that much of the world's population may be intolerant of lactose. This factor is important in the consideration of milk as a source of protein in regions of widespread malnutrition. The reduction or complete withdrawal of lactose from the diet is necessary to alleviate symptoms. Replacement therapy with lactase is not feasible or practical.

The withdrawal of other sugars from the diet may be crucial in rare instances. A genetically transmitted combined deficiency of intestinal sucrase and isomaltase produces an intolerance to table sugar, which must be withdrawn from the diet (Nordio and Lamedica, 1964; Auricchio *et al.*, 1965; Jansen *et al.*, 1965). Defects in the absorption of the actively transported monosaccharides glucose and galactose also occur, particularly in children. The disorder is caused by an inherited, congenital defect in the intestinal carrier-transport system shared by glucose and galactose and responds to reduction or withdrawal of sugars containing the monosaccharides, with substitution of fructose (Lindquist and Meeuwisse, 1962; Schneider *et al.*, 1966; Meeuwisse and Dahlqvist, 1968).

Withdrawal of Food Allergens. Removal of a "sensitizing" food substance from the diet may improve gastrointestinal symptoms in patients with allergic gastroenteropathy. Although much of the evidence for gastrointestinal allergy is circumstantial, techniques for measurement of gastrointestinal protein loss, immunodiffusion assay, and intestinal biopsy have made the case more convincing. Amelioration of protein-losing enteropathy by elimination of milk from the diet has incriminated milk as an allergen (Waldmann *et al.*, 1967). The infants in this report had many typical clinical features of allergy as well as strong family histories of allergy. In some individuals, sensitivity to cow's milk protein may produce intestinal bleeding (Wilson *et al.*, 1964), colitis (Gryboski *et al.*, 1966, 1968), intolerance to other food proteins, and intestinal malabsorption (Gryboski *et al.*, 1968; Liu *et al.*, 1968).

Although circulating antibodies to milk proteins have been found in several intestinal diseases, their relationship to gastrointestinal milk allergy is unproved. Precipitating antibodies to milk, soy, and cereal products were found in stool specimens from children with chronic idiopathic diarrhea. These patients improved after elimination of the offending dietary antigen (Self *et al.*, 1969). Although these findings must be substantiated, they suggest that coproantibodies contained in the immunoglobulin-A fraction of intestinal secretions may be important in intestinal allergy. A case of protein-losing enteropathy apparently related to several food proteins, particularly red meats, raises the possibility that many proteins may act as intestinal antigens (Greenberger *et al.*, 1967b).

Replacement of a Deficient Substance

Pancreatic Enzyme Therapy in Pancreatic Exocrine Deficiency. Although steatorrhea and azotorrhea are usually found in severe impairment of pancreatic function, carbohydrate hydrolysis is not significantly altered. Steatorrhea usually is the most important clinical problem and is due to deficient hydrolysis of long-chain triglycerides, which are relatively insoluble in bile salt micelles and therefore remain in the oil phase of the intestinal content (Krone *et al.*, 1968). Inadequate pancreatic lipase activity may be due to deficient enzyme production (resulting from advanced pancreatic damage) and/or to an abnormally depressed intraduodenal pH, which may be the result of excessive gastric acid production (as in the Zollinger-Ellison syndrome) or of deficient pancreatic bicarbonate production.

The goals of therapy with pancreatic extracts are to approximate the normal pattern of pancreatic secretion in response to meals, reduce steatorrhea, restore lost weight, and minimize diarrhea. These goals can be achieved when adequate doses of potent preparations are utilized (Jordan and Grossman, 1959; Marks *et al.*, 1963; Iber, 1968; Kalser *et al.*, 1968). The problems that remain to be elucidated are considered in an excellent review (Littman and Hanscom, 1969). The factors most important for successful therapy are the potency of the enzyme preparation (especially the lipase activity) and the dosage schedule. Until recently it has been difficult to assay accurately the lipase activity of various preparations, and the potency has often varied from one batch to another. Present evidence conflicts as to whether better results are obtained when the pancreatic supplements are given with meals or when the same amount is given at hourly intervals. Patients with marked defects in lipid absorption may respond better to hourly administration, and this method seems advisable when other schedules are unsuccessful. Some authors feel that the usually recommended dose is often inadequate and should be increased as needed to obtain clinical improvement (Marks and Bank, 1965). *Principle: It may be necessary to increase the dose until either the desired response is achieved or intolerable side effects occur.* Because adjustment and individualization of dosage are so crucial, fixed combinations of pancreatic extracts with other drugs should not be used. Many preparations include small amounts of bile salts, theoretically to enhance the activity of lipase on triglyceride substrates. However, few patients with pancreatic insufficiency have a significant deficiency of bile salts, and, even if deficiency were present, the amount of active bile salt in such preparations would probably be inadequate.

Because pancreatic lipase and trypsin are inactivated at pH 4.5 and 3.5, respectively, there is some question as to the amount of active enzyme entering the duodenum after passage through the stomach. Although no conclusive studies are available, gastric inactivation is clearly a major limiting factor (Heizer *et al.*,

1965). Enteric-coated preparations are neither reliable nor clinically more effective. The administration of antacids concomitantly may potentiate the effect of pancreatic enzymes, both by preventing gastric inactivation and by increasing the normally alkaline intraduodenal pH. The administration of sodium bicarbonate may be beneficial in selected patients (Veeger et al., 1962).

Replacement of Electrolytes, Vitamins, and Iron. *Calcium and Magnesium in Gastrointestinal Disease.* Although severe, acute diarrhea or chronic diarrhea may be associated with deficiencies of sodium, potassium, and bicarbonate, only calcium and magnesium will be considered here. Replacement of these ions may be important in treating patients with severe diarrhea and/or steatorrhea.

Although most of our information on calcium absorption has been derived from animal experiments, many of the principles apply to man and are considered in a detailed review (Wasserman, 1968). Several points are important in understanding why calcium deficiency may develop in gastrointestinal disease states. Since most dietary calcium is in bound form, its ionization is necessary prior to absorption. Many calcium salts, either dietary or formed in the intestinal tract (such as calcium carbonate and phosphate), are relatively insoluble and must be dissolved in order to be absorbed. Dissociation of complexes and dissolution of precipitates are pH dependent, in the range of pH 5 to 7. Therefore, gastric acid production is potentially important, although no direct evidence substantiates this. The lowest intestinal pH occurs in the duodenojejunum, where calcium absorption takes place at a faster rate than in the ileum, probably owing to an active transport-carrier system (Birge et al., 1969; Wensel et al., 1969). Calcium absorption decreases with advancing age, especially in women (Avioli et al., 1965). It is not surprising, therefore, that a combination of factors may lead to reduced calcium absorption and osteomalacia after gastric resection, particularly in postmenopausal women (Deller et al., 1964; Morgan et al., 1966). Surgical procedures for peptic ulcer remove gastric acid, and frequently the site of maximal calcium absorption in the duodenojejunal area is bypassed. Poor intake or malabsorption of vitamin D may also contribute to defective calcium absorption after gastrectomy (Thompson et al., 1966; Bordier et al., 1968).

Intestinal absorption of calcium is probably a two-step process: cellular uptake and transport across the cell. In both animals and man these steps depend upon the stimulating effect of vitamin D. Calcium absorption is likely to be reduced in intestinal disease states with altered mucosa, steatorrhea, and loss of vitamin D (Harrison et al., 1969; Wensel et al., 1969), resulting in low serum calcium levels with tetany and even seizures. Calcium and vitamin D replacement may be extremely important in celiac sprue, regional enteritis, short-bowel syndrome, and Whipple's disease.

Chronic diarrhea and steatorrhea may cause loss of magnesium in the stool sufficient to produce magnesium deficiency (Booth et al., 1963; Gerlach et al., 1970). This may occur in a variety of intestinal disorders, including celiac sprue (Balint and Hirschowitz, 1961; Goldman et al., 1962), radiation enteropathy (Vallee et al., 1960), short bowel (Opie et al., 1964), and intestinal or biliary fistulas (Fishman, 1965). In the above situations, replacement therapy with magnesium-free parenteral solutions may aggravate unrecognized magnesium depletion. Magnesium deficiency leads to neuromuscular dysfunction manifested by hyperexcitability, tetany, seizures, tremors, irritability, and psychotic behavior (Wacker and Parisi, 1968; Shils, 1969), which are reversed by magnesium administration. Tetany, in particular, may occur in the absence of acid-base imbalance or hypocalcemia and may be reversed promptly by administration of magnesium, but not calcium. Most patients with magnesium deficiency have other electrolyte abnormalities, especially hypocalcemia and hypokalemia. Indeed, magnesium deficiency per se may lead to these aberrations (Petersen, 1963; Shils, 1969), and magnesium replacement may be necessary to correct the hypocalcemia. Thus, oral calcium supplements, administered without correction of a coexisting magnesium deficiency, may only aggravate the latter by increasing intestinal losses of magnesium, consistent with a presumed common transport mechanism for these divalent cations (Booth et al., 1963; Petersen, 1963). *Principle: Multiple interrelated deficiencies are common in severe malabsorptive syndromes, and successful management requires attention to all factors.*

Vitamin B_{12} in Gastric Disease, Ileal Disease, and Malabsorption. The normal absorptive process for dietary vitamin B_{12} may be interrupted by various diseases at different sites in the gastrointestinal tract. An understanding of clinical syndromes leading to vitamin B_{12} deficiency requires an appreciation of normal B_{12} absorptive mechanisms (Herbert and Castle, 1964; Herbert, 1968). Most vitamin B_{12} is actively absorbed and requires the formation of a complex with intrinsic factor, which is probably produced by the gastric parietal cell

(Hoedemaeker *et al.*, 1964). Active absorption takes place only in the ileum (Stewart *et al.*, 1967), where the intrinsic factor–B$_{12}$ complex presumably attaches to a selective receptor site on the microvillus border (Donaldson *et al.*, 1967; MacKenzie *et al.*, 1968). Attachment of complex to the receptor site requires a pH above 5.6 and the presence of calcium ions. The mechanism whereby B$_{12}$ enters the mucosal cell and ultimately the portal blood (bound to alpha- and beta-globulin) is unknown.

Any disease process that results in a decreased number or function of gastric parietal cells may produce a deficiency of intrinsic factor and ultimately a deficiency of vitamin B$_{12}$. This is classically illustrated by addisonian pernicious anemia, in which atrophy of the gastric mucosa produces a deficiency of intrinsic factor. Some patients with this disease have either precipitating or blocking antibodies to intrinsic factor, making it unavailable for binding with B$_{12}$ (Fisher *et al.*, 1966; Schade *et al.*, 1966). Intrinsic factor deficiency may also occur following total or extensive gastric resection (Deller and Witts, 1962; Hines *et al.*, 1967).

Defective function of the ileum, due to disease or surgical resection, may also reduce B$_{12}$ absorption and eventually lead to pernicious anemia (Schofield, 1965; Dotevall and Kock, 1968). Regional enteritis or more generalized disorders of the gut mucosa (e.g., tropical sprue, celiac disease, and Whipple's disease) may lead to B$_{12}$ malabsorption. Tests of B$_{12}$ absorption may be useful in assessing ileal function in these conditions. Another mechanism of vitamin B$_{12}$ malabsorption is seen in the "blind-loop" syndromes, in which excessive growth of intestinal microorganisms occurs at sites of intestinal stasis. These conditions include multiple jejunal diverticula, afferent loop obstruction after partial gastrectomy and gastrojejunostomy, blind loops secondary to intestinal surgery, and strictures or fistulas of the small intestine (Cameron *et al.*, 1949). Malabsorption of vitamin B$_{12}$ results from the incorporation of the vitamin by multiplying organisms (Booth and Heath, 1962; Donaldson *et al.*, 1962), a mechanism similar to that described in patients with *Diphyllobothrium latum* infestation (Nyberg *et al.*, 1961). Pancreatic insufficiency also affects vitamin B$_{12}$ absorption (Veeger *et al.*, 1962; LeBauer *et al.*, 1968), presumably owing in part to changes in intraluminal pH. Although the administration of pancreatic enzymes and sodium bicarbonate is useful in some instances, more information is required to assess the role of the pancreas in vitamin B$_{12}$ absorption (Toskes *et al.*, 1971).

Regardless of the mechanism accounting for B$_{12}$ deficiency, a megaloblastic anemia usually results, although central nervous system dysfunction may occasionally occur in the absence of anemia. Patients with a malabsorption syndrome often have multiple deficiencies, hindering recognition of specific defects. A concomitant malabsorption of iron and/or folic acid may make interpretation of the hematologic findings difficult, unless all potential factors are kept in mind. *Principles: (1) A normal adult has sufficient body stores of B$_{12}$ (particularly in the liver) to last for 1 to 5 years. (2) In many conditions, the development of B$_{12}$ deficiency can be predicted and should be prevented by prophylactic administration of parenteral B$_{12}$. (3) Depending on the underlying condition, replacement therapy may be required indefinitely or only until the underlying intestinal defect is corrected (which can be determined by tests of B$_{12}$ absorption, such as the Schilling test). (4) If B$_{12}$ is not needed, it can serve no useful function; in the United States the drug is used much more extensively than is necessary to treat pernicious anemia.* Chapter 14 verifies the frequent use of B$_{12}$ as a placebo. Although common, the practice is expensive, therapeutically useless, and in many instances frankly dangerous.

Fat-Soluble Vitamins in Steatorrhea. Replacement of fat-soluble vitamins may be therapeutically important in some patients with steatorrhea. These vitamins (A, D, K, and E) are aromatic compounds that may be lost in the stool in sufficient quantities to produce deficiency in patients with moderate-to-severe steatorrhea.

Vitamin A is an alcohol and forms esters with fatty acids. Although fish liver oils are rich in this vitamin, the carotenoids found in green vegetables are the major dietary source. Carotene itself possesses no vitamin A activity but is converted, probably in the intestinal mucosal cell, to vitamin A. As carotenes are also lipid soluble, they may be poorly absorbed in patients with steatorrhea. Characteristic signs of vitamin A deficiency are impairment of dark adaptation by the retina and the presence of hyperkeratotic papules around hair follicles. However, prominent signs of vitamin A deficiency accompanying steatorrhea are unusual, except in patients with the rare condition a-beta-lipoproteinemia (acanthocytosis), who have intermittent steatorrhea and a very low or absent plasma beta-lipoprotein. Low vitamin A stores may account for the "night blindness" experienced by many of these patients (Isselbacher *et al.*, 1964).

Vitamin D is a steroid that exists in at least two active forms, ergocalciferol (D$_2$) and cholecalciferol (D$_3$), the natural vitamin. These active forms are derived from the ultraviolet light irradiation of the inactive precursor sterols, ergosterol and 7-dehydrocholesterol, respectively. Fish liver oils are a rich natural source of vitamin D, but milk and other foods have been treated (either by irradiation or with vitamin D additives) to provide additional dietary sources. In most parts of the world vitamin D is provided largely by activation of sterols in the skin by sunlight. Malabsorption of vitamin D is relatively common in disorders causing steatorrhea, such as celiac sprue and postgastrectomy states, and is a major cause of calcium malabsorption. Vitamin D therapy and calcium administration may be necessary to avoid hypocalcemia and defective bone formation, particularly in those diseases with no effective treatment of the underlying defect.

Vitamin K is a substituted naphthoquinone. Although this substance is found in alfalfa and fish meal, deficiency in man does not result from dietary lack because it is constantly synthesized by intestinal bacteria. Antibiotic administration in rats may so alter the intestinal flora that signs of vitamin K deficiency may develop, but in man other factors are necessary. Normal synthesis of prothrombin by the liver requires vitamin K, and a deficiency is manifested by hypoprothrombinemia and impairment of blood clotting. Vitamin K deficiency is a common defect in steatorrhea caused by celiac sprue, pancreatic insufficiency, biliary obstruction, and blind-loop syndrome. Oral or parenteral administration of a water-soluble derivative of vitamin K usually corrects the deficiency rapidly. Adequacy of therapy can be assessed by serial determinations of the prothrombin concentration in plasma.

Vitamin E is an aromatic substance of the tocopherol family. A deficiency of this vitamin in rats and guinea pigs may produce infertility, renal tubule damage, hemolysis, and muscular dystrophy. Although low serum concentrations of tocopherol may be found in some patients with steatorrhea, the deficiency in man has no definite adverse effects (Binder et al., 1965).

Principle: Of the vitamin deficiencies mentioned, that of vitamin D is by far the most important long-term problem in patients with gastrointestinal disorders. Unfortunately, the postgastrectomy patient or the patient with long-standing steatorrhea is too often allowed to develop clinically important bone disease before the vitamin D deficiency is treated (Crooks et al., 1965). An area for fruitful preventive medicine is thereby neglected.

Iron in Gastrointestinal Disease. Perhaps one of the most common forms of replacement therapy is iron administration to correct (or prevent) iron-deficiency anemia. Iron deficiency may result from inadequate dietary intake, nonavailability of dietary iron, blood loss, or malabsorption.

The average person ingests 10 to 20 mg of iron daily, but only about 10% of this is available for absorption, as most iron in food is chemically bound to substances (such as phytates and phosphates) that either are insoluble or prevent the iron from being absorbed. Iron in animal hemoglobin and porphyrin is particularly well absorbed and appears to enter the intestinal cell as part of the heme molecule (Turnbull et al., 1962; Conrad et al., 1966; Weintraub et al., 1968). Ferrous salts are more readily assimilated than ferric salts. Insoluble ferric hydroxide precipitates at the alkaline pH of the lower duodenum, and the iron is unavailable for absorption. Hydrochloric acid enhances the absorption of ferric iron, but not of hemoglobin or ferrous iron (Choudhury and Williams, 1959; Jacobs et al., 1964). Ascorbic acid from dietary or endogenous sources (such as bile) can form a chelate with ferric salts, which maintains the iron in a soluble form over a pH range of 2 to 11 (Conrad and Schade, 1968; Schade et al., 1968), thus ensuring solubility at duodenal pH and enhancing absorption. The chemical reaction between ferric salts and ascorbic acid must be initiated at an acid pH, probably in the stomach, to ensure the formation of soluble iron chelate. Ferrous salts, on the other hand, may combine with ascorbate at pHs found in the duodenum; therefore, the role of hydrochloric acid is less important in this reaction. In addition to ascorbic acid, certain sugars, polyols, and amino acids may also bind iron to form chelates, which remain soluble at an alkaline pH and increase iron absorption (Charley et al., 1963; Kroe et al., 1963). Active absorption of iron is probably a two-step process: mucosal uptake from the lumen and mucosal transfer of iron to other depots (Wheby et al., 1964). Body stores of iron (in particular, the iron content of the intestinal epithelium) are important in regulating absorption (Conrad et al., 1964). Absorption of food iron is thus limited by several factors, and iron balance is normally maintained within a narrow range.

Mechanisms by which iron deficiency occurs in gastrointestinal disorders include (1) blood loss, particularly chronic; (2) reduction in the availability of absorbable iron at the absorptive cell; and (3) defective mucosal function. Two of these mechanisms are operative after gastric resection (Baird et al., 1957; Hines et al., 1967). These patients frequently lose blood, ingest marginal diets, have decreased or absent hydrochloric acid, and, in addition, often have a surgical bypass of the duodenum, where the active transport mechanism of iron absorption is maximal (Wheby *et al.*, 1964). In the presence of diseases that affect the intestinal mucosa (e.g., celiac disease, tropical sprue, radiation enteropathy, and Whipple's disease) the lumen-to-mucosa transfer of iron may be impaired. Because the mucosal lesion in celiac disease is maximal in the proximal small bowel, iron-deficiency anemia may be the *only* detectable absorptive defect in some patients (McGuigan and Volwiler, 1964).

In all the conditions mentioned, iron replacement with ferrous salts is usually sufficient to restore body iron and correct the anemia. There is little evidence to support the widespread belief that inorganic iron compounds cause undesirable intestinal symptoms (Kerr and Davidson, 1958), and there is little scientific or practical justification for the use of "sustained-release" iron preparations (Middleton *et al.*, 1966). In rare situations in which oral iron therapy is not successful (often owing to unreliable administration or noncompliance), parenteral iron may be given in the form of iron dextran. The latter may be particularly useful in children, in whom iron absorption may be diminished as a result of mucosal dysfunction induced by the iron deficiency itself (Kimber and Weintraub, 1968).

Gamma Globulin in the Treatment of Hypogammaglobulinemia Associated with Gastrointestinal Manifestations. Some patients with immunoglobulin deficiencies may develop diarrhea and malabsorption (Allen and Hadden, 1964; Waldmann and Laster, 1964; Collins and Ellis, 1965). The pathogenesis of the malabsorption, however, has eluded classification. Jejunal biopsies either have been normal (Waldmann and Laster, 1964; McCarthy *et al.*, 1965) or have shown definite villous atrophy (Waldmann and Laster, 1964; Collins and Ellis, 1965). The diarrhea and steatorrhea have responded to a gluten-free diet in only a few individuals. Gastrointestinal symptoms have also been associated with nodular lymphoid hyperplasia of the small intestine, deficiencies of IgA and IgM (Hermans *et al.*, 1966; Hermans, 1967; Kirkpatrick *et al.*, 1968), and thymoma (Conn and Quintiliani, 1966; Sherman *et al.*, 1966). These syndromes and the relationship of immune responses to the gut have been reviewed (Watson, 1969).

Interference with or Antagonism of a Normal or Exaggerated Physiologic Process

Antacid Therapy in Peptic Ulcer Disease. The etiology of peptic ulcer disease, one of the most common afflictions of Western civilization, is still unknown (Kirsner, 1968b). The relative importance of psychic and emotional stress, mucosal resistance, ingested irritants, the rate of gastric acid and pepsin production, and a host of other factors is not clear. Spontaneous remission is so common that the efficacy of medical treatment is difficult to prove. However, one established fact has led to the use of antacids as the keystone of therapy, namely, "no acid, no ulcer." Patients with achlorhydria do not, except rarely, form benign ulcers, presumably because pepsin is not active at a pH above 4.0. Gastric acid secretion is required for the formation and persistence of the lesion. A more practical reason for the widespread use of antacids in the therapy of ulcer disease is that they *are* effective in relieving pain (Lawrence, 1952). As a result, over 600 nonprescription and 160 prescription antacid preparations were available on the American market in 1967 (Kirsner, 1968a).

Despite a reasonably good rationale for the use of antacids in the therapy of benign peptic ulcer, convincing evidence that the rate of healing is accelerated, or that recurrences are prevented, is lacking (Baume and Hunt, 1969). However, if one accepts the desirability of neutralizing gastric acid, antacids can accomplish this goal when used appropriately (Dotevall and Walan, 1967). Cost, palatability, and side effects are important considerations in choosing an antacid for a therapeutic program. The most popular antacids are calcium carbonate, aluminum hydroxide, and magnesium hydroxide, oxide, and trisilicate. The magnesium compounds are often added to overcome the constipating effects of aluminum hydroxide. Despite its widespread use, aluminum hydroxide alone is a weak antacid and in tablet form is particularly impotent (Piper and Fenton, 1964).

How should antacids be used to treat ulcer disease? *If the goal of treatment is continuing neutralization of gastric acidity, the major limiting factor in antacid therapy is the rate of gastric emptying; therefore, the frequency of antacid administration is the most important aspect of rational therapy.* Indeed, gastric emptying is so predominant in determining the duration of neutralization that such factors as gastric acid production and the dose of the antacid are of less importance. For example, a single 4-g dose of $CaCO_3$ is sufficient, *in vitro*, to neutralize the entire daily output of hydrochloric acid in many patients. In contrast, such a dose *in vivo* has a neutralizing effect for only 30 to 40 minutes in the fasting state. The difference is due to gastric emptying. It is therefore ludicrous to prescribe antacids three or four times a day. *If the goal of significant neutralization of gastric acid is to be* seriously pursued, the antacid chosen must be given at frequent intervals. It may be optimal to have the patient suck antacid tablets constantly during waking hours, but in practice the patient usually takes the antacid every hour between meals while awake. Recent studies lend support to the choice of this latter interval between doses (Dotevall and Walan, 1967; Morrissey et al., 1967). It may be particularly important to take the antacid approximately 1 hour after meals, when the drug has a much longer effect owing to slower gastric emptying and "acid rebound" is prevented (Fordtran and Collyns, 1966).

Liquid or powder forms of antacid are generally more effective than tablets, presumably owing to more rapid dispersion (see Chapter 2). In vitro tests have demonstrated that tablet forms have a lower neutralizing efficiency than liquid preparations of the same antacid (Brody and Bachrach, 1959; Piper and Fenton, 1964). (Indeed, aluminum hydroxide in tablet form is virtually inert as an antacid!) If tablets are used, they should be chewed before swallowing, or merely sucked. A minimum dose of the hydroxide gels is 30 ml (Kirsner and Palmer, 1940; Brody and Bachrach, 1959). The standard dose of $CaCO_3$ is 2 to 4 g dispersed in water or chewed before swallowing. If the patient does not respond to these doses given hourly, it is preferable to give the same dose more frequently rather than to increase the dose. *Principle: Ulcer therapy is inadequate unless pain is prevented and not merely relieved when it occurs* (Kirsner, 1968b). If the patient responds to the antacid program with relief of symptoms, how long should the strict hourly program be continued? Gastric ulcers must be treated rigorously until complete radiologic healing takes place. However, in the case of duodenal ulcer, serial radiographic evaluation is neither desirable nor rewarding. As symptoms usually disappear long before the ulcer is completely healed, a satisfactory antacid program must be continued long after the patient is asymptomatic. *Principle: Chronic administration of a drug is often neglected by patients whose symptoms have remitted.* Nearly all adequately treated duodenal ulcers heal within 1 to 3 months; thus, it seems desirable to continue the antacid program for that time (Grossman, 1962). Many physicians then instruct the patient to take the antacid three or four times a day.

Antacids have many potential side effects. Calcium carbonate and aluminum hydroxide gels may be constipating, particularly when given to elderly patients or when there is associated upper intestinal bleeding; intestinal obstruction may occur (Havens, 1939; Brettschneider et al., 1965; Potyk, 1970). Nearly all

the hydroxide gel compounds contain sodium, so that an hourly antacid regimen may provide 500 to 2500 mg of additional dietary sodium, an important factor in patients with edema (Rimer and Frankland, 1960). Urinary calculi of silica may occur after prolonged ingestion of antacids containing magnesium trisilicate (Herman and Goldberg, 1960). Various aluminum compounds may adsorb organic and inorganic substances (e.g., tetracycline antibiotics). The use of $Al(OH)_3$ antacids to treat upper intestinal symptoms may lead to significantly lower blood levels of tetracyclines (Paul and Harrington, 1952). Certain anticholinergics, including atropine, may be similarly adsorbed (Grote and Woods, 1953). Aluminum hydroxide binds inorganic phosphate in the intestinal lumen, leading to increased fecal phosphate excretion and decreased serum phosphate concentrations. This property of $Al(OH)_3$ is sometimes utilized in the treatment of uremia, when it also may be important to avoid magnesium-containing antacids because of the danger of hypermagnesemia. Because of phosphate binding in the gut, chronic ingestion of these antacids may lead to abnormal bone metabolism and osteomalacia (Bloom and Flinchum, 1960). The possibility of a clinically important "phosphorus depletion syndrome" has been discussed (Lotz et al., 1968).

Although $CaCO_3$ is the cheapest and most potent antacid, one drawback to its use is the occasional occurrence of clinically significant hypercalcemia. Radioactive tracer studies have demonstrated that the calcium in $CaCO_3$ is absorbed to the same degree as the calcium in the soluble salt calcium gluconate, that is, 9 to 37% (Ivanovich et al., 1967). As hypercalcemia is common when $CaCO_3$ is used in effective doses (Stiel et al., 1967), it seems prudent to determine the serum calcium at periodic intervals and to avoid the use of this agent in patients with renal disease. When marked hypercalcemia occurs, increased epigastric pain, nausea, vomiting, polyuria, alkalosis, and eventually azotemia due to nephrocalcinosis may result, a picture referred to as the "milk alkali syndrome" (McMillan and Freeman, 1965). Presumably, patients who absorb large amounts of calcium develop alkalosis because the net loss of hydrogen ions in the stomach (net gain of HCO_3^-) is no longer balanced by the binding of HCO_3^- (net loss of HCO_3^-) in the upper small intestine by unabsorbed calcium (Schroeder, 1969). A high milk intake may further deplete calcium in the duodenum by binding it as calcium phosphate.

In summary, the use of antacids in the treatment of peptic ulcer disease has a logical theoretic basis. Proper use of these drugs can at least partially accomplish the goal of neutralization of gastric contents, and symptoms improve in the vast majority of patients. However, there is no conclusive evidence that the natural history of the ulcer is altered, although an adequately designed study has never been conducted. This fact, plus the inability or unwillingness of many patients to conform to a rigorous antacid program, has led to an increasing interest in other approaches to the therapy of ulcer disease.

Miscellaneous Agents in Peptic Ulcer Disease. Attempts to find more satisfactory means of healing ulcers have led to such measures as stilbestrol treatment in men (Truelove, 1960b), gastrin antagonists (Connell *et al.*, 1968), and pepsin inhibitors (Zimmon *et al.*, 1969). The latter two approaches are promising but require further clinical testing. The use of carbenoxolone sodium has been effective in the treatment of *gastric* ulcers in several controlled trials in Europe (McHardy, 1969). Although the mode of action of this compound is uncertain, enhancement of mucus secretion by gastric mucosa may be involved. The drug is synthesized from glycyrrhizinic acid, a glycoside extracted from licorice. Because it is absorbed from the stomach, a position-release capsule has been developed for its use in the treatment of duodenal ulcers, with as yet unproved efficacy (Montgomery *et al.*, 1968). Because of the aldosterone-like side effects of carbenoxolone, a deglycyrrhizinated preparation (Caved-S) has been developed and appears to be equally effective in the treatment of gastric ulcer (Turpie *et al,*, 1969). More carefully designed, controlled studies of this agent are justified.

Anticholinergic Drugs in Gastrointestinal Disorders. Aside from tranquilizers and sedatives, anticholinergic (antimuscarinic) agents are most widely prescribed for intestinal disorders. Parasympathetic activity is of paramount importance in the extrinsic nervous control of the gut, as it enhances both tone and motility. In addition, vagal parasympathetic impulses stimulate gastric and pancreatic secretions. Anticholinergic therapy may be efficacious in many common disorders. Unfortunately, the exact role of these drugs in therapy is still debatable (Ingelfinger, 1963).

The prototypical anticholinergic drug is atropine, the principal ingredient of belladonna. Despite numerous attempts to find equally effective drugs with minimal side effects, few drugs are more effective than atropine or belladonna (Grossman, 1962; Friend, 1963). With all anticholinergic drugs, the dosage must usually be increased to the point of side effects

in order to achieve consistent, measurable pharmacologic effects on the target organ. Mild side effects (dry mouth, blurring of vision, etc.) should be produced to ensure adequate dosage for the desired pharmacologic effect. *Principle: When doses of any anticholinergic drug are large enough to be effective (other than as a placebo), almost invariably they cause one or more typical atropinic side effects.* Given the necessity to individualize the dose, combinations of these drugs with various sedatives and tranquilizers in fixed dosage is patently irrational. Their extensive use is sad commentary on both the pharmaceutical industry and the medical profession!

Anticholinergic Drugs and Peptic Ulcer Disease. The pathogenesis of peptic ulcer disease is poorly understood, but gastric acid production appears to play an important role, whether active or permissive. Vagal impulses mediate the "cephalic phase" of gastric secretion, stimulate gastrin release, and potentiate the effects of gastrin (Grossman, 1966). In effective doses, anticholinergic drugs reduce acid production and gastric motility and slow emptying, thereby reducing pain and prolonging the neutralizing effect of food or antacids. *Basal* acid secretion can be significantly reduced (Mitchell *et al.*, 1962; Bitsch and Kristensen, 1966), but the effect on *stimulated* gastric acid secretion and on gastric emptying time is less consistently demonstrable (Fordtran and Collyns, 1966; Morrissey *et al.*, 1967; Konturek *et al.*, 1968). Given evidence that the desired action of the drug can be achieved, the question of clinical usefulness must still be answered. Although *chronic* anticholinergic therapy may be beneficial in the management of duodenal ulcer, the overall course has not been significantly altered in most instances (Cayer, 1956; Lennard-Jones, 1961; Ruffin and Cayer, 1962). One double-blind controlled study stands out as a major exception to the usual reports (Sun, 1964). In this study, the long-term use of an individualized optimal dose of glycopyrrolate led to a markedly lower incidence of clinical recurrences of duodenal ulcer over a minimum observation time of 18 months. This striking result needs confirmation. It is difficult to convince patients to take medications chronically when side effects are common and the disorder is asymptomatic. In addition, long-term therapy with anticholinergic drugs may mask or alter symptoms so as to delay recognition of recurrences (Roth *et al.*, 1956). In the *short-term* management of ulcer disease, anticholinergic drugs may help reduce gastric acidity (particularly during the night when the patient does not take antacids), prolong the effect of antacids

(Dotevall and Walan, 1967), and reduce gastric motility. (However, reduction in gastric motility might have the undesirable effect of stimulating the gastrin mechanism.) There are numerous contraindications to the use of these agents, including glaucoma, prostatic disease, gastric outlet obstruction, and reflux esophagitis. The latter may be worsened by decreased gastric emptying and decreased lower esophageal sphincter pressure (Bettarello *et al.*, 1960; Skinner and Camp, 1968).

In selected cases of the Zollinger-Ellison syndrome, a marked reduction in acid secretion has been achieved over long periods of time, demonstrating that anticholinergic drugs *do* reduce gastric acid output when properly used (Shimoda and Rubin, 1968).

Anticholinergic Drugs and Other Gastrointestinal Disorders. Anticholinergic therapy has been widely applied in the management of acute pancreatitis. Although the exact pathogenesis of this disorder is still poorly understood, therapy should be directed at "putting the pancreas to rest." Anticholinergic agents have a significant inhibitory effect on the basal and hormonally stimulated pancreatic secretion of fluid, electrolytes, and enzymes (Dreiling and Janowitz, 1960; Bock *et al.*, 1968). However, there is no good evidence that such therapy is of clinical value in treatment. Although side effects are less important in the management of a life-threatening, acute illness, an undesirable pharmacologic effect is the suppression or elimination of intestinal peristaltic activity, which is ordinarily used as a sign of activity of the disease. Pancreatitis may be mimicked by several acute surgical disorders of the abdomen, and the presence of a drug-induced paralytic ileus complicates diagnosis and management. *Principle: Undesirable side effects often outweigh benefits of a drug and nullify its usefulness.*

Perhaps the most common cause of gastrointestinal symptoms is the irritable colon syndrome, and anticholinergic therapy is often used to reduce intestinal motility and "spasm" (Ingelfinger, 1943). Controlled studies have shown a beneficial *initial* effect on symptoms, but the evidence is far from convincing (Connell and Kellock, 1959; Kasich and Rafsky, 1959; McHardy *et al.*, 1968).

In summary, anticholinergic drug therapy has a logical place in the management of many gastrointestinal disorders, based on the ability of these drugs (when given at maximal tolerable dosage) to reduce the tone and motility of the gut and the secretion of acid and pancreatic juice. Properly used, they can accomplish the desired effect on the target organ. However, the frequency and virtual necessity of annoying side effects, the fact that other aspects of treatment seem more important, and the lack of convincing evidence of *clinical* value have led to a general lack of enthusiasm for their routine use.

Dumping Syndrome. A constellation of symptoms occurring up to 20 minutes after meals in occasional postgastrectomy patients is known as the dumping syndrome. These can be divided into intestinal symptoms (hyperperistalsis, bloating, discomfort, cramps, nausea, and diarrhea) and vasomotor symptoms (weakness, pallor, tachycardia, flushing, sweating, palpitations, etc.). The syndrome is caused by the sudden "dumping" of a hypertonic solution into the jejunum, with resultant excessive intestinal secretion and distention (Machella, 1950). In some uncertain way, this produces peripheral vasodilation, decreased effective plasma volume, and postural hypotension. Patients with the severe form of this syndrome often exhibit marked weight loss and poor nutrition (they are afraid to eat!), presenting a difficult problem in management. Dietary therapy has been the most effective means of treatment, and all but the most severe "dumpers" improve when they use a diet low in carbohydrate and omit fluids at mealtimes (Robinson and Pittman, 1957). This approach prevents solutions with high osmolar content from abruptly reaching the jejunum. Efforts to devise pharmacologic means of controlling at least some of the symptoms have been stimulated by the evidence that humoral factors may be important in pathogenesis. Following preliminary evidence for the existence of a transfusible "dumping factor" (in dogs), it was demonstrated that peripheral plasma concentrations of serotonin and bradykinin are increased in patients with the dumping syndrome at the time of typical vasomotor symptoms (Johnson and Jesseph, 1961; Zeitlin and Smith, 1966; Reichle *et al.*, 1967; MacDonald *et al.*, 1969). The possible role of bradykinin is particularly attractive because of the ability of this peptide to cause vasodilation and flushing in patients with the carcinoid syndrome. This ability, plus the presence of argentaffin cells in the jejunum, has led to the working hypothesis that the sudden jejunal distention leads to the release of vasoactive peptides into the portal vein in quantities sufficient to elude hepatic detoxification, reach the systemic circulation, and elicit the vasomotor abnormalities. In preliminary uncontrolled experiments, use of the serotonin antagonists cyproheptadine and methysergide has led to apparent improvement in vasomotor symptoms and diarrhea (Johnson *et al.*, 1962; Peskin and Miller, 1965). There is as yet insufficient experience to reach any conclusions, but carefully controlled and randomized studies with antagonists of serotonin and bradykinin may lead to a better understanding of this occasionally disabling syndrome.

Antimicrobial Agents

Salicylazosulfapyridine in the Treatment of Ulcerative Colitis. The etiology of chronic ulcerative colitis is unknown, although bacterial pathogens may have a causative role. Investigations of fecal flora in patients with this disease have not demonstrated significant deviations from normal (Cooke, 1967; Gorbach et al., 1968). Salicylazosulfapyridine, a compound resulting from the diazotation of sulfapyridine and coupling of the diazonium salt with salicylic acid, appears effective in the treatment of mild-to-moderate ulcerative colitis (Baron et al., 1962; Dick et al., 1964) and reduces the incidence of relapse (Misiewicz et al., 1965). Although unpleasant side effects often occur, they are dose related and minimal with daily doses of 1 to 2 g. The benefits of the drug often are not evident for a considerable time, unlike the frequently dramatic effects of corticosteroids.

The mechanism of action of salicylazosulfapyridine is unknown. It works best in mild-to-moderate disease in which bacterial flora is not altered, and careful studies have not shown a significant change in flora after successful treatment (Gorbach et al., 1968; Cooke, 1969). Thus, there is no evidence for an antibacterial mechanism of action. The drug has a strong affinity for connective tissue, and part of the absorbed compound is apparently stored in collagen and elastic tissue, including that of the colon (Hanngren et al., 1963). Some alteration in the tissue response to inflammation therefore may be important in its mechanism of action (see Chapter 9).

Antimicrobial Agents in the Treatment of Diverticulitis. Acute diverticulitis is often associated with fever, leukocytosis, and septicemia. Perforation of the inflamed diverticula, with pericolonic abscess formation, is a frequent complication. Antimicrobial agents have a logical place in therapy, and the question is mainly choice of agent. Both nonabsorbable and absorbable antibiotics and sulfas have been advocated, although unfortunately no controlled studies have assessed their relative value. The choice lies between achieving a high intraluminal concentration of the antimicrobial agent and obtaining high blood and tissue concentration. Although pertinent information is not available, the latter approach seems more logical in patients with systemic signs of infection.

Blind-Loop Syndrome. Overgrowth of small-bowel bacteria may complicate several disorders of the small intestine involving stasis of the intestinal contents. These include afferent loop stasis following gastrectomy (Wirts and Goldstein, 1963; Mortimer et al., 1964; Tabaqchali and Booth, 1966), jejunal diverticulosis (Cooke et al., 1963), enteroenteric anastomosis (Siurala and Kaupainen, 1953), and visceral neuropathy in diabetes, amyloid disease, and scleroderma (Malins and French, 1957; Sumi and Finlay, 1961; Kahn et al., 1966; Solen et al., 1966). In these diseases, bacterial counts in the intestinal fluid may be greater than 10^8 or 10^9 organisms per milliliter and may consist of a variety of organisms, including *Escherichia coli*, *Neisseria*, *Bacteroides*, *Lactobacillus*, and *Clostridium* (Rosenberg et al., 1967; Tabaqchali and Booth, 1967; Krone et al., 1968; Polter et al., 1968). *Bacteroides* may be the most abundant organism when appropriate culture techniques are utilized (Hill and Drasar, 1968).

Malabsorption is frequently associated with bacterial overgrowth. When bacterial proliferation is primarily limited to the ileum (such as in surgical blind loops of the distal bowel, ileal strictures, and fistulas), only the absorption of vitamin B_{12} may be impaired. When bacterial overgrowth occurs in the more proximal regions of the intestine (as in afferent loop stasis, proximal blind loops and jejunal diverticula), malabsorption of fat may also be present. The reduction of steatorrhea by treatment with "broad-spectrum" antibiotics gives further evidence that bacterial overgrowth in these disorders is causally related to malabsorption (Badenoch, 1960; Doig and Girdwood, 1960; Cooke et al., 1963; Wirts and Goldstein, 1963; Paulk and Farrar, 1964; Kahn et al., 1966). Some strains of *Bacteroides*, as well as *Streptococcus faecalis* and clostridia, are now known to be capable of hydrolytic deconjugation of glucuronide from normal bile acids (Norman and Grubb, 1955; Drasar et al., 1966). Intestinal fluid recovered from patients with blind loops contains increased amounts of free bile acids (Donaldson, 1965; Tabaqchali and Booth, 1966; Rosenberg et al., 1967; Tabaqchali et al., 1968), a state that may be reversed by antibiotic therapy. Two mechanisms have been proposed to relate the altered bile acid metabolism to the steatorrhea. The unconjugated bile acids may exert a direct toxic effect on the intestinal mucosa, or, as most of the evidence suggests, the reduced amounts of conjugated bile acids may impair micelle formation in the bowel lumen (Kim et al., 1966; Krone et al., 1968; Rosenberg, 1969). Although treatment with antibiotics may dramatically improve fat absorption, the results are often transient, and surgical correction of the blind-loop stasis is the treatment of choice.

The blind-loop syndromes illustrate how the success of a logical mode of therapy (i.e., antibiotics to suppress bacterial overgrowth) stimulated investigation of the mechanisms involved, leading in turn to increased understanding of bacterial and bile acid metabolism. *Principle: The success of a therapeutic method may precede and stimulate knowledge of its mechanism of action* (see Chapter 18).

Tropical Sprue. This well-known malabsorption syndrome occurs in tropical and subtropical areas, although it may persist in individuals who subsequently move to temperate zones. Although histologic changes in the intestine may resemble those found in celiac disease, they are usually less severe, and treatment with a gluten-free diet is ineffective. The pathogenesis of this disease is unknown, but the clinical, biochemical, and histologic improvement after "broad-spectrum" antibiotic therapy suggests that an enteric infection or altered intestinal flora may be responsible (Sheehy and Perez-Santiago, 1961; Klipstein and Falaiye, 1969). No specific agents (viral, bacterial, or parasitic) have been isolated. Folic acid therapy alone has produced clinical remissions (Sheehy *et al.*, 1965), although malabsorption is not known to be caused by folic acid deficiency per se. Further studies of small-bowel flora, bile acid metabolism, and micelle formation may provide an explanation for the success of antibiotic therapy. A comprehensive review of this disorder has been published (Klipstein, 1968).

Whipple's Disease. Whipple's disease is an excellent example of a primary intestinal malabsorptive disease that responds to antibiotic therapy. Until the use of antibiotics, this disease was invariably fatal. "Broad-spectrum" antibiotic therapy (e.g., tetracycline) abolishes the malabsorption and, when maintained for periods of months to years, restores the patient to health in most instances (Kuntz *et al.*, 1962; Davis *et al.*, 1963; Trier *et al.*, 1965; Laster *et al.*, 1966). Bacilliform bodies have been found in the intestinal mucosa, a finding specific for this disease (Haubrich *et al.*, 1960; Chears and Ashworth, 1961; Hollenberg and Jennings, 1962; Kuntz *et al.*, 1962). Electron micrographs have shown these bacilli in various stages of degeneration in cytoplasmic inclusions within large macrophages located in the lamina propria (Trier *et al.*, 1965; Dobbins and Ruffin, 1967). The response to antibiotic therapy and the observation that the bacilli disappear during successful therapy and reappear during relapse (Ashworth *et al.*, 1964; Trier *et al.*, 1965; Ruffin *et al.*, 1966) suggest that this is an infectious disease, although attempts to culture a specific organism have been only partially successful. Cytochemical, histochemical, and electron microscopic studies confirm the bacterial structure of the "organisms" and suggest that they resemble a gram-negative species of *Hemophilus* (Sobel, 1966). Once again, the success of a method of treatment stimulated intensive research directed at the pathophysiology of a disease.

"Prophylactic" Use of Antibiotics in Colonic Surgery. Antibiotics are commonly utilized in preparing patients for colonic surgery. The objective is a significant reduction in the colonic bacterial flora and the prevention of postoperative abdominal infection. Poorly absorbed drugs, such as neomycin, kanamycin, or nonabsorbable sulfas, are the most widely used agents and are given for 3 to 5 days prior to surgery, combined with purgation. In many instances, systemic antibiotics are also given postoperatively as routine "prophylaxis," even in the absence of any suspected spillage or contamination of the peritoneal cavity during surgery. These applications of "prophylactic" antimicrobial therapy, despite wide acceptance (in the case of preoperative use), are of unproved merit, possibly because they are based on unsound assumptions. Vigorous mechanical cleansing of the bowel *itself* effects a drastic reduction in the total intestinal bacterial population, independent of any antibiotic effect. In this instance, the *qualitative* makeup of the flora is relatively unchanged. Although antimicrobial agents can reduce susceptible organisms, rapid growth of resistant organisms often occurs, leading to a radical change in the qualitative composition of the flora (Gaylor *et al.*, 1960). Thus, intestinal antisepsis more often than not results in an altered microflora, rather than in a significant numerical reduction (Tyson and Spaulding, 1966). Elimination of vulnerable coliforms often leads to rapid colonization with resistant *Klebsiella, Proteus, Pseudomonas, Candida*, and especially *Staph. aureus* (Gaylor *et al.*, 1960; Tyson and Spaulding, 1966). Furthermore, it often takes 7 to 10 days for recolonization with normal flora to occur after withdrawal of antimicrobial therapy, allowing ample time for development of postoperative infections with highly resistant organisms (Gaylor *et al.*, 1960). Retrospective studies now indicate an increased risk of significant postoperative infections when patients having bowel surgery are given routine preoperative antimicrobial agents (Polacek and Sanfelippo, 1968). A carefully controlled, prospective, double-blind study (Gaylor *et al.*, 1960) revealed a significantly lower incidence of postoperative infections in a placebo-treated group than in patients treated with four different antibiotic regimens. Staphylococcal enterocolitis and wound infections are distinctly more common in antibiotic-treated patients, particularly when *postoperative* antibiotics are also utilized "prophylactically" (Polacek and Sanfelippo, 1968; Azar and Drapanas, 1968). Thus, despite continuing enthusiasm for "prophylactic" antimicrobial therapy (Cohn, 1966), there is an urgent need for more carefully controlled, prospective trials to elucidate the problem. With the evidence at hand, it seems unwarranted to continue this practice in routine cases. *Principle: Whenever prophylaxis is directed at the elimination or reduction of all types of microorganisms, as distinct from the prevention of infection by a specific organism, failure is the rule* (Weinstein, 1964).

Anti-inflammatory and "Immunosuppressive" Drugs (see also Chapter 9)

Corticosteroid Therapy of Inflammatory Bowel Disease. Steroid therapy was introduced early in the management of the common idiopathic inflammatory diseases of the bowel. The justification for their use, then as now, was that patients with ulcerative colitis or Crohn's disease were often desperately sick due to inflammation in the gut, and corticosteroids had potent anti-inflammatory properties. An autoimmune pathogenesis has also been a theoretic rationale for steroid therapy. Steroids did produce clear-cut beneficial effects in the treatment of idiopathic ulcerative colitis, and several carefully designed controlled studies have documented their effectiveness. On the other hand, the role of steroids in the management of Crohn's disease is still debatable.

The following facts have been established regarding the use of corticosteroids to treat ulcerative colitis: (1) patients on systemic cortisone therapy have a higher incidence of remission (particularly in first attacks) than do controls (Truelove and Witts, 1955); (2) in mild-to-moderate attacks, nightly administration of hydrocortisone hemisuccinate per rectum (Truelove, 1958; Watkinson, 1958) or retention enemas containing prednisolone-21-phosphate (Matts, 1960) lead to significantly more remissions than do placebos; and (3) in mild-to-moderate attacks, a combination of moderate doses of oral prednisolone and hydrocortisone hemisuccinate given per rectum is more effective than either mode of therapy alone (Truelove, 1960a). Because of the effectiveness of rectally administered steroids in this disease, it is of some interest to speculate on the mechanism of action. Does the steroid work topically, or is the pharmacologic action due to absorption of the drug through the inflamed mucosa? Rectal administration does lead to significant absorption of the drug in some instances, depending in part upon the preparation utilized (Nabarro *et al.*, 1957). Even in normal subjects, significant pituitary-adrenal suppression may occur with the use of soluble steroid enemas (Sparberg *et al.*, 1967); acute adrenal insufficiency may follow stress in patients treated in this manner. On the other hand, a topical action seems likely and is probably more important. Rectal administration of the minimally absorbed steroid preparation, hydrocortisone hemisuccinate, is significantly beneficial (Schwartz *et al.*, 1958). The physician is not merely treating the distal few inches of colon when using enemas or rectal drips. For example, contrast material, when given as a small retention enema or as a suppository, often spreads proximally as far as the mid-transverse colon (Matts, 1960; Parker and Siegelman, 1965).

The usefulness of corticosteroid therapy in the treatment of severe, fulminant attacks of ulcerative colitis is more difficult to assess, and, in view of the efficacy of treatment in mild-to-moderate cases, controlled studies are ethically contraindicated. Most gastroenterologists feel that large doses of steroids or ACTH are sometimes lifesaving in patients with severe attacks, allowing time for medical management or elective (as opposed to emergency) surgical intervention (Korelitz and Lindner, 1964). Owing to the life-threatening nature of the disease in such patients, large parenteral doses of steroid should be used. Once the disease is controlled, slow tapering of the drug should be carried out as tolerated, until the smallest effective maintenance dose is reached. If there is no clear-cut beneficial response within a few days, this form of therapy is unlikely to be successful and other steps should be considered. The hazards and side effects of long-term steroid therapy are impressive (Goldstein *et al.*, 1967) (see Chapter 9); for this reason intermittent therapy has been tried, with some success, but only after a partial remission has already been achieved (Cocco and Mendeloff, 1967).

There are as yet no good, prospective, double-blind studies on the effect of steroids on the course of Crohn's disease (regional enteritis), although this form of treatment is frequently used. Uncontrolled retrospective studies have suggested that the initial response to steroids is usually good, although the long-term course of the disease is probably not modified (Jones and Lennard-Jones, 1966; Sparberg and Kirsner, 1966; Law, 1969). Some authors prefer to initiate therapy with an infusion of ACTH, later switching to oral steroids (Hanson *et al.*, 1969).

"Immunosuppressive" Therapy in Inflammatory Bowel Disorders. "Immunosuppressive" drugs, particularly azathioprine, are now the fashionable treatment for ulcerative colitis and Crohn's disease. Uncontrolled experience has suggested possible benefit, particularly in Crohn's disease (Bowen *et al.*, 1966; Brooke *et al.*, 1969; Brooke *et al.*, 1970); hopefully, controlled prospective studies will be forthcoming.

Dietary Therapy

Most patients, with or without intestinal disease, have firmly entrenched notions that certain foods regularly and reproducibly cause disturbing symptoms (Koch and Donaldson, 1964). Patients therefore *want* special dietary instructions and are usually skeptical if the physician de-emphasizes their importance. If dietary restrictions are not imposed by the physician, they are usually self-imposed by the patient, assisted by his relatives and friends. Consequently, the physician should provide guidance in this aspect of therapy, utilizing scientifically demonstrable facts when possible, and preventing the adoption of unsound, nutritionally inadequate, or unnecessarily expensive and tedious maneuvers. *Principle: Dietary instructions cannot be ignored or avoided; if the physician does not provide a special diet, the patient will!*

If a food is to produce or allay intestinal symptoms, it presumably must alter the motility, secretions, or structure (including vascularity) of the organ in question. As there is little information concerning these effects (Weinstein *et al.*, 1961), most current practices are based on unsubstantiated opinion and tradition. Even the classification of foods, such as high or low "residue," is influenced by local dietary habits and prejudices (Kramer, 1964).

Several principles of dietary therapy are generally accepted. *Principles: (1) The diet should be nutritionally complete. (2) As symptoms attributed to specific foods tend to be unique for the patient, not the underlying disease, the diet must be adapted to the patient as well as to the disease. (3) Undue stress on scientifically unproved measures should be avoided at all costs so as not to cause dietary invalidism, a condition frequently much worse than the original disorder* (Bircher and Haemmerli, 1967; Salter, 1969).

The few special diets of proven merit in gastroenterology include (1) gluten-free diet in celiac sprue, (2) withdrawal of the offending sugar in disaccharide and monosaccharide intolerance, (3) fat restriction in patients with symptomatic steatorrhea, (4) protein restriction in patients with portosystemic encephalopathy,

and (5) avoidance of osmotically potent foods in the dumping syndrome. Of theoretically sound but unproven value are "low-roughage" or "low-residue" diets in patients with a critically narrowed intestinal lumen (e.g., in Crohn's disease) and low-fat diets in patients with symptomatic cholelithiasis or pancreatitis (Koch and Donaldson, 1964; Taggart and Billington, 1966). More controversial is the use of "bland" and/or "low-residue" diets in the management of peptic ulcer, diverticular disease of the colon, inflammatory bowel disease, and irritable colon syndrome; there are no controlled studies showing the value of such therapy.

The role of dietary therapy in peptic ulcer disease deserves additional comment. Advocates of special diets (frequently graded according to the stage of the ulcer disease being treated) emphasize the following goals: (1) reduction in gastric acid production by eliminating gastric secretogogues; (2) frequent small feedings to prevent distention of the antrum (with its consequent release of gastrin) and to avoid hunger contractions; (3) relatively high fat content in order to stimulate enterogastrone release from the duodenum, thereby slowing gastric motility; and (4) prevention of abrasion of the ulcer crater by elimination of "high-residue" foods (Roth, 1966). These considerations have led to the widespread use of frequent milk and cream feedings in the patient with an active ulcer, with progression to a more liberal "bland diet" in the second or third week of treatment. Although strictly double-blind studies are not possible in the evaluation of such therapy, there is much evidence that regimens varying from continuous milk drips to more liberal bland diets do *not* reduce intragastric acidity or enhance healing (Doll *et al.*, 1956; Lennard-Jones and Babouris, 1965). Furthermore, the chronic ingestion of large quantities of milk and cream carries the potential danger of undue weight gain and possibly an increased incidence of coronary atherosclerosis (Briggs *et al.*, 1960; Brooks *et al.*, 1963). Even if everyone agreed as to what constitutes a "bland diet" ("blandness" is a somewhat nebulous quality), there is no evidence that "nonbland" foods are harmful to the gastric or duodenal mucosa or to an ulcer crater. Given this relative lack of information, and despite the theoretic advantages stated above, many have concluded that except for elimination of proven secretogogues such as caffeine and alcohol, the patient with an ulcer should be allowed to eat whatever he can tolerate, and that the therapeutic program should emphasize frequent and regular administration of antacids (Ingelfinger, 1966). Advocates of both methods can quote extensive personal experience illustrating the merit of their approach. The skeptic might argue that this is because the active ulcer tends to heal under the most varied regimens imaginable; this may be another reason to keep therapy as uncomplicated as possible.

Medium-Chain Triglyceride Therapy

A promising new development in the dietary therapy of gastrointestinal disorders is a preparation of medium-chain triglycerides (MCT). MCT preparations contain triglycerides whose fatty acids (mainly octanoic and decanoic) have chain lengths varying from 6 to 12 carbon atoms. In contrast to long-chain triglycerides, MCT are rapidly hydrolyzed in the gut lumen, are apparently less dependent on both bile salts and pancreatic lipase for absorption, and appear in the portal vein as free fatty acids (rather than being incorporated into chylomicron triglyceride). MCT are metabolized differently from long-chain fats, being rapidly catabolized in the liver to carbon dioxide and ketone bodies. MCT have therefore been advocated in a variety of conditions, with encouraging early experiences. Conditions potentially amenable to MCT therapy include disorders of intestinal lymphatic drainage, malabsorptive disorders (due to intestinal mucosal disease, short-bowel syndrome, pancreatic exocrine insufficiency, bile salt deficiency, etc.), and perhaps fat-induced hypertriglyceridemias (Zurier *et al.*, 1966; Greenberger *et al.*, 1967a; Holt, 1968; Greenberger and Skillman, 1969). Since about half the carbohydrate in MCT powder is lactose, patients with intestinal lactase deficiency may develop a worsening of diarrhea with this form of therapy. Much remains to be learned about MCT as a therapeutic approach, including its specific areas of usefulness, possible hazards, and such practical aspects as palatability.

New Approaches in the Treatment of Cholera

Recent advances in the management of patients with cholera provide an excellent example of the application of physiologic principles to the treatment of a disease. In this disorder, an enterotoxin produced by the organism *Vibrio comma* significantly alters small-bowel water, as well as sodium and bicarbonate fluxes, producing a severe, acute diarrhea. If untreated, these patients develop a severe metabolic acidosis, hypovolemia, and shock associated with a high mortality (Gordon *et al.*, 1966). The epithelial surface of the small-bowel mucosa remains anatomically intact (Gangarosa *et al.*, 1960), but the reaction to the cholera enterotoxin produces a markedly increased capillary permeability with an outpouring of fluid into the lamina propria and the lumen. The major therapeutic problem has been adequate and rapid replacement of the massive losses of fluid and electrolytes. The enterotoxin does not alter normal sodium transport mechanisms, at least in the ileum (Grady *et al.*, 1967), nor does it affect glucose absorption (Pierce *et al.*, 1968). As in normal man (Malawar *et al.*, 1965), glucose absorption enhances sodium and water absorption in patients with cholera (Nablin *et al.*, 1968; Pierce *et al.*, 1968; Carpenter, 1971; Chen *et al.*, 1971; Field, 1971). Therefore, treatment of cholera with oral electrolyte solutions containing glucose may reduce intravenous fluid requirements and make replacement therapy available to a greater number of patients.

USE OF DRUGS AND THERAPEUTIC MEASURES IN DIAGNOSIS

Therapeutic Trials

Gluten-Free Diet. Patients with celiac sprue have a "toxic" reaction to gluten and some of its derivatives. Strict withdrawal of gluten from the diet is usually followed by a reduction in steatorrhea and ultimately by normal absorption. In fact, a well-documented response to a gluten-free diet is one of two prerequisites for the diagnosis of celiac sprue, the other being compatible histopathology (loss of villi). This is one of the most vital therapeutic trials in gastroenterology.

"Milk-Free" Diet. Patients with intestinal symptoms due to lactase deficiency improve when milk and milk products are withdrawn from the diet. However, several points should be emphasized in the interpretation of a therapeutic trial with milk-free diet: (1) milk intolerance is relatively common in patients without lactase deficiency (Koch and Donaldson, 1964); (2) not all patients with lactase deficiency give a clear history of an association between symptoms and milk ingestion (Haemmerli *et al.*, 1965; Peternel, 1965); and (3) the amount of milk tolerated by lactase-deficient patients may vary according to gastric emptying rate and the relative degree of enzyme deficiency. Thus, a lactose tolerance test, with or without actual mucosal enzyme determinations, is required for a definitive diagnosis (McGill and Newcomer, 1967).

D-*Xylose Tolerance Test*

D-Xylose, a pentose sugar, is utilized in a useful screening test for intestinal malabsorption (Benson *et al.*, 1957; Christiansen *et al.*, 1959; Fordtran *et al.*, 1962). This substance is absorbed by active transport (Csaky and Lassen, 1964; Cocco *et al.*, 1965) and, contrary to initial impressions, is partly metabolized in man to CO_2 (Segal and Foley, 1959). However, most D-xylose is rapidly excreted in the urine; this is the basis of its use as a diagnostic test of absorption. The drug is taken orally, and its excretion in the urine over the next 5 hours is measured (blood levels may also be assayed during this period). The urinary excretion after a 25-g oral dose usually separates patients with malabsorption due to intestinal mucosal disease from normal subjects (Rinaldo and Gluckmann, 1964). Several factors may lead to a falsely abnormal test: severe diarrhea after ingestion of the drug; massive fluid retention, especially ascites (Marin et al., 1968); renal insufficiency; thyroid disease (Broitman et al., 1964); and upper intestinal stasis (Goldstein et al., 1970).

Secretogogues

Qualitative and quantitative measurements of gastric acid production have long been utilized in clinical medicine, although their differential diagnostic usefulness has often been exaggerated (Wormsley and Grossman, 1965). Increasingly potent stimulants of acid secretion have been used, and with the chemical identification and synthesis of gastrin and pentagastrin, these natural gastric secretogogues may supplant all other agents. Histamine, betazole, gastrin, and pentagastrin apparently have similar potencies (when used in appropriate dosage) in terms of peak acid response (Isenberg et al., 1968; Jepson et al., 1968). For gastric secretory studies to have any clinical value, control values must be established within a given institution, using the same method of stimulation and collection, and the same index of output. When unpurified hormones, including secretin, pancreozymin, and cholecystokinin, are utilized in diagnostic tests, the same considerations apply (Sun, 1965). *Principle: Controlled observations are just as crucial when drugs are used as diagnostic tools as when they are used therapeutically.*

ROLE OF THE ALIMENTARY TRACT IN THE ABSORPTION AND EXCRETION OF DRUGS

Unfortunately, there is little documented information concerning the mechanisms of intestinal absorption for most commonly used drugs (see Chapter 2). Most drugs are absorbed by passive diffusion, with the nonionized lipid-soluble moiety crossing the lipid membrane of the absorptive cell (Levine and Pelikan, 1964; Brodie, 1967). The lipid membrane concept is therefore crucial in explaining drug absorption and distribution. However, certain naturally occurring substances, such as iron and vitamin B_{12}, are absorbed by "facilitated diffusion," in which transfer across the cell is mediated by temporary combination with a "carrier" (this reaction being rate limiting), and some foreign compounds may be absorbed by similar mechanisms.

Many physiologic factors are involved in the absorption of drugs from the intestine (Smyth, 1964; Levine, 1970). The site of absorption is important; drugs absorbed high in the intestinal tract (such as in the mouth or stomach) have a more rapid onset of action than drugs absorbed farther down. Regional differences in absorptive capacity for exogenous drugs may exist, owing to specific "carriers" or differences in intraluminal environment. The rate of gastric emptying and intestinal motility may affect drug absorption, depending somewhat on the site of most rapid absorption. Thus, rapid gastric emptying may reduce overall absorption of drugs more dependent on the small intestine. Rapid peristalsis may increase overall absorption by promoting better contact between drug and absorptive cell or may decrease absorption by reducing the critical time required. Changes in intestinal blood flow may affect drug absorption, although little is known about this factor. Digestive secretions, by means of enzymatic action and effects on intraluminal pH, may greatly influence drug absorption and metabolism. (A few examples have been discussed earlier, such as the effect of gastric pH on salicylate absorption, or the inactivation in the stomach of orally administered bile salts or pancreatic enzyme preparations.) The structure and continuity of the intestinal tract are crucial. Finally, the administration of other drugs may influence the absorption of the agent in question (see Chapter 16).

One drug can affect the absorption of another by a variety of mechanisms, both simple and complex. A cathartic-induced diarrhea may lead to decreased absorption of other substances, owing simply to excessive "intestinal hurry." Certain drugs may decrease the availability of other drugs for absorption. For example, cholestyramine may bind several commonly used drugs, retarding or reducing absorption (Gallo et al., 1965). Antacid gels may chelate other drugs, especially the tetracyclines. Neomycin-induced malabsorption affects the absorption of other drugs, such as penicillin (Cheng and White, 1962), owing at least in part to effects on the absorptive cell. The megaloblastic anemia sometimes seen in patients receiving diphenylhydantoin has been traced to malabsorption of folic acid owing to inhibition of an intestinal enzyme needed for normal folate absorption (Hoffbrand and Necheles, 1968). PAS inhibits folic acid absorption, which in turn may interfere with normal B_{12} absorption (Palva *et al.*, 1966). Drug interactions do not necessarily affect absorption adversely. For example, the alteration of intraluminal pH by one drug may favor the absorption of another.

Little is known about the mechanisms of drug absorption, but still less information is available regarding the excretion of drugs into the gut or the metabolism of drugs by the gut. Although passage across the bowel wall into the lumen occurs in some instances, the biliary tract is probably the major route by which systemically absorbed drugs enter the intestine (Stowe and Plaa, 1968). Drugs or their metabolites entering the gut lumen may be reabsorbed via the enterohepatic circulation, thus prolonging their duration of action. Biotransformation of drugs by intestinal microorganisms may produce compounds of greater biologic activity or toxicity (Scheline, 1968). As the intestinal flora may be of great significance in determining the metabolic fate of drugs, there is an urgent need for more information in this area.

EFFECT OF INTESTINAL DISEASE ON PLANNING DRUG THERAPY

How does the presence of intestinal disease influence the use of drugs in the treatment of *any* disorder? A patient with gastric retention and/or frequent vomiting, or with upper intestinal obstruction, must be given all drugs parenterally. The same is true for the patient with a gastrocolic fistula. The patient with gross steatorrhea absorbs fat-soluble vitamins poorly. Aside from these examples, one is quickly handicapped by inadequate information about drug absorption and metabolism in the presence of intestinal disease. Many investigations have dealt with the absorption of various nutrients, minerals, and vitamins in various disorders, but almost none with drug absorption. What, for example, is the influence of diffuse small intestinal mucosal disease, such as celiac sprue, on the absorption of drugs? Cortisol (Schedl and Clifton, 1963), folic acid (Hepner *et al.*, 1968), phenoxymethyl penicillin (Davis and Pirola, 1968), and thyroxine (Collins, 1966; Hays, 1968) may be poorly absorbed in such patients, and many other commonly used drugs may be similarly affected. Whether malabsorption of drugs in these patients is of clinically significant magnitude is not known. The reserve capacity for absorption of drugs may be sufficient to render differences between normal and diseased bowel clinically unimportant in most instances (Mlynaryk and Kirsner, 1963). If this is true, one explanation may be that most drugs are absorbed at least in part by passive diffusion,

requiring no cellular energy (Levine and Pelikan, 1964). *Principle: Until more is known about gastrointestinal absorption of drugs, parenterally administered agents should be used to treat any acute process (e.g., infection or congestive heart failure) in patients with diffuse small-bowel disease, or whenever the patient does not respond to therapy in the expected manner.*

REFERENCES

Aach, R. D.: Corticosteroids and bilirubin metabolism. *Gastroenterology*, **56**:363–66, 1969.

Abouna, G. M.; Kirkley, J. R.; Hull, C. J.; Kerr, D. N. S.; and Ashcroft T.: Treatment of heptatic coma by extracorporeal pig liver perfusion. *Lancet*, **1**:64–68, 1969.

Acocella, G.; Muttiussi, R.; Nicolis, F. B.; Pallanza, R.; and Tenconi, L. T.: Biliary excretion of antibiotics in man. *Gut*, **9**:536–45, 1968.

Alexander, R. W.; Berman, E.; and Balfour, D. C., Jr.: Relationship of glutamic acid and blood ammonia to hepatic coma. *Gastroenterology*, **29**:711–18, 1955.

Allen, G. E., and Hadden, D. R.: Congenital hypogammaglobulinaemia with steatorrhoea in two adult brothers. *Brit. Med. J.*, **2**:486–90, 1964.

Anderson, P., and Popper, H.: Change in hepatic structure in Wilson's disease. *Amer. J. Path.*, **36**:483–97, 1960.

Artman, E. L., and Wise, R. A.: Hypokalemia in liver cell failure. *Amer. J. Med.*, **15**:459–67, 1953.

Artz, S. S.; Paes, I. C.; and Falloon, W. W.: Hypokalemia-induced hepatic coma in cirrhosis: occurrence despite neomycin therapy. *Gastroenterology*, **51**:1046–53, 1966.

Ashworth, C. T.; Douglas, F. C.; Reynolds, R. C.; and Thomas, P. J.: Bacillus-like bodies in Whipple's disease: disappearance with clinical remission after antibiotic therapy. *Amer. J. Med.*, **37**:481–90, 1964.

Atkinson, M., and Losowsky, M. S.: The mechanism of ascites formation in chronic liver disease. *Quart. J. Med.*, **30**:153–66, 1961.

Atkinson, M.; Nordin, B. E. C.; and Sherlock, S.: Malabsorption and bone disease in prolonged obstructive jaundice. *Quart. J. Med.*, **25**:299–312, 1956.

Auricchio, S.; Rubino, A.; Prader, A.; Rey, J.; Jos, J.; Frézal, J.; and Davidson, M.: Intestinal glycosidase activities in congenital malabsorption of disaccharides. *J. Pediat.*, **66**:555–64, 1965.

Avioli, L. V.; McDonald, J. E.; and Lee, S. W.: The influence of age on the intestinal absorption of ^{47}Ca in women and its relation to ^{47}Ca absorption in postmenopausal osteoporosis. *J. Clin. Invest.*, **44**:1960–67, 1965.

Ayliffe, G. A. J., and Davies, A.: Ampicillin levels in human bile. *Brit. J. Pharmacol.*, **24**:189–93, 1965.

Azar, H., and Drapanas, T.: Relationship of antibiotics to wound infection and enterocolitis in colon surgery. *Amer. J. Surg.*, **115**:209–17, 1968.

Badenoch, J.: Steatorrhoea in the adult. *Brit. Med. J.*, **2**:963–74, 1960.

Baertl, J. M., and Gabuzda, G. J.: Metabolic effects of glutamate and arginine administration and protein restriction in patients with liver disease. *Gastroenterology*, **37**:617–36, 1959.

Baertl, J. M.; Sancetta, S. M.; and Gabuzda, G. J.: Relation of acute potassium depletion to renal ammonium metabolism in patients with cirrhosis. *J. Clin. Invest.*, **42**:696–706, 1963.

Baird, I. McL.; Podmore, D. A.; and Wilson, G. M.: Changes in iron metabolism following gastrectomy and other surgical operations. *Clin. Sci.*, **16**:463–73, 1957.

Baldus, W. P.; Feichter, R. N.; and Summerskill, W. H. J.: The kidney in cirrhosis: I. The clinical and biochemical features of azotemia in hepatic failure. *Ann. Intern. Med.*, **60**:353–65, 1964a.

Baldus, W. P.; Summerskill, W. H. J.; Hunt, J. C.; and Maher, F. T.: Renal circulation in cirrhosis: observations based on catheterization of renal vein. *J. Clin. Invest.*, **43**:1090–97, 1964b.

Balint, J. A., and Hirschowitz, B. I.: Hypomagnesia with tetany in nontropical sprue. *New Eng. J. Med.*, **265**: 631–33, 1961.

Baraona, E.; Orrego, H.; Fernandez, O.; Amenabar, E.; Maldonado, E.; Tag, F.; and Salinas, A.: Absorptive function of the small intestine in liver cirrhosis. *Amer. J. Dig. Dis.*, **7**:318–30, 1962.

Baron, J. J.; Connell, A. M.; Lennard-Jones, J. E.; and Jones, F. A.: Sulphasalazine (azulfidine) and salicylazosulphadimidine in ulcerative colitis. *Lancet*, **1**:1094–96, 1962.

Baume, P. E., and Hunt, J. H.: Failure of potent antacid therapy to hasten healing in chronic gastric ulcers. *Aust. Ann. Med.*, **18**:113–16, 1969.

Bayless, T. M., and Huang, S. S.: Inadequate intestinal digestion of lactose. *Amer. J. Clin. Nutr.*, **22**:250–56, 1969.

Bayless, T. M., and Rosensweig, N. S.: A racial difference in incidence of lactase deficiency: a survey of milk intolerance and lactase deficiency in healthy adult males. *J.A.M.A.*, **197**:968–72, 1966.

Bearn, A. G.: Wilson's disease. In Stanbury, J. B.; Wyndgaarden, J. B.; and Fredrickson, D. S. (eds.): *The Metabolic Basis of Inherited Disease*, 2nd ed. McGraw-Hill Book Co., New York, 1966.

Becker, C. E.: The clinical pharmacology of alcohol. *Calif. Med.*, **113**:37–45, 1970.

Beecher, H. K.: The powerful placebo. *J.A.M.A.*, **159**:1602–06, 1955.

Beeken, W. L.: Effect of five salicylate-containing compounds upon loss of 51-chromium-labeled erythrocytes from the gastrointestinal tract of normal man. *Gut*, **9**:475–79, 1968.

Benson, G. D.; Kowlessar, O. D.; and Sleisenger, M. H.: Adult celiac disease, with emphasis upon response to gluten-free diet. *Medicine (Balt.)*, **43**:1–40, 1964.

Benson, J. A., Jr.; Culver, P. J.; Ragland, S.; Jones, C. M.; Drummey, G. D.; and Bougas, E.: The D-xylose absorption test in malabsorption syndromes. *New Eng. J. Med.*, **256**:335–39, 1957.

Berger, R. L.; Stanton, J. R.; Liversage, R. M.; Goldrick, D. M.; Graham, J. H.; and Stohlman, F., Jr.: Blood exchange in the treatment of hepatic coma. *J.A.M.A.*, **202**:267–74, 1967.

Berk, D. P., and Chalmers, T.: Deafness complicating antibiotic therapy of hepatic encephalopathy. *Ann. Intern. Med.*, **73**:393–96, 1970.

Bessman, A. N., and Hawkins, R.: The relative effects of enterically administered plasma and packed cells on circulating blood ammonia. *Gastroenterology*, **45**.368–73, 1963.

Bessman, A. N.; Mirick, G. S.; and Hawkins, R.: Blood ammonia levels following the ingestion of casein and whole blood. *J. Clin. Invest.*, **37**:990–98, 1958.

Bettarello, A.; Tuttle, S. G.; and Grossman, M. I.: Effect of autonomic drugs on gastroesophageal reflux. *Gastroenterology*, **39**:340–46, 1960.

Billing, B. H.: The disposal of bilirubin. In Popper, H., and Schaffner, F. (eds.): *Progress in Liver Diseases*, Vol. 2. Grune & Stratton, Inc., New York, 1965, pp. 1–14.

Binder, H. J.; Herting, D. C.; Hurst, V.; Finch, S. C.; and Spiro, H. M.: Tocopherol deficiency in man. *New Eng. J. Med.*, **273**:1289–97, 1965.

Bircher, J., and Haemmerli, U. P.: Diet therapy of gastrointestinal disorders—attempt at critical evaluation. *Schweiz. Med. Wschr.*, **97**:1687–96, 1967.

Bircher, J.; Müller, J.; Guggenheim, P.; and Haemmerli, U. P.: Treatment of chronic portal-systemic encephalopathy with lactulose. *Lancet*, **1**:890–92, 1966.

Birge, S. J.; Peck, W. S.; Berman, M.; and Whedon, G. D.: Study of calcium absorption in man: a kinetic analysis and physiologic model. *J. Clin. Invest.*, **48**: 1705–13, 1969.

Bitsch, V., and Kristensen, M.: Determination of peptic activity and acid in the gastric juice of patients with peptic disease before and after administration of glycopyrrolate. *Acta Med. Scand.*, **180**:385–93, 1966.

Block, M.; Moore, G.; Wasi, P.; and Haiby, G.: Histogenesis of the hepatic lesion in primary hemochromatosis: with consideration of the pseudo-iron deficient state produced by phlebotomies. *Amer. J. Path.*, **47**:89–123, 1965.

Bloom, W. L., and Flinchum, D.: Osteomalacia with pseudofractures caused by the ingestion of aluminum hydroxide. *J.A.M.A.*, **174**:1327–30, 1960.

Bock, O. A. A.; Bank, S.; Marks, I. N.; Moshal, M. G.; Groll, A.; Loxton, A.; and Dines, M.: Effect of propantheline bromide and pipenzolate bromide upon exocrine pancreatic secretion. *Gastroenterology*, **55**: 199–203, 1968.

Boley, S. J.; Schultz, L.; Krieger, H.; Schwartz, S.; Elquezabal, A.; and Allen, A. C.: Experimental evaluation of thiazides and potassium as a cause of small-bowel ulcer. *J.A.M.A.*, **192**:763–68, 1965.

Bolt, R. J.; Dillon, R. S.; and Pollard, H. M.: Interference with bilirubin excretion by a gall-bladder dye (Bunamiodyl). *New Eng. J. Med.*, **265**:1043–45, 1961.

Booth, C. C.; Babouris, N.; Hanna, S.; Babouris, N.; and MacIntyre, I.: Incidence of hypomagnesaemia in intestinal malabsorption. *Brit. Med. J.*, **2**:141–44, 1963.

Booth, C. C., and Heath, J.: The effect of E. coli on the absorption of vitamin B_{12}. *Gut*, **3**:70–73, 1962.

Bordier, P.; Matrajt, H.; Hioco, D.; Hepner, G. W.; Thompson, G. R.; and Booth, C. C.: Subclinical vitamin D deficiency following gastric surgery: histological evidence in bone. *Lancet*, **1**:437–40, 1968.

Bosman, S. C. W.; Terblanche, J.; Saunders, S. J.; and Harrison, G. G.: Cross-circulation between man and baboon. *Lancet*, **2**:583–85, 1968.

Bowen, G. E.; Irons, G. V., Jr.; Rhodes, J. B.; and Kirsner, J. B.: Early experiences with azathioprine in ulcerative colitis: a note of caution. *J.A.M.A.*, **195**:460–64, 1966.

Boyer, J. L., and Klatskin, G.: Pattern of necrosis in acute viral hepatitis. Prognostic value of bridging (subacute hepatic necrosis). *New Eng. J. Med.*, **283**:1063–71, 1970.

Brette, R.; Lambert, R.; and Trachot, R.: Biliary excretion of antibiotics. In Taylor, W. (ed.): *The Biliary System*. F. A. Davis Co., Philadelphia, 1965.

Brettschneider, L.; Monafo, W.; and Osborne, D. P.: Intestinal obstruction due to antacid gels: complication of medical therapy for gastrointestinal bleeding. *Gastroenterology*, **49**:291–94, 1965.

Briggs, R. D.; Rubenberg, M. L.; O'Neal, R. M.; Thomas, W. A.; and Hartroft, W. S.: Myocardial infarction in patients treated with sippy and other high-milk diets: an autopsy study of fifteen hospitals in the U.S.A. and Great Britain. *Circulation*, **21**:538–42, 1960.

Britton, R. C., and Nakamoto, S.: Intravenous infusion of dialyzed, autogenous, ascitic fluid in the management of cirrhotic ascites. *Cleveland Clin. Quart.*, **27**:82–87, 1960.

Brodie, B. B.: Physiochemical and biochemical aspects of pharmacology. *J.A.M.A.*, **202**:600–609, 1967.

Brodie, B. B.; Burns, J. J.; and Weiner, M.: Metabolism of drugs in subjects with Laennec's cirrhosis. *Med. Exp.* (*Basel*), 1:290–92, 1959.

Brody, J., and McKenzie, D.: Therapeutic phlebotomies in idiopathic hemachromatosis. *Amer. J. Med. Sci.*, 244:575–86, 1962.

Brody, M., and Bachrach, W. H.: Antacids. I. Comparative biochemical and economic considerations. *Amer. J. Dig. Dis.*, 4:435–60, 1959.

Broitman, S. A.; Bondy, D. C.; Yachnin, I.; Hoskins, L. C.; Ingbar, S.; and Zamcheck, N.: Absorption and disposition of D-xylose in thyrotoxicosis and myxedema. *New Eng. J. Med.*, 270:333–37, 1964.

Brooke, B. N.; Hoffman, D. C.; and Swarbrick, E. T.: Azathioprine for Crohn's disease. *Lancet*, 2:612–14, 1969.

Brooke, B. N.; Javett, S. L.; and Davison, O. W.: Further experience with azathioprine for Crohn's disease. *Lancet*, 2:1050–53, 1970.

Brooks, F. P.; Sandweiss, D. J.; and Long, J. F.: The relationship between peptic ulcer and coronary occlusion. *Amer. J. Med. Sci.*, 245:277–82, 1963.

Brown, H., and Englert, E.: Corticosteroid metabolism in liver disease. *Arch. Intern. Med.* (*Chicago*), 107:778–83, 1961.

Brown, H.; Trey, C.; and McDermott, V., Jr.: Lactulose treatment of hepatic encephalopathy in outpatients. *Arch. Surg.*, 102:25–27, 1971.

Brown, M.; McDermott, W. V.; and Brown, M. E.: Blood ammonia. *J.A.M.A.*, 199:473, 1967.

Buchan, D. J., and Houston, C. S.: Small bowel ulceration associated with enteric-coated potassium chloride and hydrochlorthiazide. *Canad. Med. Ass. J.*, 92:176–79, 1965.

Bunton, G. L., and Cameron, R.: Regeneration of liver after biliary cirrhosis. *Ann. N.Y. Acad. Sci.*, 111:412–21, 1963.

Burke, V., and Danks, D. M.: Medium-chain triglyceride diet: its use in treatment of liver disease. *Brit. Med. J.*, 2:1050–51, 1966.

Burnell, J. M.; Dawborn, J. K.; Epstein, R. B.; Gutman, R. A.; Leinbach, G. E.; Thomas, E. D.; and Volwiler W.: Acute hepatic coma treated by cross-circulation or exchange transfusion. *New Eng. J. Med.*, 276:935–43, 1967.

Cain, G. D.; Reiner, E. B.; and Patterson, M.: Effects of neomycin on disaccharidase activity of the small bowel. *Arch. Intern. Med.* (*Chicago*), 122:311–14, 1968.

Cameron, D. G.; Watson, G. M.; and Witts, L. J.: Clinical association of macrocytic anemia with intestinal stricture and anastomosis. *Blood*, 4:793–802, 1949.

Carbone, J. V., and Matthews, H. H.: The use of prednisone to initiate or potentiate diuresis in chronic hepatic disease with ascites. *Gastroenterology*, 38:52–59, 1960.

Carey, J. B.: The serum trihydroxy-dihydroxy bile acid ratio in liver and biliary tract disease. *J. Clin. Invest.*, 37:1494–1503, 1958.

Carman, C. T., and Giansiracusa, J. E.: Effect of steroid therapy on the clinical and laboratory features of primary biliary cirrhosis. *Gastroenterology*, 28:193–215, 1955.

Carpenter, C. C. J., Jr.: Cholera enterotoxin—recent investigations yield insights into transport processes. *Amer. J. Med.*, 50:1–7, 1971.

Cayer, D.: Use of methionine and vitamin supplements in treatment of hepatic disease. *Arch. Intern. Med.* (*Chicago*), 80:644–54, 1947.

———: Prolonged anticholinergic therapy of duodenal ulcer. *Amer. J. Dig. Dis.*, 1:301–309, 1956.

Cayer, D., and Cornatzer, W. E.: Radioactive phosphorus as an indicator of the rate of phospholipid formation in patients with liver disease. *Gastroenterology*, 14:1–10, 1950.

Chadwick, D. A., and Jennings, R. C.: Massive hepatic necrosis associated with halothane anesthesia. *Lancet*, 1:793–95, 1964.

Chalmers, T. C.: An evaluation of dietary protein in the treatment of liver disease. *Ann. Intern. Med.*, 48:320–29, 1958.

———: Pathogenesis and treatment of hepatic failure. *New Eng. J. Med.*, 263:23–30, 1960.

———: The management of hepatic coma: a continuing problem. *Med. Clin. N. Amer.*, 52:1475–81, 1968.

Chalmers, T. C.; Eckhardt, R. D.; Reynolds, W. E.; Cigarroa, J. G., Jr.; Deane, N.; Reifenstein, R. W.; Smith, C. W.; and Davidson, C. S.: The treatment of acute infectious hepatitis: controlled studies of the effects of diet, rest and physical reconditioning on the acute course of the disease and on the incidence of relapses and residual abnormalities. *J. Clin. Invest.*, 34:1163–1235, 1955.

Charley, P. J.; Sarkar, B.; Stitt, C. F.; and Saltman, P.: Chelation of iron by sugars. *Biochim. Biophys. Acta*, 69:313–21, 1963.

Chears, W. C., Jr., and Ashworth, C. T.: Electron microscopic study of the intestinal mucosa in Whipple's disease: demonstration of encapsulated bacilliform bodies in the lesion. *Gastroenterology*, 41:129–38, 1961.

Chen, L. C.; Rohde, J. E.; and Sharp, G. W. G.: Intestinal adenyl-cyclase activity in human cholera. *Lancet*, 1:939–40, 1971.

Cheng, S. H., and White, A.: Effect of orally administered neomycin on the absorption of pencillin V. *New Eng. J. Med.*, 267:1296–97, 1962.

Choudhury, M. R., and Williams, J.: Iron absorption and gastric operations. *Clin. Sci.*, 18:527–32, 1959.

Christiansen, P. A.; Kirsner, J. B.; and Ablaza, J.: D-Xylose and its use in the diagnosis of malabsorptive states. *Amer. J. Med.*, 27:443–53, 1959.

Cocco, A. E., and Mendeloff, A. I.: An evaluation of intermittent corticosteroid therapy in the management of ulcerative colitis. *Johns Hopkins Med. J.*, 120:162–69, 1967.

Cocco, A. E.; Rosensweig, N. S.; and Hendrix, T. R.: Absorption of xylose against a concentration gradient *in vivo. Clin. Res.*, 13:252, 1965.

Cohen, M. I.; Wilson, P. R.; and Boley, S. J.: Intestinal obstruction associated with cholestyramine therapy. *New Eng. J. Med.*, 280:1285–86, 1969.

Cohen, S.; Ohta, G.; Singer, E. J.; and Popper, H.: Immunocytochemical study of gamma globulin in liver in hepatitis and postnecrotic cirrhosis. *J. Exp. Med.*, 111:285–94, 1960.

Cohn, H. J.; Perlmutter, M.; Silverstein, J. N.; and Numeroff, M.: Prolonged hypoglycemia in response to intravenous tolbutamide in a patient with Laennec's cirrhosis and severe malnutrition. *J. Clin. Endocr.*, 24:28–34, 1964.

Cohn, I., Jr.: Kanamycin as an intestinal antiseptic and in the treatment of peritonitis: resume of clinical experience. *Ann. N.Y. Acad. Sci.*, 132:860–69, 1966.

Collins, J. R.: Celiac disease in elderly patients. Report of 13 cases, with a note concerning drug absorption. *Amer. J. Dig. Dis.*, 11:564–71, 1966.

Collins, J. R., and Ellis, D. S.: Agammaglobulinemia, malabsorption and rheumatoid-like arthritis. *Amer. J. Med.*, 39:476–82, 1965.

Combes, B.; Shibata, H.; Adams, R.; Mitchell, B. D.; and Trammell, V.: Alterations in sulfobromophthalein sodium-removal mechanisms from blood during normal pregnancy. *J. Clin. Invest.*, 42:1431–42, 1963.

Conn, H. O.: A rational program for the management of hepatic coma. *Gastroenterology*, 57:715–23, 1969.

Conn, H. O., and Dalessio, D. J.: Multiple infusions of posterior pituitary extract in the treatment of bleeding esophageal varices. *Ann. Intern. Med.*, 57:804–809, 1962.

Conn, H. O., and Quintiliani, R.: Severe diarrhea controlled by gammaglobulin in a patient with agammaglobulinemia, amyloidosis, and thymoma. *Ann. Intern. Med.*, 65:528–41, 1966.

Conn, H. O., and Simpson, J. A.: Excessive mortality associated with balloon tamponade of bleeding varices. *J.A.M.A.*, 202:587–91, 1967.

————: A rational program for diagnosis and treatment of bleeding esophageal varices. *Med. Clin. N. Amer.*, 52:1457–74, 1968.

Connell, A. M.; Hill, R. A.; Macleod, I. B.; Sircus, W.; and Thomson, C. G.: Effects of SC 15396 on gastric secretion. *Gut*, 9:641–54, 1968.

Connell, A. M., and Kellock, T. D.: Treatment of chronic nonspecific diarrhea: a clinical comparison. *Brit. Med. J.*, 1:151–53, 1959.

Conney, A. H.: Pharmacological implications of microsomal enzyme induction. *Pharmacol. Rev.*, 19:317–66, 1967.

Conrad, M. E., and Schade, S. G.: Ascorbic acid chelates in iron absorption: a role for hydrochloric acid and bile. *Gastroenterology*, 55:35–45, 1968.

Conrad, M. E.; Weintraub, L. R.; and Crosby, W. H.: The role of the intestine in iron kinetics. *J. Clin. Invest.*, 43:963–74, 1964.

Conrad, M. E.; Weintraub, L. R.; Sears, D. A.; and Crosby, W. H.: Absorption of hemoglobin iron. *Amer. J. Physiol.*, 211:1123–30, 1966.

Cook, G. C., and Kajubi, S. K.: Tribal incidence of lactase deficiency in Uganda. *Lancet*, 1:725–29, 1966.

Cook, G. C.; Velasco, M.; and Sherlock, S.: The effect of corticosteroid therapy on bromsulphthalein excretion in active chronic hepatitis. *Gut*, 9:270–83, 1968.

Cooke, A. R.: Corticosteroids and peptic ulcer: is there a relationship? *Amer. J. Dig. Dis.*, 12:323–29, 1967.

Cooke, A. R., and Hunt, J. N.: Absorption of acetylsalicylic acid from unbuffered and buffered gastric contents. *Amer. J. Dig. Dis.*, 15:95–102, 1970.

Cooke, E. M.: A quantitative comparison of the faecal flora of patients with ulcerative colitis and that of normal persons. *J. Path. Bact.*, 94:439–44, 1967.

————: Faecal flora of patients with ulcerative colitis during treatment with salicylazosulphapyridine. *Gut*, 10:565–68, 1969.

Cooke, W. T.; Cox, E. V.; Fone, D. J.; Meynell, M. J.; and Gaddie, R.: Clinical and metabolic significance of jejunal diverticula. *Gut*, 4:115–31, 1963.

Copenhagen Study Group: Effect of prednisone on the survival of patients with cirrhosis of the liver. *Lancet*, 1:119–21, 1969.

Crews, R. H., and Faloon, W. W.: The fallacy of a low fat diet in liver disease. *J.A.M.A.*, 181:754–59, 1962.

Crigler, J. F., Jr., Gold, N. I.; and Janeway, C. A.: Effect of sodium phenobarbital on metabolism of bilirubin ^{3}H and ^{14}C in an infant with congenital nonhemolytic jaundice and kernicterus. *J. Clin. Invest.*, 46:1047, 1967.

Crooks, J.; Clark, C. G.; Amar, S. S.; and Coull, D. C.: Preventive medicine and the gastrectomized patient. *Lancet*, 2:943–45, 1965.

Csaky, T. Z., and Lassen, U. V.: Active intestinal transport of D-xylose. *Biochim. Biophys. Acta*, 82:215–17, 1964.

Datta, D. V., and Sherlock, S.: Cholestyramine for long term relief of the pruritus complicating intrahepatic cholestasis. *Gastroenterology*, 50:322–32, 1966.

Davenport, H. W.: Salicylate damage to the gastric mucosal barrier. *New Eng. J. Med.* 276:1307–12, 1967.

————: Gastric mucosal hemorrhage in dogs: effects of acid, aspirin, and alcohol. *Gastroenterology*, 56:439–49, 1969.

Davidson, C. S.: Hepatic coma. *D.M.: Disease-a-Month*, January 1964.

————: Is life worth living? It depends on the liver. *New Eng. J. Med.*, 274:894–96, 1966.

Davis, A. E., and Bolin, J.: Lactose intolerance in Asians. *Nature (London)*, 216:1244–45, 1967.

Davis, A. E., and Pirola, R. C.: Absorption of phenoxymethyl penicillin in patients with steatorrhea. *Aust. Ann. Med.*, 17:63–65, 1968.

Davis, T. D., Jr.; McBee, J. W.; Borland, J. L., Jr.; Kurtz, S. M.; and Ruffin, J. M.: The effect of antibiotic and steroid therapy in Whipple's disease. *Gastroenterology*, 44:112–16, 1963.

Dawson, A. M.; McLaren, J.; and Sherlock, S.: Neomycin in the treatment of hepatic coma. *Lancet*, 2:1262–68, 1957.

Dawson, J. L.: Acute post-operative renal failure in obstructive jaundice. *Ann. Roy. Coll. Surg. Eng.*, 42:163–68, 1968.

Delaney, J. P.; Goodale, R. L.; Cheng, J.; and Wangensteen, O. W.: The influence of vasopressin on upper gastrointestinal blood flow. *Surgery*, 59:397–400, 1966.

Deller, D. J.; Begely, M. D.; Edwards, R. G.; and Addison, M.: Metabolic effects of partial gastrectomy with special reference to calcium and folic acid. I. Changes in calcium metabolism and the bones. *Gut*, 5:218–25, 1964.

Deller, D. J., and Witts, L. J.: Changes in the blood after partial gastrectomy with special reference to vitamin B_{12}. I. Serum vitamin B_{12}, haemoglobin, serum iron, and bone marrow. *Quart. J. Med.*, 31:71–88, 1962.

DeMatteis, F.: Disturbances of liver porphyric metabolism caused by drugs. *Pharmacol. Rev.*, 19:523–57, 1967.

Denny-Brown, D.: Hepatolenticular degeneration (Wilson's disease). *New Eng. J. Med.*, 270:1149–56, 1964.

DePalma, R. G.; Hartman, P. H.; Levy, S.; and Hubay, C. A.: Bile acids and serum cholesterol following T-tube drainage. *Arch. Surg. (Chicago)*, 94:271–76, 1967.

Dick, A. P.; Grayson, N. J.; Carpenter, R. G.; and Pelrie, A.: Controlled trial of sulphasalazine in the treatment of ulcerative colitis. *Gut*, 5:437–42, 1964.

Dicke, W. K.; Weijers, H. A.; and van de Kamer, J. H.: Coeliac disease: presence in wheat of a factor having deleterious effect in cases of coeliac disease. *Acta Paediat. Scand.*, 42:34–42, 1953.

Dobbins, W. O.: Drug-induced steatorrhea. *Gastroenterology*, 54:1193–95, 1968.

Dobbins, W. O., and Ruffin, J. M.: A light and electron-microscopic study of bacterial invasion in Whipple's disease. *Amer. J. Path*, 51:225–42, 1967.

Doig, A., and Girdwood, R. H.: Absorption of folic acid and labeled cyanocobalamin in intestinal malabsorption. *Quart. J. Med.*, 29:333–74, 1960.

Doll, R.; Friedlander, P.; and Pygott, F.: Dietetic treatment of peptic ulcer. *Lancet*, 1:5–9, 1956.

Donaldson, R. M., Jr.: Studies on the pathogenesis of steatorrhea in the blind-loop syndrome. *J. Clin. Invest.*, 44:1815–25, 1965.

Donaldson, R. M., Jr.; Corrigan, H.; and Natsios, G.: Malabsorption of Co^{60}-labeled cyanocobalamin in rats with intestinal diverticula. II. Studies on contents of the diverticula. *Gastroenterology*, 43:282–90, 1962.

Donaldson, R. M., Jr.; Mackenzie, I. L.; and Trier, J. S.: Intrinsic factor-mediated attachment of vitamin B_{12}

to brush borders and microvillous membranes of hamster intestine. *J. Clin. Invest.* **46**:1215–28, 1967.

Doniach, D., and Walker, J. G.: A unified concept of autoimmune hepatitis. *Lancet*, **1**:813–15, 1969.

Dotevall, G., and Kock, N. G.: Absorption studies in regional enterocolitis (Mb. Crohn). *Scand. J. Gastroent.* **3**:293–98, 1968.

Dotevall, G., and Walan, A.: Antacids in the treatment of peptic ulcer. *Acta Med. Scand.*, **182**:529–37, 1967.

Douvres, P. A.: Effect of high parenteral doses of vitamin-K analogs and serum albumin on the prothrombin level and liver function in alcoholic cirrhosis. *Amer. J. Dig. Dis.*, **10**:635–42, 1965.

Drasar, B. S.; Hill, M. J.; and Shiner, M.: The deconjugation of bile salts by human intestinal bacteria. *Lancet*, **1**:1237–38, 1966.

Dreiling, D. A., and Janowitz, H. D.: Inhibitory effect of new anticholinergics on the basal and secretin-stimulated pancreatic secretion in patients with and without pancreatic disease. *Amer. J. Dig. Dis.*, **5**:639–54, 1960.

Duffy, T. J., and Meister, L.: Hemochromatosis: report of a case followed for seven years with repeated phlebotomies and liver biopsies. *Amer. J. Med.*, **35**:434–38, 1963.

Eckhardt, R. D.; Zamcheck, N.; Sidman, R. L.; Gabuzda, G. J.; and Davidson, C. S.: Effect of protein starvation and of protein feeding on the clinical course, liver function, and liver histochemistry of three patients with active fatty alcoholic cirrhosis. *J. Clin. Invest.*, **29**:227–37, 1950.

Editorial: Editor's choice, Wilson's disease. *New Eng. J. Med.*, **278**:392–93, 1968.

Eiseman, B.: Hepatic perfusion. In *Colston Papers: Liver Diseases.* Butterworth Scientific Publications, London, 1967.

Eisner, G. M., and Levitt, M. F.: The cirrhotic nephropathy. In Popper, H., and Schaffner, F. (eds.): *Progress in Liver Diseases.* Grune & Stratton, Inc., New York, 1961.

Elkington, S. G.; Floch, M. H.; and Conn, H. O.: Lactulose in the treatment of chronic portal-systemic encephalopathy: a double-blind clinical trial. *New Eng. J. Med.*, **281**:408–12, 1969.

Engel, F. L.: Addison's disease and peptic ulcer. *J. Clin. Endocr.*, **15**:1300–1307, 1955.

Enquist, I. F.; Golding, M. R.; Aiello, R. G.; Fierst, S. M.; and Solomon, N. A.: The effect of portal hypertension on intestinal absorption. *Surg. Gynec. Obstet.*, **120**:87–91, 1965.

Erenoglu, E.; Edreira, J. G.; and Patek, A. J., Jr.: Observations on patients with Laennec's cirrhosis receiving alcohol while on controlled diets. *Ann. Intern. Med.*, **60**:814–23, 1964.

Evans, A. F.; Sprinz, H.; and Nelson, R. S.: Adrenal hormone therapy in viral hepatitis: the effect of ACTH in the acute disease. *Ann. Intern. Med.*, **38**:1115–59, 1953.

Fallon, H. J., and Woods, J. W.: Response of hyperlipoproteinemia to cholestyramine resin. *J.A.M.A.*, **204**:1161–64, 1968.

Faloon, W. W.; Eckhardt, R. D.; Murphy, T. L.; Cooper, A. M.; and Davidson, C. S.: An evaluation of human serum albumin in the treatment of cirrhosis of the liver. *J. Clin. Invest.*, **28**:583–94, 1949.

Faloon, W. W.; Paes, I. C.; Woolfolk, D.; Nankin, H.; Wallace, K.; and Haro, E. N.: Effect of neomycin and kanamycin upon intestinal absorption. *Ann. N.Y. Acad. Sci.*, **132**:879–87, 1966.

Fast, B.; Wolfe, S. J.; Stormont, J.; and Davidson, C. S.: Antibiotic therapy in the management of hepatic coma. *Arch. Intern. Med. (Chicago)*, **101**:467–75, 1958.

Fekety, F. R.: Gastrointestinal complications of antibiotic therapy. *J.A.M.A.*, **203**:210–12, 1968.

Fenster, L. F.: The non-efficacy of short-term anabolic therapy in alcoholic liver disease. *Ann. Intern. Med.*, **65**:738–44, 1966.

Field, M.: Intestinal secretion: Effects of cyclic AMP and its role in cholera. *New Eng. J. Med.*, **284**:1137–44, 1971.

Finkel, M. J.: Vitamin K_1 and vitamin K analogues. *Clin. Pharmacol. Ther.*, **2**:794–814, 1961.

Fishbein, W. N.; Carbone, P. P.; and Hochstein, H. D.: Acetohydroxamate: bacterial urease inhibitor with therapeutic potential in hyperammonaemic states. *Nature (London)*, **208**:46–48, 1965.

Fisher, C. J., and Faloon, W. W.: Blood ammonia levels in hepatic cirrhosis. *New Eng. J. Med.*, **256**:1030–35, 1957.

Fisher, J. M.; Rees, C.; and Taylor, K. B.: Intrinsic factor antibodies in gastric juice of pernicious-anaemia patients. *Lancet*, **2**:88–89, 1966.

Fishman, R. A.: Neurological aspects of magnesium metabolism. *Arch. Neurol. (Chicago)*, **12**:562–69, 1965.

Fleischer, N.; Brown, H.; Graham, D. Y.; and Delena, S.: Chronic laxative-induced hyperaldosteronism and hypokalemia simulating Bartter's syndrome. *Ann. Intern. Med.*, **70**:791–98, 1969.

Fordtran, J. S., and Collyns, J. A. H.: Antacid pharmacology in duodenal ulcer—effect of antacids on postcibal gastric acidity and peptic activity. *New Eng. J. Med.*, **274**:921–27, 1966.

Fordtran, J. S.; Soergel, K. H.; and Ingelfinger, F. J.: Intestinal absorption of D-xylose in man. *New Eng. J. Med.*, **267**:274–79, 1962.

French, J. M.; Hawkins, C. F.; and Smith, N.: The effect of wheat-gluten-free diet in adult idiopathic steatorrhea, a study of 22 cases. *Quart. J. Med.*, **26**:481–99, 1957.

Friend, D. G.: Gastrointestinal anticholinergic drugs. *Clin. Pharmacol. Ther.*, **4**:559–68, 1963.

Gabuzda, G. J.; Eckhart, R. D.; and Davidson, C. S.: Effect of choline and methionine, testosterone propionate and dietary protein on nitrogen balance in patients with liver disease. *J. Clin. Invest.*, **29**:566–76, 1950.

Gallo, D. G.; Bailey, K. R.; and Sheffner, A. L.: The interaction between cholestyramine and drugs. *Proc. Soc. Exp. Biol. Med.*, **120**:60–65, 1965.

Gangarosa, E. J.; Beisel, W. R.; Benyajati, C.; Sprinz, H.; and Piyaratn, P.: The nature of the gastrointestinal lesion in Asiatic cholera and its relation to pathogenesis: a biopsy study. *Amer. J. Trop. Med.*, **9**:125–35, 1960.

Gantt, C. L.; Ecklund, R. E.; and Dyniewicz, C. M.: Significance of aldosterone antagonism in the treatment of edema and ascites. *Amer. J. Med.*, **33**:490–500, 1962.

Gartner, L. M., and Arias, I. M.: Formation, transport, metabolism and excretion of bilirubin. *New Eng. J. Med.*, **280**:1339–45, 1969.

Gaylor, D. W.; Clark, J. S.; Kudinoff, Z.; and Finegold, S. M.: Preoperative bowel "sterilization"—a double blind study comparing kanamycin, neomycin, and placebo. *Antimicrob. Agents Ann.*, 1960, pp. 392–403.

Geenen, J. E.; Hensley, G. T.; and Winship, D. H.: Chronic active hepatitis treated with 6-mercaptopurine—sustained remission. *Ann. Intern. Med.*, **65**:1277–83, 1966.

Gelzayd, E. A., and Kirsner, J. B.: Immunological aspects of chronic active hepatitis in young people. *Amer. J. Med. Sci.*, **253**:98–109, 1967.

Gerlach, K.; Morowitz, D. A.; and Kirsner, J. B.: Symptomatic hypomagnesemia complicating regional enteritis. *Gastroenterology*, **59**:567–74, 1970.

Goldberg, L., and Smith, J. P.: Iron overloading and

hepatic vulnerability. *Amer. J. Path.*, **36**:125–49, 1960.

Goldgraber, M. G., and Kirsner, J. B.: Corticotropin (ACTH) and adrenal steroids in liver disease. *Arch. Intern. Med. (Chicago)*, **104**:469–80, 1959.

Goldman, A. S.; Van Fossan, D. D.; and Baird, E. E.: Magnesium deficiency in celiac disease. *Pediatrics*, **29**:948–52, 1962.

Goldstein, F.; Karacadag, S.; Wirts, C. W.; and Kowlessar, O. D.: Intraluminal small-intestinal utilization of D-xylose by bacteria. A limitation of the D-xylose absorption test. *Gastroenterology*, **59**:380–86, 1970.

Goldstein, M. J.; Gelzayd, E. A.; and Kirsner, J. B.: Some observations on the hazards of corticosteroid therapy in patients with inflammatory bowel disease. *Trans. Amer. Acad. Ophthal. Otolaryng.*, **71**:254–61, 1967.

Goodman, L. S., and Gilman, A.: *The Pharmacological Basis of Therapeutics*, 4th ed. The Macmillan Co., New York, 1970.

Gorbach, S. S.; Nahas, L.; Plaut, A. G.; Weinstein, L.; Patterson, J. F.; and Levitan, R.: Studies of intestinal microflora. V. Fecal microbial ecology in ulcerative colitis and regional enteritis: relationship to severity of disease and chemotherapy. *Gastroenterology*, **54**:575–87, 1968.

Gordon, R. S., Jr.; Feelay, J. C.; Greenough, W. B.; Sprinz, H.; and Oseasohn, R.: Cholera: combined clinical staff conference at the National Institutes of Health. *Ann. Intern. Med.*, **64**:1328–51, 1966.

Grady, G. F.: The prevention of (viral) hepatitis. *D.M.: Disease-a-Month*, July, 1968.

Grady, G. F., and Bennett, A. J. E.: Prevention of post-transfusion hepatitis by γ-globulin. Preliminary report. *J.A.M.A.*, **214**:140–42, 1970.

Grady, G. F.; Madoff, M. A.; Duhawel, R. C.; Moore, E. W.; and Chalmers, T. C.: Sodium transport by human ileum *in vitro* and its response to cholera enterotoxin. *Gastroenterlogy*, **53**:737–44, 1967.

Greenberger, N. J.; Ruppert, R. D.; and Tzagournis, M.: Use of medium-chain triglycerides in malabsorption. *Ann. Intern. Med.*, **66**:727–34, 1967a.

Greenberger, N. J., and Skillman, T. G.: Medium-chain triglycerides—physiologic considerations and clinical implications. *New Eng. J. Med.*, **280**:1045–58, 1969.

Greenberger, N. J.; Tennenbaum, J. I.; and Ruppert, R. D.: Protein-losing enteropathy associated with gastrointestinal allergy. *Amer. J. Med.*, **43**:777–84, 1967b.

Grosberg, S. J.: Hemochromatosis and heart failure: presentation of a case with survival after three years' treatment by repeated venesection. *Ann. Intern. Med.*, **54**:550–59, 1961.

Gross, L., and Brotman, M.: Hypoprothrombinemia and hemorrhage associated with cholestyramine therapy. *Ann. Intern. Med.*, **72**:95–96, 1970.

Grossman, J., and Yalow, A. A.: Effects of anabolic steroids on albumin metabolism. *J. Clin. Endocr.*, **25**:698–707, 1965.

Grossman, M. I.: Physiologic approach to medical management of duodenal ulcer. In McHardy, G. (ed.): *Current Gastroenterology*. Paul B. Hoeber, Inc., New York, 1962, pp. 303–14.

———: Gastrin. *Ann. Intern. Med.*, **64**:212–16, 1966.

Grossman, M. I.; Janowitz, H. D.; Ralston, H.; and Kim, K. S.: The effect of secretin on bile formation in man. *Gastroenterology*, **12**:133–38, 1949.

Grossman, M. I.; Matsumoto, K. K.; and Lichter, R. J.: Fecal blood loss produced by oral and intravenous administration of various salicylates. *Gastroenterology*, **40**:383–88, 1961.

Grote, I. W., and Woods, M.: Studies on antacids. IV. Adsorption effects of various aluminum antacids upon

simultaneously administered anticholinergic drugs. *J. Amer. Pharm. Ass.*, **42**:319–20, 1953.

Gryboski, J. D.; Burkle, F.; and Hillman, R.: Milk induced colitis in an infant. *Pediatrics*, **38**:299–302, 1966.

Gryboski, J. D.; Katz, J.; Reynolds, D.; and Herskovic, T.: Gluten intolerance following cow's milk sensitivity: two cases with coproantibodies to milk and wheat proteins. *Ann. Allerg.*, **26**:33–39, 1968.

Györy, A. Z., and Stiel, J. N.: Effect of particle size on aspirin-induced gastrointestinal bleeding. *Lancet*, **2**:300–302, 1968.

Haemmerli, U. P.; Kistler, H.; Ammann, R.; Marthaler, T.; Semenza, G.; Aurricchio, S.; and Prader, A.: Acquired milk intolerance in the adult caused by lactose malabsorption due to a selective deficiency of intestinal lactase activity. *Amer. J. Med.*, **38**:17–30, 1965.

Hammond, J. B., and Griffiths, R. S.: Factors effecting the absorption and biliary excretion of erythromycin and two of its derivatives in humans. *Clin. Pharmacol. Ther.*, **2**:308–12, 1961.

Hanngren, Å.; Hansson, E.; Svartz, N.; and Ullberg, S.: Distribution and metabolism of salicylazosulfapyridine. *Acta Med. Scand.*, **173**:61–72, 391–99, 1963.

Hanson, K. C.; Maizel, H.; and Ruffin, J. M.: The effect of ACTH upon patients having regional enteritis. *Southern Med. J.*, **62**:532–34, 1969.

Hardison, G. M., and Rosenberg, I. H.: Bile salt deficiency in the steatorrhea following resection of the ileum and proximal colon. *New Eng. J. Med.*, **277**:337–42, 1967.

Hargreaves, T.: *The Liver and Bile Metabolism*. Appleton-Century-Crofts, Inc., New York, 1968.

Harker, L. A.; Funk, D. D.; and Finch, C. A.; Evaluation of storage iron by chelates. *Amer. J. Med.*, **45**:105–15, 1968.

Harrison, J. E.; Hitchman, A. J. W.; Finlay, J. M.; and McNeil, K. G.: Calcium kinetic studies in patients with malabsorption syndrome. *Gastroenterology*, **56**:751–57, 1969.

Harvey, S. C.: Gastric anatacids and digestants. In Goodman, L. S., and Gilman, A. (eds.): *The Pharmacological Basis of Therapeutics*, 3rd ed. The Macmillan Co., New York, 1965, pp. 990–1007.

Haubrich, W. S.; Watson, J. H. L.; and Sieracki, J. C.: Unique morphologic features of Whipple's disease: a study in light and electron microscopy. *Gastroenterology*, **39**:454–68, 1960.

Havens, W. P.: Intestinal obstruction caused by colloidal aluminum hydroxide. *J.A.M.A.*, **113**:1564–65, 1939.

Havens, W. P., and Bluemle, L. W.: The effect of human serum albumin and mercurial diuretics on ascites in patients with hepatic cirrhosis. *Gastroenterology*, **16**:455–65, 1950.

Hays, M. T.: Absorption of oral thyroxine in man. *J. Clin. Endocr.*, **28**:749–56, 1968.

Heaton, K. W.; Austad, W. I.; Lack, L.; and Tyor, M. P.: Entero-hepatic circulation of C^{14}-labeled bile salts in disorders of the distal small bowel. *Gastroenterology*, **55**:5–16, 1968.

Heimburger, I.; Teramoto, S.; and Shumacker, H. B.: Effect of surgical pituitrin upon portal and hepatic circulation. *Surgery*, **48**:706–15, 1960.

Heinemann, H. O., and Emirgil, C.: Hypokalemia in liver disease. *Metabolism*, **9**:869–79, 1960.

Heizer, W. D.; Cleaveland, C. R.; and Iber, F. L.: Gastric inactivation of pancreatic supplements. *Bull. Johns Hopkins Hosp.*, **116**:261–70, 1965.

Heizer, W. D.; Warshaw, A. L.; Waldmann, T. A.; and Laster, L.: Protein-losing gastroenteropathy and malabsorption associated with factitious diarrhea. *Ann. Intern. Med.*, **68**:839–52, 1968.

Helman, R. A.; Temko, M. H.; Nye, S. W.; and Fallon, H. J.: Alcoholic hepatitis. Natural history and evaluation of prednisolone therapy. *Ann. Intern. Med.*, 74:311–21, 1971.

Henley, K. S.; Streeten, M. D.; and Pollard, H. M.: Hyperaldosteronism in liver disease. *Gastroenterology*, 36:681–89, 1960.

Hepner, G. W.; Booth, C. C.; Cowan, J.; Hoffbrand, A. V.; and Mollin, D. L.: Absorption of crystalline folic acid in man. *Lancet*, 2:302–306, 1968.

Herbert, V.: Absorption of vitamin B_{12} and folic acid. *Gastroenterology*, 54:110–15, 1968.

Herbert, V., and Castle, W. B.: Intrinsic factor. *New Eng. J. Med.*, 270:1181–85, 1964.

Herman, J. R., and Goldberg, A. S.: New type of urinary calculus caused by antacid therapy. *J.A.M.A.*, 174:1206–1207, 1960.

Hermans, P. E.: Nodular lymphoid hyperplasia of the small intestine and hypogammaglobulinemia: theoretical and practical considerations. *Fed. Proc.*, 26:1606–11, 1967.

Hermans, P. E.; Huizenga, K. A.; Hoffman, H. N.; Brown, A. L., Jr.; and Markovitz, H.: Dysgammaglobulinemia associated with nodular lymphoid hyperplasia of the small intestine. *Amer. J. Med.*, 40:78–89, 1966.

Hill, M. J., and Drasar, B. S.: Degradation of bile salts by human intestinal bacteria. *Gut*, 9:22–27, 1968.

Hines, J. D.; Hoffbrand, A. V.; and Mollin, D. L.: The hematologic complications following partial gastrectomy: a study of 292 patients. *Amer. J. Med.*, 43:555–69, 1967.

Hoedemaeker, P. J.; Abels, J., Jr.; Wachters, J. J.; Arends, A.; and Niewig, H. O.: Investigations about the site of production of Castle's gastric intrinsic factor. *Lab. Invest.*, 13:1394–99, 1964.

Hoffbrand, A. V., and Necheles, T. F.: Mechanism of folate deficiency in patients receiving phenytoin. *Lancet*, 2:528–30, 1968.

Hofmann, A. F.: Clinical implications of physicochemical studies on bile salts. *Gastroenterology*, 48:484–94, 1965.

———: The syndrome of ileal disease and the broken enteropathic circulation: cholerheic enteropathy. *Ibid.*, 52:752–57, 1967.

Hofmann, A. F., and Poley, J. R.: Cholestyramine treatment of diarrhea associated with ileal resection. *New Eng. J. Med.*, 281:397–402, 1969.

Holland, P. V.; Rubinson, R. M.; Morrow, A. G.; and Schmidt, P. J.: Gamma globulin in the prophylaxis of post transfusion hepatitis. *J.A.M.A.*, 196:471–74, 1966.

Hollenberg, M., and Jennings, B.: Whipple's disease: a case report, with enzyme histochemical and electron microscopic findings. *Amer. J. Med.*, 32:448–59, 1962.

Holt, P. R.: Medium-chain triglycerides: their absorption, metabolism, and clinical applications. In Glass, G. B. J. (ed.): *Progress in Gastroenterology*, Vol. 1. Grune and Stratton, Inc., New York, 1968, pp. 277–98.

Huang, S. S., and Bayless, T. M.: Milk and lactose intolerance in healthy Orientals. *Science*, 160:83–84, 1968.

Hwang, Y. F., and Brown, E. B.: Evaluation of desferoxamine in iron overload. *Arch. Intern. Med. (Chicago)*, 114:741–53, 1964.

Iber, F. L.: Topics in clinical medicine: treatment of pancreatic insufficiency. *Johns Hopkins Med. J.*, 22:172–79, 1968.

Ingelfinger, F. J.: The modification of intestinal motility by drugs. *New Eng. J. Med.*, 229:114–22, 1943.

———: Anticholinergic therapy of gastrointestinal disorders. *Ibid.*, 268:1454–57, 1963.

———: Let the ulcer patient enjoy his food. In Ingelfinger, F. J.; Relman, A. S.; and Finland, M. (eds.): *Controversy in Internal Medicine.* W. B. Saunders Co., Philadelphia, 1966, pp. 171–79.

Isenberg, J. I.; Brooks, A. M.; and Grossman, M. I.: Pentagastrin vs. betazole as stimulant of gastric secretion: comparative study in man. *J.A.M.A.*, 206:2897–98, 1968.

Isselbacher, K. J.; Scheig, R.; Plotkin, G. R.; and Caulfield, J. B.: Congenital β-lipoprotein deficiency: an hereditary disorder involving a defect in the absorption and transport of lipids. *Medicine (Balt.)*, 43:347–61, 1964.

Ivanovich, P.; Fellows, H.; and Rich, C.: The absorption of calcium carbonate. *Ann. Intern. Med.*, 66:917–23, 1967.

Ivy, A. C.: Cholecystagogues, choleretics and cholpoietics. *Gastroenterology*, 3:54–57, 1944.

Jabbari, M., and Leevy, C. M.: Protein anabolism and fatty liver of the alcoholic. *Medicine (Balt.)*, 46:131–39, 1967.

Jacobs, P.; Bothwell, T.; and Charlton, R. W.: Role of hydrochloric acid in iron absorption. *J. Appl. Physiol.*, 19:187–88, 1964.

Jacobs, W. H.: Unusual fatal infectious complications of steriod-treated liver disease. *Gastroenterology*, 44:519–26, 1963.

Jacobson, E. D.; Chodos, R. B.; and Faloon, W. W.: An experimental malabsorption syndrome induced by neomycin. *Amer. J. Med.*, 28:524–33, 1960.

Jansen, W.; Que, G. S.; and Vegger, W.: Primary combined saccharase and isomaltose deficiency. *Arch. Intern. Med. (Chicago)*, 116:879–85, 1965.

Javitt, N. B.: Bile salt regulation of hepatic excretory function. *Gastroenterology*, 56:622–25, 1969.

Jepson, K.; Duthie, H. L.; Fawcett, A. N.; Gumpert, J. R.; Johnston, D.; Lari, J.; and Wormsley, K. G.: Acid and pepsin response to gastrin I, pentagastrin, tetragastrin, histamine, and pentagastrin snuff. *Lancet*, 2:139–41, 1968.

Johnson, L. P., and Jesseph, J. E.: Evidence for a humoral etiology of the dumping syndrome. *Surg. Forum*, 12:316–17, 1961.

Johnson, L. P.; Sloop, R. D.; Jesseph, J. E.; and Harkins, H. N.: Serotonin antagonists in experimental and clinical "dumping." *Ann. Surg.*, 156:537–49, 1962.

Jones, D. P., and Davidson, C. S.: The treatment of hepatic coma. *New Eng. J. Med.*, 267:196–98, 1962.

Jones, E. A.; Clain, D.; Clink, H. M.; MacGillivray, M.; and Sherlock, S.: Hepatic coma due to acute hepatic necrosis treated by exchange blood transfusion. *Lancet*, 2:169–72, 1967.

Jones, J. H., and Lennard-Jones, J. E.: Corticosteroids and corticotrophin in the treatment of Crohn's disease. *Gut*, 7:181–87, 1966.

Jones, R. R.; Dawson, B.; Adson, M. A.; and Summerskill, W. H. J.: Halothane and nonhalogenated anesthetic agents in patients with cirrhosis of the liver: mortality and morbidity following portal systemic venous anastomoses. *Surg. Clin. N. Amer.*, 45:983–90, 1965.

Jordan, P. H., Jr., and Grossman, M. I.: Effect of dosage schedule on the efficacy of substitution therapy in pancreatic insufficiency. *Gastroenterology*, 36:447–51, 1959.

Kahn, I. J.; Jeffries, G. H.; and Sleisenger, M. H.: Malabsorption in intestinal scleroderma: correction by antibiotics. *New Eng. J. Med.* 274:1339–44, 1966.

Kaiser, G. C.: Intravenous infusion of ascitic fluid. *Arch. Surg. (Chicago)*, 85:763–71, 1962.

Kalser, M. H.; Leite, C. A.; and Warren, W. D.: Fat assimilation after massive distal pancreatectomy. *New Eng. J. Med.*, 279:570–76, 1968.

Kappas, A., and Song, C. S.: Enzyme induction in the liver. *Gastroenterology*, **55**:731–34, 1968.

Kasich, A. M., and Rafsky, J. C.: Clinical evaluation of an anticholinergic in the irritable colon syndrome: a double-blind study of tricyclamol. *Amer. J. Gastroent.*, **31**:47–52, 1959.

Kassirer, J. P., and Schwartz, W. B.: The response of normal man to selective depletion of hydrochloric acid: factors in the genesis of persistent gastric alkalosis. *Amer. J. Med.*, **40**:10–18, 1966.

Kater, R. M. H.; Roggin. G.; Tabon, F.; Zieve, P.; and Iber, F. L.: Increased rate of clearance of drugs from circulation of alcoholics. *Amer. J. Med. Sci.*, **258**:35–39, 1969.

Katz, R.; Ducci, H.; and Alessandri, H.: Influence of cortisone and prednisolone on hyperbilirubinemia. *J. Clin. Invest.*, **36**:1370–74, 1957.

Katz, R.; Velasco, M.; Klinger, J.; and Alessandri, H.: Corticosteroids in the treatment of acute hepatitis in coma. *Gastroenterology*, **42**:258–65, 1962.

Keczkes, K.; Goldberg, D. M.; and Ferguson, A. G.: Xanthomatous biliary cirrhosis treated with cholestyramine. *Arch. Intern. Med. (Chicago)*, **114**:321–28, 1964.

Kehayoglou, A. K.; Agnew, J. E.; Holdsworth, C. D.; Whelton, M. J.; and Sherlock, S.: Bone disease and calcium absorption in primary biliary cirrhosis. *Lancet*, **1**:715–18, 1968.

Kent, G., and Popper, H.: Liver biopsy in the diagnosis of hemochromatosis. *Amer. J. Med.*, **44**:837–41, 1968.

Kent, G.; Volini, F. I.; Minick, O. T.; Orfei, E.; and de la Huerga, J.: Effect of iron loading upon the formation of collagen in the hepatic injury induced by carbon tetrachloride. *Amer. J. Path.*, **45**:129–55, 1964.

Kern, F.; Vinnik, I. E.; Struthers, J. E.; and Hill, R. B.: The treatment of chronic hepatitis with adrenal cortical hormones. *Amer. J. Med.*, **35**:310–22, 1963.

Kerr, D. N. S., and Davidson, Sir. S.: Gastrointestinal intolerance to oral iron preparations. *Lancet*, **2**:489–92, 1958.

Keynes, W. M.: Haemodialysis in the treatment of liver failure. *Lancet*, **2**:1236–38, 1968.

Khan, G. A., and Scott, A. J.: The place of rifamycin B diethylamide in the treatment of cholangitis complicating biliary obstruction. *Brit. J. Pharmacol.*, **31**:506–12, 1967.

Kiley, J. E.; Pender, J. C.; Welch, H. F.; and Welch, C. S.: Ammonia intoxication treated by hemodialysis. *New Eng. J. Med.*, **259**:1156–61, 1958.

Kim, Y. S.; Spritz, N.; Blum, M.; Terz, J.; and Sherlock, S.: The role of altered bile acid metabolism in the steatorrhea of experimental blind-loop. *J. Clin. Invest.*, **45**:956–62, 1966.

Kimber, C., and Weintraub, L. R.: Malabsorption of iron secondary to iron deficiency. *New Eng. J. Med.*, **279**:453–59, 1968.

Kirkpatrick, C. H.; Waxman, D.; Smith, O.; and Schimke, R. W.: Hypogammaglobulinemia with nodular lymphoid hyperplasia of small bowel. *Arch. Intern. Med. (Chicago)*, **121**:273–77, 1968.

Kirsner, J. B.: Controlling gastric secretion. *Postgrad. Med.*, **44**:76–79, 1968a.

———: Peptic ulcer: a review of the recent literature on various clinical aspects. *Gastroenterology*, **54**:611–41, 1968b.

Kirsner, J. B., and Palmer, W. L.: The effect of various antacids upon the hydrogen ion concentration of the gastric contents. *Amer. J. Dig. Dis.*, **7**:85–93, 1940.

Klaassen, C. D., and Plaa, G. L.: Studies on the mechanism of phenobarbital-enhanced sulfobromophthalein disappearance. *J. Pharmacol. Exp. Ther.*, **161**:361–66, 1968.

Klatskin, G.: Introduction: mechanisms of toxic and drug hepatic injury. In Fink, B. R. (ed.): *Toxicity of Anesthetics*. Williams & Williams Co., Baltimore, 1968.

———: Toxic and drug-induced hepatitis. In Schiff, L. (ed.): *Diseases of the Liver*, 3rd ed. J. B. Lippincott Co., Philadelphia, 1969.

Klatskin, G.; Krehl, W. A.; and Conn, H. O.: The effect of alcohol on choline requirement. I. Changes in rat's liver following prolonged ingestion of alcohol. *J. Exp. Med.*, **100**:605–14, 1954.

Kleiner, G. J.; Kresch, L.; and Arias, I. M.: Studies of hepatic excretory function. II. The effect of norethynodrel and mestranol on bromsulfalein sodium metabolism in women of childbearing age. *New Eng. J. Med.*, **273**:420–23, 1965.

Klipstein, F. A.: Tropical sprue. *Gastroenterology*, **54**: 275–93, 1968.

Klipstein, F. A., and Falaiye, J. M.: Tropical sprue in expatriates from the tropics living in the continental United States. *Medicine (Balt.)*, **48**:475–91, 1969.

Knauer, C. M.; Gamble, C. N.; and Monroe, L. S.: The reversal of hemochromatotic cirrhosis by multiple phlebotomies: report of a case. *Gastroenterology*, **49**:667–71, 1965.

Koch, J. P., and Donaldson, R. M., Jr.: A survey of food intolerances in hospitalized patients. *New Eng. J. Med.*, **271**:657–60, 1964.

Konturek, S. J., Oleksy, J.; and Wysocki, A.: Effect of atropine on gastric acid response to graded doses of pentagastrin and histamine in duodenal ulcer patients before and after vagotomy. *Amer. J. Dig. Dis.*, **13**:792–800, 1968.

Koppel, M. H.; Coburn, J. W.; Mims, M. M.; Goldstein, H.; Boyle, J. D.; and Rubini, M. E.: Transplantation of cadaveric kidneys from patients with hepatorenal syndrome: evidence for the functional nature of renal failure in advanced liver disease. *New Eng. J. Med.*, **280**:1367–71, 1969.

Korelitz, B. I., and Lindner, A. E.: The influence of corticotrophin and adrenal steroids on the course of ulcerative colitis: a comparison with the presteroid era. *Gastroenterology*, **46**:671–79, 1964.

Kory, R. C.; Bradley, M. H.; Callahan, R.; and Peters, B. J.: A six-month investigation of an anabolic drug—norethandrolone—in underweight persons. *Amer. J. Med.*, **26**:243–48, 1959.

Kramer, P.: The meaning of high and low residue diets. *Gastroenterology*, **47**:649–52, 1964.

Kramer, P., and Pope, C. E.: Factitious diarrhea induced by phenolphthalein. *Arch. Intern. Med. (Chicago)*, **114**:634–36, 1964.

Krawitt, E. L.; Stein, J. H.; Kirkendall, W.; and Clifton, J. A.: Mercaptopurine hepatotoxicity in a patient with chronic active hepatitis. *Arch. Intern. Med. (Chicago)*, **120**:729–34, 1967.

Kreek, M. J., and Sleisenger, M. H.: Reduction of serum-conjugated bilirubin with phenobarbitone in adult congenital non haemolytic unconjugated hyperbilirubinemia. *Lancet*, **2**:73–77, 1968.

Kreek, M. J.; Sleisenger, M. H.; and Jeffries, G. H.: Recurrent cholestatic jaundice of pregnancy with demonstrated estrogen sensitivity. *Amer. J. Med.*, **43**:795–803, 1967a.

Kreek, M. J.; Weser, E.; Sleisenger, M. H.; and Jeffries, G. H.: Idiopathic cholestasis of pregnancy: the response to challenge with the synthetic estrogen, ethinyl estradiol. *New Eng. J. Med.*, **277**:1391–95, 1967b.

Kroe, D.; Kinney, T. D.; Kaufman, H.; and Klavins, J. V.: The influence of amino acids on iron absorption. *Blood*, **21**:546–52, 1963.

Krone, C. L.; Theodor, E.; Sleisenger, M. H.; and Jeffries, G. H.: Studies on the pathogenesis of malabsorption: lipid hydrolysis and micelle formation in the intestinal lumen. *Medicine (Balt.)*, **47**:89–106, 1968.

Krugman, S.: The clinical use of gamma globulins. *New Eng. J. Med.*, **269**:195–201, 1963.

Krugman, S.; Ward, R.; Giles, J. P.; and Jacobs, A. M.: Infectious hepatitis: studies on the effect of gamma globulin and on the incidence of inapparent infection. *J.A.M.A.*, **174**:823–30, 1960.

Kunelis, C. T.; Peters, J. L.; and Edmondson, H. A.: Fatty liver of pregnancy and its relationship to tetracycline therapy. *Amer. J. Med.*, **38**:359–77, 1965.

Kunin, C. M.; Chalmers, T. C.; Leevy, C. M.; Sebastyen, S. C.; Lieber, C. S.; and Finland, M.: Absorption of orally administered neomycin and kanamycin: with special reference to patients with severe hepatic and renal disease. *New Eng. J. Med.*, **262**:380–85, 1960.

Kunin, C. M., and Finland, M.: Excretion of demethyl chlortetracycline into bile. *New Eng. J. Med.*, **261**:1069–71, 1959.

Kunin, C. M.; Glazko, A. J.; and Finland, M.: Persistence of antibiotics in blood of patients with acute renal failure. II. Chloramphenicol and its metabolic products in the blood of patients with severe renal disease or hepatic cirrhosis. *J. Clin. Invest.*, **38**:1498–1508, 1959.

Kuntz, S. M.; Davis, T. D., Jr.; and Ruffin, J. M.: Light and electron microscopic studies of Whipple's disease. *Lab. Invest.*, **11**:653–65, 1962.

Laidlaw, J.; Read, A. E.; and Sherlock, S.: Morphine tolerance in hepatic cirrhosis. *Gastroenterology*, **40**:389–96, 1961.

Lancestremere, R. G.; Davidson, P. L.; Early, L. E.; O'Brien, F. J.; and Papper, S.: Renal failure in Laennec's cirrhosis. II. Simultaneous determination of cardiac output and renal hemodynamics. *J. Clin. Invest.*, **41**:1922–27, 1962.

Laragh, J. H.: The proper use of newer diuretics. *Ann. Intern. Med.*, **67**:606–13, 1967.

Last, P., and Sherlock, S.: Systemic absorption of orally administered neomycin in liver disease. *New Eng. J. Med.*, **262**:385–89, 1960.

Laster, L.; Waldmann, T. A.; Fenster, L. F.; and Singleton, J. W.: Albumin metabolism in patients with Whipple's disease. *J. Clin. Invest.*, **45**:637–44, 1966.

Law, D. H.: Regional enteritis. *Gastroenterology*, **56**:1086–1110, 1969.

Lawrence, J. S.: Dietetic and other methods of treatment of peptic ulcer. *Lancet*, **1**:482–85, 1952.

LeBauer, E.; Smith, K.; and Greenberger, N. J.: Pancreatic insufficiency and vitamin B_{12} malabsorption. *Arch. Intern. Med. (Chicago)*, **122**:423–25, 1968.

Leevy, C. M.; Baker, H.; tenHove, W.; Frank, O.; and Cherrick, G. R.: B complex vitamins in liver disease of the alcoholic. *Amer. J. Clin. Nutr.*, **16**:339–46, 1965.

Lennard-Jones, J. E.: Experimental and clinical observations on poldine in treatment of duodenal ulcer. *Brit. Med. J.*, **1**:1071–76, 1961.

Lennard-Jones, J. E., and Babouris, N.: Effect of different foods on the acidity of the gastric contents in patients with duodenal ulcer. I. A comparison between two "therapeutic" diets and freely-chosen meals. *Gut*, **6**:113–17, 1965.

Leonards, J. R., and Levy, G.: Reduction or prevention of aspirin-induced occult gastrointestinal blood loss in man. *Clin. Pharmacol. Ther.*, **10**:571–75, 1969.

Lester, R.; Hammaker, L.; and Schmid, R.: A new therapeutic approach to unconjugated hyperbilirubinaemia. *Lancet*, **2**:1257, 1962.

Levi, A. J.: Some aspects of drug metabolism in liver disease. In McIntyre, N., and Sherlock, S. (eds.): *Therapeutic Agents and the Liver*. F. A. Davis Co., Philadelphia, 1965, pp. 51–56.

Levi, A. J.; Sherlock, S.; Scheuer, P. J.; and Cumings, J. N.: Presymptomatic Wilson's disease. *Lancet*, **2**:575–79, 1967.

Levi, A. J.; Sherlock, S.; and Walker, D.: Phenylbutazone and isoniazid metabolism in patients with liver disease in relation to previous drug therapy. *Lancet*, **1**:1275–79, 1968.

Levine, H.; Gilbert, A. J.; and Bodansky, M.: Pulmonary and urinary excretion of paraldehyde in normal dogs and dogs with liver damage. *J. Pharmacol. Exp. Ther.*, **69**:316–23, 1940.

Levine, R. R.: Factors affecting gastrointestinal absorption of drugs. *Amer. J. Dig. Dis.*, **15**:171–88, 1970.

Levine, R. R., and Pelikan, E. W.: Mechanisms of drug absorption and excretion—passage of drugs out of and into the gastrointestinal tract. *Ann. Rev. Pharmacol.*, **4**:69–84, 1964.

Levy, G., and Hayes, B. A.: Physicochemical basis of the buffered acetylsalicylic acid controversy. *New Eng. J. Med.*, **262**:1053–58, 1960.

Lewis, B. I.: A psychomedical survey of a private outpatient clinic in a university hospital. *Amer. J. Med.*, **14**:586–99, 1953.

Lieber, C. S., and Davidson, C. S.: Complications resulting from renal failure in patients with liver disease. *Arch. Intern. Med. (Chicago)*, **106**:749–52, 1960.

Lindquist, B., and Meeuwisse, G. W.: Chronic diarrhea caused by monosaccharide malabsorption. *Acta Paediat. Scand.*, **51**:674–85, 1962.

Linscheer, W. G.; Patterson, J. F.; Moore, E. W.; Clermont, R. J.; Sander, R. C.; Robins, S. J.; and Chalmers, T. C.: Medium and long chain fat absorption in patients with cirrhosis. *J. Clin. Invest.*, **45**:1317–25, 1966.

Litchfield, J. A.: Low potassium syndrome resulting from the use of purgative drugs. *Gastroenterology*, **37**:483–88, 1959.

Littman, A., and Hanscom, D. H.: Pancreatic extracts. *New Eng. J. Med.*, **218**:201–204, 1969.

Liu, H. Y.; Tsao, M. U.; Moore, B.; and Giday, Z.: Bovine milk protein-induced intestinal malabsorption of lactose and fat in infants. *Gastroenterology*, **54**:27–34, 1968.

Lloyd, H. M.; Powell, L. W.; and Thomas, M. J.: Idiopathic haemochromatosis in menstruating women: a family study, including the use of diethylene triamine penta-acetic acid. *Lancet*, **2**:555–57, 1964.

Losowsky, M. S., and Atkinson, M.: Intravenous albumin in the treatment of diuretic resistant ascites in portal cirrhosis. *Lancet*, **2**:386–89, 1961.

Losowsky, M. S., and Walker, B. E.: Liver disease and malabsorption. *Gastroenterology*, **56**:589–600, 1969.

Lottsfeldt, F. I.; Krivit, W.; Aust, J. B.; and Carcy, J. B., Jr.: Cholestyramine therapy in intrahepatic biliary atresia. *New Eng. J. Med.*, **269**:186–89, 1963.

Lotz, M.; Zisman, E.; and Bartter, F. C.: Evidence for a phosphorus-depletion syndrome in man. *New Eng. J. Med.*, **278**:409–15, 1968.

Lutz, E. E., and Margolis, A. J.: Obstetric hepatosis: treatment with cholestyramine and interim response to steroids. *Obstet. Gynec.*, **33**:64–71, 1969.

Ma, M. H.; McLeod, J. G.; and Blackburn, C. R. B.: Long term treatment of portal systemic encephalopathy with lactulose. *Aust. Ann. Med.*, **18**:117–23, 1969.

Macbeth, W. A.; Kass, E. M.; and McDermott, W. V., Jr.: Treatment of hepatic encephalopathy by alteration of intestinal flora with lactobacillus acidophilus. *Lancet*, **1**:399–403, 1965.

McCarthy, C. F.; Austad, W. I.; and Read, A. E. A.: Hypogammaglobulinemia and steatorrhea. *Amer. J. Dig. Dis.*, **10**:945–57, 1965.

MacDonald, J. M.; Webster, M. M., Jr.; Tennyson,

C. H.; and Drapanas, T.: Serotonin and bradykinin in the dumping syndrome. *Amer. J. Surg.*, **117**:204–13, 1969.

MacDonald, R. A.: Experimental pigment cirrhosis: its production in rats by feeding a choline-deficient diet with excess iron. *Amer. J. Path.*, **36**:499–519, 1960.

———: *Hemochromatosis and Hemosiderosis.* Charles C Thomas, Publisher, Springfield, Ill., 1964.

McDonald, W. C.; Brandborg, L. L.; Flick, A. L.; Trier, J. S.; and Rubin. C. E.: Studies of celiac sprue. IV. The response of the whole length of the small bowel to a gluten-free diet. *Gastroenterology*, **47**:573–89, 1964.

McGill, D. B., and Newcomer, A. D.: Comparison of venous and capillary blood samples in lactose tolerance testing. *Gastroenterology*, **53**:371–74, 1967.

McGuigan, J. E., and Volwiler, W.: Celiac-sprue: malabsorption of iron in the absence of steatorrhea. *Gastroenterology*, **47**:636–41, 1964.

McHardy, G.: What is carbenoxolone sodium? *Gastroenterology*, **56**:818–19, 1969.

McHardy, G.; Sekinger, D.; Balart, L.; and Cradic, H. E.: Chlordiazepoxideclidinium bromide in gastrointestinal disorders: controlled clinical studies. *Gastroenterology*, **54**:508–13, 1968.

Machella, T. E.: Mechanism of the postgastrectomy dumping syndrome. *Gastroenterology*, **14**:237–55, 1950.

MacKay, I. R.: Chronic hepatitis: effect of prolonged suppressive treatment and comparison of azathioprine with prednisolone. *Quart. J. Med.*, **37**:379–92, 1968.

MacKay, I. R.; Weiden, S.; and Ungar, B.: Treatment of active chronic hepatitis and lupoid hepatitis with 6-mercaptopurine and azathioprine. *Lancet*, **1**:899–902, 1964.

MacKay, I. R., and Wood, I. J.: Autoimmunity in liver disease. In Popper, H., and Schaffner, F. (eds.): *Progress in Liver Disease.* Grune & Stratton, Inc., New York, 1961.

MacKenzie, I. L.; Donaldson, R. M.; Kopp, W. L.; and Trier, J. S.: Antibodies to intestinal microvillous membranes. II. Inhibition of intrinsic factor-mediated attachment of vitamin B_{12} to hamster brush borders. *J. Exp. Med.*, **128**:375–86, 1968.

McMillan, D. E., and Freeman, R. B.: The milk-alkali syndrome: a study of the acute disorder with comments on the development of the chronic condition. *Medicine (Balt.)*, **44**:485–501, 1965.

McPhedran, N. T., and Henderson, R. D.: Pruritus and jaundice. *Canad. Med. Ass. J.*, **92**:1258–60, 1965.

Malawar, S. J.; Ewton, M.; Fordtran, J. S.; and Ingelfinger, F. J.: Interrelation between jejunal absorption of sodium, glucose, and water in man. *J. Clin. Invest.*, **44**:1072–73, 1965.

Malins, J. M., and French, J. M.: Diabetic diarrhea. *Quart. J. Med.*, **26**:467–80, 1957.

Marcus, F. I., and Kapadia, G. G.: The metabolism of tritiated digoxin in cirrhotic patients. *Gastroenterology*, **47**:517–24, 1964.

Marin, G. A.; Clark, M. L.; and Senior, J. R.: Distribution of D-xylose in sequestered fluid resulting in false-positive tests for malabsorption. *Ann. Intern. Med.*, **69**:1155–62, 1968.

Marks, I. N., and Bank, S.: Treatment of steatorrhea due to pancreatic insufficiency. *Mod. Treatm.*, **2**:326–34, 1965.

Marks, I. N.; Bank, S.; and Airth, E. M.: Pancreatic replacement therapy in the treatment of pancreatic steatorrhoea. *Gut*, **4**:217–22, 1963.

Marver, H. S., and Schmid, R.: Biotransformation in the liver: implications for human disease. *Gastroenterology*, **55**:282–89, 1968.

Matts, S. G. F.: Local treatment of ulcerative colitis with prednisolone-21-phosphate enemata. *Lancet*, **1**:517–19, 1960.

Maurer, H. M.; Wolff, J. A.; Poppers, P. J.; Finster, M.; Conney, A. H.; Pantuck, E.; and Knutzman, R.: Reduction in concentration of total serum bilirubin in offspring of women treated with phenobarbitone during pregnancy. *Lancet*, **2**:122–24, 1968.

Meeuwisse, G. W., and Dahlqvist, A.: Glucose-galactose malabsorption: a study with biopsy of the small intestinal mucosa. *Acta Paediat. Scand.*, **57**:273–80, 1968.

Mendenhall, C. L.: Anabolic steroid therapy as an adjunct to diet in alcoholic hepatic steatosis. *Amer. J. Dig. Dis.*, **13**:783–91, 1968.

Merigan, T. C.; Plotkin, G. R.; and Davidson, C. S.: Effect of intravenously administered posterior pituitary extract on hemorrhage from bleeding esophageal varices. *New Eng. J. Med.*, **266**:134–35, 1962.

Middleton, E. J.; Nagy, E.; and Morrison, A. B.: Studies on the absorption of orally administered iron from sustained-release preparations. *New Eng. J. Med.*, **274**:136–39, 1966.

Mindrum, G. M., and Schiff, L.: Use of a high-fat diet in cases of fatty liver. *Gastroenterology*, **29**:825–36, 1955.

Mirick, G. S.; Ward, R.; and McCollum, R. C.: Modification of post-transfusion hepatitis by gamma globulin. *New Eng. J. Med.*, **273**:59–65, 1965.

Misiewicz, J. J.; Lennard-Jones, J. E.; Connell, A. M.; Baron, J. H.; and Jones, F. A.: Controlled trial of sulphasalazine in maintenance therapy for ulcerative colitis. *Lancet*, **1**:185–88, 1965.

Mistilis, S. P., and Blackburn, C. R.: The treatment of active chronic hepatitis with 6-mercaptopurine and azathioprine. *Aust. Ann. Med.*, **16**:305–11, 1967.

Mistilis, S. P., and Schiff, L.: Steroid therapy in chronic hepatitis. *Arch. Intern. Med. (Chicago)*, **113**:54–62, 1964.

Mitchell, R. D.; Hunt, J. N.; and Grossman, M. I.: Inhibition of basal and postprandial gastric secretion by poldine and atropine in patients with peptic ulcer. *Gastroenterology*, **43**:400–406, 1962.

Mlynaryk, P., and Kirsner, J. B.: Absorption and excretion of 1,2,H^3-hydrocortisone in regional enteritis and ulcerative colitis, with a note on hydrocortisone production rates. *Gastroenterology*, **44**:257–60, 1963.

Moeschlin, S., and Schnider, U.: Treatment of primary and secondary hemochromatosis and acute iron poisoning with a new, potent iron-eliminating agent (desferrioxamine-B). *New Eng. J. Med.*, **269**:57–66, 1963.

Montgomery, R. D.; Lawrence, I. H.; Manton, D. J.; Mendl, K.; and Rowe, P.: A controlled trial of carbenoxolone sodium capsules in the treatment of duodenal ulcer. *Gut*, **9**:704–706, 1968.

Morgan, D. B.; Pulvertaft, C. N.; and Fourman, P.: Effects of age in the loss of bone after gastric surgery. *Lancet*, **2**:772–73, 1966.

Morrissey, J. F.; Honda, T.; Tanaka, Y.; and Perna, G.: Gastric mucosal coating and gastric emptying time of antacids—a gastrocamera study. *Arch. Intern. Med. (Chicago)*, **119**:510–17, 1967.

Mortimer, D. C.; Reed, P. I.; Vidinli, M.; and Finlay, J. M.: Role of upper gastrointestinal flora in malabsorption syndrome. *Canad. Med. Ass. J.*, **90**:559–64, 1964.

Mortimer, P. R.; Mackie, D. B.; and Haynes, S.: Ampicillin levels in human bile in the presence of biliary tract disease. *Brit. Med. J.*, **2**:88–89, 1969.

Motulsky, A. G.: The genetics of abnormal drug response. *Ann. N.Y. Acad. Sci.*, **123**:167–77, 1965.

———: Drugs and genes. *Ann. Intern. Med.*, **70**:1269–73, 1969.

Mowat, A. P., and Arias, I. M.: Liver function and oral contraceptives. *J. Reprod. Med.*, **3**:19–29, 1969.

Nabarro, J. D. N.; Moxham, A.; Walker, G.; and Slater, J. D. H.: Rectal hydrocortisone. *Brit. Med. J.*, 2:272–74, 1957.

Najarian, J. S.; Dakin, R. L.; Quinnel, C. M.; Jew, J.; Harper, H. A.; and McCorkle, H. J.: Control of ammonia production in the colon with neomycin enemas. *Arch. Surg. (Chicago)*, 78:844–50, 1959.

Najarian, J. S., and Harper, H. A.: A clinical study of the effect of arginine on blood ammonia. *Amer. J. Med.*, 21:832–42, 1956.

Nalin, D. R.; Cash, R. A.; Islam, R.; Molla, M.; and Phillips, R. A.: Oral maintenance therapy for cholera in adults. *Lancet*, 2:370–72, 1968.

Nelson, E.: Rate of metabolism of tolbutamide in test subjects with liver disease or with impaired renal function. *Amer. J. Med. Sci.*, 248:657–60, 1964.

Nienhuis, L. I.; Mulmed, E. I.; and Kelley, J. W.: Hepatic coma: treatment emphasizing merit of peritoneal dialysis. *Amer. J. Surg.*, 106:980–85, 1963.

Nordio, S., and Lamedica, G. A.: Intolerance of sucrose, maltose, isomaltose and starch. In Durand, P. (ed.): *Disorders due to Intestinal Defective Carbohydrate Digestion and Absorption.* Grune & Stratton, Inc., New York, 1964, pp. 141–87.

Norman, A., and Grubb, R.: Hydrolysis of conjugated bile acids by clostridia and enterococci. *Acta Path. Microbiol. Scand.*, 36:537–47, 1955.

Northcutt, R. C.; Stiel, J. N.; Hollifield, J. W.; and Stant, E. G.: The influence of cholestyramine on thyroxine absorption. *J.A.M.A.*, 208:1857–61, 1969.

Nyberg, W.; Saarni, M.; Gothoni, G.; and Järventie, G.: The influence of *Diphyllobothrium latum* on the complex formed between the vitamin B_{12} binding principle in human gastric juice and $^{60}Co-B_{12}$. *Acta Med. Scand.*, 170:257–62, 1961.

Ockner, R. K., and Davidson, C. S.: Hepatic effects of oral contraceptives. *New Eng. J. Med.*, 276:331–34, 1967.

Opie, L. H.; Hunt, B. G.; and Finlay, J. M.: Massive small-bowel resection with malabsorption and negative magnesium balance. *Gastroenterology*, 47:415–20, 1964.

Osborn, E. C.; Wootton, I. D.; da Silva, L. C.; and Sherlock, S.: Serum-bile acid levels in liver disease. *Lancet*, 2:1049–53, 1959.

Owen, E. E.; Tyor, M. P.; Flanagan, J. F.; and Berry, J. N.: The kidney as source of blood ammonia in patients with liver disease: the effect of acetazolamide. *J. Clin. Invest.*, 39:288–94, 1960.

Page, A. R.; Condie, R. M.; and Good, R. A.: Suppression of plasma cell hepatitis with 6-mercaptopurine. *Amer. J. Med.*, 36:200–13, 1964.

Page, A. R., and Good, R. A.: Plasma-cell hepatitis, with special attention to steroid therapy. *Amer. J. Dis. Child.*, 99:288–314, 1960.

Palmer, R. H., and Hruban, Z.: Production of bile duct hyperplasia and gallstones by lithocholic acid. *J. Clin. Invest.*, 45:1255–67, 1966.

Palva, I. P.; Heinivaara, O.; and Mattila, M.: Drug-induced malabsorption of vitamin B_{12}. III. Interference of PAS and folic acid in the absorption of vitamin B_{12}. *Scand. J. Haemat.*, 3:149–53, 1966.

Papper, S., and Vaamonde, C. A.: Renal failure in cirrhosis—role of plasma volume. *Ann. Intern. Med.*, 68:958–59, 1968.

Parker, J. G., and Siegelman, S.: Retrograde spread of contrast medium released from suppositories—a partial explanation for the efficacy of therapeutic suppositories. *Amer. J. Dig. Dis.*, 10:463–66, 1965.

Parry, D. J., and Wood, P. H. N.: Relationship between aspirin-taking and gastroduodenal hemorrhage. *Gut*, 9:301–307, 1967.

Paul, H. E., and Harrington, C. M.: Adsorption characteristics of Aureomycin and Terramycin on aluminum hydroxide gel and on a bismuth subsalicylate preparation. *J. Amer. Pharm. Ass.*, 41:50 1952.

Paulk, E. A., Jr., and Farrar, W. E., Jr.: Diverticulosis of the small intestine and megaloblastic anemia: intestinal microflora and absorption before and after tetracycline administration. *Amer. J. Med.*, 37:473–80, 1964.

Peskin, G. W., and Miller, L. D.: The use of serotonin antagonists in postgastrectomy syndromes. *Amer. J. Surg.*, 109:7–13, 1965.

Peternel, W. W.: Lactose tolerance in relation to intestinal activity. *Gastroenterology*, 48:299–306, 1965.

Peters, R. L.; Edmondson, H. A.; Mikkelsen, W. P.; and Tatter, D.: Tetracycline-induced fatty liver in nonpregnant patients: a report of six cases. *Amer. J. Surg.*, 113:622–32, 1967.

Petersen, V. P.: Metabolic studies in clinical magnesium deficiency. *Acta Med. Scand.*, 173:285–98, 1963.

Phear, E. A., and Ruebner, B.: *In vitro* production of ammonium and amines by intestinal bacteria in relation to nitrogen toxicity as a factor in hepatic coma. *Brit. J. Exp. Path.*, 37:253–62, 1956.

Phillips, R. A.; Love, A. H. G.; Mitchell, T. G.; and Neptune, E. M., Jr.: Cathartics and the sodium pump. In Bushnell, O. A., and Brookhyser, C. E. (eds.): *Proceedings of the Cholera Research Symposium, Honolulu, 1965.* Dept. of Health, Education, and Welfare, Public Health Service. U.S. Government Printing Office, Washington, D.C., 1965, pp. 85–86.

Pierce, N. F.; Banwell, J. G.; Rupak, C. M.; Caranosos, G. J.; Keimowitz, R. I.; Mondal, A.; and Manji, P. M.: Effect of intragastric glucose-electrolyte infusion upon water and electrolyte balance in Asiatic cholera. *Gastroenterology*, 55:333–43, 1968.

Piper, D. W., and Fenton, B. H.: An evaluation of antacids *in vitro*. *Gut*, 5:585–89, 1964.

Polacek, M. W., and Sanfelippo, P.: Oral antibiotic bowel preparation and complications in colon surgery. *Arch. Surg. (Chicago)*, 97:412–17, 1968.

Polter, D. E.; Boyle, J. D.; Miller, L. G.; and Finegold, S. M.: Anaerobic bacteria as cause of the blind-loop syndrome: a case report with observations on response to antibacterial agents. *Gastroenterology*, 54:1148–54, 1968.

Popoff, N.; Budzilovich, G.; Goodgold, A.; and Feigin, I.: Hepatocerebral degeneration: its occurrence in the presence and in the absence of abnormal copper metabolism. *Neurology (Minneap.)*, 15:919–30, 1965.

Popper, H.; Paronetto, F.; and Schaffner, F.: Immune processes in the pathogenesis of liver disease. *Ann. N.Y. Acad. Sci.*, 124:781–99, 1965a.

Popper, H.; Rubin, E.; Gardiol, D.; Schaffner, F.; and Paronetto, F.: Drug-induced liver disease. *Arch. Intern. Med. (Chicago)*, 115:128–36, 1965b.

Porter, H. P.; Simon, F. R.; Pope, C. E., II; Volwiler, W.; and Fenster, L. F.: Corticosteroid therapy in severe alcoholic hepatitis: a double-blind drug trial. *New Eng. J. Med.*, in press, 1971.

Post, J.; Rose, J. V.; and Shore, S. M.: Intravenous use of salt-poor human albumin. *Arch. Intern. Med. (Chicago)*, 87:775–88, 1951.

Potyk, D.: Intestinal obstruction from impacted antacid tablets. *New Eng. J. Med.*, 283:134–35, 1970.

Powell, W. J., and Klatskin, G.: Duration of survival in patients with Laennec's cirrhosis. *Amer. J. Med.*, 44:406–20, 1968.

Preston, F. W.; Silverman, M.; Henegar, G. C.; and Neveril, E.: The excretion of kanamycin in bile and pancreatic fluid. *Antibiot. Ann.*, 1959–1960, pp. 857–61.

Price, J. B., Jr.; McCullough, W.; Peterson, L.; Britton, R. C.; and Voorhees, A. B., Jr.: Effects of portal systemic shunting on intestinal absorption in the dog and man. *Surg. Gynec. Obstet.*, 125:305–10, 1967.

Pruzanski, W.: The influence of steroids on serum bilirubin, leucine, aminopeptidase, and alkaline phosphatase in extrahepatic obstructive jaundice: the possible diagnostic importance. *Amer. J. Med. Sci.*, 251:685–89, 1966.

Pulaski, E. J., and Fusillo, M. H.: Gall bladder bile concentration of the major antibiotics following intravenous administration. *Surg. Gynec. Obstet.*, 100:571–74, 1955.

Ramboer, C.; Thompson, R. P. H.; and Williams, R.: Controlled trials of phenobarbitone therapy in neonatal jaundice. *Lancet*, 1:966–68, 1969.

Rawson, M. D.: Cathartic colon. *Lancet*, 1:1121–24, 1966.

Read, A. E.; Laidlaw, J.; Haslam, R. M.; and Sherlock, S.: Neuropsychiatric complications following chlorothiazide therapy in patients with hepatic cirrhosis: possible relation to hypokalemia. *Clin. Sci.*, 18:409–23, 1959.

Read, A. E.; McCarthy, C. F.; Heaton, K. W.; and Laidlaw, J.: *Lactobacillus acidophilus* (Enpac) in the treatment of hepatic encephalopathy. *Brit. Med. J.*, 1:1267–69, 1966.

Redeker, A. C.; Kuzma, O. T.; and Reynolds, T. B.: Effective treatment of refractory ascites in cirrhosis of the liver. *Arch. Intern. Med. (Chicago)*, 105:594–600, 1960.

Reichle, F. A.; Brigham, M. P.; and Rosemond, G. P.: Serotonin and the dumping syndrome. *J.A.M.A.*, 199:914–16, 1967.

Reisner, E. H.; Norman, J.; Field, W. W.; and Brown, R.: The effect of liver dysfunction on the response to Dicumarol. *Amer. J. Med. Sci.*, 217:445–47, 1949.

Reynolds, T. B.: Exchange transfusion in fulminant hepatic failure. *Gastroenterology*, 56:170–72, 1969.

Reynolds, T. B.; Lieberman, F. L.; and Redeker, A. G.: Functional renal failure with cirrhosis: the effect of plasma expansion therapy. *Medicine (Balt.)*, 46:191–96, 1967.

Reynolds, T. B.; Redeker, A. G.; and Davis, P.: A controlled study of the effects of L-arginine on hepatic encephalopathy. *Amer. J. Med.*, 25:359–67, 1958.

Reynolds, T. B.; Redeker, A. G.; and Kuzma, O. T.: Role of alcohol in pathogenesis of alcoholic cirrhosis. In McIntyre, N., and Sherlock, S. (eds.): *Therapeutic Agents and the Liver*. F. A. Davis Co., Philadelphia, 1965, pp. 131–42.

Rimer, D. G., and Frankland, M.: Sodium content of antacids. *J.A.M.A.*, 173:995–98, 1960.

Rinaldo, J. A., Jr., and Gluckmann, R. F.: Maximal absorption capacity for xylose in nontropical sprue. *Gastroenterology*, 47:248–50, 1964.

Robinson, F. W., and Pittman, A. C.: Dietary management of postgastrectomy dumping syndrome. *Surg. Gynec. Obstet.*, 104:529–34, 1957.

Rosenberg, I. H.: Influence of intestinal bacteria on bile-acid metabolism and fat absorption: contributions from studies of blind-loop syndrome. *Amer. J. Clin. Nutr.*, 22:284–91, 1969.

Rosenberg, I. H.; Hardison, W. G.; and Bull, D. M.: Abnormal bile-salt patterns and intestinal bacterial overgrowth associated with malabsorption. *New Eng. J. Med.*, 276:1391–97, 1967.

Roth, J. L. A.: The ulcer patient should watch his diet. In Ingelfinger, F. J.; Relman, A. S.; and Finland, M. (eds.): *Controversy in Internal Medicine*. W. B. Saunders Co., Philadelphia, 1966, pp. 161–70.

Roth, J. L. A.; Wechsler, R. L.; and Bockus, H. L.: Hazards in the use of anticholinergic drugs in the management of peptic ulcer disease. *Gastroenterology*, 31:493–99, 1956.

Rubin, C. E.; Brandborg, L. L.; Flick, A. L.; Phelps, C.; Parmentier, C.; and Van Niel, S.: Studies of celiac sprue. III. The effect of repeated wheat instillation into the proximal ileum of patients on a gluten-free diet. *Gastroenterology*, 43:621–41, 1962.

Rubin, E.; Gang, H.; Misra, P. S.; and Lieber, C. S.: Inhibition of drug metabolism by acute ethanol intoxication. A hepatic microsomal mechanism. *Amer. J. Med.*, 49:801–806, 1970.

Rubin, E.; Hutterer, F.; and Lieber, C. S.: Ethanol increases hepatic smooth endoplasmic reticulum and drug-metabolizing enzymes. *Science*, 159:1469–70, 1968.

Rubin, E., and Lieber, C. S.: Malnutrition and liver disease—an over-emphasized relationship. *Amer. J. Med.*, 45:1–6, 1968a.

———: Alcohol, other drugs, and the liver. *Ann. Intern. Med.*, 69:1063–67, 1968b.

———: Hepatic microsomal enzymes in man and rat: induction and inhibition by ethanol. *Science*, 162:690–91, 1968c.

Ruffin, J. M., and Cayer, D.: The role of anticholinergic drugs in treatment of peptic-ulcer disease. *Ann. N.Y. Acad. Sci.*, 99:179–89, 1962.

Ruffin, J. M.; Kurtz, S. M.; and Roufail, W. M.: Intestinal lipodystrophy (Whipple's disease). *J.A.M.A.*, 195:476–78, 1966.

Salter, R. H.: What should the patient eat? *Lancet*, 1:879–80, 1969.

Schade, S. G.; Cohen, R. J.; and Conrad, M. E.: Effect of hydrochloric acid on iron absorption. *New Eng. J. Med.*, 279:672–74, 1968.

Schade, S. G.; Muckerheide, M.; Feick, P.; and Schilling, R. F.: Occurrence in gastric juice of antibody to a complex of intrinsic factor and vitamin B_{12}. *New Eng. J. Med.*, 275:528–31, 1966.

Schaffner, F.: The effect of oral contraceptives on the liver. *J.A.M.A.*, 198:1019–21, 1966.

Schaffner, F.; Klion, F. M.; and Latuff, A. J.: The long term use of cholestyramine in the treatment of primary biliary cirrhosis. *Gastroenterology*, 48:293–98, 1965.

Schedl, H. P., and Bartter, F. C.: An explanation for and experimental correction of the abnormal water diuresis in cirrhosis. *J. Clin. Invest.*, 39:248–61, 1960.

Schedl, H. P., and Clifton, J. A.: Cortisol absorption in man. *Gastroenterology*, 44:134–45, 1963.

Scheinberg, I. H., and Sternlieb, I.: The liver in Wilson's disease. *Gastroenterology*, 37:550–64, 1959.

Scheline, R. R.: Drug metabolism by intestinal microorganisms. *J. Pharm. Sci.*, 57:2021–37, 1968.

Schmidt, C. R.; Beazell, J. M.; Atkinson, A. J.; and Ivy, A. C.: The effect of therapeutic agents on volume and constituents of bile. *Amer. J. Dig. Dis.*, 5:613–17, 1938.

Schneider, A. J.; Kinter, W. B.; and Stirling, C. E.: Glucose-galactose malabsorption: report of a case with autoradiographic studies of a mucosal biopsy. *New Eng. J. Med.*, 274:305–12, 1966.

Schofield, P. F.: The natural history and treatment of Crohn's disease. *Ann. Roy. Coll. Surg. Eng.*, 36:258–79, 1965.

Schrier, R. W., and Bulger, R. J.: Steroid-induced pancreatitis. *J.A.M.A.*, 194:564–65, 1965.

Schroeder, E. T.: Alkalosis resulting from combined administration of a "nonsystemic" antacid and a cation-exchange resin. *Gastroenterology*, 56:868–74, 1969.

Schultz, J. C.; Adamson, J. S., Jr.; Workman, W. W.; and Norman, T. O.: Fatal liver disease after intravenous administration of tetracycline in high dosage. *New Eng. J. Med.*, 269:999–1004, 1963.

Schwartz, I. R.: A clinical evaluation of a choleretic

with special emphasis on its effect on blood cholesterol. *Amer. J. Gastroent.*, 37:442–51, 1962.

Schwartz, R. D.; Cohn, G. L.; Bondy, P. K.; Brodoff, M.; Upton, G. V.; and Spiro, H. M.: Absorption of cortisol from the colon in ulcerative colitis. *Proc. Soc. Exp. Biol. Med.*, 97:648–50, 1958.

Scott, J. T.; Porter, I. H.; Lewis, S. M.; and Dixon, A. St. J.: Studies of gastrointestinal bleeding caused by corticosteroids, salicylates, and other analgesics. *Quart. J. Med.*, 30:167–88, 1961.

Segal, S., and Foley, J. B.: The metabolic fate of C^{14}-labeled pentoses in man. *J. Clin. Invest.*, 38:407–13, 1959.

Self, T. W.; Herskovic, T.; Czapek, E.; Caplan, D.; Schonberger, T.; and Gryboski, J.: Gastrointestinal protein allergy: immunologic considerations. *J.A.M.A.*, 207:2393–96, 1969.

Sen, P. K.; Bhalero, R. A.; Parulkar, G. P.; Samsi, A. B.; Shah, B. K.; and Kinare, S. G.: Use of isolated perfused cadaveric liver in the management of hepatic failure. *Surgery*, 59:774–81, 1966.

Sessions, J. T.; Minkel, H. P.; Bullard, J. C.; and Ingelfinger, F. J.: The effect of barbiturates in patients with liver disease. *J. Clin. Invest.*, 33:1116–27, 1954.

Shaldon, S.; Dolle, W.; Guevang, L.; Iber, F. L.; and Sherlock, S.: Effect of pitressin on splanchnic circulation in man. *Circulation*, 24:797–807, 1961.

Shaldon, S., and Sherlock, S.: The use of vasopressin (Pitressin) in the control of bleeding from esophageal varices. *Lancet*, 2:222–25, 1960.

Shear, L.; Bonkowsky, H. L.; and Gabuzda, G. J.: Renal tubular acidosis in cirrhosis: a determinant of susceptibility to recurrent hepatic precoma. *New Eng. J. Med.*, 280:1–7, 1969.

Shear, L.; Kleinerman, J.; and Gabuzda, G. J.: Renal failure in patients with cirrhosis of the liver. *Amer. J. Med.*, 39:184–209, 1965.

Sheehy, T. W.; Cohen, W. C.; Wallace, D. K.; and Legters, L. J.: Tropical sprue in North Americans. *J.A.M.A.*, 194:1069–76, 1965.

Sheehy, T. W., and Perez-Santiago, E.: Antibiotic therapy in tropical sprue. *Gastroenterology*, 41:208–14, 1961.

Sherlock, S.: *Diseases of the Liver*, 3rd ed. F. A. Davis Co., Philadelphia, 1963a.

———: The aetiology and mangement of ascites in patients with hepatic cirrhosis. *Gut*, 4:95–105, 1963b.

———: Haematemesis in portal hypertension. *Brit. J. Surg.*, 51:746–49, 1964.

———: Hepatic reactions to therapeutic agents. *Ann. Rev. Pharmacol.*, 5:429–46, 1965.

———: Prediction of hepatotoxicity due to therapeutic agents in man. *Medicine (Balt.)*, 45:453–58, 1966.

———: *Diseases of the Liver*, 4th ed. F. A. Davis Co., Philadelphia, 1968.

Sherlock, S.; Senewiratne, B.; Scott, A.; and Walker, J. G.: Complications of diuretic therapy in hepatic cirrhosis. *Lancet*, 1:1049–52, 1966.

Sherman, J. D.; Banas, J. S., Jr.; Edwards, T. L.; Mac-Mahon, H. E.; and Patterson, J. F.: A syndrome of diarrhea, thymoma, and hypogammaglobulinemia. *Gastroenterology*, 51:681–88, 1966.

Shils, M. E.: Experimental human magnesium depletion. *Medicine (Balt.)*, 48:61–85, 1969.

Shimoda, S. S., and Rubin, C. E.: The Zollinger-Ellison syndrome with steatorrhea. I. Anticholinergic treatment followed by total gastrectomy and colonic interposition. *Gastroenterology*, 55:695–704, 1968.

Silverberg, M., and Gellis, S. S.: The liver in juvenile Wilson's disease. *Pediatrics*, 30:402–13, 1962.

Simpson, D. P.: Hepatic regeneration and hyperplasia. *Med. Clin. N. Amer.*, 47:765–77, 1963.

Siurala, M., and Kaupainen, W. J.: Intestinal megalo-

blastic anemia. *Acta Med. Scand.*, 147:197–201, 1953.

Sjöberg, K. H., and Welin, G.: Treatment of active chronic hepatitis with 6-mercaptopurine. *Acta Hepato-splen. (Stuttgart)*, 14:157–62, 1967.

Sjövall, K., and Sjövall, J.: Serum bile acid levels in pregnancy with pruritus. *Clin. Chim. Acta*, 13:207–11, 1966.

Skinner, D. B., and Camp, T. F., Jr.: Relation of esophageal reflux to lower esophageal sphincter pressures decreased by atropine. *Gastroenterology*, 54:543–51, 1968.

Smith, P. M.; Miller, J. P. G.; Pitcher, C. S.; Lestas, A. N.; Dymock, I. W.; and Williams, R.: The differential ferrioxamine test in the management of idiopathic haemochromatosis. *Lancet*, 2:402–405, 1969.

Smyth, D. H.: Alimentary absorption of drugs: physiological considerations. In Binns, T. B. (ed.): *Absorption and Distribution of Drugs*. E. & S. Livingstone, Ltd., London, 1964, pp. 1–15.

Sobel, H. J.: The histogenesis of Whipple's disease: a cytochemical, electron microscopic, and histochemical study. *Bull. N. Y. Acad. Med.*, 42:514–15, 1966.

Soehring, K., and Schuppel, R.: Interactions between alcohol and drugs. *Deutsch. Med. Wschr.*, 91:1892–96, 1966.

Solen, G.; Goldstein, F.; and Wirts, C. W.: Malabsorption in intestinal scleroderma, relation to bacterial flora and treatment with antibiotics. *Ann. Intern. Med.*, 64:834–41, 1966.

Sparberg, M.; Jensen, R.; Beering, S. C.; and Shannon, I.: Pituitary-adrenal suppression following intrarectal administration of dexamethasone-21-phosphate. *Gastroenterology*, 52:519–20, 1967.

Sparberg, M., and Kirsner, J. B.: Long-term corticosteroid therapy for regional enteritis: an analysis of 58 courses in 54 patients. *Amer. J. Dig. Dis.*, 11:865–80, 1966.

Spiegel, E. L.; Schubert, W.; Perrin, E.; and Schiff, L.: Benign recurrent intrahepatic cholestasis with response to cholestyramine. *Amer. J. Med.*, 39:682–88, 1965.

Spiro, H. M., and Milles, S. S.: Clinical and physiologic implications of the steroid-induced peptic ulcer. *New Eng. J. Med.*, 263:286–94, 1960.

Steigmann, F.; Schrifter, H.; Yiotsas, Z. D.; and Pamukcu, F.: Vitamin K therapy in liver disease—need for a reevaluation. *Amer. J. Gastroent.*, 31:369–75, 1959.

Stephens, F. O.; Milverton, E. J.; Hambly, C. J.; and van der Ven, E. K.: The effects of food on aspirin-induced gastrointestinal blood loss. *Digestion*, 1:267–76, 1968.

Sternlieb, I., and Scheinberg, I. H.: Penicillamine therapy for hepatolenticular degeneration. *J.A.M.A.*, 189:748–54, 1964.

———: Prevention of Wilson's disease in asymptomatic patients. *New Eng. J. Med.*, 278:352–59, 1968.

Stewart, J. S.; Pollack, D. J.; Hoffbrand, A. V.; Mollin, D. L.; and Booth, C. C.: A study of proximal and distal intestinal structure and absorptive function in idiopathic steatorrhoea. *Quart. J. Med.*, 36:425–44, 1967.

Stiel, J. N.; Mitchell, C. A.; Radcliff, F. J.; and Piper, D. W.: Hypercalcemia in patients with peptic ulceration receiving large doses of calcium carbonate. *Gastroenterology*, 53:900–904, 1967.

Stowe, C. M., and Plaa, G. L.: Extrarenal excretion of drugs and chemicals. *Ann. Rev. Pharmacol.*, 8:337–56, 1968.

Strickland, R. G.; Fisher, J. M.; and Taylor, K. B.: Effect of prednisolone on gastric function and structure in man. *Gastroenterology*, 56:675–86, 1969.

Suhrland, L. G., and Weisberger, A. S.: Chloramphenicol toxicity in liver and renal disease. *Arch. Intern. Med. (Chicago)*, **112**:747–54, 1963.

Sumi, S. M., and Finley, J. M.: On the pathogenesis of diabetic steatorrhea. *Ann. Intern. Med.*, **55**:994–97, 1961.

Summerskill, W. H. J.; Clowdus, B. F.; Bollman, J. L.; and Fleisher, G. A.: Clinical and experimental studies on the effect of corticotropin and steroid drugs on bilirubin. *Amer. J. Med. Sci.*, **241**:555–62, 1961.

Summerskill, W. H. J.; Thorsell, F.; Feinberg, J. H.; and Aldrete, J. S.: The effects of urease inhibition in hyperammonemia: clinical and experimental studies with acetohydroxamic acid. *Gastroenterology*, **54**:20–26 1968.

Sun, D. C. H.: Long-term anticholinergic therapy for prevention of recurrences in duodenal ulcer. *Amer. J. Dig. Dis.*, **9**:706–16, 1964.

———: Diagnostic tests for chronic pancreatic disease. *Arch. Intern. Med. (Chicago)*, **115**:57–61, 1965.

———: Effect of corticotropin on gastric acid, pepsin, and mucus secretion in dogs with fistulas. *Amer. J. Dig. Dis.*, **14**:107–12, 1969.

Swell, L., and Bell, C. C.: Influence of bile acids on biliary lipid excretion in man. *Amer. J. Dig. Dis.*, **13**:1077–80, 1968.

Tabaqchali, S., and Booth, C. C.: Jejunal bacteriology and bile salt metabolism in patients with intestinal malabsorption. *Lancet*, **2**:12–15, 1966.

———: Relationship of the intestinal bacterial flora to absorption. *Brit. Med. Bull.*, **23**:285–90, 1967.

Tabaqchali, S.; Hatzioannou, J.; and Booth, C. C.: Bile-salt deconjugation and steatorrhoea in patients with the stagnant-loop syndrome. *Lancet*, **2**:12–16, 1968.

Taggart, D., and Billington, B. P.: Fatty foods and dyspepsia. *Lancet*, **2**:464–66, 1966.

Thistle, J. L., and Schoenfield, L. J.: Lithogenic bile among young Indian women. Lithogenic potential decreased with chenodeoxycholic acid. *New Eng. J. Med.*, **284**:177–81, 1971.

Thompson, A., and Holmes, A. W.: Immune inhibition of urea breakdown in patients with cirrhosis. *Gastroenterology*, **52**:14–17, 1967.

Thompson, G. R.; Neale, G.; Watts, J. M.; and Booth, C. C.: Detection of vitamin D deficiency after partial gastrectomy. *Lancet*, **1**:623–26, 1966.

Thompson, R. P. H.; Stathers, G. M.; Pilcher, G. W. T.; McLean, A. E. M.; Robinson, J.; and Williams, R.: Treatment of unconjugated jaundice with dicophane. *Lancet*, **2**:4–6, 1969.

Thompson, R. P. H., and Williams, R.: Treatment of chronic intrahepatic cholestasis with phenobarbitone. *Lancet*, **2**:646–48, 1967.

Thorling, L.: Jaundice in pregnancy: clinical study. *Acta Med. Scand.*, **151** (Suppl. 302):1–123, 1955.

Thorsen, W. B.; Western, D.; Tanaka, Y.; and Morrissey, J. F.: Aspirin injury to the gastric mucosa—gastrocamera observations of the effect of pH. *Arch. Intern. Med. (Chicago)*, **121**:499–506, 1968.

Tisdale, W. A.: Clinical and pathological features of subacute hepatitis. *Medicine (Balt.)*, **45**:557–63, 1966.

Tisdale, W. A.; Fenster, L. F.; and Klatskin, G.: Acute staphylococcal enterocolitis complicating oral neomycin therapy in cirrhosis. *New Eng. J. Med.*, **263**:1014–16, 1960.

Topuzlu, C., and Stahl, W. M.: Effect of bile infusion on the dog kidney. *New Eng. J. Med.*, **274**:760–63, 1966.

Toskes, P. P.; Hansell, J.; Cerda, J.; and Deren, J. J.: Vitamin B_{12} malabsorption in chronic pancreatic insufficiency. Studies suggesting the presence of a pancreatic "intrinsic factor." *New Eng. J. Med.*, **284**:627–32, 1971.

Trey, C.; Burns, D. G.; and Saunders, S. J.: Treatment of hepatic coma by exchange blood transfusion. *New Eng. J. Med.*, **274**:473–81, 1966.

Trey, C.; Lipworth, L.; Chalmers, T. C.; Davidson, C. S.; Gottlieb, L. S.; Popper, H.; and Saunders, S. J.: Fulminant hepatic failure: presumable contribution of halothane. *New Eng. J. Med.*, **279**:798–801, 1968.

Trier, J. S.; Phelps, P. C.; Erdelman, S.; and Rubin, C. E.: Whipple's disease: light and electron microscopic correlation of jejunal mucosal histology with antibiotic treatment and clinical status. *Gastroenterology*, **48**:684–707, 1965.

Tristani, F. E., and Cohn, J. N.: Systemic and renal hemodynamics in oliguric hepatic failure: effect of volume expansion. *J. Clin. Invest.*, **46**:1894–1906, 1967.

Trolle, D.: Decrease of total serum bilirubin concentration in newborn infants after phenobarbitone treatment. *Lancet*, **2**:705–708, 1968.

Truelove, S. C.: Treatment of ulcerative colitis with local hydrocortisone hemisuccinate sodium: a report on a controlled therapeutic trial. *Brit. Med. J.*, **2**:1072–77, 1958.

———: Systemic and local corticosteroid therapy in ulcerative colitis. *Brit. Med. J.*, **1**:464–67, 1960a.

———: Stilboestrol, phenobarbitone and diet in chronic duodenal ulcer: a factorial therapeutic trial. *Brit. Med. J.*, **2**:559–66, 1960b.

Truelove, S. C., and Witts, L. J.: Cortisone in ulcerative colitis: final reports on a therapeutic trial. *Brit. Med. J.*, **2**:1041–48, 1955.

Truelove, S. C., and Wright, R.: The controlled therapeutic trial in gastroenterology. *Amer. J. Dig. Dis.*, **9**:1–30, 1964.

Tucci, J. R., and Martin, M. M.: Effect of liver disease upon adrenocortical ACTH and metyrapone responsiveness in man. *Gastroenterology*, **51**:515–23, 1966.

Turnbull, A.; Cleton, F.; and Finch, C. A.: Iron absorption. IV. The absorption of hemoglobin iron. *J. Clin. Invest.*, **41**:1897–1907, 1962.

Turpie, A. G. G.; Runcie, J.; and Thomson, T. J.: Clinical trial of deglycirrhizinized licorice in gastric ulcer. *Gut*, **10**:299–302, 1969.

Twiss, J. R.; Gillette, L.; Berger, W. V.; Aronson, A. R.; and Siegel, L.: The role of antibiotics in infections of the biliary tract: studies in sensitivity and biliary tract excretion. *Ann. Surg.*, **144**:1008–12, 1956.

Tyson, R. R., and Spaulding, E. H.: Antibiotic preparation of the bowel—a chimera. In Ingelfinger, F. J.; Relman, A. S.; and Finland, M. (eds.): *Controversy in Internal Medicine.* W. B. Saunders Co., Philadelphia, 1966.

Unger, P. N., and Shapiro, S.: The prothrombin response to parenteral administration of large doses of vitamin K in subjects with normal liver function and in cases of liver disease: a standardized test for estimation of hepatic function. *J. Clin. Invest.*, **27**:39–47, 1948.

Urban, E.; Frank, B. W.; and Kern, F, J,: Liver dysfunction with mestranol but not with norethynodrel in a patient with Enovid-induced jaundice. *Ann. Intern. Med.*, **68**:598–602, 1968.

Vakil, B. J.; Iyer, S. N.; Shah, S. C.; Gadgil, R. K; and Wagholikar, U. N.: A controlled trial of prednisolone in the treatment of infective hepatitis. *J. Indian Med. Ass.*, **45**:357–64, 1965.

Vallee, B. L.; Wacker, W. E. C.; and Ulmer, D. D.: Magnesium-deficiency tetany syndrome in man. *New Eng. J. Med.*, **262**:155–61, 1960.

Van Itallie, T. B., and Hashim, S. A.: Clinical and experimental aspects of bile acid metabolism. *Med. Clin. N. Amer.*, **47**:629–48, 1963.

Van Itallie, T. B.; Hashim, S. A.; Crampton, R. S.; and Tennent, D. M.: The treatment of pruritus and hypercholesteremia of primary biliary cirrhosis with cholestyramine. *New Eng. J. Med.*, **265**:469–74, 1961.

Veeger, W.; Abels, J.; Hellemans, N.; and Nieweg, H. O.: Effect of sodium bicarbonate and pancreatin on the absorption of vitamin B_{12} and fat in pancreatic insufficiency. *New Eng. J. Med.*, **267**:1341–44, 1962.

Victor, M.; Adams, R. D.; and Cole, M.: The acquired (non-Wilsonian) type of chronic hepatocerebral degeneration. *Medicine (Balt.)*, **5**:345–96, 1964.

Vlahcevic, Z. R.; Adham, N. F.; Chalmers, T. C.; Clermont, R. J.; Moore, E. W.; Jick, H.; Curtis, G. W.; and Morrison, R. S.: Intravenous therapy of massive ascites in patients with cirrhosis. *Gastroenterology*, **53**:211–28, 1967.

Wacker, W. E. C., and Parisi, A.: Magnesium metabolism. *New Eng. J. Med.*, **278**:658–63, 712–17, 772–76, 1968.

Waitman, A. M.; Dyck, W. P.; and Janowitz, H. D.: Effect of secretin and acetazolamide on the volume and electrolyte composition of hepatic bile in man. *Gastroenterology*, **56**:286–94, 1969.

Waldmann, T. A., and Laster, L.: Abnormalities of albumin metabolism in patients with hypogammaglobulinemia. *J. Clin. Invest.*, **43**:1025–35, 1964.

Waldmann, T. A.; Wochner, R. D.; Laster, L.; and Gordon, R. S., Jr.: Allergic gastroenteropathy: a cause of excessive protein loss. *New Eng. J. Med.*, **276**:761–69, 1967.

Walser, M., and Bodenlos, L. J.: Urea metabolism in man. *J. Clin. Invest.*, **38**:1617–26, 1959.

Walsh, J. R.; Mass, R. E.; Smith, F. W.; and Lange, V.: Desferrioxamine effect on iron excretion in hemochromatosis. *Arch. Intern. Med. (Chicago)*, **113**:435–41, 1964.

Walshe, J. M.: Effect of glutamic acid on the coma of hepatic failure. *Lancet*, **1**:1075–77, 1953.

Warren, K. S.; Iber, F. L.; Dolle, W.; and Sherlock, S.: Effects of alterations in blood pH on distribution of ammonia from blood to cerebrospinal fluid in patients in hepatic coma. *J. Lab. Clin. Med.*, **56**:687–94, 1960.

Wasserman, R. H.: Calcium transport by the intestine: a model and comment on vitamin D action. *Calc. Tiss. Res.*, **2**:301–13, 1968.

Watkinson, G.: Treatment of ulcerative colitis with topical hydrocortisone hemisuccinate sodium: a controlled trial employing restricted sequential analysis. *Brit. Med. J.*, **2**:1077–82, 1958.

Watson, D. W.: Immune responses and the gut. *Gastroenterology*, **56**:944–65, 1969.

Webster, L. T.: Hepatic coma—a biochemical disorder of the brain. *Gastroenterology*, **49**:698–702, 1965.

Webster, L. T., and Gabuzda, G. J.: Relation of azotemia to blood "ammonium" in patients with hepatic cirrhosis. *Arch. Intern. Med. (Chicago)*, **103**:15–22, 1959.

Weiner, M.; Chenkin, T.; and Burns, J. J.: Observations on the metabolic transformation and effects of phenylbutazone in subjects with hepatic disease. *Amer. J. Med. Sci.*, **228**:36–39, 1954.

Weinstein, L.: Superinfection: a complication of antimicrobial therapy and prophylaxis. *Amer. J. Surg.*, **107**:704–709, 1964.

Weinstein, L., and Dalton, A. C.: Host determinants of response to anti-microbial agents. *New Eng. J. Med.*, **279**:524–31, 1968.

Weinstein, L.; Olson, R. E.; Van Itallie, T. B.; Caso, E.; Johnson, D.; and Ingelfinger, F. J.: Diet as related to gastrointestinal function, *J.A.M.A.*, **176**:935–41, 1961.

Weintraub, L. R.; Conrad, M. E.; and Crosby, W. H.: The treatment of hemochromatosis by phlebotomy. *Med. Clin. N. Amer.*, **50**:1579–90, 1966.

Weintraub, L. R.; Weinstein, M. B.; Huser, H.; and

Rafal, S.: Absorption of hemoglobin iron: the role of a heme-splitting substance in the intestinal mucosa. *J. Clin. Invest.*, **47**:531–39, 1968.

Wells, R.: Prednisolone and testosterone propionate in cirrhosis of the liver: a controlled trial. *Lancet*, **2**:1416–19, 1960.

Wensel, R. H.; Rich, C.; Brown, A. C.; and Volwiler, W.: Absorption of calcium measured by intubation and perfusion of the intact human small intestine. *J. Clin. Invest.*, **48**:1768–75, 1969.

Whalley, P. J.; Adams, R. H.; and Combes, B.: Tetracycline toxicity in pregnancy. *J.A.M.A.*, **189**:357–62, 1964.

Wheby, M. S.; Jones, L. G.; and Crosby, W. H.: Studies on iron absorption: intestinal regulatory mechanisms. *J. Clin. Invest.*, **43**:1433–42, 1964.

Wheeler, H. O.: The flow and ionic composition of bile. *Arch. Intern. Med. (Chicago)*, **108**:156–62, 1961.

———: The function of the biliary tract. In Popper, H., and Schaffner, F. (eds.): *Progress in Liver Diseases*, Vol. 2. Grune & Stratton, Inc., New York, 1965.

Whelton, M. J.; Allaway, A.; Stewart, A.; and Kreel, L.: Ergot poisoning in acute hepatic necrosis. *Gut*, **9**:287–89, 1968a.

Whelton, M. J.; Krustev, L. P.; and Billing, B. H.: Reduction in serum bilirubin by phenobarbital in adult unconjugated hyperbilirubinaemia. *Amer. J. Med.*, **45**:160–64, 1968b.

Wilkinson, P., and Sherlock, S.: The effect of repeated albumin infusion in patients with cirrhosis. *Lancet*, **2**:1125–29, 1962.

Williams, R., and Billing, B. H.: Action of steroid therapy in jaundice. *Lancet*, **2**:392–96, 1961.

Williams, R. D.; Elliott, D. W.; and Zollinger, R. M.: The effect of hypotension in obstructive jaundice. *Arch. Surg. (Chicago)*, **81**:334–40, 1960.

Williams, R. T.; Milburn, P.; and Smith, R. L.: The influence of the enterohepatic circulation on the toxicity of drugs. *Ann. N.Y. Acad. Sci.*, **123**:110–24, 1965.

Wilson, J. F.; Heiner, D. C.; and Lakey, M. E.: Milk-induced gastrointestinal bleeding in infants with hypochromic microcytic anemia. *J.A.M.A.*, **189**:568–72, 1964.

Wirts, C. W., and Goldstein, F.: Studies of the mechanism of postgastrectomy steatorrhea. *Ann. Intern. Med.*, **58**:25–36, 1963.

Wormsley, K. G., and Grossman, M. I.: Maximal histalog test in control subjects and patients with peptic ulcer. *Gut*, **6**:427–35, 1965.

Wruble, L. D.; Kalser, M. H.; Jones, R. H.; Vloedman, D.; and Bachorik, P.: Jaundice: value of five-day steroid test in differential diagnosis. *J.A.M.A.*, **195**:184–88, 1966.

Wu, C.; Bollman, J.; and Butt, H. R.; Changes in free amino acids in the plasma during hepatic coma. *J. Clin. Invest.*, **34**:845–49, 1955.

Yaffee, S. J.; Levy, G.; Matsuzawa, T.; and Ballah, T.: Enhancement of glucuronide conjugating capacity in a hyperbilirubinemic infant due to apparent enzyme induction by phenobaribital. *New Eng. J. Med.*, **275**:1461–66, 1966.

Yamahiro, H. S., and Reynolds, T. B.: Effects of ascitic fluid infusion on sodium excretion, blood volume and creatinine in cirrhosis. *Gastroenterology*, **40**:497–503, 1961.

Zeitlin, I. J., and Smith, A. N.: 5-Hydroxindoles and kinins in the carcinoid and dumping syndromes. *Lancet*, **2**:986–91, 1966.

Zieve, L.: Pathogenesis of hepatic coma. *Arch. Intern. Med. (Chicago)*, **118**:211–23, 1966.

Zimmerman, H. J.: Drugs and the liver. *D.M.: Disease-a-Month*, May, 1963.

Zimmerman, T. S.; McMillin, J. M.; and Watson, C. J.: Onset of manifestations of hepatic porphyria in relation to the influence of female sex hormones. *Arch. Intern. Med. (Chicago)*, 118:229–40, 1966.

Zimmon, D. S.; Miller, G.; Cox, G.; and Tesler, M. A.: Specific inhibition of gastric pepsin in the treatment of gastric ulcer. *Gastroenterology*, 56:19–23, 1969.

Zinneman, H. H.; Seal, U. S.; and Doe, R. P.: Plasma and urinary amino acids in Laennec's cirrhosis. *Amer. J. Dig. Dis.*, 14:118–26, 1969.

Ziter, F. M. H.: Cathartic colon. *New York J. Med.*, 67:546–49, 1967.

Zurier, R. B.; Campbell, R. G.; Hashim, S. A.; and Van Itallie, T. B.: Use of medium-chain triglyceride in management of patients with massive resection of the small intestine. *New Eng. J. Med.*, 274:490–93, 1966.

Chapter 5

CARDIOVASCULAR DISORDERS

Alan S. Nies

I. ALTERATION OF ARTERIAL PRESSURE AND REGIONAL BLOOD FLOW

GENERAL PATHOPHYSIOLOGIC CONSIDERATIONS

Determinants of Arterial Pressure and Blood Flow to Tissues

The cardiovascular system's physiologic role is to deliver oxygen and nutrients to the tissues and to transport carbon dioxide and metabolic wastes from the tissues to the major organs of excretion and detoxification (lungs, kidney, and liver). The vital task of providing adequate blood flow is accomplished primarily by the myocardium, which must develop sufficient tension to overcome variable peripheral vascular resistance. Factors such as the stroke volume, systolic ejection, and arterial compliance mainly affect systolic blood pressure, whereas the state of arteriolar constriction mainly determines diastolic blood pressure. The driving force for blood flow (or mean arterial pressure) is related to blood flow and resistance as follows:

$$\text{Flow} = \frac{\text{Pressure}}{\text{Resistance}}$$

This relationship applies not only to the body as a whole but also to any individual organ. Thus, adequate blood flow to the body or to an organ can occur when arterial or perfusion pressure is low if the vascular resistance is also low. Conversely, if the peripheral vascular resistance is high, arterial pressure also must be high to maintain adequate perfusion. This simple relationship is emphasized to provide background for the rational therapy of states of either low or high arterial blood pressure. Either state may be associated with impaired blood flow to vital tissues.

Autonomic Nervous System

Autonomic nervous system activity may account for the clinical symptoms and signs of a patient with shock or hypertension. Many of the therapies of shock and hypertension depend upon pharmacologic alteration of autonomic nervous function, regardless of whether the function of the system is a primary determinant in the pathogenesis of the disease.

Organization. The parasympathetic and sympathetic nervous systems have the same basic organization. Impulses arise in the central nervous system in response to stimuli from pressure, stretch, or chemically activated peripheral sensors, or from the cerebral cortex. The impulses are carried to the autonomic ganglia and then to the postganglionic neurons. All autonomic ganglia react similarly to chemical blockers, but postganglionic neurons respond differently to drugs. At the postganglionic nerve ending, neuronal depolarization releases a humoral neurotransmitter, acetylcholine in the parasympathetic system and norepinephrine (in most cases) in the sympathetic nervous system.

Spatial and functional separation of the

adrenergic and cholinergic systems as well as inherent biochemical differences between them allows diseases or drugs to produce distinct effects in either component. The physician can use the patient's case history, physical findings, and results of physiologic and pharmacologic tests to localize defects in the function of the autonomic nervous system. With a proper approach, characteristic disorders may be recognized, the extent of autonomic dysfunction may be assessed, and unusual responses to drugs may be anticipated.

Spontaneous Responses to Hemorrhage, Sepsis, and Myocardial Infarction. Arterial hypotension usually elicits an increase in sympathetic activity. This response is predominantly mediated by baroreceptors, regularly occurs during hemorrhage (Chien, 1967) and usually follows myocardial infarction (Gazes *et al.*, 1959; Valori *et al.*, 1967). An increase in sympathetic activity is teleologically useful, because it increases cardiac output and redistributes blood flow to vital organs whose function depends on a constant supply of oxygen, glucose, or fatty acids (Forsyth *et al.*, 1970). Occasionally, in clinical or experimental myocardial infarction, the expected increase in sympathetic activity does not occur; instead parasympathetic activity may be excessive (Constantin, 1963; Shillingford and Thomas, 1967a, 1967b, 1968). *Principle: Knowledge of the usual pathophysiologic consequences of a disease helps the physician to anticipate signs and therapy, but treatment must be based on observations made at the bedside.*

During gram-negative sepsis, the response of the autonomic nervous system varies. Clinical evidence as well as studies in primates suggests that effective sympathetic stimulation does not occur during early phases of endotoxic shock when the peripheral vascular resistance is low (Wilson *et al.*, 1965, 1967; Nies *et al.*, 1968; Wyler *et al.*, 1969). In the late phases of septic shock, sympathetic activity may be appropriate (Udhoji *et al.*, 1963). *Principle: A disease process is dynamic. Therapy appropriate at one phase of the process may be inappropriate later.*

Role in Hypertension. Malfunction of the sympathetic nervous system or abnormalities of synthesis, release, or metabolism of catecholamines are not etiologically related to essential hypertension (Sjoerdsma, 1961; Editorial, 1964; Peart, 1966). Only in pheochromocytoma is an excess of circulating catecholamines important to the pathogenesis of hypertension. However, in patients with essential hypertension, pharmacologic inhibition of the sympathetic nervous system often helps to control elevated blood pressure, probably by decreasing cardiac output and/or peripheral vascular resistance; such

action forms the principal basis for current antihypertensive therapy (Nies and Melmon, 1967).

Autonomic Insufficiency and Cardiac Denervation. Autonomic insufficiency and the consequences of cardiac transplantation are clinical models that emphasize the importance of the autonomic nervous system in normal function of the cardiovascular system. Autonomic insufficiency results in a syndrome consisting of orthostatic hypotension with syncopal episodes, a slow pulse rate, impaired glucose mobilization, bowel and bladder dysfunction, impotence, and abnormalities of sweating. The syndrome can be caused by a variety of diseases affecting the central or peripheral autonomic nervous system, but commonly is the result of drugs that impair autonomic nervous system activity (e.g., the antihypertensive agents or phenothiazines). When the autonomic nervous system is being evaluated in any patient, a thorough history of drug intake is essential. *Principle: Unless careful histories of drug ingestion are obtained, important symptoms due to drugs may be falsely attributed to disease.*

Similarly, drugs can cause specific cardiac responses like those seen in the patient or animal with sympathetic denervation. Deprived of its extrinsic cardiac nerves, the heart after cardiac transplantation can still respond to circulating catecholamines and can utilize intrinsic mechanisms for increasing stroke volume and cardiac output. However, the maximal response to stress is decreased and the fine control of heart rate and inotropic state of the myocardium is lost (Cooper, 1967; Donald *et al.*, 1968; Goodwin and Oakley, 1969).

Assessment of Function. *Sympathetic System.* SYMPTOMS AND SIGNS OF DYSFUNCTION. The most commonly recognized abnormality of the sympathetic system is orthostatic hypotension, marked by dizziness, fainting, and focal neurologic signs that resolve when the patient assumes a horizontal posture. More subtle evidence is a moderate fall in orthostatic mean blood pressure without the usual 10 to 20 beat/min increase in heart rate. Failure of the pulse rate to increase when the patient stands and further failure to increase after exercise suggest dysfunction in the sympathetic-mediated cardioaccelerator mechanism.

The pupillary responses provide an index of autonomic integrity. Small fixed pupils or pupils that do not dilate when the lower lateral aspect of the neck is sharply pinched (ciliospinal reflex) suggest impaired function.

Nocturnal polyuria, a frequent complaint associated with inhibition of the sympathetic nervous system, is an exaggeration of the normal increase in the glomerular filtration rate when the patient is supine. Weakness, hunger pangs, lethargy, yawning, and muscle fasciculations may be signs of hypoglycemia due to impaired glucose mobilization.

A history of drug ingestion is of particular importance since many drugs interfere with the sympathetic system. Common offenders include the antihypertensive drugs. Other drugs that influence the autonomic nervous system, but are not used for that purpose, include the phenothiazines, which have alpha-adrenergic blocking activity; imipramine, which has anticholinergic and antiadrenergic activity; amphetamines; and antibiotics such as furazolidone (monoamine oxidase inhibitors). The symptoms of an underlying primary disease may dominate those of autonomic insufficiency.

PHYSIOLOGIC TESTING. Perhaps the most useful test for autonomic integrity is Valsalva's maneuver (Figure 5–1). The patient is instructed to exhale against a closed glottis or into a manometer for 20 to 30 seconds. This creates a positive intrathoracic pressure of about 40 mm Hg, which markedly reduces venous return. In subjects with intact sympathetic pathways, there is a brief increase and then a precipitous fall in mean arterial pressure and pulse pressure, accompanied by an increase in heart rate. When the systemic pressure falls, pressure receptors in the aorta and the carotid sinus initiate the increase in heart rate and peripheral vasoconstriction. After release of intrathoracic pressure, there is a bounding overshoot of systolic and diastolic blood and pulse pressures as venous return becomes supranormal and stroke volume suddenly increases. Para-

sympathetic influence then predominates, resulting in bradycardia. The normal response depends on an intact reflex arc, including baroreceptors, afferent pathways, vasomotor centers, sympathetic and parasympathetic outflow, and responsive end-organs (arteriolar bed, venous capacitance bed, heart). Autonomic dysfunction may be reflected by several abnormal response patterns. If impairment is due to disease of the sympathetics, the response is altered so that the heart rate fails to increase during the phase of positive intrathoracic pressure, and overshoot of diastolic and systolic pressures is absent. (Blood pressure overshoot may also be absent in heart failure and hypovolemia.) Parasympathetic dysfunction may be manifest by failure of the heart rate to slow during the period of blood pressure overshoot.

The cold-pressor test may also be used to assess sympathetic function. When normal patients place their hands in ice water for 60 seconds, their blood pressure increases (16 to 20 mm Hg systolic, 12 to 15 mm Hg diastolic). If blood pressure does not increase, the reflex arc is probably incomplete. Such a breakdown can occur in the sensory nerves, spinothalamic tracts, suprapontine and infrathalamic relays, or descending sympathetic pathways or peripheral sympathetic nerves, or at the end-organs. The combined use of the Valsalva maneuver and the cold-pressor test helps to locate the lesion. If the response to the Valsalva maneuver is abnormal and the response to the cold-pressor test is normal, the lesion is probably in either the baroreceptor or the afferent baroreceptor nerve (a defect in some diabetic and tabetic patients).

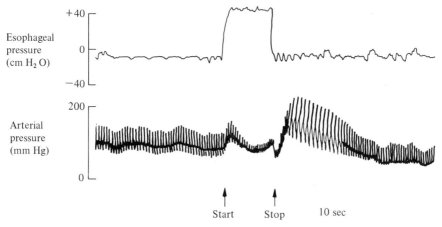

Figure 5–1. Normal blood pressure and pulse response to the Valsalva maneuver in man. The esophageal pressure reflects positive intrathoracic pressure during straining. See text for discussion. (From Thomson, P. D., and Melmon, K. L.: Clinical assessment of autonomic function. *Anesthesiology*, **29**:724–31, 1968.)

Manipulation of the patient's blood volume is useful in assessing sympathetic function. In normal patients, inflation of cuffs on the thighs to within a few mm Hg of diastolic pressures for 10 minutes causes a fall in mean blood pressure no greater than 10 mm Hg. During sympathetic impairment, such a bloodless "phlebotomy" is accompanied by an exaggerated and prolonged fall in blood pressure. Conversely, infusions of 3000 ml of 0.9% sodium chloride in 1 hour produce only minor changes in normal subjects, but result in a 20 to 35 mm Hg increase in blood pressure in patients with sympathetic impairment. During such an infusion, normal subjects excrete approximately 6 ml of urine per minute and 15 mEq of sodium per hour, but patients with sympathetic impairment excrete an average of 23 ml per minute and 80 mEq of sodium per hour. This test must not be used in patients with incipient heart failure because of the risk of producing pulmonary edema.

In healthy people the stress of mental arithmetic usually causes increases in blood pressure and pulse rate because it stimulates efferent sympathetics but does not depend on the afferent limb. The results of this stimulation and of Valsalva's maneuver give further information about the sympathetic reflex arc. An abnormal response to Valsalva's maneuver plus stable blood pressure and pulse rate during mental arithmetic suggest a lesion in the vasomotor center, efferent pathway, or end-organ.

Thus, careful integration of the patient's history and physical findings during certain maneuvers can yield information about the integrity of the afferent, central, and segmental portions of the sympathetic system. Pharmacologic tests and biochemical determinations can give more information about the efferent side.

PHARMACOLOGIC TESTS. Several tests may be used to distinguish sympathetic denervation from end-organ insensitivity to catecholamines. Conjunctival instillation of 1 or 2 drops of a 1:1000 solution of epinephrine into a normally innervated eye produces minor changes in the size of the pupil. If the postganglionic sympathetic pathway is denervated, denervation hypersensitivity occurs and the pupil dilates widely. In normal subjects, infusion of norepinephrine (0.05 μg/kg/min) increases the systolic pressure less than 23 mm Hg and the diastolic pressure less than 19 mm Hg (average, 8 to 9 mm Hg), but in patients with denervation hypersensitivity, such an infusion produces a marked pressor response. When the response is less than expected, the end-organ may be insensitive, as in amyloidosis. However, ingestion or administration of drugs that produce alpha blockade must be excluded (e.g., dibenzyline, phenothiazine, quinidine, and a variety of psychoactive agents). Before the patient undergoes surgery, it is particularly important to ascertain whether alpha blockade is present, because if it is, the patient will tend to be refractory to the usual doses of commonly used pressor agents (levarterenol, metaraminol). In this setting, drugs such as angiotensin that do not act on the alpha receptors may be more effective.

Exaggerated responses to a variety of vasoactive drugs occur during autonomic insufficiency. Sublingual nitroglycerin (0.4 mg) ordinarily produces a small decrease in blood pressure. With dysfunction of afferent pathways, the vasomotor center, sympathetic outflow, or end-organs, the blood pressure decreases more than 15 mm Hg systolic and 5 mm Hg diastolic. Exaggerated hypotensive responses to tetraethylammonium chloride and oxytocin may be equally effective signs of defective sympathetic reflexes.

The function of sweat glands other than those in the axilla depends on efferent sympathetic integrity from the hypothalamus to the skin. Normal subjects sweat when they are placed in a warm environment so that rectal temperature only rises 0.5° to 1° C (e.g., under a leg cradle with a heat lamp). If this fails to produce sweating, the defect can be further defined by assessment of axon reflex sweating. When intradermal injections of 0.1 ml of 1:10,000 acetylcholine (or 1:100,000 nicotine) result in sweating around the injection site, the local nerve supply to the sweat gland is intact. When acetylcholine has no effect, intradermal injection of 1:1000 pilocarpine may produce a wheal and local sweating. Such a response is evidence that the sweat glands are intact and capable of responding to stimuli.

Recently, tests that are particularly helpful in evaluation of function and neurotransmitter stores of the postganglionic sympathetic nerve ending have been devised. These tests are most useful when the patient is taking antiadrenergic agents (e.g., reserpine, guanethidine, methyldopa, or monoamine oxidase inhibitors) or adrenergic blocking agents (e.g., phentolamine, dibenzyline, or propranolol). Such agents interfere with autonomic activity by interrupting the function in the postganglionic nerve or by blocking the reception of the neurotransmitter at the effector site.

Tyramine, a primary phenolic amine found frequently in naturally fermented dairy and grape products, produces its major pharmacologic effect by releasing amines stored in the sympathetic nerve endings. After injection or infusion of tyramine, neurotransmitter is released and characteristic alpha and beta stimulation occurs. Normally the effects of tyramine are transient because it is rapidly oxidized by monoamine oxidase in tissue and plasma. The dose of tyramine necessary to provoke a pressor or cardioaccelerator response depends in part on the size of readily released catecholamine stores, the ease with which such amines are released from nerve endings, and the ability of tyramine to reach the nerve ending. The test may be conducted in the following manner: The patient should be supine in a quiet room. A slow intravenous infusion of 5% dextrose in water is started, and when blood pressure and pulse are stable, a placebo is injected and cardiovascular measurements are made. Then doses of tyramine are administered starting at 250 μg, increasing to 500, 1000, 1500, and 2000 μg, with higher doses given in 1000-μg increments to a limit of 6000 μg. Response is measured after each dose with a 10- to 15-minute interval between doses. A rise in systolic pressure greater than 20 mm Hg after injection of 1000 μg is an exaggerated response. Absence of blood pressure rise after 6000 μg may be considered a depressed response.

In patients with pheochromocytoma, tyramine injections result in transient but profound blood pressure increases owing to release of greater-than-normal amounts of catecholamines from the expanded stores in the nerve endings. When a patient's nerve endings are depleted of catecholamines by reserpine or guanethidine, the tyramine pressor response is diminished. The more tyramine necessary to provoke a standard pressor response, the greater is the sympathetic interference that can be attributed to these antihypertensive drugs. In addition, the more difficult it is to evoke a tyramine response, the more unlikely standard doses of pressor agents, which work primarily by release of endogenous catecholamines (metaraminol, mephentermine), are to be effective for treatment of hypotension in medical or surgical settings.

The tyramine response is complex during administration of antiadrenergic agents such as alpha-methyldopa. At least part of the antiadrenergic action of alpha-methyldopa depends on (1) its uptake into sympathetic nerve endings, (2) its decarboxylation to alpha-methyldopamine, and (3) its later conversion by dopamine beta-oxidase to the false neurotransmitter, alpha-methylnorepinephrine. A false neurotransmitter, a substance not normally found in the nerve ending, accumulates at the same site as norepinephrine and is responsive to the same physiologic and pharmacologic stimuli as norepinephrine. Alpha-methylnorepinephrine accumulates in place of norepinephrine and can be released by tyramine. However, alpha-methylnorepinephrine may be less potent than norepinephrine as a pressor or cardioaccelerator agent. The tyramine response is thus decreased during the early phase of treatment with alpha-methyldopa as nerve endings are depleted of norepinephrine but before alpha-methylnorepinephrine accumulates. During later stages of therapy, the tyramine response may return or even become exaggerated, presumably owing to larger stores and release of greater amounts of transmitter now composed primarily of alpha-methylnorepinephrine but with small amounts of norepinephrine. "Denervation hypersensitivity" is another factor that may result in an augmented tyramine response after long-standing treatment with alpha-methyldopa. Hypersensitivity can be tested by determination of an increased responsiveness to direct-acting sympathomimetic drugs (e.g., norepinephrine or phenylephrine).

When a patient is receiving monoamine oxidase inhibitors, another group of antiadrenergic drugs, tyramine response may be increased as much as 1000% to 10,000%. The principal reasons for such an exaggerated response are (1) a prolonged half-life of tyramine, which is normally metabolized by monoamine oxidase, and (2) expansion of the stores of both native transmitter (norepinephrine) and false neurotransmitter (octopamine) in the sympathetic nerve. Testing with tyramine must be approached with caution and started at low doses (e.g., 2.5 μg). With judicious use, however, the results of tyramine testing can yield information regarding the degree of MAO blockade. For a further discussion of the effects of tyramine in the nerve ending, see the discussion of false neurotransmitters below.

Alpha-adrenergic blocking agents blunt the effects of tyramine, which releases endogenous catecholamines, as well as the effects of infused exogenous catecholamines. In commonly used low doses, the blockade is competitive and can be overcome by increasing doses of catecholamines or tyramine. The amount of tyramine or norepinephrine necessary for a standard pressor response relates directly to the degree of adrenergic blockade. When using beta blocking agents (e.g., propranolol), the degree of blockade of the cardioaccelerator effects of isoproterenol or epinephrine can be used to determine the effectiveness of beta blockade.

Parasympathetic System. SYMPTOMS AND SIGNS OF DYSFUNCTION. Symptoms of abnormal parasympathetic function are usually less conspicuous than those associated with sympathetic dysfunction. The most common symptoms include impotence and impaired libido. Anorexia, incontinence of urine and feces, urinary retention, and alternation of constipation and diarrhea are encountered. The iris may be atrophic and may exhibit no pupillary response to light or accommodation; tearing is diminished after repeated corneal irritation, and the salivation response to the taste of lemon is diminished. Rapid resting heart rate becomes disproportionately increased during orthostatic change and may indicate reduced parasympathetic function. Each of the above functions depends upon an intact reflex arc that includes efferent parasympathetic fibers. Anal sphincter tone and the bulbocavernosus reflex also depend on sacral parasympathetic integrity.

The history of drug ingestion must be considered carefully. Drugs, rather than disease, frequently cause the autonomic dysfunction by their parasympatholytic action.

PHYSIOLOGIC TESTS. The results of the Valsalva maneuver are useful for determining parasympathetic insufficiency as well as sympathetic insufficiency. A slowing of the heart rate after the systolic and diastolic overshoot requires intact parasympathetic function.

Carotid sinus massage produces slowing of the heart rate in most normal patients; lack of effect may indicate interrupted parasympathetic pathways. Similar conclusions are warranted when cold (ice bag) applied to the face fails to produce bradycardia. Slowed gastrointestinal motility may bear the same connotation.

PHARMACOLOGIC TESTS. Acetylcholine is the neurohumoral transmitter at all levels in the parasympathetic system (i.e., synaptic junctions within the central nervous system, within peripheral ganglia, and at the nerve terminal and receptor organ junction). The pharmacologic tests aimed at assessing transmission at any one of these sites are almost impossible because the pharmacologic agents (atropine, acetylcholinesterase inhibitors) act at each of the sites. Atropine, however, can give useful information because it affects the receptor more than it affects the other junctions.

Use of Animal Models in Shock and Hypertension

The extrapolation of data from experimental models of shock and hypertension to the clinical setting may be dangerously misleading. Certain types of experimental hypertension, e.g., that caused by renal artery stenosis or mineralocorticoids and salt excess, seem to have their clinical counterparts, and the models have been useful in the study of pathogenesis and treatment of these diseases. Essential hypertension in man has no satisfactory animal equivalent; results obtained from animals with hypertension of various types may have little relevance to the disease in humans. Some of the drugs effective in treating essential hypertension have been discovered by their action in man (Oates et al., 1960), and only later have animal models been found that respond to the drugs. The lack of a good model means that valid studies on the pathogenesis and treatment of essential hypertension must be conducted in man.

Experimental models of shock have likewise not been entirely satisfactory. No model of cardiogenic shock has been devised that mimics the shock seen in man with myocardial infarction. The models currently in use are interesting and may provide clues, but the definitive study of the treatment of cardiogenic shock at present must be in man.

The dog is commonly utilized for the study of shock, but responds to hemorrhagic and endotoxic shock with mesenteric ischemia and necrosis of the gastrointestinal tract. These responses are not commonly seen in man (Simeone, 1961; Zweifach, 1961; Smith and Moore, 1962). The so-called "irreversible shock" seen in dogs after hemorrhage may not have a counterpart in man. Certainly no living patient should be diagnosed as having "irreversible shock" (Smith and Moore, 1962). The subhuman primate's response to shock resembles man's in terms of (1) relative resistance to hemorrhage, (2) lack of gastrointestinal necrosis after prolonged hypotension, and (3) hemodynamic responses to endotoxin and hemorrhage (Gilbert, 1960, 1962; Kuida et al., 1961; Nies et al., 1968; Forsyth et al., 1970). Data obtained from the primate are more valuable than those obtained from the dog, but confirmation of relevance to man is still necessary.

HYPERTENSION

Hypertension is defined as an elevation of arterial pressure above an age-related arbitrary norm of 140/90 to 150/90 mm Hg and is associated with premature death as a consequence of accelerated vascular disease of the brain, heart, or kidney, or of myocardial failure. Most attention is given to the diastolic pressure, but measurement of systolic and mean arterial pressure also contributes to a determination of the need for treatment (Deming, 1968). The diagnosis of hypertension may be complicated by marked fluctuation in arterial pressure. The problem of labile hypertension is included in the discussion of specific therapy.

The clinician's major diagnostic responsibility

in hypertension is to rule out a surgically treatable primary disorder, e.g., lesions of the kidney or adrenal gland and coarctation of the aorta (Table 5–1). The vast majority of hypertensive patients, however, require medical treatment.

Table 5–1. CLASSIFICATION OF HYPERTENSION

1. Renal hypertension
   a. Renal artery stenosis
   b. Renal disease
2. Neural crest hypertension
   a. Pheochromocytoma
   b. Neuroblastoma, ganglioneuroma (occasional hypertension)
3. Adrenocortical hypertension
   a. Aldosterone-producing adenoma
   b. Adrenocortical hyperplasia
   c. Cushing's syndrome
   d. Metabolic defects
      (1) 11-hydroxylase deficiency
      (2) 17α-hydroxylase deficiency
4. Coarctation of the aorta
5. Neural abnormalities (intracranial lesions, carotid sinus denervation, familial dysautonomia)
6. Eclampsia
7. Essential hypertension

Categories of Drugs Used in Hypertension

Drugs that interfere with autonomic nervous system function can lower arterial blood pressure and theoretically could act at the central nervous system, the ganglia, the nerve endings or the vascular adrenergic receptors (Figure 5–2). In addition, drugs acting directly on vascular smooth muscle without influencing the sympathetic nervous system can affect blood pressure.

Agents Altering Sympathetic Activity: Central Nervous System and Autonomic Ganglia. No drugs are currently available that decrease sympathetic outflow from the central nervous system (CNS), although reserpine and alpha-methyldopa have some effects on the CNS. Hydralazine may produce some of its effects by a central action, but it primarily acts directly on peripheral vessels (Moyer, 1953).

Drugs that block the autonomic ganglia are effective hypotensive agents. These drugs stabilize both the sympathetic and parasympathetic ganglia to the effects of acetylcholine, interrupting autonomic transmission. Because both parasympathetic and sympathetic functions are blocked, side effects such as dry mouth, blurred vision, ileus, impotence, and urinary retention occur. These side effects have limited the usefulness of ganglionic blocking drugs, except as immediate therapy for selected patients during hypertensive emergencies and as adjunctive therapy when other drugs are insufficient.

Drugs Altering the Postganglionic Sympathetic

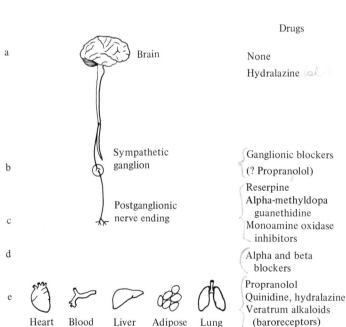

Drugs

a — Brain — None
Hydralazine (?)

b — Sympathetic ganglion — Ganglionic blockers (? Propranolol)

c — Postganglionic nerve ending — Reserpine, Alpha-methyldopa, guanethidine, Monoamine oxidase inhibitors

d — Alpha and beta blockers

e — Heart, Blood vessels, Liver, Adipose, Lung — Propranolol, Quinidine, hydralazine, Veratrum alkaloids (baroreceptors), Thiazides

Receptor Sites

Figure 5–2. Schematic representation of various anatomic levels at which antihypertensive drugs affecting the nervous system may work. *a*, Central nervous system; *b*, sympathetic and parasympathetic ganglia; *c*, postganglionic nerve body; *d*, postganglionic nerve ending; *e*, effector site for catecholamines. (From Nies, A. S., and Melmon, K. L.: Recent concepts in the clinical pharmacology of antihypertensive drugs. *Calif. Med.*, **106**:388–99, 1967.)

Nerve Endings. Modern antihypertensive therapy began with the discovery that reserpine in clinically useful doses can deplete tissues of catecholamines (Chidsey et al., 1963), specifically inhibit sympathetic reflexes (Mason and Braunwald, 1964a), and lower blood pressure. This discovery led to an understanding of the function of the sympathetic postganglionic nerve ending and its alteration by drugs.

The postganglionic nerve ending is the site of synthesis, storage, and release of the neurotransmitter, norepinephrine (Figure 5–3). The amino acid tyrosine is actively transported into the sympathetic neuron and hydroxylated in the mitochondria to dihydroxyphenylalanine (dopa) (Nagatsu et al., 1964). Dopa is decarboxylated to dopamine in the cytoplasm; dopamine is then taken up by a specialized granule where it is hydroxylated and stored as norepinephrine (Von Euler and Hillarp, 1956; Wurtman, 1965; Nies and Melmon, 1967). In the adrenal medulla and organ of Zuckerkandl a cytoplasmic enzyme methylates norepinephrine, producing epinephrine, which is also stored in granules (Axelrod, 1962).

Under normal circumstances, the first hydroxylation (① in Figure 5–3) is rate limiting, and norepinephrine or other catecholamines may inhibit synthesis by end product inhibition at this step (Alousi and Weiner, 1966; Udenfriend, 1966; Spector et al., 1967; De Quattro and Sjoerdsma, 1968; Sedvall et al., 1968). An experimental drug, alpha-methylparatyrosine, effectively inhibits tyrosine hydroxylase. As much as 80% inhibition of catecholamine synthesis, as measured by catecholamine metabolite excretion, has been accomplished with alpha-methylparatyrosine in man (Engelman et al., 1968a, 1968b). The drug is most successful in ameliorating the symptoms due to production of excess catecholamines by pheochromocytoma. Selected patients with essential hypertension also respond favorably to the drug. However, side effects (sedation, anxiety, tremor, diarrhea, and crystalluria) limit clinical use of alpha-methylparatyrosine (Engelman et al., 1968a, 1968b).

Disulfiram inhibits dopamine β-oxidase, another potential rate-limiting step, and results in increased tissue content of dopamine, depleted stores of norepinephrine, and hypotension (Goldstein et al., 1964; Musacchio et al., 1966b; Goldstein and Nakajima, 1967; Thoenen et al., 1967). Use of disulfiram has not been reported for the treatment of essential hypertension or pheochromocytoma.

Fortunately for therapists, the nerve ending is relatively indiscriminate in that foreign substances may be taken up by active transport at the nerve membrane, then stored or utilized as substrates by the enzymes involved in norepinephrine synthesis. Likewise, the storage granules accept other amines if they have a β-hydroxyl or a dihydroxyphenyl (catechol) group (Figure 5–4) (Musacchio et al., 1966a).

The storage granules normally protect amines from catabolism, but in some pathologic states or during drug treatment (e.g., with reserpine) the amines are released from the granules and are oxidized by intracellular monoamine oxidase (Kopin, 1964; Dahlström et al., 1965; Wurtman, 1965; Carlsson, 1966; de Champlain et al., 1969). The biologically inactive product is then released from the cell (Figure 5–5). By depleting norepinephrine in the sympathetic nerve ending, reserpine produces a "pharmacologic" denervation (Chidsey et al., 1963).

The mechanism by which a nerve impulse releases stored catecholamines from the nerve ending is unknown. One hypothesis is that acetylcholine synthesized and stored within the nerve ending allows an increased entry of calcium into the postganglionic neuron, which in turn discharges the contents of norepinephrine from some of the granules (Burn and Rand, 1965; Ferry, 1966). The evidence for this mechanism is attractive but can conservatively be viewed as inconclusive.

Epinephrine and norepinephrine are metabolized by two enzymes, catechol-o-methyltransferase (COMT) and monoamine oxidase (MAO). Circulating catecholamines are first methylated by COMT, and inhibition of this enzyme prolongs the action of infused or endogenously released catecholamines (Bacq et al., 1959). Catecholamines released into the cytoplasm of the nerve ending but kept from the circulation are oxidized by intraneuronal MAO. Although inhibition of MAO alters the intraneuronal stores of catecholamine (see False Neurotransmitters, below), it does not alter the responses to infused catecholamines (Kopin, 1964). The final catabolic products are shown in Figure 5–5.

The biologic inactivation of norepinephrine occurs largely by reuptake of the amine into the adrenergic neuron and restorage in the specialized granules and the cytoplasm (Ferry, 1967). The membrane pump for norepinephrine also transports foreign compounds such as guanethidine, amphetamine, and tyramine, and is blocked by cocaine, imipramine and its derivatives, and the alpha-adrenergic blocking agents phenoxybenzamine and phentolamine (Hertting et al., 1961; Ferry, 1967). Uptake into the storage granules is inhibited by reserpine,

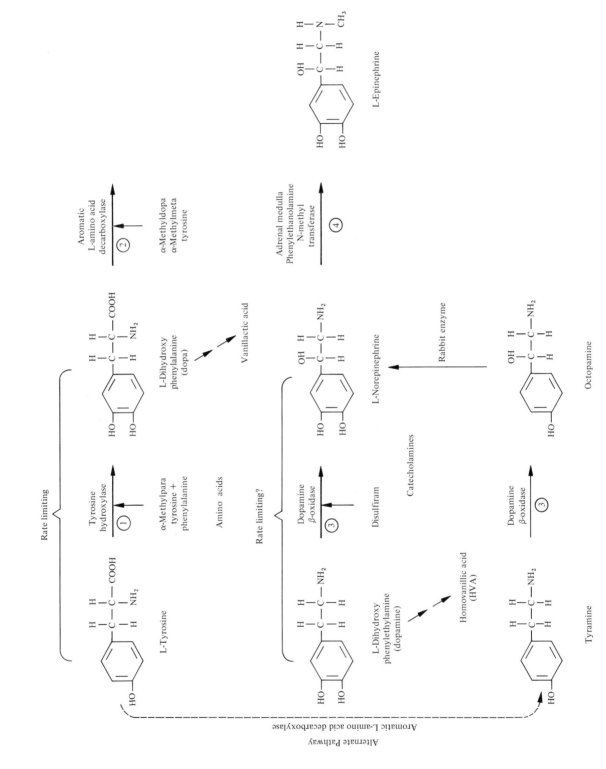

Catechol

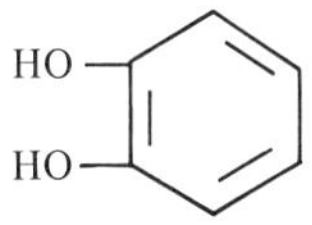

Catecholamines

Dihydroxybenzene

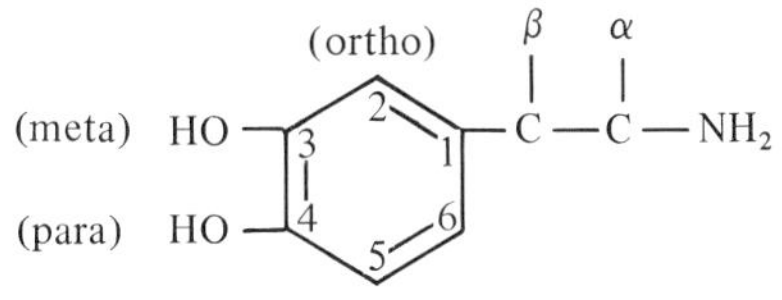

3,4-Dihydroxyphenylethylamine
(dopamine)

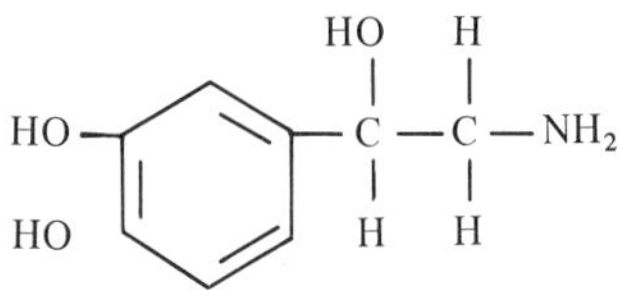

Norepinephrine

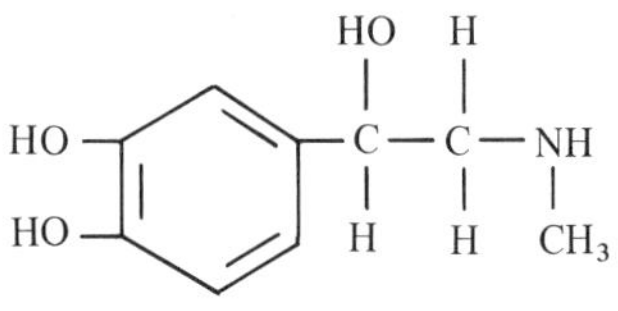

Epinephrine

Figure 5–4. Chemical structure of a catechol (left) and of the endogenous catecholamines (right). The phenolic ring and carbon chain positions are indicated on the dopamine structure. (From Nies, A. S., and Melmon, K. L.: Recent concepts in the clinical pharmacology of antihypertensive drugs. *Calif. Med.*, **106**:388–99, 1967.)

guanethidine, and destruction of the nerve endings by drugs like 6-hydroxydopamine.

Inhibition of catecholamine uptake results in exaggerated and prolonged action of infused or released catecholamine unless the catecholamine receptor is also blocked (e.g., by phentolamine or phenoxybenzamine) (Figure 5–6).

False Neurotransmitters. *Alpha-Methyldopa (Methyldopa) and Alpha-Methylnorepinephrine.* Methyldopa was first studied as an antihypertensive drug because it was known to inhibit L-amino acid decarboxylase *in vitro*. The effects in animals were discouraging, but Oates and co-workers found that the L-isomer inhibited decarboxylase, decreased tissue stores of norepinephrine, and lowered arterial pressure in patients with essential hypertension (Oates et al., 1960). These actions were considered to be related to diminished catecholamine synthesis by drug-induced inhibition of the conversion of dopa to dopamine until it was discovered that (1) norepinephrine depletion produced by methyldopa exceeds the duration of decarboxylase inhibition; (2) metabolism of catecholamines as reflected by vanilmandelic acid excretion in urine was not significantly

changed after administration of methyldopa; and (3) agents producing more profound decarboxylase inhibition did not alter the rates of synthesis, size of stores, or turnover of catecholamines, nor did they affect arterial blood pressure. Decarboxylation was not a rate-limiting step, and its inhibition could not be expected to affect the synthesis of the end product (Levine and Sjoerdsma, 1964). Often theories derived from the observation of drug effects *in vitro* are uncritically applied to the more complex events they cause *in vivo*. The therapist should be skeptical of the wide applicability of such theories and should always be willing to test them. If the concept of inhibition of synthesis of catecholamines were not questioned in relation to methyldopa, the unifying, convenient, and clinically helpful hypothesis of drugs acting as false neurotransmitters would not have been brought to light. Critical observations testing hypotheses often reveal important new facts or theories. The new theories too must be tested rigorously with proper experimental design.

From the observations on methyldopa and other drugs, including monoamine oxidase, the

Figure 5–3. Biosynthetic pathways for catecholamine production. The bold arrows indicate major steps in synthesis. Light arrows indicate steps of minor or unestablished importance in man. Possible excretion products of catecholamines or their precursors of minor importance are indicated by diagonal arrows. (From Melmon, K. L.: Catecholamines and the adrenal medulla. In Williams, R. H. [ed.]: *Textbook of Endocrinology*, 4th ed. W. B. Saunders Co., Philadelphia, 1968.)

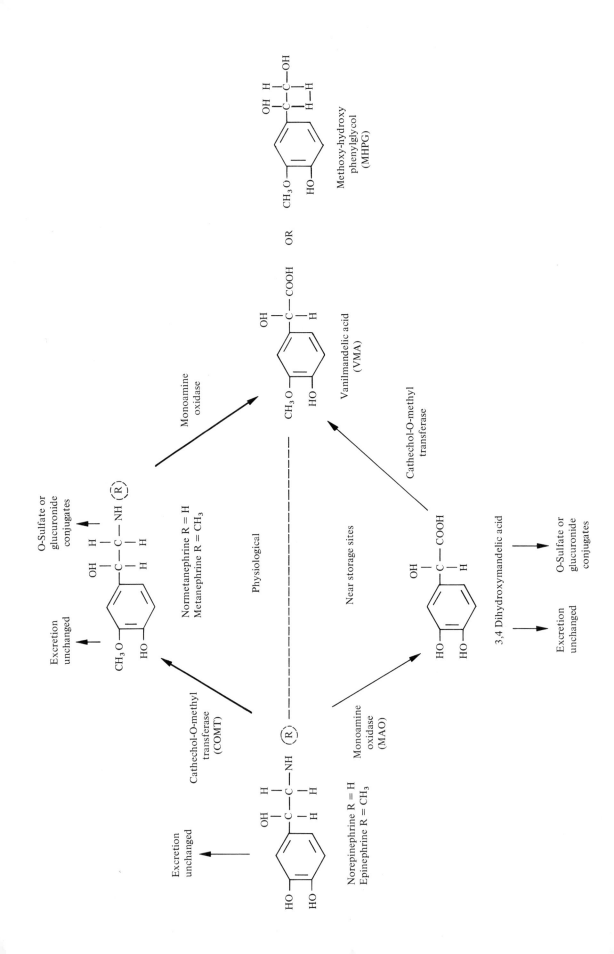

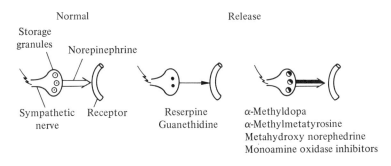

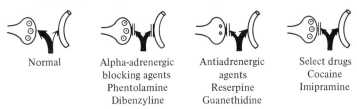

Figure 5–6. Schematic diagram of the mechanics by which pharmacologic agents alter the effect of exogenous catecholamines. Some agents (top) act by diminishing the stores of catecholamines in the nerve endings (reserpine, guanethidine), by promoting formation of false neurotransmitters (methyldopa), or by being accumulated themselves as false neurotransmitters (metahydroxynorephedrine). Other agents (bottom) act by inhibiting uptake of catecholamines into storage sites or into both storage and effector sites (phentolamine, dibenzyline). When uptake into storage sites is blocked (reserpine, imipramine), uptake into effector sites is greatly increased. (From Melmon, K. L.: Catecholamines and the adrenal medulla. In Williams, R. H. [ed.]: *Textbook of Endocrinology*, 4th ed. W. B. Saunders Co., Philadelphia, 1968.)

concept of a false neurotransmitter arose. As originally designed, the false neurotransmitter (1) is not normally present in nerve endings, (2) accumulates in the same sites as the physiologic transmitter, (3) can be released by the same pharmacologic and physiologic stimuli that release norepinephrine, and (4) is less potent than norepinephrine (Kopin *et al.*, 1965; Kopin, 1968). However, as the facts about the false neurotransmitter concept expanded, the definition was extended to include substances that (5) may be equipotent to norepinephrine, (6) may produce effects by inhibition of enzyme action, and (7) may produce their antihypertensive effects by other mechanisms (Nies and Melmon, 1967).

Tracing the history of the evaluation of methyldopa contributes to an understanding of the evolution of this "new" concept. After effective doses of methyldopa were administered to animals, alpha-methylnorepinephrine was found in brain tissue. The amino acid drug had been taken into the sympathetic neurons, decarboxylated, and subsequently β-hydroxylated to alpha-methylnorepinephrine by the same enzymes that convert dopa to norepinephrine (Carlsson and Lindqvist, 1962) (Figure 5–7). The newly formed alpha-methylnorepinephrine displaced norepinephrine, was stored in the storage granules, and was released in place of norepinephrine by nerve stimulation (Muscholl and Maitre, 1963; Day and Rand, 1964). Therefore alpha-methylnorepinephrine is a false neurotransmitter.

The biochemical mechanism by which methyl dopa produces its antihypertensive effects is not completely understood. Alpha-methylnorepinephrine is nearly as potent a vasoconstrictor and cardioaccelerating agent as norepinephrine when tested in many animals (Muscholl and

Figure 5–5. Biochemical pathways for the metabolism of catecholamines. Heavy diagonal arrows indicate the major sequence of metabolism of catecholamines released into the circulation. Light diagonal arrows indicate the sequence of metabolism of catecholamines released intracellularly. Vertical arrows indicate minor mechanism of excretion or metabolism of specific intermediary products. (From Melmon, K. L.: Catecholamines and the adrenal medulla. In Williams, R. H. [ed.]: *Textbook of Endocrinology*, 4th ed. W. B. Saunders Co., Philadelphia, 1968.)

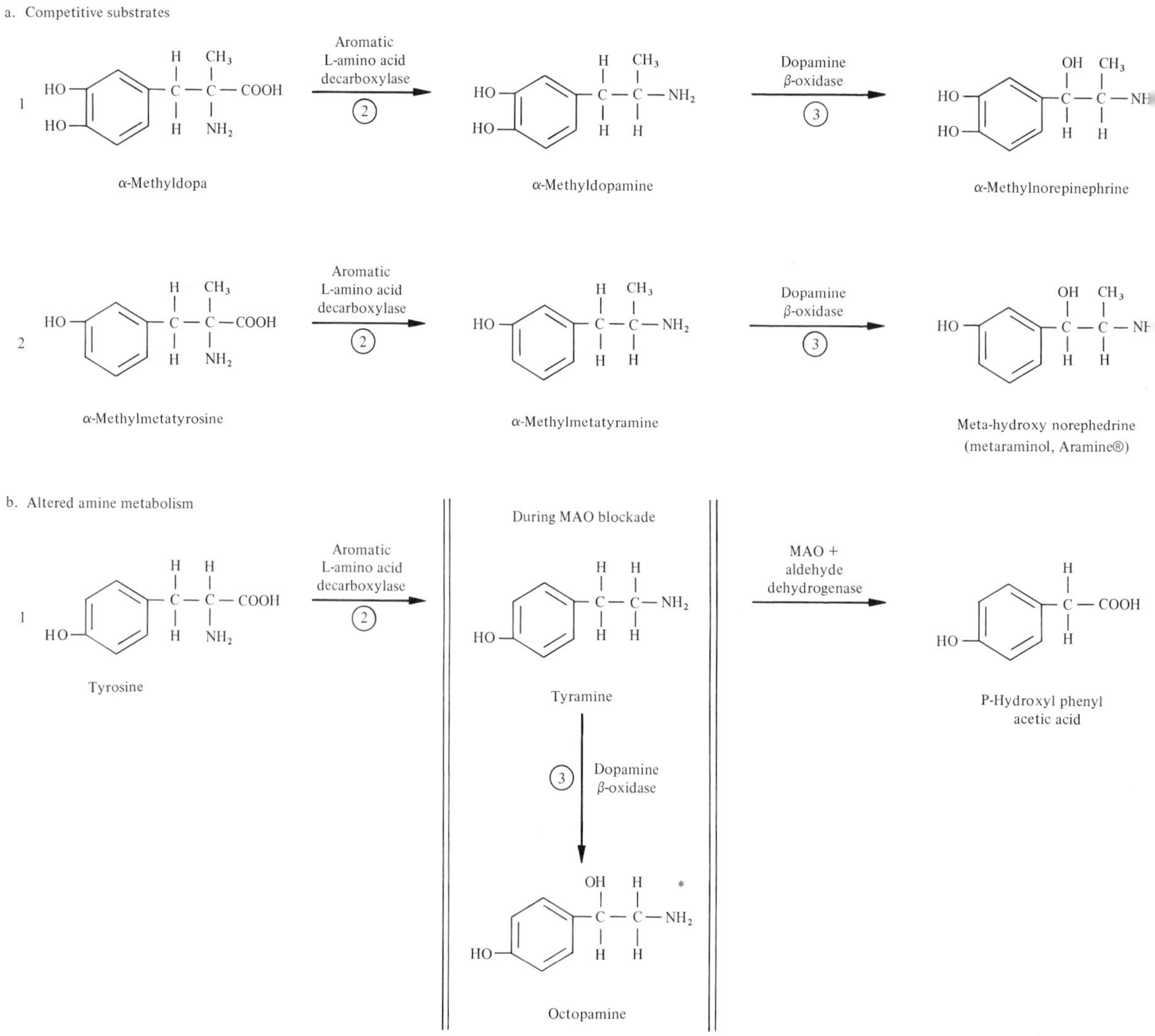

Figure 5–7. Formation of false neurotransmitters. The false neurotransmitters (starred) are formed from amino acid substrates by the same enzymes utilized in the synthesis of norepinephrine. The numbered reactions refer to similar steps in Figure 5–3. (From Nies, A. S., and Melmon, K. L.: Recent concepts in the clinical pharmacology of antihypertensive drugs. *Calif. Med.*, **106**:388–99, 1967.)

Maitre, 1963; Conradi *et al.*, 1965; Haefely *et al.*, 1966), but it may be somewhat less potent than norepinephrine in man (Kopin, 1968). The sympathetic blockade produced by methyldopa may be related to inhibition of tyrosine hydroxylase in the nerve ending by alpha-methylnorepinephrine. Inhibition of this rate-limiting step in the synthesis of catecholamines results in a decrease in the synthesis of norepinephrine and in the amount of transmitter available for release (Kopin, 1968). Another possibility is that alpha-methylnorepinephrine may be less available for release by nerve stimulation, yet capable of displacing the native neurotransmitters from binding sites within the cell. Neither of these explanations is proved and the actual mechanism is unknown. Indeed, there is some evidence that methyldopa has important effects on arterial blood pressure through direct dilation of peripheral vessels (Mohammed *et al.*, 1968a), through inhibition of the secretion of renin (Gaffney *et al.*, 1969), or through an action on the central nervous system. *Principle: A theory may be correct without offering a comprehensive explanation of the mechanism of action of a drug.*

Alpha-Methylmetatyrosine and Metaraminol.
Following the discovery that alpha-methyl-norepinephrine suited the false neurotransmitter hypothesis, the breadth of the concept was tested in a prospective manner. Additional analogs of tyrosine, dopa, dopamine, and norepinephrine were fruitfully investigated. Alpha-methylmetatyrosine was found to be transported into the nerve endings and brain and transformed into meta-hydroxynorephedrine (metaraminol) by the same enzymes that form norepinephrine from tyrosine (Figure 5–7). The endogenously formed metaraminol is a false neurotransmitter; it stoichiometrically displaces norepinephrine from the storage sites; and it is released by stimulation of nerves (Carlsson and Lindqvist, 1962; Gessa *et al.*, 1962; Anden, 1964; Shore *et al.*, 1964; Cohen, R. A., *et al.*, 1966). Such findings emphasize the assets of a hypothesis in helping to design prospective studies on the mechanism of action of a drug.

Infused metaraminol is taken up by the adrenergic neuron and directly displaces norepinephrine from the granules. When clinically useful doses are infused rapidly, metaraminol is initially an effective pressor agent. However, tachyphylaxis to the pressor effects of metaraminol occurs later, an effect that can be explained by the false neurotransmitter hypothesis. Metaraminol has less than 5% of the potency of norepinephrine; when most of the norepinephrine in the nerve ending has been replaced, stimulation of the nerve results in minimal release of native transmitters, and a partial blockade of the sympathetic nervous system has been established. Further doses of metaraminol fail to release adequate amounts of the potent neurotransmitter, resulting not only in refractory responses to metaraminol but also in the appearance of a new drug effect: hypotension (Figure 5–8). Metaraminol given in repeated small doses does not produce hypertension, because the quantity of catecholamines released after a single dose is small, but eventually the cumulative effects can seriously deplete stores of catecholamines and reduce the blood pressure of patients with essential hypertension. Although we do not advocate the use of metaraminol as an antihypertensive drug, knowledge of its mechanism of action can help explain an otherwise paradoxical response. Patients treated with metaraminol have large concentrations of the drug in their sympathetic tissues (Crout, 1966b). An infusion of norepinephrine re-establishes the stores of norepinephrine and restores the hypertensive response to metaraminol. Both metaraminol and alpha-methylmetatyrosine therefore can be antihypertensive agents in man (Horwitz and Sjoerdsma, 1964; Cohen, R. A., *et al.*, 1966; Crout, 1966b). *Principle: A valid hypothesis not only may explain an observed effect but also may predict what future observations will be (regardless of how unexpected they may seem).*

If the hypothesis fails to predict a response, either the hypothesis or the observations are incorrect. Usually the hypothesis is most vulnerable. In the case of metaraminol, the hypothesis has allowed a useful explanation of the mode of action and development of tachyphylaxis to the drug and has even provided a basis for predicting the antihypertensive effects of a drug classically considered a pressor. The real value of a hypothesis is that it forms the basis for future investigations.

Observations of the effects of metaraminol allow us to refine the false neurotransmitter hypothesis: (1) Metaraminol does not cross the blood-brain barrier; therefore, attention can be focused entirely upon peripheral mechanisms of sympathetic blockade, which do not differ from the effects of agents that also act on the central nervous system. (2) Metaraminol has only one hydroxyl group on the aromatic ring, proving that the catechol (dihydroxyphenyl) structure is not a requisite for a false neurotransmitter.

Monoamine Oxidase Inhibitors. Originally used as antidepressants, monoamine oxidase inhibitors were found to produce postural hypotension that correlated with the degree of *in vivo* inhibition of MAO (Orvis *et al.*, 1963). Although the enzyme is not primarily responsible for the inactivation of circulating catecholamines, monoamine oxidase does metabolize amines that are accessible to it in the cell's cytoplasm (Kopin, 1964). When MAO is blocked, the stores of norepinephrine as well as of other amines (e.g., octopamine) increase in the storage granules. When these amines enter the granule, they become potential false neurotransmitters that compete with norepinephrine for release. Octopamine is a key false neurotransmitter during MAO inhibition. It is formed by β-hydroxylation of tyramine, the product of decarboxylation of tyrosine, and is less than 1% as potent as norepinephrine (Figure 5–7). Normally tyramine and octopamine are rapidly destroyed by MAO. However, when protected from oxidation during MAO inhibition, octopamine can accumulate. Thus, after any standard nerve stimulation a finite amount of transmitter leaves the nerve ending, but the amount of potent transmitter is diluted by the impotent false neurotransmitter, octopamine (Figures 5–6 and 5–7). The resulting sympathetic blockade accounts for the antihypertensive action of MAO inhibition (Fischer *et al.*, 1965; Kopin *et al.*, 1965).

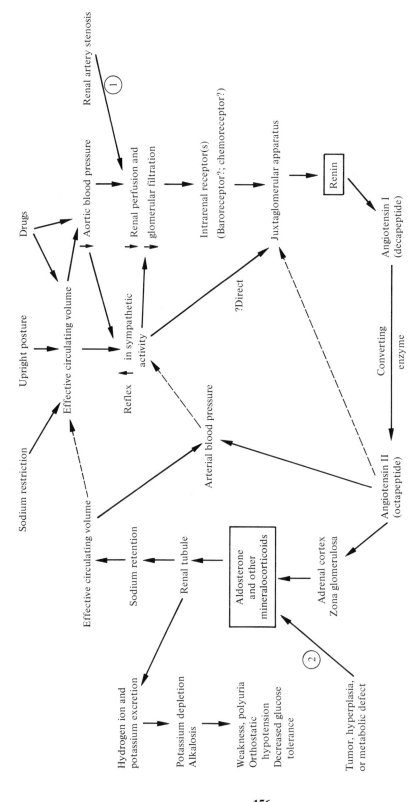

Figure 5–8. The renin-angiotensin system. Renin is secreted from the juxtaglomerular apparatus in response to a decreased renal perfusion. Renin forms angiotensin from a substrate in plasma. Angiotensin stimulates the adrenal cortex to secrete aldosterone. Aldosterone causes an increase in blood volume that acts as a negative feedback (-----→) to renin secretion. Angiotensin also decreases renin secretion directly. Increased sympathetic nervous system activity also increases renin release.

Pathologic changes in this complex system can cause hypertension. At ① renal artery stenosis is a persistent stimulus to renin release and is additive to other physiologic and pharmacologic stimuli.

At ② tumors, hyperplasia, or metabolic abnormalities of the adrenal cortex cause a persistent secretion of aldosterone or other mineralocorticoids.

Tyramine is also important in the untoward effects of MAO inhibition. In normal persons, infused tyramine releases norepinephrine from nerve endings and results in a brief rise of arterial pressure. Because tyramine is rapidly destroyed by MAO, its effects are transient. When catecholamine stores are increased, as in patients with pheochromocytoma, an infusion of tyramine produces a brief but exaggerated rise of arterial blood pressure. During MAO inhibition not only are the stores of catecholamines increased, but tyramine is protected from destruction and relatively small amounts can provoke both severe and prolonged hypertensive reactions. Under such circumstances the tyramine absorbed through the intestine is not metabolized and produces a pressor effect. Hypertensive reactions have been reported after ingestion of tyramine-containing foods including aged cheese, wine, beer, marmite, pickled herring, broad beans, or chicken liver (Hodge and Nye, 1964; Horwitz et al., 1964; Hedberg et al., 1966; Pettinger and Oates, 1968). In addition to tyramine-containing foods, commonly used catecholamine-releasing drugs (amphetamine, ephedrine, phenylpropanolamine, mephentermine, metaraminol, methylphenidate, and phenmetrazine) can produce hypertensive reactions during MAO inhibition (Brownlee and Williams, 1963; Oates and Doctor, 1965; Oates, 1967). Considerable information about the mechanism of the changed effect can be derived from measurements of the amount of change in blood pressure and the duration of change after tyramine infusions. *Principle: The concept of changes in dose-response relationships induced by disease or other drugs is not new. When the changes are specific for a disease state, the response can be used as evidence for the presence of the disease.*

Guanethidine. Guanethidine has many properties in common with the false neurotransmitters but probably acts in a unique manner. Guanethidine is actively transported into the nerve ending by the transport system for norepinephrine. Likewise, the uptake of guanethidine is blocked by the same drugs that block norepinephrine uptake (cocaine, imipramine and derivatives, amphetamine) (Day and Rand, 1963; Leishman et al., 1963; Brodie et al., 1965; Mitchell et al., 1967). Guanethidine is bound to the norepinephrine storage sites (Chang et al., 1965); it releases norepinephrine from the nerve ending (Cass et al., 1960). Guanethidine can be released by reserpine (Chang et al., 1964, 1965) or by nerve stimulation (Boullin et al., 1966), and its effects can be prevented or reversed by imipramines, cocaine, ephedrine, amphetamine, tyramine, or metaram-

inol, drugs that also release or block the uptake of norepinephrine (Brodie et al., 1965; Gulati et al., 1966; Mitchell et al., 1970).

However, in spite of the similarity to "classic" false neurotransmitters, guanethidine produces sympathetic inhibition prior to major decreases in catecholamine stores and disappears before the amine content is noticeably repleted (Cass and Spriggs, 1961; Sanan and Vogt, 1962). Guanethidine probably acts by interfering with the release of norepinephrine during physiologic stimulus of the nerve as well as by depleting norepinephrine. Perhaps guanethidine causes a persistent and direct depolarization of the sympathetic nerve ending, which causes the initial discharge of catecholamines and results in adrenergic inhibition (Brodie et al., 1965; Chang et al., 1965). This hypothesis is consistent with the observation that large parenteral doses of guanethidine release enough norepinephrine to induce hypertension while simultaneously blocking the response to postganglionic nerve stimulation (Brodie et al., 1965). Hypertensive response to agents that deplete adrenergic neuronal stores of norepinephrine should not be unexpected, particularly in patients with expanded stores of catecholamines (e.g., caused by pheochromocytoma, neuroblastoma, or monoamine oxidase inhibitors), and should be treated when necessary with the most specific therapy known: alpha-adrenergic blocking agents.

Adrenergic Receptor Blocking Drugs. The cardiovascular adrenergic receptors are classified into two types (Table 5–2): (1) alpha-receptor stimulation produces vasoconstriction of small arterioles and venules; and (2) beta-receptor stimulation dilates arteries and arterioles primarily in skeletal muscle, increases the rate and force of contraction of the heart, and dilates bronchi. Both alpha and beta stimulation cause diminished motility of the bowel and metabolic effects. Alpha (α) stimulation inhibits whereas beta (β) stimulation increases insulin release. Beta stimulation also promotes glycogenolysis and lipolysis (Porte, 1967, 1969). In general, sympathomimetic agents vary only quantitatively in their action on receptors. Large doses of alpha-stimulators can produce effects usually attributed to beta stimulation. Conversely, receptor blocking agents can produce relatively selective inhibition of the effects of circulating norepinephrine or isoproterenol. Peripheral competitive blocking agents are evaluated either in *in vitro* test systems or in specific organ systems affected by the agonist. Blocking drugs often are congeners of the agonist; it should not be surprising that they may block the effects of the agonist. In patients with a pheochromo-

Table 5–2.   CLASSIFICATION OF THE MAJOR ALPHA- AND BETA-ADRENERGIC RESPONSES

ORGAN	EFFECT	ALPHA	BETA
Blood vessels	a. Constrict arterioles and venules	+	0
	b. Dilate arterioles, especially in skeletal muscle	0	+
Heart	a. Increase rate of sinoatrial node discharge	0	+
	b. Increase contractility	0	+
	c. Increase conduction velocity in atrium, AV node, and ventricle	0	+
	d. Increase ventricular automaticity	0	+
Lungs	a. Dilate bronchial musculature	0	+
Gastrointestinal tract	a. Inhibit peristalsis	+	+
Metabolic effects	a. Lipolysis	0	+
	b. Block insulin release	+	0
	c. Stimulate insulin release	0	+
	d. Stimulate formation of cyclic 3′,5′-AMP	0	+
	e. Increase fasting blood sugar	±	+

cytoma and excessive circulating norepinephrine, blood pressure and heart rate changes, and even metabolic changes associated with the disease and produced by norepinephrine, are blocked by phentolamine. Competitive blockade means what it implies. There can be no standard dose of such drugs; requirements must be assessed in each patient and must be determined by the amount of circulating catecholamines. Because pheochromocytomas secrete varying amounts of catecholamines at different times, adequate doses of short-acting drugs (e.g., phentolamine) may be more difficult to use than effective doses of a longer-acting drug (e.g., phenoxybenzamine).

Because the adrenergic blocking agents antagonize only extracellular catecholamines and because these catecholamines have no obvious role in essential hypertension, alpha-adrenergic blocking drugs are not effective in the treatment of essential hypertension.

The short-acting alpha-adrenergic blocker phentolamine is important in the evaluation and management of patients with hypertension. Guanethidine, parenteral reserpine, and methyldopa release stored catecholamines and may produce serious hypertension if given to patients with pheochromocytoma. Hypertensive crises may be produced by excessive release of catecholamines in patients who also are taking MAO blocking drugs.

If a patient has a hypertensive crisis, the response to a dose of 1 to 5 mg of phentolamine often helps the therapist to decide whether the hypertension is due to catecholamine excess. A significant decrease in arterial blood pressure following the administration of phentolamine indicates both that catecholamine release is substantially contributing to the hypertension and that phentolamine can be continued as a therapeutic agent. If phentolamine produces little or no decrease in blood pressure, it is fairly safe to proceed with therapy that includes the use of catecholamine releasing agents. In any case, if the blood pressure rises after the use of such agents, alpha-adrenergic blocking drugs may be necessary.

The role of beta-adrenergic blocking agents in the treatment of hypertension is still disputed. Some hypertensive patients respond to propranolol, the only commercially available β-blocking agent (Prichard and Gillam, 1964; Patterson and Dollery, 1966; Waal, 1966). However, propranolol has many effects; some are related to its β-blocking action, but some are not (e.g., it produces nonspecific depression of myocardial contractility). The predominant effect of propranolol during chronic therapy of hypertension is to lower cardiac output; total peripheral resistance is unchanged or actually rises slightly (Epstein and Braunwald, 1966a, 1967b; Frohlich et al., 1968; Ulrych et al., 1968; Prichard et al., 1970). There is no evidence in support of "resetting of baroreceptors" suggested by some investigators (Prichard and Gillam, 1966). The use of propranolol is rational in those patients whose cardiac output is elevated and whose arterial blood pressure is labile or sustained at high levels (Eich et al., 1962, 1966; Finkielman et al., 1965). That some patients have very sensitive β-adrenergic receptors (Da Costa, 1871; Gorlin, 1962; Frohlich et al., 1966, 1969; Warkentin and Cunningham, 1968), resulting in high cardiac outputs and hypertension, is debatable (Bourne et al., 1970; Frohlich et al., 1970). If such a group could be unequivocally identified, they might respond favorably to propranolol. A well-controlled study is needed to establish the identification and treatment of such patients.

The potentially dangerous aspects of propranolol include worsening of heart failure (see page 192), precipitation of asthma, and constriction of coronary arteries. The drug has not yet been used long enough to ascertain its long-term effects, or in enough patients to establish the incidence of uncommon side effects (Epstein and Braunwald, 1966a; Zaid and Beall, 1966; Whitsitt and Lucchesi, 1967). A new drug should not be used without previous examination of the data. The high doses of propranolol required to lower arterial pressure decrease cardiac output and increase peripheral vascular resistance. In addition, an important mechanism for increasing cardiac output during stress is blocked, and a patient who requires maximum myocardial reserve while taking propranolol may be at a significant disadvantage.

Thiazides. The precise mechanism whereby thiazides and other oral diuretics lower arterial pressure is unknown. The initial hypotensive effect is due to a diminished blood volume with a consequent decrease in cardiac output. After a few weeks of therapy the cardiac output and blood volume return almost to normal but a persistent deficit in extracellular water and plasma volume can be detected during chronic thiazide administration (Leth et al., 1970; Tarazi et al., 1970). The effectiveness may be in part related to a depletion or redistribution of body sodium. Strict sodium restriction can lower the arterial pressure in essential hypertension (Kempner, 1948), and a large intake of salt or an infusion of saline, but not dextran, can completely reverse the hypotensive effects of thiazide diuretics (Winer, 1961; Finnerty et al., 1968). The thiazides may act in part by direct arteriolar dilation (Peters, 1966; Tobian, 1967). Diazoxide, an investigational, sodium-*retaining* thiazide, is a rapidly acting, potent antihypertensive agent and seems to have a direct effect on arterioles (Finnerty, 1968; Hamby et al., 1968).

A major benefit of the thiazide diuretics is their ability to potentiate the hypotensive action of other drugs, possibly by adding their effects on the peripheral vascular resistance to the decrease in cardiac output caused by other agents. Thiazides acutely decrease cardiac output by their known diuretic action. The chronic effects of thiazides, however, are due to some other action that has not been so fully demonstrated. *Principle: Early studies to define the mechanism of action of a drug may not give valid data regarding the chronic effects of the drug.*

Hydralazine. Hydralazine dilates arterioles without producing a significant antisympathetic effect. The lower peripheral resistance results in a fall in arterial pressure, an increase in cardiac output by baroreceptor reflex mechanisms, and an increase in flow to the renal, splanchnic, and coronary circulation (Rowe et al., 1955; Freis, 1962). In these respects hydralazine seems to be an ideal drug. Unfortunately, tolerance commonly develops, angina or congestive heart failure may be precipitated, and in high doses a lupus erythematosus-like syndrome may occur (Alarcon-Segovia et al., 1967; Condemi et al., 1967). Hydralazine is useful parenterally in malignant hypertension and in low doses as adjunctive therapy in mild to relatively severe hypertension. The antihypertensive effects of a vasodilator drug are most apparent when other drugs are used to block the sympathetic nervous system to prevent compensatory tachycardia and increases in cardiac output (Gilmore et al., 1970).

Diagnosis and Therapy of Hypertension

The initial step in managing a hypertensive patient is to establish the presence and severity of hypertension. In patients with severe hypertension this is not difficult; the blood pressure is markedly elevated and there are often signs of target organ damage in the kidney, retina, or heart. However, in patients with blood pressures above the arbitrary norm of 140/90 without vascular disease, some attempt must be made to establish how consistently the blood pressure is elevated during each day. This can be accomplished with varying degrees of success by multiple casual blood pressure determinations in the clinic over a period of several weeks, blood pressures obtained during hospitalization, or blood pressures taken at home by the patient or with an automatic portable blood pressure device. Blood pressures taken at home for several days are a better index of the severity of hypertension and correlate better with hypertensive complications than do casually obtained blood pressures (Kain et al., 1964; Sokolow et al., 1966). Blood pressures measured during hospitalization are often significantly lower than the average ambulatory blood pressures and cannot be used for the definitive diagnosis of hypertension or for establishing optimum therapy for an ambulatory hypertensive patient (Moutsos et al., 1967).

The rationale for the therapy of hypertension is based on the fact that (1) patients with hypertension have premature atherosclerosis and develop the typical "hypertensive complications" of cerebrovascular hemorrhage, uremia, left ventricular hypertrophy, and dissecting aortic aneurysm (Kannel et al., 1961; Freis,

1962, 1969; Stamler, 1962); (2) the life expectancy of hypertensive patients decreases as their blood pressure increases; and (3) experimental evidence links hypertension with the development of vascular damage.

The value of antihypertensive therapy was most easily established for severe hypertension (Dustan *et al.*, 1958; Mohler and Freis, 1960; Sokolow and Perloff, 1960). The value of treatment for moderate hypertension (diastolic BP > 115 to 130) has been established recently (Wolff and Lindeman, 1966; Veterans Administration, 1967). Treatment in this group lowers the incidence of hypertensive complications and improves survival; but the accelerated rate of development of atherosclerotic coronary artery disease has not been slowed. A recent study has established that antihypertensive therapy is of value for patients with diastolic pressures of 90 to 115 mm Hg (Veterans Administration, 1970; Freis, 1971a, b). Although a long-term study is in progress, for the present it seems rational to offer young patients with sustained diastolic pressures > 90 mm Hg the most aggressive therapy. Patients over 60 years old with mild or labile hypertension probably do not warrant aggressive therapy, lest ischemia of the brain or myocardium be induced.

The patient with severe hypertension and renal failure poses a special problem in management. Early observations showed that renal function deteriorated shortly after therapy was begun, and it was feared that continued antihypertensive therapy would further impair renal function. However, it is now clear that effective control of the arterial pressure halts the progression of renal damage and that long-term survival is improved (McCormack *et al.*, 1958). Even in patients with severe renal failure some improvement is possible (Woods and Blythe, 1967). Since one cannot predict which patients will be improved and since hypertension is known to affect renal function adversely, therapy must be given to benefit those who are able to respond favorably.

The duration of therapy is lifelong in most patients, but occasional patients have stopped taking medication and have remained normotensive. The incidence of this resetting of the "barostats" is not known but probably is not common (Thurm and Smith, 1967; Dustan *et al.*, 1968). Once the presence of hypertension is established, the patient should be evaluated for curable forms of hypertension (Table 5–1).

Renovascular Hypertension. *Pathophysiology.* Kidney function is critical in the control of blood pressure and vascular volume. Control mechanisms for renin synthesis and release are a matter of some debate (Skinner *et al.*, 1964;

Gordon *et al.*, 1967; Vander, 1967; Wood, 1967). Classic experiments (Goldblatt *et al.*, 1934) demonstrated that elevated arterial pressure can result from renal arterial lesions. Similar situations exist in man. A generally accepted scheme for the renin-angiotensin-aldosterone system is outlined in Figure 5–8. A decrease in renal arterial pressure due to a lesion of the renal artery produces a decrease in effective blood flow that stimulates the juxtaglomerular cells to secrete renin (① in Figure 5–8) (Crocker *et al.*, 1962). Renin is a proteolytic enzyme that forms angiotensin I from an alpha-2-globulin. Converting enzymes in the plasma and especially in the lung convert the decapeptide to the more active angiotensin II, an octapeptide. Angiotensin II is both a potent vasoconstrictor and a major physiologic regulator of aldosterone secretion (Laragh *et al.*, 1960). Aldosterone increases effective circulatory volume by causing sodium retention and potassium excretion in the renal tubule. The direct vascular effects of angiotensin II and the sodium retention induced by aldosterone summate to raise arterial pressure. During renal artery stenosis, hypertension is a consequence of a moderate elevation of both cardiac output and peripheral vascular resistance, as might be indicated by the pharmacology of angiotensin (Frohlich *et al.*, 1967). Although attractive, this explanation cannot account for all the pathophysiologic observations seen during renal artery stenosis. Plasma renin is not consistently elevated during chronic renovascular hypertension; renin, angiotensin, and aldosterone concentrations in plasma may be elevated without hypertension. Undefined factors must be important during hypertension of this etiology (Bartter *et al.*, 1962; Gordon, 1966; Creditor and Loschky, 1967; Brackett *et al.*, 1968; Haber, 1969a,b).

Physiologic Diagnostic Tests. Although the diagnosis of renovascular hypertension may be suspected when a bruit is heard in the flank or abdomen, for practical purposes the history and physical examination usually do not establish the diagnosis (Julius and Stewart, 1967). The diagnosis is based on procedures that (1) demonstrate a functional impairment of the involved kidney (e.g., rapid-sequence intravenous pyelogram, the accumulation and excretion of radioactive substances, or renal function studies of each kidney), (2) demonstrate arterial stenosis by arteriography, and (3) assay the renal venous plasma for renin activity. The advantages, hazards, and accuracy of these procedures have been reviewed (Kaufman *et al.*, 1966; Kirkendall *et al.*, 1967; Brest, 1968; Harrington *et al.*, 1968; Foster *et al.*, 1969; Hunt *et al.*, 1969). The presence of a surgically correctable stenosis depends on demonstration of an arterial lesion (Holley *et al.*, 1964). However, functional significance of the stenosis usually is assessed by split renal function tests (Howard *et al.*, 1953; Stamey, 1961; Howard and Connor, 1962) and measurement of the differential in renal venous plasma renin activities (McPhaul *et al.*, 1965; Michelakis *et al.*, 1967; Woods and Michelakis, 1968; Amsterdam *et al.*, 1969). The upright posture is a physiologic stimulus to renin release (Cohen, E. L., *et al.*, 1966), and when patients are in a standing position the difference in renin activity from the two kidneys is maximal (Foster *et al.*, 1969; Michelakis *et al.*, 1969). Although some authorities suggest a bilateral renal biopsy to rule out lesions of the "uninvolved kidney" (Vertes *et al.*, 1964), this procedure is not generally done and indeed some degree of nephrosclerosis does not necessarily forecast a poor surgical result (Strickler, 1965).

Pharmacologic Diagnostic Tests. Infusion of angiotensin II is used as a test for renovascular hypertension on the basis that patients with renovascular hypertension have elevated endogenous levels of angiotensin II and might be less responsive to a small amount of exogenously administered peptide (Kaplan and Silah, 1964a, 1964b). Although most patients with renovascular hypertension are somewhat less responsive to the infusion of angiotensin than patients with essential hypertension, patients with renovascular hypertension or accelerated hypertension and normal individuals react similarly. The abnormality appears to be an excessive response to angiotensin in patients with essential hypertension. Patients with essential hypertension also overreact to a variety of other stimuli, including vasopressin, norepinephrine, and exogenous stress, whereas patients with renovascular hypertension respond like normals (Editorial, 1966; Nicotero *et al.*, 1966). The differences in response to angiotensin, however, are too small and inconsistent to be of much value, and this agent has caused uncontrollable hypertension and death in sensitive individuals (Genest, 1968). *Principle: Provocative pharmacologic tests are often relatively dangerous and are of value only if other diagnostic methods fail.* In the case of renovascular hypertension, the angiotensin infusion test is based on sound reasoning, but the results are difficult to interpret and the test is of little value.

Treatment. When a diagnosis of functionally significant renal artery stenosis is made, a major decision remains regarding treatment: Will surgery be adequate to correct the hypertension and are the risks of surgery justified? Review of surgical experience for the treatment of this disease suggests that surgery gives the best results in patients who are under 55 years old, have no evidence of generalized vascular disease, and retain good function in the "uninvolved kidney" (Shapiro *et al.*, 1969). Whether the risks of surgery are justified has not been answered. Medical treatment may be effective, but the involved kidney may deteriorate owing to progressive ischemia beyond the arterial stenosis (Sheps *et al.*, 1965). A long-term controlled study comparing surgical and medical therapy is needed to answer this question. Such a study would certainly be ethical, particularly in patients over 55 who show relatively poor results from surgery compared with the good results of antihypertensive drug therapy (Shapiro *et al.*, 1969). Surgical therapy may not be indicated in a majority of these patients. As Stamey has said, "We are in an era of romance with renal artery stenosis. When the hue and cry is over, there will be far less enthusiasm for the surgical repair of even the functionally significant atherosclerotic occlusions of the renal artery" (Stamey, 1963). Romance cannot be used as a basis for therapy and must be separated from fact. A treatment program can be relied upon only after it compares favorably with standard and effective methods.

Hypertension Produced by Intrinsic Renal Disease. The hypertension associated with renal failure is related to excessive retention of sodium and production of renin, along with other ill-defined factors. Some patients undergoing dialysis are rendered normotensive when their sodium intake is controlled, but other patients require antihypertensive medication. Excessive production of renin has been found in some patients with refractory hypertension that can be corrected only by bilateral nephrectomy (Page, 1969; Vertes *et al.*, 1969). Special therapeutic considerations of a proper antihypertensive drug for patients with impaired renal function must take into account the potential alterations in the drug's absorption, distribution, metabolism, and excretion.

Hypertension and Excessive Secretion of Mineralocorticoids. The adrenal cortex may produce excessive amounts of mineralocorticoids, resulting in hypertension (Davis *et al.*, 1967; Katz, F. H., 1967; Biglieri *et al.*, 1968). The most common type of adrenocortical endocrine hypertension is primary aldosteronism resulting from an adenoma or hyperplasia of the adrenals. However, the hypertension of Cushing's syndrome (Biglieri *et al.*, 1968) and of congenital adrenal hyperplasia (17- and 11-hydroxylase deficiencies) (Bongiovanni and Root, 1963; Biglieri *et al.*, 1966; Goldsmith *et al.*, 1967) results from excessive secretion of

Table 5–3. RENIN–ALDOSTERONE AND BLOOD VOLUME DURING HYPERTENSION

| | | SECRETION OF | | | | | |
| | | RENIN | | | ALDOSTERONE | | |
		EssHT	RvHT	Aldo	EssHT	RvHT	Aldo
Increase circulating volume	High-salt intake (100 µg/day) DOCA 20 mg/day × 3	↓	± ↑	↓ ↓	↓	↑	↑
Decrease circulating volume	Low-salt intake (10 µg/day) Upright posture	↑	↑ ↑*	↓	↑	↑	↑

* Renin secretion by the involved kidney ≫ uninvolved kidney during these maneuvers.
EssHt = Essential hypertension
RvHT = Renovascular hypertension
Aldo = Aldosteronism

mineralocorticoids in addition to or other than aldosterone.

Diagnosis. As with other hormone-producing tumors, the diagnosis is based on the high concentration of the suspected hormone in the urine or blood and on the autonomy of mineralocorticoid production (②) in Figure 5–8). In primary aldosteronism, aldosterone secretion rate is not decreased by expansion of plasma volume, and renin concentrations in blood remain subnormal at all times (Table 5–3, Figure 5–8). Thus, a low renin activity in the presence of a persistently elevated aldosterone secretion rate is a *sine qua non* of primary aldosteronism.

Aldosterone excess may be detected by measurement of its secretory rate or, more commonly, by its effects on sodium and potassium balance (Lauler, 1966; Editorial, 1967f; Espiner *et al.*, 1967; Conn *et al.*, 1969). Despite excessive aldosterone secretion, a high-salt intake usually is not associated with edema, for reasons that are unclear (Earley and Daugharty, 1969). However, increasing dietary sodium does enhance potassium excretion as larger amounts of sodium reach the site in the distal tubule under the control of aldosterone. In this instance sodium is reabsorbed at the expense of potassium loss (see Chapter 3). The resulting hypokalemia contributes to the weakness, polyuria, orthostatic hypotension, and impaired glucose tolerance that are clues to the presence of hypokalemia and mineralocorticoid excess (Conn, J. W., 1965; Biglieri and McIlroy, 1966). Hypokalemia, however, is not present in all cases (Conn *et al.*, 1966), and if the patient is on a diet restricted in sodium, serum potassium concentration is likely to revert to normal. Therefore, a patient suspected of having aldosteronism must be given a diet high in salt for several days before the concentration of

potassium in serum is a reliable index of aldosterone effect.

Low renin activity in the plasma of patients on low-sodium diets is another major clue to the diagnosis, but this may also be found in patients with essential hypertension (Helmer and Judson, 1968; Channick *et al.*, 1969; Jose and Kaplan, 1969; Streeten *et al.*, 1969; Woods *et al.*, 1969).

Normally, a fall in arterial pressure decreases renal perfusion and increases sympathetic activity and renin output (Figure 5–8). In primary hyperaldosteronism this response is not present. Drugs that cause a fall in pressure without interfering with the sympathetic nervous system (diazoxide, hydralazine, and sodium nitroprusside) have been used to test the integrity of the renin-angiotensin system in an attempt to distinguish primary aldosteronism from other types of hypertension (Kaneko *et al.*, 1967; Küchel *et al.*, 1967; Ueda *et al.*, 1968). These drugs are no more useful than upright posture together with a low-sodium diet as a stimulus for renin release.

The suggestion has been made that patients who develop hypokalemia while taking thiazide diuretics are likely to have primary aldosteronism (Conn *et al.*, 1965). However, this diagnostic maneuver is invalid (Kaplan, 1967).

The response to administration of 400 mg per day of the aldosterone antagonist spironolactone may distinguish primary from secondary aldosteronism (Spark and Melby, 1968). The hypertension of patients with primary aldosteronism is controlled within 3 to 5 weeks, whereas the hypertension of secondary aldosteronism is not. More patients should be studied to determine the discriminating ability of this pharmacologic test.

A rare cause of hypertension is licorice ingestion. Licorice contains an aldosterone-like substance that can deplete exchangeable potassium and can therefore mimic the signs and symptoms of aldosteronism; however, aldosterone secretion rate is actually decreased (Koster and David, 1968). Clearly surgical intervention is not indicated. *Principle: Accurate diagnosis must be made before definitive treatment of a primary cause of hypertension is contemplated.*

Treatment. Removal of an aldosterone-secreting tumor acutely relieves the hypertension, but the blood pressure often increases after several years (Biglieri *et al.*, 1970). Adenomatous adrenal hyperplasia occurs in hypertensive patients, and clinical findings may be similar to those seen in patients with adrenal tumors, but the hypertension is unlikely to be improved by surgery. Adrenal venous angiograms may allow radiologic discovery of very small adrenal tumors and may distinguish the disease from adrenal hyperplasia. Thus, patients may be rationally selected for surgery. As in the treatment of renovascular hypertension, controlled trials are needed to compare medical with surgical treatment of adenomatous adrenal hyperplasia or even of adrenal adenomas.

Pheochromocytoma. Pheochromocytoma is a rare tumor of the adrenal medulla or of other cells of neural crest origin. Pheochromocytoma and related tumors can cause surgically curable hypertension (Figure 5–9). The blood pressure of the patient with pheochromocytoma may be of almost any value. Most symptoms and signs can be related to the effects of circulating catecholamines secreted by the tumor, and the patient's history often strongly suggests the diagnosis. However, a mistaken diagnosis is not uncommon because the symptoms may also mimic those of more common disorders such as thyrotoxicosis, anxiety, diabetes mellitus, or hyperventilation (Table 5–4) (Melmon, 1968).

Biochemical Diagnostic Tests. The definitive diagnosis of pheochromocytoma is made by measuring the urinary excretion of catecholamines and their metabolites (Table 5–5, Figure 5–5). Urinary excretion of vanilmandelic acid and metanephrine plus normetanephrine is elevated in 90% and 95%, respectively, of patients with pheochromocytoma, regardless of the patient's blood pressure during the collection period. Urinary excretion of catecholamines is abnormal in greater than 95% of cases (Sjoerdsma *et al.*, 1966). An increase of up to twice normal in urinary excretion of catecholamines and metabolites may be produced by any stress that stimulates sympathetic activity. Thus hypotension, myocardial infarction, surgery, and severe exercise may result in a mistaken diagnosis if the biochemical tests are misinterpreted. False positives may also occur for other reasons; methyldopa (which forms a fluorophor), sympathomimetic nosedrops or bronchodilators, and fluorescent compounds (tetracycline, quinidine, quinine) interfere with accurate catecholamine determinations (Sjoerdsma *et al.*, 1966; Melmon, 1968). Monoamine oxidase inhibitors, by interfering with catecholamine metabolism (Figure 5–5), may increase the excretion of metanephrine and normetanephrine and decrease the formation and excretion of vanilmandelic acid. The determination of vanilmandelic acid may be falsely elevated by dietary phenolic acids (as in vanilla and coffee), particularly if a simple screening test is used (Medical Letter, 1967c).

Any one of the biochemical tests will suffice for most cases, but urinary vanilmandelic acid

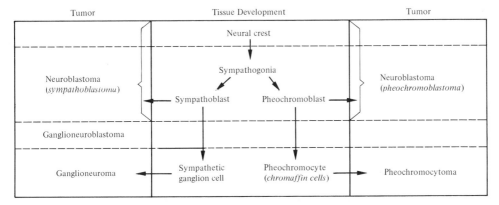

Figure 5–9. Embryologic derivation of endocrinologically functioning tumors of neural crest origin. The ganglioneuroblastoma is derived from cell types intermediate between those of the neuroblastoma and pheochromocytoma. (From Melmon, K. L.: Catecholamines and the adrenal medulla. In Williams, R. H. [ed.]: *Textbook of Endocrinology*, 4th ed. W. B. Saunders Co., Philadelphia, 1968.)

Table 5–4. COMMON MANIFESTATIONS OF PHEOCHROMOCYTOMA AND UNUSUAL COMBINATIONS OF SYMPTOMS LEADING TO ERRONEOUS DIAGNOSIS*†

SIGNS AND SYMPTOMS ATTRIBUTABLE TO CATECHOLAMINE SECRETION	
Hypertension Sweating Paroxysmal attacks of blanching or flushing Palpitations and tachycardia Headache Anorexia, weight loss, psychic changes Evidence of hypermetabolism, increased fasting blood glucose level Decreased gastrointestinal motility Postural hypotension	Commonly found in pheochromocytoma
Increased fasting blood glucose level and abnormal results in glucose tolerance tests	Suggesting diabetes mellitus
Psychosis, tremulousness, increased respiratory rate	Suggesting functional hyperventilation
Decreased gastrointestinal motility and resultant constipation	Suggesting Hirschsprung's disease
Increased basal metabolic rate, increased oxygen consumption, weight loss, psychosis, tremulousness, increased respiratory rate	Suggesting thyrotoxicosis

* From Melmon, K. L.: Catecholamines and the adrenal medulla. In Williams, R. H. (ed.): *Textbook of Endocrinology*, 4th ed. W. B. Saunders Co., Philadelphia, 1968.
† Data obtained from review of 50 consecutive patients with pheochromocytoma seen recently at the University of California Medical Center.

or metanephrine and normetanephrine can usually be determined more readily than catecholamines (Crout, 1966a). *Principle: No single laboratory test can be accepted as diagnostic or pathognomonic without an adequate history and examination to rule out the pathologic, physiologic, pharmacologic, or technical reasons for abnormal tests that can obscure the correct diagnosis.*

Pharmacologic Diagnostic Tests. Pharmacologic tests for pheochromocytoma have only two indications: (1) in a patient with severe hypertension who requires therapy before a diagnosis can be made, and (2) in a patient with an intermittently secreting tumor who has normal urinary excretion of catecholamines and metabolites. The routine use of pharmacologic tests is less rewarding than the use of biochemical tests.

The drugs used in the diagnosis of pheochromocytoma either block the action of circulating catecholamines or release catecholamines from increased stores. Phentolamine is the alpha-adrenergic blocking drug most commonly used as an intravenous test. In a patient with pheochromocytoma, doses as little as 1 mg may lead to a profound fall in arterial pressure. A positive response is a fall in blood pressure of 35/25 lasting at least 4 minutes. A simultaneous fall in blood sugar also is seen in positive tests (Spergel *et al.*, 1970).

Occasionally a patient with a paroxysmally secreting pheochromocytoma may show normal urinary excretion of catecholamines and metabolites; in this patient a provocative test is useful. The test should include not only physiologic measurements of arterial pressure but also determination of plasma catecholamines or a 2-hour urine collection for catecholamines (not metabolites) prior to and after the stimulation test. Histamine and tyramine release catecholamines from nerve endings. The histamine test may produce dangerous elevations in blood pressure, even with small doses; consequently phentolamine should be readily available in case of a large rise in blood pressure. The tyramine test is safer than histamine but less sensitive (produces more false-negative results). Other provocative tests using glucagon or

Table 5–5. NORMAL RANGE OF CATECHOLAMINE AND METABOLITE CONCENTRATIONS*†

Urine	
Catecholamines‡	
Norepinephrine:	10–70 µg/24 hr
Epinephrine:	0–20 µg/24 hr
Normetanephrine and metanephrine:	
< 1.3 mg/24 hr	
Vanilmandelic acid:	1.8–9.0 mg/24 hr
Dopamine:	< 200 µg/24 hr
Blood	
Catecholamines:	< 1 µg per liter
Adrenal medulla	
Norepinephrine:	0.04–0.16 mg/g
Epinephrine:	0.22–0.84 mg/g

* From Melmon, K. L.: Catecholamines and the adrenal medulla. In Williams, R. H. (ed.): *Textbook of Endocrinology*, 4th ed. W. B. Saunders Co., Philadelphia, 1968.
† Since the values obtained in different laboratories vary considerably, only a general range can be given.
‡ In most patients with pheochromocytomas, total catecholamine excretion is > 300 µg per day.

physiologic stimuli such as tilting are variations on a common theme. More experience is required in patients with a variety of diseases, including pheochromocytoma with normal urinary excretion, before the efficacy of these studies can be determined (Editorial, 1967a; Harrison et al., 1967; Lawrence, 1967). The accuracy of any of the pharmacologic tests for pheochromocytoma is at best 75 to 85% (Melmon, 1968).

Once the diagnosis of pheochromocytoma has been made, careful examination of the pattern of urinary catecholamines and metabolites can help to localize and define the size, and possibly the malignancy, of the tumor. The adrenal medulla and organ of Zuckerkandl are the only organs normally capable of forming epinephrine from norepinephrine (④ in Figure 5–3) (Axelrod, 1962). When urinary epinephrine composes more than 20% of the total catecholamines, the tumor is, with rare exceptions, in one of these locations (Crout and Sjoerdsma, 1960; Engelman and Hammond, 1968). When epinephrine accounts for less than 20% of the urinary catecholamines, the tumor is found in an extra-adrenal site in 20% of cases.

The urinary vanilmandelic acid/catecholamine ratio may help to determine the size of the tumor (Crout and Sjoerdsma, 1964). Tumors secreting large amounts of epinephrine and norepinephrine into the circulation usually produce symptoms early and weigh less than 50 g. Because they are small, they may not be easy to discover by routine diagnostic procedures before surgery or even during surgery. When a small tumor is suspected, the diagnostic workup should be aggressive enough to allow determination of its approximate location. Such tumors bind catecholamines poorly in their granules, and very little of the active catecholamine is metabolized within the tumor. The high concentration of free catecholamines is reflected in a low urinary vanilmandelic acid/catecholamine ratio. Patients whose tumors bind catecholamines well and metabolize them to pharmacologically inactive products prior to release from the tumor tend to be relatively asymptomatic. By the time these tumors are discovered they are large (greater than 50 g) and produce a high vanilmandelic acid/catecholamine ratio. These large tumors are easily located during surgery or in preoperative diagnostic procedures.

The urinary excretion of norepinephrine precursors, dopa, dopamine, and their metabolites (homovanillic acid and 3-methoxytyramine), is common in neuroblastomas and suggests a more primitive cell type, incapable of producing norepinephrine. Malignant pheochromocytomas may, in some instances, also secrete dopa, dopamine and their metabolites. The urinary excretion of these substances thus may be used as a biochemical indicator of malignancy. The number of cases in which these metabolites have been measured is so few that much more experience is necessary to make a firm generalization about malignant and benign pheochromocytomas (Anton et al., 1967). Careful examination of available tests may give much more information than mere confirmation of the diagnosis of a pheochromocytoma. Proper interpretation may aid the surgeon in determining the size, the location, and possibly the malignancy of the tumor.

Treatment. The ultimate treatment consists of surgical removal of the tumor, but this is preceded by therapy with catecholamine blocking drugs. Either phentolamine, the short-acting, competitive alpha-adrenergic blocking drug, or phenoxybenzamine, the long-acting drug that can produce a nonequilibrium blockade, may be used. The pharmacologic effect of oral phentolamine lasts only 3 to 6 hours, necessitating frequent administration, even awakening the patient at night to effect a continuous alpha-adrenergic blockade. Frequent oral administration of phentolamine also elicits nausea, diarrhea, and/or tachycardia in some patients. Errors in drug administration, even in hospitalized patients, are more common when several drugs are prescribed, or if multiple doses of a single drug are compared to single-dose administration (see Chapter 17). To avoid the problems associated with oral phentolamine, many therapists use phenoxybenzamine (Sjoerdsma et al., 1966; Melmon, 1968). This drug is metabolized to an alkylating agent, which is the active compound. The effects are not immediate but are long lasting, and control of symptoms of a pheochromocytoma is generally excellent.

The effectiveness of therapy can be judged clinically by disappearance of symptoms and by return of catecholamine-induced laboratory abnormalities to normal. Thus the patient becomes normotensive, does not perspire excessively, and loses his palpitations or orthostatic hypotension. The elevated fasting blood sugar and free fatty acid concentrations usually fall to normal values. If the blood volume was reduced prior to treatment, it returns to normal; prior signs of cardiomyopathy are no longer apparent.

In some patients with high concentrations of circulating epinephrine, phenoxybenzamine does not reverse all the cardiac, metabolic, or gastrointestinal effects of the pheochromocytoma. In these people, a beta-adrenergic blocking drug may be helpful (Dornhorst and Laurence, 1963; Wilson and Theilen, 1967).

Another approach to the preoperative therapy of a pheochromocytoma or the therapy of a malignant pheochromocytoma is the use of an inhibitor of catecholamine synthesis. Alpha-methyltyrosine is an experimental drug that competitively inhibits tyrosine hydroxylation (① in Figure 5–3), the rate-limiting step in catecholamine synthesis (Engelman *et al.*, 1968a,b), and effectively decreases the excretion of catecholamines and their metabolites.

Since catecholamines that are released still produce their effects, alpha- and beta-blocking drugs must be available at surgery (Jones *et al.*, 1968). It is logical and efficacious to use an inhibitor of synthesis with an alpha-adrenergic blocking drug if either agent alone given in maximally tolerable doses does not control the symptoms or signs preoperatively.

The duration of preoperative therapy is variable. In patients without evidence of cardiomyopathy, the circulatory and metabolic abnormalities usually return to normal within 2 weeks. However, if cardiac damage is evident clinically or by the presence of arrhythmias or nonspecific changes in the ST-T vectors on the electrocardiogram, medical therapy should be continued until maximal improvement has occurred prior to surgery; this may take several months (Engelman and Sjoerdsma, 1964; Sjoerdsma *et al.*, 1966).

Patients with metastatic pheochromocytomas can usually be controlled symptomatically with the same medical management used for preoperative control of the symptoms and signs of catecholamine excess. Antitumor agents have generally not been effective (Engelman and Sjoerdsma, 1964).

The operative management of pheochromocytoma requires the use of a rapidly acting, competitive alpha-adrenergic blocking drug intravenously to control hypertension, sometimes a beta-adrenergic blocking drug to control catecholamine-induced arrhythmias, and, often, blood or plasma to control hypotension after the tumor is removed. Pressor agents are generally not needed after the tumor is removed if previous blood volume expansion has been adequate. If an occasion to use a pressor arises, however, and if norepinephrine fails, angiotensin, which vasoconstricts via receptors other than adrenergic, is a reasonable choice, considering the variable levels of circulating catecholamines and the varying degrees of adrenergic receptor blockade.

The choice of an anesthetic is important. Halothane has been used successfully in combination with intermittent use of a beta-adrenergic blocking agent to control cardiac arrhythmias (Cooperman *et al.*, 1967), which

are probably due to the increased myocardial irritability to catecholamines produced by halothane anesthesia (Hall and Norris, 1958; Andersen and Johansen, 1963). Nitrous oxide–oxygen has been suggested as an alternative that would be less likely to sensitize the heart to catecholamines (Melmon, 1968).

Principle: Knowledge of the pathogenesis of a disease should not lead to complacency about its therapy. We treat pheochromocytoma with surgery, alpha- and sometimes beta-adrenergic blocking agents, or drugs that prevent the synthesis of catecholamines. Only surgery is definitive, and medical treatment sometimes fails. When a patient with neuroblastoma is considered, the principle is even better illustrated. Although metabolic products of catecholamines are excreted in excess, there is little evidence that circulating catecholamines are abnormal. Yet surgical removal of the tumor reverses the hypertension commonly associated with neuroblastoma (indicating that a substance from the tumor was responsible). Adrenergic blocking agents in patients with neuroblastoma may be useless in reversing the hypertension. Discrepancies between assumed pathogenesis and therapeutic results should suggest the need for study in both areas.

Essential Hypertension. Essential hypertension is a diagnosis made by exclusion, but accounts for more than 80% of all hypertensives in the United States. The principal physiologic abnormality in essential hypertension is usually an elevated peripheral vascular resistance that is *not* due to sympathomimetic overactivity. In some patients with labile hypertension, the major abnormality may be an elevation of cardiac output (Eich *et al.*, 1962, 1966; Finkielman *et al.*, 1965; Editorial, 1968a). The therapy of patients with labile hypertension (if any is needed) requires further study of both the natural history of this disease and the actual effects of lowering the blood pressure.

The therapist should pay special attention to any disease classified as "essential" or "idiopathic." Such a title openly advertises our ignorance of the pathogenesis of the disease; therefore, we cannot determine whether any therapy directly antagonizes the pathophysiologic factors. Empiric therapy may be efficacious and is proper until it can be compared to more specific therapy when the pathogenesis is defined. All hypertension was considered "essential" prior to the discovery of distinct entities that may respond to specific and effective therapy. However, the cure of renovascular lesions may not always be the best way of managing renovascular hypertension. The older individual with extensive vascular complications related to hypertension may be effectively treated by medical means when the risk of surgical correction is too great. Some antihypertensive drugs exacerbate hypertension if misused in selected patients. Any drug that can release catecholamines from the postganglionic nerve ending may produce paradoxical hypertension if given inadvertently to a patient with pheochromocytoma who has expanded stores of norepinephrine in nerve endings. The same event can also occur when inordinately large doses of guanethidine or alpha-methyldopa are given to hypertensive patients without pheochromocytoma. Rapidly acting alpha-adrenergic blocking agents can counter this complication of therapy. If phentolamine were given (and had lowered blood pressure) before use of drugs operative on the postganglionic nerve fiber, the increased blood pressure would be correctly attributed to catecholamine excess and the paradoxical rise could be anticipated and avoided by withholding the catecholamine-releasing drugs.

Treatment of Mild Hypertension (*Blood Pressure 140/90 to 160/100 Without Complications*). Reserpine and the oral diuretics are used to treat mild hypertension. Therapy is best started with a thiazide; many patients require no further treatment. The mechanism of the antihypertensive effects of thiazides is to decrease peripheral vascular resistance perhaps independent of blood volume depletion or action on the sympathetic nervous system. Thus the drug can be used successfully with antiadrenergic agents or even with drugs like hydralazine, because the mechanisms of action are different. More important, the use of the thiazides may allow a decrease in the dose of the often more potent but also more toxic drugs used to lower supine blood pressure. *Principle: Drug combinations may be used rationally to decrease the chances of toxicity of either drug and to make therapy more practical.*

Despite claims of superiority of different products by advertising agencies, all thiazide diuretics produce similar therapeutic and side effects. Only the dosage varies; this is of little importance in the use of any drug since such statements of "relative potency" reveal nothing about maximum effect (Gaffney *et al.*, 1969). *Principle: Do not be confused by statements regarding relative potency of drugs. The important factors are the maximum effect that can be produced and the relationship of the effective dose to the toxic dose.*

Thiazides with a duration of action of 6 to 8 hours (e.g., chlorothiazide and hydrochlorothiazide) should be given in divided doses, whereas others with a longer duration of action (e.g., bendroflumethiazide and polythiazide) can be given once daily. Potassium depletion with metabolic alkalosis may be produced by chronic thiazide administration, but the incidence is low in patients with mild hypertension alone (Smith *et al.*, 1966). However, patients who are seen infrequently or who are taking digitalis should receive supplemental potassium chloride solution or tablets (Kaplan, 1967; Schwartz *et al.*, 1968). Enteric-coated potassium chloride tablets are variably absorbed (see Chapter 2), may cause serious or fatal ulceration of the small bowel, and must be avoided (Lawrason *et al.*, 1965). Hyperglycemia and hyperuricemia with or without gout are common side effects of thiazide therapy; pancreatitis, vasculitis, jaundice, photosensitivity, skin rashes, and bone marrow depression occur rarely.

Reserpine or rauwolfia alkaloids may be added if the response to a thiazide alone is inadequate. The combination of reserpine (or its equivalent, rauwolfia) and a thiazide is effective in almost all cases of mild hypertension and in most patients with moderate hypertension (Smith, W. M., *et al.*, 1964, 1966, 1969). The dose of reserpine is limited by the appearance of toxicity after daily doses exceed 0.5 mg. The most dangerous complication of chronic administration of reserpine is a psychotic depression and suicide. Other side effects include increased gastric acid secretion and mucosal ulceration, diarrhea, abdominal cramps, and nasal stuffiness, most of which are due to the sympathetic blockade with relative parasympathetic overactivity. If side effects of reserpine are tolerated poorly, small doses of hydralazine, methyldopa or guanethidine may be useful.

Treatment of Moderate Hypertension (*Blood Pressure 160/100 to 200/120 with or Without Left Ventricular Hypertrophy and Grade II Retinopathy Without Other Complications*) *and Severe Hypertension* (*Blood Pressure Greater than 200/120 or Complications of Cardiac or Renal Damage*). Many patients with moderate hypertension respond to oral diuretics and reserpine. In some patients, more effective drugs including methyldopa, guanethidine, monoamine oxidase inhibitors (MAOI), or ganglionic blocking drugs are needed to control the blood pressure.

Methyldopa is a useful antihypertensive agent in this clinical setting. During effective therapy, cardiac output is well maintained, and the reduction in blood pressure may result from a fall in peripheral vascular resistance due either to the direct effect of the drug on blood vessels, to its partial interference with the sympathetic nervous system, or to its ill-defined action on the central nervous system (Sannerstedt *et al.*, 1962;

Dollery, 1965). Therefore, methyldopa, con-trasted with pargyline and guanethidine, usually produces a considerably greater decrease in supine arterial pressure for a given decrease in standing arterial pressure and results in less symptomatic orthostatic hypotension for any given lowering of blood pressure in the supine position (Oates *et al.*, 1965). This beneficial effect may occur because the sympathetic blockade is less complete with methyldopa, but it also tends to confirm studies that methyldopa has modes of action other than sympathetic blockade (Mohammed *et al.*, 1968a; Gaffney *et al.*, 1969). This conclusion is also suggested by data that show that renal blood flow is maintained despite reduction in renal artery pressure; hence renal vascular resistance is decreased (Luke and Kennedy, 1964; Morin *et al.*, 1964; Mohammed *et al.*, 1968b). The drug is especially valuable in hypertensive patients with compromised renal function.

Oral absorption of methyldopa is variable, and effective daily doses range from 500 to 3000 mg. Maximum effects are seen in 4 to 8 hours after an oral dose or in 4 hours after intravenous administration. The duration of effect of the oral dose is usually no longer than 48 hours. Common side effects are transient drowsiness and fatigue, fever with or without abnormalities in liver function, diarrhea or constipation, and skin rash (Horwitz *et al.*, 1967; Glontz and Saslaw, 1968). Unusual effects are lactation (Pettinger *et al.*, 1963) and, after several months of therapy, development of reversible positive direct Coombs test with or without hemolytic anemia (Smith *et al.*, 1966; LoBuglio and Jandl, 1967). Unfortunately, some patients become tolerant to methyldopa after prolonged treatment, necessitating a change in medication (Prescott *et al.*, 1966).

Guanethidine is most helpful in moderate-to-severe hypertension, but may be used in small doses in patients with mild hypertension who are not controlled by or cannot tolerate other drugs. The hypotensive effect of guanethidine is pre-dominantly due to venous pooling of blood that decreases cardiac output; postural hypotension may be pronounced, particularly during exercise. However, in patients with cardiac failure and hypertension, the cardiac output may increase because of the decreased work load on the heart after blood pressure is lowered. Renal blood flow and glomerular filtration rate are decreased by guanethidine (Freis, 1965). Effective doses range from 10 to 400 mg daily. The maximum cumulative effect of a given dose may not be seen for 4 to 10 days, and effects may last for a similar period after the drug is discontinued. Because of the long duration of the drug's effect, dosages

should be adjusted in outpatients only after being given for several days at the same level. Hospitalized patients can be given more aggressive therapy, beginning with an oral loading dose if more rapid control of arterial pressure is required. One experimental approach for hastening the control of blood pressure has been to give guanethidine intramuscularly (Leishman and Sandler, 1965). However, the variability of individual responses combined with the prolonged action of the drug makes this method of treatment potentially dangerous. As with other drugs that block the sympathetic nervous system, undesirable effects generally represent extensions of the therapeutic effects. Thus, orthostatic dizziness or syncope (especially in the morning or after exercise), diarrhea, failure to ejaculate, dry mouth, nasal stuffiness, and bradycardia are common.

Although monoamine oxidase inhibitors are not commonly used as antihypertensive drugs, pargyline is selected most often. The onset of action is slow, requiring 1 to 3 weeks for appearance of maximum effects, and effects last for up to 3 weeks after the drug has been dis-continued. Cardiac output is maintained, peripheral vascular resistance is decreased (Brest *et al.*, 1963), and mood-elevating effects are prominent. The undesirable effects are considerable and severely limit the usefulness of this class of drug. Adverse effects include symptoms of sympathetic blockade (sympto-matic orthostatic hypotension and increased gastrointestinal motility); excessive central ner-vous system stimulation, resulting in insomnia, nightmares, and muscular twitching; and an impressive number of drug and food interactions (see Chapter 16).

The most serious side effect is the precipitation of hypertensive crises by drugs that release norepinephrine or by tyramine-containing foods. These crises should be treated with the alpha-adrenergic blocking drug phentolamine. In addition, undesirable effects may be produced by narcotics, antihistamines, other MAO inhibitors, imipramine and its derivatives, seda-tives, and hypoglycemic drugs when added to a MAO inhibitor. *Principle: All therapeutic decisions must weigh risks vs. benefits. The risks of MAO inhibitors seem to outweigh their benefits for most patients.*

Ganglionic blocking drugs are used infre-quently in chronic therapy. The most com-monly used agents are pentolinium tartrate, chlorisondamine, and mecamylamine. Side effects resulting from autonomic blockade include dry mouth, blurred vision, constipation or paralytic ileus, impotence, and urinary retention. Some of the effects related to lack of parasympathetic action can be mitigated at times with small doses of directly acting para-sympathomimetics such as pilocarpine or bethanechol.

Mecamylamine, a secondary amine, is more completely absorbed by the oral route than are the other ganglionic blocking drugs, which are quaternary amines. Because it is a weak base, mecamylamine's distribution and excretion depends to a large extent on the pH of urine and blood. If the plasma becomes more acid, mecamylamine redistributes to extracellular fluid (where it exerts its action) and ganglionic block-ade increases (Payne and Rowe, 1957). If the urine is acid, the drug is more rapidly excreted (Peters, 1960). The effects of pH on the action of this drug have clinical importance and alter the effective dose and frequency of administration necessary to achieve a desired and stable effect.

In the treatment of hypertension, drugs must be used to achieve predetermined specific goals. Often a patient is labeled "refractory" to standard antihypertensive agents or sensitive to a "normal" dose because of undesirable side effects. Many such patients, when properly treated, respond satisfactorily to the very drugs to which they have been termed "refractory." For example, in treating a patient who is refractory to 100 mg of guanethidine daily, the physician must decide whether guanethidine is producing pharmacologic effects. That is, is there evidence of sympathetic blockade such as orthostatic hypotension, a fixed pulse rate during orthostatic hypotension, or an absent overshoot in blood pressure after Valsalva's maneuver ("square wave" response) (Thomson and Melmon, 1968)? If no evidence of sym-pathetic blockade exists, the dose of the drug can be safely increased to an amount that gives evidence of pharmacologic action. If there is evidence of sympathetic blockade, but satis-factory control of the blood pressure cannot be obtained without intolerable side effects, another drug or combination of drugs may be helpful. *Principle: Drugs must be used in the dose required to obtain the desired response unless intolerable "toxicity" or side effects supervene.*

With some drugs, data indicate that beyond a certain dose, very little therapeutic benefit is obtained in most patients. This is true of methyldopa (3 g daily) and the thiazides (100 mg of hydrochlorothiazide daily). With other drugs (e.g., hydralazine and reserpine) serious toxicity may limit the dose that can be safely given, even though further therapeutic effects may be found at higher doses (Gaffney et al., 1969). Finally, with many drugs (e.g., guanethidine and the ganglionic blocking agents) true toxicity is uncommon; the side effects are

primarily an extension of predictable pharmaco-logic actions, and the dose can be increased as much as necessary (see Chapter 15). Only when pharmacologic effect is seen (i.e., sympathetic blockade) is there evidence that the patient is receiving enough drug.

Drug Combinations. The most useful and commonly used combination is a thiazide plus a sympathetic blocking drug. Clinical experience has shown that for the moderate-to-severe hypertensive patient thiazides alone do not suffice for adequate therapy. Many of the drugs that interfere with the sympathetic nervous system result in fluid retention, which may account for "tolerance" to the antihypertensive effect or even congestive heart failure. The combination of thiazides with other anti-hypertensive drugs counteracts the fluid reten-tion, increases the antihypertensive effects, and allows the use of smaller doses of the more potent drugs, with better control of blood pressure and fewer side effects. For this reason thiazides should be a part of all antihypertensive regimens. The routine use of other combinations, however, cannot be recommended. There are few data on the pharmacology of drug combina-tions to guide the clinician. On the basis of the known mechanisms of action of the drugs, combinations can be tried in the patient who does not respond adequately to single drugs. The combination of reserpine, a thiazide, and small doses of oral hydralazine has been efficacious in many patients with moderate hypertension who do not respond adequately to reserpine and an oral diuretic. The divergent mechanisms of action of these drugs make their combination rational. The doses of reserpine and hydralazine are limited, however, by their toxicity.

Guanethidine and methyldopa both act at the postganglionic nerve ending but in a different manner. This combination may be helpful in some cases (Leonard et al., 1965), but the incidence of adverse side effects is high. The addition of a small dose of a ganglionic blocking drug to guanethidine may allow control of the blood pressure with fewer side effects such as diarrhea or ileus than with either drug alone. The combination of a vasodilator drug with a beta-adrenergic receptor blocking agent also has shown promise (Gilmore et al., 1970). *Principle: The physician using triple combinations of drugs in treating hypertension should have first tried the combination of a thiazide and an adrenergic blocker to its limit, must be thoroughly familiar with the pharmacology of the individual drugs and their possible and reported interactions, must outline his therapeutic goals, and must know how to evaluate the drug effects. If there is not a large clinical experience or experimental data to support his selections, he is experimenting and must therefore be very careful in observing the patient and recording the observations accurately.*

The Hypertensive Emergency. The patient who presents with grade IV retinopathy, neurologic signs and symptoms, or severe heart failure needs therapy prior to complete hypertensive evaluation. In approaching such a patient, the physician must decide how quickly the pressure must be reduced. This decision is based on the history of abruptness of pressure rise and on the presence of life-threatening cardiac or central nervous system complications. Prior to any treatment, a thorough history of previous drug therapy must be obtained, searching for drugs such as antihypertensives, psychoactive agents, monoamine oxidase inhibitors, or pressors, which can precipitate a hypertensive crisis or modify the response to therapy. An evaluation of coexisting diseases also helps to determine the choice and rapidity of therapy. In the presence of angina, acute deterioration of renal function, acute heart failure, or central nervous system signs, the decision is usually made to lower the arterial pressure within 30 minutes to diastolic pressures of 100 to 105 mm Hg. Acutely decreasing the pressure may decrease flow to vital organs, and central nervous system function, electrocardiogram, and urine volumes must be monitored to ensure adequate tissue perfusion. Before any therapy, a phentolamine test should be done to rule out hypertension due to excess circulating catecholamines from a pheochromocytoma or due to prior drug therapy. If small doses (1 to 5 mg) of phentolamine decrease blood pressure for prolonged periods, release of catecholamines for whatever reason is contributing substantially to the change in blood pressure. In such a setting it would be foolish to use antihypertensive drugs that act on the postganglionic nerve ending to further release catecholamines. While the underlying reason for catechol excess is being investigated, phentolamine or dibenzyline may be useful to manage the hypertension.

If the phentolamine test is negative, the ganglionic blockers are available for rapid and predictable control of blood pressure; trimethaphan camphorsulfonate is the most rapidly acting agent. The effect can be varied from minute to minute via an intravenous drip. Pentolinium tartrate has a longer duration of activity and is also useful in the emergency management of hypertension. The hypotension produced by drugs that block the sympathetic nervous system is potentiated in the upright position, as the effect of gravity increases venous pooling. Accordingly, the patient should be placed in the reverse Trendelenburg position with the head of the bed on blocks; elevation of the head half of the bed is not sufficient. Predictable side effects such as ileus may occur and should be recognized as drug induced.

Parenteral hydralazine is another useful drug for hypertensive crises, but unless it is combined with antiadrenergic drugs, large doses likely to cause angina or increasing heart failure are commonly needed to reduce the blood pressure satisfactorily.

The experimental thiazide diazoxide has been widely acclaimed as valuable in the acute management of the patient with malignant hypertension (Finnerty et al., 1963; Finnerty, 1968; Hamby et al., 1968). This drug can be rapidly administered intravenously, resulting in a rapid and prolonged antihypertensive effect. The hyperglycemia and sodium retention that may ensue is of little consequence in the acute situation.

Most patients with malignant hypertension can be treated as subacute emergencies. Methyldopa is a safe, effective, and predictable agent for such patients. Intravenous doses of 500 to 1000 mg promote a smooth lowering of systolic and diastolic pressures, usually beginning within 2 hours. Rarely, a paradoxical rise in arterial pressure occurs after parenteral administration of methyldopa. These increases in arterial pressure are effectively treated with phentolamine (Levine and Strauch, 1966).

Intravenous or intramuscular reserpine, in doses up to 5 mg, has been recommended for the treatment of malignant hypertension. Administered by this route, reserpine not only depletes catecholamines but also has direct vasodilating effects on arterioles (Parks et al., 1961). However, the onset, severity, and duration of the effects of parenteral reserpine are unpredictable and occasionally dangerously dramatic (Hughes et al., 1955; Fletcher, 1963; Leonberg et al., 1964). Controlling the profound hypotension that may occur after as little as 0.1 mg may not be easy. Sympathomimetic drugs that depend on release of stored catecholamines (e.g., metaraminol) have unpredictable effects because the stores are compromised by reserpine treatment. Directly acting sympathomimetic drugs (e.g., norepinephrine) have an enhanced effect because reserpine prevents their entrance into storage granules. Phenylephrine is a reasonable drug to use because it has moderately weak but direct sympathomimetic effects. Since more predictable agents are now available to lower pressure acutely, the value of parenteral reserpine is limited.

Tachyphylaxis develops promptly to trimethaphan camphorsulfonate and to parenteral hydralazine, in part owing to fluid retention. Potent oral antihypertensive therapy should be initiated as soon as possible, even if initial blood pressure control is adequate, to preclude later loss of blood pressure control. The choice of drugs is the same as for moderate-to-severe hypertension. If guanethidine is used, the patient requires additional therapy for several days until its full effects are manifest. *Principle: A hypertensive emergency may be satisfactorily treated only to find the patient relapsing because potent, long-term therapy was not started concomitantly with or shortly after the initiation of emergency treatment.*

SHOCK

Shock is an all-inclusive term for inadequate tissue perfusion (primarily of the heart, brain, and kidney) produced by a number of diseases. A clinical mistake is made in diagnosis of shock if one waits until the arterial blood pressure is low. Inadequate delivery of oxygen and nutrients to the tissues need not be associated with hypotension. In addition, cardiac output can be normal but individual tissues may suffer from inadequate flow because of a relative increase in regional vascular resistance. The diagnosis of shock must not be based on the level of arterial pressure, but should take into consideration signs of inadequate perfusion of critical organs. As blood flow to the kidney decreases, urine flow is diminished. A clouded sensorium, a change in myocardial performance, or the appearance of an arrhythmia may herald poor perfusion in the brain or heart. Often biochemical evidence of anaerobic metabolism becomes apparent when large masses of tissues are poorly perfused and lactate production, acidemia, and hyperkalemia develop. The hemodynamic abnormality underlying the defective perfusion must be discovered and reversed even if the blood pressure is normal (Figure 5–10, Table 5–6). Sequential changes in the indices of tissue perfusion serve as the basis for evaluating therapy. If tissue perfusion is normal, needless therapy only exposes the patient to the risk of drug toxicity. *Principle: When it is determined that therapy is needed, the specific pathogenetic abnormalities should be assessed to determine what therapeutic steps are necessary. Then specific goals must be established and measurements made frequently to determine whether the abnormalities are being corrected.*

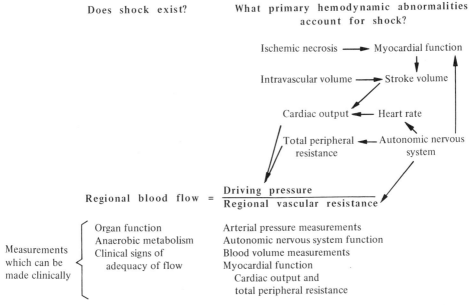

Figure 5–10. A diagrammatic representation of the determinants of shock. Decreased tissue perfusion is requisite for the diagnosis of shock. Once shock is diagnosed, the primary hemodynamic abnormalities must be assessed. Therapy is then directed toward correction of the hemodynamic abnormalities (right side of diagram). The efficacy of therapy is assessed by changes in organ function or tissue metabolism or by other evidence of changing regional blood flow (left side of diagram). (From Nies, A. S., and Melmon, K. L.: The rational management of cardiogenic shock. In Brest, A. N. [ed.]: *Cardiovascular Therapy*, Vol. 1. F. A. Davis Co., Philadelphia, 1969.)

Table 5–6. INDICATORS OF THE STATE OF TISSUE PERFUSION AND MYOCARDIAL AND AUTONOMIC NERVOUS SYSTEM FUNCTION*

DIAGNOSIS OF SHOCK AND EFFICACY OF THERAPY		PRIMARY HEMODYNAMIC ABNORMALITY AND TARGET OF THERAPY	
Function Assessed	*Variable Monitored*	*Function Assessed*	*Variable Monitored*
Tissue perfusion	AV oxygen difference Central venous oxygen saturation Skin temperature	Autonomic nervous system ↑ Sympathetic activity	Pallor Pupillary dilation ↑ Heart rate ↓ Bowel sounds ↑ Sweating Dry mouth Clinical evidence of vaso- constriction
Organ function Kidney Brain Heart	Urine output Mental function Chest pain, cardiac rhythm Central venous pressure†		
Anaerobic metabolism	↑ Lactate/pyruvate ↓ pCO₂ ↓ pH Serum electrolytes Hyperkalemia Increased respiratory rate Decreased response to catecholamines	↓ Sympathetic and ↑ parasympathetic activity	Pupillary constriction ↓ Heart rate Sinus bradycardia Heart block Absence of vasoconstriction ↑ Bowel sounds Salivation
		Blood volume	Central venous pressure† Dilution methods, e.g., RISA
		Myocardial function	Responses to volume load Central venous pressure† Cardiac output
		Cardiac output and total peripheral resistance	Dye dilution techniques Fick principle Changes in central venous oxygen saturation Intra-arterial pressure recording

* From Nies, A. S., and Melmon, K. L.: The rational management of cardiogenic shock. In Brest, A. N. (ed.): *Cardio-vascular Therapy*, Vol. 1. F. A. Davis Co., Philadelphia, 1969.
† Note that central venous pressure is monitored to assess three functions.

Drugs Used in Shock

Drugs commonly used in shock can be classified by their mechanism of action and their effects (Table 5–7). By proper selection of drugs, the physician can devise a therapeutic plan to alter peripheral resistance, increase force and rate of cardiac contraction, or alter autonomic activity in an attempt to counter the hemo-dynamic abnormalities in the patient without undue toxicity. Thus when a patient has signs of poor tissue perfusion, digitalis would not improve his cardiac output if hypovolemia were a major determinant of his shock. *Principle: Drugs administered in response to a sign or symptom without consideration of pathophysio-logy or pharmacology are not likely to be efficacious and may be truly dangerous.*

Agents Used to Increase Cardiac Output. *Blood Volume Expanders.* Blood volume expansion increases cardiac output in patients with inadequate venous return to the heart. Intra-vascular volume should be assessed early in shock. If the volume is decreased, replacement with blood, plasma, or saline is rational and physiologically sound (Bishop *et al.*, 1964) and may be strikingly effective as sole or adjunctive therapy (Cohn, J. N., *et al.*, 1967). Over-replacement of intravascular volume may continue to increase cardiac output by increasing diastolic myocardial fiber length (Starling's law) (Figure 5–11). Even in cardiogenic shock, when myocardial function is depressed, the increment in output after volume replacement may be substantial (Sarnoff and Berglund, 1954). Eventually, hydrostatic pressure in the capil-laries exceeds plasma oncotic pressure and edema results. For this reason central venous or pulmonary arterial diastolic pressure must be continuously monitored during volume admin-istration to avoid precipitation of overt con-gestive heart failure (Cohn, 1967).

Inotropic Agents. Prolonged shock of any

etiology may result in cardiac decompensation (Sarnoff et al., 1954; Duff et al., 1965); in such cases inotropic agents are indicated.

The cardiac glycosides and beta-mimetic adrenergic drugs have some properties in common. Both types of drugs shift the ventricular function curve upward and to the left (Figure 5–11), increase the velocity of contraction (Krasnow et al., 1964; Lyon and DeGraff, 1966c; Mason and Braunwald, 1968), and increase myocardial oxygen utilization (Covell et al., 1966; Braunwald, 1967).

The major determinants of the oxygen demand by the myocardium are the velocity of fiber shortening, heart rate, and the intra-

myocardial (wall) tension (Covell et al., 1966; Mason et al., 1969a). Since tension is a function of intracardiac pressure and ventricular size, inotropic agents can lower the intramyocardial tension by decreasing heart size. Overall oxygen requirement may actually be decreased by digitalis or isoproterenol, since the decrease in wall tension can balance the increased oxygen requirement owing to the direct effect of the drugs on velocity of myocardial fiber shortening (Covell et al., 1966; Mason et al., 1969a).

Beta-adrenergic stimulating drugs (Table 5–2) have important additional actions that must be considered in the choice of an inotropic agent. These drugs dilate arterioles and decrease

Table 5–7. DRUGS USED IN SHOCK *

PHARMACOLOGICAL ALTERATION OF HEMODYNAMIC ABNORMALITY	AGENT	SITE OF ACTION	REMARKS
Increase cardiac output	Volume expanders	Myocardial fiber stretch (Starling's Law)	Useful adjunct to other therapy —often the first drug considered
	β-adrenergic stimulant (isoproterenol)	β-adrenergic receptor (inotropic and chronotropic effect)	Also dilates arterioles in skeletal muscle and has metabolic effects
	Cardiac glycosides	Direct myocardial effect (inotropic)	Also constricts peripheral arterioles and veins
Increase peripheral resistance	α-adrenergic stimulant (methoxamine, phenylephrine)	α-adrenergic receptor	Reflex effects tend to lower cardiac output
	Angiotensin	Direct vascular stimulant	Reflex effects tend to lower cardiac output. Under all circumstances, increasing resistance increases cardiac work load
Mixed effects	Direct sympathomimetics (norepinephrine)	α- and β-adrenergic receptor	
	Indirect sympathomimetics (metaraminol, mephentermine)	Postganglionic sympathetic nerve ending	Releases norepinephrine. May be affected by prior therapy
	Dopamine	α- and β-adrenergic receptors	
Decrease sympathetic action	α blockers (phentolamine, phenoxybenzamine)	Blocks α-receptor stimulation	Potentially harmful
	β blockers	Blocks β-receptor stimulation	Potentially harmful
Decrease parasympathetic action	Atropine	Competitively blocks acetylcholine receptors	Side effects may limit usefulness
Miscellaneous	Oxygen	Increases peripheral resistance	May be effective to increase cardiac output if tissue oxygenation can be significantly improved, but should always be monitored for its efficacy
	Morphine	Arterial and venous dilation. Histamine release. Vestibular sensitization. Chemoreceptor trigger zone stimulation. Pain sensation decreased	Must be used sparingly with monitoring
	Corticosteroids (pharmacologic doses)	Myocardial stimulation. Decrease peripheral resistance. Cellular effects	Other agents are more predictable

* From Nies, A. S., and Melmon, K. L.: The rational management of cardiogenic shock. In Brest, A. N. (ed.): *Cardiovascular Therapy*, Vol. 1.   F. A. Davis Co., Philadelphia, 1969.

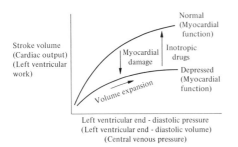

Figure 5–11. Schematic representation of two left ventricular function curves. (From Nies, A. S., and Melmon, K. L.: The rational management of cardiogenic shock. In Brest, A. N. [ed.]: *Cardiovascular Therapy*, Vol. 1. F. A. Davis Co., Philadelphia, 1969.)

peripheral vascular resistance. Whether or not a fall in arterial pressure occurs depends on the extent of the increase in cardiac output produced by the same dose. Isoproterenol can dilate the coronary arteries (Klocke *et al.*, 1965; Pitt *et al.*, 1967), but this effect is not important in cardiogenic shock when coronary vessels are already maximally dilated. In addition to inotropic effects, isoproterenol increases the rate of contraction and ventricular excitability; the drug can be used with benefit in patients with heart block (Benchimol *et al.*, 1965), but must be used with caution in patients who already have arrhythmias.

A cardiac glycoside may be the inotropic agent of choice in some instances. The inotropic effects occur in both normal and failing hearts and do not depend upon the condition of the sympathetic nervous system (Spann *et al.*, 1966). The maximum inotropic effect reached prior to toxicity is less with the cardiac glycosides than with isoproterenol (Beiser *et al.*, 1968a).

Digitalis has important peripheral effects that differ from those of isoproterenol. Digitalis directly constricts arterioles and veins (Mason and Braunwald, 1964b). In the absence of congestive failure this action increases total peripheral resistance and restricts venous return to the heart; consequently, cardiac output remains stable or decreases. In congestive heart failure, the direct effects of digitalis on peripheral vessels are overshadowed by the digitalis-induced increase in cardiac output and reflex diminution of sympathetic activity that decreases arteriolar and venous tone. The best results of digitalis therapy in shock are found in patients with congestive heart failure (Gorlin and Robin, 1955; Kuhn, 1967a, 1967b).

In the absence of congestive heart failure, the peripheral effects of digitalis may limit its usefulness. Rapid digitalization may increase

peripheral resistance without augmenting cardiac output (Malmcrona *et al.*, 1966; Balcon *et al.*, 1968); this elevated afterload can result in a raised left ventricular end-diastolic pressure and occasionally precipitates frank pulmonary edema (Cohn and Tristani, 1967). In addition, the hypoxemia, acidosis, and electrolyte abnormalities that occur in shock can alter the therapeutic and toxic responses to digitalis (Williams *et al.*, 1968; Donlon and Yu, 1969; Mason *et al.*, 1969a) and limit its clinical usefulness and safety. In the absence of congestive failure, isoproterenol has more predictable effects, can produce maximum inotropic effects, can be titrated accurately, and probably is the inotropic agent of choice. The cardiac glycosides are discussed further on pages 181–83.

Agents Used to Increase Peripheral Vascular Resistance. Agents used solely to increase peripheral vascular resistance are uncommonly required in shock (West *et al.*, 1962; Gunnar *et al.*, 1966; Dietzman *et al.*, 1967). The peptide angiotensin and the alpha-adrenergic stimulators methoxamine and phenylephrine raise peripheral resistance and have little if any direct effect on myocardial function. However, baroreceptor reflexes and the increase in afterload may further depress cardiac contractility and output, particularly in patients with myocardial infarction (Puri and Bing, 1968). Overemphasis on restoration of normal blood pressure may be detrimental to the patient. Vasoconstrictors can increase pressure, but often do so at the expense of decreasing blood flow to tissues, and dramatically increase the work of the heart at any stroke volume.

Agents with Mixed Effects. In contrast to the "pure" vasoconstricting agents, drugs that can raise both resistance and cardiac output may have some utility in shock. These drugs include sympathomimetics, which stimulate both the alpha and beta receptors (e.g., norepinephrine and epinephrine), and drugs that release neurotransmitter from the nerve endings (e.g., metaraminol and mephentermine). The effectiveness of sympathomimetics depends in part on the chemical state of the sympathetic nerve ending (see discussion of antihypertensive agents acting at the nerve endings, page 148, and Table 5–8). Patients who have been treated with norepinephrine-depleting agents (reserpine or guanethidine) or agents that act as false neurotransmitters (metaraminol or methyldopa) may be resistant to or may develop rapid tachyphylaxis to indirectly acting pressors. Unusually large responses may be obtained from the use of indirectly acting sympathomimetics in patients treated with MAO inhibitors, including drugs used for hypertension, angina, depression, infection, or malignancy (Stern et al., 1967; Pettinger et al., 1968). Because of these alterations in response, an accurate drug history must be obtained prior to the use of any of these agents (Table 5–8).

Dopamine is a catecholamine precursor of norepinephrine (Figures 5–3 and 5–4) that has direct actions on adrenergic receptors as well as indirect actions due to norepinephrine release (Goldberg et al., 1969). Dopamine increases myocardial contractility (beta), has weak vasoconstrictor (alpha) effects on most peripheral vessels, and appears to dilate renal and mesenteric vessels by mechanisms not requiring alpha- or beta-adrenergic receptors (McNay and Goldberg, 1966; Meyer et al., 1967). It is an experimental drug, but its unique property of increasing cardiac output and renal blood flow without greatly altering peripheral vascular resistance makes it potentially useful (Goldberg et al., 1966; Gunnar et al., 1968; Carvalho et al., 1969; Talley et al., 1969).

Blockade of Autonomic Receptors. Blockade of the autonomic receptors may be helpful in certain situations. Atropine competitively blocks the muscarinic actions of acetylcholine and is beneficial in some patients with cardiogenic shock with evidence of excessive vagal activity (the most important clinical signs are sinus bradycardia and increasing atrioventricular blockade) (Thomas and Woodgate, 1966; Shillingford and Thomas, 1968).

The actions of alpha- and beta-adrenergic blocking agents have been discussed. The proposed rationale for the use of alpha-adrenergic blockade in shock is that the sympathetic response to hypotension reduces flow to and may damage tissues (Lillehei et al., 1964). Alpha-adrenergic blocking agents inhibit norepinephrine-induced vasoconstriction and presumably may increase tissue perfusion. They may also reduce the relatively pronounced venoconstriction, which increases transudation across capillaries, promotes trapping of blood in the microcirculation, and results in plasma loss in some animals in shock. In experimental settings, alpha-adrenergic blocking agents have improved survival (Nickerson and Gourzis, 1962; Nickerson, 1965; Chien, 1967; Dietzman and Lillehei, 1968a). However, animal models of shock often have little relevance to man (Smith and Moore, 1962). In addition, excessive sympathetic activity may be an asset during shock and may be responsible for maintaining and

Table 5–8. COMMONLY USED DRUGS ALTERING THE FUNCTION OF THE SYMPATHETIC NERVOUS SYSTEM*

DRUG	MECHANISM	RESPONSES TO SYMPATHOMIMETICS	
		Indirect	*Direct*
Antihypertensives			
Alpha-methyldopa	Displaces norepinephine by false neurotransmitter	± ↓	↑
Guanethidine	Blocks physiological release of norepinephrine	↓ ↓	↑
	Depletes norepinephrine stores		
Reserpine	Depletes norepinephrine stores	↓ ↓	↑
Monoamine oxidase inhibitors (pargyline)	Abnormal accumulation of amines	↑ ↑ ↑	↑
Indirect pressors			
Metaraminol	Displaces norepinephrine	↓	±
Mephentermine		↓	±
Psychoactive agents			
Monoamine oxidase inhibitors	Abnormal accumulation of amines	↑ ↑ ↑	↑
Imipramine	Blocks entry of other agents into nerve ending	↓	↑
Phenothiazines	Blocks alpha adrenergic receptor	↓	↑
Antibiotics			
Furazolidone	Monoamine oxidase inhibitor	↑ ↑ ↑	↑
Cancer chemotherapeutic agents			
Procarbazine	Monoamine oxidase inhibitor	↑ ↑ ↑	↑

* Modified from Nies, A. S., and Melmon, K. L.: The rational management of cardiogenic shock. In Brest, A. N. (ed.): *Cardiovascular Therapy*, Vol. 1. F. A. Davis Co., Philadelphia, 1969.

redistributing cardiac output to preserve flow to vital areas such as brain and heart (Hoffbrand et al., 1968). Even when volume replacement is adequate, alpha-adrenergic blocking agents may produce severe hypotension and may decrease flow to vital organs. At the present time the value of alpha-adrenergic blocking agents has not been studied in a controlled manner in man, and their clinical value remains undefined; however, existing evidence indicates that these agents are infrequently useful clinically (Wilson, R. F., et al., 1964; Goldberg, 1968; Perlroth and Harrison, 1969). The beta-adrenergic blocking agent propranolol has no known role in the treatment of clinical shock. Its negative inotropic effects may precipitate heart failure (Epstein and Braunwald, 1967b).

Agents Used to Alter the Secondary Manifestations of Shock. *Oxygen.* Arterial hypoxemia is common in shock following myocardial infarction and can be related to pulmonary arteriovenous shunting of up to 25% of the cardiac output (MacKenzie et al., 1964; Storstein and Rasmussen, 1968). Other types of shock are not usually associated with low arterial pO_2. In patients with hypoxemia, oxygen therapy may increase myocardial and peripheral tissue oxygenation and may be a critical therapeutic factor in improving the clinical state of the patient. However, oxygen should not be given indiscriminately to all patients in shock. Oxygen may cause pulmonary toxicity or myocardial depression and directly increases peripheral vascular resistance; the increased afterload and baroreceptor reflexes may result in decreased cardiac output (MacKenzie et al., 1964; Thomas et al., 1965a; Shillingford and Thomas, 1967a; Kenmure et al., 1968). The use of hyperbaric oxygen is still experimental; its benefits and hazards need further definition (Cameron et al., 1966; Whalen and Salzman, 1968). *Principle: There is no drug, including oxygen, that is devoid of harmful effects. The goals of therapy must be defined and the course of the patient must be carefully followed.*

Alkali. Lactic acid production is common in shock, reflecting diminished tissue perfusion and increased anaerobic glycolysis (Broder and Weil, 1964; Peretz et al., 1965). Acidosis reduces the effectiveness of sympathomimetic drugs and endogenous catecholamines and thereby reduces response to therapy (Burget and Visscher, 1927; Thrower et al., 1961). Appropriate therapy for this acidosis is almost always sodium bicarbonate. Lactate buffers are available, but their use is not recommended in view of their high osmolar activity and their relatively weak alkalinizing action compared to bicarbonate. Lactate is metabolized aerobically to bicarbonate; during tissue hypoxia metabolism of lactate does not occur and no effective buffering occurs, excluding this as a form of therapy.

Other Agents. Massive doses of adrenal corticosteroids can increase cardiac output and decrease peripheral vascular resistance (Sambhi et al., 1965; Dietzman and Lillehei, 1968b). In addition, corticosteroids have cellular effects, such as lysosomal stabilization, which may be potentially valuable in treating shock (Weissmann and Thomas, 1962, 1964a, 1964b; Janoff and Zeligs, 1968). However, there is no convincing clinical evidence that shock of any etiology is greatly helped by corticosteroids, and their routine use cannot be recommended until more careful studies define their role. The use of adrenal corticosteroids as "medical last rites" is based more on the physician's frustration at being unable to halt relentless deterioration than on experimental or clinical observation.

Phenothiazines have been used in shock because of their modest alpha-adrenergic blocking properties (Dietzman and Lillehei, 1968a). These drugs have antihistamine, antiserotonin, and antibradykinin properties as well as central nervous system effects. Their value has not been shown clinically, and the use of such drugs without any defined therapeutic goals or critical evaluation of response is not recommended.

Of theoretic interest in the treatment of septic shock are agents that interfere with the formation or action of the vasoactive mediators thought to be pathogenetically important. These agents include anticomplement drugs, antihistamines, salicylates, and possibly corticosteroids. These drugs are considered briefly in the discussion of septic shock.

Therapy of Shock

The abnormality common to all types of shock is poor tissue perfusion. Poor perfusion may result from inadequate cardiac output (due to decreased venous return to the heart or impaired myocardial contractility) or from altered peripheral vascular resistance or autonomic function due to drugs or disease (Figure 5–10). Before therapy is considered, the hemodynamic abnormalities must be carefully analyzed and therapy tailored to correct them.

Physiologic Monitoring (Table 5–6). The patient in shock should be monitored in an intensive-care or coronary-care unit, although some critical observations can be made in any hospital ward. The function of the autonomic nervous system and the adequacy of tissue perfusion can be assessed (Joly and Weil, 1969). The blood volume may be measured by radioactive albumin distribution or estimated by changes in hematocrit in the absence of blood loss. Central venous pressure is a guide to the status of the blood volume as well as to myocardial function, but may be misleading in the presence of chronic lung disease or severe, acute left ventricular failure (e.g., after myocardial infarction) (Cohn, 1967; Prout, 1968; Hamosh and Cohn, 1971). The change in central venous pressure (CVP) (ordinarily not to exceed 15 cm of saline) with intravenous fluid therapy is an indication of myocardial function. In cases of acute left ventricular failure, however, central venous pressure may not be elevated. A flow-directed pulmonary artery catheter has been used experimentally to estimate left ventricular end-diastolic pressure (Scheinman et al., 1969a).

The cardiac output should be measured by standard techniques. Changes in cardiac output can be estimated by changes in mixed venous oxygen saturation, best obtained from the right atrium, right ventricle, or pulmonary artery (Goldman et al., 1968a, 1968b; Scheinman et al., 1969b). Increased cardiac output is reflected by an increased oxygen saturation, assuming that the oxygen concentration in inspired air remains constant. Most important, the physician should do repeated physical examinations, determine the fluid and electrolyte abnormalities and correct them, and use the changes in the electrocardiogram as an index of potential arrhythmias.

In the treatment of shock, drugs should be administered intravenously. During low and variable tissue perfusion, drug absorption from subcutaneous and intramuscular sites is unpredictable (see Chapter 2). *Principle: The early and adequate replacement of fluids, electrolytes, and oxygen may make the response to drugs more predictable and may possibly obviate the need for them.*

Hypovolemic Shock. The major hemodynamic abnormality is decreased venous return to the heart and consequent low cardiac output. The subsequent change in regional vascular resistance favors maintenance of blood flow to vital organs, even though the total peripheral vascular resistance may be normal (Chien, 1967; Forsyth et al., 1970). Effective therapy consists of appropriate fluid replacement using saline, plasma, or blood. If fluid volume is replaced early, no other therapy may be necessary. Whether an "irreversible" stage of shock exists is unknown (Smith and Moore, 1962). It seems logical, however, that cardiac damage may occur during a prolonged period of hypovolemia, perpetuating a low cardiac output and inadequate perfusion of tissues even after volume replacement (Crowell and Guyton, 1962). If cardiac output and tissue flow do not increase when the intravascular volume is replaced, and if an elevated central venous or pulmonary artery pressure indicates myocardial depression, therapy should include agents to treat cardiogenic shock.

Cardiogenic Shock. Therapy of cardiogenic shock is presently inadequate. The mortality rate of the disease is about 75% (Cronin et al., 1965). We have learned more about shock following myocardial infarction by careful monitoring of physiologic variables in patients in coronary-care units. Although low cardiac output and elevated peripheral resistance are common and can lead to poor tissue perfusion, many patients have a normal or low peripheral resistance and variable autonomic responses (Malmcrona and Varnauskas, 1964; Thomas, M., et al., 1966; Kuhn, 1967a; Shillingford and Thomas, 1967a, 1967b). Therapy probably decreases mortality if peripheral and coronary artery perfusion can be returned to adequate levels without unduly increasing myocardial oxygen demand (Braunwald, 1967; Ross, 1967). Much of our confusion related to therapy of cardiogenic shock has been created by conflicts in the literature, probably due to inadequate selection of patients for study. Unless the variable patterns of cardiogenic shock are appreciated and patients are divided into study groups depending on important identifiable and different hemodynamic abnormalities, the results of therapeutic trials will remain uninterpretable (see Chapter 1).

When the patient's disease is characterized by high peripheral resistance and low cardiac output, first-line therapeutic maneuvers are correction of fluid, electrolyte, and acid-base abnormalities. Fluid should be given intravenously until the central venous pressure rises, ordinarily not to exceed 15 cm of saline. The rate of fluid administration can be critical. If small (100-ml) volumes are given rapidly (15 to 30 minutes), and if the central venous pressure rises significantly and only slowly returns to normal, further fluid administration may be dangerous. Such test bolus administration can help to prevent serious and irreversible fluid overload that may occur if infusion rates are slow and prolonged. When replacement of volume is adequate, mental alertness, skin temperature, and arterial pH may revert rapidly to normal. Return of urine volume may be considerably delayed even after blood volume and renal perfusion are normal. Very often, fluid replacement alone is insufficient. In a patient with low cardiac output and elevated peripheral vascular resistance, the choice of isoproterenol is logical, but neither animal studies nor clinical reports have shown unequivocal benefit from isoproterenol (Cronin, 1967; Eichna, 1967; Gunnar et al., 1967; Hood et al., 1967, 1969;

Kuhn *et al.*, 1967; Morse *et al.*, 1967; Smith *et al.*, 1967; Fearon, 1968). Infusion of 1 to 10 μg of isoproterenol per minute should increase the force and rate of cardiac contraction and cardiac output, decrease peripheral vascular resistance and ventricular filling pressures, and restore tissue perfusion. A sinus tachycardia of approximately 130 or increasing ventricular irritability during constant infusions is an indication of the maximum tolerable dose. At times the fall in peripheral vascular resistance produced by isoproterenol is disproportionate to the increase in cardiac output, and arterial pressure cannot be restored sufficiently by fluid replacement to maintain peripheral and coronary artery flow. In such cases it is necessary to increase aortic pressure by using mixed alpha- and beta-stimulating drugs like norepinephrine alone, or in addition to isoproterenol.

Heart failure is an indication for cautious digitalization, but the routine use of cardiac glycosides, although advocated by some (Braunwald, 1967; Mason *et al.*, 1969a), is not recommended because the rapidly changing electrolyte and acid-base balance accompanying shock enhances the probability of digitalis toxicity. In addition, more prompt, more easily controlled, and greater inotropic effects can be obtained with isoproterenol (Beiser *et al.*, 1968a; Selzer, 1968).

Oxygen should be used to increase the arterial pO_2 to normal. Further increasing the pO_2 may be detrimental owing to the direct vascular effects of oxygen. Frequent assessment of the patient's hemodynamic and tissue flow status indicates whether oxygen should be continued.

Morphine is discussed in the section on pulmonary edema, but its routine use in cardiogenic shock is to be discouraged, as it may, by its pharmacologic action, induce hypotension and increase cardiac damage (Thomas *et al.*, 1965b).

When cardiac output is low and peripheral resistance is normal, dopamine seems to be an ideal drug to use after volume deficiencies and electrolyte abnormalities have been corrected (Talley *et al.*, 1969). Until this drug becomes generally available and is carefully tested, however, isoproterenol or isoproterenol plus norepinephrine are good choices.

Atropine is indicated in most patients who have low cardiac outputs, bradycardia, and hypotension. Intravenous administration of 0.4 to 1.5 mg every 3 to 4 hours is the average dose, but low doses may intensify bradycardia owing to atropine's central nervous system effects. Therapy should be discontinued only if there is no desirable effect on cardiac output and tissue flow at a time when there is other evidence of atropine effects, or if intolerable side effects occur in addition to therapeutic effects. Electrical pacing or isoproterenol then become useful. A further discussion of electrical pacing appears on page 208.

When a patient is hypotensive but shows no evidence of decreased tissue perfusion, shock is not present. If peripheral vascular resistance becomes so low that flow to vital organs is decreased, fluid replacement and atropine and/ or norepinephrine therapy may be beneficial. ***Principle: Treatment of the patient with cardiogenic shock must be based on the measured abnormalities present at any specific time. Therapy must be adjusted to the changing hemodynamic state of each individual. A cookbook approach is clearly inadequate. Better understanding of the pathophysiology of a disorder allows greater likelihood of successful treatment.***

Even with the best drug therapy possible, many patients die because a severely damaged myocardium is not able to support the circulation. Mechanical aids to the circulation, though experimental, are the most promising type of nonpharmacologic therapy (Soroff *et al.*, 1969). If the damaged myocardium can be supported by means of drugs or mechanical devices for the first few critical days after infarction, survival rates can be expected to rise.

Septic Shock. Shock associated with gram-negative bacteremia has a complex pathogenesis. It is probably due to the release of endogenous vasoactive peptides (e.g., bradykinin) and amines (e.g., histamine), as well as to direct cellular effects of endotoxin (Hinshaw *et al.*, 1961; Weissmann and Thomas, 1964b; Hjort and Rapaport, 1965; Cline *et al.*, 1968; Nies *et al.*, 1968). Antigen-antibody reactions and activation of complement are important in some of the actions of endotoxin (Cline *et al.*, 1968; Nies and Melmon, 1971; Nies *et al.*, 1971). The early phase of endotoxic shock is characterized by a low peripheral resistance and an essentially normal cardiac output and is a "warm shock" (Hopkins *et al.*, 1965; Wilson *et al.*, 1965, 1967; Nies *et al.*, 1968). Later, as the cardiac output falls and the peripheral resistance rises, the hemodynamic pattern resembles classic cardiogenic shock (Udhoji *et al.*, 1963; Nies *et al.*, 1968). Therapy depends on which phase of shock is being treated, although there have been no studies to prove this. Of established therapeutic value are antibiotics (Weil *et al.*, 1964), volume expansion to tolerance, careful control of acid-base balance, and isoproterenol (du Toit *et al.*, 1966; Kardos, 1966), the latter being most useful in the late phases when cardiac output is low and total peripheral resistance is high.

Rational therapy of the early phase of septic

shock requires further knowledge of the pathogenetic mediators involved. Of value in experimental endotoxic shock but not proved clinically are adrenal corticosteroids, salicylates, antihistamines, and anticomplement drugs, all aimed at trying to prevent the release or the effects of vasoactive mediators of shock. Steroids also have other potentially useful actions, as discussed above. The use of alpha-adrenergic blocking agents or phenothiazines has experimental support, but adequate clinical data are lacking.

Principle: The treatment of all varieties of shock is aimed at increasing tissue perfusion and nutrient capillary blood flow, and not at increasing the blood pressure per se. Accomplishment of the goal is predicted on first clearly defining hemodynamic abnormalities accounting for poor tissue flow; correcting fluid, electrolyte, and acid-base abnormalities; and then choosing a drug whose action will reverse the observed abnormalities. The drug is given until evidence of effect is seen and continued if the effect is salutary. Otherwise therapy must be changed.

UNUSUAL RESPONSES TO CATECHOLAMINES OR ANTIHYPERTENSIVES

Some drug-drug and drug-disease interactions have been mentioned; others are discussed in Chapter 16. Several points deserve re-emphasis. During some disease states, catecholamines may produce effects that are abnormally large or small or qualitatively different from normal (Table 5-9) (Melmon, 1968). The conditions associated with increased sensitivity are due to an alteration of the adrenergic receptors or to a decrease in catecholamine reuptake into nerve endings. In many instances the mechanism is unknown.

A decrease in sensitivity to catecholamines is associated with acidosis, myxedema, or Addison's disease. A defect in receptor responsivity seems likely. In patients with the carcinoid syndrome or in patients taking alpha-adrenergic blocking drugs (e.g., phenothiazines), vasodepressor responses to catecholamines may be seen. The carcinoid tumor may release vasodilator peptides and the alpha-adrenergic blockade can prevent all but the beta-stimulating effects of catecholamines, resulting in a fall in pressure.

The response to antihypertensive drugs varies markedly from person to person. Genetic factors may be important; there is evidence that Negroes respond to therapy less well than

Caucasians (Howard and Tiedeman, 1967). Drugs can diminish the response to some antihypertensive agents by blocking entry to receptors or by displacing them from the site of action, as has been discussed for guanethidine.

Table 5-9. SOME CONDITIONS CHARACTERIZED BY ALTERED SENSITIVITY TO CATECHOLAMINES*

Conditions associated with increased sensitivity

Cardiomegaly
   Congestive heart failure
   Hypertrophy—secondary to physical obstruction
      or increase in peripheral vascular resistance
   Myocardiopathy of various etiologies
Thyrotoxicosis
Sympathetic denervation
   Diabetes mellitus
   Surgical or anesthetic procedures
   Orthostatic hypotension
Nutritional abnormalities
   Scurvy
Unclassified diseases
   Familial dysautonomia
Drugs
   Imipramine
   Some antiadrenergic drugs (e.g., guanethidine and
      reserpine)

Conditions associated with decreased sensitivity

Acidosis—metabolic or respiratory
Myxedema
Adrenal insufficiency

Conditions associated with paradoxical effects

Diseases
   Carcinoid syndrome
Drug administration
   Phenothiazine and congeners

* From Melmon, K. L.: Catecholamines and the adrenal medulla. In Williams, R. H. (ed.): *Textbook of Endocrinology*, 4th ed. W. B. Saunders Co., Philadelphia, 1968.

Patients with central nervous system lesions may experience a greater-than-usual response to parenteral reserpine (Leonberg *et al.*, 1964), and hypovolemic, hypertensive patients may go into shock after small doses of antihypertensive drugs (Cohn, 1966).

Principle: In treating shock and hypertension, there is no standard dose or regimen that always works; each patient must be evaluated individually and treated as a therapeutic experiment (see Chapter 1). *Only in this way can patients who require more or less drug or a different drug than the "usual patient" be adequately and safely treated.*

II. ALTERATION OF CARDIAC FUNCTION WITHOUT SHOCK

CHARACTERISTICS OF THE DISEASE STATE

Congestive Heart Failure

The clinical syndrome of congestive heart failure results from an inability of the heart to pump sufficient blood to satisfy the body's needs (Stead et al., 1948). Although the fundamental cause of myocardial failure is unknown, the biochemical defect involves an abnormal conversion of chemical energy (as adenosine triphosphate) to mechanical work (Braunwald et al., 1966; Weissler, 1968).

Volume Loading. When the heart begins to fail as a pump, compensatory mechanisms to maintain cardiac output appear. Renal sodium and water retention occurs early in heart failure, the kidney responding as if excessive aldosterone and antidiuretic hormone were being secreted. This response is associated with an increase in blood volume. The augmented intravascular blood volume increases venous return, which lengthens the myocardial fibers at end diastole and increases stroke volume (Starling's law) (Figure 5–11, page 174). The pathophysiologic basis for sodium and water retention during congestive heart failure could be a response to increased sympathetic nervous system activity and to intrarenal redistribution of blood flow to glomeruli associated with long tubules, where relatively long tubular transit times would favor reabsorption (Barger, 1966; Wolff et al., 1966; Earley and Daugharty, 1969) (see Chapter 3). The relative roles and interplay of hormonal and sympathetic nervous system mechanisms in the disordered fluid and electrolyte balance of congestive heart failure are not yet known.

Adrenergic Stimulation. Another major mechanism of compensation for the failing heart is an augmentation of sympathetic nervous activity (as shown by tachycardia, vasoconstriction, and sweating), with increased plasma concentrations of norepinephrine during stress and increased urinary excretion of norepinephrine at rest (Chidsey et al., 1962, 1965). Catecholamines increase cardiac output by augmenting myocardial contractility (positive inotropic effects) (Figure 5–11, page 174), and by increasing cardiac rate (positive chronotropic effects). During chronic heart failure, cardiac norepinephrine stores become depleted but cardiac responsiveness to catecholamines may be enhanced (Chidsey et al., 1965; Shaffer and Katz, 1967; Vogel et al., 1968), and the function of the sympathetic nervous system remains critical in maintaining cardiac output. Interference with the adrenergic support of myocardial contractility by reserpine, guanethidine, or beta-adrenergic blockade may significantly worsen congestive heart failure (Gaffney and Braunwald 1963; Epstein and Braunwald, 1966b).

The symptoms of congestive heart failure are infrequently due to diminished cardiac output. During the early phases of heart failure, the cardiac output is not greatly reduced, and the symptoms are related to the "side effects" of the compensatory mechanisms. Sodium and water retention leads to elevated venous pressure, pulmonary vascular congestion, and peripheral edema. The increased sympathetic activity produces tachycardia, sweating, and vasoconstriction. Treatment of these symptoms of compensation without improving myocardial function (e.g., treating arrhythmias with myocardial depressants, mild increased peripheral resistance with antiadrenergic agents, or pulmonary vascular congestion with diuretics) may decrease cardiac output, eliciting symptoms of weakness and fatigability (Stampfer et al., 1968). *Principle: Treatment of congestive heart failure should improve cardiac function without undermining the compensatory mechanisms of the body.*

Acute Pulmonary Edema

Acute pulmonary edema usually occurs in the presence of underlying heart disease and is precipitated by an event that causes either an acute decrease in left ventricular output or a rapid increase in venous return or right ventricular output (Table 5–10). The result is to

Table 5–10. COMMON EVENTS PRECIPITATING PULMONARY EDEMA

1. Acute myocardial infarction, ruptured chorda tendineae
2. Cardiac arrhythmias
3. Acute fluid or salt overload
4. Acute hypertension
5. Exercise
6. Drugs
   a. Cardiac depressants (quinidine)
   b. Sympatholytics (beta blockers, guanethidine)
   c. Alpha-adrenergic stimulators (norepinephrine, methoxamine, phenylephrine)
7. Pulmonary emboli
8. Infection

increase pulmonary capillary hydrostatic pressure above a critical level (25 to 40 mm Hg). This level is determined by plasma oncotic pressure, the permeability of the pulmonary capillaries, tissue resistance to edema formation, and the capacity of pulmonary lymphatics to remove fluid. Fluid escapes from the capillaries, collects in interstitial spaces surrounding vessels and airways, and is returned to the general circulation by the pulmonary lymphatics. With increased transudation of fluid, the resorptive capacity of the lymphatics is overwhelmed and fluid begins to collect in the alveoli, producing the characteristic signs and symptoms of pulmonary edema (Luisada, 1964; Staub et al., 1967; Hultgren and Flamm, 1969). In chronic pulmonary capillary hypertension (e.g., in mitral stenosis), extensive perivascular fibrosis leads to increased tissue resistance to edema formation or to a greater capacity for lymphatic removal of fluid, accounting for tolerance of relatively high pulmonary venous pressures without pulmonary edema.

CATEGORIES OF DRUGS AND THERAPEUTIC PRINCIPLES

Cardiac Glycosides

Inotropic and Extracardiac Effects. Digitalis exerts positive inotropic effects in both normal and diseased hearts. The effect on cardiac output, however, is modulated by the extracardiac effects of digitalis as well as by normal homeostatic mechanisms. In the normal subject, arteriolar and venous constriction is produced by digitalis, and the increased peripheral vascular resistance and bradycardia tend to negate the effects of increased contractility. The cardiac output in normals thus may remain steady or may actually fall. Vasoconstriction is not a prominent effect of digitalis in patients with heart failure because vascular tone is already increased by adrenergic activity. Moreover, reflex vasodilation appears to counter the primary vascular effects of digitalis in patients with heart failure (Mason and Braunwald, 1964b, 1968; Mason et al., 1969a). Thus, although patients with congestive heart failure respond to digitalis with increased cardiac output, the result depends on the interplay of cardiac and extracardiac effects of the glycosides. Experimentally the inotropic effects of digitalis increase linearly with increasing dose (Williams et al., 1966; Helfant et al., 1967c). However, the near maximum increases in contractility can precede severe loss of intracellular potassium, usually associated with evidence of conduction abnormalities such as ventricular premature beats. Since there is no "threshold" for the contractile effects of digitalis, the inotropic effects seen at low doses may be sufficient clinically without risking toxicity. Therefore, the use of digitalis for its positive inotropic effects usually does not require the induction of arrhythmias, as is supposed by some clinicians who feel the "need" to increase doses until toxic effects are seen in the patient. The proper use of digitalis was well described over 150 years ago:

> The proper dose of a medicine is undoubtedly that quantity which produces the effect required, whatever be its numerical denomination. A full dose of foxglove is, therefore, merely a relative term.
>
> To one patient one-half grain may be a full dose; to another, six or eight grains may be given, not only without inconvenience, but without producing any sensible effect.
>
> These varieties of sensibility and habit can only be ascertained by beginning with the lowest dose and increasing it with the most scrupulous care.
>
> The patient's pulse must be examined from hour to hour, and on its first tendency to flag, or on the slightest indication of sickness, the exhibition of the medicine must be suspended (Ferriar, 1816).

Principle: Measure the therapeutic responses such as changes in venous pressure, pulse rate, diastolic gallop rhythm, and diuresis as guidelines to adequacy of digitalization. Patients are quite variable in response to digitalis, and digitalis toxicity is dangerous.

Effect of Digitalis on Heart Rate. Digitalis can slow ventricular heart rates during normal sinus rhythm or during supraventricular tachy-arrhythmias by several mechanisms. Sinus tachycardia is common during congestive heart failure because of enhanced sympathetic nervous system activity. Because digitalis improves myocardial function and cardiac output in these patients, the general reflex sympathetic activity decreases, as does nerve discharge to the sino-atrial node. This mechanism of cardiac slowing is indirect and does not occur if the sinus tachycardia is due to some other cause. Thyro-toxic patients, for example, continue to have tachycardia even when fully digitalized; they become digitalis intoxicated if restoration of normal heart rate is the sole criterion of administration of the drug.

Digitalis indirectly slows the heart by a second mechanism, that is, increasing cardiac sensitivity to vagal stimulation. This "vagotonic" action of digitalis seems to be more prominent in animals than in man (Modell, 1966). Nonetheless, vagolytic drugs such as atropine are useful in the treatment of bradycardias induced by digitalis.

Another mechanism for cardiac slowing involves the direct action of digitalis to depress atrioventricular (AV) nodal conductivity (dro-motropic effect). Digitalis decreases AV con-duction velocity and lengthens the refractory period of the AV node. Therapeutic doses of digitalis may prolong the P-R interval, but this effect is not ordinarily of clinical consequence. Larger doses can cause second- or third-degree heart block, which is undesirable during normal sinus rhythm but therapeutic in supraventricular tachycardias with rapid ventricular response. In atrial fibrillation with rapid ventricular response, the dromotropic effect of digitalis on the AV node slows the ventricular response and may be the major therapeutic effect. This is particularly true in patients with mitral stenosis; slowing the ventricular rate greatly enhances diastolic filling of the left ventricle and increases cardiac output (Beiser et al., 1968b). Digitalis toxicity is a relative term. At the same dosage, digitalis may produce a major therapeutic effect in slowing the ventricular response during a supraventricular tachyarrhythmia, but may produce dangerous and deleterious AV block during normal sinus rhythm. Literally one man's cure becomes another's poison; a cure in one circumstance can be a poison in another.

Atrioventricular conductivity is further de-pressed by vagal stimulation and severe hyper-kalemia, whereas sympathetic stimulation facili-tates AV conduction (Linhart et al., 1965; Ogden et al., 1969). Thus multiple factors affecting AV nodal conductivity are operative clinically. For example, in the patient with atrial fibrillation, congestive heart failure, and excess sympathetic

stimulation, digitalis can decrease the ventricu-lar response both by directly depressing AV conduction and by indirectly decreasing sympathetic stimulation as the congestive heart failure is corrected. In the treatment of digitalis-induced heart block, isoproterenol may im-prove AV conduction, whereas potassium administration may induce hyperkalemia, which may increase the degree of heart block. The AV node is subject to multiple influences. The expected effects of digitalis can be modulated by the autonomic nervous system, serum potassium concentrations, and the presence of other drugs.

Cellular Effects. Considerable information is available on the cellular effects of digitalis and the relationship of these effects to the inotropic and toxic manifestations of the drug. The earliest observations on the cellular actions of digitalis were related to the inhibition by toxic doses of sodium- and potassium-activated adenosine triphosphatase at the cell membrane, resulting in a loss of intracellular potassium and an increase in intracellular sodium (Glynn, 1957, 1964). This action of digitalis *in vitro* is reversed by increasing the extracellular potassium ion concentration (Palmer and Nechay, 1964) and may account for some of the electrophysiologic changes and clinical arrhythmias seen with toxic doses of digitalis (see page 190). Consistent with this hypothesis is the observation that *in vivo* digitalis toxicity is associated with myocardial potassium loss. Administration of potassium ion, quinidine, diphenylhydantoin, or large doses of pronethalol, or the induction of hypo-thermia not only protects against digitalis toxic arrhythmias but also prevents the digitalis-induced myocardial potassium loss (Williams et al., 1966; Damato, 1969; El-Fiky and Katzung, 1969). The major known biochemical defect in digitalis intoxication is intracellular potassium depletion. Correction of this defect should be the major concern of the clinician. Antiarrhythmic drugs may be of some assistance, but potassium replacement is a more desirable and specific intervention. Potassium must be given with care, however, lest hyperkalemia be produced.

The cellular basis for the inotropic effects of digitalis is probably enhancement of excitation-contraction coupling, that process by which chemical energy is converted into mechanical energy when triggered by membrane depolariza-tion. Most evidence relates this process to entry of calcium ions into the cell during depolariza-tion of the membrane and/or to release of calcium from intracellular binding sites on the sarcoplasmic reticulum. The free calcium ion mediates the interaction of actin and myosin, and contraction results. Digitalis may increase the net influx of calcium into the cell and may release calcium from the intracellular binding sites. Whether the effects of digitalis on calcium ion are related to the membrane effects on sodium and potassium is subject to debate (Glynn, 1964; Govier and Holland, 1965; Lyon and DeGraff, 1966a; Weatherall, 1966; Izquierdo and Izquierdo, 1967; Koch-Weser, 1967; Moran, 1967; Mason and Braunwald, 1968; Mason et al., 1969a). Calcium ion and digitalis have additive inotropic and toxic effects. Calcium administration is contra-indicated during digitalis toxicity, and digitalis administration is dangerous during hyper-calcemia.

Uptake of Digitalis by the Myocardium. The inotropic (contractile) effects of digitalis are not dependent upon myocardial catecholamine stores (Spann et al., 1964). Reserpine, however, diminishes the myocardial response to digitalis in experimental animals (Tanz, 1964), probably by decreasing the myocardial uptake of digitalis (Marcus et al., 1968). Whether this effect of reserpine is due to altered hemodynamics or to alteration of binding sites for digitalis is un-known. Clinically, doses of reserpine used for the chronic treatment of hypertension have no discernible effect on the inotropic response to digitalis (Marcus et al., 1968). Sinus brady-cardia may be seen, however, when reserpine or guanethidine is given with digitalis, the blunting of sympathetic activity apparently unmasking the relatively weak vagomimetic action of digitalis.

The concentration of sodium and potassium ions in serum alters the myocardial concentra-tion of radiolabeled (^{3}H) digoxin. Hypo-natremia and hyperkalemia reduce the myo-cardial concentration of digoxin, whereas hypokalemia increases the concentration of digoxin in the heart (Cohn, K. E., et al., 1967; Marcus et al., 1967a; Harrison and Wakim, 1969). These findings merit consideration in predicting, avoiding, and treating digitalis toxicity.

Metabolism. Pharmacokinetic data have been difficult to obtain, because a good assay for the glycosides has been lacking until the recent development of an immunoassay (Smith, T. W., et al., 1969). Many of the data have been ob-tained using ^{3}H- or ^{14}C-labeled materials and require confirmation by the more specific assays. The glycosides vary widely in their water solubility, gastrointestinal absorption, extent of metabolism, and excretion (Lyon and DeGraff, 1966b; Doherty, 1968; Wilson, 1969). Digitoxin, a nonpolar (lipid-soluble) compound, is com-pletely absorbed orally, bound to plasma proteins, and extensively metabolized by the liver to active (digoxin) and inactive chemicals. The approximate biologic half-life ($t_{1/2}$) for digitoxin in the body is 7 days, and effects may persist for weeks (Okita et al., 1955). Digoxin is more polar, 80 to 90% absorbed orally, not bound to plasma proteins, and excreted largely unchanged in the urine. The biologic half-life for digoxin averages 1.5 days (Doherty et al., 1961; Marcus et al., 1966, 1967b; Jelliffe, 1968). An occasional patient may eliminate digoxin rapidly or may absorb it poorly from the gastro-intestinal tract and is thus resistant to the therapeutic action of conventional doses (Luchi and Gruber, 1968). Renal failure increases the $t_{1/2}$ of digoxin, a fact that is important clinically (Doherty et al., 1964; Jelliffe, 1968). Con-versely, hepatectomy in rodents increases the $t_{1/2}$ of digitoxin (St. George et al., 1952), suggesting the need for caution in patients with liver disease.

Studies in man have emphasized the im-portance of the concentration of the drug in plasma and of the biochemical half-life of the drug in plasma (Smith and Haber, 1970; Doherty, 1971). It is assumed that drug con-centration in tissues is more important than the concentration in plasma, but that the concen-tration in tissues is related to the plasma level when a steady state had been established. This assumption has experimental support; in dogs the half-times of disappearance of digoxin from blood, kidney, urine, liver, and myocardium are similar (Doherty and Perkins, 1966a).

Interaction with Thyroid Disease. Thyroid disease alters the patient's response to digitalis. Hyperthyroid patients are relatively resistant to cardiac glycosides; hypothyroid patients are very sensitive to these drugs and readily develop arrhythmias. Two experimental observations help to explain these clinical findings. First, after a standard dose the concentrations of tritiated digoxin in serum are inversely related to thyroid activity; hypothyroid patients have the highest concentrations and hyperthyroid patients the lowest (Doherty and Perkins, 1966b). Second, the inotropic response of the isolated cat papillary muscle to digitalis is inversely related to thyroid activity (Buccino et al., 1967). The reasons for the altered inotropic effect found in vitro are unknown, but the findings may have important clinical implications when digitalis is given to patients with thyroid disease.

Other Agents Acting in Heart Failure

Diuretics. The actions of the diuretics and the principles of their use, singly and in com-bination, are discussed in Chapter 3. Some of the special considerations in the treatment of heart failure are discussed later in this section.

Opium Alkaloids. Morphine is efficacious in the management of acute pulmonary edema. Its beneficial effects are related to its direct vasodilator action; in monkeys and probably in man it can selectively increase blood flow to the brain and coronary blood vessels while decreasing actual flow only to bronchial vessels and the diaphragm (Miller *et al.*, 1970). Arteriolar and venous dilation causes pooling of blood in the peripheral circulation, thereby decreasing venous return, cardiac work, and pulmonary venous pressure and shifting blood from the central to the peripheral circulation (Henney *et al.*, 1966). The inotropic effect of morphine, sometimes seen in experimental animals, is an indirect effect related to release of catecholamines (Vasko *et al.*, 1966). Morphine should be used carefully in patients with myocardial infarction (Thomas *et al.*, 1965b) or limited myocardial contractile reserve, since a marked fall in cardiac output and blood pressure may attend the drug-induced peripheral vasodilation and bradycardia. Such falls in blood pressure were previously attributed to release of histamine by morphine, but recent data cast some doubt on this theory and point to the direct effect of morphine in redistributing blood flow even before gross changes in hemodynamics can be measured.

Sensitization of the vestibular apparatus by morphine may lead to nausea and vomiting, and histamine release by morphine may trigger bronchospasm in asthmatic individuals (Comroe and Dripps, 1948; Eckenhoff and Oech, 1960). The effects of morphine on the blood pressure and vestibular apparatus are most obvious when the patient is in the upright position, which is favored for the treatment of pulmonary edema (Drew *et al.*, 1946; Comroe and Dripps, 1948). *Principle: The adverse effects of a drug may have to be tolerated in order to gain maximum therapeutic efficacy.*

Xanthines. Combination of a xanthine (theophylline) with ethylenediamine is aminophylline. The beneficial actions of the xanthines on the cardiovascular system are: (1) they have a cardiac inotropic effect; and (2) they dilate arterioles and veins, leading to a reduction of peripheral vascular resistance and to venous pooling with decreased venous return. These events summate and shift blood from the central to the peripheral circulation, thus decreasing cardiac work. (3) They dilate bronchi and relieve bronchospasm, which may occur during acute pulmonary congestion; and (4) they produce a diuresis by increasing cardiac output and glomerular filtration rate owing to a direct dilating action on the efferent arterioles of the kidneys. In most instances, amino-

phylline is used for its cardiac and vascular effects. Occasionally, it may be useful as an adjunct or synergist to other diuretic therapy. However, since the introduction of the potent diuretics, furosemide and ethacrynic acid, the diuretic properties of aminophylline are rarely needed (see Chapter 3).

Intravenous aminophylline must be given slowly, particularly when a patient is in shock or has severe mitral stenosis or aortic stenosis. Theophylline is insoluble in water at physiologic pH; the ethylenediamine is added as a solubilizer. Rapid injection may cause theophylline to precipitate, and some of the toxic effects of rapid injection may be due to precipitation within the vascular system and to subsequent embolization.

Mechanical Methods. The acutely elevated pulmonary capillary pressure in pulmonary edema can be very quickly altered by mechanical means rather than or in addition to pharmacologic maneuvers. The upright position and the use of limb tourniquets trap blood in the peripheral circulation. Rapid removal of 200 to 600 ml of blood from a large vein acutely lowers venous return to the right heart and thus decreases the central blood volume. Often these simple procedures can be extremely effective and relatively safe and should not be dismissed in favor of potent, dangerous drugs that may accomplish the same end. *Principle: Time-honored, safe, simple procedures may be more effective and less risky than potent and potentially dangerous drugs.*

Intermittent positive pressure breathing (IPPB) may be valuable. IPPB increases intrathoracic pressure, thereby decreasing venous return and right-heart output. In addition, when pulmonary intra-alveolar pressure is increased, fluid transudation from the capillaries is decreased (Miller and Sproule, 1959). *Principle: When therapy is beneficial, the more conservative the approach and the more tolerable the gradual improvement, the less likely a complication of therapy is to occur.*

CLINICAL THERAPY

Treatment of Congestive Heart Failure

The goal of therapy is to improve myocardial function so that the compensatory mechanisms are no longer required, while maintaining or restoring to normal the cardiac output and tissue perfusion. When congestive heart failure first appears in a patient or when a steady state of compensation deteriorates, an intensive search for underlying mechanisms is mandatory. Several conditions or diseases can cause or aggravate congestive heart failure. The most common include voluntary omission of medication, dietary indiscretion leading to increased salt and water ingestion, increased physical activity, a silent but acute myocardial infarction, a pulmonary embolus, an intercurrent infection, hypoxia, or a sudden arrhythmia. A more inclusive list of conditions that must be considered in all patients who are refractory to therapy or who develop increasing heart failure without obvious cause appears in Table 5–11.

Table 5–11. DISEASE CAUSING OR AGGRAVATING CONGESTIVE HEART FAILURE

1. *Increased demand for blood flow*
   a. Cirrhosis of the liver
   b. Hyperthyroidism
   c. Anemia
   d. Pregnancy
   e. Arteriovenous fistula
   f. Beriberi heart disease (thiamine deficiency)
   g. Paget's disease
   h. Intracardiac shunts
   i. Intercurrent infection including pneumonia leading to hypoxia
2. *Obstruction to flow*
   a. Extracardiac
      (1) Hypertension
      (2) Pulmonary vascular obstruction
         (a) Chronic emphysema
         (b) Acute or multiple pulmonary emboli
         (c) Primary vascular disease
         (d) Other (foreign material, i.e., in drug addicts; parasites)
   b. Cardiac
      (1) Valvular stenosis
      (2) Supravalvular or subvalvular stenosis
      (3) Constrictive pericarditis
3. *Fluid retention*
   a. Acute nephritis
   b. Hyperadrenocorticism
4. *Myocardial lesions*
   a. Myocardial infarction
      (1) Arrhythmia
      (2) Ventricular aneurysm
      (3) Papillary muscle dysfunction
   b. Bacterial endocarditis
   c. Acute rheumatic fever
   d. Alcoholic myocardiopathy
   e. Idiopathic myocardiopathy
   f. Toxic—diphtheria
   g. Collagen disease
   h. Catecholamine myocardiopathy—pheochromocytoma or prolonged therapy with catecholamines
   i. Parasites—Chagas' disease
   j. Infiltrative—scleroderma, hemochromatosis, amyloidosis, endomyocardial fibrosis

Treatment of the underlying disease may partially or completely correct the heart failure. Most patients, however, require medical therapy to improve myocardial function. The response to medical therapy can often be predicted by the type of lesion producing failure. Heart failure due to obstructive lesions, which mechanically limit flow, does not respond unless ventricular disease is also present (which is usually the case except in pure mitral stenosis, when pulmonary congestion rather than heart failure may be prominent), and maximum response cannot be obtained until the obstruction (valvular or pericardial constriction) is relieved. Patients without obstructive lesions may respond well. However, even during initial therapy, those with infiltrative cardiomyopathies or idiopathic cardiomyopathies may respond poorly to digitalis. Eventually all patients with congestive heart failure respond poorly to digitalis, because the drug does not act on the primary pathophysiologic process. *Principle: The pathophysiologic basis of the patient's symptoms, as well as the severity and stage of the disease, profoundly influences the choice of therapy and the expected results of any procedure. If possible, treat the cause of a disease rather than its manifestations.*

Digitalis Glycosides. Digitalis, bed rest, and salt restriction are the time-honored and primary therapeutic interventions for treating heart failure. The use of diuretics has been added recently. Only digitalis can directly increase myocardial contractility; other measures may be important but are nonspecific (see Chapter 14). Diuretics are first-line drugs only when gross volume overload is apparent, and in most cases diuretics alone do not increase cardiac output. If possible, diuretics should not be used unless the full effect from digitalis has been obtained, cardiac failure persists, and the patient is uncomfortable because of volume overload (experiences dyspnea on exertion, paroxysmal nocturnal dyspnea, ascites, or peripheral edema). If these drugs are used only when necessary, the problems of volume depletion, electrolyte abnormalities, and the considerable toxicity of diuretics are avoided. In addition, the adequacy of digitalization can be judged with greater precision when diuretics have not been used.

Choice of Preparation. The choice of a preparation of digitalis should depend on the need for rapid effects, the available route of administration, and the desired duration of action for the particular patient. The most frequently used preparations are lanatoside C and ouabain when intravenous preparations are necessary and rapid onset and short duration of action are desirable. Digoxin is commonly given either intravenously or orally; it has a moderately rapid onset of effect and a medium duration of action. Digitoxin and digitalis leaf are given orally but have a slow onset and a long duration of action. The difference between these latter two drugs probably is substantial. Digitoxin is a pure substance and can be relied upon to produce consistent effects if the clinical situation remains stable. However, digitalis leaf is standardized by methods that do not necessarily depend on the effects of the pill's content of digitalis glycoside. In addition, different batches of the preparation may have varying ratios of active glycosides. Therefore, this preparation cannot be relied upon to give predictable results when different batches are used or when the disease state changes. In some ways the choice between the leaf preparation and the pure drug is analogous to the choice between desiccated thyroid and either synthetic triiodothyronine or thyroxine (see Chapter 7). Since digoxin can be used intravenously and orally, and since its duration of action or toxicity is relatively short compared with that of digitoxin, digoxin is commonly used in many circumstances for initial digitalization and maintenance therapy, especially in patients with unstable features in their disease.

Loading Dose. To obtain a rapid onset of action, a large initial dose of digitalis is followed by smaller maintenance doses. The advantages and dangers of a loading dose are discussed in Chapter 2. The initial dose is designed to rapidly achieve high concentrations of the drug in blood and tissues; the maintenance dose is a fraction of the loading dose equal to the daily loss rate of digitalis from the body. Since the disappearance of digitalis glycosides from the body follows first-order kinetics, the amount excreted per day is a fixed percentage of the amount in the body. Approximately 35% of the digoxin and 10% of the digitoxin in the body are excreted per day (Modell, 1966; Jelliffe, 1968). If the loading dose is chosen correctly, the daily dose to maintain a constant amount of drug in the body is 35% of the loading dose for digoxin and 10% of the loading dose for digitoxin. However, no matter what loading dose is chosen, over a long period (exceeding five half-lives) the final concentration of drug in the body is determined by the daily maintenance dose (Figure 5–12). This fact has led some authors to advocate digitalization without a loading dose (Marcus *et al.,* 1967b). Theoretically greater than 90% of the final drug concentration is achieved in four half-lives of the drug and 96% in five half-lives. For a drug with a short half-life (e.g., digoxin $t_{1/2} = 1.5$ days), the maximum concentration of drug in blood and tissue is achieved in 6 to 8 days in the absence of a loading dose. These predictions conform to experimental observations in man. For many patients, the accumulation interval may be too long. However, since the inotropic effects of

digitalis are essentially linear, some effect occurs even at low blood and tissue concentrations (Williams *et al.,* 1966). Given a drug with a long half-life (e.g., digitoxin $t_{1/2} = 7$ days) a digitalizing dose most often is necessary because administration of maintenance doses would not achieve maximum therapeutic effects for a month or more (Figure 5–12).

During renal failure, the half-life of digoxin is lengthened. If conventional maintenance doses are given, therapeutic effect is seen earlier, but digitalis toxicity almost inevitably ensues if a standard maintenance dose of digoxin is continued.

Implicit in the above discussion is the assumption that the necessary loading or maintenance dose can be accurately estimated. Unfortunately, this is not the case, as too many other variables (e.g., different etiologies of heart failure, electrolyte balance, thyroid function, duration of disease, etc.) influence response. Despite advances in the knowledge of cardioactive glycosides, it has not been possible to elucidate all the mechanisms or variations in patients that account for the wide range of digitalizing and maintenance doses. The "average dose" as given in texts of pharmacology was derived from empiric observations of the response to ventricular rate in atrial fibrillation and of the occurrence of frank toxicity produced by "single doses." These dose ranges are applicable to a population of patients, but may be inappropriate for a given case. In hospitalized patients, these "conventional doses" result in a high (20%) incidence of toxic manifestations (Rodensky and Wassermann, 1961). When the drug is given with undue timidity, incomplete digitalization and ineffective levels are obtained. The only way to properly digitalize a patient is to individualize the dose and carefully observe the responses. Keep your eye on the patient and not on the "series." One of the most dangerous logical fallacies that confounds the therapist is the concept of "conventional dose." A patient may be placed in a series, but the therapist may not apply probability data from a series to a given patient unless he is willing to accept gross error rates, randomly determined.

Evaluation of Degree of Digitalization. There is no simple test specific for digitalis effects. The most reliable way to follow a patient's digitalization is by careful, repeated physical examinations. Disappearance of a ventricular gallop, a decrease in hepatic and cardiac size, relief of elevated venous pressure, and disappearance of peripheral edema and pulmonary congestion are signs of effective therapy. Daily measurements of weight, urine volume, and urinary sodium excretion are helpful. Valsalva's maneu-

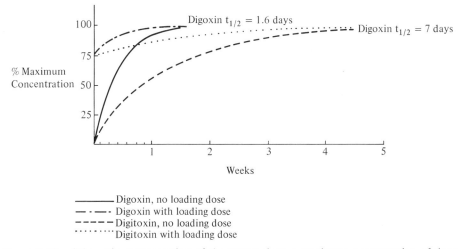

Figure 5–12. Schematic representation of the approach to a maximum concentration of drug in the body. The maximum concentration is 90% attained by four half-lives, 6.4 days with digoxin and 4 weeks with digitoxin. If too large a maintenance dose is used, toxicity may be slow to develop because of the gradual accumulation of drug. If a loading dose is used to rapidly establish 75% of the maximum concentration, final equilibrium is still reached over a period of four half-lives, but therapeutic or toxic concentrations may be attained much more rapidly (see Chapter 2 also).

ver may be utilized to follow the resolution of failure in the patient with a normal autonomic nervous system (Figure 5–1, page 144). The characteristic square-wave response observed during congestive failure is due to a constant cardiac output during the straining phase, which results from the large central blood volume necessary to maintain increased atrial and ventricular filling pressures. Because the volume is expanded, cardiac output does not drop during the straining phase and baroreceptors are not activated; therefore, no vasoconstriction occurs. When the high intrathoracic pressure is released, stroke volume does not increase suddenly against a constricted peripheral vasculature, and neither overshoot of blood pressure nor bradycardia ensues (Sharpey-Schafer, 1953; Judson et al., 1955; Stone et al., 1965). With a total evaluation of the patient, the progress of digitalization can usually be satisfactorily followed. Another end point that cannot always be avoided is the appearance of early toxicity. This is an indication to withhold digitalis and is discussed later (page 190).

The only direct indications of the effect of digitalis are an increase in force of contraction as measured by a strain gauge sutured to the heart, the rate of rise of pressure (dp/dt) measured during systole with an intracardiac pressure transducer, or the rate of change of myocardial fiber length during systole (dl/dt) measured by cineangiography. Although these measurements have been made in man, they are not yet clinically applicable. A recent report suggests using the systolic ejection time as measured by an external-carotid-pulse-wave recording device. Shortening of the time from the beginning of the pulse to the dicrotic notch, corrected for heart rate, is said to correlate with digitalis effect (Weissler et al., 1966). Broader experience with this test is necessary to determine its clinical usefulness.

Maintenance Dose. As Modell (1966) has pointed out, the digitalizing dose is usually chosen with much thought, discussion, and observation of the patient, but after the initial response, the patient is placed on a standard maintenance dose and put on the "back burner." Since the maintenance dose ultimately determines the concentration of drug in tissues, choice of this dose is all-important. When the wrong choice has been made, the full effects may not be apparent for 7 to 30 days depending on the half-life of the preparation used. It is easy for the patient who is "already digitalized" to gradually become under- or overdigitalized on the basis of a wrong maintenance dose, even without the additive effect of electrolyte shifts. Despite these precautions, some patients become digitalis toxic since in their case the therapeutic effects are seen at doses near toxicity. The appearance of digitalis intoxication requires explanation, and the reason can usually be clarified by investigation of the patient. The entire history of digitalis administration should be reviewed to determine whether the maintenance dose was too large or whether the toxicity was due entirely or in part to electrolyte or acid-base disturbance, changing renal function, other drugs, a worsening of chronic lung disease, or other predisposing factors. If no precipitating cause for toxicity is found, the maintenance dose was probably too large. Patients must not repeatedly be made digitalis toxic by using "standard," "textbook-ordained" maintenance doses, and patients should be carefully observed for at least three to five half-lives of the drug after each change in dose. The incidence of digitalis toxicity is high and its consequences are costly. Every effort should be made to avoid digitalis toxity in man, as it is associated with a high incidence of mortality (see Chapter 15). *Principle: More than any other commonly used drug, digitalis must be used only in the doses necessary to achieve a predetermined goal.* Only in this way can the high incidence of serious digitalis toxicity be reduced.

Diuretics. *Therapeutic Goals.* Many physicians prescribe a diuretic for initial treatment of heart failure without defining their therapeutic aims. Often diuretics are not needed, but if the response to digitalis and salt restriction is insufficient, diuretics are valuable adjunctive therapy. What is the therapeutic goal? Edema fluid is unsightly, but peripheral edema is no hazard to the patient. The effect presumably desired is to decrease the blood volume and in this way to decrease pulmonary vascular congestion, peripheral edema, and symptoms due to the edema.

Many physicians think that diuretic therapy increases cardiac output. This misconception stems from experimental observations that overloading the heart eventually decreases cardiac output. Cardiac function curves obtained experimentally show that beyond a certain point, further myocardial fiber stretch decreases the force of contraction: the descending limb of the Starling curve (Braunwald *et al.*, 1966, 1969). In chronic congestive heart failure in man, however, the descending limb of the Starling curve is never seen. A careful study in nine patients of the effects of diuretics on exercise capacity showed that diuresis was associated with a *decrease* in cadiac output in all nine, but with an improvement in symptoms and exercise tolerance in eight (Stampfer *et al.*, 1968). One patient became significantly worse. The beneficial effects of diuretics, therefore, seem to be related to a decrease in pulmonary venous pressure during exercise and to a decrease in cardiac size, cardiac output, and systemic and pulmonary arterial pressure, resulting in a decrease in cardiac work. The effects of diuretics contrast with those of digitalis,

which increase the cardiac output at rest and exercise and thus improve the function of the heart as a pump (Braunwald *et al.*, 1969).

Patients can be made worse by diuretics. In such patients, the decrease in blood volume and cardiac output dominates the clinical picture, causing symptoms of malaise, listlessness, and postural hypotension, and signs of diminished tissue perfusion such as mental confusion and prerenal azotemia. Patients with these symptoms or signs may be at "dry weight," but they feel and perform better with a larger blood volume and even with some peripheral edema (Braunwald *et al.*, 1969). *Principle: Diuretic therapy to rid patients of all traces of edema is not necessary and may be harmful.*

Choice of Drug. For those patients who require diuretic therapy, one of the benzothiadiazides may be most useful. Intermittent injections of mercurials may be helpful in some cases, particularly when renal freewater clearance is compromised, as manifested by hyponatremia and relatively concentrated urine. The use of the very potent diuretics ethacrynic acid or furosemide as initial diuretic therapy in mild disease states is to be condemned. Volume depletion and significant electrolyte abnormalities can occur with astonishing rapidity in a sensitive patient.

If a patient is refractory to therapy with digitalis and benzothiadiazides, the physician should again review the etiology of the heart failure to see if any correctable conditions exist. In addition to the conditions listed in Table 5–11, constrictive pericarditis or pericardial tamponade may give symptoms mimicking those of heart failure (Magidson, 1967).

Truly refractory failure requires therapy with furosemide, ethacrynic acid, or a combination of a mercurial with aminophylline. Some patients retain sodium so avidly that any increased sodium delivered to the distal tubule is exchanged at that site for potassium ion, which increases excretion of potassium in the urine. In these patients, the addition of spironolactone, triamterene, or amiloride to one of the diuretics acting at a more proximal site may effectively increase sodium excretion and decrease potassium excretion. Amiloride and triamterene do not require the presence of increased amounts of aldosterone and are synergistic with the effects of spironolactone. Spironolactone competes with aldosterone, and doses sufficient to block aldosterone effect may be quite large. The daily urinary content of sodium and potassium is a convenient and probably essential guide to adequate dosage of spironolactone. The onset and offset of spironolactone effect may be delayed, as it acts indirectly (see Chapter 3).

Spironolactone in effective doses plus triamterene, with or without a benzothiadiazide, is so potent a combination that appearance of volume depletion or hyperkalemia may limit its use. *Principle: There are many degrees of severity and chronicity in congestive heart failure. Proper therapy takes into consideration factors that may initiate or aggravate the congested state.*

Potency of a diuretic need not guarantee its efficacy in advanced congestive heart failure, when secondary hyperaldosteronism or changes in intrarenal blood flow may necessitate use of agents to block sodium-potassium exchange. There are no intrinsic merits of milligram potency, short duration of action, or rapid onset of action in subacute or chronic disease states in which symptoms may be gradually reversed with greater safety.

Potassium Depletion. Potassium depletion is a frequent sequela of diuretic therapy in heart failure. All diuretics, except those acting on the sodium-potassium exchange mechanism in the distal tubules, can cause potassium depletion because of increased delivery of sodium to the distal tubule. Potassium depletion is particularly serious in the digitalized patient because it predisposes to digitalis toxicity. Two ways to avoid potassium depletion are to give intermittent courses of diuretic therapy or to give adequate amounts of potassium chloride as a dietary supplement. The form of potassium used for supplementation must be the chloride salt, since potassium depletion is frequently associated with a hypochloremic alkalosis. Chloride ion as well as potassium ion is required for potassium retention, bicarbonate excretion, and correction of the alkalosis (Schwartz et al., 1968). A liquid preparation of the salt is reasonably well tolerated and avoids the high local concentrations caused by enteric-coated formulations, which may be responsible for serious or fatal small-bowel ulcerations or strictures.

Another way to avoid the problem of potassium depletion is to use a combination of diuretics, one of which blocks sodium reabsorption proximally (mercurials, thiazides, ethacrynic acid, furosemide), and one of which blocks the sodium-potassium exchange mechanism either directly (amiloride, triamterene) or by blocking the action of aldosterone (spironolactone). If this combination of diuretics is used, the patient's serum and urinary electrolytes must be determined frequently, because the response to each of the two diuretics may be variable and hyperkalemia or hypokalemia may result (Cohen, 1966; Hansen and Bender, 1967). The available fixed-ratio combinations of these drugs are much less desirable

than individualized doses of each drug as determined by a patient's response to each of them.

Potassium depletion, when diagnosed, may be remarkably large (1 to 10 mEq/kg). Hypokalemia is but one of the serum electrolyte abnormalities suggesting this diagnosis. Hyponatremia or hypochloremic alkalosis may be the only abnormality in moderate potassium depletion. The hyponatremia may occur because the potassium is lost primarily from cells, decreasing intracellular osmolality. Since intracellular and extracellular osmolality must be equal, and since sodium is the major determinant of extracellular osmolality, water shifting from cells would dilute the sodium and cause hyponatremia. An alternative mechanism for the hyponatremia would be a defect in renal free-water clearance induced by potassium depletion. Kaliopenic nephropathy, however, is characterized by vasopressin-resistant isosthenuria (Relman and Schwartz, 1958). Treatment with potassium chloride increases the serum sodium concentration or corrects the alkalosis if the abnormalities are due to potassium depletion. Potassium depletion is a frequent sequela to diuretic therapy in advanced congestive heart failure. It is more common in severe congestive heart failure than in mild cases. It can be detected and even prevented by using readily available laboratory procedures to guide the judicious use of diuretics and potassium supplements.

Treatment of Pulmonary Edema

Acute pulmonary edema is a true medical emergency, but it usually responds promptly to therapy unless shock is present. Initial therapy is directed at decreasing the central blood volume: The patient should sit with legs dependent, limb tourniquets may be applied, and a phlebotomy with a blood donor set may be helpful. Morphine sulfate is often effective; it is traditionally administered subcutaneously or intramuscularly, but for the true emergency, which might include cutaneous vasoconstriction and variable blood flow in muscle, intravenous therapy is preferred. A small intravenous dose can be repeated if the response is inadequate and if there are no signs of respiratory or cardiovascular depression. Aminophylline may also be given intravenously over 30 minutes with careful measurement of the vital signs. Inhalation of increased concentrations of oxygen is helpful for hypoxemic patients because of the barrier to diffusion created by the alveolar fluid. Arterial oxygen concentrations greater than normal should be avoided, however, because this induces further systemic vasoconstriction, which increases the work of the left heart and increases central blood volume.

If the above procedures are not quickly successful, intermittent positive-pressure breathing may be an effective addition.

The immediate administration of intravenous digitalis glycosides is usually advocated, but since the onset and maximal effect of most preparations occur long after symptoms have been controlled by other means, digitalis is probably best used as prophylaxis against recurrence. During acute pulmonary edema, a major therapeutic objective is to diminish the central blood volume and lessen the chances of transudation through the pulmonary capillaries, regardless of the filling pressure of the right atrium or ventricle. This tendency to transudation must be corrected first. Then if digitalis is needed to treat the primary disease, it can be given safely in less dynamic settings. In patients with rapid supraventricular arrhythmias who have not been previously digitalized, digitalis glycosides are probably indicated. This is particularly true of patients with mitral stenosis, who may benefit dramatically from control of the ventricular rate and increased diastolic filling time. Digoxin is usually chosen, since the speed of ouabain is not needed and direct extracardiac effects may be detrimental. The intravenous digitalizing dose should be small and given slowly (over 10 to 15 minutes) to avoid direct arteriolar vasoconstriction or disproportionate stimulation of the right ventricle, causing a worsening of the pulmonary edema. In the absence of arrhythmias, the use of digitalis is debatable. Most people who present with pulmonary edema due to left ventricular disease eventually require digitalis and can be "slowly" digitalized intravenously. However, patients with mitral stenosis without arrhythmias may not improve with digitalis if their ventricular failure is a "compensatory" complication of the disease, reducing flow to the pulmonary vessels. Pulmonary edema in patients at this stage of mitral stenosis may be precipitated or worsened by digitalis (Luisada, 1964).

Beta-stimulating catecholamines might be useful, since they decrease peripheral vascular resistance and increase cardiac output. Both changes are desirable but usually not necessary for reversing pulmonary edema. Since clinical experience with the beta-mimetic catecholamines in acute pulmonary edema is limited, these agents are best reserved for acutely ill patients with a shock syndrome, who are resistant to the more conventional and efficacious therapeutic interventions.

Although previously available diuretics have not been helpful in the emergency management of pulmonary edema, the availability of a parenteral form of ethacrynic acid and furosemide, rapidly acting, potent diuretics, has renewed interest in the value of rapid and profound diuresis in lowering intravascular volume. However, a controlled study showed no better results with ethacrynic acid than with a mercurial diuretic, and the patients had largely improved by the time the diuresis occurred with either agent (Fine and Levy, 1965; Rosenberg *et al.*, 1965; Editorial, 1968c; Lesch *et al.*, 1968). Thus, a diuretic is only rarely needed for the emergency management of pulmonary edema. In fact, the hazards of potent diuretic therapy (potassium losses and excessive volume depletion) argue against vigorous early diuresis. *Principle: Even the most attractive theories in therapeutics must be verified by carefully controlled clinical trials before their widespread adoption is warranted. All known forms of therapy entail risks. The therapist cannot afford to expose any patient to any risk, unless the benefit to be accrued by the therapy is well documented.*

UNWANTED RESPONSES TO THERAPEUTIC AGENTS

Digitalis Toxicity

Digitalis intoxication, the most common of the serious iatrogenic diseases, has increased in incidence and severity since Withering's early descriptions (Friend, 1962) (see Chapter 15). Digitalis toxicity can manifest itself in a variety of unusual ways and must be considered in *every* patient receiving the drug. The toxic manifestations can be grouped into cardiac and extracardiac effects (Table 5–12). Upper gastrointestinal symptoms are the most common presenting complaint with early toxicity, but they are not always present and may occur after serious cardiac toxicity. Diarrhea or abdominal pain is unusual. The neurologic manifestations should be kept in mind, since they may be prominent but are not often linked with digitalis toxicity (Batterman and Gutner, 1948; Church and Marriott, 1959; Lyon and DeGraff, 1963; Dubnow and Burchell, 1965). The visual symptoms usually are not volunteered, and careful questioning of the patient may be required.

The appearance of gynecomastia during digitalis administration is usually attributed correctly to the drug, even when the gynecomastia is unilateral. Abnormally low urinary follicle-stimulating hormone (FSH) excretion rates in postmenopausal women receiving digitalis are a more recent finding and may be due to an estrogen-like activity of the glycoside that inhibits the pituitary (Burckhardt *et al.*, 1968).

Table 5–12. THE TOXIC MANIFESTATIONS OF DIGITALIS

TOXICITY	FREQUENCY IN PATIENTS WITH TOXICITY
Cardiac toxicity	
Arrhythmias	30%
Increasing congestive heart failure	5–10%
Extracardiac toxicity	
Neurologic	5–40%
Blurred, dancing, flashing, cloudy, or colored vision	
Headaches, drowsiness, dizziness, weakness	
Psychosis or disorientation	
Paresthesias	
Gastrointestinal	75%
Nausea	
Anorexia, paradoxical anorexia	
Vomiting	
Diarrhea	
Abdominal pain	
Allergic	0–5%
Urticaria or other rashes	
Eosinophilia	
Thrombocytopenia	
Endocrinologic	
Gynecomastia	
Suppression of FSH secretion	

Cardiac toxicity is the most serious adverse effect of digitalis and may be manifested by arrhythmias or by increasing heart failure. Arrhythmias of virtually any type may occur, but the most common are ventricular premature beats, atrial tachycardia with or without block, nodal tachycardia, and various types of atrioventricular block. Atrial fibrillation or flutter is unusual but may occur as a manifestation of digitalis intoxication (Shrager, 1957; Lown et al., 1959; Delman and Stein, 1964; Dubnow and Burchell, 1965). Recognition of digitalis toxicity may be particularly difficult in patients with chronic atrial fibrillation who develop non-paroxysmal nodal tachycardia with varying degrees of exit block, leading to an irregular ventricular response rate (Kastor and Yurchak, 1967) (see below for the pathogenetic factors in digitalis-induced arrhythmias and logical countermeasures).

Worsening of congestive heart failure is a poorly appreciated manifestation of digitalis toxicity. It is particularly dangerous since the physician may be tempted to use even higher doses of digitalis, precipitating a fatal arrhythmia. In a study of patients made repeatedly toxic with the same or different preparations of digitalis, different signs and symptoms occurred with each episode of toxicity. There was no difference in the types of toxicity seen with different preparations (Church et al., 1962).

Clinical Situations Predisposing to Digitalis Toxicity. *Cardiopulmonary Disease.* The status of the myocardium contributes to the problems encountered with digitalis. Experimentally, myocardial infarction decreases the dose of digitalis required to produce toxic arrhythmias, but no study has shown this to be clearly important in clinical situations (Askey, 1951; Morris et al., 1969). Many patients with cardiomyopathies respond poorly to the inotropic effects of digitalis and seem quite sensitive to its toxic effects (Friend, 1962; Brandt et al., 1968). In hypertrophic subaortic stenosis, digitalis and other agents that produce positive inotropic effects are contraindicated. The positive inotropic effects increase the degree of outflow tract obstruction in systole and significantly increase signs and symptoms. If the physician uses the drug for such an abnormality, he can expect to produce toxicity because the efficacious effects of the drug cannot possibly appear.

Cor pulmonale, with hypoxemia and acidosis, requires special caution in digitalis therapy (Williams et al., 1968). The increased sensitivity to digitalis is probably related to the hypoxia and the acid-base and electrolyte abnormalities, since digoxin kinetics seem to be normal in patients with cor pulmonale (Doherty, 1968).

Disease of Other Organs. Renal disease, with a reduced creatinine clearance, delays the excretion of digoxin and can reduce the maintenance dose requirements to 40 to 50% of the usual dose (Doherty et al., 1964; Bloom et al., 1966; Doherty, 1968; Jelliffe, 1968). Digitoxin is largely metabolized by the liver, but one of the metabolites, digoxin, is excreted by the kidney. However, the effect of renal failure on shifting the requirements for digitoxin seems small, probably because the digoxin makes up a relatively small proportion of the metabolites of digitoxin. Dialysis removes very little digitalis but may greatly alter the concentration of electrolytes in serum as well as acid-base balance, precipitating digitalis toxicity (Ackerman et al., 1967). Severe liver failure might impair the metabolism of digitoxin, but this effect has not been demonstrated clinically. Cirrhosis of the liver does not change the $t_{1/2}$ of digoxin (Marcus and Kapadia, 1964).

The alterations of cardiac sensitivity and metabolism of digitalis in thyroid disease have already been discussed. Hyperthyroidism decreases cardiac sensitivity to the inotropic effects of digitalis and is associated with lower concentrations of digoxin in plasma, whereas marked sensitivity is the rule in hypothyroidism.

The age of the patient can predispose to digitalis toxicity (Dall, 1965). Whether this effect is due to some decrease in renal function, altered distribution of the drug, or an increased sensitivity of the myocardium is unknown.

Interaction with Drugs. Digitalis-induced arrhythmias are potentiated by catecholamines (Roberts *et al.*, 1963) and lessened by catecholamine depletion by reserpine or cardiac sympathectomy (Méndez *et al.*, 1961; Erlij and Méndez, 1963; Roberts *et al.*, 1963). Some "beta-adrenergic blocking" drugs reduce the incidence of digitalis-induced arrhythmias. The major protective effect of the beta-adrenergic receptor blocking agents, however, seems to be related to a quinidine-type effect rather than to beta-adrenergic receptor blockade (Sekiya and Vaughan Williams, 1963; Lucchesi, 1965; Somani *et al.*, 1966; Lucchesi *et al.*, 1967) (see page 205). Other investigators have experimentally reversed digitalis toxic arrhythmias with catecholamines (Ogden *et al.*, 1969). Clinically, reserpine treatment precipitates some toxic arrhythmias (Lown *et al.*, 1961). These divergent and confusing findings on the interaction of catecholamines and digitalis in producing arrhythmias are probably related to the multiple electrophysiologic and autonomic effects each exerts on the heart and to the models chosen for study (see page 147).

Electrolyte Status. In a previously stable patient, the most common cause of digitalis toxicity is a change in electrolyte concentration in plasma. Potassium depletion, hypomagnesemia, hypercalcemia, and disturbances of acid-base balance (predominantly alkalosis) predispose to digitalis toxicity. The most common among these is potassium depletion, usually due to the use of diuretics. Potassium depletion must be considered in all patients receiving diuretics, even if the serum potassium is normal (see Chapter 3).

Treatment of Digitalis Toxicity. *Potassium.* In most cases conservative management is safest and most successful. If the patient is severely toxic he should be placed in an intensive-care unit where he can be carefully followed. Digitalis glycosides and diuretics should be withheld. Potassium chloride should be given unless complete heart block or hyperkalemia is present. Oral administration of potassium chloride is usually sufficient unless severe arrhythmias are present, in which case an intravenous infusion of potassium chloride may be necessary. Potassium infusions require constant vigil and revision based on the changes either in the electrocardiogram or in the concentration of potassium in serum. Such a statement is based on the fact that digitalis inhibits

potassium uptake by cells, and dangerous hyperkalemia may occur with relatively small doses of potassium. Renal insufficiency and potassium-retaining diuretics also favor appearance of hyperkalemia and modify the ordinarily allowable doses of potassium. Hyperkalemia can occur during oral replacement therapy, but intermittent electrocardiograms and assay of serum concentrations of potassium ordinarily suffice as guides to therapy.

Antiarrhythmic Drugs. Potassium chloride is sufficient to reverse digitalis-induced arrhythmias in most cases, but its action may be too slow for certain life-threatening arrhythmias. Only in these instances should more aggressive therapy with lidocaine, diphenylhydantoin, propranolol, or other drugs be used. Quinidine, procainamide, and propranolol depress contractility and produce similar electrophysiologic effects. In the presence of AV block these drugs precipitate complete heart block. Because they also depress automaticity, they may prevent takeover by an idioventricular pacemaker and thus may precipitate a cardiac arrest. Thus AV block is a contraindication to the use of these drugs unless a pacemaker wire is positioned in the right ventricle to counteract possible cardiac standstill.

Diphenylhydantoin has proved to be helpful in the treatment of digitalis arrhythmias. It depresses ventricular automaticity and thus is effective in eliminating ventricular premature beats, but has little depressant effect on myocardial contractility (Helfant *et al.*, 1967b, 1967c). Occasionally the ventricular response is slowed by diphenylhydantoin (Rosati *et al.*, 1967; Rosen *et al.*, 1967; Ungar and Sklaroff, 1967). Slowing of the ventricular rate could be due to facilitated AV conduction, the entry of additional impulses resulting in decremental conduction (Damato, 1969). The unique action of diphenylhydantoin and its clinical promise make the drug worthy of further clinical study (the use of diphenylhydantoin in arrhythmias is discussed below, page 204).

Calcium and Magnesium. Digitalis toxicity can be accentuated by calcium infusions and ameliorated by calcium chelation. Intravenous ethylenediaminetetraacetic acid (EDTA) has been successfully used for the treatment of digitalis toxicity (Gubner and Kallman, 1957), but remains an experimental maneuver because the extent of chelation is difficult to control and because EDTA can produce renal toxicity.

The cardiac effects of magnesium infusions are similar to the effects of potassium infusions, and this treatment may abolish digitalis-induced ventricular extrasystoles (Sodeman, 1965). However, because of its extracardiac (central nervous system and peripheral vascular) effects and the difficulty in controlling concentration of the drug in blood, magnesium is rarely used to treat digitalis toxicity and can be recommended only when hypomagnesemia exists.

Cardioversion. Digitalis lowers the threshold to electrically produced ventricular arrhythmias in animals (Lown *et al.*, 1965; Helfant *et al.*, 1968a, 1968b) and in man (Gilbert and Cuddy, 1965; Kleiger and Lown, 1966; Castellanos *et al.*, 1967). Digitalis toxic arrhythmias may not be corrected by cardioversion and may be converted to a more serious arrhythmia (Lown *et al.*, 1965; Ten Eick *et al.*, 1967). For these reasons, electrical cardioversion should be used with caution if digitalis toxicity is known to be present. If cardioversion is to be tried in an arrhythmia that might be due to digitalis, a low "dose" of electricity should be used first and increased gradually. If digitalis toxicity is present abnormal ventricular irritability may become manifest even at low-level DC discharge (Castellanos *et al.*, 1967).

Pacing. Rapid ventricular pacing ("electrical overdrive") can suppress ventricular arrhythmias arising from any cause (Mason *et al.*, 1969a). The clinical utility of cardiac pacing during digitalis toxicity is unknown. During digitalis toxicity, passage of a pacing wire alone or subsequent electrical stimulation may induce serious arrhythmias. In this condition, ventricular overdrive represents a dangerous therapeutic maneuver. It should be used only when medical therapy fails and then probably in combination with administration of diphenylhydantoin or lidocaine, which can protect against electrically induced arrhythmias (Helfant *et al.*, 1968a, 1968b; Vassaux and Lown, 1969). *Principle: When a dangerous therapeutic measure becomes necessary, knowledge of its potential adverse effects can be used to provide ready access to or simultaneous use of an antidote.*

Treatment of Complete Heart Block. Complete heart block induced by digitalis is the only digitalis-induced arrhythmia in which potassium is contraindicated (Fisch *et al.*, 1964). Patients with this arrhythmia should be placed in an intensive-care unit. The principles of management are discussed on pages 211–13. Because the abnormality is transient, medical management is usually successful, but a pacemaker wire should ordinarily be placed and ready to use. Should a ventricular tachyarrhythmia appear in such a patient, the drug treatment of choice might be diphenylhydantoin, since it may improve AV conduction as well as suppress the arrhythmia (Helfant *et al.*, 1967a, 1967b, 1967c, 1968a); even then a pacemaking wire would be necessary in the event diphenylhydantoin caused asystole (Damato, 1969).

Problems of Multiple-Drug Therapy

Patients with congestive heart failure often need a combination of drugs for proper therapy. However, no new drug should be added without specific indications. It may be gratifying to see a rapid diuresis after an initial combination of drugs until one realizes that the patient is dehydrated, hypotensive, comatose, potassium depleted, digitalis toxic, or dead. *Principle: As with all therapy, the fewer drugs required, the less likely there will be trouble* (see Chapter 16).

Fixed combinations of drugs have no role in the therapy of the cardiac patient. Combinations of thiazide diuretics and potassium salts are available, but such combinations contain too little potassium to be of value but enough to cause serious or fatal intestinal ulcerations when provided in enteric-coated formulations. Combinations of a fixed dose of a thiazide and a potassium-sparing diuretic may cause severe electrolyte abnormalities. Such combinations are all the more dangerous because the physician may be lulled into a false sense of security and may become careless.

Principle: The therapy of congestive heart failure must be individualized in order to obtain the best results without toxicity. Fixed drug combinations do not allow effective or safe therapy.

III. ARRHYTHMIAS

Effective therapy of cardiac arrhythmias requires an accurate electrocardiographic and pathophysiologic diagnosis and the use of a drug or a sequence of drugs chosen on the basis either of their pharmacologic actions or of valid empiric observations of their clinical effects. Studies of the pathogenesis of arrhythmias and the mechanisms of action of the antiarrhythmic drugs have shown that (1) arrhythmias of similar electrocardiographic appearance can have different etiologies, (2) the pharmacologic actions of antiarrhythmic drugs vary, and (3) the effects produced by a drug are dependent in part on the underlying state of the cardiac cells.

Rational therapy of cardiac arrhythmias must take these considerations into account. Techniques are being developed to characterize cardiac electrophysiologic behavior (rates of atrioventricular or intraventricular conduction and the duration of the refractory period) in man. The data obtained from pioneer investigations in animals must eventually be clinically explored to determine their applicability to patient care.

Currently, the physician uses empiric observations of clinical effects, but he should try to reconcile these observations as a basis for therapy with the available information on the

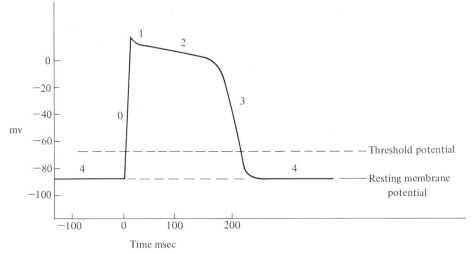

Figure 5–13. The action potential of a single myocardial cell. Any process that lowers the membrane potential to the threshold potential causes rapid depolarization (phase 0). Repolarization (phases 1 to 3) restores the transmembrane potential to the resting level (phase 4).

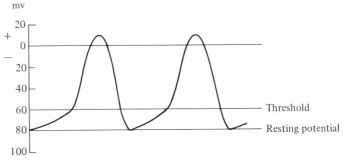

Figure 5–14. The action potential of an automatic cell. Spontaneous diastolic depolarization during phase 4 occurs in specialized cardiac conductive tissues. When the threshold potential is reached, the action potential is initiated. Repolarization restores the maximum diastolic (resting) potential.

pathophysiologic etiology of arrhythmias and the actions of drugs. This approach to therapy is superior to treatment based on the generalities solely derived from empiric experience. At the very least, a basic understanding of the pathophysiology of disease and the pharmacology of drugs should stimulate the physician to think, rather than to react, when treating arrhythmias.

CARDIAC ELECTROPHYSIOLOGY

All cardiac cells maintain a resting membrane potential and are excitable. Some cells spontaneously depolarize slowly from their resting membrane potential until, at a threshold potential, an action potential results. This sequence is divided into four phases (Figure 5–13). The following discussion emphasizes the period of slow spontaneous depolarization (phase 4) and the action potential (phase 0).

Automaticity

The generation of the cardiac impulses is normally confined to specialized tissues in the heart that spontaneously depolarize during phase 4. Slow spontaneous depolarization proceeds to a threshold, at which an action potential is initiated and propagated through the cardiac conduction system to the muscle cells (Figure 5–14). Cells capable of slow diastolic depolarization have the property of automaticity and are called automatic cells (Hoffman and Cranefield, 1964). The most rapidly discharging cells in the heart are normally located in the sinoatrial node. Automatic cells that discharge more slowly than the cardiac pacemaker are depolarized by a propagated impulse before they spontaneously reach their threshold potential. Such automatic cells are "latent pacemakers" (Figure 5–15) (Hoffman *et al.*, 1966) and may become cardiac pacemakers if their rate of phase 4 depolarization is increased relative to other automatic cells.

The spontaneous discharge rate of the automatic cells can be altered by changing either (1) the slope of phase 4 spontaneous depolarization, (2) the resting membrane potential, or (3) the threshold potential (Figures 5–16, 5–17, and 5–18; Table 5–13). The discharge rate is increased by increasing the slope of phase 4, by decreasing (making less negative) the resting membrane potential, or by increasing (making more negative) the threshold potential. Opposite changes in these variables slow the frequency of spontaneous discharges. If the normal pace-

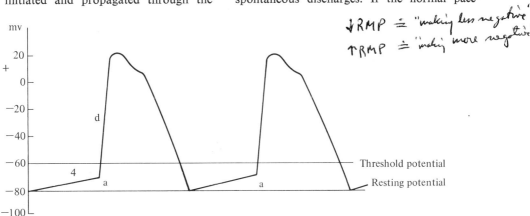

Figure 5–15. A "latent pacemaker" cell. This automatic cell undergoes spontaneous phase 4 depolarization more slowly than the cardiac pacemaker. The spontaneous depolarization is interrupted by a propagated impulse at point *a* arising from the cardiac pacemaker. If the normal cardiac pacemaker were to be slowed, this cell could take over the pacemaker function.

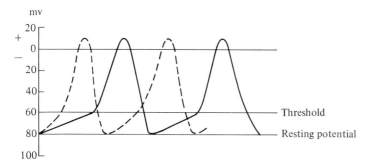

Figure 5–16. The effect of changes in the rate of slow-phase diastolic repolarization on the spontaneous discharge rate of automatic cells. The dotted lines represent rapid diastolic depolarization leading to rapid rates of firing. The solid line shows that the lower slope of phase 4 diastolic depolarization leads to fewer action potentials in the same time interval.

maker is suppressed or if latent pacemakers are stimulated so that the normal pacemaker no longer discharges at the fastest rate, an ectopic focus becomes the dominant pacemaker.

Table 5–13. CONDITIONS OR DRUGS AFFECTING DIASTOLIC DEPOLARIZATION

FAVORING RAPID DEPOLARIZATION	FAVORING SLOW DEPOLARIZATION
Ischemia	Quinidine
Digitalis	Procainamide
Catecholamines	Hyperkalemia
Atropine	Acetylcholine
Hypokalemia	Lidocaine
Myocardial stretch	Diphenylhydantoin
Heat	Propranolol
Myocardial trauma	Edrophonium
Profound hypocalcemia	Cold
Respiratory acidosis	

Ischemia, myocardial stretch, acidosis, or catecholamine excess may cause arrhythmias by increasing the discharge rate of latent pacemakers. Enhanced vagal activity, acetylcholine, or cardiac depressant drugs can decrease the rate of discharge of the SA node and permit ectopic foci to dominate the cardiac rhythm (Table 5–13).

Conduction

Another important property of excitable tissue is its ability to conduct an impulse.

Conduction velocity is a function of the amplitude of the action potential and its rate of rise (expressed as dv/dt of phase 0, or membrane responsiveness) (Singer *et al.*, 1967b). Both of these variables are predictably related to the membrane potential present at the onset of the action potential (Figure 5–19) (Weidmann, 1955a). A smaller (less negative) membrane potential results in a decrease in the amplitude of the action potential, a decrease in the slope of phase 0, and decreased conduction velocity. Decreases in the membrane potential are present if the cell is discharged prior to complete repolarization in phase 3 (Figure 5–20, *b*), if slow spontaneous depolarization occurs during phase 4 prior to phase 0 discharge (Figure 5–20, *c*), or if the resting membrane potential is decreased by drugs or pathologic states (Figure 5–20, *d*). A decrease in intraventricular conduction may be reflected in the electrocardiogram by a widening of the QRS complex. A decrease in AV conduction is indicated by a prolonged P-R interval.

When an impulse traverses tissue that offers high electrical resistance, a progressive decrease in the rate of rise and amplitude of the action potential occurs until the impulse can no longer be propagated. This phenomenon is called decremental conduction (Hoffman and Cranefield, 1964). "Functional block" is not due to mechanical interruption of the conduction system but fluctuates with changes in heart rate, drugs, or pathologic factors that influence the rate of repolarization, the slope of phase 4, the level of the membrane potential, or the relation-

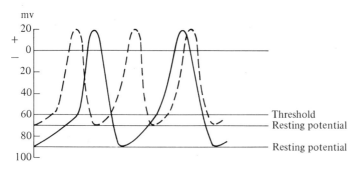

Figure 5–17. Effect of alteration in maximum diastolic potential on the rate of discharge of automatic tissue. As the maximum potential becomes larger, the rate becomes slower. High extracellular potassium, respiratory acidosis, and myocardial stretch decrease the maximum diastolic potential. A rapid decrease in plasma potassium increases this potential.

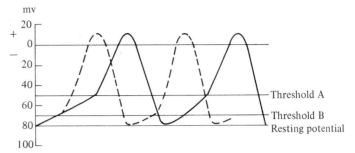

Figure 5–18. Shifts in the threshold potential may alter discharge rates. When the threshold is shifted to *A*, a slower rate results than that seen at threshold *B*. Hypercalcemia would shift the threshold toward *A*, whereas hypocalcemia reverses the process (*B*).

ship between the slope of phase 0 and the membrane potential. The functional block produced by decremental conduction can be unidirectional. A variable block over short distances or a unidirectional block may result in coupled beats or even a self-sustained ectopic focus (Figure 5–21). In the *a* portion of Figure 5–21, conduction is slowed through a portion of the conduction tissue (cross-hatched). When the slowly conducted impulse arrives at normal tissue again, a second action potential can occur if the normal tissue has repolarized from the

response elicited by the first impulse. In the *b* portion of Figure 5–21, a similar mechanism can account for a self-sustained ectopic focus owing to the impulse's repeatedly traversing a circular path. This type of impaired conductivity may account for some instances of ventricular bigeminy or ventricular tachycardia (Hoffman *et al.*, 1966) and probably is an important factor in chronic atrial fibrillation (Singer *et al.*, 1967a). AV block and many instances of bundle block in the His-Purkinje system may be accounted for by decremental conduction (Hoffman *et al.*, 1966).

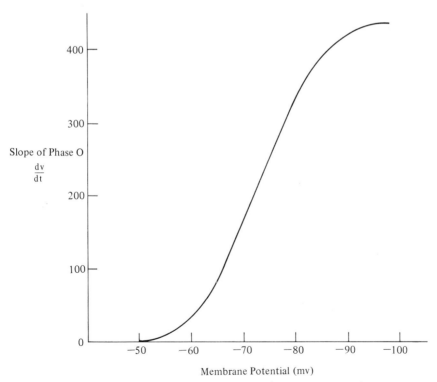

Figure 5–19. The relationship of the slope of phase 0 (membrane responsiveness) to membrane potential at the moment of depolarization. The maximum slope occurs at membrane potentials greater than (more negative than) −90 mv, with the cell becoming unresponsive below −60 mv. Conduction velocity increases with higher slopes of phase 0, and vice versa. Depressant drugs, quinidine, propranolol, procainamide, and lidocaine shift the curve to the right. Calcium and diphenylhydantoin shift the curve to the left.

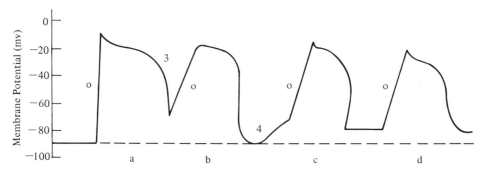

Figure 5–20. The slope of phase 0 and magnitude of the action potential depend upon the membrane potential at the time of depolarization. A normal action potential is shown in *a*. Discharge prior to complete repolarization (*b*) or during phase 4 depolarization (*c*) can decrease the amplitude of the action potential and the slope of phase 0. A similar action potential occurs if the resting membrane potential is made smaller by drugs or environmental influences (*d*). All three abnormal action potentials (*b, c, d,*) are conducted at a slower velocity than normal (*a*).

Repolarization

Drugs can alter both the rate of repolarization and the relationship of the duration of the action potential to the refractoriness of the cell. A cell can be stimulated prior to complete repolarization (at the end of the effective refractory period), but excitation then begins at a less negative membrane potential, and conduction is slowed (Figure 5–20, *b*). Most antiarrhythmic agents alter the repolarization phase of the action potential. A shortened repolarization phase (indicated in the electrocardiogram by a shortened QT interval as seen with digitalis) renders the cell responsive sooner than normal and thus more susceptible to ectopic or premature stimuli. A lengthened repolarization phase (as seen with quinidine) has the opposite effect and may interrupt premature stimuli.

Drugs may also change the duration of the effective refractory period without altering the rate of repolarization. A change that renders the cell refractory until repolarization is more

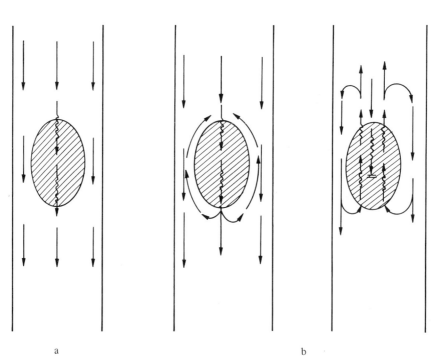

Figure 5–21. A partial conduction block in *a* can retard a portion of the total impulse to such an extent that the tissue beyond the block repolarizes, and when the impulse emerges a coupled beat can result. In *b* a block is illustrated that can account for a self-sustaining ectopic focus.

complete (i.e., membrane potential is more negative) prevents stimuli from propagating at low membrane potentials and thereby decreases the chance of decremental conduction. Such a change in refractoriness can be independent of the actual duration of the action potential and is theoretically an asset of an antiarrhythmic drug (Bigger *et al.*, 1968a; Singer and Ten Eick, 1969).

CLASSIFICATION OF DRUGS

Drugs That Depress the Myocardium

Quinidine and Procainamide. *Electrophysiology.* Quinidine and procainamide have similar electrophysiologic effects on the heart (Table 5–14). Both decrease the slope of phase 4 depolarization and therefore depress automaticity. This probably accounts for the effectiveness of these drugs in arrhythmias arising from an ischemic myocardium (Conn and Luchi, 1964).

In addition, both drugs possess other important properties that can affect arrhythmias. They increase the effective refractory period and shift the curve of dv/dt versus membrane potential (Figure 5–19) to the right, so that the cells are less responsive at any level of membrane potential (Weidmann, 1955b). This latter action accounts for a decrease in conduction velocity that is independent of the changes produced in phase 4 depolarization.

The mechanism of action of an antiarrhythmic agent can be complex. For example, because of the relationship between membrane potential, slope of phase 0, and conduction velocity, it has been suggested that depressant drugs can paradoxically increase conduction velocity in some circumstances (Singer and Ten Eick, 1969). Since these drugs depress spontaneous diastolic depolarization in all automatic fibers, a propagated impulse arriving at tissues so influenced meets fibers with a relatively increased membrane potential. If this effect on the membrane potential of the automatic fibers is greater than the effect on membrane responsiveness (Figure 5–19), the rate of rise and amplitude of the action potential increase, conduction improves, and re-entrant rhythms may be suppressed (Singer *et al.*, 1967b). In other circumstances quinidine may cause an overall decrease in conduction velocity, and the beneficial effects may be due to the decreased responsiveness, the altered refractory period, or the suppression of abnormal automaticity (Sokolow and Perloff, 1961). Recognition that quinidine can, under some circumstances, enhance membrane responsiveness and conduction velocity has allowed prediction that drugs such as diphenylhydantoin, which regularly increases responsiveness and conduction velocity, may be good antiarrhythmic agents. At any time, the predominant effect of an antiarrhythmic agent is dependent on the state of the cardiac cells. Knowledge of the unicellular electropotential changes that occur in physiologic and pathologic conditions and in states influenced by drugs has diminished empiricism in antiarrhythmic therapy and has allowed a priori selection of antiarrhythmic agents (e.g., catecholamines for the treatment of ventricular tachyarrhythmias produced by quinidine). The changes in unicellular potential are not, however, the sole determinants of the presence of an arrhythmia or even the major indicator of the most efficacious drug. As we learn more about conductivity and other basic factors of membrane physiology, other factors may emerge that will help to determine therapeutic choice.

Quinidine and procainamide depress myocardial contractility and dilate peripheral vessels (particularly when the drugs are given intravenously) and therefore may produce hypotension (Conn and Luchi, 1964). Both drugs also have vagolytic action that enhances conduction through the AV node and may in certain instances increase the ventricular response to rapid atrial arrhythmias. *Principle: The effect of a drug in any arrhythmia depends on many factors, including the state of the myocardium and conductive tissue and the relative effects of the drug on the phases of cellular electrophysiology. The effect may also depend on the extracardiac effects of the drug and the general state of the vascular system.*

Pharmacokinetics. The half-life of both quinidine and procainamide in serum is about four hours. Following oral administration, peak concentrations in plasma occur in 2 to 4 hours with quinidine and in 1 to 1 1/2 hours with procainamide (Sokolow and Perloff, 1961; Bigger and Heissenbuttel, 1969). Renal excretion accounts for about 60% of elimination of a dose of procainamide and 10 to 30% of elimination of a dose of quinidine. Urinary pH may markedly alter the renal clearance of quinidine, a weak base with pK_a of 8.57. Excretion of the drug increases as the urine becomes more acidic and the drug becomes ionized (Gerhardt *et al.*, 1969) (see Chapter 2). Decreased renal function requires that dosage of both drugs be decreased (Bellet *et al.*, 1971; Koch-Weser and Klein, 1971). The concentration in serum of either drug roughly correlates with either the pharmacologic effect or toxicity. The therapeutic range for both drugs is 3 to 8 μg/ml of blood, and myocardial toxicity is likely to occur at the higher concentrations. A low concentration of drug in serum does not rule out toxicity, since some patients seem to be very sensitive to the effects of quinidine and procainamide (Selzer and Wray, 1964).

Toxicity. The cardiac toxicity of these drugs includes atrioventricular and intraventricular block, ventricular tachyarrhythmias, and depression of myocardial contractility. With the exception of the last effect, these potential catastrophes are often heralded by a prolongation of the QRS interval of 50% above control values, a manifestation of the decreased intraventricular conduction velocity. The toxic tachyarrhythmias may be related to the marked depression of intraventricular conduction allowing re-entry phenomena and the establishment of an ectopic focus (Figure 5–21). Toxic doses of either drug may paradoxically enhance automaticity by lowering the resting membrane potential and by occasionally increasing the slope of phase 4 (Hoffman and Singer, 1967; Bigger and Heissenbuttel, 1969; Singer and Ten Eick, 1969). Fortunately both drugs have a short half-life, and toxicity can usually be treated by simply withdrawing the drug and supporting the patient. If more than supportive therapy is required, treatment with electrical means or drugs that counteract some of the known electrophysiologic effects of quinidine and procainamide is rational (Linenthal and Zoll, 1963). Catecholamines may improve depressed intraventricular conduction as the resting membrane potential and the rate of rise of the action potential increase; this effect might interrupt re-entrant arrhythmias. Automaticity may be affected variably; the increased slope of phase 4, usually produced by catecholamines, may be prevented by toxic doses of procainamide or quinidine. If the predominant effect of the catecholamines is to increase the resting membrane potential, automaticity diminishes (Hoffman and Singer, 1967).

Decreasing the serum potassium concentration has been suggested as therapy for intoxication with quinidine or procainamide. A reduction of external potassium increases resting membrane potential and thereby may enhance conductivity. Quinidine interferes with potassium efflux from the myocardial cell; hypokalemia may also counteract this effect (Watanabe et al., 1963). The empiric use of sodium lactate or bicarbonate to treat quinidine toxicity has some theoretic support, since alkalosis induces potassium shifts from extracellular to intracellular sites. The alkalosis can undesirably result in a decreased urinary excretion of the weak base quinidine (Bellet et al., 1959a, 1959b; Bailey, 1960). Diphenylhydantoin might reverse toxicity to quinidine or procainamide because it can experimentally reverse the conduction abnormalities caused by quinidine (Bigger et al.,

1968a). *Principle: Few drugs, if any, have a single pharmacologic effect, and few maneuvers to counteract a drug's effect or toxicity to a drug are simple.*

Other manifestations of quinidine toxicity include cinchonism, symptoms of gastrointestinal malfunction, hypersensitivity reactions, and occasional depression in the concentration of the formed elements in the blood, particularly platelets. Procainamide can also produce hypersensitivity reactions and may induce a usually reversible lupus erythematosus syndrome that may be related to the total amount of drug ingested (Fakhro et al., 1967; Blomgren et al., 1969).

Lidocaine. *Electrophysiology.* Lidocaine has recently become a very popular and useful agent. The cardiac electrophysiologic actions have not been entirely clarified (Table 5–14). It was initially believed that the action of lidocaine was similar to that of quinidine. However, lidocaine differs in important ways. Therapeutic serum concentrations of lidocaine (2 to 5 μg/ml) suppress phase 4 depolarization, but have little effect on conduction velocity and cardiac output (Harrison et al., 1963), and may enhance repolarization (Bigger and Heissenbuttel, 1969). Lidocaine does not have the vagolytic properties of quinidine and procainamide. High doses of lidocaine depress conduction velocity and have a negative inotropic effect, similar to that of quinidine and procainamide (Wallace et al., 1966; Sugimoto et al., 1969).

Pharmacokinetics. Lidocaine is usually administered intravenously. The drug is metabolized by the liver, with only a small percentage of the dose being excreted unchanged in the urine (Thomson et al., 1969a, 1971). After an intravenous bolus of 50 to 100 mg, plasma concentration of lidocaine falls rapidly (half-time of 15 to 20 minutes) as the drug is distributed into tissues. This rapid phase of distribution correlates with the clinically apparent brief (20-minute) duration of action after injections of lidocaine. However, the true (chemical) half-life of the drug is actually about 2 hours (Figure 5–22). If similar amounts of the drug are administered repeatedly (as they are likely to be in many clinical settings) at equal intervals of less than 2 hours, the drug accumulates in plasma and tissues for 8 to 10 hours before the mean plasma concentration reaches a plateau. Constant intravenous infusions following a bolus injection, however, can quickly achieve a constant plasma concentration of lidocaine (Thomson et al., 1970) (see Chapter 2). *Principle: Toxicity appearing after prolonged administration of a drug is likely to last longer than toxicity occurring after the first or second dose.*

Therapy of toxicity should be managed accordingly.

Because lidocaine is metabolized almost entirely by the liver, hepatic disease may be associated with lower-than-normal clearance of the drug. Usually, liver disease is not associated with changes in the volume of distribution of the drug (Thomson *et al.*, 1969b, 1971). However, during congestive heart failure both the volume of distribution and the clearance of lidocaine are decreased. After any given dose of lidocaine, patients with congestive heart failure have plasma concentrations two to three times higher than patients without heart failure, and drug toxicity may result. The requirement for lidocaine in these patients is decreased (Stenson *et al.*, 1971). The half-life of lidocaine in patients with congestive heart failure is not significantly different from the normal value, and its use alone is not helpful in predicting the need for a decrease in dosage (Thomson *et al.*, 1969a). *Principle: The half-life is only one pharmacokinetic determinant of importance in therapy. Significant changes in the volume of distribution and the clearance of a drug may make dosage adjustments mandatory.*

Toxicity. Although lidocaine is a relatively safe drug, toxicity occurs and is usually expressed in the central nervous system (somnolence, convulsions, behavioral disturbances, or increased irritability) or by changes in myocardial function resembling the toxic effects of quinidine or procainamide (heart block, induction of ventricular tachyarrhythmias, and widening of the QRS complex). Toxicity may be mistakenly interpreted as an extension of the underlying disease, particularly when ventricular arrhythmias are the manifestation. Because of the short half-life of lidocaine, toxicity is usually treated adequately by discontinuing the drug. *Principle: Toxicity of a drug can be predicted by knowledge of its pharmacology. Special precautions must be taken when toxic effects can mimic aspects of the disease and can be interpreted as extensions of the disease state. Unless the physician is particularly sensitive to this problem he may continue to administer the drug and to increase toxicity without realizing that he has been responsible for the adverse course of the patient* (see discussion of drug combinations, page 213).

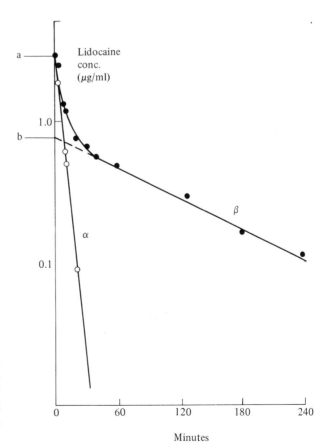

Figure 5–22. The disappearance of lidocaine from the plasma after an intravenous injection is biphasic. The half-time of disappearance for the tissue distribution phase is 15 to 20 minutes (α). The half-time of disappearance for the slower metabolic phase (β) is about 2 hours.

Table 5-14. PERTINENT CHARACTERISTICS OF SELECTED ANTIARRHYTHMIC AGENTS

AGENT	SLOW SPONTANEOUS DEPOLARIZATION (PHASE 4)	SLOPE AND AMPLITUDE OF PHASE 0	CONDUCTION	REPOLARIZATION	RELATIONSHIPS OF SLOPE OF PHASE 0 (dv/dt) TO MEMBRANE POTENTIAL	MAXIMUM (RESTING) DIASTOLIC POTENTIAL	PHARMACOKINETICS	OTHER EFFECTS
Quinidine and procainamide	Decreases slope	Usually decreases	Usually decreases in atria, AV node, and intraventricular (HIS) system, but vagolytic effects may increase AV nodal conduction at low doses	Lengthens the time course of repolarization and increases effective refractory period	Decreases slope of phase 0 at any given membrane potential (shifts curve to the right)	Decreases at high doses	$T_{1/2}$ approx. 4 hours. Quinidine excreted 10–30% unchanged in urine. Procainamide excreted 50–60% unchanged. Effective concentration approx. 3–8 $\mu g/ml$	Direct depression of myocardial contractility and arteriolar vasodilation, particularly if administered intravenously. Electrocardiogram shows prolongation of P-R, QRS, and QT intervals
Lidocaine	Decreases slope	Usually little effect (high doses decrease)	Usually little effect, but high doses can decrease conduction, particularly if depressed. May increase block at AV node in patients with supraventricular tachyarrhythmias (see text)	Shortens time course of repolarization to a greater extent than the effective refractory period	Unchanged at low doses. Probably shifts curve to right (similar to quinidine) in toxic doses	Little effect but toxic doses probably decrease	$T_{1/2} = 2$ hours (see text). Less than 5% excreted in urine unchanged. Effective concentration 2–5 $\mu g/ml$	Little effect on myocardial contractility or peripheral vasculature, even when given intravenously. No vagolytic properties. Rapid intravenous injections can depress myocardial contractility
Diphenylhydantoin	Decreases slope	Little effect in normal fibers but increases in depressed fibers	Enhances AV and intraventricular conduction, particularly if depressed. May increase block at AV node in patients with supraventricular tachyarrhythmias (see text)	Shortens time course of repolarization to a greater extent than the effective refractory period	Increases slope of phase 0 at any given membrane potential (shifts curve to the left), particularly in abnormal fibers	Increases if abnormally low	$T_{1/2}$ probably about 24 hours. Very little excreted unchanged in urine. Metabolism affected by other drugs (see text). Effective concentration 10–18 $\mu g/ml$	Little effect on myocardial contractility or peripheral vasculature. Occasional depression of myocardial contractility seen after rapid intravenous injections; effect is partly due to the commercial solvent
Propranolol	Decreases slope	Usually decreases	Usually decreases AV and intraventricular conduction. Blocks effects of catecholamines	Shortens time course of repolarization to a greater extent than the effective refractory period	Decreases slope of phase 0 at any given membrane potential (shifts to right)	Decreases at high doses	$T_{1/2}$ probably about 3 hours. Effective blood levels for β-blockade are ~ 100 $\mu g/ml$	Has negative inotropic effects that are independent of the beta-adrenergic blocking effects
Digitalis	Direct effect is to increase slope, but the vagotonic effects cause a decreased slope, particularly in the sinus node. At toxic doses the direct effects of digitalis predominate	Decreases	Therapeutic doses increase intraventricular conduction and decrease AV conduction. Toxic doses decrease AV and intraventricular conduction	Shortens time course of repolarization in atria and ventricle, but lengthens time course of repolarization in AV node	Little effect. Toxic doses of one preparation (acetylstrophanthidin) can shift curve to the right	Decreases	Depends on preparation (see text)	Inotropic myocardial effects. Electrocardiogram shows a shortened QT interval and may show a prolonged P-R interval even at therapeutic doses

Acetylcholine	Decreases slope	Minimal effect in Purkinje system	Enhances conduction in atria, little effect in ventricle. Depresses conduction in AV node	Shortens time course of repolarization in atria and lengthens in AV node	Little effect	Increases	
Beta-adrenergic sympathomimetics	Usually increases slope except in very abnormal fibers (see text)	Little effect in normal but increases if depressed	Increases particularly if depressed. Increases AV nodal conduction more than intraventricular conduction	Shortens time course of repolarization and shortens effective refractory period	No effect	Increases if partially depolarized, otherwise no effect	Many of the electrophysiologic effects oppose the effects of quinidine
Hypokalemia	Increases slope	Increases	Increases AV and intraventricular conduction	Prolongs repolarization, particularly phase 3	No effect	Acute hypokalemia increases	Enhances the increased automaticity caused by digitalis toxicity. Electrocardiogram shows flat T waves and prominent U waves that reflect the changes in phase 3 of the action potential
Hyperkalemia	Decreases slope	Usually decreases (see text)	Usually decreases AV and intraventricular conduction	Shortens time course of repolarization, particularly phase 3	No effect	Decreases	Electrocardiographic changes include peaked tall T waves, reflecting changes in repolarization. Prolonged P-R and QRS intervals may be seen with high potassium concentrations. Many of the toxic effects of hyperkalemia are countered by calcium
Hypocalcemia	Profound decreases in calcium can increase slope	Decreases	Decreases AV and intraventricular conduction	Lengthens time course of repolarization	Decreases slope of phase 0 at any given membrane potential (shifts curve to right)	No change	Increases diastolic threshold (more negative) and thereby enhances automaticity. Electrocardiogram shows a lengthened QT interval
Hypercalcemia	No change	Increases	Increases AV and intraventricular conduction	Shortens time course of repolarization	Increases slope of phase 0 at any given membrane potential (shifts curve to left)	No change	Decreases diastolic threshold (less negative) and thereby decreases automaticity. Electrocardiogram shows a shortened QT interval

Diphenylhydantoin

Electrophysiology. Diphenylhydantoin is qualitatively different from the quinidine-like drugs and supports the concept that an effective antiarrhythmic drug need not be a cardiac depressant at efficacious doses. The electrophysiologic effects of diphenylhydantoin depend in part on the underlying status of the myocardium (Table 5–14). In normal automatic fibers the drug depresses the slope of diastolic depolarization, does not alter the slope or amplitude of the action potential, and shortens the duration of the action potential more than the duration of the effective refractory period (Bigger *et al.*, 1968a).

In fibers that have an abnormally low resting membrane potential with depressed conduction (e.g., after toxic doses of procainamide or digitalis), diphenylhydantoin increases resting membrane potential toward normal, increases the slope of phase 0 (rate of rise of the action potential, dv/dt), and thus increases conduction velocity (Bigger *et al.*, 1970). The improvement in conduction velocity and the responsiveness of the membrane contrasts with the usual depressant effects of quinidine and procainamide (Figure 5–19). Diphenylhydantoin improves conduction in depressed fibers (1) by increasing resting membrane potential, (2) by decreasing automaticity and thus increasing the membrane potential of conducting tissues at the time of their activation, and (3) by increasing membrane responsiveness. In suppressing automaticity diphenylhydantoin resembles quinidine; in all other respects, diphenylhydantoin counteracts the effects of quinidine-like drugs (Helfant *et al.*, 1967a, 1967b, 1967c). Arrhythmias that may be due to unidirectional block and re-entry, such as some instances of digitalis or quinidine toxicity, may be improved by diphenylhydantoin (Helfant *et al.*, 1967b, 1969). *Principle: When different drugs can be used for a similar clinical effect but have different mechanisms of action, they may be used together if one fails or if lower doses of both prevent the toxicity of either. In some instances each may be used to counter the toxicity of the other.*

Pharmacokinetics. The effects of diphenylhydantoin are related to its concentration in plasma (Bigger *et al.*, 1968b, 1969). The pharmacokinetics of diphenylhydantoin have recently been studied in man. After tissue distribution, the half-life of diphenylhydantoin in plasma may be 24 hours or longer (Bigger *et al.*, 1968b). The drug does exhibit dose dependency of its metabolism with clinically useful doses, so that first-order kinetics are not applicable. At higher plasma levels, therefore, the drug disappears from

the plasma at a slower rate than at lower plasma levels (Arnold and Gerber, 1970). Appropriate intravenous therapy can rapidly produce effective concentrations in plasma ($> 10\ \mu g/ml$); however, if conventional oral doses are used, 6 to 10 days may be required before a plateau concentration is reached. Therapy should usually be initiated with intravenous injections of 100 mg every 5 minutes until a therapeutic effect is seen, until toxicity appears, or until 1000 mg has been given (Bigger *et al.*, 1969). Oral therapy, if used, is begun with a loading dose of 1000 mg in the first day to shorten the time necessary to reach therapeutic concentrations (Bigger *et al.*, 1968b).

Diphenylhydantoin is metabolized by hydroxylating microsomal enzymes in the liver. Its metabolism can be increased and its pharmacologic effect decreased by drugs such as phenobarbital that induce increased activity of hepatic microsomal enzymes (Cucinell *et al.*, 1965). Drugs that appear to decrease diphenylhydantoin metabolism include bishydroxycoumarin (Hansen *et al.*, 1966) and isonicotinic acid hydrazide (Kutt *et al.*, 1966); if these drugs are used in a patient taking stable doses of diphenylhydantoin, or in a patient predisposed to a toxic reaction, they may precipitate toxicity. *Principle: A carefully taken history can sometimes make the difference between efficacious use of a drug and either toxicity or lack of a therapeutic effect* (see Chapter 16).

Toxicity. Acute toxicity is usually manifested by central nervous system effects, including nystagmus, when concentrations in plasma exceed 20 $\mu g/ml$ of diphenylhydantoin. Cardiac toxicity has not been prominent (Bassett *et al.*, 1967), and some of the depressant effects observed may have been due to the diluent used with the commercial preparation of diphenylhydantoin (40% propylene glycol and 10% ethanol) (Louis *et al.*, 1967; Bigger *et al.*, 1968a). Nonetheless, a transient negative inotropic effect occurs after rapid intravenous administration of clinically available diphenylhydantoin (Lieberson *et al.*, 1967; Boyd and Williams, 1969), and although the drug usually does not alter cardiac output or pulmonary or systemic arterial pressures if infused at 25 to 50 mg/min (Conn *et al.*, 1967), hypotension has occurred even during slow injections (Karliner, 1967; Rosen *et al.*, 1967).

Treatment of patients with atrial tachyarrhythmias with diphenylhydantoin has occasionally resulted in an increased AV block (Conn, R. D., 1965; Helfant *et al.*, 1967a, Mercer and Osborne, 1967; Rosen *et al.*, 1967; Damato, 1969). The drug ordinarily increases AV conduction, but this paradoxical effect may be due to enhanced entry of stimuli into the AV node with decremental conduction (Damato, 1969). One study has shown that diphenylhydantoin is capable of slowing AV conduction in a denervated canine heart (Rosati *et al.*, 1967). The potential induction of high degrees of atrioventricular block should be considered before giving the drug, but the incidence is low; a transvenous percutaneous ventricular pacemaker should be readily available but need not be placed prior to the use of the drug. *Principle: Anticipation of potentially dangerous toxicity is the first requisite to safe and effective drug therapy.*

Drugs Affecting the Autonomic Nervous System

Parasympathetic (Cholinergic). Acetylcholine decreases automaticity by depressing the slope of phase 4 (spontaneous diastolic depolarization) and increasing the resting membrane potential (Table 5–14). Automatic cells vary in their sensitivity to acetylcholine and in their proximity to the vagal nerve endings. Vagal stimulation affects the sinus node more than automatic cells in other parts of the atrium and affects the His-Purkinje system least. As a consequence, vagal activation can shift the pacemaker from the sinus node to another atrial site or even to latent pacemakers in the His-Purkinje system, which produces the "vagal escape" rhythm (Trautwein, 1963; Hoffman and Cranefield, 1964). Acetylcholine slows conduction through the AV node, prolongs its refractory period, and can produce atrioventricular block.

Vagal activation is induced by reflexes after carotid sinus baroreceptor stimulation (by hypertension or by massage), in some patients with myocardial infarction, or by a variety of medical-surgical procedures, including intubation of the trachea, stomach or rectum, or visceral manipulation. Sometimes maneuvers that stimulate vagal activity are useful diagnostically or therapeutically (e.g., application of carotid sinus pressure, Valsalva maneuver, and self-induced gagging, or vomiting). Pharmacologically, cholinesterase inhibitors (e.g., edrophonium, organophosphate insecticides) prevent acetylcholine destruction and enhance vagal activity (Moss and Aledort, 1966). The reversible, short-acting cholinesterase inhibitor, edrophonium, may be useful in slowing (in order to aid diagnosis) or converting supraventricular arrhythmias.

Anticholinergic drugs such as atropine block the effects of vagal stimulation and are useful as premedication to protect against the bradyarrhythmias, and to treat some bradycardias associated with myocardial infarction (Cooper and Frieden, 1969). *Principle: If vagal activity is*

likely to be enhanced by a diagnostic or therapeutic maneuver, prophylactic use of atropine is rational.

Quinidine has an anticholinergic action that may increase the sinus rate and facilitate AV conduction, an undesirable property if the drug is being used to treat atrial tachyarrhythmia with rapid ventricular response. Likewise, therapeutic maneuvers to increase vagal discharge may be unsuccessful in the presence of quinidine (Sokolow and Perloff, 1961). *Principle: A valuable drug may be harmful if it is used without regard for all of its pharmacologic effects.*

Sympathetic (Adrenergic). In normal automatic fibers, beta-adrenergic stimulation increases the slope of phase 4 (spontaneous diastolic) depolarization without altering the resting membrane potential or the relationship between membrane potential and membrane responsiveness (Figure 5–19, Table 5–14) (Hoffman and Singer, 1967). The result usually is an increase in sinus rate, but occasionally there is a shift in pacemaker locus, particularly during intense stimulation. Conduction velocity in normal fibers is usually unchanged.

In fibers that are partly depolarized by drugs (digitalis, quinidine-like drugs) or pathologic states (hypoxia, stretch), catecholamines increase maximum diastolic potential and thereby increase the slope of phase 0 and the amplitude of the action potential. Hence, the conduction velocity is also increased (Hoffman and Singer, 1967). The refractory period is shortened by catecholamines and the slope of phase 4 is usually increased. These effects correlate with the tachyarrhythmias induced by catecholamines as well as their beneficial effects in treating AV block.

In highly abnormal fibers, catecholamines can improve conduction and increase transmembrane potential without further increasing the slope of phase 4 and thus can terminate arrhythmias due to decremental conduction, unidirectional block, and re-entry. These conditions probably exist in many patients with atrial and ventricular fibrillation, and in some patients with ventricular bigeminy or tachycardia (Singer and Ten Eick, 1969). Clinically, there has been an understandable reluctance to use catecholamines for the treatment of tachyarrhythmias. Excess of catecholamines can precipitate or aggravate many of these abnormal rhythms. When the abnormal electrophysiology of various arrhythmias is further defined, the catecholamines may be found useful for treating rhythms produced by partly depolarized fibers, decremental conduction, and re-entry (as is probably the case with quinidine toxicity). These drugs will probably not be indicated in similar rhythms due to enhanced automaticity (e.g., myocardial infarction, hypoxia, alkalosis) without heart block (Hoffman and Singer, 1967; Singer and Ten Eick, 1969). *Principle: Cardiac arrhythmias of identical electrocardiographic appearance may have different pathophysiologic bases. As clinical tests become available to detect these differences in etiology, therapy of arrhythmias will become more rational and hopefully more efficacious.*

Beta-adrenergic receptor blocking drugs may clinically have profound effects on the electrophysiology of the heart, but only a part of their action is due to adrenergic receptor blockade (Epstein and Braunwald, 1967a, 1967b; Hoffman and Singer, 1967; Lucchesi *et al.*, 1967; Parmley and Braunwald, 1967; Lucchesi and Iwami, 1968; Gibson and Sowton, 1969; Pitt and Ross, 1969). In addition to its beta-adrenergic receptor blocking action, D,L-propranolol is a cardiac depressant (like quinidine.) The quinidine-like activity may be responsible for some of the drug's effects. Some observers have attributed the efficacy of propranolol to beta-adrenergic blockade alone, when in fact the two actions are separable. Beta-adrenergic blocking drugs without quinidine-like effects are useful in arrhythmias produced by catecholamines alone or by catecholamines plus inhalation anesthetics, but are ineffective in most other circumstances (Somani and Watson, 1968). D-Propranolol, on the other hand, has an antiarrhythmic spectrum similar to quinidine but has relatively little beta-adrenergic receptor blocking effect. L-Propranolol (Inderal) combines quinidine-like action and beta-adrenergic receptor blockade. However, at doses of D,L-propranolol usually employed clinically, the plasma levels attained are well below the concentrations associated with the nonspecific, quinidine-like effects (Shand *et al.*, 1970; Coltart *et al.*, 1971). Propranolol lacks the vagolytic action of quinidine and differs from quinidine in its effect on the duration of the action potential (Table 5–14) (Davis and Tempte, 1968; Bigger and Heissenbuttel, 1969). *Principle: Drug labels may obscure or confuse interpretation of important pharmacologic effects. Beta-adrenergic blockade may be only one of the actions of "beta-adrenergic blocking drugs."* "other-like effects..."

The clinical role of propranolol is as yet undefined; controlled clinical trials are needed to compare this drug to standard therapy. Propranolol can slow the ventricular response to atrial fibrillation by altering AV conduction (Harrison *et al.*, 1965). The effect on the AV node may also be responsible for the efficacy of propranolol in some cases of paroxysmal supraventricular tachycardias (Gettes and Yoshonis, 1970). Digitalis-induced arrhythmias are respon-

sive to propranolol (Taylor *et al.*, 1964; Gianelly *et al.*, 1967b; Irons *et al.*, 1967). Propranolol is an effective antianginal agent but is not cleared by the FDA for this purpose (see Chapter 2). Propranolol is claimed by some to be "synergistic" with quinidine (Stern, 1966; Visioli and Bertaccini, 1968; Stern and Eisenberg, 1969). One case of presumed quinidine toxicity has been successfully treated with propranolol (Seaton, 1966). However, in spite of these few reports, the electrophysiologic effects of propranolol and quinidine are so similar that one would expect many of their therapeutic and toxic effects to be essentially additive. Until more information is available, the two drugs should not be used together with the expectation of more than additive effects. *Principle: Knowledge of the pharmacology of different drugs can lead to predictions concerning the effects and probable usefulness of their combined use.*

Electrolytes

Potassium. The resting membrane potential is a function of the ratio of intracellular potassium/extracellular potassium. Lowering the extracellular potassium increases maximum diastolic potential, phase 4 depolarization, and conduction velocity and may cause a shift of the pacemaker to normally latent sites. The electrophysiologic effects of hypokalemia are opposite to those of quinidine and may account for the efficacy of alkaline solutions (by lowering serum potassium) in the treatment of quinidine toxicity. The use of adrenal corticosteroids to alter the intracellular concentration of electrolytes and the use of diuretics to achieve hypokalemia have had some success in the treatment of heart block (Criscitiello, 1968). The effects of steroids are complex and in some cases beneficial effects may be related to their anti-inflammatory actions (Dall, 1964) (see Chapter 9).

Hyperkalemia lowers the resting membrane potential, decreases the slope of phase 4 depolarization and thus decreases conduction velocity in normal fibers. However, the effect of extracellular potassium on conduction in abnormal fibers depends on the state of the cardiac cell. Theoretically, conduction can be enhanced if the effect on depression of phase 4 is greater than the decrease in the resting membrane potential, so that activation occurs at a higher membrane potential (Figure 5–23). The beneficial effect of potassium in digitalis toxicity is probably due not only to the decrease in automaticity but also to an enhancement of conduction in the digitalis toxic fibers (Hoffman and Cranefield, 1964; Hoffman and Singer, 1964). However, hyperkalemia per se can cause

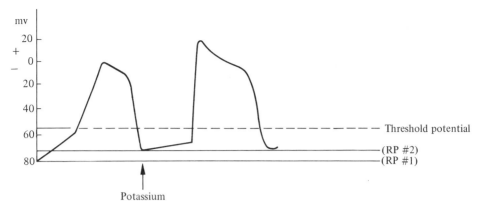

Figure 5–23. Under some conditions, potassium administration can increase conductivity. The first action potential is in an automatic fiber with rapid spontaneous depolarization, which is excited by a propagated stimulus before the phase 4 depolarization reaches the threshold potential (*TP*). Administration of potassium shifts the maximum diastolic (resting) potential from *RP #1* to *RP #2*. Normally this decrease in potential would result in a decrease in amplitude of the action, slope of phase 0, and conduction velocity. However, in this fiber, which has a rapid spontaneous diastolic depolarization, potassium acts to stabilize the membrane potential and to decrease the slope of phase 4. As a consequence, the latent pacemaker is excited by a propagated stimulus at a higher potential after potassium, and conduction velocity, slope of phase 0, and action potential amplitude are increased.

abnormalities in sinoventricular conduction, SA or AV block, or ventricular standstill.

Calcium. Calcium alters cardiac rhythm largely by changing the threshold potential. Hypercalcemia shifts the threshold potential toward zero and thereby decreases automaticity (Figure 5–18). Calcium also shifts the curve relating responsiveness and membrane potential to the left (increased membrane responsiveness) and shortens the action potential and the effective refractory period (Weidmann, 1955b). These effects may partly explain the therapeutic value of calcium in cardiac arrest by increasing the likelihood that an impulse will be conducted. Calcium also increases myocardial contractility. Digitalis and calcium ion are synergistic in their inotropic and toxic effects; digitalization in hypercalcemic states is therefore hazardous. Hypocalcemia has effects opposite to those of hypercalcemia and in addition can increase the slope of diastolic depolarization and enhance automaticity. Because automatic cells vary in sensitivity to the effects of hypocalcemia, shifts in pacemaker may occur (Singer and Ten Eick, 1969).

Magnesium. Magnesium affects the heart much like potassium. In magnesium depletion states there is an associated potassium deficit in cardiac cells. Hypermagnesemia causes electrocardiographic changes similar to those of hyperkalemia, but the extracardiac clinical effects resemble those of hypercalcemia (Randall *et al.*, 1964). A sodium-potassium pump may be dependent on magnesium, but the predominant cellular basis for magnesium's action has not been clearly defined.

Digitalis

Many of the effects of digitalis have been discussed in earlier sections. Digitalis in toxic doses increases automaticity by decreasing the maximum diastolic potential and by increasing the slope of phase 4 (Table 5–14). As a consequence of the decreased membrane potential at the time of activation, conduction velocity is slowed by toxic doses of digitalis, reflected by an increased P-R or QRS interval on the electrocardiogram (Kosowsky *et al.*, 1968). (Therapeutic doses may increase conductivity in the ventricle.) The effective refractory period in the AV node is increased by all doses of digitalis but is decreased by therapeutic doses in the atrium and ventricle (as reflected by a shortened QT in the electrocardiogram). The therapeutic and toxic atrioventricular block that occurs is due to the effects of digitalis on conduction and refractoriness of the AV node, whereas the tachyarrhythmias due to digitalis toxicity are a combination of enhanced automaticity and conduction disturbances giving rise to unidirectional block and re-entry (Hoffman and Singer, 1964). Ventricular arrhythmias in heart failure due to myocardial stretch or hypoxia may improve with digitalis because the drug improves contractility, decreases stretch, and increases cardiac output and coronary flow. Digitalis increases the effects of vagal stimulation, an action that may be useful during treatment of supraventricular arrhythmias (Theilen *et al.*, 1964).

Electricity

Cardioversion. Cardioversion and pacing are useful measures for countering arrhythmias. Cardioversion depolarizes all cardiac cells, allowing restoration of synchrony and domination of the rhythm by normal pacemaker tissue. The use of antiarrhythmic agents in addition to cardioversion is usually necessary to maintain normal rhythm (Lown, 1964; Morris *et al.*, 1966). Cardioversion, like any drug, has its drawbacks, and if the patient has been taking digitalis the cardioversion may produce serious arrhythmias. To decrease the chance of inducing arrhythmias, the cardioversion is performed with low levels of energy and the watt-seconds are built up to higher "doses" only if necessary. The reasons for toxicity of cardioversion in the presence of digitalis are unknown, but toxicity may be related to intracellular potassium loss and to release of acetylcholine and catecholamines caused by the electrical energy (Regan *et al.*, 1969). The electricity-digitalis-induced rhythms usually respond well to lidocaine (Szekely *et al.*, 1969; Vassaux and Lown, 1969; Wittenberg and Lown, 1969). *Principle: Adverse reactions increase with the use of polypharmacy. Cardioversion can be considered a drug. Therefore, when patients are likely candidates for both cardioversion and digitalis, the risk of either can be reduced by using cardioversion first.* If digitalis must be used before cardioversion, then fewer watt-seconds of electricity should be tried.

Pacemakers. Electrical pacemakers are used to treat AV block and may also be used to control other arrhythmias (Humphries, 1964; Harthorne *et al.*, 1967; Sowton, 1967; Hollingsworth *et al.*, 1969; Lown and Kosowsky, 1970). In "electrical overdrive" the electrical pacemaker is set at a rate fast enough to dominate the rhythm of the heart (Greenfield and Orgain, 1967; Kastor *et al.*, 1967; Sowton, 1967; Moss *et al.*, 1968; Zeft *et al.*, 1969b). Conduction velocity is improved at the faster rate, since less time is allowed for phase 4 depolarization, and cardiac activation occurs at a time when the membrane potential is greater (more negative). The negativity enhances the rate of rise and amplitude of the action potential. Usually, electrical pacemakers are used to treat rapid arrhythmias only after drug therapy and cardioversion have failed. Pacemakers may be used in combination with drugs that suppress automaticity (Cohen *et al.*, 1967). *Principle: Knowledge of cardiac electrophysiology and pharmacology allows the physician to tailor therapy for particularly vexing arrhythmias in individual patients.*

CLINICAL THERAPY

Goals of Therapy

The pathophysiologic effects of an arrhythmia often dictate the aggressiveness of therapy. Arrhythmias may be lethal (ventricular fibrillation), may seriously compromise cardiac output (rapid heart rate in mitral stenosis), or may herald more dangerous rhythms (e.g., premature ventricular systoles in myocardial infarction), and thus may require rapid and effective therapy. Conversely, many arrhythmias do not greatly alter cardiac function or influence prognosis, and therapy may be unnecessary. In the latter setting, therapy can be expectant and potentially toxic drugs may not be justified (Hurst and Myerburg, 1968). *Principle: "Benign" arrhythmias should not be treated with "malignant" drugs. A harmless arrhythmia can be transformed into a serious case of drug toxicity by well-meaning but overzealous therapy.*

Tachyarrhythmias

Diagnosis. An accurate diagnosis of the arrhythmia is mandatory if therapy is to be rational, safe, and maximally efficacious. A rapid rhythm with a broad QRS complex and no visible P waves on the standard electrocardiogram leads can be due to at least six rhythms, each requiring differing and specific intervention (Morrelli and Melmon, 1967) (Figure 5–24).

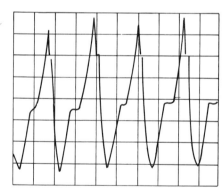

Figure 5–24. The electrocardiogram of a patient shows a rapid rate that appears to be regular. The following disturbances in cardiac mechanism could produce this pattern: ventricular tachycardia with atrioventricular dissociation, atrial fibrillation with complete heart block and independent ventricular tachycardia, paroxysmal atrial tachycardia with aberrant intraventricular conduction, nodal tachycardia with aberrant intraventricular conduction, atrial flutter with 2:1 atrioventricular block and aberrant intraventricular conduction, sinus tachycardia with aberrant conduction, or ventricular tachycardia without AV block.

The standard electrocardiogram may not be sufficient for accurate diagnosis. In many instances, carotid sinus massage slows the rhythm sufficiently to aid in defining the supraventricular arrhythmia, but often esophageal or intra-atrial leads are necessary to define the relationship of atrial (P waves) to ventricular (QRS) activity. *Principle: Do not guess (basis: a nondiagnostic standard electrocardiogram) when you can be certain (basis: esophageal or intraatrial leads). Drug therapy based on an improper diagnosis may be ineffective and dangerous.*

Pathogenesis. Detecting the underlying cause of the arrhythmia is extremely important before choosing therapy. The same arrhythmia can result from a variety of etiologies. For example, myocardial infarction, congestive heart failure, digitalis toxicity, quinidine toxicity, hypokalemia, hyperkalemia, or azotemia may produce ventricular tachycardia. Ideally, specific etiologies may be identified and specifically reversed. Many causes of arrhythmias are readily reversed (e.g., drugs, congestive heart failure, electrolyte imbalance, changes in pH, and hypoxia) (Ayres and Grace, 1969). Some are not so obvious. Frequently a catheter placed in the right ventricle to measure the central venous pressure or to function as a pacemaker can mechanically stimulate the ventricle and cause an arrhythmia. The specific therapy for this abnormality is to withdraw the catheter rather than to administer antiarrhythmic drugs. *Principle: An accurate electrocardiographic diagnosis is only the first step in rational choice of antiarrhythmic drugs. The different pathophysiologic etiologies for the arrhythmia must be considered and approached with a drug selected to counter the suspected abnormal state. If initial therapy fails, the physician must re-evaluate his decision-making process entirely and must proceed in a logical manner to other approaches. Avoid use of drugs based on reflex rather than thought; treat the patient, not his arrhythmia.*

Rational Choice of Drugs. *Ventricular Tachyarrhythmias.* After defining the type of arrhythmia and the most likely etiology, the physician is in a position to decide whether the arrhythmia can be treated with specific therapy (e.g., electrolytes or oxygen for deficiencies, digitalis for congestive heart failure) or whether it requires an antiarrhythmic drug. If an antiarrhythmic drug is required, previous drug therapy and the status of the myocardium must be carefully considered. When ventricular tachycardia is identified, a call for standby defibrillatory equipment is mandatory.

Digitalis excess results in loss of myocardial potassium and is ordinarily best treated with potassium chloride. Even though the serum potassium is usually within the normal range (Beller et al., 1971), great care is necessary to prevent hyperkalemia. Other drugs may be required in acutely life-threatening arrhythmias. Diphenylhydantoin and lidocaine have been effective in digitalis-induced ventricular arrhythmias (Gianelly et al., 1967c; Damato, 1969). Diphenylhydantoin seems to be an especially attractive choice, since the known electrophysiologic effects of the two drugs counteract each other (Table 5–14), and since the proper mode of administration has been determined (Bigger et al., 1968b). Quinidine, procainamide, and propranolol (quinidine-like drugs) may also be effective (Gianelly et al., 1967b), but their cardiac depressant effects are generally unwelcome. Their efficacy in relation to potassium chloride, diphenylhydantoin, or lidocaine has not been demonstrated.

When paroxysmal ventricular tachycardia complicates AV block, all drugs that depress automaticity are contraindicated unless a ventricular pacemaker wire has been inserted. Isoproterenol, when cautiously administered, may be effective by enhancing AV and/or intraventricular conduction. However, because it also enhances automaticity, isoproterenol has rarely been used during ventricular tachycardia, but may be effective if the arrhythmia is due to impaired conductivity. Access to defibrillation equipment is mandatory if isoproterenol is used.

If rational drug selection is impossible, the safest procedure may be cardioversion or ventricular overdrive with an electrical pacemaker. The use of the pacemaker may allow time for further analysis of the patient and appropriate selection of drug or other therapeutic maneuver.

Ventricular tachycardia due to toxicity with quinidine-like drugs, including the phenothiazines (Madan and Pendse, 1963; Schoonmaker et al., 1966; Lippmann and Wishnick, 1967; Fletcher et al., 1969), presents an interesting therapeutic problem. Based on the known electrophysiologic action of quinidine, isoproterenol or diphenylhydantoin may be helpful. Treatment of such an arrhythmia with another quinidine-like drug might succeed by impairing conduction so completely that re-entry is blocked, but is less rational than other options and probably would increase the toxicity. Agents that lower extracellular potassium, such as alkaline solutions, glucose, insulin, or diuretics, may be useful by improving conductivity.

Ventricular arrhythmias not produced by a specifically remediable cause such as congestive heart failure, and not associated with drugs or complete heart block, are effectively treated with the quinidine-like drugs or lidocaine. The choice of the agent depends on the need for rapid therapy. For intravenous use, lidocaine has become the drug of choice (Gianelly et al., 1967c). If cardiac output is relatively well maintained, procainamide can be used intramuscularly or orally every 3 to 4 hours (Koch-Weser and Klein, 1971). Quinidine is best used orally. The experience with propranolol is limited, but logically it is the drug of choice only for therapy of suspected catecholamine-induced ventricular tachyarrhythmias (e.g., in pheochromocytoma, as a result of overdosage or drug interactions, or during release or enhanced effect of catecholamines by anesthesia). Since propranolol may precipitate or worsen congestive heart failure, it must be selected judiciously and used cautiously.

Atrial Tachyarrhythmias. Similar considerations apply to atrial as to ventricular arrhythmias except that atrial arrhythmias usually are not life threatening. Some supraventricular arrhythmias, such as atrial fibrillation or flutter, do not have a readily discerned etiology. Diffuse fibrosis in the atria may impair conductivity and may favor the appearance or recurrence of arrhythmias (Bailey et al., 1968). Electrical countershock combined with a quinidine-like drug may be the preferred therapy of these arrhythmias if emergency therapy is necessary or if drug therapy is unsuccessful. Digitalis may convert rapid atrial arrhythmias to normal sinus rhythm, but even if the arrhythmia persists, digitalis is useful in controlling the rate of ventricular response and in improving cardiac output. When the digitalis regimen is stable, quinidine-like drugs can be added as an adjunct for cardioversion. After conversion to normal sinus rhythm, quinidine or procainamide may be continued in an attempt to maintain sinus rhythm (Lown, 1964).

The condition of the patient is important in determining therapy of atrial arrhythmias. A young, healthy patient may need no other therapy than mild sedation, whereas an elderly patient or a patient with mitral stenosis may require dangerous emergency procedures. If the arrhythmia occurs infrequently, as in some patients with paroxysmal atrial tachycardia, carotid sinus massage or other maneuvers to increase vagal activity may be the only treatment needed to convert the arrhythmia to normal sinus rhythm. These arrhythmias may spontaneously revert to normal. If therapy is required, digitalis alone may control the ventricular rate.

Other supraventricular arrhythmias, notably paroxysmal atrial tachycardia with AV block (Lown et al., 1959) or nonparoxysmal nodal tachycardia with or without exit block (Kastor and Yurchak, 1967), are frequently associated with digitalis intoxication, commonly during depletion of total body potassium. There is no close correlation between serum potassium concentration and intracellular potassium concentration (Moore et al., 1954; Edelman and Liebman, 1959) (see Chapter 3). Therapy of these arrhythmias, in addition to discontinuation of the digitalis preparation, should include administration of potassium chloride. Appropriate measurements of potassium and its effects should be made frequently, and pacemaking equipment should be on hand in case high degrees of AV block occur.

Treatment of supraventricular arrhythmias in patients with thyrotoxicosis merits additional comment. Although the metabolism of digitalis is accelerated during thyrotoxicosis (Doherty and Perkins, 1966b), the heart is alleged to be "sensitive" to digitalis during hyperthyroidism. This may be due in part to overly zealous attempts to bring the ventricular response rate in atrial fibrillation to a level appropriate for the normal patient (i.e., 60 to 90/min), when in fact some degree of tachycardia is appropriate to support the hypermetabolic state.

Some authors have claimed that catecholamine-depleting agents such as reserpine or guanethidine are useful for the treatment of arrhythmias associated with thyrotoxicosis (Canary et al., 1957; Lee et al., 1962; Dillon et al., 1970). The results are difficult to interpret, however, since antithyroid drugs were used simultaneously, and since the antiarrhythmic effect occurred at a time appropriate for control of the thyrotoxicosis. Recently beta-adrenergic receptor blocking drugs have been tried in thyrotoxic arrhythmias (Wilson, W. R., et al., 1964; Rowlands et al., 1965; Das and Krieger, 1969; Riddle and Schwartz, 1970). Although they usually slow the heart rate in thyrotoxicosis, beta-adrenergic receptor blocking drugs may precipitate congestive heart failure. Since appropriate antithyroid therapy is effective within hours to days, the use of the beta-adrenergic blocking drugs as *sole* therapy or for a long term is hard to justify. If these drugs are used acutely, baseline studies of arteriovenous oxygen differences or central venous lactate determinations should be compared to those obtained after therapy, to ensure that the alterations of adrenergic function are more beneficial than harmful.

Bradyarrhythmias

Complete AV block with a slow ventricular rhythm can occur as an acute manifestation of drug toxicity or myocardial infarction or may be a chronic problem due to an anatomic abnormality in the conduction system. In patients whose arrhythmia is likely to be transient, drug therapy is warranted (e.g., in patients whose rhythms are due to drug toxicity or myocardial infarction). In these situations atropine and isoproterenol are useful. The drugs should be given in the smallest doses that increase the cardiac output to maintain adequate perfusion of vital organs, even if the rate remains rather slow. Atropine in doses of 0.5 to 1.5 mg every 4 to 6 hours may decrease the block. The side effects of this therapy may limit its duration to short courses. When isoproterenol is used, it must be given intravenously. Doses of 1 to 10 μg per minute usually suffice to increase heart rate and cardiac output without undue toxicity.

Any patient with chronic AV block who has syncope, persistent symptoms of low cardiac output, heart failure, or ventricular irritability probably should be treated with a permanent pacemaker rather than with drugs. Patients with myocardial infarction who develop complete heart block should first be treated with drugs until a temporary transvenous pacemaker is placed. Patients with anterior myocardial infarctions and bundle-branch block are particularly prone to develop sudden complete heart block, and many cardiologists now advocate prophylactic insertion of a pacemaker at the onset of bundle-branch block (Lown and Kosowsky, 1970). The therapy of second-degree heart block in myocardial infarction is debated, but the prophylactic insertion of a transvenous pacemaker is advocated by most authorities (Stanzler, 1966; Criscitiello, 1968). The presence of first-degree heart block or the Wenckebach phenomenon occurring after an inferior myocardial infarction can usually be monitored, since higher degrees of heart block occur slowly enough to permit insertion of a pacemaker before complete block occurs. Adrenocortical steroids may be effective in acute myocardial infarction with AV block, but more clinical data on their use are required, and pacing is undoubtedly more certain.

Cardiac Arrest

Therapy of cardiac arrest must be rapid and definitive. Although a proper diagnosis of the arrhythmia is eventually required, immediate resuscitative procedures must be initiated. When a physician is not present, other trained personnel should summon help and begin resuscitation.

Initial Resuscitation. If the patient is in a coronary-care or intensive-care unit that has an operating electrical defibrillator *immediately* available, electrical defibrillation should be attempted within 30 seconds. Lacking a defibrillator, the resuscitator should administer a sharp blow to the chest. If cardiac action is not restored, cardiopulmonary resuscitation must begin at once (Messer, 1966).

Cardiopulmonary resuscitation consists of assuring a patent airway, ventilating the lungs, and restoring a circulation adequate to maintain viability of the brain and heart. Endotracheal intubation usually is not required immediately and wastes precious time; ventilation can be accomplished with a mask and self-inflating bag or by mouth-to-mouth artificial respiration. *Principle: Time spent searching for an endotracheal tube and laryngoscope may cost the patient his life. In severe emergencies use expedient measures even if they are not optimal.*

Artificial circulation is begun simultaneously with or shortly after artificial ventilation. External cardiac compression ordinarily is the procedure of choice and is performed on a noncompressible surface such as a bed board or the floor (Kouwenhoven *et al.*, 1960). Pressure is applied to the lower sternum with the heel of the hand approximately 60 times a minute. A circulation of about 1 liter per minute can be produced with external cardiac compression, and arterial pO_2 can be maintained in the normal range (Del Guercio *et al.*, 1965; Hansen and Sandoe, 1966; Grossman and Rubin, 1969a). By avoiding compression of the rib cage and xiphoid process, the resuscitator can minimize the risk of hepatic lacerations and rib fractures. Bone marrow or fat emboli occur in 30 to 50% of autopsied cases (Himmelhoch *et al.*, 1964).

"Definitive" Therapy. Once artificial ventilation and circulation have begun, diagnosis and definitive therapy can be pursued. One member of the resuscitating team should insert an intravenous catheter while another obtains an electrocardiogram. With adequate help and with one person directing the resuscitation, procedures can be performed efficiently. *Principle: Cardiopulmonary resuscitation must be coordinated to ensure execution of important details and to decrease the time spent on nonessentials.*

The etiology of the cardiac arrest may be suspected from the events preceding the arrest and may suggest relatively specific therapy. If digitalis intoxication is the cause of ventricular fibrillation, potassium ion is helpful and calcium infusions should be avoided. If hyperkalemia is the cause, calcium infusions can reverse much of the abnormal electrophysiology and may be lifesaving while measures to lower serum potassium are being instituted. *Principle: Even in the emergency of cardiac arrest, the patient's history of prior illness and drug administration is key to the choice of appropriate therapy and the avoidance of harmful agents.*

Acidosis. Acidosis complicates cardiac arrest in any arrhythmia and often is a combination of metabolic (lactic) and respiratory components (Ledingham and Norman, 1962; Chazan *et al.*, 1968). Since acidosis decreases myocardial contractility, the effect of sympathomimetics, and the threshold for induction of ventricular fibrillation, therapy of the acidosis is necessary for maximum success of the resuscitative effort. The respiratory component of the acidosis is treated by adequate ventilation. Sodium bicarbonate is most useful to neutralize the metabolic acidosis. Since arterial pH and plasma bicarbonate concentration cannot usually be obtained immediately, the empiric intravenous administration of 45 mEq of sodium bicarbonate (one ampul) after 5 minutes of resuscitation and every 8 to 10 minutes thereafter is recommended. Occasionally, dramatic clinical responses have been reported with the use of bicarbonate (Stewart *et al.*, 1962), and experimentally, bicarbonate increases the effectiveness of epinephrine in resuscitation (Redding and Pearson, 1968).

Ventricular Fibrillation. Ventricular fibrillation is present in most patients seen with cardiac arrest (Grossman and Rubin, 1969b). Ventricular fibrillation rarely reverts spontaneously to an effective rhythm. Electrical defibrillation is usually required. However, in spite of repeated electrical discharges the arrhythmia may persist. There are essentially no clinical data that critically evaluate drugs in refractory ventricular fibrillation. In the dog, epinephrine, phenylephrine, or methoxamine is effective in aiding defibrillation (Redding and Pearson, 1963, 1968). The common effective mechanism of these drugs is related to peripheral vasoconstriction, which provides a higher diastolic pressure during external cardiac compression and thus increases coronary and cerebral blood flow. Epinephrine also has electrophysiologic effects (Table 5–14) that favor improved conduction and increased automaticity. Because of the enhanced automaticity, caution has been used in giving epinephrine to patients with ventricular fibrillation. However, there is no experimental or clinical evidence that defibrillation is aided by withholding epinephrine or that recurrence of fibrillation is more common in patients given epinephrine.

The route of drug administration must be either intracardiac or intravenous. Experimentally, these two routes give the same results (Redding *et al.*, 1967). The choice depends on the availability of an intravenous route. Drug administration by either route must be followed by continuation of artificial ventilation and circulation in order to distribute the drug to the cardiac and extracardiac receptor sites (Pearson and Redding, 1963a, 1963b).

The impressive experimental effectiveness of sympathomimetics in both ventricular fibrillation and asystole argues for the empiric use of epinephrine as initial therapy after institution of artificial ventilation and circulation. Little would be lost and much might be gained by such an approach (Messer, 1966).

Calcium chloride may be helpful in refractory fibrillation by increasing conduction and thereby suppressing arrhythmias arising from decremental conduction and conduction delays (Weidmann, 1955b; Singer and Ten Eick, 1969). Calcium infusions must not be given if the patient has digitalis toxicity.

Intravenous or intracardiac lidocaine may be useful in aiding defibrillation or in preventing a recurrence of fibrillation (Grossman and Rubin, 1969b). Experimentally, lidocaine increases the effectiveness of epinephrine in aiding defibrillation, but there is no increase in ultimate survival with or without lidocaine (Redding and Pearson, 1968).

Asystole. Ventricular asystole is less common than ventricular fibrillation. Epinephrine may restore an effective rhythm, or may convert ventricular asystole to ventricular fibrillation that can be defibrillated. Electrophysiologically, epinephrine enhances automaticity and conduction, thereby favoring the effective propagation of an action potential. Epinephrine in the doses used (0.5 to 1.0 mg) also causes peripheral vasoconstriction. Isoproterenol experimentally is no more effective and probably less effective than epinephrine in ventricular asystole (Pearson and Redding, 1963a, 1963b; Warner, 1967). The fact that pure alpha-adrenergic sympathomimetics are effective indicates that extracardiac effects are important, and the beneficial cardiac effects of isoproterenol are counterbalanced by the peripheral vasodilation that distributes blood away from the heart and brain. *Principle: The total action of a drug must be considered. For ventricular standstill, the cardiac effects of isoproterenol are beneficial but the peripheral effects are detrimental.*

Electrical pacing may be effective in restoring cardiac action. Unfortunately the results of external cardiac pacing are disappointing. Internal cardiac pacing via a transvenous pacemaker is more effective but also more difficult to use in an emergency. However, in patients with asystole refractory to drugs and external pacing, a trial of internal pacing should be considered. The pacemaker must be inserted during the continuation of artificial ventilation and circulation.

Termination. When is a resuscitation attempt stopped? This decision must be made by the physician in charge. Patients have successfully been resuscitated after several hours of external cardiac massage. Contraction of the pupils with the artificial ventilation and circulation indicates that the central nervous system is being perfused adequately and that resuscitation attempts should continue. However, dilated pupils are not an absolute indication of failure. Pupillary dilation may be the result of alpha-adrenergic stimulation from the sympathomimetics used in the resuscitation. Complete recovery of patients with dilated pupils is possible. Even post-resuscitative coma or decerebrate posturing may be transient (Stemmler, 1965; Hansen and Sandoe, 1966).

Postresuscitation Care. After a successful resuscitation, recurrent cardiac arrests are common. The number of patients initially resuscitated is five to ten times greater than the number of long-term survivors. The number alive 24 hours after the arrest is three times greater than the number of long-term survivors (Stemmler, 1965; Grossman and Rubin, 1969b). The patient must be placed in an intensive-care unit where cardiac action is monitored, electrical defibrillation is immediately available, and excellent nursing care is offered. Intravenous infusions of lidocaine or sympathomimetics, internal cardiac pacemaking, or assisted ventilation may have to be continued. The etiology of the cardiac arrest must be vigorously sought and corrected. *Principle: An initially successful resuscitation is only the first step. Ultimate survival of the patient depends on continued and effective intensive care.*

The higher success rate of resuscitations performed in an operating room or in a coronary-care unit than in other circumstances indicates that the speed of initiation of treatment is a critical determinant of success. For this reason it is unwise to restrict the use of resuscitative techniques to physicians. Nurses must be capable of cardiac resuscitation, including electrical defibrillation. Nonmedical personnel employed in hazardous occupations (e.g., electrical workers, lifeguards, and firemen) should be able to correctly administer mouth-to-mouth ventilation and closed-chest cardiac compression (Holling, 1965). *Principle: Time is the enemy in cardiopulmonary resuscitation. The sooner the resuscitation is begun, the greater the possibility of success.*

Combinations of Drugs

In the treatment of cardiac disease, drug combinations should be used only if absolutely necessary. The incidence of drug toxicity is high in patients treated with a single drug and is compounded by the use of multiple agents (see Chapters 15 and 16). Arrhythmias resulting from multiple-drug use (e.g., digitalis and quinidine) are very difficult to treat and require a careful history to discern the probable offending agent. *Principle: An arrhythmia in a patient taking a drug combination could be due to the disease, one drug, or both drugs. A dilemma is difficult to resolve, a "trilemma" virtually impossible. Therefore, the necessity for multiple drugs must be compelling in order to justify their use.*

If multiple drugs are needed, two drugs from the same class by the same route of administration (e.g., quinidine plus procainamide) generally have no advantage over the use of a single drug. Lidocaine is often combined with an oral agent such as procainamide with the expectation that the parenteral drug can eventually be discontinued. The use of two drugs for this reason is rational.

If the quinidine-like drugs are not effective and another drug is needed, the second drug is best given alone to ascertain its individual effects. If both drugs are individually ineffective and work by different mechanisms (i.e., diphenylhydantoin and quinidine), combinations may rationally be used cautiously. As with many other drug combinations used in cardiovascular disease, there are few experimental or clinical data to rely on and the physician is an experimenter. Therefore, he should be particularly careful and observant.

ALTERATIONS IN PHARMACOLOGIC RESPONSE INDUCED BY CARDIOVASCULAR DISEASE*

The cardiovascular system plays a key role in the distribution of drugs. Alterations in cardiovascular function may significantly affect rates of absorption, distribution, metabolism, and excretion, thereby influencing the intensity and duration of a pharmacologic effect of a standard dose of drug. In addition to hemodynamic factors that influence the disposition of drugs, the diseased myocardium may change in sensitivity to the therapeutic as well as the toxic effects of drugs. Systemic metabolic changes due to impaired circulation may further influence the type and magnitude of pharmacologic response in various tissues.

Altered Drug Disposition

The role of the cardiovascular system in the absorption of drugs is better appreciated

---

* This portion of Chapter 5 (Section III) is written by Pate D. Thomson.

clinically than is its role in distribution, metabolism, and excretion. Therapists seldom administer urgently needed drugs orally, intramuscularly, or subcutaneously when the patient is in shock, in a malignant phase of hypertension, or in severe congestive heart failure, because absorption may be erratic and slow at a time when a predictable and rapid effect of drug is mandatory. Slow and unpredictable absorption from the gut, muscle, or a subcutaneous depot may make it difficult to decide whether enough drug has been administered, if the patient is unresponsive to the drug, or if the correct drug has been selected. Failure to observe the desired response may lead the physician to administer a larger dose by the same route. When the therapeutic effect is finally achieved, perfusion of the site of administration may suddenly improve, leading to rapid absorption and an overshoot in the intended pharmacologic effect. The consequences of such an overshoot may be fatal. To avoid unnecessary confusion and risk, urgently needed drugs should be administered by the intravenous route. In addition, abnormalities of cardiac function can produce anomalies in the disposition of a drug independent of its absorption or the route of administration. Data from studies of lidocaine (Thomson et al.,1969a, 1969b; Thomson, 1971), thiopental (Price, 1960; Price et al., 1960), and quinidine (Brown et al., 1953; Ditlefsen, 1957) suggest that the circulation plays an important role in influencing dose-blood level and dose-response relationships. The importance of distribution and subsequent competition among body tissues for uptake of thiopental has been demonstrated (Price et al., 1960). The competition between body tissues for a drug determines the changing concentration of the drug in brain and therefore the duration and depth of narcosis. Competition between tissues may be modulated by alterations in perfusion of tissue produced by or subsequent to reflex events associated with hemorrhage, congestive heart failure, or drug administration (including vasoactive agents that significantly alter regional systemic perfusion). The increased sensitivity to thiopental observed in patients who have hemorrhaged and in patients with heart failure may be accounted for by the reduced perfusion of noncritical tissues (i.e., fat, muscle, viscera) that ordinarily take up large amounts of the drug. When these large but noncritical tissue masses are not being perfused, tissues such as the heart and brain receive a greater fraction of the total blood flow and therefore a greater proportion of the administered drug. The result is reflected by a greater depth and duration of anesthesia or by a more profound cardiovascular depression than is seen with equivalent doses of thiopental in patients without heart failure or hemorrhage.

Increased sensitivity to therapeutic and toxic effects of intravenous lidocaine, a widely used antiarrhythmic drug, has been observed in patients with congestive heart failure (Anderson and Pitt, 1969; Thomson et al., 1969a, 1969b; Stenson et al., 1971; Thomson, 1971) and with syndromes associated with low cardiac output (Thomson et al., 1969a, 1969b; Thomson, 1971). Concentration of drug in the blood of these patients is two to three times higher than in normals after a single intravenous dose (Figure 5–25). Alterations in total blood flow and regional distribution of flow result in a smaller pool for drug distribution and in a reduced plasma clearance of lidocaine. These alterations account for the unusual concentrations of drug in blood. The reduced plasma clearance of lidocaine may reflect reduced total hepatic blood flow, as the liver is thought to rapidly extract lidocaine from the perfusing blood (see Chapter 2). Similarly, quinidine blood levels may be higher in patients with heart failure (Bellet et al., 1971); when the disease has been effectively treated, the dose-blood level relationships return to normal (Brown et al., 1953). Whether or not patients with heart failure are more susceptible to the toxic effects of quinidine is uncertain.

The evidence pointing to the importance of the circulatory status as a modifying factor influencing the delivery of drugs to critical tissues, thereby modifying the observed pharmacologic response, warrants further study, but these effects should be anticipated by the physician.

Alterations in Cardiac Muscle Responsiveness

The state of the heart may profoundly influence observed pharmacologic responses. In acute myocardial infarction, the tendency of digitalis to cause arrhythmias is augmented (Morris et al., 1969). Ischemic areas may produce electrophysiologic disturbances that increase automaticity and disturb conduction, but the pathophysiologic disturbance alone may not be of sufficient magnitude to produce an arrhythmia. A drug known to produce electrophysiologic changes similar to ischemia may summate with the disease process, increasing automaticity and/or decreasing conduction to a critical level. Then the appearance or aggravation of an arrhythmia is likely. Other disease-related factors increase automaticity. *Principle: In patients with cardiac disease, many common disorders induce pathophysiologic changes that may summate with the pharmacologic effects of digitalis to cause arrhythmias.*

The response to drugs that have myocardial-

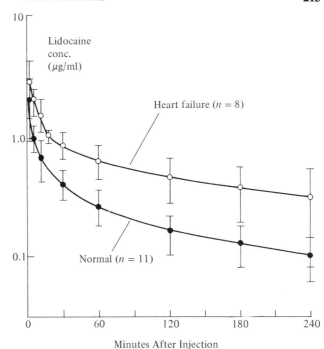

Figure 5–25. Shown are mean values (± one standard deviation) for plasma levels of lidocaine after a 50-mg intravenous bolus in ten normal subjects and eight patients with documented heart failure. The concentrations of lidocaine in the blood of patients in congestive heart failure are significantly higher than in controls.

depressant properties may be influenced by the functional capacity of the diseased myocardium. Figure 5–26 illustrates this point. Curves *a*, *b*, and *c* show decreasing degrees of myocardial contractility. Given a drug with potent myocardial depressant properties, a normal subject may shift from curve *a* (point 1) to curve *b* (point 2) but he would compensate by altering ventricular function as described by moving along the ventricular function curve to point 3. The ventricular performance is restored to normal, and clinical evidence of pulmonary or systemic congestion is not seen because ample reserves exist to compensate for ventricular depression. However, if the patient initially has impaired contractility (curve *b*, point 2) and a drug adds to his myocardial depression, shifting his ventricular function curve to *c*, the attempts to compensate (by moving from 4 to 5) are inadequate, ventricular performance is not maintained, the myocardial function deteriorates, and signs and symptoms of inadequate perfusion and pulmonary and systemic congestion develop. This phenomenon is particularly important when some antiarrhythmic drugs that depress contractility are used. These drugs are often required in patients with heart disease who have intrinsically depressed myocardial function.

Altered pharmacologic response to inotropic drugs may be seen in acute myocardial ischemia or infarction. The ability of the heart to generate

a detectable hemodynamic response depends on functioning of the ventricle as a coordinated unit. Asynergy of contraction or systolic expansion of part of the ventricle may occur in myocardial infarction (Tennant, 1935; Tatooles and Randall, 1961). Similarly, papillary muscle dysfunction in this setting may result in mitral regurgitation. These processes absorb and dissipate any potential hemodynamic advantage provided by drug-induced increases in contractility of normally functioning tissue. Metabolic disturbances in ischemic or infarcted tissue may exert a negative inotropic effect on all or part of the ventricular muscle (Katz and Hecht, 1969). During acute ischemia or infarction, digitalis may be incapable of improving the circulatory status. At a later stage of the disease, when healing has begun to occur, the ventricle again functions as a coordinated, less depressed unit and the response to the drug may be more favorable. ***Principle: Failure of a drug to produce a response at one phase of a disease does not prevent the same drug from being effective at a later phase of the disease.***

Altered Metabolic Milieu Influencing Drug Responsiveness

An altered metabolic environment in both cardiac and extracardiac tissues may influence the response to drugs in patients with heart disease. Perhaps one of the most important

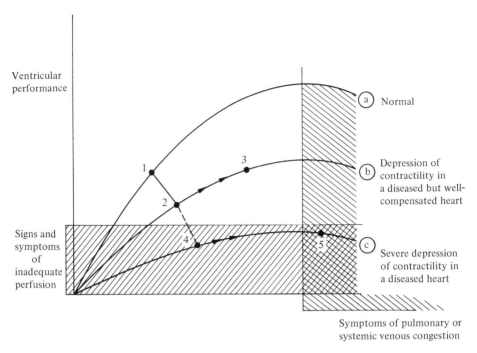

Figure 5–26. Myocardial contractility represents the ventricular performance of a given fiber length. Indices of ventricular performance include stroke volume, stroke work, and cardiac output. Parameters of fiber length include ventricular end-diastolic volume, end-diastolic pressure, ventricular circumference, and mean atrial pressure. Curves *a*, *b*, and *c* represent decreasing myocardial contractility (see text for discussion).

clinical settings in which this occurs is cardiogenic shock when systemic acidosis is likely to develop. Acidosis accompanies severely compromised cardiovascular function when delivery of oxygen to tissues is inadequate and when lactic acid production and accumulation are a consequence of anaerobic metabolism. In addition to directly depressing myocardial contractility, acidosis impairs cardiac and vascular responsiveness to endogenous and exogenous catecholamines (Nash and Heath, 1961; Nahas and Poyart, 1967). Therefore, repeated measurements of arterial blood gases are essential to the management of any patient with cardiogenic shock. The appearance of acidosis may be subtle and clinically undetected. Its development clearly demonstrates the inadequacy of the circulation and the need for therapeutic interventions. Detection and correction of the acidosis may improve the state of the circulation, and the response to catecholamines and other drugs may become dramatic.

Many other metabolic events that accompany systemic disease may alter the sensitivity of the heart to the effects of drugs. For example, hypoxia, hypercapnea (Coraboeuf and Boistel, 1953), acidosis (Hecht and Hutter, 1964), increasing myocardial stretch (Dubel and Trautwein, 1954), potassium depletion with alteration of the intracellular and extracellular potassium concentration ratio (Hoffman and Cranefield, 1964), hypocalcemia (Hoffman and Cranefield, 1964), and magnesium depletion (Seller *et al.*, 1970) increase automaticity in the heart and may summate with the arrhythmia-producing properties of digitalis.

The presence of heart disease should alert the therapist to the ways in which the disease may influence pharmacologic responses to drugs, including altered drug disposition, altered cardiac muscle responsiveness, and an altered metabolic milieu. An awareness of this potential for modification of response to a drug should stimulate the physician to improve the accuracy of his observations and may help to reduce the incidence of adverse drug reactions and to improve the quality of cardiovascular therapeutics.

IV. CORONARY ARTERY DISEASE

CHARACTERISTICS OF THE DISEASE STATE

Atherosclerotic coronary artery disease is the major health problem of Western nations (Page et al., 1966). In spite of extensive research, the etiology of coronary artery disease remains unknown, perhaps because it develops slowly in man, and because animal models do not provide good mirrors of human disease (Getz et al., 1969). Most of the information helpful in management of coronary artery disease comes from epidemiologic studies (Mann, 1969). Many of the epidemiologic clues have been partly confirmed experimentally and focus attention on possible etiologic factors.

Knowledge of the etiologic factors in coronary disease allows approaches to both prevention and treatment of ischemic heart disease. Autopsy studies of young persons dying of trauma indicate that atherosclerosis is established in many by the age of 25 (Enos et al., 1955; Viel et al., 1969). Most deaths from coronary artery disease occur within a few hours after the first acute symptoms appear, before the patient has a chance to see a physician (Stamler et al., 1966; Frank, 1968; Lown et al., 1969). Once disease of the coronary vessels becomes symptomatic, the prognosis for long-term survival is poor (Frank, 1968). Therefore, the primary therapeutic goal must be prevention of coronary disease (Master and Kuhn, 1967).

Risk Factors

The "coronary risk factors" are derived from associations noted between characteristics of a *group* and their subsequent development of coronary artery disease. The assumptions implicit in the application of data of this type to clinical treatment are unproved: (1) there is a causal relationship between the risk factors and coronary artery disease; (2) atherosclerosis can be halted, prevented, or reversed by altering the risk factors; and (3) genetic factors may be important, but in most cases environmental changes can alter the course of atherosclerotic disease. The first two assumptions are amenable to controlled clinical trials, and studies generally indicate their validity, although conclusions remain tentative. The importance of genetic versus environmental influences is unresolved (Kuo, 1968). Environmental factors are emphasized by a study comparing Japanese-Americans with native Japanese. Serum cholesterol values and coronary disease incidence in Japanese-Americans resemble those of Caucasian Americans rather than those of native Japanese (Keys et al., 1958). Genetic factors are important, as the disease in identical twins is more similar than the disease in nonidentical siblings (Sidd et al., 1966). Current views describe multiple genetic and environmental factors that interact to influence the production of atherosclerotic disease. Therapy for this disease is presently based on alteration of the environmental influence (including drugs and diet).

High-risk factors include lipid abnormalities, hypertension, diabetes mellitus, obesity, electrocardiographic abnormalities, cigarette smoking, and a positive family history of coronary artery disease. Lack of physical activity, certain behavior patterns, amount of education, and hyperuricemia may also be important, but are based on less certain evidence (Doyle et al., 1964; Cady, 1967; Friedman et al., 1968; Hinkle et al., 1968; Shekelle, 1969). Many of these factors are interrelated, and experiments to alter only one of them are difficult, if not impossible, to design. Conclusions regarding single factors are usually conditional. Nonetheless, the overall probability of the development of coronary artery disease is assumed to be related to the interplay of multiple-risk factors, and mathematical formulas have been created to express the probability (Cornfield, 1962; Kagan et al., 1963; Epstein, 1968).

Lipid Abnormalities. There is a strong correlation between elevated serum cholesterol and the risk of coronary artery disease. Large epidemiologic studies have found no concentration of serum cholesterol below which the risk of coronary disease remains constant. Thus, the definition of a "normal" concentration of cholesterol in serum for our population is not likely to be the optimal level (Stamler *et al.*, 1966). On the basis of epidemiologic studies, a serum cholesterol of less than 200 mg/100 ml may be considered "optimal" and greater than 250 mg/100 ml definitely elevated (Page and Stamler, 1968). Perhaps the population's "normal range" should be termed "characteristic range." *Principle: A population mean and standard deviation may define statistical normality, but the "normal" may not be biologically optimal for minimal risk of disease.*

Five types of hyperlipemias have been characterized by lipoprotein electrophoresis and ultracentrifugation (Table 5–15) (Brown *et al.*, 1965; Fredrickson *et al.*, 1967; Harlan *et al.*, 1967; Blankenhorn *et al.*, 1968; Falsetti *et al.*, 1968; Ostrander, 1968; Levy and Glueck, 1969). In patients with modest elevation of serum lipids, the concentration of serum cholesterol is an adequate indicator of the risk of coronary disease (Brown *et al.*, 1965; Gofman *et al.*, 1966; Stamler *et al.*, 1966; Thomas, H. E., *et al.*, 1966). In patients with severe hyperlipemia, lipoprotein analysis is essential to proper diagnosis, assessment of coronary disease risk, and appropriate therapy (Kuo, 1968; Brown 1969; Lees and Wilson, 1971).

Hypertension. Animal experiments, human autopsy studies, and prospective population studies have established hypertension as a major risk factor for coronary artery disease (Kannel *et al.*, 1961; Stamler *et al.*, 1966; Deming, 1968; Freis, 1969, 1970). There is no evidence that antihypertensive therapy stops the development of coronary artery disease in humans, but it does decrease the rate of complications in other organs (Smirk and Hodge, 1963; Berkson and Stamler, 1965; Freis, 1969, 1970). Antihypertensive therapy does reduce the development of coronary artery disease in animals (Deming *et al.*, 1961). Further long-term clinical studies are needed, with *strict control* of even moderate hypertension, to permit complete analysis of this risk factor.

Cigarette Smoking. Epidemiologic studies have firmly indicated cigarette smoking as a significant risk factor. The mechanism whereby smoking is associated with atherosclerosis is unknown, but any serious attempt at primary or secondary prevention of coronary disease must include cessation of smoking (Doyle *et al.*, 1964; U.S. Public Health Service, 1964, 1967a, 1968; Auerbach *et al.*, 1965, 1968; Sackett *et al.*, 1968; Selzer, 1968).

Physical Activity. Lack of physical activity may be important in the development of coronary disease, but the level of activity required for prevention is unknown (Morris and Crawford, 1958; Brunner and Manelis, 1960; Katz, 1967; Fox and Haskell, 1968; Mann *et al.*, 1969; Morris and Gardner, 1969). Exercise has an important psychologic effect, particularly in the patient with previous myocardial infarction or with angina pectoris. Regular exercise induces physiologic changes characterized by a slower pulse rate and lower arterial pressure at rest and at any degree of exercise, an adaptation that allows for an increase in physical work capacity (MacAlpin and Kattus, 1966; Frick and Katila, 1968; Hellerstein, 1968; Naughton *et al.*, 1969).

Obesity. Obesity as an isolated factor correlates poorly with risk, but gains importance because of its association with hypertension, diabetes, and hyperlipemia, and because of increased demands on ischemic myocardium (Kannel *et al.*, 1967, 1969; Bierman and Porte, 1968; Chiang *et al.*, 1969a).

Diagnosis

Coronary artery disease may be asymptomatic or associated with angina pectoris, myocardial infarction, or sudden death. The patient's history is particularly important in the original diagnosis of angina pectoris (Friedberg, 1967). However, because pain is subjective,

Table 5–15.   HYPERLIPIDEMIAS

CLASS	PAPER ELECTROPHORESIS	ULTRACENTRIFUGE	OTHER
I	Origin	Very low density	Chylomicronemia
II	Beta	Low density	Hypercholesterolemia
III	Broad beta	Very low density ⎫	
IV	Prebeta	Very low density ⎬	Carbohydrate sensitive
V	Origin and prebeta	Very low density ⎭	
Unclassified	Beta and prebeta	Low density and very low density	Mixed

techniques for quantitation of myocardial ischemia are needed both for diagnostic purposes and as a means of following therapy. The electrocardiogram taken at rest and during exercise, when correlated with the patient's symptoms, is the simplest and one of the best diagnostic procedures (Hultgren *et al.*, 1967). Abnormal responses to exercise increase as the severity of the exercise is increased. Maximal exercise tests may be more sensitive than standard submaximal tests, but could be more hazardous, and the interpretion of these results remains somewhat speculative (Sheffield and Reeves, 1965; Doan *et al.*, 1966; Master and Rosenfeld, 1967; Kattus *et al.*, 1968). *Principle: Whenever the sensitivity of a diagnostic test is increased, its specificity for the disease state is decreased. Extensive experience with the new test is required to establish its clinical relevance diagnostically and prognostically for the disease.*

Coronary arteriography is a valuable research procedure but causes enough mortality and morbidity to preclude its routine use. In difficult cases when coronary artery surgery is contemplated, in valvular heart disease when coronary disease may contribute to the symptoms or prognosis, or when the diagnosis is in doubt in a young patient, coronary arteriography may be indicated (Hultgren *et al.*, 1967; Ross, 1968). Myocardial lactate production has been used as an index of myocardial ischemia and may be helpful when arteriography is equivocal or negative; however, it is a research procedure with limited indications.

Patients with angina pectoris may have normal coronary arteriograms. Some of these patients have cellular hypoxia as indicated by myocardial lactate production (Likoff *et al.*, 1967; Neill *et al.*, 1968). The possibility that hemoglobin–oxygen-binding abnormalities, small coronary vessel disease, or another type of heart disease may be responsible for the pain must be considered. Pulmonary hypertension, cardiomyopathies, and valvular heart disease can cause angina pectoris. In some cases, chest pain similar to angina pectoris is produced by diseases of the gastrointestinal tract, gallbladder, cervicothoracic spine, or chest wall. Patients without heart disease must be identified to avoid a diagnosis and treatment that can produce a "cardiac cripple" (Elliot and Gorlin, 1966). *Principle: Overdiagnosis and consequent overtreatment of coronary artery disease can do as much damage as underdiagnosis.*

CLASSIFICATION OF DRUGS

Lipid-Altering Agents

Although it is not known if alterations in blood lipids affect the development of coronary artery disease (Dole *et al.*, 1963), the available evidence logically leads to the conclusion that an "optimum" serum lipid pattern, with serum cholesterol less than 200 mg/100 ml, is associated with less risk than elevated lipids (i.e., serum cholesterol greater than 250 mg/100 ml). In evaluating the lipid-altering agents, a concurrent control group is essential to help account for unexpected factors such as seasonal variation of up to 30% in serum cholesterol levels (Doyle *et al.*, 1965).

Diet. Changing the diet is an effective way to alter the serum lipid composition. Dietary alteration should be considered equivalent to drug therapy in that goals must be clearly defined and effects of therapy carefully followed. There should be no assumption that alteration of diet is free of harmful side effects. In rats, a diet high in polyunsaturated fats reduces serum cholesterol but increases the cholesterol content of the heart and aorta (Gerson *et al.*, 1961).

The goal of therapy is to prevent further atherosclerosis, not merely to lower serum lipids. No physician can be certain from his own data that lowering serum lipids is advantageous; large prospective studies are necessary. Some studies are encouraging (Christakis *et al.*, 1966; Leren, 1966, 1968; Bierenbaum *et al.*, 1967; Rinzler, 1968; Dayton *et al.*, 1969; Armstrong, 1970; Wright, 1970; Stamler, 1971), whereas others have not shown decreases in morbidity or mortality related to coronary disease, in spite of successful lowering of serum cholesterol (Research Committee, 1965; Rose *et al.*, 1965; Leading Article, 1968a; Dayton and Pearce, 1969). Many of these studies involved populations with established coronary artery disease. It is possible that established disease is little affected by dietary alterations. Other explanations for the varying results are inadequate randomization of control and treatment groups and differences in definition of therapeutic end points. Objective end points are less subject to bias than subjective end points such as the improvement of angina pectoris. A large-scale prospective study is needed; the feasibility of such a study has been discussed (National Diet Heart Study, 1968; Page and Brown, 1968).

At the present time, dietary alterations cannot be recommended for most United States citizens. However, for the high-risk group of young patients with lipid abnormalities, dietary therapy has the appeal of logic, if not of fact. Weight reduction helps to control associated hypertension or glucose intolerance and may be sufficient therapy for minimal hyperlipemia.

Modified Fat Diets. Most dietary studies have substituted polyunsaturated fat for saturated fat. These diets have a cholesterol content of less than 300 mg per day, 30 to 35% of calories from fat, 40 to 45% of calories from carbohydrate, and 20 to 25% of calories from protein. Such diets lower plasma lipids in a matter of weeks (Keys, 1968; Page and Stamler, 1968). The diets may lower cholesterol by increasing the excretion of bile acids in the feces and by decreasing cholesterol absorption (Connor et al., 1964; Wilson and Lindsey, 1965; Kuo, 1968).

Modified Carbohydrate Diets. The importance of the type and amount of dietary carbohydrate is a matter of continuing debate (McGandy et al., 1967; Kuo, 1968). The normal response to an increase in dietary carbohydrate, particularly simple sugars, is an increase in serum triglycerides (very-low-density lipoproteins or prebeta lipoproteins). Serum cholesterol concentrations may also increase with increased dietary carbohydrate but if saturated fat is restricted, the serum cholesterol concentration falls (Antonis and Bersohn, 1961, 1962; McGandy et al., 1966). If a high-carbohydrate, low-fat diet is continued for 5 to 6 months, serum triglyceride concentrations return to normal (Antonis and Bersohn, 1961). The transient nature of the triglyceride elevation may have been overlooked by short-term investigations and may account for some of the dispute about recommendations for dietary carbohydrate for relatively normal people (McGandy et al., 1967).

Some patients with moderate to large elevations of serum triglycerides are extremely sensitive to the lipogenic effects of carbohydrate. The most common type of "carbohydrate sensitive hyperlipoproteinemia" is Fredrickson's type IV (hyperprebetalipoproteinemia) with elevations of very-low-density lipoproteins (Fredrickson et al., 1967; Strisower et al., 1968). Patients with this disorder often are obese and show abnormal glucose tolerance with an excessive insulin response to a carbohydrate load. Serum triglycerides and cholesterol are elevated, and premature coronary artery disease is common (Tzagournis et al., 1967; Blankenhorn et al., 1968). Moderate reduction of dietary carbohydrate, particularly simple sugars, and attainment of ideal weight may be helpful (Bierman and Porte, 1968). A severely carbohydrate-restricted diet is often not tolerated, and a compromise diet in addition to drug therapy may be most effective.

Clofibrate. Clofibrate, estrogens, nicotinic acid, and D-thyroxine are the subjects of study by the Coronary Drug Project, a cooperative, double-blind, placebo-controlled study supported by the National Institutes of Health. This study will attempt to assess the value of drug therapy in lowering serum lipids and in preventing atherosclerotic complications in patients with a previous myocardial infarction (U.S. Public Health Service, 1967b). A study of the prevention of coronary artery disease is still necessary and will probably be forthcoming (Fredrickson, 1968). The cost of such a study is enormous, but without it, physicians will never know the value of the lipid-lowering drugs in the prevention of atherosclerotic coronary artery disease. Stratification of patients based on their serum lipoprotein analyses should be included for maximum value from the study.

Clofibrate is most effective in patients with elevated very-low-density lipoproteins in blood (broad-beta or prebetalipoproteinemia—Fredrickson type III, IV, and V). Triglycerides and often cholesterol levels in serum are elevated, and the patients usually have carbohydrate-sensitive hyperlipoproteinemia. Serum triglyceride concentration is lowered to a greater extent than serum cholesterol by clofibrate, and in some patients, the drug may induce a *rise* in the cholesterol-rich, low-density lipoproteins (beta) as it reduces the very-low-density lipoproteins (Strisower et al., 1968). The low-density lipoproteins are thought to be the most atherogenic fraction. Thus, it is critically important to follow the lipoprotein patterns closely in patients receiving clofibrate. If the low-density lipoproteins increase, the patient should be controlled with diet alone or with other drugs. Recommendations for clofibrate restrict its use to high-risk patients who are followed at monthly intervals with lipoprotein analyses (Medical Letter, 1967a). *Principle: A drug may lower total serum lipids but may increase the concentration of key atherogenic fractions and thus be potentially detrimental.*

The mechanism of action of clofibrate is not completely understood. Although it displaces thyroxine from its protein-binding sites, clofibrate probably has multiple actions including increased clearance of triglycerides, increased fecal excretion of neutral sterols, alteration of hepatic triglyceride synthesis, and inhibition of cholesterol synthesis (Hellman et al., 1963; Howard et al., 1963; Avoy et al., 1965; Azarnoff et al., 1965; Ryan and Schwartz, 1965; Mishkel and Webb, 1967; Connor, 1968; Sachs, 1968; Horlick et al., 1971).

In addition to its effects on serum lipids, clofibrate decreases the requirements for coumarin anticoagulants, perhaps owing to competition for protein binding (Oliver et al., 1963). Clofibrate also decreases platelet "stickiness," alters platelet function, increases platelet survival in some tests but not others, and lowers plasma fibrinogen (Carsen et al., 1963; Cotton *et al.*, 1963; Srivastara *et al.*, 1963; Glynn *et al.*, 1967; O'Brien, 1968). These effects on the clotting system are thought by some to be important therapeutically, but there is no firm clinical evidence to support this concept (Oliver, 1968).

Clofibrate can cause a reversible myositis with elevations of serum glutamic oxaloacetic transaminase and creatine phosphokinase, with or without symptoms (Langer and Levy, 1968). In rats, liver enlargement and ultrastructural changes occur, but this effect is not found in monkeys and there is no evidence of its occurrence in man (Svoboda and Azarnoff, 1966).

Nicotinic Acid. Nicotinic acid has long been known to lower serum cholesterol. Almost all patients, including those with type II hyperlipoproteinemia (which is poorly responsive to clofibrate), respond to this drug. Its mechanism of action is probably due to multiple effects including inhibition of cholesterol synthesis, increased cholesterol oxidation, and inhibition of hormone-sensitive lipase (Kritchevsky *et al.*, 1960; Carlson, 1963; Parsons, 1965).

The use of nicotinic acid may be limited by annoying side effects: marked flushing, pruritus, nausea, and vomiting. Gradual increments in dose usually allow effective amounts of drug to be tolerated. More worrisome side effects include reduced carbohydrate tolerance, abnormal liver function tests, and ultrastructural changes in the liver. The hepatic and metabolic abnormalities are reversible and serious sequelae have not been reported (Gurian and Adlersberg, 1959; Parsons, 1961a, 1961b, 1965). The drug has enthusiastic advocates, particularly for therapy of type II hyperlipoproteinemia.

D-Thyroxine. Both D- and L-thyroxine reduce serum cholesterol concentrations. The degree of calorigenic action of D-thyroxine at doses that lower lipids (Moyer, 1967) is disputed. One authoritative source (Medical Letter, 1967d) estimated the metabolic potency of D-thyroxine to be 10% of that of L-thyroxine. The dose of D-thyroxine used for lipid-lowering effects is ten times greater than the dose of L-thyroxine used for thyroid replacement therapy. D-Thyroxine causes nervousness, weight loss, and diarrhea as "side effects," and angina pectoris may be increased by the drug (Oliver and Boyd, 1961a; Robinson and LeBeau, 1963; Parsons, 1965; Oliver, 1967a).

The thyroid hormones decrease the concentration of the cholesterol-rich beta lipoproteins more than that of other lipid fractions, probably by causing increased hepatic metabolism of cholesterol (Rabinowitz *et al.*, 1963).

A sustained reduction in beta lipoproteins may be produced by D-thyroxine in some patients with type II lipoproteinemia (Moyer, 1967; Strisower, 1968; Cohen, 1969). However, considering the metabolic effects and the possible worsening of angina pectoris, D-thyroxine should be reserved for high-risk patients with type II hypercholesterolemia who fail to respond to other agents (Margolis and Baker, 1969). Therapy with D-thyroxine decreases the dose requirement of oral anticoagulants, and dosage adjustments must be made (Owens *et al.*, 1962).

Estrogens. The natural resistance of the female to coronary artery disease has led to the study of the effects of estrogens on serum lipids in men. Doses large enough to cause feminization lower serum beta-lipoprotein concentrations. In clinical trials, estrogens lowered serum lipids, but there was insufficient evidence that estrogens affected mortality due to coronary artery disease. The drug was poorly tolerated, and thromboembolic complications tended to increase (Oliver and Boyd, 1961b; Marmorston *et al.*, 1962; Stamler *et al.*, 1963). Perhaps some of the difficulty in interpreting the effects of estrogens may be related to varying stages of the disease in which therapy is initiated. Conceivably, estrogens could be efficacious in preventing the disease (if started when the patient is young), but are of little benefit for the patient with established anatomic abnormalities. In some patients, estrogens increase serum triglyceride concentrations (Furman *et al.*, 1967; Hazzard *et al.*, 1969). *Principle: Few drugs, if any, have predictable effects on lipids in all patients. The physician must carefully assess the effects of any drug in each patient.*

Agents Affecting Cholesterol by Reducing Bile Acid Absorption. *Cholestyramine.* Cholestyramine binds bile acids in the gastrointestinal lumen and is used mainly to prevent the pruritus of cholestatic jaundice (see Chapter 4). Since prevention of bile acid absorption increases the catabolism of cholesterol, cholestyramine lowers serum cholesterol. Binding of bile acids also decreases the absorption of cholesterol and dietary fat (Hashim and Van Itallie, 1965; Connor, 1968; Fallon and Woods, 1968).

As part of its pharmacologic action on fat absorption, cholestyramine decreases the absorption of fat-soluble vitamins; supplemental therapy is required. Cholestyramine also binds drugs and may decrease the absorption and efficacy of drugs (warfarin, digitoxin, thyroxine and probably many others) when given concomitantly with the resin (Gallo *et al.*, 1965; Caldwell and Greenberger, 1970; Gross and Brotman, 1970; Robinson *et al.*, 1971). The drug is bulky and foul tasting, causes gastrointestinal disturbances, and may be poorly tolerated.

Sitosterol. This plant sterol is thought to compete with cholesterol for absorption (Best *et al.*, 1955; Moyer, 1967). Because it is expensive and not very effective, sitosterol has little merit as a therapeutic agent.

Aminosalicylic Acid. Although not widely used, aminosalicylic acid (para-aminosalicylic acid, PAS) can lower serum cholesterol, even in difficult cases of type II hyperbetalipoproteinemia. The mechanisms of action probably involves diminished absorption of cholesterol and bile acids (Samuel and Waithe, 1961; Kerstell and Svanborg, 1966; Levine, 1968). In high doses, aminosalicylic acid can cause steatorrhea, but this is not a necessary concomitant of the lipid-lowering effect. Aminosalicylic acid may inhibit vitamin B_{12} absorption (Heinivaara and Palva, 1965). Since vitamin B_{12} and bile salts are absorbed by the distal ileum, the effect on vitamin B_{12} may resemble the sequelae of an ileal bypass operation (Buchwald and Varco, 1966).

Neomycin. This antibiotic in small doses lowers serum cholesterol and in high doses causes steatorrhea (Samuel *et al.*, 1967; Samuel and Meilman, 1967). Neomycin precipitates bile salts *in vitro*, and its hypocholesterolemic action may be related in part to this effect (Faloon *et al.*, 1966; Thompson *et al.*, 1971). This drug has been used for several years without significant toxicity in a few patients. Although neomycin is poorly absorbed, it may cause systemic toxicity if given for prolonged periods of time (Berk and Chalmers, 1970).

Anticoagulants

Blood clotting has been implicated both as a primary cause of coronary thrombosis and as a secondary factor producing occlusion of a coronary artery narrowed by an atherosclerotic plaque. These considerations have led to the use of anticoagulants to prevent recurrence of myocardial infarction. Anticoagulants are also used to prevent thromboembolic complications in selected patients with acute myocardial infarction. The choice of anticoagulants is discussed on pages 231–36. This section presents the rationale for the use of anticoagulants in myocardial infarction.

Short-Term Anticoagulation. Few topics in therapy have been so controversial and resistant to resolution as the issue of anticoagulant therapy for acute myocardial infarction. Early studies strongly supported the short-term use of anticoagulants (Wright *et al.*, 1948, 1954). The treatment appeared to decrease the incidence of thromboembolic complications and mortality;

thus began an era in which the standard treatment of myocardial infarction included anticoagulants. Residual skepticism about efficacy led to further studies that, although well conducted, have clouded the issue. Several studies support (Toohey, 1958; Griffith *et al.*, 1962) and several refute the efficacy of anticoagulants (Hilden *et al.*, 1961; Wasserman *et al.*, 1966; British Medical Research Council, 1969a). The disparate results may be partly due to different degrees of anticoagulation of patients (Wasserman, 1969; Wright, 1969a, 1969b, 1969c), but significant differences in study design and elimination of bias seem equally important. The differences betweeen studies and the influence of their deficiencies on results have recently been reviewed (Gifford and Feinstein, 1969). A consensus of the studies shows little benefit from anticoagulation in terms of mortality, but thromboembolic complications may be decreased. Each physician must make a decision *pro* or *con*, depending upon emotional bias or the flip of a coin, but upon his knowledge of the physiology of the heart and the clotting system. The individual patient's clinical status is a more important determinant than any data found in the literature. If the patient has evidence of complicating features such as venous stasis, previous history of excessive clotting, or congestive heart failure, anticoagulants are potentially helpful. However, if the patient has any previous contraindications for anticoagulation, the drugs should be withheld.

The varying results of investigations using anticoagulants emphasize the importance of proper experimental design in demonstrating small differences between control and treated groups. No one has conclusively proved the value of anticoagulants in acute myocardial infarction. *Principle: When large differences exist between control and experimental groups, as in penicillin treatment of pneumococcal pneumonia, proper study design is not so crucial as when the groups differ very little or not at all. In the latter case, an improperly designed study is worse than useless because it may be misleading* (Chapter 1).

Long-Term Anticoagulation. Anticoagulation after hospitalization for myocardial infarction is also controversial. Well-designed cooperative studies indicate a slight reduction in mortality during the first few years after infarction, but this benefit is lost in 5 to 6 years (Aspenström and Korsan-Bengtsen, 1964; Conrad *et al.*, 1964; Lovell *et al.*, 1967; Borchgrevink *et al.*, 1968; British Medical Research Council, 1969a, 1969b; Ebert *et al.*, 1969; Seaman *et al.*, 1969). The differences are so small that large studies are necessary to detect them. On discontinuing anticoagulation, there is no evidence of "rebound" (i.e., an increased incidence of infarction) (Michaels and Beamish, 1967; Kamath and Thorne, 1969).

Other Alterations of the Coagulation System. Several drugs reduce platelet adhesiveness and interfere with normal platelet function *in vitro* (O'Brien, 1966). Among these drugs are aspirin, dipyridamole, and clofibrate (Chakrabarti *et al.*, 1968; Gent *et al.*, 1968; Oliver, 1968; Sullivan *et al.*, 1968; Sahud and Aggeler, 1969). Whether these agents have any effect on preventing myocardial infarctions is unknown. If the coagulation system is etiologically involved in acute myocardial infarction, platelet thrombus formation is undoubtedly an important initial event. Clinically used amounts of heparin and warfarin do not halt formation of platelet thrombi, and inhibition of the platelet's function would be theoretically attractive. Impeccably designed and executed clinical trials are needed to evaluate this approach.

Agents for Relief of Angina Pectoris

Ischemic myocardial pain results from an imbalance between the oxygen supply and the oxygen demand of the myocardium. The mechanism whereby ischemia evokes pain is unknown. Oxygen delivery may be inadequate because of diminished caliber of the coronary vessels, decreased perfusion pressure, arterial hypoxia, decreased oxygen-carrying capacity of the blood, increased affinity of the hemoglobin for oxygen, or a decreased flow of blood due to high blood viscosity. Myocardial oxygen demand is increased by inotropic agents (e.g., catecholamines), increased heart rate, or increased myocardial wall tension. Myocardial wall tension is a function of intraventricular pressure and ventricular radius (i.e., myocardial fiber length) (Haddy, 1969). Angina pectoris is often preceded by a rise in systemic pressure and/or heart rate, hence an increased oxygen demand (Roughgarden and Newman, 1966; Robinson, 1967). Accordingly, therapy to relieve cardiac pain is aimed at reducing ischemia by increasing oxygen supply or by decreasing cardiac work (oxygen demand).

Vasodilator Drugs. *Nitrates.* Nitroglycerin is the prototype organic nitrate used to treat patients with angina pectoris. The mechanism of action of nitroglycerin is unclear. In normal man or experimental animals, nitroglycerin increases coronary blood flow (Essex *et al.*, 1940; Brachfeld *et al.*, 1959; Cohen *et al.*, 1965). In contrast, an increase in coronary flow has *not* been a consistent effect of nitroglycerin in patients with coronary artery disease (Gorlin *et al.*, 1959; Ross *et al.*, 1964). Recent studies have partly revived the coronary flow theory

(Fam and McGregor, 1964, 1968; Winbury *et al.*, 1969; Becker *et al.*, 1971; Winbury, 1971). Experimentally, nitroglycerin redistributes blood flow within the coronary vascular tree to favor ischemic tissue without increasing total flow. The results suggest that this action, which is unique among vasodilators studied, including dipyridamole and isoproterenol, is a major reason for the the effectiveness of nitrates. Whether this effect occurs in man is unknown (Cowan *et al.*, 1969).

Numerous studies have considered the peripheral actions of nitrates in an attempt to explain their therapeutic action. Arterial pressure and peripheral vascular resistance fall, and the heart volume decreases as blood shifts from the central to the peripheral circulation. These effects decrease myocardial oxygen demands by decreasing wall tension and myocardial work (Gorlin *et al.*, 1959; Christensson *et al.*, 1965; Mason and Braunwald, 1965; Williams *et al.*, 1965; Robin *et al.*, 1967b; Frick *et al.*, 1968; Graham *et al.*, 1968; Robinson, 1968; Weisse and Regan, 1969).

The principal action of nitrates has not been delineated, but an experimental effect of a drug may not represent its most important effect in a given therapeutic setting. Patients with angina pectoris have different pathophysiologic bases for their symptoms. If coronary "vasodilators" fail to relieve symptoms, agents that decrease cardiac work may be used, and vice versa, or combinations may be used.

Long-acting nitrates have been disappointingly ineffective in the treatment of angina pectoris (Oram and Sowton, 1961; Weisse and Regan, 1969). In addition, cross-tolerance to the effects of organic nitrates may develop in patients taking long-acting nitrates, making nitroglycerin less effective when it is needed (Schelling and Lasagna, 1967). *Principle: The futility of using a nonefficacious drug is magnified when this preparation's major action is to nullify the effects of a very useful drug.* Nitrates should be avoided in acute cardiac infarction, as their peripheral actions may produce significant hypotension and further cardiac damage.

Other Vasodilators. Several potent coronary vasodilators (e.g., cyanide, dipyridamole, and hydralazine) are effective but impractical. There is little evidence that angina pectoris is improved by the drugs (Kinsella *et al.*, 1962; DeGraff and Lyon, 1963; Rowe, 1966, 1968). Whether long-term administration of coronary vasodilators has a beneficial influence on development of coronary collaterals in humans has not been determined. Animal experiments indicating a beneficial effect on development of collaterals cannot necessarily be applied to man. *Principle: Care must be taken in extrapolating the claims of efficacy in animals to man. Coronary artery disease is a disease of humans.*

Alteration of the Sympathetic Nervous System. Angina pectoris can be precipitated by emotion, exertion, or other circumstances that increase sympathetic nervous system activity. Sympathetic stimulation increases myocardial oxygen demand by increasing the arterial pressure, heart rate, cardiac inotropic state, and oxidative metabolism. The relief of angina pectoris by carotid sinus massage has long been noted (Lown and Levine, 1961; Levine, 1962). Carotid massage elicits a reflex inhibition of the sympathetic nervous system with a decrease in heart rate, arterial pressure, and myocardial contractility (Epstein and Braunwald, 1968). Electrical stimulation of the carotid sinus nerves relieves anginal attacks and increases exercise tolerance (Braunwald et al., 1967; Epstein et al., 1969a, 1969b). *Principle: Major departures from standard therapy come either by serendipity or by a thorough understanding of the pathophysiology of disease. The latter is more satisfying and reliable.*

A beta-adrenergic blocking agent, propranolol, accomplishes sympathetic blockade less dramatically than does electrical stimulation of the carotid sinus nerves (see discussion of sympathetic nervous system, page 142). Reports on propranolol have generally been favorable (Epstein and Braunwald, 1966a, 1968; Gianelly et al., 1967b, 1969; Leading Article, 1969; Zeft et al., 1969a). The beneficial effect of propranolol is due to a decrease in oxygen demand and not to an increase in coronary blood flow (Dwyer et al., 1968). Propranolol's effect in angina pectoris may not be entirely due to beta-adrenergic blockade, since doses required to give relief are often much higher than doses needed for adequate beta blockade. In high doses, propranolol decreases heart rate and arterial pressure and directly depresses myocardial contractility (Epstein et al., 1965; Åström, 1968; Parker et al., 1968). These effects decrease cardiac work and myocardial oxygen requirements. Thus, the drug acts as a governor of the myocardial response to exercise and stress.

Propranolol may cause an increase in heart size (Chamberlain, 1966; Epstein and Braunwald, 1968) and may prolong systolic ejection time (Sowton and Hamer, 1966; Lewis and Brink, 1968), effects that increase cardiac work and myocardial requirements for oxygen. Propranolol also decreases coronary blood flow and may increase coronary arteriovenous oxygen differences (Gaal et al., 1966; McKenna et al., 1966; Wolfson and Gorlin, 1969). Some have attributed the effect on coronary flow to interference with autoregulatory systems as a

consequence of decreased myocardial oxygen demand (Whitsitt and Lucchesi, 1967; Lewis and Brink, 1968). Others have suggested that propranolol either directly increases coronary resistance or allows unopposed alpha-adrenergic-mediated coronary artery vasoconstriction (Parratt and Grayson, 1966a, 1966b; Wolfson et al., 1966; Feigl, 1967; Parratt, 1967). Propranolol's action in angina is delicately balanced between effects that decrease oxygen requirements and other effects that increase oxygen demand or decrease oxygen delivery (Table 5–16). Patients may react differently to propranolol because of individual variations in the way propranolol alters the balance of oxygen supply and demand (Gianelly et al., 1967b; Robin et al., 1967a; Mason et al., 1969b). *Principle: It is not always possible to know a priori if a drug will be beneficial in an individual patient with angina pectoris because of the varying pathophysiology and the multiple effects of drugs on oxygen supply and demand.*

Table 5–16. EFFECTS OF PROPRANOLOL IN ANGINA PECTORIS

DETRIMENTAL	BENEFICIAL
Increases myocardial demand	*Decreases myocardial oxygen demand*
Increases cardiac volume	Decreases myocardial contractility
Prolongs systolic ejection time	Decreases heart rate
May decrease oxygen delivery	Decreases arterial pressure
Increases coronary AV oxygen difference	Decreases effects of sympathetic stimulation

One theoretically interesting property of propranolol is its effect on the blood clotting system. Sympathetic stimulation and exercise increase fibrinolytic activity and concentrations of factor VIII in blood. Propranolol blocks the rise in factor VIII but not the rise in fibrinolytic activity. This observation is of unknown significance but may be important in the long-term use of the drug (Cohen et al., 1968; Leading Article, 1968b).

The combination of propranolol and nitrates might have additive effects, since the drugs have different mechanisms of action (Mason et al., 1969b). Unless the doses are correctly chosen and their effects adequately assessed so that doses of the drug can be adjusted, the combination of a vasodilator and a beta-adrenergic blocking agent might result in marked hypotension and subsequent reduction in blood flow in the coronary vessels. These effects, due to sympathetic inhibition by propranolol, interfere with responses to baroreceptor stimulation and result in an inability to increase heart rate and stroke output in response to vasodilation. Clinical trials with the combination of a nitrate and propranolol are somewhat encouraging but await further evaluation (Russek, 1968; Aronow and Kaplan, 1969; Battock et al., 1969; Wiener et al., 1969). Differences in the studies reported may be due to several factors, including experimental design, severity and type of disease, dose of medications, and methods of evaluating response (Harrison, 1969; Leading Article, 1969). Further studies are needed to define the patients likely to respond to a given drug or drug combination.

Propranolol can produce serious side effects, including precipitation of congestive heart failure (Epstein and Braunwald, 1966a, 1966b; Vogel and Chidsey, 1969), asthma (Zaid and Beall, 1966), and hypoglycemia (Kotler et al., 1966; Jenkins, 1967). In addition, several problems may become apparent after the long-term use of propranolol at high doses (Elliot and Stone, 1969). (1) If a patient taking propranolol had a myocardial infarction, he would probably be at a disadvantage because one of the important compensatory mechanisms, increased sympathetic activity, is blocked. (2) If propranolol's effect on coronary vasoconstriction is greater than the diminished oxygen requirement of the heart, myocardial damage may result (Robin et al., 1967a). (3) Prolonged use of propranolol in high doses causes cardiac damage in mice (Sun et al., 1967).

Other Drugs Used in Angina

Other drugs are uncommonly used in angina pectoris. However, the myocardial depressant activity of propranolol is shared by other drugs, including quinidine and procainamide (see page 228). Whether these compounds are effective antianginal drugs is untested. An important difference between these drugs and propranolol is that the latter consistently slows the heart at rest and during exercise. This reduces the overall myocardial requirement for oxygen. Other antiarrhythmic agents either have little effect on the resting or postexercise heart rate (e.g., lidocaine) or actually increase the heart rate by blocking vagal action (e.g., quinidine). The increase in heart rate caused by quinidine is probably responsible for the observation that the drug increases myocardial oxygen consumption and coronary blood flow (Rowe, 1968).

If the patient has congestive heart failure, digitalis may decrease the frequency of angina attacks as the heart size and rate decrease and as cardiac output increases. These changes reduce myocardial requirements for oxygen and/or increase coronary blood flow. In the absence of congestive heart failure, digitalis has no demonstrable beneficial effect on angina pectoris (Parker et al., 1969).

CLINICAL THERAPY

Coronary Artery Disease

Therapy of a population predisposed to coronary artery atherosclerosis is more like genetic counseling than treatment of a disease like pneumococcal pneumonia. We do not know the pathogenesis of the disease; risk factors are determined but their etiologic relationship to the disease is uncertain; the extent of either the assets or the liabilities of altering the risk factors in patients is unknown; and the risk factors are not entirely identified. Therapeutic management of isolated manifestations of the established disease is not curative nor does it substantially prolong life (treatment of hypertension may be an exception); the disease can be silent but well established by the second or third decade of life (Enos et al., 1955; Viel et al., 1969); if a significant impact is to be made on the public health of this country, preventive measures must be discovered and effectively applied in young people. Physicians must proceed pending definitive studies, but must also recognize the limited evidence that is available. We should avoid substantial and unpalatable therapeutic programs that may force those patients who comply with our prescriptions to alter their way of life significantly for relatively little gain. Stringent measures that are not efficacious can only lead to suffering and noncompliance. *Principle: Do not make the patient worse by therapy.* As an unlikely example, some have suggested that the adrenal glands might be removed in all patients to lower blood pressure and to reduce the risks of hypertension and atherosclerosis. Likewise some authorities (we hope with tongue in cheek) have suggested that all women should undergo prophylactic mastectomies to prevent breast cancer. Probably both suggestions are logical and valid and would be to some extent efficacious. However, the population is not sophisticated enough for the mastectomies, and physicians are not sufficiently sophisticated or knowledgeable to manage all the complications of the adrenalectomies. In both examples the price to the patient and the public is simply too great to balance the risk. This imbalance also characterizes many suggestions for therapy of atherosclerosis. In addition, in contrast to the two rather facetious analogies, there is almost no way of predicting the beneficial effects of countering risk factors in the majority of the population.

For the present, the treatment of the high-risk patient must be reasonable and feasible. All coronary risk factors that are present should be treated, including reduction of serum lipids, blood pressure, obesity, glucose intolerance, smoking, and physical inactivity. Many of these therapies are nonpharmacologic and require co-operation of the patient. Lowering of serum lipids can be justified only if the serum lipids are high. A serum cholesterol of less than 200 mg/100 ml and a serum triglyceride of less than 140 mg/100 ml have been suggested as optimal, although higher levels are "normal" for our population (Page and Stamler, 1968). Dietary therapy with maintenance of ideal weight is primary. Use of a carbohydrate-restricted or a fat-altered diet depends on the type of hyper-lipidemia present (U.S. Public Health Service, 1970). Drugs might be added if dietary control is insufficient, but the efficacy of drugs that suppress the appetite is low and the risk often high (Edison, 1971). The choice of drugs to lower the concentration of cholesterol or triglycerides in serum is largely made by trial and error. Determination of the lipoprotein pattern may make the choice less arbitrary. Clofibrate is most helpful in Fredrickson type III and IV hyperlipemias, and there is evidence that control of hyperlipidemia can improve peripheral vascular disease in these patients (Zellis et al., 1970). For type II hyper-cholesterolemia, nicotinic acid, cholestyramine or D-thyroxine, para-aminosalicylic acid, or neomycin may be effective.

Some of the problems in evaluating therapy of hyperlipemia are illustrated by the drug MER-29 (triparanol), which was introduced in the late 1950s as a promising cholesterol-lowering agent. Serum cholesterol could be consistently lowered by this agent, which blocked the last step in cholesterol synthesis (the conversion of desmosterol to cholesterol) (Parsons, 1965). This drug was taken off the market when it was found to cause cataracts. It was also discovered that desmosterol accumulated in atherosclerotic plaques and was at least as destructive to arteries as cholesterol. Hence, a drug that clearly lowered serum cholesterol was not helpful and was perhaps harmful to patients by accelerating plaque formation. Although none of the currently used drugs block cholesterol synthesis at a late step, they may have other obscure deleterious effects. Herein lies a paradox: If a drug lowered cholesterol by causing lipid to deposit in atherosclerotic plaques, it might be widely praised for its therapeutic efficacy in lowering serum cholesterol but the primary goal of halting coronary artery disease would be adversely affected. *Principle: Only by clearly defining the goals of therapy can the physician evaluate the effects of treatment. A decrease in serum cholesterol is of value only if the incidence of coronary artery disease is reduced.*

Angina Pectoris

The goal of therapy in patients with angina pectoris is to decrease the frequency and severity of attacks to allow a more useful if not a longer life. Evaluation of drug efficacy in patients with angina is difficult. No matter how vigorous the effort to obtain quantitative and objective data, angina pectoris remains a subjective symptom. Coronary arteriograms and exercise tests may give valuable information regarding myocardial ischemia and coronary blood flow, but only the patient's interpretation of his pain determines whether the therapy is efficacious.

The placebo effect in therapy of angina pectoris is prominent; there is a characteristic rapport period during initiation of therapy (Figure 5–27) (Beecher, 1955; Cole et al., 1958) (see Chapter 14). In evaluating the literature on antianginal drugs, one must be certain that appropriate controls were used. A double-blind, randomly sampled, placebo-controlled study is essential for valid results. Some investigators claim that the placebo responders can be separated from nonresponders by coronary angiographic studies (Amsterdam et al., 1969), but insufficient data exist to validate this claim. Crossover studies may or may not give meaningful results because of the variability of the course of the disease (Figure 5–27) (see Chapter 1). Following the "rapport" period there is often a plateau in response, succeeded by worsening or further improvement. If a drug is tested during the rapport period, it may be deemed falsely effective, and the drug would have an advantage or a disadvantage to its comparison depending on the time of the drug crossover. *Principle: Unrecognized therapeutic measures are extremely critical when subjective responses are the main criteria of efficacy.*

The usual history of newly introduced anti-anginal drugs is an initial enthusiasm based on uncontrolled studies and testimonials. Well-controlled studies follow, with such disappointing results that the drug is discarded as valueless. The only drugs that have withstood the tests of time and critical scrutiny are the short-acting nitrates and nitrites; they remain the mainstay of therapy for angina pectoris. Nitroglycerin given sublingually is effective in terminating an attack, and in preventing attacks expected within 30 minutes. However, the dose used and the interval between doses are important. Some people are more sensitive to the drug than others.

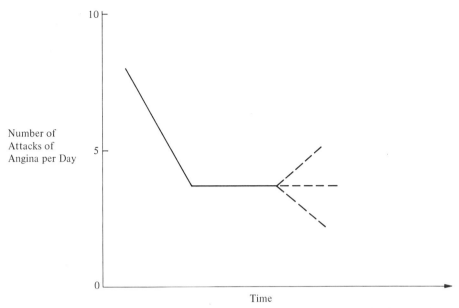

Figure 5–27. The course of angina pectoris. At the initiation of therapy there is often a period of improvement without specific therapy (the rapport period), after which the severity of the disease plateaus. The course of the disease may then worsen, remain constant, or further improve. The difficulties of evaluating therapy are related to the unpredictable natural history of angina pectoris.

Too small a dose is ineffective; too large a dose causes excessive hypotension and may compromise the coronary circulation. A patient who fails to respond to nitroglycerin may need more *or less* drug. A hypotensive reaction to the drug can often be identified by the faintness, severe headache, or dimming of vision. A patient with *no* subjective response such as "pounding in the head" probably needs a larger dose. Nitroglycerin tablets deteriorate with age, and they must fragment readily to permit sublingual absorption at a therapeutic rate. Tolerance appears to develop on chronic excessive use, and sensitivity may be restored by interruptions in therapy. *Principle: The reasons for failure of a therapeutic regimen may include lack of availability of the drug to the patient. Several commercial preparations of the same chemical may have identical content but may produce varying therapeutic effects in the same patient. The argument of the desirability of generic versus brand name enters into consideration when responses vary from prescription to prescription* (see Chapter 1).

Propranolol may be tried in patients who require large amounts of nitroglycerin for normal daily activities, as long as congestive heart failure has not occurred. As with other drugs that alter cardiovascular physiology, propranolol is difficult to test "double blind" because in adequate doses it slows the heart rate

significantly. The end point often used in an individual case is slowing of the pulse by 20 beats per minute while the patient is standing (Battock *et al.*, 1969), a mean of 60 beats per minute when the patient is resting (Harrison, 1969), or the appearance of side effects. The side effects are predictable and may be serious. During propranolol therapy, nitroglycerin should be continued and the number of tablets required recorded as an indication of the severity of the angina and the effectiveness of the propranolol. A smaller dose of nitroglycerin may be needed when a patient is taking propranolol, since the hypotension induced by a standard dose of nitroglycerin may be greater than usual during beta-adrenergic receptor blockade.

The value of propranolol plus a long- or intermediate-acting nitrate is not yet established. If a clinician chooses to use such a combination, he must attempt to critically evaluate the effect of therapy. Combinations should not be used unless simple methods fail.

Equally important to pharmacologic therapy is the prevention of factors that precipitate angina, such as exposure to cold (Epstein *et al.*, 1969c) and cigarette smoking (Aronow *et al.*, 1968; Aronow and Swanson, 1969). The patient should attain ideal weight, and a program of graded physical exercise may allow a patient to live a more productive life. Whether or not exercise increases the development of coronary collateral circulation, physical exercise does increase cardiovascular efficiency and allows more exercise to be done at a fixed demand for oxygen by the myocardium (Fox and Skinner, 1964; Fox and Haskell, 1968; Kattus *et al.*, 1968; Taylor, 1968; Clausen *et al.*, 1969; Frick, 1969).

Most patients can be managed satisfactorily when exercise is used as a therapeutic agent, smoking is eliminated, cold is avoided, and nitroglycerin is used as needed. Propranolol may be added in those who have an unsatisfactory response. Combination drug therapy may then be tried in patients who are refractory to standard treatment. The use of surgical procedures for carotid sinus stimulation or for myocardial revascularization is still highly experimental, must have extraordinary placebo effect, and should be reserved for patients incapacitated by angina unresponsive to medical therapy.

The steps in therapy recommended here have not been carefully compared to totally random drug administration. Awaiting unequivocal demonstration of unique advantages of a known or new therapeutic approach, the physician should use an initially conservative approach, hoping to compensate for "type II" errors in clinical studies through painstaking evaluation of the patient.

Myocardial Infarction

The two major life-threatening problems of myocardial infarction, arrhythmias and shock, have been discussed. A few additional points unique to myocardial infarction require emphasis.

Immediate Therapy. The immediate goal of therapy during acute myocardial infarction is to maintain the patient's life so that healing of the myocardium can occur. Studies performed in coronary-care units show that 70 to 90% of patients have arrhythmias in the first 3 days after myocardial infarction (Spann *et al.*, 1964; Yu *et al.*, 1965; Bashour *et al.*, 1967; Mounsey, 1967; Stock *et al.*, 1967; Stock, 1968). The greatest success in preventing serious arrhythmias is achieved when intensive monitoring of the rhythm and factors that influence arrhythmias is combined with aggressive prophylactic therapy of ventricular arrhythmias (Lown *et al.*, 1967, 1969; Lown and Vassaux, 1968). Intravenous lidocaine is instituted for ventricular premature beats if they interrupt the T wave (since the ventricles' tendency to arrhythmias are greatest late in repolarization), occur in runs of two or more, are multifocal, or occur at a rate greater than five per minute. Ventricular

tachycardia is usually treated with intravenous lidocaine. Ventricular premature beats can be treated by intravenous lidocaine, oral procainamide, or quinidine, depending on the urgency of the situation, considerations of the hypotensive effects of parenteral procainamide or quinidine, and other less critical but unique features (e.g., the capacity of procainamide to induce a lupus erythematosus-like syndrome and of quinidine to induce cinchonism or thrombocytopenia). *Principle: Aggressive early treatment of common, but potentially serious, arrhythmias is the key to successful prevention of fatal ventricular arrhythmias.*

Patients who develop ventricular fibrillation require immediate electrical defibrillation. This emergency treatment usually is in the hands of nurses and ancillary staff who are in the coronary-care unit at all times (Killip and Kimball, 1967; Kimball and Killip, 1968). All other therapy of arrhythmias follows the principles discussed on pages 225–28.

Prophylactic antiarrhythmic therapy after myocardial infarction would be an attractive way to decrease serious arrhythmias if a safe drug were available and if adequate doses of drug could be given (Killip, 1969). A recent study with prophylactic procainamide is encouraging (Koch-Weser *et al.*, 1969), but assay of the drug in plasma is required for adequate and safe therapy. The concept of prophylaxis, however, seems valid if assays of the drug are available or if a safe antiarrhythmic agent free of myocardial depressant actions can be developed.

Propranolol has been tried as a prophylactic antiarrhythmic drug in acute myocardial infarction (Snow, 1965; Multicentre Trial, 1966; Norris *et al.*, 1968). It does not reduce the incidence of arrhythmias and has no influence on mortality of myocardial infarction (Sowton, 1968); however, as might be expected from the drug's pharmacology, cardiac failure and hypotension may be found more frequently in those patients receiving propranolol (Multicentre Trial, 1966; Sowton, 1968).

Experimental therapies such as potassium, insulin, and glucose infusions are not convincingly effective, and the risk of causing electrolyte abnormalities or hypoglycemia is great (Malach, 1967; Surawicz, 1968).

Supraventricular tachyarrhythmias in the modern coronary-care unit have as poor a prognosis as do ventricular arrhythmias (Stock, 1968; Jewitt *et al.*, 1969; Lown *et al.*, 1969). Supraventricular arrhythmias often reflect cardiac failure or cardiogenic shock, and the patient dies of "pump failure." Many ventricular tachyarrhythmias are not associated with heart failure, but are due to electrical instability of the heart, a transient, eminently treatable condition.

Sinus bradycardia, first-degree atrioventricular block, and the Wenckebach phenomenon are usually reversed with drugs. Fixed second-degree block or a complete heart block requires a pacemaker. If the complete heart block has progressed from first- or second-degree block, its prognosis is good and recovery without persisting block can be expected in 75% of the patients. If the heart block had no antecedent abnormality in AV conduction but was heralded by a bundle-branch block, the prognosis is poor; 75% of these patients die (Lown et al., 1969). *Principle: In evaluating the therapeutic literature, the physician must consider the natural history of the disease without therapy. A comparison of pacemaker versus drug therapy for complete heart block is of little value if one group includes more patients with antecedent bundle-branch block than the other group.*

In spite of the success of the coronary-care unit, the overall reduction of deaths due to acute myocardial infarction is small. Most deaths occur within 4 hours after the onset of symptoms (Bainton and Peterson, 1963; Pell and D'Alonzo, 1964; Pantridge and Geddes, 1967), and it is estimated that *less than 35%* of these patients live long enough to reach a hospital; survival is even less with younger patients (Kuller et al., 1966; Julian, 1968; Lown et al., 1969). One approach to this problem is the mobile coronary-care unit, pioneered in Ireland and Scotland (Pantridge and Geddes, 1967; Cooper et al., 1969). The usefulness of such units depends on how quickly they can reach the patient, how many lives they can save, and their cost. Another approach is to administer an antiarrhythmic agent when the patient is first seen in his home (Lown and Vassaux, 1968; Lown et al., 1969). The effectiveness of lidocaine given intramuscularly is unknown. If lidocaine is as effective as has been recently claimed in preventing early deaths due to arrhythmias, its efficacy would be easy to prove by an experimental trial. If, however, the drug is ineffective, prophylactic antiarrhythmic agents given without proper supervision are potentially dangerous. In any event, a controlled trial is necessary to establish the value of this treatment. A patient who reaches the coronary-care unit is a "selected patient" with a good prognosis. The larger problem is the treatment of those patients who would otherwise die before reaching a hospital.

Long-Term Care. Evidence in favor of long-term anticoagulants has been cited. The best studies show a decrease in mortality for the first few years following an infarction but no difference in mortality after 5 years. If there is no contraindication to anticoagulants, and if the patient can be seen frequently and is conscientious, anticoagulant therapy can be used (Lovell, 1969). The effect of the anticoagulant, however, is not great enough to justify its use in patients who have medical contraindications or who are unreliable.

As with angina pectoris, a program of physical fitness (Naughton et al., 1969) and correction of known risk factors has the appeal of logic and some experimental support (Leren, 1966).

The incidence of sudden death is unaffected by anticoagulants or other known therapies. Sudden death may occur more commonly in patients who have had serious arrhythmias during their first infarction (Lovell, 1969) or who have ventricular premature systoles outside the hospital (Chiang et al., 1969b). If appropriate future clinical trials prove encouraging, these patients may be candidates for long-term prophylactic antiarrhythmic therapy.

In summary, the overall mortality from coronary artery disease will be improved little by further refinement of an acute attack in the coronary-care unit. The hope for the future lies in primary prevention of coronary disease, prophylactic treatment of high-risk patients, effective treatment of patients within the first minutes of an attack, and effective secondary prevention of heart attacks once coronary disease is established. *Principle: A physician can rationally use the data currently available to guide his treatment of individual patients and can follow the important studies in progress on primary and secondary prevention of coronary artery disease, in the hope that more definitive therapies will be forthcoming.*

V. PULMONARY EMBOLISM

CHARACTERISTICS OF THE DISEASE STATE

Although pulmonary embolic disease continues to be an important cause of death in hospitalized patients, the diagnosis is often not considered seriously or early enough to allow institution of aggressive and effective therapy (see Chapter 6). Advances in diagnostic techniques have been helpful, but probably the most critical determinant of morbidity and mortality of the disease is its suspicion by the doctor. Studies will probably indicate that the earlier the diagnosis of this common disease is made, the more favorable its outcome will be.

Clinical Circumstances Predisposing to Pulmonary Embolic Disease

Thrombi in the pelvic or leg veins or in the right atrium are the usual sources of pulmonary emboli. The single most important factor predisposing to thrombus formation is stasis of blood in large veins. Intrinsic disease of the valves in the vein commonly slows the flow of blood and initiates clotting. Other important factors include physical damage to or inflammation of the vein or perivenous tissues, and hypercoagulability. Diseases that require strict bed rest or immobilization of a limb, or are associated with pre-existing venous disease, congestive heart failure, atrial fibrillation, or depletion of plasma volume, are potential causes of stasis (Dalen and Dexter, 1967). The probabilities of thrombosis are increased when surgery, trauma, burns, or infection involves a vein. Surgery, malignancy, pregnancy, oral contraceptives, and estrogens are associated with an increased incidence of thromboembolism, and "hypercoagulability" has been implicated in an increased incidence of thrombosis (Wessler, 1963; Bailar, 1967; Oliver, 1967b; Vessey, 1969). However, "hypercoag-ulability" is not adequately defined and there are currently no clinically useful tests for the state (Owen, 1965). *Principle: Prompt and accurate diagnosis often may be the critical determinant of ultimate survival. Effective therapeutic measures may be useless if they are not applied or are given in adequate amounts at inappropriate times.*

Diagnosis

If a physician waits for the appearance of classical clinical roentgenologic and cardiographic signs of a pulmonary embolus before considering the diagnosis, he will fail to detect a large majority of the cases. Subtle changes such as unexplained tachypnea, tachycardia, or fever may be the only clue to the presence of an embolus. The patient may gradually or acutely develop heart failure that is unresponsive to therapy with digitalis. Hypotension, cardiac arrest, pleural effusion, an elevated diaphragm, or dyspnea with or without wheezing is consistent with the presence of pulmonary embolism. *Principle: Pulmonary embolism must be suspected in all hospitalized patients with a complicated course.*

If suspected clinically, the diagnosis can often be confirmed by appropriate tests. Pulmonary angiography, "lung scanning," and an arterial pO_2 are of particular value in confirming the diagnosis and following the response to therapy; these tests and the ratio of VD/VT may also be used to evaluate the effects of new drugs on the natural history of pulmonary embolus (Amador and Potchen, 1966; Fred et al., 1966; Editorial, 1967c; Tauxe et al., 1967; Tow et al., 1967; Poulose et al., 1968; Dalen et al., 1969a; Murray, 1971; Szacs et al., 1971) (see Chapter 6).

Natural History

The majority (75%) of deaths from pulmonary emboli occur within 1 hour of the acute symptoms; almost all the remaining deaths occur within the first 24 hours (Donaldson *et al.*, 1963). Patients surviving the first 24 hours usually live and may completely recover.

Resolution of the actual embolus in a patient receiving anticoagulants may be complete within a few days, but most emboli that produce moderate to severe pulmonary artery obstruction require weeks to months. After a single large embolus or multiple small emboli have caused extensive pulmonary artery occlusion, pulmonary blood flow may never return to normal. Indeed, cor pulmonale can develop insidiously after repeated small pulmonary emboli that have never caused symptoms or signs of pulmonary embolism on conventional x-ray examination of the chest (Editorial, 1967d; Fleischner, 1967). Because the natural history of pulmonary embolism varies and is represented by a wide spectrum of signs and symptoms, therapeutic interventions are difficult to evaluate. The criteria for patient selection for an experimental study should be carefully defined, and then meaningful data related to survival or improvement must be sought; for example, if patients are not brought into a study until 24 to 48 hours after an acute event, survival data are meaningless unless the study is extremely well controlled and large numbers of people are studied. Likewise, crossover studies are meaningless unless embolization is chronic, persistent, and frequent and each episode is identical to the previous episodes. The response to therapy in the experimental group and to standard measures in the control group should be based on objective assessment of acute and chronic changes in measurements of pulmonary function and hemodynamics.

Hemodynamic and Respiratory Responses

Mechanical obstruction of greater than 60% of the pulmonary circulation is required to cause pulmonary hypertension. With an acute pulmonary embolus, pulmonary hypertension may seem to be more severe than that expected on the basis of simple mechanical obstruction from the arterial occlusion. Experiments in animals have shown that neurogenic reflexes or the release of vasoactive substances may be important in the pathogenesis of hemodynamic and bronchoconstrictor responses to emboli. Barium sulfate emboli in cats cause pulmonary hypertension and constriction of the terminal airways (Price *et al.*, 1955; Nadel *et al.*, 1964). Histamine has been implicated in the constriction of the airways and sympathetic nervous reflexes in the genesis of pulmonary hypertension. With embolism of other unusual substances, varying from spores to glass beads,

results have been variable. The mechanism of response to experimental pulmonary emboli may be related to the physical size of the embolic particles rather than to their chemical composition (Sasahara, 1967). Experiments that use autologous blood clots as emboli more closely resemble the clinical situation. In such experiments, serotonin is released from platelets in the lung; the amine seems to account for bronchoconstriction and may contribute to vasoconstriction (Thomas, D. P., *et al.*, 1964, 1966). Wheezing and asthma-like attacks sometimes occur in humans after pulmonary emboli, and an endogenous substance such as serotonin may be responsible (Comroe *et al.*, 1953; Webster *et al.*, 1966; Sasahara *et al.*, 1967a; Olazábal *et al.*, 1968; Dalen *et al.*, 1969b).

Another mechanism that contributes to local bronchoconstriction is hypocapnia in alveolar gas. If blood flow ceases in a segment of the lung, the pCO_2 decreases, local bronchoconstriction occurs (Severinghaus, 1964), and the alveoli may collapse as the production of pulmonary surfactant decreases (Sutnick and Soloff, 1967; Morgan, 1971).

In clinical settings, hypoxia may play a role in the pathogenesis of pulmonary hypertension, and therapy with oxygen may partly or completely reverse the pulmonary hypertension after a pulmonary embolus (Sasahara, 1967). Alveolar hypoxia causes pulmonary hypertension by an unknown mechanism. Animal studies suggest that histamine, catecholamines, or a product of anaerobic metabolism may mediate the pulmonary hypoxic response (Liljestrand, 1958; Brutsaert, 1964; Robin *et al.*, 1967b; Hauge, 1968; Hauge and Melmon, 1968; Silove and Grover, 1968). In man, the mechanism of hypoxic pulmonary hypertension is still undefined. Current data are insufficient to allow specific therapy to be directed at the mediators of pulmonary hypertension.

ALTERATION OF CLOTTING SYSTEM

Anticoagulants

Anticoagulants have firm experimental and clinical bases in the treatment of thromboembolism. Prophylactic anticoagulation decreases thrombus formation when stasis is induced experimentally or clinically, and even if a thrombus is formed, adequate anticoagulation prevents extension of the thrombus (Thomas, 1965). Anticoagulant therapy, however, does not alter the preformed clot. Relief of vascular obstruction is dependent on dissolution, fragmentation, organization, and recanalization of the clot and on formation of collateral flow (Deykin, 1969).

Heparin. Heparin is a sulfated polysaccharide and a strong acid, carries a negative charge at physiologic pH, and combines with a variety of proteins. As a result of its interaction with proteins, heparin has direct anticoagulant properties (i.e., it acts *in vitro* and *in vivo*). Heparin prevents activation of factor IX and acts in combination with a plasma protein cofactor as an antithrombin (Figure 5–28) (Porter *et al.*, 1967; Deykin, 1969). As a consequence, the thrombin-mediated formation of fibrin and the thrombin-induced aggregation of platelets are inhibited. In this way heparin prevents the thrombin in newly formed thromboemboli from catalyzing further fibrin deposition and extension of the clot. It also prevents thrombin-induced platelet aggregation with release of pharmacologically active platelet contents, including serotonin and ADP (Thomas, D. P., *et al.*, 1966). The high concentration of heparin required to inhibit thrombin-induced platelet aggregation may not be achieved clinically. Nonetheless, patients occasionally have clinically significant bronchospasm during pulmonary emboli, and heparin is claimed to be useful as immediate treatment for the wheezing (Webster *et al.*, 1966; Sasahara *et al.*, 1967a), although there is no evidence that pulmonary hypertension is lowered (Sasahara, 1967).

Since the principal pharmacologic action of heparin appears to be a simple physicochemical interaction with basic proteins, other physical or chemical combinations can be predicted. The principal antidote for heparin is protamine, a base. Other heparin antagonists formerly used to reverse its effects (toluidine blue and hexadimethrine) are also basic (but too toxic for clinical use). A variety of commonly used drugs are basic and are known *in vivo* to combine with heparin, but their clinical effects have not been fully evaluated; they include antihistamines, quinidine, quinine, phenothiazines, tetracyclines and neomycin. Gross precipitation with basic drugs may appear in intravenous solutions containing heparin. Diminished effect of both drugs may occur if a combination is given even by separate routes.

Heparin is not a uniform molecular species; hence it is prescribed in units, as opposed to weight. Some preparations containing at least 120 units/ml are marketed as "standard." The use of a standard unit/ml of preparation gives a more reproducible dose than does a prescription written for milligram quantities.

Although there is incomplete information about the disposition of heparin, only 20% appears in the urine; the remainder is probably metabolized.

The half-life of intravenously administered heparin is dose dependent, increasing with the dose of the drug (after injection of 100, 200, and 400 units/kg, half-lives of 56, 96, and 152

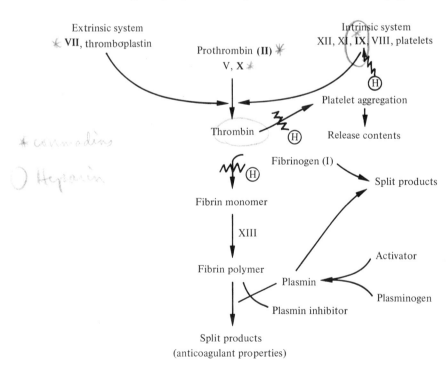

Extrinsic system
VII, thromboplastin

Prothrombin (II)
V, X

Intrinsic system
XII, XI, IX, VIII, platelets

Platelet aggregation

Thrombin (H)

Release contents

Fibrinogen (I)

Split products

Fibrin monomer

XIII

Fibrin polymer

Plasmin

Plasmin inhibitor

Activator

Plasminogen

Split products
(anticoagulant properties)

Figure 5–28. The clotting system. The intrinsic system probably is not important for intravascular thrombus formation. Heparin inhibits activation of IX and the action of thrombin (H). Oral anticoagulants decrease the production of vitamin K–dependent factors II, VII, IX, and X (in boldface type). Plasminogen activators act to form plasmin. Factors measured by prothrombin time are VII, X, V, II, and I. Factors known to be produced in the liver are I, II, V, VII, IX, and X.

minutes, respectively, are seen). This effect implies that the metabolic pathways for disposition of heparin are capable of saturation, and that at higher doses clearance by the kidney may increase (see Chapter 2).

Because heparin acts directly on coagulation factors, the kinetic data imply that unless there is a change in concentration of clotting factors due to synthesis or consumption, or a change in heparin metabolism, the peak anticoagulant effect, duration of action, and patient response are relatively constant. The short half-life of even the larger doses indicates the need for fairly frequent intravenous administration if a sustained effect is desired.

There is no uniformity of opinion concerning the optimal dose of heparin, the frequency of its administration, or the method of regulating the dose. Dosage is usually based on the clotting time of whole blood; a clotting time of at least twice control is considered therapeutic. Some recommend a continuous intravenous infusion of heparin at a rate determined by frequent assay of clotting times, a difficult procedure because it requires special nursing care to adjust the rate of infusion. However, infusion is probably the most reliable means to keep the clotting time constantly elevated when rigorous control is advisable (e.g., after multiple pulmonary emboli with borderline cardiovascular compensation, when continuing control may prevent a last fatal embolus). Others recommend giving 5,000 to 10,000 units of heparin intravenously every 4 hours, determining the clotting time initially and just prior to the next dose of heparin, adjusting the dose to maintain the clotting time no more than two to four times longer than the control. Although intermittent therapy results in peaks and troughs of anticoagulation, good results obtain. The use of intermittent intravenous heparin in large doses ($\geq 40,000$ units per day) without measuring clotting times has also produced favorable clinical results (Barritt and Jordan, 1960; Stamm, 1963; Bauer, 1964). However, since there is a considerable variation in the response to heparin between individuals and at different times in the same patient, the clotting time can help to ensure efficacy and to limit toxicity. Subcutaneous or intramuscular administration has been used, but adjustment of dosage and neutralization of effect are more difficult and bleeding into tissues at the intramuscular site is likely. Repository forms of heparin are available, but their use is hardly justifiable, because they may deliver active drug erratically, and the long duration of action of regular heparin permits relatively infrequent administration.

Side effects of heparin are largely related to hemorrhage. The incidence of hemorrhage is increased in elderly patients, particularly in women over 50 years of age (Jick et al., 1968). Drugs that inhibit platelet function, such as aspirin or dipyridamole, may provoke bleeding.

Sometimes the hemorrhage is not obvious, and its first manifestation may be a falling hematocrit or shock as a retroperitoneal hematoma develops. In addition, conditions simulating an intra-abdominal crisis and suggesting the need for surgery may in fact represent hemorrhage into the rectus abdominis, bleeding into the bowel wall or mesentery, or paralysis of a nerve due to pressure from a hematoma in a confined space (Morrison and Wurzel, 1964; Babb et al., 1965; Leatherman, 1968; Susens et al., 1968).

The anticoagulant action of heparin may be neutralized by a positively charged basic protein, protamine, but when given in excess, protamine has anticoagulant properties of its own. A 1-mg dose of protamine binds and neutralizes about 100 units of heparin. The amount of protamine required to neutralize the heparin remaining in the body can be calculated from the estimated blood volume and by the amount of protamine needed in vitro to return the clotting time of 10 ml of the patient's blood to normal. Smaller doses than estimated are used initially to avoid protamine-induced bleeding.

Heparin suppresses secretion of aldosterone and produces potassium retention (Majoor et al., 1960; Majoor, 1968). When given chronically, heparin has been associated with selective hypoaldosteronism and atrophy of the zona glomerulosa of the adrenal (Wilson and Goetz, 1964). The potential clinical importance of this effect should be considered when patients are treated even for a matter of days to weeks.

Chronic therapy with heparin (greater than 10,000 units per day for more than 6 months) causes osteoporosis and its complications (e.g., spontaneous fractures) (Annotation, 1965; Coon and Willis, 1966). *Principle: Chronic administration of a drug used for one purpose may cause profound changes in another system that outweigh the initial value of the drug.*

Uncommon side effects are alopecia, paresthesias, thrombocytopenia, urticaria, and other allergic manifestations, including anaphylactic shock (Wessler and Gaston, 1966).

Oral Anticoagulation. The two oral anticoagulants used most commonly in the United States are the coumarins warfarin and bishydroxycoumarin. Indanedione derivatives are often used in Europe. The drugs have different pharmacokinetics, but all influence the clotting mechanism similarly (Figure 5–28). The oral anticoagulants have no direct action on co-agulation, but they effectively antagonize vitamin K and thereby reduce the concentration of the clotting factors II, VII, IX, and X, which require vitamin K for their synthesis (Figure 5–28) (Aggeler, 1967; Lowenthal and Birn-baum, 1969). Factor IX is required for the intrinsic coagulation system, factor VII is required for the extrinsic coagulation system, and factors II and X are required by both systems.

Dosage of oral anticoagulants is adjusted by the changes in coagulation tests, the most widely used being the one-stage prothrombin time. A prothrombin time twice the control or a "prothrombin activity" of less than 25% is accepted as adequate anticoagulation (Wright, 1969a, 1969b). The one-stage prothrombin time is dependent on factors II, V, VII, and X; factor IX activity is not measured by this test.

The speed of onset of anticoagulant action depends on the normal catabolism of the affected clotting factors (Nagashima et al., 1969). Factor VII has a short biologic half-life of 1 1/2 to 6 hours; factor II has a half-life of 60 to 123 hours, and factors IX and X have half-lives of 20 to 40 hours (O'Reilly and Aggeler, 1968). As a consequence, when oral anti-coagulants are given, factor VII is the first to decrease and to influence the prothrombin time. Eventually the other factors fall to about the same level. However, for the first few days of therapy the lengthened prothrombin time is largely a reflection of the decrease in factor VII and does not necessarily indicate adequate anticoagulation.

Whether factor VII is important in the forma-tion of intravascular thrombi is not known, but it is probably not as important as factors II, IX, and X, which are part of the intrinsic coagulation system (Wessler, 1962). Experimental formation of intravascular thrombi has suggested that although the one-stage prothrombin time can be brought into the therapeutic range within 36 hours, the "antithrombotic" effect of bis-hydroxycoumarin is delayed for 1 week, presumably as a result of the slower catabolism of factors II, IX, and X (Deykin et al., 1960). Therefore, when anticoagulation is started with heparin and warfarin is added, heparin should be continued for several days after the warfarin-induced prothrombin time is in a desirable range. If heparin is withdrawn as soon as the changes in prothrombin time are "sufficient," the anticoagulant control is lost or at least becomes erratic.

In the past, therapy with oral anticoagulants was begun with large loading doses in order to achieve a rapid response of the prothrombin time. However, because the antithrombotic effects may not occur for 5 to 7 days, it has been suggested that smaller starting doses be used on a daily basis (O'Reilly and Aggeler, 1968). When warfarin is given in daily doses of 10 to 15 mg, the decline in concentration of factors II, IX, and X is no slower than with a large loading dose of 50 to 120 mg, although the decline in factor VII concentration is delayed. Patients receiving the smaller daily dose achieve thera-peutic prothrombin times within a week, which is the minimum time required experimentally for antithrombotic effects of coumarins to appear. Objectives must be carefully set before therapy is begun. In most instances the criteria used to assess progress directly relate to the pharmaco-logic effect of the drug as it alters the manifesta-tions of disease or its physiology. Often drugs are given for prophylaxis when the objective is maintenance of homeostasis. In such settings and in other instances when the only direct beneficial effect of drug therapy is recorded by laboratory procedures, the details of those tests and their relation to physiology should be carefully assessed and understood so that guidance provided by the test is rational and reflects the desired changes that can be produced by the drug.

Smaller daily doses are preferred to a very large loading dose because anticoagulation fluctuates less and the difference between the starting and daily maintenance doses (5 to 10 mg of warfarin) is small. Some patients with heart failure or liver disease, or who are elderly or malnourished, may be particularly sensitive to the oral anticoagulants, and a large loading dose may be especially hazardous.

If rapid anticoagulation is required, heparin should be used. Heparin affects the one-stage prothrombin time because of its antithrombin effects. Hence, when oral anticoagulants are given to a patient also taking heparin, the prothrombin time reflects the presence of both heparin and coumarin. When heparin is withdrawn, the dosage of coumarin must be adjusted. If intravenous heparin is used in-termittently every 4 to 6 hours, there is usually little effect on the prothrombin time of blood drawn just prior to the next dose (Moser and Hajjar, 1967).

The pharmacokinetics of oral anticoagulants differ. Warfarin and bishydroxycoumarin are good examples of the differences. Warfarin has a half-life of about 44 hours, and the drug dis-appears by first-order kinetics (the disappear-ance rate is constant and independent of the dose or concentration [see Chapter 2]). In contrast, bishydroxycoumarin has a biologic half-life that is dose dependent; the biologic half-life in-creases with increased doses. Thus larger doses disappear from the body more slowly (with longer half-lives) than do smaller doses. This difference is important to remember both in setting the dose for therapy and in understanding drug interactions (O'Reilly *et al.*, 1964; Nagashima *et al.*, 1968).

Unusual responses to the oral anticoagulants may be based either on genetic abnormalities or on drug interactions. Two types of resistance to warfarin unrelated to drug interaction have been reported. In one type the patients have a decreased sensitivity to high concentrations of drug in plasma; in the other type, patients metabolize the drug more rapidly than normals (O'Reilly *et al.*, 1964; Lewis *et al.*, 1967). *Principle: Acquired or genetic defects can lead to both extremes in a person's response to a drug. Often increased sensitivity is easy to diagnose because it results in expression of toxicity to the drug. However, unless clear criteria for an effect of a drug are set and the dose of the drug is increased until the effect is seen (no reliance on cookbook prescriptions), the lack of response to a drug may not be detected and the patient may be cheated by inappropriate use of an otherwise efficacious drug.*

Interactions of drugs with coumarin anticoagulants are discussed in Chapter 16. Drugs can alter the effect of coumarin by interfering with (1) protein binding (phenylbutazone), (2) metabolism (phenobarbital, glutethimide), and possibly (3) absorption (phenobarbital) or (4) receptor-site affinity for the anticoagulants (Figure 5–29) (Carter, 1965; Corn, 1966;

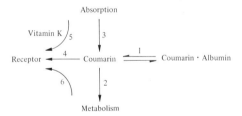

Figure 5–29. Drugs can affect the response to oral anticoagulants by (*1*) influencing protein binding, (*2*) changing the rate of metabolism, (*3*) altering absorption, or (*4*) altering receptor site affinity for the drug. (*5*) Drugs affecting the absorption or availability of vitamin K alter the response to coumarins. Other drugs (*6*) can independently compete with vitamin K and thus can be additive to the coumarin drugs.

Aggeler, 1967; Aggeler *et al.*, 1967; Medical Letter, 1967b; O'Reilly, 1967; Hunninghake and Azarnoff, 1968; MacDonald *et al.*, 1969). In addition, drugs may independently affect (5) vitamin K absorption (antibiotics, cholestyr-

amine) or (6) the vitamin-K-sensitive clotting factors (propylthiouracil, salicylates, quinidine) and thus may alter the response to the oral anticoagulants (Medical Letter, 1967b; Koch-Weser, 1968a). Sometimes the interaction is obvious but the mechanism is not (clofibrate, D-thyroxine) (Solomon and Schrogie, 1966).

Principle: Experiments in animals can be valuable, but data obtained from humans are essential for complete understanding of the effects and use of a drug. For example, barbiturates can stimulate drug-metabolizing enzymes in animals and man, and barbiturates decrease the half-life and hypoprothrombinemic effect of bishydroxycoumarin in man (Aggeler and O'Reilly, 1966). A logical but fallacious assumption might be that barbiturates stimulate enzymes that metabolize bishydroxycoumarin (Goss and Dickhaus, 1965). However, the anticoagulant effect of intravenously administered bishydroxycoumarin is not changed by barbiturates (Dayton *et al.*, 1961); therefore, enzyme induction of metabolism may not explain this drug interaction (Lewis, 1966). Barbiturates also increase the fecal excretion of orally administered bishydroxycoumarin. Since the excretion rate of bishydroxycoumarin depends on the dose of the drug in blood, the decreased half-life of orally administered bishydroxycoumarin could be the result of interference in its absorption by barbiturate. Thus the interaction of barbiturates and bishydroxycoumarin may not be due to enzyme stimulation alone, but rather to diminished absorption of the anticoagulant when it is taken orally (Aggeler, 1967). *Principle: One must be careful in extrapolating data from mouse to man, or in assuming that a single mechanism is responsible for a given effect.*

Bishydroxycoumarin can potentiate the action of both tolbutamide and diphenylhydantoin. Such potentiation may occur by inhibition of the metabolism of these two drugs by the anticoagulant (Sise, 1967; Wright, 1969c). *Principle: Interactions are probably more common than is now suspected, and clinical alertness to an unusual response is the key to their discovery.*

As with heparin, side effects of oral anticoagulants are primarily related to overt or occult bleeding. The indanedione compounds are allergenic and have been associated with agranulocytosis (Weiner, 1967). The coumarins have been associated with a peculiar necrosis of the skin and subcutaneous tissue, primarily in women (Koch-Weser, 1968b; Korbitz *et al.*, 1969). Fortunately all side effects except hemorrhage are rare, and hemorrhage represents inappropriate use of the drug that usually can be rapidly countered by transfusions with whole blood or plasma, if an immediate effect is needed, or by vitamin K_1 if the bleeding must be stopped before drug effect wanes. If a non-hemorrhagic side effect occurs, anticoagulation can be accomplished with heparin while the offending agent is withdrawn.

Vitamin K_1 counteracts the effects of the oral anticoagulants by increasing the synthesis rate of factors II, VII, IX, and X; its effects are necessarily slower than the effects of transfusion, which immediately supplies these factors. Because normal levels of these factors are not restored for several hours, the effect of vitamin K_1 on anticoagulation is not analogous to the immediate effects of protamine, i.e., antagonism of heparin effects. Vitamin K_3 (menadione) is much less effective than vitamin K_1 (mephyton) for reversal of the anticoagulant effects of the coumarins. If vitamin K_1 is used to reverse the effects of oral anticoagulation, reinstitution of anticoagulation may be difficult. Therefore, the use of vitamin K_1 for minor hemorrhage is not encouraged if the patient must be continued on effective anticoagulant therapy. Withdrawal of the oral anticoagulant for a few days or the administration of small oral doses of vitamin K_1 is usually sufficient to re-establish therapeutic control of prothrombin activity and to halt minor bleeding. Moderate-to-severe hemorrhage must be treated with vitamin K_1, which can be given parenterally

Experimental Drugs Altering Coagulation

Thrombolytic Agents. Urokinase and streptokinase are two plasminogen activators currently being tested. The aim of such therapy is to establish a controlled, tolerated, fibrinolytic state that is capable of disintegrating intravascular clots (Figure 5–28). Plasminogen is activated by urokinase and streptokinase to form plasmin, a relatively nonspecific proteolytic enzyme. A circulating plasmin inhibitor effectively counteracts the proteolytic potential of plasmin. Plasmin formed from plasminogen within a fibrin clot, however, is protected from the circulating plasmin inhibitor, is capable of fibrinolysis, and can digest the fibrin clot. In this way, controlled fibrinolysis confined to fibrin clots can be obtained (Sherry, 1968). Since plasmin digests fibrinogen as well as fibrin and since the products of digestion have anticoagulant properties, an uncontrolled fibrinolytic state causes fibrinogen depletion and anticoagulation, leaving the patient particularly vulnerable to hemorrhage (McNicol and Douglas, 1967).

Thrombolysis may be beneficial in the treatment of those patients with pulmonary emboli who survive the first hour but who would be expected to die within 24 to 48 hours. Prelim-

inary results using angiography, lung scanning, and hemodynamic measurements have suggested that pharmacologic stimulation of thrombolysis can dissolve pulmonary emboli (Editorial, 1967e; Sasahara et al., 1967b; Tow et al., 1967; Genton and Wolf, 1968; Wright, 1969c). The best results are obtained when the embolic event is recent (Genton and Wolf, 1968). Whether thrombolytic therapy followed by anticoagulation with coumarin-like drugs is superior to anticoagulant therapy alone in terms of speed of clot resolution, morbidity, or mortality is unknown, but this question is the subject of a cooperative study utilizing urokinase (Walsh et al., 1969).

Streptokinase is a streptococcal antigen and is inactivated by circulating antistreptococcal antibody present to variable extents in all patients. Therefore, the dose necessary to achieve controlled fibrinolysis also is variable, and continuing intermittent or recurrent therapy is difficult since a large amount of antibody that inactivates the drug is produced during the first course of treatment. Owing to the practical difficulty in using the drug and the presence of a pyrogen in some early preparations, streptokinase is not being investigated in the United States. European experience with a more purified preparation has been encouraging, and since the drug is relatively easy to produce, streptokinase may deserve further evaluation in the United States (Sherry, 1969).

Urokinase, a substance in human urine, is nonantigenic; therefore, its effects are more easily controlled than those of streptokinase. However, urokinase is difficult to prepare and is available to only a few investigators.

Although thrombolytic therapy is presently far from routine, the concept is attractive as a "medical embolectomy" and may be useful in selected patients (Genton and Pechet, 1968).

Malayan Pit Viper Venom's Fraction 6. Blood obtained from patients bitten by the Malayan pit viper does not clot. Venom's fraction 6 is capable of causing defibrination by forming abnormal fibrin polymers that are easily lysed to fibrin split products with antithrombin effects (Ashford et al., 1968; Reid and Chan, 1968). Plasminogen is also depleted, perhaps as a direct effect of the venom, but platelets and other clotting factors are unaltered. Patients have been treated with fraction 6; some have responded satisfactorily, and spontaneous bleeding has been uncommon. However, the fraction of venom is antigenic; tolerance to the pharmacologic effects can develop (Pitney et al., 1969) and hypersensitivity reactions are fairly common (Bell et al., 1968; Sharp et al., 1968). An instance of microangiopathic hemolytic anemia also has occurred, suggesting that fibrin is deposited in small vessels (Sharp *et al.*, 1968) and that the plasminogen depletion that occurs may protect such fibrin deposits from endogenous fibrinolysis (Editorial, 1968b). Currently, the difficulties with defibrination therapy outweigh its potential advantages, and unless therapeutic superiority over standard anticoagulants is shown, fraction 6 will remain a research tool (Editorial, 1968b). *Principle: New therapy must be proved superior to standard effective therapy. It should not be accepted merely because it is unique and theoretically attractive.*

CLINICAL THERAPY

Knowledge of the clinical settings predisposing to stasis, hypercoagulability, or vascular damage can indicate the need for prevention of pulmonary thromboembolic disease. If prevention is not hazardous it is always preferable to treatment after the fact.

Prophylactic Therapy

Prophylactic therapy in its simplest and safest form is directed at minimizing the venous stasis of bed rest. Elastic stockings, exercises, and early ambulation after surgery or disease can prevent venous thrombosis and subsequent pulmonary embolism. Simple methods such as these are often overlooked but in the long run may be more valuable than anticoagulants, thrombolytic agents, or a basketful of pit vipers.

In certain high-risk groups of patients the value of prophylactic anticoagulation is well established. These patients are unable to ambulate, are in a cast, or have veins damaged by surgery or inflammation, and are thereby susceptible to venous thrombosis. Elderly patients with fractures provide excellent examples of the value of prophylactic anticoagulation (Sevitt and Gallagher, 1959; Salzman *et al.*, 1966), and the same probably applies to all fractures of the pelvis or lower limbs requiring prolonged bed rest (Sevitt, 1962; Neu *et al.*, 1965; Thomas, 1965). In such patients the incidence of thromboembolism is reduced from 10 to 20% to about 1%, and overt venous thrombosis is also decreased. In spite of the acknowledged difficulties in diagnosis of venous thrombosis and pulmonary embolism, the striking improvement obtained with prophylactic anticoagulation seems valid.

Patients with gynecologic disease who are undergoing pelvic surgery also benefit from prophylatic anticoagulation (Bottomley *et al.*, 1964). Other good candidates for anticoagulation are patients with burns, severe congestive heart failure, and a history of thrombophlebitis.

Although the concept of prophylactic anticoagulation is sound, the need for anticoagulants in the latter conditions is not well established (Sevitt and Gallagher, 1961).

The oral anticoagulants are used most commonly for prophylaxis and are continued until the patient is able to ambulate. Heparin can also be used and is desirable if closer control or immediate anticoagulation is required. Patients with established contraindications to anticoagulants, such as current or recent severe bleeding, central nervous system surgery, and clotting disorders should not be treated. Patients with a history of peptic ulcers, colitis, minor gastrointestinal bleeding, hypertension greater than 180/100, renal or hepatic disease, or polycythemia with hemorrhagic complications should be considered at increased risk for complications, and the proposed benefits must be weighed against the dangers (Wright, 1969b). *Principle: All therapy is potentially hazardous. Contraindications to therapy are absolute only if risk outweighs the benefits.*

In the reported series, the incidence of complications from prophylactic anticoagulation is low, and major hemorrhage requiring transfusion is less than 1%. Surgery on a limb can be performed while the prothrombin time is in the therapeutic range with little increase in risk from hemorrhage (Salzman *et al.*, 1966). In summary, the evidence clearly supports the value of prophylactic anticoagulation in the high-risk groups. This form of therapy is not widely used, even in teaching hospitals, because it is difficult to persuade a physician to use therapy that has obvious potential hazards but no easily recognizable direct benefits. Such therapy, however, is the essence of preventive medicine. *Principle: Prophylactic therapy may be the most effective way to treat a disease. If controlled studies show definite benefit and minimal risk in high-risk groups of patients, prophylaxis is reasonable although direct benefit to the individual patient cannot be ascertained.*

Therapy of Acute Pulmonary Embolism

Immediate anticoagulation using intravenous heparin (usually 40,000 units per day) reduces new clot formation and the propagation of old clots and may decrease the thrombin-induced release of pharmacologically active substances from platelets. Adequate anticoagulation (greater than two times control clotting time) decreases the mortality rate of pulmonary emboli from 30% to 5% (Barritt and Jordan, 1960; Bauer, 1964). Oxygen therapy may also be of value in decreasing pulmonary vascular resistance.

The duration of therapy is arbitrary. Usually, heparin is continued for 1 to 3 weeks or until ambulation is complete and evidence of venous thrombosis or phlebitis has disappeared (De-Graff and Buchnam, 1969). Firm adherence of the clot to the wall of the vessel probably occurs by one week (Thomas, 1965). Patients who cannot be mobilized or otherwise continue to be at high risk for pulmonary emboli, as well as those who have recurrent pulmonary emboli, should be continued on anticoagulants indefinitely. Anticoagulation is begun with heparin and continued with oral anticoagulants. There is little clinical evidence that heparin offers more protection than oral anticoagulants, and the major reason to use heparin first is the immediacy of its effect.

Surgical Therapy

Venous Ligation or Plication. If pulmonary emboli recur while the patient is adequately anticoagulated, or if the patient with a pulmonary embolus cannot be anticoagulated, surgery on the affected veins is indicated. Vena caval ligation or plication followed by anticoagulation if possible is the current procedure of choice.

The mortality of the procedure varies widely in different series and depends on the general cardiac status of the patient. The morbidity (incapacitating sequelae) of the procedure varies from 0 to 50%.

In spite of the lack of a properly controlled, randomized study, venous ligation is considered to be lifesaving in selected patients with large emboli arising in the legs or pelvis. However, a properly performed operation is no guarantee of continued success, since emboli may arise in the right heart or in the cul-de-sac left in the vena cava, or may traverse dilated collateral veins to reach the lungs (Gurewich et al., 1966; Sautter, 1969). A late failure rate of surgery of as much as 20% has been reported (Gurewich et al., 1966).

Pulmonary Embolectomy. One of the most dramatic treatments in modern medicine is acute pulmonary embolectomy. The role of this procedure in treatment of pulmonary emboli is not established. Ideally, the candidates selected for embolectomy would otherwise not survive (Stansel et al., 1967). Since most of the deaths that occur take place within one hour, a very alert team must be available at all times if embolectomy is to be a practical form of therapy. Mortality of the procedure is high, and a few misdiagnoses can negate much of the benefit of therapy. Therefore, emergency pulmonary angiograms are essential. Because of the effectiveness of heparin therapy in management of pulmonary emboli and the promising experience with thrombolytic agents, pulmonary embolectomy probably will have little to offer.

In any event, the surgical procedure must be proved by a randomized series to be superior to medical management before such heroics can be generally recommended. *Principle: Dramatic therapy is not necessarily good therapy, and many surgical procedures can be considered admissions of our ignorance (hopefully temporary) of adequate medical management.*

REFERENCES

Ackerman, G. L.; Doherty, J. E.; and Flanigan, W. J.: Peritoneal dialysis and hemodialysis of tritiated digoxin. Ann. Intern. Med., 67:718–23, 1967.

Aggeler, P. M.: Blood coagulation and the coumarin anticoagulant drugs. Calif. Med., 106:255–71, 1967.

Aggeler, P. M., and O'Reilly, R. A.: The pharmacologic basis of oral anticoagulant therapy. Thromb. Diath. Haemorrh., 15 (Suppl. 21):227–56, 1966.

Aggeler, P. M.; O'Reilly, R. A.; Leong, L.; and Kowitz, P. E.: Potentiation of anticoagulant effect of warfarin by phenylbutazone. New Eng. J. Med., 276:496–501, 1967.

Alarcon-Segovia, D.; Wakim, K. G.; Worthington, J. W.; and Ward, L. E.: Clinical and experimental studies on the hydralazine syndrome and its relationship to systemic lupus erythematosus. Medicine, 46:1–33, 1967.

Alousi, A., and Weiner, N.: The regulation of norepinephrine synthesis on sympathetic nerves: effect of nerve stimulation, cocaine, and catecholamine releasing agents. Proc. Nat. Acad. Sci., 66:1491–96, 1966.

Amador, E., and Potchen, J.: Serum lactic dehydrogenase activity and radioactive lung scanning in the diagnosis of pulmonary embolism. Ann. Intern. Med., 65:1247–55, 1966.

Amsterdam, E. A.; Couch, N. P.; Christlieb, A. R.; Harrison, J. H.; Crane, C.; Dobrzinsky, S. J.; and Hickler, R. B.: Renal vein renin activity in the prognosis of surgery for renovascular hypertension. Amer. J. Med., 47:860–68, 1969.

Amsterdam, E. A.; Wolfson, S.; and Gorlin, R.: New aspects of the placebo response in angina pectoris. Amer. J. Cardiol., 24:305–306, 1969.

Anden, N. E.: On the mechanism of noradrenalin depletion by α-methyl meta-tyrosine and metaraminol. Acta Pharmacol. Toxicol., 21:260–71, 1964.

Andersen, N., and Johansen, S. H.: Incidence of catecholamine-induced arrhythmias during halothane anesthesia. Anesthesiology, 24:51–56, 1963.

Andersen, R. W.; James, P. M.; Bredenberg, C. E.; and Hardaway, R. M.: Phenoxybenzamine in septic shock. Ann. Surg., 165:341–50, 1967.

Anderson, S. T., and Pitt, A.: Lidocaine in the management of ventricular arrhythmia. Med. J. Aust., 1:208–11, 1969.

Annotation: Heparin and osteoporosis. Lancet, 2:376, 1965.

Anton, A. H.; Greer, M.; Sayre, D. F.; and Williams, C. F.: Dihydroxyphenylalanine secretion in a malignant pheochromocytoma. Amer. J. Med., 42:469–75, 1967.

Antonis, A., and Bersohn, I.: Influence of diet on serum-triglycerides in South African white and Bantu prisoners. Lancet, 1:3–9, 1961.

———: The influence of diet on serum lipids in South African white and Bantu prisoners. Amer. J. Clin. Nutr., 10:484–99, 1962.

Armstrong, M. L.; Warner, E. D.; and Connor, W. E.: Regression of coronary atheromatosis in Rhesus monkeys. Circ. Res., 27:59–67, 1970.

Arnold, K., and Gerber, N.: The rate of decline of diphenylhydantoin in human plasma. *Clin. Pharmacol. Ther.*, **11**:121–34, 1970.

Aronow, W. S., and Kaplan, M. A.: Propranolol combined with isosorbide dinitrate versus placebo in angina pectoris. *New Eng. J. Med.*, **280**:847–50, 1969.

Aronow, W. S.; Kaplan, M. A.; and Jacob, D.: Tobacco: a precipitating factor in angina pectoris. *Ann. Intern. Med.*, **69**:529–36, 1968.

Aronow, W. S., and Swanson, A. J.: Non-nicotinized cigarettes and angina pectoris. *Ann. Intern. Med.*, **70**: 1227, 1969.

Ashford, A.; Ross, J. W.; and Southgate, P.: Pharmacology and toxicology of defibrinating substance from Malayan pit viper venom. *Lancet*, **1**:486–89, 1968.

Askey, J. M.: Digitalis in acute myocardial infarction. *J.A.M.A.*, **146**:1008–10, 1951.

Aspenström, G., and Korsan-Bengtsen, K.: A double-blind study of Dicumarol prophylaxis in coronary heart disease. *Acta Med. Scand.*, **176**:563–75, 1964.

Åström, H.: Haemodynamic effects of beta-adrenergic blockade. *Brit. Heart J.*, **30**:44–49, 1968.

Auerbach, O.; Hammond, E. C.; and Garfinkel, L.: Smoking in relation to atherosclerosis of the coronary arteries. *New Eng. J. Med.*, **273**:775–79, 1965.

———: Thickening of walls of arterioles and small arteries in relation to age and smoking habits. *New Eng. J. Med.*, **278**:980–84, 1968.

Avoy, D. R.; Swyryd, E. A.; and Gould, R.: Effects of alpha-*p*-chlorophenoxy-isobutyrlethyl ester (CPIB) with and without androsterone on cholesterol biosynthesis in rat liver. *J. Lipid Res.*, **6**:369–76, 1965.

Axelrod, J.: Purification and properties of phenylethanolamine-N-methyl transferase. *J. Biol. Chem.*, **237**:1657–60, 1962.

Ayres, S. M., and Grace, W. J.: Inappropriate ventilation and hypoxemia as causes of cardiac arrhythmias. *Amer. J. Med.*, **46**:495–505, 1969.

Azarnoff, D. L.; Tucker, D. R.; and Barr, G. A.: Studies with ethyl chlorophenoxyisobutyrate (clofibrate). *Metabolism*, **14**:959–65, 1965.

Babb, R. R.; Spittell, J. A., Jr.; and Bartholomew, L. G.: Hematoma of the rectus abdominis muscle complicating anticoagulant therapy. *Mayo Clin. Proc.*, **40**:760–65, 1965.

Bacq, Z. M.; Gosselin, L.; Dresse, A.; and Renson, J.: Inhibition of *o*-methyltransferase by catechol and sensitization to epinephrine. *Science*, **130**:453–54, 1959.

Bailar, J. C.: Thromboembolism and oestrogen therapy. *Lancet*, **2**:560, 1967.

Bailey, D. J., Jr.: Cardiotoxic effects of quinidine and their treatment. *Arch. Intern. Med. (Chicago)*, **105**:13–22, 1960.

Bailey, G. W. H.; Braniff, B. A.; Hancock, E. W.; and Cohn, K. E.: Relation of left atrial pathology to atrial fibrillation in mitral valvular disease. *Ann. Intern. Med.*, **69**:13–20, 1968.

Bainton, C. R., and Peterson, D. R.: Deaths from coronary heart disease in persons fifty years of age and younger. *New Eng. J. Med.*, **268**:569–75, 1963.

Balcon, R.; Hoy, J.; and Sowton, E.: Haemodynamic effects of rapid digitalization following acute myocardial infarction. *Brit. Heart J.*, **30**:373–76, 1968.

Barger, A. C.: Renal hemodynamic factors in congestive heart failure. *Ann. N.Y. Acad. Sci.*, **139**:276–84, 1966.

Barritt, D. W., and Jordan, S. C.: Anticoagulant drugs in treatment of pulmonary embolism: a controlled trial. *Lancet*, **1**:1309–12, 1960.

Bartter, F. C.; Pronove, P.; Gill, J. R., Jr.; and MacCardle, R. C.: Hyperplasia of juxtaglomerular complex with hyperaldosteronism and hypokalemic alkalosis: a new syndrome. *Amer. J. Med.*, **33**:811–28, 1962.

Bashour, F. A.; Jones, E.; and Edmonson, R.: Cardiac arrhythmias in acute myocardial infarction. II. Incidence of the common arrhythmias with special reference to ventricular tachycardia. *Dis. Chest*, **51**:520–29, 1967.

Bassett, A. L.; Bigger, J. T.; and Hoffman, B. F.: Effects of diphenylhydantoin on cat heart muscle. *Circulation*, **36** (Suppl. II):61, 1967.

Batterman, R. C., and Gutner, L. B.: Hitherto undescribed neurological manifestations of digitalis toxicity. *Amer. Heart J.*, **36**:582–86, 1948.

Battock, D. J.; Alvarez, H.; and Chidsey, C. A.: Effects of propranolol and isosorbide dinitrate on exercise performance and adrenergic activity in patients with angina pectoris. *Circulation*, **39**:157–69, 1969.

Bauer, G.: Clinical experiences of a surgeon in the use of heparin. *Amer. J. Cardiol.*, **14**:29–35, 1964.

Becker, L. C.; Fortuin, N. J.; and Pitt, B.: Effect of ischemia and antianginal drugs on the distribution of radioactive microspheres in the canine left ventricle. *Circ. Res.*, **28**:263–69, 1971.

Beecher, H. K.: Appraisal of drugs intended to alter subjective responses, symptoms: report to Council on Pharmacy and Chemistry. *J.A.M.A.*, **158**:399–401, 1955.

Beiser, G. D.; Epstein, S. E.; Stampfer, M.; Robinson, B.; and Braunwald, E.: Studies on digitalis. XVII. Effects of ouabain on the hemodynamic response to exercise in patients with mitral stenosis in normal sinus rhythm. *New Eng. J. Med.*, **278**:131–37, 1968b.

Beiser, G. D.; Stampfer, M.; Goldstein, R. E.; Epstein, S. E.; and Braunwald, E.: Comparison of the peak inotropic effects of a catecholamine and a digitalis glycoside in the intact canine heart. *Clin. Res.*, **16**:221, 1968a.

Bell, W. R.; Pitney, W. R.; and Goodwin, J. F.: Therapeutic defibrination in treatment of thrombotic disease. *Lancet*, **1**:490–93, 1968.

Beller, G. A.; Smith, T. W.; Abelmann, W. H.; Haber, E.; and Hood, W. B.: Digitalis intoxication. A prospective clinical study with serum level correlations. *New Eng. J. Med.*, **284**:989–97, 1971.

Bellet, S.; Hamdan, G.; Somlyo, A.; and Lara, R.: The reversal of cardiotoxic effects of quinidine by molar sodium lactate: an experimental study. *Amer. J. Med. Sci.*, **237**:165–76, 1959a.

———: The reversal of cardiotoxic effects of procainamide by molar sodium lactate. *Amer. J. Med. Sci.*, **237**:177–89, 1959b.

Bellet, S.; Roman, L. R.; and Boza, A.: Relation between serum quinidine levels and renal function. Studies in normal subjects and patients with congestive failure and renal insufficiency. *Amer. J. Cardiol.*, **27**:368–71, 1971.

Benchimol, A.; Lucena, E. G.; and Dimond, E. G.: Stroke volume and peripheral resistance during infusion of isoproterenol at a constant fixed heart rate. *Circulation*, **31**:417–28, 1965.

Berk, D. P., and Chalmers, T.: Deafness complicating antibiotic therapy of hepatic encephalopathy. *Ann. Intern. Med.*, **73**:393–96, 1970.

Berkson, D. M., and Stamler, J.: Epidemiological findings on cerebrovascular diseases and their implications. *J. Atheroscler. Res.*, **5**:189–202, 1965.

Best, M. M.; Duncan, C. H.; Van Loon, E. J.; and Wathen, J. D.: Effects of sitosterol on serum lipids. *Amer. J. Med.*, **19**:61–70, 1955.

Bierenbaum, M. L.; Green, D. P.; Florin, A.; Reischman, A. I.; and Caldwell, A. B.: Modified-fat dietary management of the young male with coronary disease. *J.A.M.A.*, **202**:1119–23, 1967.

Bierman, E. L., and Porte, D., Jr.: Carbohydrate intolerance and lipemia. *Ann. Intern. Med.*, 68:926–33, 1968.

Bigger, J. T.; Bassett, A. L.; and Hoffman, B. F.: Electrophysiological effects of diphenylhydantoin on canine Purkinje fibers. *Circ. Res.*, 22:221–36, 1968a.

Bigger, J. T., and Heissenbuttel, R. H.: The use of procainamide and lidocaine in the treatment of cardiac arrhythmias. *Progr. Cardiov. Dis.*, 11:515–34, 1969.

Bigger, J. T.; Schmidt, D. H.; and Kutt, H.: Relationship between the plasma level of diphenylhydantoin and its cardiac antiarrhythmic effects. *Circulation*, 38:363–74, 1968b.

————: A method for estimation of plasma diphenylhydantoin concentration. *Amer. Heart J.*, 77:572–73, 1969.

Bigger, J. T.; Weinberg, D. I.; Kovalik, A. T.; Harris, P. D.; Cranefield, P. C.; and Hoffman, B. F.: Effects of diphenylhydantoin on excitability and automaticity in the canine heart. *Circ. Res.*, 26:1–15, 1970.

Biglieri, E. G.; Herron, M. A.; and Brust, N.: 17-Hydroxylation deficiency in man. *J. Clin. Invest.*, 15:1946–54, 1966.

Biglieri, E. G., and McIlroy, M. B.: Abnormalities of renal function and circulatory reflexes in primary aldosteronism. *Circulation*, 33:78–86, 1966.

Biglieri, E. G.; Schambelan, M.; Slaton, P. E.; and Stockigt, J.: The intercurrent hypertension of primary aldosteronism. *Circ. Res.*, 27 (Suppl I):195–202, 1970.

Biglieri, E. G.; Slaton, P. E.; Schambelan, M.; and Kronfield, S. J.: Hypermineralocorticism. *Amer. J. Med.*, 45:170–75, 1968.

Bishop, V. S.; Stone, H. L.; and Guyton, A. C.: Cardiac function curves in conscious dogs. *Amer. J. Physiol.*, 207:677–82, 1964.

Blankenhorn, D. H.; Chin, H. P.; and Lau, F. Y. K.: Ischemic heart disease in young adults: metabolic and angiographic diagnosis and the prevalence of type IV hyperlipoproteinemia. *Ann. Intern. Med.*, 69:21–33, 1968.

Blomgren, S. E.; Condemi, J. J.; Bignall, M. C.; and Vaughan, J. H.: Antinuclear antibody induced by procainamide: a prospective study. *New Eng. J. Med.*, 281:64–66, 1969.

Bloom, P. M.; Nelp, W. B.; and Tuell, S. H.: Relationship of the excretion of tritiated digoxin to renal function. *Amer. J. Med. Sci.*, 251:133–44, 1966.

Bongiovanni, A. M., and Root, A. W.: The adrenogenital syndrome. *New Eng. J. Med.*, 268:1283–89, 1342–51, 1391–99, 1963.

Borchgrevink, C. F.; Bjerkelund, C.; Abrahamsen, A. M.; Bay, A.; Borgen, P.; Grande, B.; Helle, I.; Kjörstad, H; Petersen, A. M.; Rörvik, T.; Thorsen, R.; and Ödegaard, A.: Long-term anticoagulant therapy after myocardial infarction in women. *Brit. Med. J.*, 3:571–74, 1968.

Bottomley, J. E.; Lloyd, O.; and Chalmers, D. G.: Postoperative prophylactic anticoagulants in gynaecology: a ten year study. *Lancet*, 2:835–36, 1964.

Boullin, D. J.; Costa, E.; and Brodie, B. B.: Discharge of tritium-labeled guanethidine by sympathetic nerve stimulation as evidence that guanethidine is a false transmitter. *Life. Sci.*, 5:803–808, 1966.

Bourne, H. R., and Melmon, K. L.: Guides to the pharmacologic management of essential hypertension. *Pharmacol. Physicians*, 5:1–6, 1971.

Bourne, H. R.; Thomson, P. D.; and Melmon, K. L.: Diagnosis and treatment of beta-adrenergic hyperresponsiveness: a critical appraisal. *Arch. Intern. Med.* (*Chicago*), 25:1063–66, 1970.

Boyd, D. L., and Williams, J. F., Jr.: The effect of diphenylhydantoin (Dilantin) on the positive inotropic action of digitalis. *Amer. J. Cardiol.*, 23: 712–18, 1969.

Brachfeld, N.; Bozer, J.; and Gorlin, R.: Action of nitroglycerin on coronary circulation in normal and in mild cardiac subjects. *Circulation*, 19:697–704, 1959.

Brackett, N. C., Jr.; Koppel, M.; Randall, R. E., and Nixon, W. P.: Hyperplasia of the juxtaglomerular complex with secondary aldosteronism without hypertension (Bartter's syndrome). *Amer. J. Med.*, 44:803–19 1968.

Brandt, K.; Cathcart, E. S.; and Cohen, A. S.: A clinical analysis of the course and prognosis of forty-two patients with amyloidosis. *Amer. J. Med.*, 44:955–69, 1968.

Braunwald, E.: The pathogenesis and treatment of shock in myocardial infarction. *Johns Hopkins Med. J.*, 121:421–29, 1967.

Braunwald, E.; Chidsey, C. A.; Pool, P. E.; Sonnenblick, E. H.; Ross, J. Jr.; Mason, D. T.; Spann, J. F.; and Covell, J. W.: Congestive heart failure: biochemical and physiological considerations. *Ann. Intern. Med.*, 64:904–41, 1966.

Braunwald, E.; Epstein, S. E.; Glick, G.; Wechsler, A. S.; and Braunwald, N. S.: Relief of angina pectoris by electrical stimulation of the carotid-sinus nerves. *New Eng. J. Med.*, 277:1278–83, 1967.

Braunwald, E.; Ross, J. Jr.; Gault, J. H.; Mason, D. T.; Mills, C.; Gabe, I. T.; and Epstein, S. E.: Assessment of cardiac function. *Ann. Intern. Med.*, 70:369–99, 1969.

Brest, A. N.: Renal arterial hypertension. *Amer. Heart J.*, 75:696–706, 1968.

Brest, A. N.; Onesti, G.; Heider, C.; and Moyer, J. H.: Cardiac and renal hemodynamic response to pargyline. *Ann. N. Y. Acad. Sci.*, 107:1016–22, 1963.

British Medical Research Council: Assessment of short-term anticoagulant administration after cardiac infarction: report of the working party on anticoagulant therapy in coronary thrombosis. *Brit. Med. J.*, 1: 335–42, 1969a.

————: Assessment of long-term anticoagulant administration after cardiac infarction: second report of the working party on anticoagulant therapy in coronary thrombosis. *Ibid.*, 2:837–43, 1969b.

Broder, G., and Weil, M. H.: Excess lactate: an index of reversibility of shock in human patients. *Science*, 143:1457–59, 1964.

Brodie, B. B.; Chang, C. C.; and Costa, E.: On the mechanism of action of guanethidine and bretylium. *Brit. J. Pharmacol.*, 25:171–78, 1965.

Brown, D. F.: Blood lipids and lipoproteins in atherogenesis. *Amer. J. Med.*, 46:691–704, 1969.

Brown, D. F.; Kinch, S. H.; and Doyle, J. T.: Serum triglycerides in health and in ischemic heart disease. *New Eng. J. Med.*, 273:947–52, 1965.

Brown, J. G.; Holzman, D.; and Creelman, E. W.: Serum quinidine concentration in congestive heart failure. *Amer. J. Med. Sci.*, 225:129–31, 1953.

Brownlee, G., and Williams, G. W.: Potentiation of amphetamine and pethidine by monoamine oxidase inhibitors. *Lancet*, 1:669, 1963.

Brunner, D., and Manelis, G.: Myocardial infarction among members of communal settlements in Israel. *Lancet*, 2:1049–50, 1960.

Brutsaert, D.: Influence of reserpine and of adrenolytic agents on the pulmonary arterial pressor response to hypoxia and catecholamines. *Arch. Int. Physiol.*, 72:395–412, 1964.

Buccino, R. A.; Spann, J. F., Jr.; Pool, P. E.; Sonnenblick, E. H.; and Braunwald, E.: Influence of the thyroid state on the intrinsic contractile properties and energy stores of the myocardium. *J. Clin. Invest.*, 46:1669–82, 1967.

Buchwald, H., and Varco, R. L.: Ileal bypass in patients with hypercholesterolemia and atherosclerosis: preliminary report on therapeutic potential. *J.A.M.A.*, **196**:627–30, 1966.

Burckhardt, D.; Vera, C. A.; and LaDue, J. S.: Effect of digitalis on urinary pituitary gonadotrophin excretion. *Ann. Intern. Med.*, **68**:1069–71, 1968.

Burget, G. E.; and Visscher, M. B.: Variations of the pH of the blood and the response of the vascular system to adrenalin. *Amer. J. Physiol.*, **81**:113–23, 1927.

Burn, J. H., and Rand, M. J.: Acetylcholine in adrenergic transmission. *Ann. Rev. Pharmacol.*, **5**:163–82, 1965.

Cady, L. D.: Epidemiology of coronary heart disease. *Amer. J. Cardiol.*, **20**:692–702, 1967.

Caldwell, J. H., and Greenberger, N. J.: Cholestyramine enhances digitalis excretion and protects against lethal intoxication. *J. Clin. Invest.*, **49**:16a, 1970.

Cameron, A. J. V.; Hutton, I.; Kenmure, A. C. F.; and Murdoch, W. R.: Haemodynamic and metabolic effects of hyperbaric oxygen in myocardial infarction. *Lancet*, **2**:833–37, 1966.

Canary, J. S.; Schaaf, M.; Duffy, B. J.; and Kyle, L. H.: Effects of oral and intramuscular reserpine in thyrotoxicosis. *New Eng. J. Med.*, **257**:435–42, 1957.

Carlson, L. A.: Studies of the effect of nicotinic acid on catecholamine stimulated lipolysis in adipose tissue *in vitro*. *Acta Med. Scand.*, **173**:719–22, 1963.

Carlsson, A. A.: Pharmacological depletion of catecholamine stores. *Pharmacol. Rev.*, **18**:541–49, 1966.

Carlsson, A. A., and Lindqvist, M.: *In vivo* decarboxylation of alpha-methyl-dopa and alpha-methylmetatyrosine. *Acta Physiol. Scand.*, **54**:87–94, 1962.

Carson, P.; McDonald, L.; Pickard, S.; Pilkington, T.; Davies, B.; and Love, F.: Effect of atromid on platelet stickiness. *J. Atheroscl. Res.*, **3**:619–22, 1963.

Carter, S. A.: Potentiation of the effect of orally administered anticoagulants by phenyramidol hydrochloride. *New Eng. J. Med.*, **273**:423–26, 1965.

Carvalho, M.; Vydon, J. K.; Bernstein, H.; Gold, H.; and Corday, E.: Hemodynamic effects of 3-hydroxytyramine (Dopamine) in experimentally induced shock. *Amer. J. Cardiol.*, **27**:217–23, 1969.

Cass, R.; Kuntzman, R.; and Brodie, B. B.: Norepinephrine depletion as a possible mechanism of action of guanethedine (SU 5864): a new type hypotensive agent. *Proc. Soc. Exp. Biol. Med.*, **103**:871–72, 1960.

Cass, R., and Spriggs, T. L. B.: Tissue amine levels and sympathetic blockade after guanethidine and bretylium. *Brit. J. Pharmacol.*, **17**:442–50, 1961.

Castellanos, A., Jr.; Lemberg, L.; Brown, J. P., Jr.; and Berkovits, E. E.: An electrical digitalis tolerance test. *Amer. J. Med. Sci.*, **254**:717–26, 1967.

Chakrabarti, R.; Fearnley, G. R.; and Evans, J. F.: Effects of clofibrate on fibrinolysis, platelet stickiness, plasma-fibrinogen and serum cholesterol. *Lancet*, **2**:1007–1009, 1968.

Chamberlain, D. A.: Effects of beta adrenergic blockade on heart size. *Amer. J. Cardiol.*, **18**:321–28, 1966.

Chang, C. C.; Costa, E.; and Brodie, B. B.: Reserpine-induced release of drugs from sympathetic nerve endings. *Life Sci.*, **3**:839–44, 1964.

————: Interaction of guanethidine with adrenergic neurons. *J. Pharmacol. Exp. Ther.*, **147**:303–12, 1965.

Channick, B. J.; Adlin, E. V.; and Marks, A. D.: Suppressed plasma renin activity in hypertension. *Arch. Intern. Med. (Chicago)*, **123**:131–40, 1969.

Chazan, J. A.; Stenson, R.; and Kurland, G. S.: The acidosis of cardiac arrest. *New Eng. J. Med.*, **278**:360–64, 1968.

Chiang, B. N.; Perlman, L. V.; and Epstein, F. H.: Overweight and hypertension. A review. *Circulation*, **39**:403–21, 1969a.

Chiang, B. N.; Perlman, L. V.; Ostrander, L. D.; and Epstein, F. H.: Relationship of premature systoles to coronary heart disease and sudden death in the Tecumseh epidemiologic study. *Ann. Intern. Med.*, **70**:1159–66, 1969b.

Chidsey, C. A.; Braunwald, E.; and Morrow, A. G.: Catecholamine excretion and cardiac stores of norepinephrine in congestive heart failure. *Amer. J. Med.*, **39**:442–51, 1965.

Chidsey, C. A., Braunwald, E.; Morrow, A. G.; and Mason, D. T.: Myocardial norepinephrine concentration in man: effects of reserpine and of congestive heart failure. *New Eng. J. Med.*, **269**:653–58, 1963.

Chidsey, C. A.; Harrison, D. C.; and Braunwald, E.: Augmentation of the plasma norepinephrine response to exercise in patients with congestive heart failure. *New Eng. J. Med.*, **267**:650–54, 1962.

Chien, S.: Role of the sympathetic nervous system in hemorrhage. *Physiol., Rev.*, **47**:214–88, 1967.

Christakis, G.; Rinzier, S. H.; Archer, M. S.; Winslow, G., Jampel, S.; Stephenson, J.; Friedman, G.; Fein, H.; Kraus, A.; and James, G.: The anti-coronary club: a dietary approach to the prevention of coronary heart disease: a seven year report. *Amer. J. Public Health*, **56**:299–314, 1966.

Christensson, R.; Karlefors, T.; and Westling, H.: Hemodynamic effects of nitroglycerin in patients with coronary heart disease. *Brit. Heart J.*, **27**:511–19, 1965.

Church, G., and Marriott, H. J. L.: Digitalis delerium. *Circulation*, **20**:549–53, 1959.

Church, G.; Schamroth, L.; Schwartz, N. L.; and Mariott, H. J. L.: Deliberate digitalis intoxication: a comparison of the toxic effects of four glycoside preparations. *Ann. Intern. Med.*, **57**:946–56, 1962.

Clausen, J. P.; Larsen, O. A.; and Trap-Jensen, J.: Physical training in the management of coronary artery disease. *Circulation*, **40**:143–54, 1969.

Cline, M. J.; Melmon, K. L.; Davis, W. C.; and Williams H. E.; Mechanism of endotoxin interaction with human leucocytes. *Brit. J. Haematol.*, **15**:539–47, 1968.

Cohen, A. B.: Hyperkalemic effects of triamterene. *Ann. Intern. Med.*, **65**:521–27, 1966.

Cohen, A. B.; Gallagher, J. P.; Luebs, E. D.; Varga, Z.; Yamanaka, J.; Zaleski, E. J.; Bluemchen, G.; and Bing, R. J.: The quantitative determination of coronary flow with a positron emitter (rubidium-84). *Circulation*, **32**:636–49, 1965.

Cohen, B. M.: The clinical use of dextrothyroxine in hypercholesterolemic states: an eight year appraisal. *J. Clin. Pharmacol.*, **9**:45–56, 1969.

Cohen, E. L.; Rovner, D. R.; and Conn, J. W.: Postural augmentation of plasma renin activity. *J.A.M.A.*, **197**:973–78, 1966.

Cohen, L. S.; Buccino, R. A.; Morrow, A. G.; and Braunwald, E.: Recurrent ventricular tachycardia and fibrillation treated with a combination of beta-adrenergic blockade and electrical pacing. *Ann. Intern. Med.*, **66**:945–49, 1967.

Cohen, R. A.; Kopin, I. J.; Creveling, C. R.; Musacchio, J. N.; Fischer, J. E.; Crout, J. R.; and Gill, J. R.: False neurochemical transmitters: combined clinical staff conference at the National Institutes of Health. *Ann. Intern. Med.*, **65**:347–62, 1966.

Cohen, R. J.; Cohen, L. S.; Epstein, S. E.; and Dennis, L. H.: Alterations of fibrinolysis and blood coagulation induced by exercise, and the role of adrenergic-receptor stimulation. *Lancet*, **2**:1264–66, 1968.

Cohn, J. N.: Paroxysmal hypertension and hypovolemia. *New Eng. J. Med.*, **275**:643–46, 1966.

————: Central venous pressure as a guide to volume expansion. *Ann. Intern. Med.*, **66**:1283–86, 1967.

Cohn, J. N.; Luria, M. N.; Daddario, R. C.; and Tristani, F. E.: Studies in clinical shock and hypotension. V. Hemodynamic effects of dextran. *Circulation*, **35**:316–26, 1967.

Cohn, J. N., and Tristani, F. E.: Cardiac and peripheral vascular effects of digitalis in cardiogenic shock. *Circulation* (Suppl. II) **36**:88–89, 1967.

Cohn, K. E.; Kleiger, R. E.; and Harrison, D. C.: Influence of potassium depletion on myocardial concentration of tritiated digoxin. *Circ. Res.*, **19**:473–76, 1967.

Cole, S. L.; Kaye, H.; and Griffith, G. C.: Assay of anti-anginal agents—the rapport period. *J.A.M.A.*, **168**:275–77, 1958.

Coltart, D. J.; Gibson, D. G.; and Shand, D. G.: Plasma propranolol levels associated with suppression of ventricular ectopic beats. *Brit. Med. J.*, **1**:490–91, 1971.

Comroe, J. H., and Dripps, R. D.: Reactions to morphine in ambulatory and bed patients. *Surg. Gynec. Obstet.*, **87**:221–24, 1948.

Comroe, J. H.; Van Lingen, B.; Strand, R. C.; and Roncoroni, A.: Reflex and direct cardiopulmonary effects of 5-OH-tryptamine (serotonin): their possible role in pulmonary embolism and coronary thrombosis. *Amer. J. Physiol.*, **173**:379–86, 1953.

Condemi, J. J.; Moore-Jones, D.; Vaughan, J. H.; and Perry, H. M.: Antinuclear antibodies following hydralazine toxicity. *New Eng. J. Med.*, **276**:486–91, 1967.

Conn, H. L., and Luchi, R. J.: Some cellular and metabolic considerations relating to the action of quinidine as a prototype antiarrhythmic agent. *Amer. J. Med.*, **37**:685–99, 1964.

Conn, J. W.: Hypertension, the potassium ion and impaired carbohydrate tolerance. *New Eng. J. Med.*, **273**:1135–43, 1965.

Conn, J. W.; Cohen, E. L.; Rovner, D. R.; and Nesbit, R. M.: Normokalemic primary aldosteronism: a detectable cause of curable "essential" hypertension. *J.A.M.A.*, **193**:200–206, 1965.

Conn, J. W.; Rovner, D. R.; Cohen, E. L.; Brookstein, J. J.; Cerny, J. C.; and Lucas, C. P.: Preoperative diagnosis of primary aldosteronism. *Arch. Intern. Med. (Chicago)*, **123**:113–23, 1969.

Conn, J. W.; Rovner, D. R.; Cohen, E. L., and Nesbit, R. M.: Normokalemic primary aldosteronism: its masquerade as "essential" hypertension. *J.A.M.A.*, **195**:21–26, 1966.

Conn, R. D.: Diphenylhydantoin sodium in cardiac arrhythmias. *New Eng. J. Med.*, **272**:277–82, 1965.

Conn, R. D.; Kennedy, J. W.; and Blackmon, J. R.: The hemodynamic effects of diphenylhydantoin. *Amer. Heart J.*, **73**:500–505, 1967.

Connor, W. E.: Measures to reduce the serum lipid levels in coronary heart disease. *Med. Clin. N. Amer.*, **52**:1249–60, 1968.

Connor, W. E.; Stone, D. B.; and Hodges, R. E.: Interrelated effects of dietary cholesterol and fat upon human serum lipid levels. *J. Clin. Invest.*, **43**:1691–96, 1964.

Conrad, L. L.; Kyriacopoulos, J. D.; Wiggins, C. W. and Honick, G. L.: Prevention of recurrences of myocardial infarction: a double-blind study of effectiveness of long-term anticoagulant therapy. *Arch. Intern. Med. (Chicago)*, **114**:348–58, 1964.

Conradi, E. C.; Gaffney, T. A.; Fink, D. A.; and Vangrow, J. S.: Reversal of sympathetic nerve blockade: a comparison of DOPA, dopamine and norepinephrine with their α-methylated analogues. *J. Pharmacol. Exp. Ther.*, **150**:26–33, 1965.

Constantin, L.: Extracardiac factors contributing to hypotension during coronary occlusion. *Amer. J. Cardiol.*, **11**:205–17, 1963.

Coon, W. W.; and Willis, T. W., III: Some side effects of heparin, heparinoids and their antagonists. *Clin. Pharmacol. Ther.*, **7**:379–98, 1966.

Cooper, J. A., and Frieden, J.: Atropine in the treatment of cardiac disease. *Amer. Heart J.*, **78**:124–27, 1969.

Cooper, J. K.; Steel, K.; and Christodoulou, J. P.: Mobile coronary care—a controversial innovation. *New Eng. J. Med.*, **281**:906–907, 1969.

Cooper, T.: The functional significance of the cardiac nerves. *Ann. Intern. Med.*, **66**:440–43, 1967.

Cooper, T., and Dempsey, P. J.: Assisted circulation. *Mod. Conc. Cardiov. Dis.*, **37**:95–106, 1968.

Cooperman, L. H.; Engelman, K.; and Mann, P. E. G.: Anesthetic management of pheochromocytoma employing halothane and beta adrenergic blockade. *Anesthesiology*, **28**:575–82, 1967.

Coraboeuf, E., and Boistel, J.: L'action des taux élevés de gaz carbonique sur le tissue cardiaque etudiée à l'aide de microélectrodes intracellulaires. *Compt. Rend. Soc. Biol.*, **147**:654–58, 1953.

Corn, M.: Effect of phenobarbital and glutethimide on biological half-life of warfarin. *Thromb. Diath. Haemorrh.*, **16**:606–12, 1966.

Cornfield, J.: Joint dependence of risk of coronary heart disease on serum cholesterol and systolic blood pressure: a discriminant function analysis. *Fed. Proc.*, **21**:58–61, 1962.

Cotton, R. C.; Wade, E. G., and Speller, G. W.: The effect of atromid on plasma fibrinogen and heparin resistance. *J. Atheroscler. Res.*, **3**:648–52, 1963.

Covell, J. W.; Braunwald, E., Ross, J., Jr.; and Sonnenblick, E. H.: Studies on digitalis. XVI. Effects on myocardial oxygen consumption. *J. Clin. Invest.*, **45**:1535–42, 1966.

Cowan, C.; Duran, P. V. M.; Corsini, G.; Goldschlager, N.; and Bing, R. J.: The effects of nitroglycerin on myocardial blood flow in man, measured by coincidence counting and bolus injections of 84-ribidium. *Amer. J. Cardiol.*, **24**:154–60, 1969.

Creditor, M. C., and Loschky, V. K.: Plasma renin activity in hypertension. *Amer. J. Med.*, **43**:371–82, 1967.

Criscitiello, M. G.: Therapy of atrioventricular block. *New Eng. J. Med.*, **279**:808–10, 1968.

Crocker, D. W.; Newton, R. A.; Mahoney, E. M.; and Harrison, J. H.: Hypertension due to primary renal ischemia: a correlation of juxtaglomerular cell counts with clinicopathological findings in twenty-five cases. *New Eng. J. Med.*, **267**:794–800, 1962.

Cronin, R. F. P.: Effect of isoproterenol and norepinephrine on myocardial function in experimental cardiogenic shock. *Amer. Heart J.*, **74**:387–95, 1967.

Cronin, R. F. P.; Moore, S., and Marpole, D. G.: Shock following myocardial infarction: a clinical survey of 140 cases. *Canad. Med. Ass. J.*, **93**:57–63, 1965.

Crout, J. R.: Catecholamines and the circulatory system: pheochromocytoma. *Pharmacol. Rev.*, **18**:651–57, 1966a.

———: Substitute adrenergic transmitters, a newly appreciated mechanism of antihypertensive drugs. *Circ. Res.*, **18** (Suppl. 1):120–30, 1966b.

Crout, J. R., and Sjoerdsma, A.: Catecholamines in the localization of pheochromocytoma. *Circulation*, **22**:516–25, 1960.

———: Turnover and metabolism of catecholamines in patients with pheochromocytoma. *J. Clin. Invest.*, **43**:94–102, 1964.

Crowell, J. W., and Guyton, A. C.: Further evidence favoring a cardiac mechanism in irreversible hemorrhagic shock. *Amer. J. Physiol.*, **203**:248–52, 1962.

Cucinell, S. A.; Conney, A. H.; Sansur, M.; and Burns, J. J.: Drug interactions in man. I. Lowering effect of phenobarbital on plasma levels of bishydroxycoumarin (Dicumarol) and diphenylhydantoin (Dilantin). *Clin. Pharmacol. Ther.*, **6**:420–29, 1965.

Da Costa, J. M.: On irritable heart; a clinical study of a form of functional cardiac disorder and its consequences. *Amer. J. Med. Sci.*, **61**:17–52, 1871.

Dahlström, A.; Fuxe, K., Hillarp, N.-Å.: Site of action of reserpine. *Acta Pharmacol. Toxicol.*, **22**:277–92, 1965.

Dalen, J. E.; Banas, J. S., Jr.; Brooks, H. L.; Evans, G. L., Paraskos, J. A.; and Dexter, L.: Resolution rate of acute pulmonary embolism in man. *New Eng. J. Med.*, **280**:1194–99, 1969a.

Dalen, J. E., and Dexter, L.: Diagnosis and management of massive pulmonary embolism. *D.M.: Disease-a-Month*, 1–34, August, 1967.

Dalen, J. E., Haynes, F. W.; Hoppin, F. G., Jr.; Evans, G. L.; Bhardwaj, P.; and Dexter, L.: Cardiovascular responses to experimental pulmonary embolism. *Amer. J. Cardiol.*, **20**:3–9, 1969b.

Dall, J. L. C.: The effect of steroid therapy on normal and abnormal atrio-ventricular conduction. *Brit. Heart J.*, **26**:537–43, 1964.

————: Digitalis intoxication in elderly patients. *Lancet*, **1**:194–95, 1965.

Damato, A. N.: Diphenylhydantoin: pharmacological and clinical use. *Progr. Cardiov. Dis.*, **12**:1–15, 1969.

Das, B., and Krieger, M.: Treatment of thyrotoxic storm with intravenous administration of propranolol. *Ann. Intern. Med.*, **70**:985–88, 1969.

Davis, L. D., and Tempte, J. V.: Effects of propranolol on the transmembrane potentials of ventricular muscle and Purkinje fibers of the dog. *Circ. Res.*, **22**:661–77, 1968.

Davis, W. W.; Newsome, H. H.; Wright, L. D.; Hammond, W. G.; Easton, J.; and Bartter, F. C.: Bilateral adrenal hyperplasia as a cause of primary aldosteronism with hypertension, hypokalemia and suppressed renin activity. *Amer. J. Med.*, **42**:642–47, 1967.

Day, M. D., and Rand, M. J.: Evidence for a competitive antagonism of guanethidine by dexamphetamine. *Brit. J. Pharmacol.*, **20**:17–28, 1963.

————: Some observations on the pharmacology of α-methyldopa. *Brit. J. Pharmacol.*, **22**:72–86, 1964.

Dayton, P. G.; Tarcin, Y.; Chenkin, T.; and Weiner, M.: Influence of barbiturafes on coumarin plasma levels and prothrombin response. *J. Clin. Invest.*, **40**:1797–802, 1961.

Dayton, S., and Pearce, M. L.: Prevention of coronary heart disease and other complications of atherosclerosis by modified diet. *Amer. J. Med.*, **46**:751–62, 1969.

Dayton, S.; Pearce, M. L.; Hashimoto, S.; Dixon, W.; and Tomiyasu, U.: A controlled clinical trial of a diet high in unsaturated fat in preventing complications of atherosclerosis. *Circulation*, **40** (Suppl. II):1–63, 1969.

de Champlain, J.; Mueller, R. A.; and Axelrod, J.: Subcellular localization of monoamine oxidase in rat tissue. *J. Pharmacol. Exp. Ther.*, **166**:339–45, 1969.

DeGraff, A. C., Jr., and Buchnam, C. A.: Treatment of pulmonary embolism. *Amer. Heart J.*, **77**:836–39, 1969.

DeGraff, A. C., Jr., and Lyon, A. F.: Evaluation of dipyridamole (Persantin). *Amer. Heart J.*, **65**:423–24, 1963.

Del Guercio, L. R. M.; Feins, N. R.; Cohn, J. D.; Coomaraswany, R. P.; Wollman, S. B.; and State, D.: Comparison of blood flow during external and internal cardiac massage in man. *Circulation*, **31-32** (Suppl. I):171–80, 1965.

Delman, A. J.; and Stein. E.: Atrial flutter secondary to digitalis toxicity. *Circulation*, **29**:593–97, 1964.

Deming, Q.: Blood pressure: its relation to atherosclerotic disease of the coronaries. *Bull. N.Y. Acad. Med.*, **44**:968–84, 1968.

Deming, Q.; Brun, L. M.; Kaplan, R.; Daly, M. M.;

Bloom, J.; and Schechter, M.: The effect of pharmacologic control of previously established hypertension on the development of dietary atherosclerosis in rats. In Brest, A. M. and Moyer, J. H. (eds.): *Hypertension*; *Second Hahnemann Symposium on Hypertensive Disease*, Lea & Febiger, Philadelphia, 1961, p. 160.

De Quattro, V., and Sjoerdsma, A.: Catecholamine turnover in normotensive and hypertensive men: effects of antihypertensive drugs. *J. Clin. Invest.*, **47**:2359–73, 1968.

Deykin, D.: The use of heparin. *New Eng. J. Med.*, **280**:937–38, 1969.

Deykin, D.; Wessler, S.; and Reimer, S. M.: Evidence for an antithrombotic effect of Dicumarol. *Amer. J. Physiol.*, **199**:1161–64, 1960.

Dietzman, R. H., and Lillehei, R. C.: The treatment of cardiogenic shock. IV. The use of phenoxybenzamine and chlorpromazine. *Amer. Heart J.*, **75**:136–38, 1968a.

————: The treatment of cardiogenic shock. V. The use of corticosteroids in the treatment of cardiogenic shock. *Amer. Heart J.*, **75**:274–77, 1968b.

Dietzman, R. H.; Lyons, G. W.; Block, J. H.; and Lillehei, R. C.: Relation of cardiac work to survival in cardiogenic shock in dogs. *J.A.M.A.*, **199**:825–29, 1967.

Dillon, P. T.; Babe, J.; Meloni, C. R.; and Canary, J. J.: Reserpine in thyrotoxic crisis. *New Eng. J. Med.*, **283**:1020–23, 1970.

Ditlefsen, E. L.: Quinidine concentration in blood and excretion in urine following parenteral administration as related to congestive heart failure. *Acta Med. Scand.*, **159**:105–109, 1957.

Doan, A. E.; Peterson, D. R.; Blackmon, J. R.; and Bruce, R. A.: Myocardial ischemia after maximal exercise in healthy men: one year follow-up of physically active and inactive men. *Amer. J. Cardiol.*, **17**:9–19, 1966.

Doherty, J. E.: The clinical pharmacology of the digitalis glycosides: a review. *Amer. J. Med. Sci.*, **255**:382–414, 1968.

Doherty, J. E., and Perkins, W. H.: Tissue concentration and turnover of tritiated digoxin in dogs. *Amer. J. Cardiol.*, **17**:47–52, 1966a.

————: Digitalis serum levels: clinical use. *Ann. Intern. Med.*, **74**:787–89, 1971.

————: Digoxin metabolism in hypo- and hyperthyroidism: studies with tritiated digoxin in thyroid disease. *Ann. Intern. Med.*, **64**:489–507, 1966b.

Doherty, J. E.; Perkins, W. H.; and Mitchell, G. K.: Tritiated digoxin studies in human subjects. *Arch. Intern. Med. (Chicago)*, **108**:531–39, 1961.

Doherty, J. E.; Perkins, W. H.; and Wilson, M. C.: Studies with tritiated digoxin in renal failure. *Amer. J. Med.*, **37**:536–44, 1964.

Dole, V. P.; Gordis, E.; and Bierman, E. L.: Hyperlipemia and atherosclerosis. *New Eng. J. Med.*, **269**:686–89, 1963.

Dollery, C. T.: Methyldopa in the treatment of hypertension. *Progr. Cardiov. Dis.*, **8**:278–89, 1965.

Donald, D. E.; Ferguson, D. A.; and Milburn, S. E.: Effect of beta-adrenergic receptor blockade with normal and with denervated hearts. *Circ. Res.*, **22**:127–34, 1968.

Donaldson, G. A.; Williams, C.; Scannell, J. G.; and Shaw, R. S.: A reappraisal of the application of the Trendelenberg operation to massive fatal embolism: report of a successful pulmonary artery thrombectomy using a cardiopulmonary bypass. *New Eng. J. Med.*, **268**:171–74, 1963.

Donlon, J. V.; and Yu, P. N.: Cardiovascular response of hypoxic myocardium to acetyl strophanthidin. *Amer. Heart J.*, **78**:238–44, 1969.

Dornhorst, A. C., and Laurence, D. R.: Use of pronethalol in phaeochrome tumors. *Brit. Med. J.*, **2**:1250–51, 1963.

Doyle, J. T.; Dawber, T. R.; Kannel, W. B.; Kinch, S. H.; and Kahn, H. A.: Relationship of cigarette smoking to coronary heart disease: second report of combined experience of Albany, N.Y. and Framingham, Mass. studies. *J.A.M.A.*, **190**:886–90, 1964.

Doyle, J. T.; Kinch, S. H.; and Brown, D. F.: Seasonal variation in serum cholesterol concentration. *J. Chron. Dis.*, **18**:657–64, 1965.

Drew, J. H.; Dripps, R. D.; and Comroe, J. H., Jr.: Clinical studies on morphine. II. The effect of morphine upon the circulation of man and upon the circulatory and respiratory responses to tilting. *Anesthesiology*, **7**:44–61, 1946.

Dubel, J., and Trautwein, W.: Das Aktionspotential und mechanogramm des Herzmuskels unter dem Einfluss der Dehnung. *Cardiologia*, **25**:344–62, 1954.

Dubnow, M. H., and Burchell, H. B.: A comparison of digitalis intoxication in two separate periods. *Ann. Intern. Med.*, **62**:956–65, 1965.

Duff, J. H.; Malave, G.; Peretz, D. I.; Scott, H. M.; and MacLean, L. D.: The hemodynamics of septic shock in man and in the dog. *Surgery*, **58**:174–84, 1965.

Dustan, H. P.; Page, I. H.; Tarazi, R. C.; and Frohlich, E. D.: Arterial pressure responses to discontinuing antihypertensive drugs. *Circulation*, **37**:370–79, 1968.

Dustan, H. P.; Schneckloth, R. E.; Corcoran, A. C.; and Page, I. H.: Effectiveness of long-term treatment of malignant hypertension. *Circulation*, **18**:644–51, 1958.

du Toit, H. V.; du Plessin. J. M. E.; Dommisse, J.; Rorke, M. J.; Theron, M. S.; and de Villiers, V. P.: Treatment of endotoxic shock with isoprenaline. *Lancet*, **2**:143–46, 1966.

Dwyer, E. M., Jr.; Wiener, L.; and Cox, J. W.: Effects of beta-adrenergic blockade (propranolol) on left ventricular hemodynamics and the electrocardiogram during exercise-induced angina pectoris. *Circulation*, **38**:250–60, 1968.

Earley, L. E.; and Daugharty, T. M.: Sodium metabolism. *New Eng. J. Med.*, **281**:72–86, 1969.

Ebert, R. V.; Borden, C. W.; Hipp, H. R.; Holzman, D.; Lyon, A. F.; and Schnaper, H.: Long-term anticoagulant therapy after myocardial infarction. *J.A.M.A.*, **207**:2263–67, 1969.

Eckenhoff, J. E.; and Oech, S. R.: The effects of narcotics and antagonists upon respiration and circulation in man. *Clin. Pharmacol. Ther.*, **1**:483–524, 1960.

Edelman, I. S.; and Liebman, J.: Anatomy of body water and electrolytes. *Amer. J. Med.*, **27**:256–77, 1959.

Edison, G. R.: Amphetamines: A dangerous illusion. *Ann. Intern. Med.*, **74**:605–10, 1971.

Editorial: Catecholamines and hypertension. *New Eng. J. Med.*, **271**:158–59, 1964.

Editorial: Angiotensin infusions. *New Eng. J. Med.*, **274**:1505–1506, 1966.

Editorial: Diagnosis of pheochromocytoma. *New Eng. J. Med.*, **277**:762–63, 1967a.

Editorial: Management of malignant hypertension. *New Eng. J. Med.*, **277**:102–103, 1967b.

Editorial: Natural history of pulmonary embolic disease. *New Eng. J. Med.*, **276**:1094, 1967c.

Editorial: Recurrent pulmonary embolism and cor pulmonale. *New Eng. J. Med.*, **276**:1261–62, 1967d.

Editorial: Urokinase. *New Eng. J. Med.*, **277**:1203–1204, 1967e.

Editorial: Screening hypertensive patients for hyperaldosteronism. *New Eng. J. Med.*, **277**:48–49, 1967f.

Editorial: A new look at pressor mechanisms. *New Eng. J. Med.*, **278**:1399, 1968a.

Editorial: Anticoagulation recidivans. *New Eng. J. Med.*, **278**:1231–32, 1968b.

Editorial: Diuretics and the treatment of pulmonary edema. *New Eng. J. Med.*, **279**:160, 1968c.

Eich, R. H.; Cuddy, R. P.; Smulyan, H.; and Lyons, R. H.: Hemodynamics in labile hypertension: a follow-up study. *Circulation*, **34**:299–307, 1966.

Eich, R. H.; Peters, R. J.; Cuddy, R. P.; Smulyan, H.; and Lyons, R. H.: Hemodynamics in labile hypertension. *Amer. Heart J.*, **63**:188–95, 1962.

Eichna, L. W.: The treatment of cardiogenic shock. III. The use of isoproterenol in cardiogenic shock. *Amer. Heart J.*, **74**:848–52, 1967.

El-Fiky, S. B. I., and Katzung, B. G.: Effects of hypothermia and pronethalol on ionic correlates of ouabain arrhythmias in dogs. *Circ. Res.*, **24**:43–50, 1969.

Elliot, W. C., and Gorlin, R.: The coronary circulation, myocardial ischemia and angina pectoris. *Mod. Conc. Cardiov. Dis.*, **35**:111–22, 1966.

Elliot, W. C., and Stone, J. M.: Beta-adrenergic blocking agents for the treatment of angina pectoris. *Progr. Cardiov. Dis.*, **12**:83–98, 1969.

Engelman, K., and Hammond, W. G.: Adrenalin production by an intrathoracic pheochromocytoma. *Lancet*, **1**:609–11, 1968.

Engelman, K.; Horwitz, D.; Jéquier, E.; and Sjoerdsma, A.: Biochemical and pharmacologic effects of α-methyltyrosine in man. *J. Clin. Invest.*, **47**:577–94, 1968a.

Engelman, K.; Jéquier, E.; Udenfriend, S.; and Sjoerdsma, A.: Metabolism of α-methyltyrosine in man: relationship to its potency as an inhibitor of catecholamine biosynthesis. *J. Clin. Invest.*, **47**:568–76, 1968b.

Engelman, K., and Sjoerdsma, A.: Chronic medical therapy for pheochromocytoma. *Ann. Intern. Med.*, **61**:229–41, 1964.

Enos, W. F., Jr.; Beyer, J. C.; and Holms, R. H.: Pathogenesis of coronary disease in American soldiers killed in Korea. *J.A.M.A.*, **158**:912–14, 1955.

Epstein, F. H.: Multiple risk factors and the prediction of coronary heart disease. *Bull. N.Y. Acad. Med.*, **44**:916–35, 1968.

Epstein, F. H.; Beiser, D.; Goldstein, R. E.; Redwood, D.; Rosing, D. R.; Glick, G.; Wechsler, A. S.; Stampfer, M.; Cohen, L. S.; Reis, R. L.; Braunwald, N. S.; and Braunwald, E.: Treatment of angina pectoris by electrical stimulation of the carotid-sinus nerves. *New Eng. J. Med.*, **280**:971–78, 1969a.

Epstein, F. H.; Beiser, G. D.; Goldstein, R. E.; Stampfer, M.; Wechsler, A. S.; Glick, G.; and Braunwald, E.: Circulatory effects of electrical stimulation of the carotid sinus nerves in man. *Circulation*, **40**:269–76, 1969b.

Epstein, F. H., and Braunwald, E.: Beta-adrenergic receptor blocking drugs: mechanisms of action and clinical applications. *New Eng. J. Med.*, **275**:1106–12, 1175–83, 1966a.

————: The effect of beta adrenergic blockade on patterns of urinary sodium excretion: studies in normal subjects and in patients with heart disease. *Ann. Intern. Med.*, **65**:20–27, 1966b.

————: Beta-adrenergic receptor blockade: propranolol and related drugs. *Ann. Intern. Med.*, **67**:1333–37, 1967a.

————: Clinical and hemodynamic appraisal of beta adrenergic blocking agents. *Ann. N.Y. Acad. Sci.*, **39**:952–67, 1967b.

————: Inhibition of the adrenergic nervous system in the treatment of angina pectoris. *Med. Clin. N. Amer.*, **52**:1031–39, 1968.

Epstein, F. H.; Robinson, B. F.; Kamler, R. L.; and Braunwald, E.: Effects of beta adrenergic blockade on the cardiac response to maximal and submaximal exercise in man. *J. Clin. Invest.*, **44**:1745–53, 1965.

Epstein, F. H.; Stampfer, M.; Beiser, D.; Goldstein,

R. E.; and Braunwald, E.: Effects of a reduction in environmental temperature on the circulatory response to exercise in man: implications concerning angina pectoris. *New Eng. J. Med.*, **280**:7–11, 1969c.

Erlij, D., and Méndez, R.: Modification of digitoxin intoxication by exclusion of sympathetic system. *Fed. Proc.*, **22**:184, 1963.

Espiner, E. A.; Tucci, J. R.; Jagger, P. I.; and Lauler, D. P.: Effect of saline infusions on aldosterone secretion and electrolyte excretion in normal subjects and in patients with primary aldosteronism. *New Eng. J. Med.*, **277**:1–7, 1967.

Essex, H. E.; Wegria, R. G. E.; Herrick, J. F.; and Mann, F. C.: The effect of certain drugs on the coronary blood flow of the trained dog. *Amer. Heart J.*, **19**:554–65, 1940.

Fakhro, A. M.; Ritchie, R. F.; and Lown, B.: Lupus-like syndrome induced by procainamide. *Amer. J. Cardiol.*, **20**:367–73, 1967.

Fallon, H. J., and Woods, J. W.: Response of hyperlipoproteinemia to cholestyramine resin. *J.A.M.A.*, **204**:1161–64, 1968.

Faloon, W. W.; Paes, I. C.; Woolfolk, D.; Nankin, H.; Wallace, K.; and Haro, E. N.: Effect of neomycin and kanamycin upon intestinal absorption. *Ann. N. Y. Acad. Sci.*, **132**:879–87, 1966.

Falsetti, H. L.; Schnatz, J. D.; Greene, D. G.; and Bunnell, I. L.: Lipid and carbohydrate studies in coronary artery disease. *Circulation*, **37**:184–91, 1968.

Fam, W. M., and McGregor, M.: Effect of coronary vasodilator drugs on retrograde flow in areas of chronic myocardial ischemia. *Circ. Res.*, **15**:355–65, 1964.

———: Effect of nitroglycerin and dipyridamole on regional coronary resistance. *Circ. Res.*, **22**:649–59, 1968.

Fearon, R. E.: Comparison of norepinephrine and isoproterenol in experimental coronary shock. *Amer. Heart J.*, **75**:634–48, 1968.

Feigl, E. O.: Sympathetic control of coronary circulation. *Circ. Res.*, **20**:262–71, 1967.

Ferriar, J.: *Medical History and Reflections*, Vol. II. Thomas Dobson, Philadelphia, 1816, p. 253.

Ferry, C. B.: Cholinergic link hypothesis in adrenergic neuroeffector transmission. *Physiol. Rev.*, **46**:420–56, 1966.

———: The autonomic nervous system. *Ann. Rev. Pharmacol.*, **7**:185–202, 1967.

Fine, S. L., and Levy, R. I.: Ethacrynic acid in acute pulmonary edema. *New Eng. J. Med.*, **273**:583–86, 1965.

Finkielman, S.; Worcel, M.; and Agrest, A.: Hemodynamic patterns in essential hypertension. *Circulation*, **31**:356–68, 1965.

Finnerty, F.: Hypertensive encephalopathy. *Amer. Heart. J.*, **75**:559–63, 1968.

Finnerty, F.; Davidov, M.; and Kakaviatos, N.: Relation of sodium balance to arterial pressure during drug induced saluresis. *Circulation*, **37**:175–83, 1968.

Finnerty, F.; Kakaviatos, N.; Tuckman, J.; and McGill, J.: Clinical evaluation of diazoxide: new treatment for acute hypertension. *Circulation*, **28**:203–208, 1963.

Fisch, C.; Greenspan, K.; Knoebel, S. B.; and Feigenbaum, H.: Effect of digitalis on conduction of the heart. *Progr. Cardiov. Dis.*, **6**:343–65, 1964.

Fischer, J. E.; Horst, W. D.; and Kopin, I. J.: β-hydroxylated sympathomimetic amines as false neurotransmitters. *Brit. J. Pharmacol.*, **24**:477–84, 1965.

Fleischner, F. G.: Recurrent pulmonary embolism and cor pulmonale. *New Eng. J. Med.*, **276**:1213–20, 1967.

Fletcher, G. F.: Hypotensive reactions after small doses of reserpine given parenterally. *New Eng. J. Med.*, **268**:309–10, 1963.

Fletcher, G. F.; Kazamias, T. M.; and Wenger, N. K.: Cardiotoxic effects of Mellaril: conduction disturbances and supraventricular arrhythmias. *Amer. Heart J.*, **78**:135–38, 1969.

Forsyth, R. B.; Hoffbrand, B. I.; and Melmon, K. L.: Redistribution of cardiac output during hemorrhage in the unanesthetized monkey. *Circ. Res.*, **27**:311–20, 1970.

Foster, J. H.; Rhamy, R. K.; Oates, J. A.; Klatte, E. C.; Burko, H. C.; and Michelakis, A. M.: Renovascular hypertension secondary to atherosclerosis. *Amer. J. Med.*, **46**:741–50, 1970.

Fox, S. M., and Haskell, W. L.: Physical activity and the prevention of coronary heart disease. *Bull. N.Y. Acad. Med.*, **44**:950–67, 1968.

Fox, S. M., and Skinner, J. S.: Physical activity and cardiovascular health. *Amer. J. Cardiol.*, **14**:731–46, 1964.

Frank, C. W.: The course of coronary heart disease: factors relating to prognosis. *Bull. N.Y. Acad. Med.*, **44**:900–915, 1968.

Fred, H. L.; Burdine, J. A., Jr.; Gonzalez, D. A.; Lockhart, R. W.; Peabody, C. A.; and Alexander, J. K.: Arteriographic assessment of lung scanning in the diagnosis of pulmonary thromboembolism. *New Eng. J. Med.*, **275**:1025–32, 1966.

Fredrickson, D. S.: The field trial: some thoughts on the indispensable ordeal. *Bull. N.Y. Acad. Med.*, **44**:985–93, 1968.

Fredrickson, D. S.; Levy, R. I.; and Lees, R. S.: Fat transport in lipoproteins—an integrated approach to mechanisms and disorders. *New Eng. J. Med.*, **276**:34–44; 94–103; 148–56; 215–24; 273–81, 1967.

Freis, E. D.: Current concepts in therapy. I. Antihypertensive agents. *New Eng. J. Med.*, **266**:507–509, 607–609, 775–77, 1962.

———: Guanethidine. *Progr. Cardiov. Dis.*, **8**:183–93, 1965.

———: Hypertension and atherosclerosis. *Amer. J. Med.*, **46**:735–40, 1969.

———: Effectiveness of drug therapy. A review. *Circ. Res.*, **28** (Suppl. II):70–73, 1971.

Frick, M. H.: The effect of physical training in manifest ischemic disease. *Circulation*, **42**:433–35, 1969.

Frick, M. H., Balcon, R.; Cross, D.; and Sowton, E.: Hemodynamic effects of nitroglycerin in patients with angina pectoris studied by an atrial pacing method. *Circulation*, **37**:160–68, 1968.

Frick, M. H., and Katila, M.: Hemodynamic consequences of physical training after myocardial infarction. *Circulation*, **37**:192–202, 1968.

Friedberg, C. K.: Angina pectoris. *Geriatrics*, **22**:144–55, 1967.

Friedman, M.; Rosenman, R. H.; Straus, R.; Wurm, M.; and Kositchek, R.: The relationship of behavior pattern A to the state of the coronary vasculature. *Amer. J. Med.*, **44**:525–37, 1968.

Friend, D. G.: Cardiac glycosides. *New Eng. J. Med.*, **266**:88–89; 187–89; 300–302; 402–404, 1962.

Frohlich, E. D.; Dustan, H. P.; and Page, I. H.: Hyperdynamic beta-adrenergic circulatory state. *Arch. Intern. Med. (Chicago)*, **117**:614–19, 1966.

Frohlich, E. D.; Dustan, H. P.; and Tarazi, R. C.: Hyperdynamic beta-adrenergic circulatory state. An overview. *Arch. Intern. Med. (Chicago)*, **126**:1068–69, 1970.

Frohlich, E. D.; Tarazi, R. C.; and Dustan, H. P.: Hyperdynamic beta-adrenergic circulatory state: increased beta-receptor responsiveness. *Arch. Intern. Med. (Chicago)*, **123**:1–7, 1969.

Frohlich, E. D.; Tarazi, R. C.; Dustan, H. P.; and Page, I. H.: The paradox of beta-adrenergic blockade in hypertension. *Circulation*, **37**:417–23, 1968.

Frohlich, E. D.; Ulrych, M.; Tarazi, R. C.; Dustan, H. P.; and Page, I. H.: Hemodynamic comparison of essential and renovascular hypertension: cardiac output and total peripheral resistance: supine and tilted patients. *Circulation*, 35:289–97, 1967.

Furman, R. H.; Alaupovic, P.; and Howard, R. P.: Effects of androgens and estrogens on serum lipids and composition and concentrations of serum lipoproteins in normolipidemic and hyperlipidemic states. *Progr. Biochem. Pharmacol.*, 2:215–49, 1967.

Gaal, P. G.; Kattus, A. A.; Kolin, A.; and Ross, G.: Effects of adrenalin and noradrenalin on coronary blood flow before and after beta-adrenergic blockade. *Brit. J. Pharmacol.*, 26: 713–22, 1966.

Gaffney, T. E., and Braunwald E.: Importance of the adrenergic nervous system in the support of circulatory function in patients with congestive heart failure. *Amer. J. Med.*, 34:320–24, 1963.

Gaffney, T. E.; Sigell, L. T.; Mohammed, S.; and Atkinson, A. J., Jr.: The clinical pharmacology of antihypertensive drugs. *Progr. Cardiov. Dis.*, 12:52–71, 1969.

Gallo, D. G.; Bailey, K. R.; and Sheffner, A. L.: The interaction between cholestyramine and drugs. *Proc. Soc. Exp. Biol. Med.*, 120:60–65, 1965.

Gazes, P. C.; Richardson, J. A.; and Woods, E. F.: Plasma catecholamine concentrations in myocardial infarction and angina pectoris. *Circulation*, 19:657–61, 1959.

Genest, J.: The value of the angiotension infusion test in the diagnosis of true renovascular hypertension. *Amer. Heart J.*, 76:443–44, 1968.

Gent, A. E.; Brook, C. G. D.; Foley, T. H.; and Miller, T. N.: Dipyridamole: a controlled trial of its effect in acute myocardial infarction. *Brit. Med. J.*, 4:366–68, 1968.

Genton, E., and Pechet, L.: Thrombolytic agents: a perspective. *Ann. Intern. Med.*, 69:625–28, 1968.

Genton, E., and Wolf, P. S.: Urokinase therapy in pulmonary thromboembolism. *Amer. Heart J.*, 76:628–37, 1968.

Gerhardt, R. E.; Knouss, R. F.; Thyrum, P. T.; Luchi, R. J.; and Morris, J. J.: Quinidine excretion in aciduria and alkaluria. *Ann. Intern. Med.*, 71:927–33, 1969.

Gerson, T.; Shorland, F. B.; and Adams, Y.: The effects of corn oil on the amounts of cholesterol and the excretion of sterol in the rat. *Biochem. J.*, 81:584–91, 1961.

Gessa, G. L.; Costa, E.; Kuntzman, R.; and Brodie, B. B.: On the mechanism of norepinephrine release by α-methyl-metatyrosine. *Life Sci.*, 1:353–60, 1962.

Gettes, L. S., and Yoshonis, K. F.: Rapidly recurring supraventricular tachycardia. A manifestation of reciprocating tachycardia and an indication for propranolol therapy. *Circulation*, 41:689–700, 1970.

Getz, G. S., Vesselinovitch, D., and Wissler, R. W.: A dynamic pathology of atherosclerosis. *Amer. J. Med.*, 46:657–73, 1969.

Gianelly, R. E.; Goldman, R. H.; Treister, G.; and Harrison, D. C.: Propranolol in patients with angina pectoris. *Ann. Intern. Med.*, 67:1216–25, 1967a.

Gianelly, R. E.; Griffin, J. R.; and Harrison, D. C.: Propranolol in the treatment and prevention of cardiac arrhythmias. *Ann. Intern. Med.*, 66:667–76, 1967b.

Gianelly, R. E.; Treister, B. L.; and Harrison, D. C.: The effect of propranolol on exercise-induced ischemic S-T segment depression. *Amer. J. Cardiol.*, 24:161-65, 1969.

Gianelly, R. E.; von der Groeben, J. O.; Spivack, A. P.; and Harrison, D. C.: Effect of lidocaine on ventricular arrhythmias in patients with coronary heart disease. *New Eng. J. Med.*, 277:1215–19, 1967c.

Gibson, D.; and Sowton, E.: The use of beta-adrenergic receptor blocking drugs in dysrhythmias. *Progr. Cardiovasc. Dis.*, 12:16–39, 1969.

Gifford, R. H., and Feinstein, A. R.: A critique of methodology in studies of anticoagulant therapy for acute myocardial infarction. *New Eng. J. Med.*, 280:354–57, 1969.

Gilbert, R. P.: Mechanisms of the hemodynamic effects of endotoxin. *Physiol. Rev.*, 40:245–78, 1960.

———: Endotoxin shock in the primate. *Proc. Soc. Exp. Biol. Med.*, 111:328–31, 1962.

Gilbert, R. P., and Cuddy, R. P.: Digitalis intoxication following conversion to sinus rhythm. *Circulation*, 32:58–64, 1965.

Gilmore, E.; Weil, J.; and Chidsey, C.: Treatment of hypertension with vasodilator and beta-adrenergic blockade. *New Eng. J. Med.*, 282:521–27, 1970.

Glontz, G. E., and Saslaw, S.: Methyldopa fever. *Arch. Intern. Med.*, 122:445–47, 1968.

Glynn, I. M.: The action of cardiac glycosides on sodium and potassium movements in human red cells. *J. Physiol.*, 136:148–73, 1957.

———: The action of cardiac glycosides on ion movements. *Pharmacol. Rev.*, 16:381–407, 1964.

Glynn, M. F.; Murphy, E. A.; and Mustard, J. F.: Effect of clofibrate on platelet economy in man. *Lancet*, 2:447–48, 1967.

Gofman, J. W.; Young, W.; and Tandy, R.: Ischemic heart disease, atherosclerosis, and longevity. *Circulation*, 34:679–97, 1966.

Goldberg, L. I.: The treatment of cardiogenic shock. VI. The search for an ideal drug. *Amer. Heart J.*, 75:416–20, 1968.

Goldberg, L.; MacCannell, K. L.; McNay, J. L.; and Meyer, M. B.: The use of dopamine in the treatment of hypotension and shock after myocardial infarction or cardiac surgery. *Amer. Heart J.*, 72:568–69, 1966.

Goldberg, L. I.; Talley, R. C.; and McNay, J. L.: The potential role of dopamine in the treatment of shock. *Progr. Cardiov. Dis.*, 12:40–51, 1969.

Goldblatt, H.; Lynch, J.; Hanzal, R. F.; and Summerville, W. W.: Studies on experimental hypertension. I. Production of persistent elevation of systolic blood pressure by means of renal ischemia. *J. Exp. Med.*, 59:347–79, 1934.

Goldman, R. H.; Braniff, B.; Harrison, D. C.; and Spivack, A. P.: The use of central venous oxygen saturation measurements in a coronary care unit. *Ann. Intern. Med.*, 68:1280–87, 1968a.

Goldman, R. H.; Klughaupt, M.; Metcalf, T.; Spivack, A. P.; and Harrison, D. C.: Measurements of central venous oxygen saturation in patients with myocardial infarction. *Circulation*, 38:941–46, 1968b.

Goldsmith, O.; Solomon, D. H.; and Horton, R.: Hypogonadism and mineralocorticoid excess: the 17-hydroxylase deficiency syndrome. *New Eng. J. Med.*, 277:673–77, 1967.

Goldstein, M.; Anagnoste, B.; Lauber, E.; and McKereghan, M. R.: Inhibition of dopamine-β-hydroxylase by disulfiram. *Life Sci.*, 3:763–67, 1964.

Goldstein, M., and Nakajima, K.: The effect of disulfiram on catecholamine levels in the brain. *J. Pharmacol. Exp. Ther.*, 157:96–102, 1967.

Goodwin, J. F., and Oakley, C. M.: Transplanation of the heart. *Amer. Heart J.*, 77:437–40, 1969.

Gordon, D. B.: Renin and hypertension. *Lancet*, 2:320–23, 1966.

Gordon, R. D.; Küchel, O.; Liddle, G. W.; and Island, D. P.: Role of the sympathetic nervous system in regulating renin and aldosterone production in man. *J. Clin. Invest.*, 46:599–605, 1967.

Gorlin, R.: The hyperkinetic heart syndrome. *J.A.M.A.*, 182:823–29, 1962.

Gorlin, R.; Brachfeld, N., MacLeod, C.; and Bopp, P.: Effect of nitroglycerin on coronary circulation in patients with coronary-artery disease or increased left ventricular work. *Circulation*, 19:705–18, 1959.

Gorlin, R., and Robin, E. D.: Cardiac glycosides in the treatment of cardiogenic shock. *Brit. Med. J.*, 1:937–39, 1955.

Goss, J. E., and Dickhaus, D. W.: Increased bishydroxycoumarin requirements in patients receiving phenobarbital. *New Eng. J. Med.*, 273:1094–95, 1965.

Govier, W. C., and Holland, W. C.: Relationship between atrial contractions and the effect of ouabain on contractile strength and calcium exchange in the rabbit atria. *J. Pharmacol. Exp. Ther.*, 148:284–89, 1965.

Graham, T. P., Jr.; Covell, J. W.; Sonnenblick, E. H.; Ross, J., Jr.; and Braunwald, E. Control of myocardial oxygen consumption: relative influence of contractile state and tension development. *J. Clin. Invest.*, 47:375–85, 1968.

Greenfield, J. C., Jr., and Orgain, E. S.: The control of ventricular tachyarrhythmias by internal cardiac pacing. *Ann. Intern. Med.*, 66:1017–19, 1967.

Griffith, G. C.; Leak, D.; and Hegde, B.: Conservative anticoagulant therapy of acute myocardial infarction. *Ann. Intern. Med.*, 57:254–61, 1962.

Gross, L., and Brotman, M.: Hypoprothrombinemia and hemorrhage associated with cholestyramine therapy. *Ann. Intern. Med.*, 72:95–96, 1970.

Grossman, J. I., and Rubin, I. L.: Cardiopulmonary resuscitation I. *Amer. Heart J.*, 78:569–72, 1969a.

———: Cardiopulmonary resuscitation II. *Ibid.*, 78:709–14, 1969b.

Gubner, R. S., and Kallman, H.: Treatment of digitalis toxicity by chelation of serum calcium. *Amer. J. Med. Sci.*, 234:136–44, 1957.

Gulati, O. D.; Dave, B. T.; Gokhale, S. D.; and Shah, K. M.: Antagonism of adrenergic neuron blockade in hypertensive subjects. *Clin. Pharmacol. Ther.*, 7:510–14, 1966.

Gunnar, R.; Cruz, A.; Boswell, J.; Co, B. S.; Pietras, R. J.; and Tobin, J. R., Jr.: Myocardial infarction with shock: hemodynamic studies and results of therapy. *Circulation*, 33:753–62, 1966.

Gunnar, R.; Loeb, H.; Pietras, R.; Oritz, J.; and Tobin, J., Jr.: Hemodynamic effects of dopamine compared to norepinephrine and isoproterenol in clinical shock. *Circulation*, 38 (Suppl. VI):91, 1968.

Gunnar, R.; Loeb, H. S.; Pietras, R. J.; and Tobin, J. R., Jr.: Ineffectiveness of isoproterenol in shock due to acute myocardial infarction. *J.A.M.A.*, 202:1124–31, 1967.

Gurewich, V.; Thomas, D. P.; and Rabinov, K. R.: Pulmonary embolism after ligation of the inferior vena cava. *New Eng. J. Med.*, 274:1350–54, 1966.

Gurian, H., and Adlersberg, D.: The effect of large doses of nicotinic acid on circulating lipids and on carbohydrate tolerance. *Amer. J. Med. Sci.*, 237:12–22, 1959.

Haber, E.: Recent developments in pathophysiologic studies of the renin-angiotensive system. *New Eng. J. Med.*, 280:148–55, 1969a.

———: The renin-angiotensive system in curable hypertension. *Mod. Conc. Cardiov. Dis.*, 38:17–22, 1969b.

Haddy, F. J.: Physiology and pharmacology of the coronary circulation and myocardium, particularly in relation to coronary artery disease. *Amer. J. Med.*, 47:274–86, 1969.

Haefely, N.; Hürlimann, A.; and Thoenen, H.: The effect of stimulation of sympathetic nerves in the cat treated with reserpine, α-methyldopa and α-methyl-metatyrosine. *Brit. J. Pharmacol.*, 26:172–85, 1966.

Hall, K. D., and Norris, F. H., Jr.: Fluothane sensitization of dog heart to action of epinephrine. *Anesthesiology*, 19:631–41, 1958.

Hamby, W. M.; Janowski, G. J.; Pouget, J. M.; Dunea, G.; and Gantt, C. L.: Intravenous use of diazoxide in the treatment of severe hypertension. *Circulation*, 37:169–74, 1968.

Hamosh, P., and Cohn, J. N.: Left ventricular function in acute myocardial infarction. *J. Clin. Invest.*, 50:523–33, 1971.

Hansen, J. M.; Kristensen, M.; Skovsted, L.; and Christensen, L. K.: Dicoumarol-induced diphenylhydantoin intoxication. *Lancet*, 2:265–66, 1966.

Hansen, K. B., and Bender, A. D.: Changes in serum potassium levels occurring in patients treated with triamterene and a triamterene hydrochlorothiazide combination. *Clin. Pharmacol. Ther.*, 8:392–99, 1967.

Hansen, P. F., and Sandoe, E.: Cardiac arrest: integrated treatment with drugs and countershock or pacemaker. *Acta Med. Scand.*, 180:501–11, 1966.

Harlan, W. R., Jr.; Oberman, A.; Mitchell, R. E.; and Graybiel, A.: Constitutional and environmental factors related to serum lipid and lipoprotein levels. *Ann. Intern. Med.*, 66:540–55, 1967.

Harrington, J. T.; Sommers, S. C.; and Kassirer, J. P.: Atheromatous emboli with progressive renal failure: renal arteriography as the probable inciting factor. *Ann. Intern. Med.*, 68:152–60, 1968.

Harrison, C. E., Jr.; and Wakim, K. G.: Inhibition of binding of tritiated digoxin to myocardium by sodium depletion in dogs. *Circ. Res.*, 24:263–68, 1969.

Harrison, D. C.: New drugs in the treatment of angina. *New Eng. J. Med.*, 280:895–96, 1969.

Harrison, D. C.; Griffin, J. R.; and Fiene, T. J.: Effects of beta-adrenergic blockade with propranolol in patients with atrial arrhythmias. *New Eng. J. Med.*, 273:410–15, 1965.

Harrison, D. C.; Sprouse, J. H.; and Morrow, A. G.: The antiarrhythmic properties of lidocaine and procaineamide. *Circulation*, 28:486–91, 1963.

Harrison, T. S.; Bartlett, J. D.; and Seaton, J. F.: Exaggerated urinary norepinephrine response to tilt in pheochromocytoma: diagnostic implications. *New Eng. J. Med.*, 277:725–28, 1967.

Harthorne, J. W.; Austen, W. G.; Corning, H.; McNamara, J. J.; and Sanders, C. A.: Permanent endocardial pacing in complete heart block. *Ann. Intern. Med.*, 66:831–37, 1967.

Hashim, S. A.; and Van Itallie, T. B.: Cholestyramine resin therapy for hypercholesterolemia. *J.A.M.A.*, 192:289–93, 1965.

Hauge, A.: Role of histamine in hypoxic pulmonary hypertension in rats. I. Blockade or potentiation of endogenous amines, kinins and ATP. *Circ. Res.*, 22:371–83, 1968.

Hauge, A., and Melmon, K. L.: Role of histamine in hypoxic pulmonary hypertension in the rat. II. Depletion of histamine, serotonin and catecholamine, *Circ. Res.*, 22:385–92, 1968.

Hazzard, W. R.; Spiger, M. J.; Bagdade, J. D.; and Bierman, E. L.: Studies on the mechanism of increased plasma triglyceride levels induced by oral contraceptives. *New Eng. J. Med.*, 280:471–74, 1969.

Hecht, H. H., and Hutter, O. F.: Action of pH on cardiac Purkinje fibers. *Fed. Proc.*, 23:157, 1964.

Hedberg, D. L.; Gordon, M. W.; and Glueck, B. C., Jr.: Six cases of hypertensive crises in patients on tranylcypromine after eating chicken livers. *Amer. J. Psychiat.*, 122:933–37, 1966.

Heinivaara, O., and Palva, I. P.: Malabsorption and deficiency of vitamin B$_{12}$ caused by treatment with para-aminosalicylic acid. *Acta Med. Scand.*, 177:337–41, 1965.

Helfant, R. H.; Lau, S. H.; Cohen, S., and Damato,

A. N.: Effects of diphenylhydantoin on atrioventricular conduction in man. *Circulation*, **36**:686–91, 1967a.

Helfant, R. H.; Scherlag, B. J.; and Damato, A. N.: The electrophysiological properties of diphenylhydantoin sodium as compared to procaine amide in the normal and digitalis-intoxicated heart. *Circulation*, **36**:108–18, 1967b.

———: Protection from digitalis toxicity with the prophylactic use of diphenylhydantoin sodium: an arrhythmic inotropic dissociation. *Circulation*, **36**:119–24, 1967c.

———: Electrophysiological effects of direct current countershock before and after ouabain sensitization and after diphenylhydantoin desensitization in the dog. *Circ. Res.*, **22**:615–23, 1968a.

———: Diphenylhydantoin prevention of arrhythmias in the digitalis-sensitized dog after direct-current cardioversion. *Circulation*, **37**:424–28, 1968b.

Helfant, R. H.; Seuffert, G. W.; Patton, R. D.; Stein, E.; and Damato, A. N.: The clinical use of diphenylhydantoin (Dilantin) in the treatment and prevention of cardiac arrhythmias. *Amer. Heart J.*, **77**:315–23, 1969.

Hellerstein, H. K.: Exercise therapy in coronary disease. *Bull. N.Y. Acad. Med.*, **44**:1028–47, 1968.

Hellman, L.; Zumoff, B.; Kessler, G.; Kara, E., Rubin, I. L.; and Rosenfeld, R. S.: Reduction of cholesterol and lipids in man by ethyl-*p*-chlorophenoxyisobutyrate. *Ann. Intern. Med.*, **59**:477–94, 1963.

Helmer, O. M., and Judson, W. E.: Metabolic studies on hypertensive patients with suppressed plasma renin activity not due to hyperaldosteronism. *Circulation*, **38**:965–76, 1968.

Henney, R. P.; Vasko, J. S.; Brawley, R. J.; Oldham, H. N.; and Morrow, A. G.: Effects of morphine on resistance and capacitance vessels of the peripheral circulation. *Amer. Heart J.*, **72**:242–50, 1966.

Hertting, G.; Axelrod, J.; and Whitby, L. G.: Effect of drugs on the uptake and metabolism of H³-norepinephrine. *J. Pharmacol. Exp. Ther.*, **134**:146–53, 1961.

Hilden, T.; Iverson, K.; Raaschou, F.; and Schwartz, M.: Anticoagulants in acute myocardial infarction. *Lancet*, **2**:327–31, 1961.

Himmelhoch, S. R.; Dekker, A.; Gazzaniga, A. B.; and Like, A. A.: Closed-chest cardiac resuscitation: a prospective clinical and pathological study. *New Eng. J. Med.*, **270**:118–22, 1964.

Hinkle, L. E., Jr.; Whitney, L. H.; Lehman, E. W.; Dunn, J.; Benjamin, B.; King, R.; Plakun, A.; and Flehinger, B.: Occupation, education, and coronary heart disease. *Science*, **161**:238–46, 1968.

Hinshaw, L. B.; Jordan, M. M.; and Vick, J. A.: Histamine release and endotoxin shock in the primate. *J. Clin. Invest.*, **40**:1631–37, 1961.

Hjort, P. F., and Rapaport, S. I.: The Shwartzman reaction: pathogenetic mechanism and clinical manifestations. *Ann. Rev. Med.*, **16**:135–68, 1965.

Hodge, J. V., and Nye, E. R.: Monoamine oxidase inhibition, broadbeans and hypertension. *Lancet*, **1**:1108, 1964.

Hoffman, B. F., and Cranefield, P. F.: The physiological basis of cardiac arrhythmias. *Amer. J. Med.*, **37**:670–84, 1964.

Hoffman, B. F.; Cranefield, P. F.; and Wallace, A. G.: Physiological basis of cardiac arrhythmias. I and II. *Mod. Conc. Cardiov. Dis.*, **35**:103–10, 1966.

Hoffman, B. F., and Singer, D. H.: Effects of digitalis on electrical activity of cardiac fibers. *Progr. Cardiov. Dis.*, **7**:226–60, 1964.

———: Appraisal of the effects of catecholamines on cardiac electrical activity. *Ann. N.Y. Acad. Sci.*, **139**:914–39, 1967.

Holley, K. E.; Hunt, J. C.; Brown, A. L., Jr.; Kincaid, O. W.; and Sheps, S. G.: Renal artery stenosis: a clinical-pathological study in normotensive and hypertensive patients. *Amer. J. Med.*, **37**:14–22, 1964.

Holling, H. E.: Closed chest resuscitation. *Ann. Intern. Med.*, **63**:719–21, 1965.

Hollingsworth, J. H.; Muller, W. H.; Beckwith, J. R.; and McGuire, L. B.: Patient selection for permanent cardiac pacing. *Ann. Intern. Med.*, **70**:263–67, 1969.

Hood, W. B., Jr.; McCarthy, B.; and Lown, B.: Myocardial infarction following coronary ligation in dogs: hemodynamic effects of isoproterenol and acetylstrophanthidin. *Circ. Res.*, **21**:191–99, 1967.

———: Aortic pressure loading in dogs with myocardial infarction. *Amer. Heart J.*, **77**:55–62, 1969.

Hopkins, R. W.; Sabga, G.; Penn, I.; and Simeone, F. A.: Hemodynamic aspects of hemorrhagic and septic shock. *J.A.M.A.*, **191**:731–35, 1965.

Horlick, L.; Kudchodkar, B. J.; and Sodhi, H. S.: Mode of action of chlorphenoxyisobutyric acid on cholesterol metabolism in man. *Circulation*, **53**:299–309, 1971.

Horwitz, D.; Lovenberg, W.; Engelman, K.; and Sjoerdsma, A.: Monoamine oxidase inhibitors, tyramine and cheese. *J.A.M.A.*, **188**:1108–10, 1964.

Horwitz, D.; Pettinger, W. A.; Orvis, H.; and Sjoerdsma, A.: Effects of methyldopa in fifty hypertensive patients. *Clin. Pharmacol. Ther.*, **8**:224–34, 1967.

Horwitz, D., and Sjoerdsma, A.: Effects of alpha-methyl-meta-tyrosine intravenously in man. *Life Sci.*, **3**:41–48, 1964.

Howard, J.; Bethrong, M. D.; Sloan, R. D.; and Yandt, E. R.: Relief of malignant hypertension by nephrectomy in four patients with unilateral renal vascular disease. *Trans. Ass. Amer. Physicians*, **66**:164–69, 1953.

Howard, J., and Connor, T. B.: Hypertension produced by unilateral renal disease. *Arch. Intern. Med. (Chicago)*, **109**:8–17, 1962.

Howard, J., and Tiedeman, G.: The relative effectiveness of antihypertensive drugs in caucasians and negroes. *Clin. Pharmacol. Exp. Ther.*, **8**:502–20, 1967.

Howard, R. P.; Alaupovic, P.; Brusco, W.; and Furman, R. H.: Effects of ethylchlorophenoxyisobutyrate alone or with androsterone (Atromid) on serum lipids, lipoproteins and related metabolic parameters in normal and hyperlipidemic subjects. *J. Atheroscler. Res.*, **3**:482–99, 1963.

Hughes, W. M.; Moyer, J. H.; and Daeschner, W. C., Jr.: Parenteral reserpine in treatment of hypertensive emergencies. *Arch. Intern. Med. (Chicago)*, **95**:563–77, 1955.

Hultgren, H.; Calciano, A.; Platt, F.; and Abrams, H.: A clinical evaluation of coronary arteriography. *Amer. J. Med.*, **42**:228–47, 1967.

Hultgren, H., and Flamm, M. D.: Pulmonary edema. *Mod. Conc. Cardiov. Dis.*, **38**:1–6, 1969.

Humphries, J. O.: Treatment of heart block with artificial pacemakers. *Mod. Conc. Cardiov. Dis.*, **33**:857–62, 1964.

Hunninghake, O. B., and Azarnoff, D. L.: Drug interactions with warfarin. *Arch. Intern. Med.*, **121**:349–52, 1968.

Hunt, J. C.; Strong, C. G.; Sheps, S. G.; and Bernatz, P. E.: Diagnosis and management of renovascular hypertension. *Amer. J. Cardiol.*, **23**:434–45, 1969.

Hurst, J. W., and Myerburg, R. J.: Cardiac arrhythmias: evolving concepts. *Mod. Conc. Cardiov. Dis.*, **37**:73–84, 1968.

Irons, G. V., Jr.; Ginn, W. N.; and Orgain, E. S.: Use of a beta adrenergic receptor blocking agent (propranolol) in the treatment of cardiac arrhythmias. *Amer. J. Med.*, **43**:161–70, 1967.

Izquierdo, J. A., and Izquierdo, I.: Electrolytes and excitable tissues. *Ann. Rev. Pharmacol.*, **7**:125–44, 1967.

Janoff, A., and Zeligs, J. D.: Vascular injury and lysis of basement membrane *in vitro* by neutral protease of human leukocytes. *Science*, **161**:702–704, 1968.

Jelliffe, R. W.: An improved method of digoxin therapy. *Ann. Intern. Med.*, **69**:703–17, 1968.

Jenkins, D. J. A.: Propranolol and hypoglycemia. *Lancet*, **1**:164, 1967.

Jewitt, D. E.; Balcon, R.; Raftery, E. B.; and Oram, S.: Incidence and management of supraventricular arrhythmias after acute myocardial infarction. *Amer. Heart J.*, **77**:290–93, 1969.

Jick, H., Stone, D.; Borda, I. T.; and Shapiro, S.: Efficacy and toxicity of heparin in relation to age and sex. *New Eng. J. Med.*, **279**:284–86, 1968.

Joly, H. R., and Weil, M. H.: Temperature of the great toe as an indication of the severity of shock. *Circulation*, **39**:131–38, 1969.

Jones, N. F.; Walker, G.; Ruthven, C. R. J.; and Sandler, M.: Alpha-methyl-*p*-tyrosine in the management of phaeochromocytoma. *Lancet*, **2**:1105–1109, 1968.

Jose, A., and Kaplan, N. M.: Plasma renin activity in the diagnosis of primary aldosteronism: failure to distinguish primary aldosteronism from essential hypertension. *Arch. Intern. Med. (Chicago)*, **123**:141–46, 1969.

Judson, W. E.; Hatcher, J. D.; and Wilkins, R. W.: Blood pressure responses to the Valsalva maneuver in cardiac patients with and without congestive heart failure. *Circulation*, **11**:889–99, 1955.

Julian, D. G.: Coronary care and the community. *Ann. Intern. Med.*, **69**:607–13, 1968.

Julius, S., and Stewart, B. H.: Diagnostic significance of abdominal murmurs. *New Eng. J. Med.*, **276**:1175–78, 1967.

Kagan, A.; Kannel, W. B.; Dawber, T. R.; and Revotskie, N.: The coronary profile. *Ann. N.Y. Acad. Sci.*, **97**: 883–94, 1963.

Kain, H. K.; Hinman, A. T.; and Sokolow, M.: Arterial blood pressure measurements with a portable recorder in hypertensive patients. I. Variability and correlation with "casual" pressures. *Circulation*, **30**:882–92, 1964.

Kamath, V. R., and Thorne, M. G.: Ischaemic heart disease and withdrawal of anticoagulant therapy. *Lancet*, **1**:1025–27, 1969.

Kaneko, Y.; Ikeda, T.; Takeda, T.; and Ueda, H.: Renin release during acute reduction of arterial pressure in normotensive subjects and patients with renovascular hypertension. *J. Clin. Invest.*, **46**:705–16, 1967.

Kannel, W. B.; Brand, N.; Skinner, J. J., Jr.; Dawber, T. R.; and McNamara, P. M.: The relation of adiposity to blood pressure and development of hypertension. *Ann. Intern. Med.*, **67**:48–59, 1967.

Kannel, W. B.; Dawber, T. R.; Kagan, A.; Revotskie, N.; and Stokes, J., III.: Factors of risk in the development of coronary heart disease: six year follow-up experience. The Framingham study. *Ann. Intern. Med.*, **55**:33–50, 1961.

Kannel, W. B.; LeBauer, J.; Dawber, T. R.; and McNamara, P. M.: Relation of body weight to development of coronary heart disease. *Circulation*, **35**:734–44, 1969.

Kaplan, N. M.: Hypokalemia in the hypertensive patient, with observations on the incidence of primary aldosteronism. *Ann. Intern. Med.*, **66**:1079–89, 1967.

Kaplan, N. M., and Silah, J. G.: Effect of angiotensin on blood pressure in humans with hypertensive disease. *J. Clin. Invest.*, **43**:659–69, 1964a.

————: The angiotensin infusion test: a new approach to the differential diagnosis of renovascular hypertension. *New Eng. J. Med.*, **271**:536–41, 1964b.

Kardos, G. G.: Isoproterenol in the treatment of shock due to bacteremia with gram-negative pathogens. *New Eng. J. Med.*, **274**:868–73, 1966.

Karliner, J. S.: Intravenous diphenylhydantoin sodium (Dilantin) in cardiac arrhythmias. *Dis. Chest*, **51**:256–68, 1967.

Kastor, J. A.; DeSanctis, R. W.; Harthorne, J. W.; and Schwartz, G. H.: Transvenous atrial pacing in the treatment of refractory ventricular irritability. *Ann. Intern. Med.*, **66**:939–45, 1967.

Kastor, J. A., and Yurchak, P. M.: Recognition of digitalis intoxication in the presence of atrial fibrillation. *Ann. Intern. Med.*, **67**:1045–54, 1967.

Kattus, A. A., Jr.; Hanafee, W. N.; Longmire, W. P., Jr.; McAlpin, R.; and Rivin, A. U.: Diagnosis, medical and surgical management of coronary insufficiency. *Ann. Intern. Med.*, **69**:115–36, 1968.

Katz, A. M., and Hecht, H. H.: The early "pump" failure of the ischemic heart. *Amer. J. Med.*, **47**:497–502, 1969.

Katz, F. H.: Primary aldosteronism with suppressed plasma renin activity due to bilateral nodular adrenocortical hyperplasia. *Ann. Intern. Med.*, **67**:1035–42, 1967.

Katz, L. N.: Physical fitness and coronary heart disease: some basic views. *Circulation*, **35**:405–14, 1967.

Kaufman, J. J.; Moloney, P. J.; and Maxwell, M. H.: Urinary blockade after bilateral catheterization. *New Eng. J. Med.*, **275**:412–16, 1966.

Kempner, W.: Treatment of hypertensive vascular disease with rice diet. *Amer. J. Med.*, **4**:545–77, 1948.

Kenmure, A. C. F.; Murdoch, W. R.; Beattie, A. D.; Marshall, J. C. B.; and Cameron, A. J. V.: Circulatory and metabolic effects of oxygen in myocardial infarction. *Brit. Med. J.*, **4**:360–64, 1968.

Kerstell, J., and Svanborg, A.: Treatment of hypercholesterolemia with para-aminosalicylic acid. *Acta Med. Scand.*, **182**:283–87, 1966.

Keys, A.: Prevention of coronary heart disease: official recommendations from Scandinavia. *Circulation*, **38**:227–28, 1968.

Keys, A.; Kimura, N.; Kusukawa, A.; Bronte-Stewart, B.; Larsen, N.; and Keys, M. H.: Lessons from serum cholesterol studies in Japan, Hawaii and Los Angeles. *Ann. Intern. Med.*, **48**:83–94, 1958.

Killip, T.: Dysrhythmia prophylaxis. *New Eng. J. Med.*, **281**:1034–35, 1969.

Killip, T., and Kimball, J. T.: Treatment of myocardial infarction in a coronary care unit: a two year experience with 250 patients. *Amer. J. Cardiol.*, **20**:457–64, 1967.

Kimball, J. T., and Killip, T.: Aggressive treatment of arrhythmias in acute myocardial infarction: procedures and results. *Progr. Cardiov. Dis.*, **10**:483–504, 1968.

Kinsella, D.; Troup, W.; and MacGregor, M.: Studies with a new coronary vasodilator drug. *Amer. Heart J.* **63**:146–51, 1962.

Kirkendall, W. M.; Fitz, A. E.; and Lawrence, M. S.: Renal hypertension: diagnosis and surgical treatment. *New Eng. J. Med.*, **276**:479–85, 1967.

Kleiger, R., and Lown, B.: Cardioversion and digitalis. II. Clinical studies. *Circulation*, **33**:878–87, 1966.

Klocke, F. J.; Kaiser, G. A.; Ross, J., Jr.; and Braunwald, E.: An intrinsic adrenergic vasodilator mechanism in the coronary vascular bed of the dog. *Circ. Res.*, **16**:376–82, 1965.

Koch-Weser, J.: Mechanism of digitalis action on the heart. *New Eng. J. Med.*, **277**:417–19, 469–71, 1967.

————: Quinidine-induced hypoprothrombinemic hemorrhage in patients on chronic warfarin therapy. *Ann. Intern. Med.*, **68**:511–17, 1968a.

————: Coumarin necrosis. *Ann. Intern. Med.*, **68**: 1365–67, 1968b.

Koch-Weser, J., and Klein, S. W.: Procainamide

dosage schedules, plasma concentrations, and clinical effects. *J.A.M.A.*, **215**:1454–60, 1971.

Koch-Weser, J.; Klein, S. W.; Foo-Canto, L. L.; Kastor, J. A.; and DeSanctis, R.: Antiarrhythmic prophylaxis with procainamide in acute myocardial infarction. *New Eng. J. Med.*, **281**:1253–60, 1969.

Kopin, I.: Storage and metabolism of catecholamines: the role of monoamine oxidase. *Pharmacol. Rev.*, **16**:179–91, 1964.

———: False adrenergic transmitters. *Ann. Rev. Pharmacol.*, **8**:377–94, 1968.

Kopin, I.; Fischer, J. E.; Musacchio, J. M.; Horst, W. D.; and Weise, V. K.: False neurochemical transmitters and the mechanism of sympathetic blockade by monoamine oxidase inhibitors. *J. Pharmacol. Exp. Ther.*, **147**:186–93, 1965.

Korbitz, B. D.; Ramirez, G.; Mackman, S.; and Davis, H. L., Jr.: Coumarin-induced skin necrosis in a sixteen year old girl. *Amer. J. Cardiol.*, **24**:420–25, 1969.

Kosowsky, B. D.; Haft, J. I.; Lau, S. H.; Stein, E.; and Damato, A. N.: The effects of digitalis on atrioventricular conduction in man. *Amer. Heart J.*, **75**:736–42, 1968.

Koster, M., and David, G. K.: Reversible severe hypertension due to licorice ingestion. *New Eng. J. Med.*, **278**:1381–83, 1968.

Kotler, M. N.; Berman, L.; and Rubenstein, A. H.: Hypoglycemia precipitated by propranolol. *Lancet*, **2**:1389–90, 1966.

Kouwenhoven, W. B.; Jude, J. R.; and Knickerbocker, G. G.: Closed-chest cardiac massage. *J.A.M.A.*, **173**:1064–67, 1960.

Krasnow, N.; Rolett, E. L.; Yurchak, P. M.; Hood, W. B., Jr.; and Gorlin, R.: Isoproterenol and cardiovascular performance. *Amer. J. Med.*, **37**:514–25, 1964.

Kritchevsky, D.; Whitehouse, M. W.; Staple, E.: Oxidation of cholesterol-26-C^{14} by rat liver mitochondria: effect of nicotinic acid. *J. Lipid Res.*, **1**:154–58, 1960.

Küchel, O.; Fishman, L. M.; Liddle, G. W.; and Michelalis, A.: Effect of diazoxide on plasma renin activity in hypertensive patients. *Ann. Intern. Med.*, **67**:791–99, 1967.

Kuhn, L. A.: The treatment of cardiogenic shock. I. The nature of cardiogenic shock. *Amer. Heart J.*, **74**:578–81, 1967a.

———: Changing treatment of shock following acute myocardial infarction: a critical evaluation. *Amer. J. Cardiol.*, **20**:757–64, 1967b.

Kuhn, L. A.; Kline, H. J.; Richmond, S.; and Klein, L.: Comparison of the hemodynamic and cardiac metabolic effects of isoproterenol and norepinephrine in experimental acute myocardial infarction with shock. *Circulation*, **36** (Suppl. II):166, 1967.

Kuida, H.; Gilbert, R. P.; Hinshaw, L. E.; Brunson, J. G.; and Visscher, M. B.: Species differences in effect of gram-negative endotoxin on circulation. *Amer. J. Physiol.*, **200**:1197–1202, 1961.

Kuller, L.; Lilienfield, A.; and Fisher, R.: Epidemiological study of sudden and unexpected deaths due to arteriosclerotic heart disease. *Circulation*, **34**:1056–68, 1966.

Kuo, P. T.: Current metabolic-genetic interrelationship in human atherosclerosis. *Ann. Intern. Med.*, **68**:449–66, 1968.

Kutt, H.; Winters, W.; and McDowell, R. H.: Depression of parahydroxylation of diphenylhydantoin by antituberculosis chemotherapy. *Neurology*, **16**:594–602, 1966.

Langer, T., and Levy, R. I.: Acute muscular syndrome associated with administration of clofibrate. *New Eng. J. Med.*, **279**:856–58, 1968.

Laragh, J. H.; Angers, M.; Kelly, W. G.; and Lieberman, S.: Hypotensive agents and pressor substances: the effect of epinephrine, norepinephrine, angiotension II, and others on the secretory rate of aldosterone in man. *J.A.M.A.*, **174**:234, 1960.

Lauler, D. P.: Preoperative diagnosis of primary aldosteronism. *Amer. J. Med.*, **41**:855–63, 1966.

Lawrason, F. D.; Albert, E.; Mohr, F. L.; and MacMahon, F. G.: Ulcerative obstructive lesions of the small intestine. *J.A.M.A.*, **191**:641–44, 1965.

Lawrence, A. M.: Glucagon provocative test for pheochromocytoma. *Ann. Intern. Med.*, **66**:1091–96, 1967.

Leading Article: Unsaturated fats and coronary heart disease. *Lancet*, **2**, 901–902, 1968a.

Leading Article: Fibrinolysis exercise and propranolol. *Lancet*, **2**:1283, 1968b.

Leading Article: Propranolol in angina pectoris. *Lancet*, **1**:1135, 1969.

Leatherman, L. L.: Intestinal obstruction caused by anticoagulants. *Amer. Heart J.*, **76**:534–37, 1968.

Ledingham, I. McA., and Norman, J. N.: Acid-base studies in experimental circulatory arrest. *Lancet*, **2**:967–69, 1962.

Lee, W. Y.; Bronsky, D.; and Waldstein, S. S.: Studies of the thyroid and sympathetic nervous system interrelationship. II. Effect of guanethidine on manifestations of hyperthyroidism. *J. Clin. Endocr. Metab.*, **22**:879–85, 1962.

Lees, R. S., and Wilson, D. E.: The treatment of hyperlipidemia. *New Eng. J. Med.*, **284**:186–95, 1971.

Leishman, A. W. D.; Mathews, H. L., and Smith, A. J.: Antagonism of guanethidine by imipramine. *Lancet*, **1**:112, 1963.

Leishman, A. W. D., and Sandler, G.: Hastening the control of blood pressure by guanethidine. *Lancet*, **1**:668–70, 1965.

Leonard, J. W.; Gifford, R. W.; and Humphrey, D. C.: Treatment of hypertension with methyldopa alone or combined with diuretics and/or guanethidine. *Amer. Heart J.*, **69**:610–18, 1965.

Leonberg, S. C.; Green, J. B.; and Elliott, F. A.: The response of stroke patients to very small doses of parenteral reserpine. *Ann. Intern. Med.*, **60**:866–70, 1964.

Leren, P.: The effect of plasma cholesterol lowering diet in male survivors of myocardial infarction: a controlled clinical trial. *Acta Med. Scand.* 466 (Suppl.): 1–92, 1966.

———: The effect of plasma-cholesterol-lowering diet in male survivors of myocardial infarction. *Bull. N. Y. Acad. Med.*, **44**:1012–20, 1968.

Lesch, M.; Caranasos, G. J.; Mulholland, J. H.; and Osler Medical House Staff: Controlled study comparing ethacrynic acid to mercaptomerin in the treatment of acute pulmonary edema. *New Eng. J. Med.*, **279**:115–22, 1968.

Leth, A.: Changes in plasma and extracellular fluid volumes in patients with essential hypertension during long-term treatment with hydrochlorothiazide. *Circulation*, **42**:479–85, 1970.

Levine, R. A.: Steatorrhea induced by para-aminosalicylic acid. *Ann. Intern. Med.*, **68**:1265–70, 1968.

Levine, R. J., and Sjoerdsma, A.: Dissociation of the decarboxylase-inhibiting and norepinephrine-depleting effects of α-methyl-dopa, α-ethyl-dopa, 4-bromo-3-hydroxy-benzyloxy amine and related substances. *J. Pharmacol. Exp. Ther.*, **146**:42–47, 1964.

Levine, R. J., and Strauch, B. S.: Hypertensive responses to methyldopa. *New Eng. J. Med.*, **275**:946–48, 1966.

Levine, S. A.: Carotid sinus massage: new diagnostic test for angina pectoris. *J.A.M.A.*, **182**:1332–34, 1962.

Levy, R. I., and Glueck, G. J.: Hypertriglyceridemia, diabetes mellitus and coronary vessel disease. *Arch. Intern. Med. (Chicago)*, 123:220–28, 1969.

Lewis, C. M., and Brink, A. J.: Beta adrenergic blockade, hemodynamics and myocardial energy metabolism in patients with ischemic heart disease. *Amer. J. Cardiol.*, 21:846–59, 1968.

Lewis, R. J.: Effect of barbiturates on anticoagulant therapy. *New Eng. J. Med.*, 274:110, 1966.

Lewis, R. J.; Spivack, M.; and Spaet, T. H.: Warfarin resistance. *Amer. J. Med.*, 42:620–24, 1967.

Lieberson, A. D.; Schumacher, R. R.; Childress, R. H.; Boyd, D. L.; and Williams, J. F.: Effects of diphenyl-hydantoin on left ventricular function in patients with heart disease. *Circulation*, 36:692–99, 1967.

Likoff, W.; Segal, B. L.; and Kasparian, H.: Paradox of normal selective coronary arteriograms in patients considered to have unmistakable coronary heart disease. *New Eng. J. Med.*, 276:1063–66, 1967.

Liljestrand, G.: Chemical control of the distribution of the pulmonary blood flow. *Acta Physiol. Scand.*, 44:216–40, 1958.

Lillehei, R. C.; Longerbeam, J. K.; Bloch, J. H.; and Manax, W.: The nature of irreversible shock: experimental and clinical observations. *Ann. Surg.*, 160:682–710, 1964.

Linenthal, A. J., and Zoll, P. M.: Prevention of ventricular tachycardia and ventricular fibrillation by intravenous isoproterenol and epinephrine. *Circulation*, 27:5–11, 1963.

Linhart, J. W.; Braunwald, E.; and Ross, J., Jr.: Determinants of the duration of the refractory period of the atrioventricular nodal system in man. *J. Clin. Invest.*, 44:883–90, 1965.

Lippmann, W., and Wishnick, M.: Effects of methotrimeprazine, other phenothiazines and related compounds on the levels of norepinephrine in the mouse heart. *J. Pharmacol. Exp. Ther.*, 157:363–70, 1967.

LoBuglio, A. F., and Jandl, J. H.: Nature of alpha-methyldopa red-cell antibody. *New Eng. J. Med.*, 276:658–65, 1967.

Louis, S.; Kutt, H.; and McDowell, F.: The cardio-circulatory changes caused by intravenous Dilantin and its solvent. *Amer. Heart J.*, 74:523–29, 1967.

Lovell, R. R.; Denborough, M. A.; Nestel, P.; and Goble, A. J.: Controlled trial of long-term treatment with anticoagulants in 412 male patients after myocardial infarction. *Med. J. Aust.*, 2:97–104, 1967.

Lovell, R. R. H.: The prevention of late deaths after myocardial infarction. *Amer. Heart J.*, 78:1–3, 1969.

Lowenthal, J., and Birnbaum, H.: Vitamin K and coumarin anticoagulants: dependence of anticoagulant effect on inhibition of vitamin K transport. *Science*, 164:181–83, 1969.

Lown, B.: Cardioversion of arrhythmias. *Mod. Conc. Cardiov. Dis.*, 33:863–74, 1964.

Lown, B.; Ehrlich, L.; Lipschultz, B.; and Blade, J.: Effects of digitalis in patients receiving reserpine. *Circulation*, 24:1185–91, 1961.

Lown, B.; Fakhro, A. M.; Hood, W. B., Jr.; and Thorne, G. W.: The coronary care unit: new perspectives and directions. *J.A.M.A.*, 199:188–98, 1967.

Lown, B.; Kleiger, R.; and Williams, J.: Cardioversion and digitalis drugs: changed threshold to electric shock in digitalized animals. *Circ. Res.*, 17:519–31, 1965.

Lown, B.; Klein, M. D.; and Hershberg, P. I.: Coronary and precoronary care. *Amer. J. Med.*, 46:705–24, 1969.

Lown, B., and Kosowsky, B. D.: Artificial cardiac pacemakers. *New Eng. J. Med.*, 283:907–16, 971–77, 1023–31, 1970.

Lown, B., and Levine, S.: The carotid sinus: clinical value of its stimulation. *Circulation*, 23:766–89, 1961.

Lown, B.; Marcus, F.; and Levine, H. D.: Digitalis and atrial tachycardia with block: a year's experience. *New Eng. J. Med.*, 260:301–309, 1959.

Lown, B., and Vassaux, C.: Lidocaine in acute myocardial infarction. *Amer. Heart J.*, 76:586–87, 1968.

Lucchesi, B. R.: Effects of pronethanol and its dextro isomer upon experimental cardiac arrhythmias. *J. Pharmacol. Exp. Ther.*, 148:94–99, 1965.

Lucchesi, B. R., and Iwami, T.: The antiarrhythmic properties of ICI 46037, a quarternary analog of propranolol. *J. Pharmacol. Exp. Ther.*, 162:49–59, 1968.

Lucchesi, B. R.; Whitsett, L. S.; and Stickney, J. L.: Antiarrhythmic effects of beta adrenergic blocking agents. *Ann. N.Y. Acad. Sci.*, 139:940–51, 1967.

Luchi, R. J., and Gruber, J. W.: Unusually large digitalis requirements. *Amer. J. Med.*, 45:322–28, 1968.

Luisada, A. A.: Therapy and management of paroxysmal pulmonary edema. *Clin. Pharmacol. Ther.*, 5:628–44, 1964.

Luke, R. G., and Kennedy, A. C.: Methyldopa in treatment of hypertension due to chronic renal disease. *Brit. Med. J.*, 1:27–30, 1964.

Lyon, A. F., and DeGraff, A. C.: The neurologic effects of digitalis. *Amer. Heart J.*, 65:839–40, 1963.

———: Reappraisal of digitalis. Digitalis action at the cellular level. *Amer. Heart J.*, 72:414–18, 1966a.

———: Reappraisal of digitalis. II. Hemodynamic effects of the cardiac glycosides. *Amer. Heart J.*, 72:565–67, 1966b.

———: Reappraisal of digitalis. IV. Metabolism of the cardiac glycosides. *Amer. Heart J.*, 72:838–40, 1966c.

MacAlpin, R. N., and Kattus, A. A.: Adaptation to exercise in angina pectoris: the electrocardiogram during treadmill walking and coronary angiographic findings. *Circulation*, 33:183–201, 1966.

McCormack, L. J.; Biland, J. E.; Schneckloth, R. E.; and Corcoran, A. C.: Effects of antihypertensive treatment on the evolution of the renal lesions in malignant nephrosclerosis. *Amer. J. Path.*, 34:1011–19, 1958.

MacDonald, M. G.; Robinson, D. S.; Sylwester, D.; and Jaffe, J. J.: The effects of phenobarbital, chloral, betaine, and glutethimide administration on warfarin plasma levels and hypoprothrombinemic responses in man. *Clin. Pharmacol. Ther.*, 10:80–84, 1969.

McGandy, R. B.; Hegstedt, D. M.; Meyers, M. L.; and Stare, F. J.: Dietary carbohydrate and serum cholesterol levels in man. *Amer. J. Clin. Nutr.*, 18:237–42, 1966.

McGandy, R. B.; Hegstedt, D. M.; and Stare, F. J.: Dietary fats, carbohydrates and atherosclerotic vascular disease. *New Eng. J. Med.*, 277:186–92, 242–47, 1967.

McKenna, D. H.; Corliss, R. J.; Sialer, S.; Zarnstoff, W. C.; Crumpton, C. W.; and Rowe, G. G.: Effect of propranolol on systemic and coronary hemodynamics at rest and during simulated exercise. *Circ. Res.*, 19:520–27, 1966.

MacKenzie, G. J.; Taylor, S. H.; Flenley, D. C.; McDonald, A. H.; Stanton, H. P.; and Donald, K. W.: Circulatory and respiratory studies in myocardial infarction and cardiogenic shock. *Lancet*, 2:825–32, 1964.

McNay, J. L., and Goldberg, L. I.: Comparison of the effects of dopamine, isoproterenol, norepinephrine and bradykinin on canine renal and femoral blood flow. *J. Pharmacol. Exp. Ther.*, 151:23–31, 1966.

McNicol, G. P., and Douglas, A. S.: Fibrinolytic mechanisms and present trends in the therapeutic use of fibrinolytic agents and of fibrinolytic inhibitors. In Fulton, W. F. M. (ed.): *Modern Trends in Pharmacology and Therapeutics.* Appleton-Century-Crofts, New York, 1967, pp. 244–80.

McPhaul, J. J., Jr.; McIntosh, D. A.; Williams, L. F.; Gritti, E. J.; Malette, W. G.; and Grollman, A.: Remediable hypertension due to unilateral renal disease: correlation of split renal-function tests and pressor assays of renal venous blood in hypertensive patients. *Arch. Intern. Med.* (*Chicago*), **115**:644–51, 1965.

Madan, B. R., and Pendse, V. K.: Antiarrhythmic activity of thioridazine hydrochloride (Mellaril). *Amer. J. Cardiol.*, **11**:78–81, 1963.

Magidson, O.: Refractory heart failure. *Geriatrics*, **22**:132–40, 1967.

Majoor, C. L. H.: Aldosterone suppression by heparin. *New Eng. J. Med.*, **279**:1172–73, 1968.

Majoor, C. L. H.; Schlatmann, R. J. A. F. M.; Jansen, A. P.; and Prenen, H.: Excretion pattern and mechanism of diuresis induced by heparin. *Clin. Chim. Acta*, **5**:591–606, 1960.

Malach, M.: Polarizing solution in acute myocardial infarction. *Amer. J. Cardiol.*, **20**:363–66, 1967.

Malmcrona, R.; Schroder, G.; and Werko, L.: Hemodynamic effects of digitalis in acute myocardial infarction. *Acta Med. Scand.*, **180**:55–63, 1966.

Malmcrona, R., and Varnauskas, E.: Haemodynamics in acute myocardial infarction. *Acta Med. Scand.*, **175**:1–18, 1964.

Mann, G. V.: Symposium on atherosclerosis, foreword. *Amer. J. Med.*, **46**:655–56, 1969.

Mann, G. V.; Garrett, H. L.; Farhi, A.; Murray, H.; and Billings, F. T.: Exercise to prevent coronary heart disease: an experimental study of the effects of training on risk factors for coronary disease in man. *Amer. J. Med.*, **46**:12–27, 1969.

Marcus, F. I.; Burkhalter, L.; Cuccia, C.; Pavlovich, J.; and Kapadia, G. G.: Administration of tritiated digoxin with and without a loading dose: a metabolic study. *Circulation*, **34**:865–74, 1966.

Marcus, F. I., and Kapadia, G. G.: The metabolism of tritiated digoxin in cirrhotic patients. *Gastroenterology*, **47**:517–24, 1964.

Marcus, F. I.; Kapadia, G. G.; and Goldsmith, C.: Inhibition of myocardial uptake of tritiated digoxin by acute hyperkalemia in the dog. *Clin. Res.*, **15**:28, 1967a.

Marcus, F. I.; Pavlovich, J.; Burkhalter, L.; and Cuccia, C.: The metabolic fate of tritiated digoxin in the dog: a comparison of digitalis administration with and without a "loading dose." *J. Pharmacol. Exp. Ther.*, **156**:548–56, 1967b.

Marcus, F. I.; Pavlovich, J.; Lullin, M.; and Kapadia, G.: The effect of reserpine on the metabolism of tritiated digoxin in the dog and man. *J. Pharmacol. Exp. Ther.*, **159**:314–23, 1968.

Margolis, S., and Baker, B. M.: Control of coronary heart disease—treatment of hyperlipidemia. *Johns Hopkins Med. J.*, **124**:224–30, 1969.

Marmorston, J.; Moore, F. J.; Hopkins, C. E.; Kuzma, O. T.; and Weiner, J.: Clinical studies of long-term estrogen therapy in men with myocardial infarction. *Proc. Soc. Exp. Biol. Med.*, **110**:400–408, 1962.

Mason, D. T., and Braunwald, E.: Effects of guanethidine, reserpine and methyldopa on reflex venous and aterial constriction in man. *J. Clin. Invest.*, **43**:1449–63, 1964a.

———: Studies on digitalis. X. Effects of ouabain on forearm vascular resistance and venous tone in normal subjects and in patients with congestive failure. *J. Clin. Invest.*, **43**:532–43, 1964b.

———: The effects of nitroglycerin and amyl nitrite on arteriolar and venous tone in the human forearm. *Circulation*, **32**:755–66, 1965.

———: Digitalis: new facts about an old drug. *Amer. J. Cardiol.*, **22**:151–61, 1968.

Mason, D. T.; Spann, J. F.; and Zelis, R.: New developments in the understanding of the actions of digitalis glycosides. *Progr. Cardiov. Dis.*, **11**:443–78, 1969a.

Mason, D. T.; Spann, J. F.; Zelis, R., and Amsterdam, E. A.: Physiologic approach to the treatment of angina pectoris. *New Eng. J. Med.*, **281**:1225–28, 1969b.

Master, A. M., and Kuhn, L. A.: Coronary disease— 45 years ago and now. *Clin. Pharmacol. Ther.*, **8**:603–14, 1967.

Master, A. M., and Rosenfeld, I.: Two-step exercise test: current status after twenty-five years. *Mod. Conc. Cardiov. Dis.*, **36**:19–24, 1967.

Medical Letter: Atromid-S for the reduction of plasma lipids, **9**:45–47, 1967a.

———: Interactions of oral anticoagulants with other drugs. **9**:97, 1967b.

———: Pheochromocytoma. **9**:34–36, 1967c.

———: Sodium dextrothyroxin (Choloxin). **9**:103–104, 1967d.

Melmon, K. L.: Catecholamines and the adrenal medulla. In Williams, R. H. (ed.): *Textbook of Endocrinology*, 4th ed. W. B. Saunders Co., Philadelphia, 1968, pp. 379–403.

Méndez, C.; Aceves, J.; and Méndez, R.: Antiadrenergic action of digitalis on refractory period of A-V transmission system. *J. Pharmacol. Exp. Ther.*, **131**:199–204, 1961.

Mercer, E. N., and Osborne, J. A.: The current status of diphenylhydantoin in heart disease. *Ann. Intern. Med.*, **67**:1084–1107, 1967.

Messer, J. V.: Management of emergencies. XIV. Cardiac arrest. *New Eng. J. Med.*, **275**:35–39, 1966.

Meyer, M. B.; McNay, J. L.; and Goldberg, L. I.: Effects of dopamine on renal function and hemodynamics in the dog. *J. Pharmacol. Exp. Ther.*, **156**:186–92, 1967.

Michaels, L., and Beamish, R. E.: Relapses of thromboembolic disease after discontinued anticoagulant therapy: a comparison of the incidence after abrupt and after gradual termination of treatment. *Amer. J. Cardiol.*, **20**:670–73, 1967.

Michelakis, A. M.; Foster, J. H.; Liddle, G. W.; Rhamy, R. K.; Kuchel, O.; and Gordon, R. D.: Measurement of renin in both renal veins: its use in diagnosis of renovascular hypertension. *Arch. Intern. Med.* (*Chicago*), **120**:444–48, 1967.

Michelakis, A. M.; Woods, J. W.; Liddle, G. W.; and Klatte, E. C.: A predictable error in use of renal vein renin in diagnosing hypertension. *Arch. Intern. Med.* (*Chicago*), **123**:359–61, 1969.

Miller, R. L.; Forsyth, R.; McCord, C.; and Melmon, K. L.: The selective changes in regional blood flow (RBF) produced by morphine. *Clin. Res.*, **20**:341, 1970.

Miller, W. F., and Sproule, B. J.: Studies on the role of intermittent inspiratory positive pressure oxygen breathing (IPPB/I-O_2) in the treatment of pulmonary edema. *Dis. Chest*, **35**:469–79, 1959.

Mishkel, M. A., and Webb, W. F.: The mechanisms underlying the hypolipidemic effects of atromid-S, nicotinic acid and benzmalecene-1. *Biochem. Pharmacol.*, **16**:897–905, 1967.

Mitchell, J. R.; Arias, L.; and Oates, J. A.: Antagonism of the antihypertensive action of guanethidine sulfate by desipramine hydrochloride. *J.A.M.A.*, **202**:973–76, 1967.

Mitchell, J. R.; Cavanaugh, J. H.; Arias, L.; and Oates, J. A.: Guanethidine and related agents. III. Antagonism by drugs which inhibit the norepinephrine pump in man. *J. Clin. Invest.*, **49**:1596–1604, 1970.

Modell, W.: The pharmacologic basis of the use of

digitalis in congestive heart failure. *Pharmacol. for Physicians*, 1:1-6, 1966.

Mohammed, S.; Gaffney, T. E.; Yard, A. C.; and Gomez, H.: Effect of methyldopa, reserpine and guanethidine on hindleg vascular resistance. *J. Pharmacol. Exp. Ther.*, 160:300-307, 1968a.

Mohammed, S.; Hanenson, I. B.; Magenheim, H. G.; and Gaffney, T. E.: The effects of alpha-methyldopa on renal function in hypertensive patients. *Amer. Heart J.*, 76:21-27, 1968b.

Mohler, E. R., and Freis, E. D.: Five-year survival of patients with malignant hypertension treated with antihypertensive agents. *Amer. Heart J.*, 60:329-35, 1960.

Moore, F. D.; Edelman, I. S.; Olvey, J. M.; James, A. H.; Brooks, L.; and Wilson, G. M.: Body sodium and potassium. III. Inter-related trends in alimentary renal and cardiovascular disease; lack of correlation between body stores and plasma concentration. *Metabolism*, 3:334-50, 1954.

Moran, N. C.: Contraction dependency of the positive inotropic actions of cardiac glycosides. *Circ. Res.*, 21: 727-40, 1967.

Morgan, T. E.: Pulmonary surfactant. *New Eng. J. Med.* 283:1185-93, 1971.

Morin, Y.; Turmel, L.; and Fortier, J.: Methyldopa: clinical studies in arterial hypertension. *Amer. J. Med. Sci.*, 248:633-39, 1964.

Morrelli, H. F., and Melmon, K. L.: Pharmacologic basis for the clinical use of antiarrhythmic drugs. *Pharmacol. for Physicians*, 1:1-8, 1967.

Morris, J. J., Jr.; Peter, A. H.; and McIntosh, H. D.: Electrical conversion of atrial fibrillation: immediate and long-term results and selection of patients. *Ann. Intern. Med.*, 65:216-31, 1966.

Morris, J. J., Jr.; Taft, C. V.; Whalen, R. E.; and McIntosh, H. D.: Digitalis and experimental myocardial infarction. *Amer. Heart J.*, 77:342-55, 1969.

Morris, J. N., and Crawford, M. D.: Coronary heart disease and physical activity of work. *Brit. Med. J.*, 2:1485-96, 1958.

Morris, J. N., and Gardner, M. J.: Epidemiology of ischaemic heart disease. *Amer. J. Med.*, 46:674-83, 1969.

Morrison, F. S., and Wurzel, H. A.: Retroperitoneal hemorrhage during heparin therapy. *Amer. J. Cardiol.*, 13:329-32, 1964.

Morse, B. W.; Danzig, R.; and Swan, H. J. C.: Effect of isoproterenol in shock associated with acute myocardial infarction. *Circulation*, 36 (Suppl. II):192, 1967.

Moser, K. M., and Hajjar, G. C.: Effect of heparin on the one-stage prothrombin time: source of artifactual "resistance" to prothrombinopenic therapy. *Ann. Intern. Med.*, 66:1207-13, 1967.

Moss, A. J., and Aledort, L. M.: Use of edrophonium (Tensilon) in evaluation of supraventricular tachycardias. *Amer. J. Cardiol.*, 17:58-62, 1966.

Moss, A. J.; Rivers, R. J.; Griffith, L. S. C.; Carmel, J. A.; and Millard, E. B.: Transvenous left atrial pacing for the control of recurrent ventricular fibrillation. *New Eng. J. Med.*, 278:928-31, 1968.

Mounsey, P.: Intensive coronary care: arrhythmias after acute myocardial infarction. *Amer. J. Cardiol.*, 20:475-83, 1967.

Moutsos, S. E.; Sapira, J. D.; Scheib, E. T.; and Shapiro, A. P.: An analysis of the placebo effect on hospitalized hypertensive patients. *Clin. Pharmacol. Ther.*, 8:676-83, 1967.

Moyer, J. H.: Hydralazine (Apresoline) hydrochloride: pharmacological observations and clinical results in the therapy of hypertension. *Arch. Intern. Med. (Chicago)*, 91:419-39, 1953.

———: A current appraisal of drug therapy of atherosclerosis. *Arch. Environ. Health (Chicago)*, 14:337-47, 1967.

Multicentre Trial: Propranolol in acute myocardial infarction. *Lancet*, 2:1435-37, 1966.

Murray, J. F.: The pathogenesis, diagnosis, and treatment of pulmonary embolus. *Calif. Med.*, 114:36-43, 1971.

Musacchio, J. M.; Fischer, J. E.; and Kopin, I. J.: Subcellular distribution and release by sympathetic nerve stimulation of dopamine and α-methyldopamine. *J. Pharmacol. Exp. Ther.*, 152:51-55, 1966a.

Musacchio, J. M.; Goldstein, M.; Anagnoste, B.; Poch, G.; and Kopin, I. J.: Inhibition of dopamine β-hydroxylase by disulfiram in vivo. *J. Pharmacol. Exp. Ther.*, 152:56-61, 1966b.

Muscholl, E., and Maitre, L.: Release by sympathetic stimulation of α-methylnoradrenaline stored in the heart after administration of α-methyldopa. *Experientia*, 19:658-59, 1963.

Nadel, J. A.; Colebatch, H. J. H.; and Olsen, C. R.: Location and mechanism of airway constriction after barium sulfate microembolism. *J. Appl. Physiol.*, 19: 387-94, 1964.

Nagashima, R.; Levy, G.; and O'Reilly, R. A.: Comparative pharmacokinetics of coumarin anticoagulants. IV. Application of a three compartmental model to the analysis of the dose dependent kinetics of bishydroxycoumarin elimination. *J. Pharm. Sci.*, 57:1888-95, 1968.

Nagashima, R.; O'Reilly, R. A.; and Levy, G.: Kinetics of pharmacologic effects in man: the anticoagulant action of warfarin. *Clin. Pharmacol. Ther.*, 10:22-35, 1969.

Nagatsu, T.; Levitt, M.; and Udenfriend, S.: Tyrosine hydoxylase: the initial step in norepinephrine biosynthesis. *J. Biol. Chem.*, 239:2910-17, 1964.

Nahas, G. G., and Poyart, C.: Effect of arterial pH alterations on metabolic activity of norepinephrine. *Amer. J. Physiol.*, 212:765-72, 1967.

Nash, C. W., and Heath, C.: Vascular responses to catecholamines during respiratory changes in pH. *Amer. J. Physiol.*, 200:755-58, 1961.

National Diet Heart Study: Final report. *Circulation*, 37 (Suppl. I):1-428, 1968.

Naughton, J.; Bruhn, J.; Lategola, M. T.; and Whitsett, T.: Rehabilitation following myocardial infarction. *Amer. J. Med.*, 46:725-34, 1969.

Neill, W. A.; Kassebaum, D. G.; and Judkins, M. P.: Myocardial hypoxia as the basis for angina pectoris in a patient with normal coronary arteriograms. *New Eng. J. Med.*, 279:789-92, 1968.

Neu, L. T.; Waterfield, J. R.; and Ash, C. J.: Prophylactic anticoagulation in the orthopedic patient. *Ann. Intern. Med.*, 62:463-67, 1965.

Nickerson, M.: Drugs inhibiting adrenergic nerves and structures innervated by them. In Goodman, L. S., and Gilman, A. (eds.): *The Pharmacological Basis of Therapeutics*. Macmillan Co., New York, 1965, pp. 546-63.

Nickerson, M., and Gourzis, J.: Blockade of sympathetic vasoconstriction in the treatment of shock. *J. Trauma*, 2:399-411, 1962.

Nicotero, J. A.; Moutsos, S. E.; Perez-Stable, E.; Turrian, H. E.; and Shapiro, A. P.: Diagnostic and physiologic implications of the angiotensin infusion test. *New Eng. J. Med.*, 274:1464-68, 1966.

Nies, A. S.; Forsyth, R. P.; Williams, H. E.; and Melmon, K. L.: Contribution of kinins to endotoxin shock in unanesthetized rhesus monkeys. *Circ. Res.*, 22:155-64, 1968.

Nies, A. S.; Greineder, D. K.; Cline, M. J.; and Melmon, K. L.: The divergent effect of endotoxin fractions on human plasma and leukocytes. *Biochem. Pharmacol.*, **20**:39–46, 1971.

Nies, A. S., and Melmon, K. L.: Recent concepts in the clinical pharmacology of antihypertensive drugs. *Calif. Med.*, **106**:388–99, 1967.

————: Mechanism of endotoxin-induced kinin production in human plasma. *Biochem. Pharmacol.*, **20**:29–37, 1971.

Norris, R.; Caughey, D. E.; and Scott, P. J.: Trial of propranolol in acute myocardial infarction. *Brit. Med. J.*, **2**:398–400, 1968.

Oates, J. A.: Antihypertensive drugs that impair adrenergic neuron function. *Pharmacol. for Physicians*, **1**:1–8, 1967.

Oates, J. A., and Doctor, R. B.: Antihypertensive agents which impair adrenergic neuron transmission. *Postgrad. Med.*, **37**:58–64, 1965.

Oates, J. A.; Gillespie, L.; Udenfriend, S.; and Sjoerdsma, A.: Decarboxylase inhibition and blood pressure reduction by α-methyl-3,4-dihydroxy-*d,l*-phenylalanine. *Science*, **131**:1890–91, 1960.

Oates, J. A.; Seligman, A. W.; Clark, M. A.; Rousseau, P.; and Lee, R. E.: The relative efficacy of guanethidine, methyldopa and pargyline as antihypertensive agents. *New Eng. J. Med.*, **273**:729–34, 1965.

O'Brien, J. R.: Platelet stickiness. *Ann. Rev. Med.*, **17**:275–90, 1966.

————: Platelet function tests and clofibrate. *Lancet*, **2**:1143–44, 1968.

Ogden, P. C.; Selzer, A.; and Cohn, K. E.: The relationship between the inotropic and dromotropic effects of digitalis: the modulation of these effects by autonomic influences. *Amer. Heart J.*, **77**:628–35, 1969.

Okita, G. T.; Talso, P. J.; Curry, J. H., Jr.; Smith, F. D., Jr.; and Geiling, E. M. K.: Metabolic fate of radioactive digitoxin in human subjects. *J. Pharmacol. Exp. Ther.*, **115**:371–79, 1955.

Olazábal, F.; Román-Irizarry, L. A.; Oms, J. D.; Conde, L.; and Marchand, E. J.: Pulmonary emboli masquerading as asthma. *New Eng. J. Med.*, **278**:999–1001, 1968.

Oliver, M. F.: Control of hyperlipidemia. In Fulton, W. F. M. (ed.): *Modern Trends in Pharmacology and Therapeutics.* Appleton-Century-Crofts, New York, 1967a, pp. 221–43.

————: Thrombosis and oestrogens. *Lancet*, **2**:510–11, 1967b.

————: The primary prevention of ischemic heart disease by means of atromid-S (Clofibrate). *Bull. N. Y. Acad. Med.*, **44**:1021–27, 1968.

Oliver, M. F., and Boyd, G. S.: Reduction of serum cholesterol by dextrothyroxine in man with coronary heart disease. *Lancet*, **1**:783–94, 1961a.

————: Influence of reduction of serum lipids on prognosis of coronary heart disease: a five-year study using oestrogen. *Lancet*, **2**:499–505, 1961b.

Oliver, M. F.; Roberts, S. D.; Hayes, D.; Pantridge, J. F.; Suzman, M. M.; and Bersohn, I.: Effect of atromid and ethylchlorophenoxyisobutyrate on anticoagulant requirements. *Lancet*, **1**:143–44, 1963.

Oram, S., and Sowton, E.: Failure of propatylnitrate and pentaerythritol tetranitrate to prevent attacks of angina pectoris. *Brit. Med. J.*, **2**:1745–46, 1961.

O'Reilly, R. A.: Studies on the coumarin anticoagulant drugs: interaction of human plasma albumin and warfarin sodium. *J. Clin. Invest.*, **46**:829–37, 1967.

O'Reilly, R. A., and Aggeler, P. M.: Studies on coumarin anticoagulant drugs: initiation of warfarin therapy without a loading dose. *Circulation*, **38**:169–77, 1968.

O'Reilly, R. A.; Aggeler, P. M.; Hoag, M. S.; Leong, L. S.; and Kropatkin, M. L.: Hereditary transmission of exceptional resistance to coumarin anticoagulant drugs: the first reported kindred. *New Eng. J. Med.*, **271**:809–15, 1964.

O'Reilly, R. A.; Aggeler, P. M.; and Leong, L. S.: Studies on the coumarin anticoagulant drugs: a comparison of the pharmacodynamics of Dicumarol and warfarin in man. *Thromb. Diath. Haemorrh.*, **11**:1–22, 1964.

Orvis, H. H.; Tamanga, I. G.; Horwitz, D.; and Thomas, R.: Correlation of hypotensive effects and urinary tryptamine levels during pargyline therapy. *Ann. N. Y. Acad. Sci.*, **107**:958–65, 1963.

Ostrander, L. D., Jr.: Alterations of factors predisposing to coronary heart disease. *Ann. Intern. Med.*, **68**:1072–77, 1968.

Owen, C. A., Jr.: Hypercoagulability and thrombosis. *Mayo Clin. Proc.*, **40**:830–33, 1965.

Owens, J. C.; Neely, W. B.; and Owen, W. R.: Effect of sodium dextrothyroxine in patients receiving anticoagulants. *New Eng. J. Med.*, **266**:76–79, 1962.

Page, I. H., and Brown, H. B.: Some observations on the national diet-heart study. *Circulation*, **37**:313–15, 1968.

Page, I. H.; Green, J. G.; and Robertson, A. L.: The physicians incompleat guide to atherosclerosis. *Ann. Intern. Med.*, **64**:189–203, 1966.

Page, I. H., and Stamler, J.: Diet and coronary heart disease. I and II. *Mod. Conc. Cardiov. Dis.*, **37**:119–30, 1968.

Page, L. B.: Hypertension in end-stage renal disease. *New Eng. J. Med.*, **280**:1018, 1969.

Palmer, R. F., and Nechay, B. R.: Biphasic renal effects of ouabain in the chicken: correlation with a microsomal Na^+–K^+ stimulated ATP-ase. *J. Pharmacol. Exp. Ther.*, **146**:92–98, 1964.

Pantridge, J. F., and Geddes, J. S.: A mobile intensive care unit in the management of myocardial infarction. *Lancet*, **2**:271–73, 1967.

Parker, J. O.; West, R. O.; and DiGiorgi, S.: Hemodynamic effects of propranolol in coronary heart disease. *Amer. J. Cardiol.*, **21**:11–19, 1968.

Parker, J. O.; West, R. O.; Ledwich, J. R.; and DiGiorgi, S.: The effect of acute digitalization on the hemodynamic response to exercise in coronary artery disease. *Circulation*, **40**:453–62, 1969.

Parks, V. J.; Sandison, A. G.; Skinner, S. L.; and Whelan, R. F.: The mechanisms of the vasodilator action of reserpine in man. *Clin. Sci.*, **20**:289–95, 1961.

Parmley, W. W., and Braunwald, E.: Comparative myocardial depressant and antiarrhythmic properties of *d*-propranolol and *dl*-propranolol and quinidine. *J. Pharmacol. Exp. Ther.*, **158**:11–21, 1967.

Parratt, J. R.: Adrenergic receptors in the coronary circulation. *Amer. Heart J.*, **73**:137–40, 1967.

Parratt, J. R., and Grayson, J.: Myocardial vascular reactivity after beta-adrenergic blockade. *Lancet*, **1**:338–40, 1966a.

————: Myocardial vascular reactivity. *Lancet*, **1**:819, 1966b.

Parsons, W. B., Jr.: Treatment of hypercholesterolemia by nicotinic acid. *Arch. Intern. Med. (Chicago)*, **107**:639–52, 1961a.

————: Studies in nicotinic acid use in hypercholesterolemia: changes in hepatic function, carbohydrate tolerance and uric acid metabolism. *Arch. Intern. Med. (Chicago)*, **107**:653–67, 1961b.

————: Chemotherapy of hyperlipidemia. *Mayo Clin. Proc.*, **40**:822–29, 1965.

Patterson, J. W., and Dollery, C. T.: Effect of propranolol in mild hypertension. *Lancet*, **2**:1148–50, 1966.

Payne, J. P., and Rowe, G. G.: The effects of mecamylamine in the cat as modified by the administration of carbon dioxide. *Brit. J. Pharmacol.*, **12**:457–60, 1957.

Pearson, J. W., and Redding, J. S.: Epinephrine in cardiac resuscitation. *Amer. Heart J.*, **66**:210–14, 1963a.

————: The role of epinephrine in cardiac resuscitation. *Anesth. Analg.*, **42**:599–606, 1963b.

Peart, W. S.: Catecholamines and hypertension. *Pharmacol. Rev.*, **18**:667–72, 1966.

Pell, S., and D'Alonzo, C. A.: Immediate mortality and five year survival of employed men with a first myocardial infarction. *New Eng. J. Med.*, **270**:915–22, 1964.

Peretz, D. I.; Scott, H. M.; Duff, J.; Dosseter, J. B.; MacLean, L. D.; and McGregor, M.: The significance of lacticacidemia in the shock syndrome. *Ann. N.Y. Acad. Sci.*, **119**:1133–41, 1965.

Perlroth, M., and Harrison, D. C.: Cardiogenic shock: a review. *Clin. Pharmacol. Ther.*, **10**:449–67, 1969.

Peters, L.: Renal tubular excretion of organic bases. *Pharmacol. Rev.*, **12**:1–35, 1960.

Peters, W. G.: Pharmacology of diuretics. In Gross, F. (ed.): *Antihypertensive Therapy, Principles and Practices: An International Symposium.* Springer-Verlag, Berlin, 1966, pp. 31–57.

Pettinger, W. A.; Horwitz, D.; and Sjoersdma, A.: Lactation due to methyldopa. *Brit. Med. J.*, **1**:1460, 1963.

Pettinger, W. A., and Oates, J. A.: Supersensitivity to tyramine during monoamine oxidase inhibition in man: mechanism at the level of the adrenergic neuron. *Clin. Pharmacol. Ther.*, **9**:341–44, 1968.

Pettinger, W. A.; Soyangco, F. G., and Oates, J. A.: Inhibition of monoamine oxidase in man by furazolidone *Clin. Pharmacol. Ther.*, **9**:442–47, 1968.

Pitney, H.; Holt, P. J. L.; Bray, C.; and Bolton, G.: Acquired resistance to treatment with Arvin. *Lancet*, **1**:79–81. 1969.

Pitt, B., Elliot, E. C.; and Gregg, D. E.: Adrenergic receptor activity in the coronary arteries of the unanesthetized dog. *Circ. Res.*, **21**:75–84, 1967.

Pitt, B., and Ross, R. S.: Beta adrenergic blockade in cardiovascular therapy. *Mod. Conc. Cardiov. Dis.*, **38**:47–54, 1969.

Porte, D., Jr.: A receptor mechanism for the inhibition of insulin release by epinephrine in man. *J. Clin. Invest.*, **46**:86–94, 1967.

————: Sympathetic regulation of insulin excretion: its relation to diabetes mellitus. *Arch. Intern. Med.* (*Chicago*), **123**:252–60, 1969.

Porter, P.; Porter, M. C.; and Shanberg, J. N.: Interaction of heparin with the plasma proteins in relation to its antithrombin activity. *Biochemistry*, **6**:1854–63, 1967.

Poulose, K.; Reba, R. C.; and Wagner, H. N.: Characterization of the shape and location of perfusion defects in certain pulmonary diseases. *New Eng. J. Med.*, **278**:1020–25, 1968.

Prescott, L. E.; Buhs, R. P.; Beattie, J. O.; Speth, O. C.; Trenner, N. R.; and Lasagna, L.: Combined clinical and metabolic study of the effects of alpha-methyldopa on hypertensive patients. *Circulation*, **34**:308–21, 1966.

Price, H. L.: A dynamic concept of the distribution of thiopental in the human body. *Anesthesiology*, **21**:40–45, 1960.

Price, H. L.; Kovnat, P. J.; Safer, J. N.; Conner, E. H.; and Price, M. L.: The uptake of thiopental by body tissues and its relation to the duration of narcosis. *Clin. Pharmacol. Ther.*, **1**:16–22, 1960.

Price, K. C.; Hata, D.; and Smith, J. R.: Pulmonary vasomotion resulting from miliary embolism of the lungs. *Amer. J. Physiol.*, **182**:183–90, 1955.

Prichard, B. N. C., and Gillam, P. M. S.: Use of propranolol in treatment of hypertension. *Brit. Med. J.*, **2**:725, 1964.

————: Propranolol in hypertension. *Amer. J. Cardiol.*, **18**:387–93, 1966.

Prichard, B. N. C.; Shinebourne, E.; Fleming, J.; and Hamer, J.: Haemodynamic studies in hypertensive patients treated by oral propranolol. *Brit. Heart J.*, **32**:236–40, 1970.

Prout, W. G.: Relative value of central venous pressure monitoring and blood-volume measurement in the management of shock. *Lancet*, **1**:1108–12, 1968.

Puri, P. S., and Bing, R. J.: Effect of drugs on myocardial contractility in the intact dog and in experimental myocardial infarction: basis for their use in cardiogenic shock. *Amer. J. Cardiol.*, **21**:886–93, 1968.

Rabinowitz, J. L.; Rodman, T.; and Myerson, R. M.: Effect of dextrothyroxine in metabolism of C^{14}-labeled cholesterol and tripalmitin. *J.A.M.A.*, **183**:758–60, 1963.

Randall, R. E., Jr.; Cohen, M. D.; Spray, C. C., Jr.; Rossmeid, E. C.: Hypermagnesemia in renal failure: etiology and toxic manifestations. *Ann. Intern. Med.*, **61**:73–88, 1964.

Redding, J. S.; Asuncion, J. S.; and Pearson, J. W.: Effective routes of drug administration during cardiac arrest. *Anesth. Analg.*, **46**:253–58, 1967.

Redding, J. S., and Pearson, J. W.: Evaluation of drugs for cardiac resuscitation. *Anesthesiology*, **24**:203–207, 1963.

————: Resuscitation from ventricular fibrillation: drug therapy. *J.A.M.A.*, **203**:255–60, 1968.

Regan, T. J.; Markor, A.; Oldewurtel, N. A.; and Harman, M. A.: Myocardial K^+ loss after counter-shock and the relation to ventricular arrhythmias after non-toxic doses of acetylstrophanthidin. *Amer. Heart J.*, **77**:367–71, 1969.

Reid, H. A., and Chan, K. E.: The paradox in therapeutic defibrination. *Lancet*, **1**:485–89, 1968.

Relman, A. S., and Schwartz, W. B.: The kidney in potassium depletion. *Amer. J. Med.*, **24**:764–73, 1958.

Research Committee of the Edgewood General, the West Middlesex and St. George's Hospitals, London: Low fat diet on myocardial infarction: a controlled trial. *Lancet*, **2**:501–504, 1965.

Riddle, M. C., and Schwartz, T. B.: New tactics for hyperthyroidism: sympathetic blockade. *Ann. Intern. Med.*, **72**:749–50, 1970.

Rinzler, S. H.: Primary prevention of coronary heart disease by diet. *Bull. N.Y. Acad. Med.*, **44**:936–49, 1968.

Roberts, J.; Ryuta, I.; Reilly, J.; and Cairoli, V. J.: Influence of reserpine and β TM10 on digitalis induced ventricular arrhythmias. *Circ. Res.*, **13**:149–58, 1963.

Robin, E.; Cowan, C.; Puri, P.; Ganguly, S.; DeBoynie, E.; Martinez, M.; Stock, T.; and Bing, R. J.: A comparative study of nitroglycerin and propranolol. *Circulation*, **36**:178–86, 1967a.

Robin. E.; Cross, C. E.; Miller, J. E.; and Murdough, H. V., Jr.: Humoral agent from calf lung producing pulmonary arterial vasoconstriction. *Science*, **156**:827–30, 1967b.

Robinson, B. F.: The relation of heart rate and systolic blood pressure to the onset of pain in angina pectoris. *Circulation*, **35**:1073–83, 1967.

————: Mode of action of nitroglycerin in angina pectoris. *Brit. Heart J.*, **30**:295–302, 1968.

Robinson, D. S.; Benjamin, D. M.; and McCormack, J. J.: Interaction of warfarin and nonsystemic gastrointestinal drugs. *Clin. Pharmacol. Ther.*, **12**:491–95, 1971.

Robinson, R. W., and LeBeau, R. J.: Dextro-thyroxine as a cholesterol lowering agent in patients with angina pectoris. *Circulation*, **28**:531–35, 1963.

Rodensky, D. L., and Wassermann, F.: Observations on digitalis intoxication. *Arch. Intern. Med.* (*Chicago*), **108**:171–88, 1961.

Rosati, R. A.; Alexander, J. A.; Schaal, S. F.; and Wallace, A. G.: Influence of diphenylhydantoin on electrophysiological properties of the canine heart. *Circ. Res.*, **21**:757–65, 1967.

Rose, G. A.; Thomson, W. B.; and Williams, R. T.: Corn oil in treatment of ischemic heart disease. *Brit. Med. J.*, **1**:1531–33, 1965.

Rosen, M.; Lisak, R.; and Rubin, I. L.: Diphenylhydantoin in cardiac arrhythmias. *Amer. J. Cardiol.*, **20**:674–78, 1967.

Rosenberg, B.; Dobkin, G.; and Rubin, R.: Intravenous use of ethacrynic acid in the management of acute pulmonary edema. *Amer. Heart J.*, **70**:333–36, 1965.

Ross, J., Jr.: Left ventricular contraction and the therapy of cardiogenic shock. *Circulation*, **35**:611–13, 1967.

Ross, R. S.; Ueda, K.; Lichtlen, P. R.; and Rees, J. R.: Measurement of myocardial flow in animals and man by selective injection of radioactive inert gas into the coronary arteries. *Circ. Res.*, **15**:28–41, 1964.

Ross, R. S.: Coronary arteriography. *Circulation*, **37**(Suppl. III):67–73, 1968.

Roughgarden, J. W., and Newman, E. V.: Circulatory changes during the pain of angina pectoris. *Amer. J. Med.*, **41**:935–46, 1966.

Rowe, G. G.: Effects of drugs on the coronary circulation of man. *Clin. Pharmacol. Ther.*, **7**:547–57, 1966.

———: Pharmacology of the coronary circulation. *Ann. Rev. Pharmacol.*, **8**:95–112, 1968.

Rowe, G. G.; Huston, J. H.; Maxwell, G. M.; Crosley, A. P., Jr.; and Crumpton, C. W.: Hemodynamic effects of 1-hydrazinopthalazine in patients with arterial hypertension. *J. Clin. Invest.*, **34**:115–20, 1955.

Rowlands, D. J.; Howitt, G.; and Markman, P.: Propranolol (Inderal) in disturbance of cardiac rhythm. *Brit. Med. J.*, **1**:891–94, 1965.

Russek, H. I.: Propranolol and isosorbide dinitrate synergism in angina pectoris. *Amer. J. Cardiol.*, **21**:44–54, 1968.

Ryan, W. G., and Schwartz, T. B.: Dynamics of plasma triglyceride turnover in man. *Metabolism*, **14**:1243–54, 1965.

Sachs, B. A.: Appraisal of clofibrate as a hypolipidemic agent. *Amer. Heart J.*, **75**:707–10, 1968.

Sackett, D. L.; Gibson, R. W.; Bross, I. D. J.; and Pickran, J. W.: Relation between aortic atherosclerosis and the use of cigarettes and alcohol. *New Eng. J. Med.*, **279**:1413–20, 1968.

Sahud, M. A., and Aggeler, P. M.: Platelet dysfunction: differentiation of a newly recognized primary type from that produced by aspirin. *New Eng. J. Med.*, **280**:453–59, 1969.

St. George, S.; Bine, R.; and Friedman, M.: Role of the liver in the excretion and destruction of digitoxin. *Circulation*, **6**:661–65, 1952.

Salzman, E. W.; Harris, W. H.; and DeSanctis, R. W.: Anticoagulation for prevention of thromboembolism following fractures of the hip. *New Eng. J. Med.*, **275**:122–30, 1966.

Sambhi, M. P.; Weil, M. H.; and Udhoji, V. N.: Acute pharmacodynamic effects of glucocorticoids: cardiac output and related hemodynamic changes in normal subjects and patients in shock. *Circulation*, **31**:523–30, 1965.

Samuel, P.; Holtzman, C. M.; and Goldstein, B. S.: Long-term reduction of serum cholesterol levels of patients with atherosclerosis by small doses of neomycin. *Circulation*, **35**:938–45, 1967.

Samuel, P., and Meilman, E.: Dietary lipids and reduction of serum cholesterol levels by neomycin in man. *J. Lab. Clin. Med.*, **70**:471–79, 1967.

Samuel, P., and Waithe, W. I.: Reduction of serum cholesterol concentrations by neomycin, paraamino salicylic acid, and other antibacterial drugs in man. *Circulation*, **24**:578–91, 1961.

Sanan, S., and Vogt, M.: Effect of drugs on the noradrenalin content of brain and peripheral tissue and its significance. *Brit. J. Pharmacol.*, **18**:109–27, 1962.

Sannerstedt, R.; Varnauskas, E.; and Werko, L.: Hemodynamic effects of methyldopa (Aldomet) at rest and during exercise in patients with arterial hypertension. *Acta Med. Scand.*, **171**:75–82, 1962.

Sarnoff, S. J., and Berglund, E.: Ventricular function. I. Starling's law of the heart studied by means of right and left ventricular function curves in the dog. *Circulation*, **9**:706–18, 1954.

Sarnoff, S. J.; Case, R. B.; Waithe, P. E.; and Issacs, J. P.: Insufficient coronary flow and myocardial failure as a complicating factor in late hemorrhagic shock. *Amer. J. Physiol.*, **176**:439–44, 1954.

Sasahara, A. A.: Pulmonary vascular responses to thromboembolism. *Mod. Conc. Cardiov. Dis.*, **36**:55–60, 1967.

Sasahara, A. A.; Cannilla, J. E.; Belko, J. S.; Morse, R. L.; and Criss, A. J.: Urokinase therapy in clinical pulmonary embolism: a new thrombolytic agent. *New Eng. J. Med.*, **277**:1168–73, 1967b.

Sasahara, A. A.; Cannilla, J. E.; Morse, R. L.; Sidd, J. J.; and Tremblay, G. M.: Clinical and physiologic studies in pulmonary thromboembolism. *Amer. J. Cardiol.*, **20**:10–20, 1967a.

Sautter, R. D.: Recanalization of the inferior vena cava after ligation. *New Eng. J. Med.*, **281**:780–81, 1969.

Scheinman, M. M.; Abbot, J. A.; and Rapaport, E.: Clinical use of a flow directed right heart catheter. *Arch. Intern. Med.* (*Chicago*), **124**:19–24, 1969a.

Scheinman, M. M.; Brown, M. A.; and Rapaport, E.: Critical assessment of use of central venous oxygen saturation as a mirror of mixed venous oxygen in severely ill cardiac patients. *Circulation*, **40**:165–72, 1969b.

Schelling, J. L., and Lasagna, L.: A study of cross-tolerance to circulatory effects of organic nitrates. *Clin. Pharmacol. Ther.*, **8**:256–60, 1967.

Schoonmaker, F. N.; Osteen, R. T.; and Greenfield, J. C., Jr.: Thioridazine (Mellaril)-induced ventricular tachycardia controlled with an artificial pacemaker. *Ann. Intern. Med.*, **65**:1076–78, 1966.

Schwartz, W. B.; van Ypersele de Strihou, C.; and Kassirer, J. P.: Role of anions in metabolic alkalosis and potassium deficiency. *New Eng. J. Med.*, **279**:630–39, 1968.

Seaman, A. J.; Griswold, H. E.; Reaume, R. B.; and Ritzmann, L.: Long-term anticoagulant prophylaxis after myocardial infarction. *New Eng. J. Med.*, **281**:115–19, 1969.

Seaton, A.: Quinidine-induced paroxysmal ventricular fibrillation treated with propranolol. *Brit. Med. J.*, **1**:1522–23, 1966.

Sedvall, G. C.; Weise, V. K.; and Kopin, I. J.: The rate of norepinephrine synthesis measured *in vivo* during short intervals: influence of adrenergic nerve impulse activity. *J. Pharmacol. Exp. Ther.*, **159**:274–82, 1968.

Sekiya, A., and Vaughan Williams, E. M.: A comparison of the antifibrillatory actions and effects on intracellular cardiac potentials of pronethalol, disopyramide and quinidine. *Brit. J. Pharmacol.*, **21**:473–81, 1963.

Seller, R. H.; Cangiano, J.; Kim, K. E.; Mendelssahn, S.; Brest, A. N.; and Swartz, C.: Digitalis toxicity and hypomagnesemia. *Amer. Heart J.*, **79**:57–68, 1970.

Selzer, A.: The use of digitalis in acute myocardial infarction. *Progr. Cardiov. Dis.*, **10**:518–27, 1968.

Selzer, A., and Wray, H. W.: Quinidine syncope. *Circulation*, **30**:17–26, 1964.

Selzer, C. C.: An evaluation of the effect of smoking on coronary heart disease. I. Epidemiological evidence. *J.A.M.A.*, **203**:193–200, 1968.

Severinghaus, J. W.: Bronchial muscle control. *Acta Anaesth. Scand.*, (Suppl. 15):48–51, 1964.

Sevitt, S.: Venous thrombosis and pulmonary embolism: their prevention by oral anticoagulants. *Amer. J. Med.*, **33**:703–16, 1962.

Sevitt, S., and Gallagher, N. G.: Prevention of venous thrombosis and pulmonary embolism in injured patients: a trial of anticoagulant prophylaxis with phenindione with middle-aged and elderly patients with fractured necks of femur. *Lancet*, **2**:981–89, 1959.

———: Venous thrombosis and pulmonary embolism: clinico-pathological study in injured and burned patients. *Brit. J. Surg.*, **48**:475–89, 1961.

Shaffer, A. B., and Katz, L. N.: Hemodynamic alterations in congestive heart failure. *New Eng. J. Med.*, **276**:853–57, 1967.

Shand, D. G.; Nuckolls, E. M.; and Oates, J. A.: Plasma propranolol levels in adults. With observations in four children. *Clin. Pharmacol. Ther.*, **11**:112–20, 1970.

Shapiro, A. P.; Perez-Stable, E., Scheib, E. T.; Bron, K.; Montsos, S. E.; Berg, G.; and Misage, J. R.: Renal artery stenosis and hypertension: observations on current status of therapy from a study of 115 patients. *Amer. J. Med.*, **47**:175–93, 1969.

Sharp, A. A.; Warren, B. A.; Paxton, W. M.; and Allington, M. J.: Anticoagulant therapy with purified fraction of Malayan pit viper venom. *Lancet*, **1**:493–99, 1968.

Sharpey-Schafer, E. P.: Effects of coughing on intra-thoracic pressure, arterial pressure and peripheral flow. *J. Physiol.*, **122**:351–57, 1953.

Sheffield, L. T., and Reeves, T. J.: Gradual exercise in the diagnosis of angina pectoris. *Mod. Conc. Cardiov. Dis.*, **34**:1–6, 1965.

Shekelle, R. B.: Educational status and risk of coronary heart disease. *Science*, **163**:97–98, 1969.

Sheps, S. G.; Osmundson, P. J.; Hunt, J. C.; Schirger, A.; and Farrbairn, J. F.: Hypertension and renal artery stenosis: serial observations on 54 patients treated medically. *Clin. Pharmacol. Ther.*, **6**:700–709, 1965.

Sheps, S. G.; Tyce, G. M.; Flock, E. V.; and Maher, F. T.: Current experience on the diagnosis of pheochromocytoma. *Circulation*, **34**:473–83, 1966.

Sherry, S.: Urokinase. *Ann. Intern. Med.*, **69**:415–25, 1968.

———: Streptokinase. *New Eng. J. Med.*, **280**:723–24, 1969.

Shillingford, J. P., and Thomas, M.: Cardiovascular and pulmonary changes in patients with myocardial infarction treated in an intensive care research unit. *Amer. J. Cardiol.*, **20**:484–93, 1967a.

———: Hemodynamic effects of acute myocardial infarction in man. *Progr. Cardiov. Dis.*, **9**:571–93, 1967b.

———: Treatment of bradycardia and hypotension syndrome in patients with acute myocardial infarction. *Amer. Heart J.*, **75**:843–44, 1968.

Shore, P. A.; Busfield, D.; and Alpers, H. S.: Binding and release of metaraminol: mechanism of nor-epinephrine depletion by methylmetatyrosine and related agents. *J. Pharmacol. Exp. Ther.*, **146**:194–99, 1964.

Shrager, M. W.: Digitalis intoxication: a review and report of 40 cases, with emphasis on etiology. *Arch. Intern. Med. (Chicago)*, **100**:881–93, 1957.

Sidd, J. J.; Sasahara, A. A.; and Littmann, D. Coronary-artery disease in identical twins: a family study. *New Eng. J. Med.*, **274**:55–60, 1966.

Silove, E. D., and Grover, R. T.: Effects of alpha adrenergic blockade and tissue catecholamine de-pletion on pulmonary vascular response to hypoxia. *J. Clin. Invest.*, **47**:274–85, 1968.

Simeone, F. A.: Critical analysis of models for the study of experimental shock. *Fed. Proc.*, **20** (Suppl. 9): 193–200, 1961.

Singer, D. H.; Harris, P. D.; Malm, J. R.; and Hoffman, B. F.: Electrophysiological basis of chronic atrial fibrillation. *Circulation*, **36** (Suppl. II):239, 1967a.

Singer, D. H.; Lazzara, R.; and Hoffman, B. F.: Inter-relationships between automaticity and conduction in purkinje fibers. *Circ. Res.*, **21**:537–58, 1967b.

Singer, D. H., and Ten Eick, R. E.: Pharmacology of cardiac arrhythmias. *Progr. Cardiov. Dis.*, **11**:488–514, 1969.

Sise, H. S.: Potentiation of tolbutamide by Dicumarol. *Ann. Intern. Med.*, **67**:460–61, 1967.

Sjoerdsma, A.: Relationship between alterations in amine metabolism and blood pressure. *Circ. Res.*, **9**:734–45, 1961.

Sjoerdsma, A.; Engelman, K.; Waldmann, T. A.; Cooperman, L. H.; and Hammond, W. G.: Pheo-chromocytoma: current concepts of diagnosis and treatment. *Ann. Intern. Med.*, **65**:1302–26, 1966.

Skinner, S. L.; McCubbin, J. W.; and Page, I. H.: Control of renin secretion. *Circ. Res.*, **15**:64–76, 1964.

Smirk, H., and Hodge, J.: Causes of death in treated hypertensive patients. *Brit. Med. J.*, **2**:1221–25, 1963.

Smith, H. J.; Oriol, A.; Morch, J.; and McGregor, M.: Hemodynamic studies in cardiogenic shock: treatment with isoproterenol and metaraminol. *Circulation*, **35**: 1084–91, 1967.

Smith, L. L., and Moore, F. D.: Refractory hypo-tension in man—is this irreversible shock? Clinical and biochemical observations. *New Eng. J. Med.*, **267**:733–42, 1962.

Smith, T. W.; Butler, V. P., Jr.; and Haber, E.: Deter-mination of therapeutic and toxic serum digoxin concentrations by radioimmunoassay. *New Eng. J. Med.*, **281**:1212–16, 1969.

Smith, T. W., and Haber, E.: Digoxin intoxication: the relationship of clinical presentation to serum digoxin concentration. *J. Clin. Invest.*, **49**:2377–86, 1970.

Smith, W. M.; Bachman, B.; Galante, J. G.; Hanowell, E. G.; Johnson, W. P.; Koch, C. E., Jr.; Korfmacher, S. D.; Thurm, R. H.; and Bromer, L.: Cooperative clinical trial of alpha-methyldopa. *Ann. Intern. Med.*, **65**:657–71, 1966.

Smith, W. M.; Damato, A. N.; Galluzzi, N. S.; Garfield, C. F.; Hanowell, E. G.; Shinson, W. M.; Thurm, R. H.; Walsh, J. J.; and Bromer, L.: The evaluation of anti-hypertensive therapy: cooperative clinical trial method. *Ann. Intern. Med.*, **61**:829–46, 1964.

Smith, W. M.; Thurm, R. H.; and Bromer, L. A.: Comparative evaluation of Rauwolfia whole root and reserpine. *Clin. Pharmacol. Ther.*, **10**:338–43, 1969.

Snow, P. J. D.: Effect of propranolol in myocardial infarction. *Lancet*, **2**:551–53, 1965.

Sodeman, W. A.: Diagnosis and treatment of digitalis toxicity. *New Eng. J. Med.*, **273**:35–37; 93–95, 1965.

Sokolow, M., and Perloff, D.: Five-year survival of consecutive patients with malignant hypertension treated with antihypertensive agents. *Amer. J. Cardiol.*, **6**:858–63, 1960.

———: The clinical pharmacology and use of quinidine. *Progr. Cardiov. Dis.*, **3**:316–30, 1961.

Sokolow, M.; Werdegar, D.; Kain, H. K.; and Hinman, A.: Relationship between level of blood pressure measured casually and by portable recorder and severity of complications in essential hypertension. *Circulation*, **34**:279–98, 1966.

Solomon, H. M., and Schrogie, J. J.: Change in receptor site affinity: a proposed explanation for the potentiating effect of D-thyroxine on the anticoagulant response to warfarin. *Clin. Pharmacol. Ther.*, **8**:797–99, 1966.

Somani, P.; Fleming, J. G.; Chan, G. K.; and Lum, B. K. B.: Antagonism of epinephrine induced cardiac arrhythmias by 4-(2-isopropylamino-1-hydroxyethyl)-methane-sulfonanilide (MJ-1999). *J. Pharmacol. Exp. Ther.*, **151**:32–37, 1966.

Somani, P., and Watson, D. L.: Antiarrhythmic activity of the dextro- and levo-rotary isomers of 4-(2-isopropylamino-1-hydroxyethyl) methane-sulfonanilide (MJ-1999). *J. Pharmacol. Exp. Ther.*, **164**:317–25, 1968.

Soroff, H. S.; Giron, F.; Ruiz, U.; Birtwell, W. C.; Hirsch, L. J.; and Dieterling, R. A., Jr.: Physiologic support of heart action. *New Eng. J. Med.*, **280**:693–704, 1969.

Sowton, E.: Cardiac pacemakers and pacing. *Mod. Conc. Cardiov. Dis.*, **36**:31–36, 1967.

————: Beta-adrenergic blockade in cardiac infarction. *Progr. Cardiov. Dis.*, **10**:561–72, 1968.

Sowton, E., and Hamer, J.: Hemodynamic changes after beta-adrenergic blockade. *Amer. J. Cardiol.*, **18**:317–20, 1966.

Spann, J. F., Jr.; Moellering, R. C., Jr.; Haber, E.; and Wheeler, E.: Arrhythmias in acute myocardial infarction: a study utilizing an electrocardiographic monitor for automatic detection and recording of arrhythmias. *New Eng. J. Med.*, **271**:427–31, 1964.

Spann, J. F., Jr.; Sonnenblick, E. H.; Cooper, T.; Chidsey, C. A.; Willman, V. L.; and Braunwald, E.: Studies on digitalis. XIV. Influence of cardiac norepinephrine stores on the response of heart muscle to digitalis. *Circ. Res.*, **19**:326–31, 1966.

Spark, R. F., and Melby, J. C.: Aldosteronism in hypertension: the spironolactone response test. *Ann. Intern. Med.*, **69**:685–91, 1968.

Spector, S.; Gordon, R.; Sjoerdsma, A.; and Udenfriend, S.: End-product inhibition of tyrosine hydroxylase as a possible mechanism for regulation of norepinephrine synthesis. *Molec. Pharmacol.*, **3**:549–55, 1967.

Spergel, G.; Levy, L. J.; Chowdhury, F. R.; Rodman, H. M.; Ertel, N. H.; and Bleicher, S. J.: A modified phentolamine test for the diagnosis of pheochromocytoma. *J.A.M.A.*, **211**:266–69, 1970.

Srivastara, S. C.; Smith, M. J.; and Dewar, H. A.: The effect of atromid on fibrinolytic activity of patients with ischaemic heart disease and hypercholesterolemia. *J. Atheroscler. Res.*, **3**:640–47, 1963.

Stamey, T. A.: Diagnosis of curable unilateral renal hypertension by ureteral catheterization. *Postgrad. Med.*, **29**:496–512, 1961.

————: *Renovascular Hypertension.* Williams and Wilkins Co., Baltimore, 1963, p. 200.

Stamler, J.: Interrelationships between the two diseases, hypertension and atherosclerosis. *Amer. J. Cardiol.*, **9**:743–47, 1962.

————: Acute myocardial infarction—progress in primary prevention. *Brit. Heart J.*, **33**(Suppl.):145–64, 1971.

Stamler, J.; Berkson, D. M.; Lindberg, H. A.; Hall, Y.; Miller, W.; Mojonnier, L.; Levinson, M.; Cohen, D. B.; and Young, Q. D.: Coronary risk factors: their impact and their therapy in the prevention of coronary heart disease. *Med. Clin. N. Amer.*, **50**:229–54, 1966.

Stamler, J.; Pick, R.; Katz, L. V.; Pick, A.; Kaplan, B. M.; Berkson, D. M.; and Century, D.: Effectiveness of estrogens for therapy of myocardial infarction in middle-aged men. *J.A.M.A.*, **183**:632–38, 1963.

Stamm, H.: Current use of heparin in venous thrombosis. *Thromb. Diath. Haemorrh.*, **3** (Suppl. II): 61–68, 1963.

Stampfer, M.; Epstein, S. E.; Beiser, G. D.; and Braunwald, E.: Hemodynamic effects of diuresis at rest and during intense upright exercise in patients with impaired cardiac function. *Circulation*, **37**:900–11, 1968.

Stansel, H. C., Jr.; Hume, M.; and Glenn, W. W. L.: Pulmonary embolectomy: results in ten patients. *New Eng. J. Med.*, **276**:717–21, 1967.

Stanzler, R. M.: Management of emergencies. X. Cardiac arrhythmias. *New Eng. J. Med.*, **274**:1307–11, 1966.

Staub, N. C.; Nagano, H.; and Pearce, M.L.: Pulmonary edema in dogs, especially the sequence of fluid accumulation in lungs. *J. Appl. Physiol.*, **22**:227–40, 1967.

Stead, E. A., Jr.; Warren, J. V.; and Brannon, E. S.: Cardiac output in congestive heart failure. *Amer. Heart J.*, **35**:529–41, 1948.

Stemmler, E. J.: Cardiac resuscitation: a 1-year study of patients resuscitated within a University Hospital. *Ann. Intern. Med.*, **63**:613–18, 1965.

Stenson, R. E.; Constantino, R. T.; and Harrison, D. C.: Interrelationships of hepatic blood flow, cardiac output, and blood levels of lidocaine in man. *Circulation*, **43**:205–11, 1971.

Stern, I. J.; Hollifield, R. D.; Wilk, S.; and Buzard, J. A.: The antimonoamine oxidase effects of furazolidone. *J. Pharmacol. Exp. Ther.*, **156**:492–99, 1967.

Stern, S.: Synergistic action of propranolol with quinidine. *Amer. Heart J.*, **72**:569–70, 1966.

Stern, S., and Eisenberg, S.: The effect of propranolol (Inderal) on the electrocardiogram of normal subjects. *Amer. Heart J.*, **77**:192–95, 1969.

Stewart, J. S. S.; Stewart, W. K.; and Gillies, H. G.: Cardiac arrest and acidosis. *Lancet*, **2**:964–66, 1962.

Stock, E.: Arrhythmias after myocardial infarction. *Amer. Heart J.*, **75**:435–38, 1968.

Stock, E.; Gable, A.; and Sloman, G.: Assessment of arrhythmias in myocardial infarction. *Brit. Med. J.*, **2**:719–23, 1967.

Stone, D. J.; Lyon, A. F.; and Tierstein, A. S.: A reappraisal of the circulatory effects of the valsalva maneuver. *Amer. J. Med.*, **39**:923–33, 1965.

Storsten, O., and Rasmussen, K.: The cause of arterial hypoxemia in acute myocardial infarction. *Acta Med. Scand.*, **183**:193–96, 1968.

Streeten, D. H. P.; Schletter, F. E.; Clift, G. V.; Stevenson, C. T.; and Dalakos, T. G.: Studies of the renin-angiotensin-aldosterone system in patients with hypertension and in normal subjects. *Amer. J. Med.*, **46**:844–61, 1969.

Strickler, W. L.: Surgical case of malignant hypertension with intrarenal arteriosclerosis. *J.A.M.A.*, **194**:233–36, 1965.

Strisower, E. H.; Adamson, G.; and Strisower, B.: Treatment of hyperlipidemias. *Amer. J. Med.*, **45**:488–501, 1968.

Sugarman, S. R.; Margolius, H. S.; Gaffney, T. E.; and Mohammed, S.: Effect of methyldopa on chronotropic response to cardioaccelerator nerve stimulation in dogs. *J. Pharmacol. Exp. Ther.*, **162**:115–20, 1968.

Sugimoto, T.; Schaal, S. F.; Dunn, N. M.; and Wallace, A. G.: Electrophysiologic effects of lidocaine in awake dogs. *J. Pharmacol. Exp. Ther.*, **166**:146–50, 1969.

Sullivan, J. M.; Kagnoff, A.; and Gorlin, R.: Reduction of platelet adhesiveness in patients with coronary artery disease. *Amer. J. Med. Sci.*, **255**:292–95, 1968.

Sun, S. C.; Burch, G. E.; and DePasquale, N. P.: Histochemical and electron microscopic study of heart muscle after beta-adrenergic blockade. *Amer. Heart J.*, **74**:340–50, 1967.

Surawicz, B.: Evaluation of treatment of acute myocardial infarction with potassium, glucose and insulin. *Progr. Cardiov. Dis.*, 10:545–60, 1968.

Susens, G. P.; Hendrickson, C. G.; Mulder, M. J.; and Sams, B.: Femoral nerve entrapment secondary to a heparin hematoma. *Ann. Intern. Med.*, 69:575–79, 1968.

Sutnick, A. I., and Soloff, L. A.: Pulmonary arterial occlusion and surfactant production in humans. *Ann. Intern. Med.*, 67:549–55, 1967.

Svoboda, D. J., and Azarnoff, D. L.: Response of hepatic microbodies to a hypolipidemic agent, ethyl chlorophenoxyisobutyrate (CPIB). *J. Cell. Biol.*, 30: 442–50, 1966.

Szekely, P.; Wynne, N. A.; Pearson, D. T.; Balson, G. A.; and Sideris, D. A.: Direct current shock and digitalis: a clinical and experimental study. *Brit. Heart J.*, 31:91–96, 1969.

Szucs, M. M., Jr.; Brooks, H. L.; Grossman, W.; Banas, J. S., Jr.; Meister, S. G.; Dexter, L.; and Dalen, J. E.: Diagnostic sensitivity of laboratory findings in acute pulmonary embolism. *Ann. Intern. Med.*, 74:161–66, 1971.

Talley, R. C.; Goldberg, L. I.; Johnson, C. E.; and McNay, J. L.: A hemodynamic comparison of dopamine and isoproterenol in patients in shock. *Circulation*, 39:361–78, 1969.

Tanz, R. D.: The action of ouabain in cardiac muscle treated with reserpine and dichlorisoproterenol. *J. Pharmacol. Exp. Ther.*, 144:205–13, 1964.

Tarazi, R. C.; Dustan, H. P.; and Frohlich, E. D.: Long term thiazide therapy in essential hypertension. Evidence for persistent alteration in plasma volume and renin activity. *Circulation*, 41:709–17, 1970.

Tatooles, C. J., and Randall, W. C.: Local ventricular bulging after acute coronary occlusion. *Amer. J. Physiol.*, 201:451–56, 1961.

Tauxe, W. N.; Burchell, H. B.; and Black, L. F.: Clinical applications of lung scanning. *Mayo Clin. Proc.*, 42:473–87, 1967.

Taylor, H. L.: The effects of rest in bed and of exercise on cardiovascular function. *Circulation*, 38:1016–17, 1968.

Taylor, R. R.; Johnston, C. I.; and Jose, A. D.: Reversal of digitalis intoxication by beta-adrenergic blockade with pronethalol. *New Eng. J. Med.*, 271:877–82, 1964.

Ten Eick, R. E.; Wyte, S. R.; Ross, S. M.; and Hoffman, B. F.: Post-countershock arrhythmias in untreated and digitalized dogs. *Circ. Res.*, 21:375–90, 1967.

Tennant, R.: Factors concerned in the arrest of contraction in an ischemic myocardial area. *Amer. J. Physiol.*, 113:677–82, 1935.

Theilen, E. O.; Warkentin, D. L.; and January, L. E.: The use of digitalis in arrhythmias. *Progr. Cardiov. Dis.*, 7:261–72, 1964.

Thoenen, H.; Haefely, W.; Gey, K. F.; and Huerlimann, A.: Quantitative aspects of the replacement of norepinephrine by dopamine as a sympathetic transmitter after inhibition of dopamine-β-hydroxylase by disulfiram. *J. Pharmacol. Exp. Ther.*, 156:246–51, 1967.

Thomas, D. P.: Treatment of pulmonary embolic disease: a critical review of some aspects of current therapy. *New Eng. J. Med.*, 273:885–92, 1965.

Thomas, D. P.; Gurewich, V.; and Ashford, T. P.: Platelet adherance to thromboemboli in relation to the pathogenesis and treatment of pulmonary embolism. *New Eng. J. Med.*, 274:953–56, 1966.

Thomas, D. P.; Stein, M.; Tanabe, G.; Rege, V.; and Wessler, S.: Mechanism of bronchoconstriction produced by thromboemboli in dogs. *Amer. J. Physiol.*, 206:1207–12, 1964.

Thomas, H. E., Jr.; Kannel, W. B.; Dawber, T. R.; and McNamara, P. M.: Cholesterol-phospholipid ratio

in the prediction of coronary heart disease: the Framingham study. *New Eng. J. Med.*, 274:701–705, 1966.

Thomas, M.; Malmcrona, R.; Fillmore, S.; and Shillingford, J.: Hemodynamic effects of morphine in patients with acute myocardial infarction. *Brit. Heart J.*, 27:863–85, 1965b.

Thomas, M.; Malmcrona, R.; and Shillingford, J.: Hemodynamic effects of oxygen in patients with acute myocardial infarction. *Brit. Heart J.*, 27:401–407, 1965a.

———: Circulatory changes associated with systemic hypotension in patients with acute myocardial infarction. *Brit. Heart J.*, 28:108–17, 1966.

Thomas, M., and Woodgate, D.: Effect of atropine on bradycardia and hypotension in acute myocardial infarction. *Brit. Heart J.*, 28:409–13, 1966.

Thompson, G. R.; Barrowman, J.; Gutierrez, L.; and Dowling, R. H.: Action of neomycin on the intraluminal phase of lipid absorption. *J. Clin. Invest.*, 50:319–23, 1971.

Thomson, P. D.; Cohn, K.; Steinbrunn, W.; Rowland, M.; and Melmon, K. L.: The influence of heart failure and liver disease on plasma concentration and clearance of lidocaine in man. *Circulation*, 40 (Suppl. III):203, 1969b.

Thomson, P. D., and Melmon, K. L.: Clinical assessment of autonomic function. *Anesthesiology*, 29:724–31, 1968.

Thomson, P. D.; Rowland, M.; Cohn, K.; Steinbrunn, W.; and Melmon, K. L.: Critical differences in the pharmacokinetics of lidocaine between normal and congestive heart failure patients. *Clin. Res.*, 17:140, 1969a.

———: The effects of heart failure on the pharmacokinetics of lidocaine. *Amer. Heart J.*, in press, 1971.

Thrower, W. B.; Darby, T. D.; and Aldinger, E. E.: Acid-base derangements and myocardial contractility: effects as a complication of shock. *Arch. Surg. (Chicago)*, 82:56–65, 1961.

Thurm, R. H., and Smith, W. M.: On resetting of "barostats" in hypertensive patients. *J.A.M.A.*, 201:301–304, 1967.

Tobian, L.: Why do thiazide diuretics lower blood pressure in essential hypertension? *Ann. Rev. Pharmacol.*, 7:399–408, 1967.

Toohey, M.: Anticoagulants in myocardial infarction *Brit. Med. J.*, 1:252–55, 1958.

Tow, D. E.; Wagner, H. N., Jr.; and Holmes, R. A.: Urokinase in pulmonary embolism. *New Eng. J. Med.*, 277:1161–67, 1967.

Trautwein, W.: Generation and conduction of impulses in the heart as affected by drugs. *Pharmacol. Rev.*, 15:277–32, 1963.

Tzagournis, M.; Seidensticker, J. F.; and Hamwi, G. J.: Serum insulin, carbohydrate, and lipid abnormalities with premature coronary heart disease. *Ann. Intern. Med.*, 67:42 47, 1967.

Udenfriend, S.: Tyrosine hydroxylase. *Pharmacol. Rev.*, 18:43–52, 1966.

Udhoji, V. N.; Weil, M. H.; Sambhi, M. P.; and Rosoff, L.: Hemodynamic studies on clinical shock associated with infection. *Amer. J. Med.*, 34:461–69, 1963.

Ueda, H.; Yagi, S.; and Kaneko, Y.: Hydralazine and plasma renin activity. *Arch. Intern. Med. (Chicago)*, 122:387–91, 1968.

Ulrych, M.; Frohlich, E. D.; Dustan, H. P.; and Page, I. H.: Immediate hemodynamic effects of beta-adrenergic blockade with propranolol in normotensive and hypertensive men. *Circulation*, 37:411–16, 1968.

Ungar, A. H., and Sklaroff, H. J.: Fatalities following intravenous use of sodium diphenylhydantoin for cardiac arrhythmias. *J.A.M.A.*, 200:335–36, 1967.

United States Public Health Service: *Smoking and Health: Report of the Advisory Committee to the Surgeon General of the Public Health Service.* Public Health Service Publication #1113. U.S. Government Printing Office, Washington, D.C., 1964.

————: *The Health Consequences of Smoking: A Public Health Service Review, 1967.* Public Health Service Publication #1696. U.S. Government Printing Office, Washington, D.C., 1967a.

————: *The Coronary Drug Project.* Public Health Service Publication #1695. U.S. Government Printing Office, Washington, D.C., 1967b.

————: *The Health Consequences of Smoking: 1968 Supplement to the 1967 Public Health Service Review.* 1968 Supplement to Public Health Service Publication #1696. U.S. Government Printing Office, Washington, D.C., 1968.

————: *The Dietary Management of Hyperlipoproteinemia. A Handbook for Physicians.* National Heart and Lung Institute, July, 1970.

Valori, C.; Thomas, M.; and Shillingford, J.: Free noradrenaline and adrenaline excretion in relation to clinical syndromes following myocardial infarction. *Amer. J. Cardiol.,* 20:605–17, 1967.

Vander, A. J.: Control of renin release. *Physiol. Rev.* 47:359–82, 1967.

Vasko, J. S.; Henney, R. P.; Brawley, R. K.; Oldham, H. N.; and Morrow, A. G.: Effects of morphine on ventricular function and myocardial contractile force. *Amer. J. Physiol.,* 210:329–34, 1966.

Vassaux, C., and Lown, B.: Cardioversion of supraventricular tachycardias. *Circulation,* 39:791–802, 1969.

Vertes, V.; Cangiano, J. L.; Berman, L. B.; and Gould, A.: Hypertension in end-stage renal disease. *New Eng. J. Med.,* 280:978–81, 1969.

Vertes, V.; Grauel, T. A.; and Goldblatt, H.: Renal arteriography, separate renal-function studies and renal biopsy in human hypertension: selection of patients for surgical treatment. *New Eng. J. Med.,* 270:656–59, 1964.

Vessey, M. P.: Oral contraceptives and thromboembolic disease. *Amer. Heart J.,* 77:153–57, 1969.

Veterans Administration Cooperative Study Group on Antihypertensive Agents: Effect of treatment on morbidity in hypertension: results in patients with diastolic blood pressures averaging 115 through 129 mm Hg. *J.A.M.A.,* 202:1028–34, 1967.

————: Effect of treatment on morbidity in hypertension. II. Results in patients with diastolic blood pressure averaging 90 through 144 mm Hg. *J.A.M.A.,* 213:1143–52, 1970.

Viel, B.; Donoso, S.; and Salcedo, D.: Coronary atherosclerosis in persons dying violently. *Arch. Intern. Med. (Chicago),* 122:97–103, 1969.

Visioli, O., and Bertaccini, G.: Combined propranolol and quinidine treatment in cardiac arrhythmias. *Amer. Heart J.,* 75:719, 1968.

Vogel, J. H. R.: Distribution of norepinephrine in the failing bovine heart. Correlation of chemical analysis and fluorescence microscopy. *Circ. Res.,* 24:71–84, 1969.

Vogel, J. H. R., and Chidsey, C. A.: Cardiac adrenergic activity in experimental heart failure assessed with beta receptor blockade. *Amer. J. Cardiol.,* 24:198–208, 1969.

Vogel, J. H. R.; Jacobowitz, D.; and Chidsey, C. A.: Chemical and morphologic studies of adrenergic nerves in the failing heart. *Clin. Res.,* 16:111, 1968.

Von Euler, U. S., and Hillarp, N.-Å.: Evidence for the presence of noradrenaline in submicroscopic structures of adrenergic axons. *Nature,* 177:44, 1956.

Waal, H. J.: Hypotensive action of propranolol. *Clin. Pharmacol. Ther.,* 7:588–98, 1966.

Wallace, A. G.; Cline, R. E.; Sealy, W. C.; Young, W. G.; and Troyer, W. G.: Electrophysiologic effects of quinidine: studies using chronically implanted electrodes in awake dogs with and without cardiac denervation. *Circ. Res.,* 19:960–69, 1966.

Walsh, P. N.; Stengle, J.; and Sherry, S.: The urokinase-pulmonary embolism trial. *Circulation,* 39:153–56, 1969.

Warkentin, D. L., and Cunningham, R. J.: Beta-adrenergic blocking agents and hyperdynamic cardiovascular states. *Med. Clin. N. Amer.,* 52:1045–48, 1968.

Warner, W. A.: Intracardiac epinephrine versus isoproterenol in cardiac arrest. *Anesth. Analg.,* 46:201–205, 1967.

Wasserman, A. J.: Anticoagulants in acute myocardial infarction: the last (?) word. *Ann. Intern. Med.,* 65:855–56, 1969.

Wasserman, A. J.; Gutterman, L. A.; Yoe, K. B.; Kemp, V. E., Jr.; and Richardson, D. W.: Anticoagulants in acute myocardial infarction: the failure of anticoagulants to alter mortality in a randomized series. *Amer. Heart J.,* 71:43–49, 1966.

Watanabe, Y.; Dreifus, L. S.; and Likoff, W.: Electrophysiologic antagonism and synergism of potassium and antiarrhythmic agents. *Amer. J. Cardiol.,* 12:702–10, 1963.

Weatherall, M.: Ions and the action of digitalis. *Brit. Heart J.,* 28:497–504, 1966.

Webster, J. R., Jr.; Saadeh, G. B.; Eggum, P. R.; and Suker, J. R.: Wheezing due to pulmonary embolism: treatment with heparin. *New Eng. J. Med.,* 274:931–33, 1966.

Weidmann, S.: The effect of the cardiac membrane potential on the rapid availability of the sodium-carrying system. *J. Physiol.,* 127:213–24, 1955a.

————: Effects of calcium ions and local anesthetics on electrical properties of Purkinje fibers. *J. Physiol.,* 129:568–82, 1955b.

Weil, M. H.; Shubin, H.; and Biddle, M.: Shock caused by gram-negative microorganisms: analysis of 169 cases. *Ann. Intern. Med.,* 60:384–400, 1964.

Weiner, M.: The rational use of anticoagulants. *Pharmacol. for Physicians,* 1:1–7, 1967.

Weisse, A. B., and Regan, T. J.: The current status of nitrites in the treatment of coronary artery disease. *Progr. Cardiov. Dis.,* 12:72–82, 1969.

Weissler, A. M.: The heart in heart failure. *Ann. Intern. Med.,* 69:929–40, 1968.

Weissler, A. M.; Snyder, J. R.; Schoenfeld, C. D.; and Cohen, S.: Assay of digitalis glycosides in man. *Amer. J. Cardiol.,* 17:768–780, 1966.

Weissmann, G., and Thomas, L.: Studies on lysosomes. I. The effects of endotoxin, endotoxin tolerance, and cortisone on the release of acid hydrolases from a granular fraction of rabbit liver. *J. Exp. Med.,* 116:433–50, 1962.

————: The effects of corticosteroids upon connective tissue and lysosomes. *Recent Progr. Hormone Res.,* 20:215–39, 1964a.

————: On the mechanism of tissue damage by bacterial endotoxin. In Landy, M., and Braun, W. (eds.): *Bacterial Endotoxins; Proceedings of a Symposium held at the Institute of Microbiology of Rutgers.* Institute of Microbiology, New Brunswick, N.J., 1964b, pp. 602–609.

Wessler, S.: Thombosis in the presence of vascular stasis. *Amer. J. Med.,* 33:648–66, 1962.

————: Stasis, hypercoagulability and thrombosis. *Fed. Proc.,* 22:1366–70, 1963.

Wessler, S., and Gaston, L. W.: Pharmacologic and clinical aspects of heparin therapy. *Anesthesiology,* 27:475–82, 1966.

West, J. W.; Faulk, A. T.; and Guzman, S. V.: Comparative study of levarterenol and methoxamine in shock associated with acute myocardial ischemia in dogs. *Circ. Res.*, 10:712–21, 1962.

Whalen, R. E., and Salzman, H. A.: Hyperbaric oxygenation in the treatment of acute myocardial infarction. *Progr. Cardiov. Dis.*, 10:575–83, 1968.

Whitsitt, L. S., and Lucchesi, B. R.: Effects of propranolol and its stereoisomers upon coronary vascular resistance. *Circ. Res.*, 21:305–17, 1967.

Wiener, L.; Dwyer, E. M.; and Cox, J. W.: Hemodynamic effects of nitroglycerin, propranolol and their combination in coronary heart disease. *Circulation*, 39:623–32, 1969.

Williams, J. F., Jr.; Boyd, D. L.; and Border, J. F.: Effect of acute hypoxia and hypercapnic acidosis on the development of acetylstrophanthidin-induced arrhythmias. *J. Clin. Invest.*, 46:1885–94, 1968.

Williams, J. F., Jr.; Glick, G.; and Braunwald, E.: Studies on cardiac dimensions in intact unanesthetized man. V. Effects of nitroglycerin. *Circulation*, 32:767–71, 1965.

Williams, J. F., Jr.; Klocke, F. J.; and Braunwald, E.: Studies on digitalis. XIII. Comparison of the effects of potassium on the inotropic and arrhythmic-producing actions of ouabain. *J. Clin. Invest.*, 45:346–52, 1966.

Wilson, I. D., and Goetz, F. C.: Selective hypoaldosteronism after prolonged heparin administration. *Amer. J. Med.*, 36:635–40, 1964.

Wilson, J. D., and Lindsey, C. A., Jr.: Studies on influence of dietary cholesterol on cholesterol metabolism in the isotopic steady state in man. *J. Clin. Invest.*, 44:1805–14, 1965.

Wilson, R. F.; Chiscano, A. D.; Quadros, E.; and Tarver, M.: Some observations on 132 patients with septic shock. *Anesth. Analg.*, 46:751–63, 1967.

Wilson, R. F.; Jablonski, D. V.; and Thal, A. P.: The usage of Dibenzyline in clinical shock. *Surgery*, 56:172–83, 1964.

Wilson, R. F.; Thal, A. P.; Kindling, P. H.; Grifka, T.; and Ackerman, E.: Hemodynamic measurements in septic shock. *Arch. Surg.* (*Chicago*), 91:121–29, 1965.

Wilson, W. R., and Theilen, E. D.: Beta-adrenergic receptor blocking drugs as physiologic tools in clinical medicine. *Ann. N.Y. Acad. Sci.*, 139:981–96, 1967.

Wilson, W. R.; Theilen, E. D.; and Fletcher, F. W.: Pharmacodynamic effects of beta-adrenergic receptor blockade in patients with hyperthyroidism. *J. Clin. Invest.*, 43:1697–1703, 1964.

Wilson, W. S.: Metabolism of digitalis. *Progr. Cardiov. Dis.*, 11:479–87, 1969.

Winbury, M. M.: Redistribution of left ventricular blood flow produced by nitroglycerin. An example of integration of the macro- and microcirculation. *Circ. Res.*, 28(Suppl. I):140–47, 1971.

Winbury, M. M.; Howe, B. B.; and Hefner, M. A.: Effect of nitrate and other coronary dilators on large and small coronary vessels: an hypothesis for the mechanism of action of nitrates. *J. Pharmacol. Exp. Ther.*, 168:70–95, 1969.

Winer, B. M.: The antihypertensive actions of benzothiadiazines. *Circulation*, 23:211–18, 1961.

Wittenberg, S. M., and Lown, B.: Cardioversion and digitalis. IV. Effect of beta-adrenergic blockade. *Circulation*, 39:29–37, 1969.

Wolff, F. W., and Lindeman, R. D.: Effects of treatment in hypertension: results of a controlled study. *J. Chron. Dis.*, 19:227–40, 1966.

Wolff, H. P.; Blaise, L. B. H.; Düsterdieck, G.; Jahnecke, J.; Kobayashi, T.; Krück, F.; Lommer, D.; and Schieffer, H.: Role of aldosterone in edema formation. *Ann. N.Y. Acad. Sci.*, 139:285–94, 1966.

Wolfson, S., and Gorlin, R.: Cardiovascular pharmacology of propranolol in man. *Circulation*, 40:501–11, 1969.

Wolfson, S.; Heinle, R. A.; Herman, M. V.; Kemp, H. G.; Sullivan, J. M.; and Gorlin, R.: Propranolol and angina pectoris. *Amer. J. Cardiol.*, 18:345–53, 1966.

Wood, J. E.: Renin mechanisms and hypertension. *Circ. Res.*, 21 (Suppl. II):1–186, 1967.

Woods, J. W., and Blythe, W. B.: Management of malignant hypertension complicated by renal insufficiency. *New Eng. J. Med.*, 277:57–61, 1967.

Woods, J. W.; Liddle, G. W.; Stant, E. G., Jr.; Michelakis, A. M.; and Brill, A. B.: Effect of an adrenal inhibitor in hypertensive patients with suppressed renin. *Arch. Intern. Med.* (*Chicago*), 123:366–70, 1969.

Woods, J. W., and Michelakis, A. M.: Renal vein renin in renovascular hypertension. *Arch. Intern. Med.* (*Chicago*), 122:392–93, 1968.

Wright, I. S.: Anticoagulant therapy in myocardial infarction. *New Eng. J. Med.*, 281:737, 1969a.

——: Anticoagulant therapy—practical management. *Amer. Heart J.*, 77:280–86, 1969b.

——: Recent developments in antithrombotic therapy. *Ann. Intern. Med.*, 71:823–31, 1969c.

Wright, I. S., and Fredrickson, D. T.: Report of Inter-Society Commission on Heart Disease Resources. *Circulation*, 42:A55–A95, 1970.

Wright, I. S.; Marple, C. D.; and Beck, D. F.: Report of committee for evaluation of anticoagulants in treatment of coronary thrombosis with myocardial infarction: progress report on statistical analysis of first 800 cases studied by this committee. *Amer. Heart J.*, 36:801–15, 1948.

——: *Myocardial Infarction: Report of the Anticoagulant Committee of the American Heart Association.* Grune & Stratton, Inc., New York, 1954.

Wurtman, R. J.: Catecholamines. *New Eng. J. Med.*, 273:637–46, 693–700, 746–53, 1965.

Wyler, F.; Forsyth, R. P.; Nies, A. S.; Neutze, J. M.; and Melmon, K. L.: Endotoxin-induced regional circulatory changes in the unanesthetized monkey. *Circ. Res.*, 24:777–86, 1969.

Yu, P. N.; Fox, S. M.; Imboden, C. A., Jr.; and Killip, T.: Coronary care unit. I. A specialized intensive care unit for acute myocardial infarction. *Mod. Conc. Cardiov. Dis.*, 34:23–26, 1965.

Zaid, G., and Beall, G. N.: Bronchial response to beta-adrenergic blockade. *New Eng. J. Med.*, 275:580–84, 1966.

Zeft, H. J.; Cobb, F. R.; Waxman, M. B.; Hunt, N. C.; and Morris, J. J., Jr.: Right atrial stimulation in the treatment of atrial flutter. *Ann. Intern. Med.*, 70:447–56, 1969b.

Zeft, H. J.; Patterson, S.; and Orgain, E. S.: The effect of propranolol in the long-term treatment of angina pectoris. *Arch. Intern. Med.* (*Chicago*), 124:578–84, 1969a.

Zelis, R.; Mason, D. T.; Braunwald, E.; and Levy, R. I.: Effects of hyperlipoproteinemias and their treatment on the peripheral circulation. *J. Clin. Invest.*, 49:1007–15, 1970.

Zweifach, B. W.: Aspects of comparative physiology of laboratory animals relative to the problem of experimental shock. *Fed. Proc.*, 20 (Suppl. 9):18–29, 1961.

Chapter 6

RESPIRATORY DISORDERS

Pate D. Thomson and *Allen B. Cohen*

Rational therapeutics can be stressed in the treatment of pulmonary disease, because small changes in many pathogenic processes are accurately reflected by easily performed tests of pulmonary function. Such tests quantitate an abnormality. These data form a solid base for making a therapeutic choice and assessing whether it is appropriate. Since pulmonary function testing has assumed a new diagnostic and therapeutic importance, the first section of this chapter emphasizes some key definitions, selected aspects of normal and abnormal pulmonary physiology, their clinical assessment, and their relevance to therapeutics.

NORMAL PHYSIOLOGY

Respiration (i.e., arterialization of mixed venous blood) is performed by the lung, employing three interrelated mechanisms: ventilation, diffusion, and pulmonary capillary blood flow (Figure 6–1). Ventilation is the cyclic process of inspiration and expiration that transports air from the environment to alveoli and from alveoli to the environment. Alveolar ventilation ($\dot{V}_A$) is that volume of gas entering adequately perfused alveoli per minute and is defined by:

Total ventilation = Alveolar ventilation
+ dead space ventilation

and

Alveolar ventilation = (Tidal volume − dead space)
× respiratory rate

The tidal volume is the volume of gas inspired or expired during each breath; the physiologic dead space or wasted ventilation is the volume of gas entering the lungs that does not participate in gas exchange. Ventilation of alveoli requires work by the muscles of respiration. Many factors may influence the process of ventilation, including changes in the mechanical properties of the lung (e.g., increasing airway resistance—the hallmark of obstructive airway disease, or increasing stiffness of lung parenchyma—the hallmark of restrictive lung disease). During severe restrictive lung disease, lung volumes may become so reduced that an adequate $\dot{V}_A$ cannot be maintained. Uneven changes in airway resistance and in distensibility (compliance) of the lung result in uneven distribution of inspired air and compromised alveolar ventilation.

Diffusion is the process by which gases are transferred between alveoli and capillary blood. Tests of diffusing capacity measure the rate of uptake of carbon monoxide (CO) or oxygen (O_2) from the lung. Within the alveolus, many factors influence the rate of uptake of the gas—for example, the distance separating alveolar gas from the capillary, the resistance to diffusion across the alveolar capillary and red-cell membranes, the rate of chemical reaction between the test gas and hemoglobin, the capillary blood volume, and the concentration of hemoglobin in blood. Within the lung as a whole, diffusing capacity is dependent not only

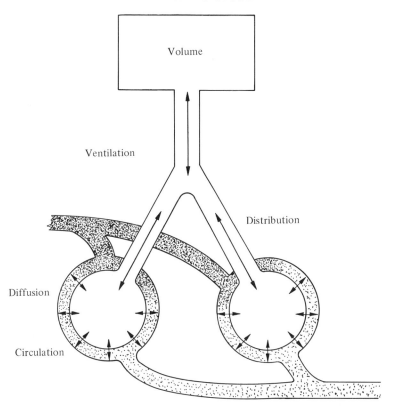

Figure 6–1. Processes in pulmonary gas exchange. The alveoli are depicted by the circular areas. Leading into these are the conducting airways or anatomic dead space. The rectangular block indicates minute volume of breathing. The arrows entering the alveoli show distribution of inspired gas. The small arrows crossing alveolar walls indicate diffusion of oxygen and carbon dioxide. The shaded channel surrounding the alveolus is the pulmonary capillary, and the mixed venous blood (shaded dark) emerges arterialized (light). (Modified from Comroe, J. H.; Forster, R. E.; Dubois, A. B.; Briscoe, W. A.; and Carlsen, E.: *The Lung: Clinical Physiology and Pulmonary Function Tests*, 2nd ed. Year Book Medical Publishers, Inc., Chicago, 1962.)

on the anatomic features of the alveolus but also on the number of alveoli present and the uniformity of distribution of the test gas (particularly when the single-breath method is used for testing) (Bates and Christie, 1964). Measurements of diffusing capacity are probably best considered as measurements of the pulmonary capillary blood volume, which reflects the surface area for diffusion and the characteristics of the available alveolar capillary membrane.

Pulmonary capillary blood flow describes the volume of mixed venous blood reaching the capillaries per unit time. The volume of blood reaching the capillaries is determined by the cardiac output, provided that no significant shunting occurs. The work required of the right ventricle to maintain its output may be influenced by changes in the mechanical properties of the vascular bed. Increasing vascular resist-

ance due to obstruction or constriction of the vascular bed may increase the work of the heart. In addition, localized changes in resistance and distensibility of the pulmonary vascular bed may result in unequal distribution of the pulmonary blood flow.

The normal lung provides the essential milieu for diffusion of gas across the capillary and alveolus by matching the alveolar ventilation to pulmonary capillary blood flow. An important impairment in respiratory function occurs when the normal balance between ventilation ($\dot{V}$) and perfusion ($\dot{Q}$) is disturbed. A small imbalance is normal and increases with age.

PATHOPHYSIOLOGY

We can measure clinically important disturbances in lung physiology that predominantly affect either ventilation, diffusing capacity, or pulmonary capillary blood flow. Rarely does a

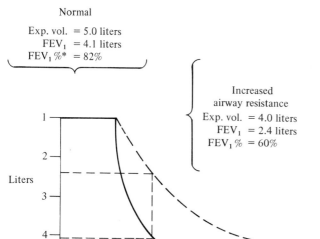

*Normal value for FEV$_1$% is greater than 81%.

Figure 6-2. Timed measurement of the forced expiratory volume. A maximally rapid expiration is made after a full inspiration. The FEV$_1$ is recorded by measuring the volume expired in the first second. The FEV$_1$% = (volume expired during the first second of a forced expiration/forced expiratory volume) × 100. The patient with increased airway resistance (broken line) demonstrates a prolonged forced expiration and a reduced timed forced vital capacity.

disease state produce an abnormality that influences only one component of respiration without directly or indirectly influencing the others. Therefore, separation of the functional disturbances tends to be somewhat artificial but provides a useful framework for discussion.

Obstructive Airway Disease

Obstruction of airways is the most common abnormality in lung disease, occurring in circumstances as diverse as tracheal stenosis, endobronchial tumors, inhalation of foreign bodies, asthma, chronic bronchitis, and emphysema.

Hyperinflation of the chest and wheezing on expiration characterize generalized airway obstruction. Wheezing on inspiration (stridor) is characteristic of extrathoracic airway obstruction. However, wheezing may disappear and breath sounds may diminish when obstruction is so severe that small volumes of air move too slowly to generate sound. A more subtle indication of airway obstruction can be elicited by timing the duration of expiration by auscultation. If expiration is longer than 4 seconds, clinically significant obstruction is present. These bedside maneuvers are useful but insensitive; it is desirable to obtain a record of the patient's ventilation from which permanent and quantitative information can be derived.

Maximum expiratory efforts may be quantitated in several ways. The most commonly used measurement is the forced expiratory volume in 1 second expressed as a percentage of the forced vital capacity (FEV$_1$%) (Figure 6-2). A forced expiratory maneuver is largely limited by physical forces beyond the control of the patient (Fry and Hyatt, 1960) and in cooperative patients is an objective and repeatable test of pulmonary function. To assess both progress of the disease and response to a therapeutic regimen, tests of bronchial obstruction can be performed with a simple inexpensive spirometer.

In general, if wheezing is present or expiration is prolonged, an abnormal FEV$_1$% can be recorded. Although this test is sensitive and reliable for diagnosing increased resistance to airflow in most patients, some patients have symptoms that do not correlate well with the FEV$_1$% tests. For example, obstruction of the smallest conducting airways may not be measured by the forced expiratory maneuver (Macklem and Mead, 1967). In this circumstance the history is more useful than the spirometer.

Increased airway resistance defines a disturbance in physiology, but does not indicate its pathogenesis or etiology. The pathogenesis of airway obstruction may vary with the phase or nature of the underlying disease. Even during different phases of the same disease, bronchial secretions, constriction of bronchial smooth muscle, edema of bronchial mucosa, anatomic narrowing of airways due to fibrosis or infiltration, airway collapse during expiratory effort, and decreased elastic recoil may contribute to obstruction of airways (Duffell et al., 1970). The response to therapeutic agents (e.g., sympathomimetic drugs) is in part determined by the predominant mechanism of obstruction (Table 6–1).

Table 6–1. CAUSES OF AIRWAY OBSTRUCTION*

1. Secretions
2. Spasm of bronchial musculature
3. Edema
4. Foreign bodies and tumors
5. Decrease in radial traction in collapsible airways
6. Expiratory effort that results in collapse of airways
7. Anatomic narrowing of airways due to fibrosis and infiltration

* Causes 1 to 4 may be readily influenced by therapeutic intervention. Decreased radial traction gradually reverts to normal in asthmatic patients when obstruction is relieved (Gold et al., 1967; Nadel et al., 1968), as does expiratory effort-induced collapse. In emphysema, results are less gratifying. Cause 6 is not generally a reversible form of obstruction.

Pulmonary function testing that includes the response to bronchodilators may help to define the type or stage of a disease process. For example, the emphysematous patient may be distinguished from an asthmatic patient by spirometric recordings of forced vital capacity; improvement may be dramatic in asthmatics but rarely occurs in patients with emphysema. While the diagnosis is being made, the efficacy of the bronchodilator may be assessed. If the patient is responsive to the drug, a useful therapeutic agent has been identified. However, disease processes resulting in increased airway resistance may be dynamic (e.g., accumulated secretions may account for the obstruction at one stage of an asthma attack and bronchospasm may predominate at another). Therefore, a patient unresponsive to bronchodilators at one stage may be responsive at another.

Increases in airway resistance may affect other physiologic processes. The work of breathing may increase, and the distribution of inspired air may become uneven. If an imbalance between ventilation and perfusion occurs, abnormal blood gas composition results. The uneven distribution of inspired air may be important in therapeutics, because it can produce uneven distribution of an inhaled bronchodilator or other aerosol. Thus, an aerosolized drug may be preferentially inhaled into well-ventilated portions of lung but may never reach the poorly ventilated areas where it is most needed. If the drug is an adrenergic bronchodilator, it may be absorbed from the well-ventilated and perfused areas, effecting an increase in pulmonary blood flow and further aggravating $\dot{V}:\dot{Q}$ imbalance by increasing perfusion of poorly ventilated alveoli. The mild increases in hypoxemia seen in asthmatic patients given isoproterenol may be explained by such a sequence (Palmer and Diament, 1967; Gazioglu et al., 1971).

Distribution of the drug may be improved by making certain that the patient takes a deep breath with each inhalation and holds it for a few seconds to allow the inspired air to reach slowly ventilated areas. Occasionally, a patient who is unresponsive to an aerosol bronchodilator improves when the drug is administered intravenously, presumably because this route of administration produces a more even distribution of the agent in the lung. Poorly ventilated areas are reached by the drug and ventilation improves.

Restrictive Respiratory Disease

Restrictive pulmonary disease is characterized by limited expansion of the lungs, as a result of diffuse pulmonary disease, pleural thickening or effusion, pneumothorax, or an abnormality of the chest wall. Pulmonary function testing should be performed to define a restrictive disease, to quantitate the severity of the abnormality, and to provide an objective measurement for assessment of the natural history of the disease and the impact of therapy. In restrictive diseases, the spirometer tracings show a decreased vital capacity, normal to elevated maximal flow rate, and a normal to elevated $FEV_1\%$ (unless the functional abnormality is complicated by the presence of obstructive airway disease). Measurement of a normal $FEV_1\%$ in the presence of a reduced vital capacity excludes obstruction of large- or medium-sized airways and implicates restrictive airway disease as the cause of the reduced vital capacity. Total lung capacity is reduced, and the ratio of residual volume (the volume of gas remaining in the lungs at the end of maximal expiration) to total lung capacity (the volume of gas contained in the lung at maximal inspiration) may be high or normal. Alveolar ventilation is usually normal until the restriction becomes severe. The diffusing capacity is usually reduced if a disease obliterates pulmonary capillaries. Roentgenographic changes do not necessarily parallel the pulmonary function disturbance (see Sarcoidosis, page 281).

If a disease involves only the pleura, chest cage, or diaphragm, the diffusing capacity is normal. Abnormalities in blood gas concentrations occur if there is mismatching of ventilation and perfusion, or if restriction is so severe that hypoventilation occurs (Comroe et al., 1962).

The choice of the function tests used to follow the course of the patient depends on the pattern of the abnormality detected by an initial thorough evaluation of pulmonary function and on the type of disease being treated. Usually, measurement of vital capacity and maximal flow rates are sufficient to follow the progress of the patient; periodically, however, more complete evaluation of pulmonary function may be indicated.

Abnormalities in Diffusion

When pulmonary disease is associated with a reduced diffusing capacity, the therapist must not equate the pulmonary function abnormality with a distinct anatomic lesion. There are many determinants affecting measurements of diffusion, and any one or some combination of these factors may be operative in a clinical setting. For example, the "alveolar capillary block syndrome" occurs in diseases characterized by diffuse interstitial lesions of the lung (e.g., sarcoidosis, diffuse interstitial fibrosis, berylliosis, asbestosis, pulmonary scleroderma, and diffuse spread of carcinoma). The typical patient with advanced disease has dyspnea, tachypnea, and signs of restrictive lung disease. Lung volumes are reduced, but the $FEV_1\%$ is normal. Arterial oxygen may be normal or low at rest, but characteristically decreases during exercise. A reduced diffusing capacity of carbon monoxide (D_LCO) correlates well with the severity of the disease, but reduced diffusion of carbon monoxide is not solely related to thickening of the alveolar capillary membrane. Patients with the alveolar capillary block syndrome may have uniformly normal alveolar capillary membranes (Gracey et al., 1968). The hypoxemia that occurs at rest in patients with advanced disease is not due to compromised membrane diffusion but to mismatching of ventilation with perfusion (Finley et al., 1962). The disease processes mentioned above may destroy alveolar-capillary units with a resultant decrease in D_LCO. In spite of the $\dot{V}_A:Q$ changes in asthma and bronchitis the D_LCO is maintained normally. Such an observation might be helpful to differentiate the two types of disease from emphysema. Therefore D_LCO is a useful measurement with which to detect disease and follow therapy, but it does not define the histopathology or the etiology of the process. The test is useful because the factors that decrease the uptake of carbon monoxide also cause the hypoxemia that occurs during exercise

in the patients mentioned above (Emergil et al., 1971).

If the variables that influence D_LCO are understood, it is easy to explain the reduced diffusing capacity in emphysema (destruction of alveolar capillary units), pulmonary embolic disease (obstruction of capillary bed), anemia (reduced hemoglobin concentration in the capillary blood), space-occupying lesions (reduced number of alveolar capillary units), and a number of other pathologic states. *Principle: If tests are to be used as a basis for therapeutic decisions, the therapist must understand the determinants of changes in a test and the relationship of these determinants to the pathophysiology of the disease.*

Abnormalities of Pulmonary Blood Vessels

One of the most difficult abnormalities to diagnose early is disease of the smaller pulmonary vessels. In the early stages of slowly progressive pulmonary vascular obstruction, the patient may have no complaints or only those of dyspnea. The disease is usually undiagnosed until pulmonary hypertension has developed. Only then do the physical, roentgenologic, and electrocardiographic findings of pulmonary hypertension become apparent. Several techniques have been devised to aid in the early diagnosis of diseases of large and small pulmonary vessels.

Obstruction of large- and intermediate-sized vessels may be identified by pulmonary angiography and radioisotopic scanning. These techniques may be helpful in selected cases of pulmonary embolism, but they can give false-negative results. Approximately 85% of pulmonary emboli are located in vessels less than 1 mm in diameter (Smith et al., 1964).

A number of diseases (e.g., systemic lupus erythematosus [Gold and Jennings, 1966], schistosomiasis, periarteritis nodosa, primary pulmonary hypertension, sometimes scleroderma [Naeye, 1963], pneumoconiosis [Schepers, 1955], and polycythemia vera [Burgess and Bishop, 1963]) obstruct only small pulmonary arteries. Techniques useful in demonstrating obstruction of small pulmonary vessels have been described (Nadel et al., 1968). Figure 6–3 illustrates the effects of vascular occlusion. The capillary to alveolus A has been obstructed, and alveolus B receives normal or increased blood flow. If there are no changes in ventilation (local obstruction of airways), expired CO_2 from the nonperfused alveolus A mixes with CO_2 from the perfused alveolus B. The mixed expired pCO_2 then falls ($PA_{CO_2} = 27$), and a difference between PA_{CO_2} and Pa_{CO_2} can be measured. In effect, the nonperfused alveolus acts as an

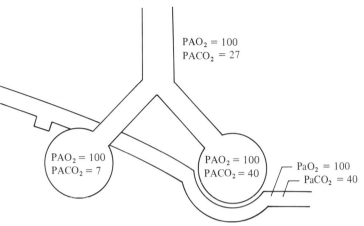

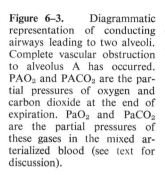

Figure 6–3. Diagrammatic representation of conducting airways leading to two alveoli. Complete vascular obstruction to alveolus A has occurred. PAO_2 and $PACO_2$ are the partial pressures of oxygen and carbon dioxide at the end of expiration. PaO_2 and $PaCO_2$ are the partial pressures of these gases in the mixed arterialized blood (see text for discussion).

extension of the anatomic dead space (airways filled with gas that do not come into contact with functioning alveolar capillaries). The increased wasted ventilation may be calculated from measurements of alveolar-arterial pCO_2 differences. Changes in the ratio of wasted ventilation (V_D) to tidal volume (V_T) help to identify areas of decreased perfusion in relation to ventilation, especially when evaluated during exercise (Severinghaus and Stupfel, 1957; Nadel et al., 1968). Indeed, when this measurement is made at rest and during exercise, the ratio of V_D/V_T does rise in some patients despite the presence of normal pulmonary artery pressure, pulmonary vascular resistance, arteriograms, and lung scans. These patients have histologically proven evidence of obstructive pulmonary vascular disease and usually a reduced capillary blood volume (demonstrated by carbon monoxide "diffusing capacity"). When studied by cardiac catheterization, they fail to exhibit a normal fall in pulmonary vascular resistance during exercise (Nadel et al., 1968).

Obstruction of large vessels may be detected by radioisotopic and angiographic methods. Small-vessel disease, which should be considered in any patient with unexplained dyspnea, may be diagnosed in the pulmonary function laboratory by measuring a rise in the ratio of V_D/V_T during exercise and a reduced carbon monoxide diffusing capacity. Although these tests require a well-equipped laboratory and some necessitate arterial catheterization, they are useful in following the course and response of the disease to treatment in selected patients with embolism or other forms of disease of the small pulmonary vessels.

OXYGEN AND CARBON DIOXIDE TRANSPORT

The most important principle in treating the distressed or unconscious patient is to maintain an open airway. If critical tissues such as the heart and brain are deprived of oxygen for 5 to 10 minutes, all other therapeutic maneuvers are useless. Transport of gas in the upper airways is the first of a complex series of steps that ensure that tissues receive and eliminate gases in order to conduct their metabolic processes. The upper airway is not, however, the only portion of the system that can be influenced by therapeutic intervention. If any part of the respiratory or cardiovascular system fails to provide tissues with sufficient oxygenated blood, organ dysfunction is inevitable. The development and use of O_2, CO_2, and pH electrodes and the routine use of arterial puncture have greatly facilitated the detection of abnormalities in pulmonary and cardiovascular physiology and the proper selection of therapeutic interventions. The recent decline in mortality in patients treated for respiratory failure no doubt relates to the liberal and accurate use of arterial blood gas measurements to assist in both diagnosis and treatment (see page 285).

Oxygen Transport and Hypoxia

A functional clinical definition of hypoxia is a reduction of oxygen supply to an organ, sufficient to impair organ function. The morbidity produced by hypoxia may be immediate if a vital organ such as the heart is concerned, or delayed if less vital tissues (e.g., skeletal muscle) are predominantly affected.

Normally the upper airway is exposed to about 760 mm Hg gas pressure at sea level, of which about 150 mm Hg is oxygen. When inspired air is mixed with alveolar air, the alveolar capillary is exposed to a pO_2 of about 100 mm Hg. A small amount of blood is shunted past alveoli owing to ventilation-perfusion imbalance and a smaller amount via the bronchial and Thebesian vessels. Therefore, a normal pO_2 in arterial blood is about 95 mm Hg.

When physical signs or symptoms suggest severe lung disease or hypoxia, arterial pO_2 should be measured. If it is low, consider the following:

1. Is blood being shunted from the right to the left side of the heart without passing through aerated parts of the lung? Shunting is present when arterial pO_2 cannot be brought to at least 580 mm Hg while the patient breathes 100% oxygen. Shunts may occur within the heart (e.g., pulmonary hypertension with a patent foramen ovale) or within the lung (e.g., atelectasis).

2. Does the patient have alveolar hypoventilation? This is diagnosed when arterial pCO_2 is high. It may be caused by decreased total ventilation or by severe ventilation-perfusion imbalance. Decreased total ventilation can be caused by depression of central nervous system respiratory control (sedative or narcotic overdose, or narcosis produced by hypercarbia), by respiratory muscle paralysis (myasthenia gravis, polio, or administration of drugs such as succinylcholine), or by an improperly set mechanical ventilator (e.g., inadequate tidal volume or respiratory rate) or subsequent to acid-base abnormalities (Tuller and Mehdi, 1971).

3. Is impaired diffusion a factor? This is probably not a cause of resting hypoxia, but may cause hypoxia in an exercising patient.

4. Is there decreased inspired oxygen concentration? This must be considered if any mechanical device is being employed to assist or control ventilation. Is the patient rebreathing with a high added deadspace from a long tube attached to a ventilator? Has the patient been using the wrong gas mixture? Has the oxygen flow into an oxygen tent stopped? Are you standing on his oxygen line?

The oxygen supplied to an organ is extracted from the capillary blood. The amount of oxygen available to an organ depends on (1) the amount of oxygen carried in each unit volume of blood and (2) the arterial blood flow to the organ. The oxygen content of arterial blood is determined by the amount of oxygen supplied by the lung (reflected by the arterial pO_2) and the capacity of the blood to accept oxygen. The oxygen-carrying capacity of the blood is largely dependent on the amount of hemoglobin and on factors that alter the ability of hemoglobin to bind oxygen.

The second determinant of tissue oxygenation is blood flow:

O$_2$ carried in the blood × blood flow
  = O$_2$ carried to the tissues

Despite a low concentration of hemoglobin in blood, an organ need not be hypoxic if blood flow to that organ increases sufficiently or if the organ's demand for oxygen is reduced.

The final factor influencing adequacy of oxygenation is the metabolic demand of the tissue. Factors affecting the development of hypoxia are summarized in Table 6-2. When

Table 6-2. FACTORS THAT CONTROL ADEQUACY OF OXYGEN DELIVERY TO TISSUES

Ability of the lung to equilibrate blood from the right side of the heart with oxygen in inspired air (total lung function)
Oxygen-carrying capacity of blood
  pO_2
  Hemoglobin concentration
  Shape of the oxygen-hemoglobin dissociation curve and factors that affect the shape of this curve
Blood flow to the body (cardiac output) or organ (regional perfusion)
Oxygen requirement of the tissues

any of these factors are adversely affected, the physician should look for signs of organ hypoxia. Conversely, when signs of generalized hypoxia are present (e.g., restlessness, tachycardia, metabolic acidosis), all the links in the oxygen-transport chain should be evaluated to establish the most direct and effective method of correcting the hypoxia (see Chapter 5).

Tolerance to hypoxia varies widely among tissues and individuals. It is influenced by (1) the capacity of the heart to increase flow in response to stress, (2) the ability of the autonomic nervous system to redistribute flow to critical organs, (3) the presence of vascular disease in critical organs, (4) the presence of anemia or abnormal hemoglobin (e.g., methemoglobin, sulfhemoglobin, carbon monoxide-hemoglobin), (5) the metabolic demands of the tissue, and (6) the pH or pCO_2 in tissues. In general, if the arterial pO_2 falls below 30 mm Hg in man, signs of ischemia begin to appear (Bendixen and Laver, 1965). With abnormalities in any of the above listed processes, signs of inadequate oxygenation may appear at an arterial pO_2 substantially higher than 30 mm Hg.

Carbon Dioxide Transport

Carbon dioxide is normally transported in plasma and red blood cells either as bicarbonate ion or dissolved carbon dioxide, or in combination with hemoglobin. The arterial pCO_2 is directly related to the metabolic production of CO_2 ($\dot{V}CO_2$) and inversely related to the amount of CO_2 eliminated by alveolar ventilation ($\dot{V}_A$):

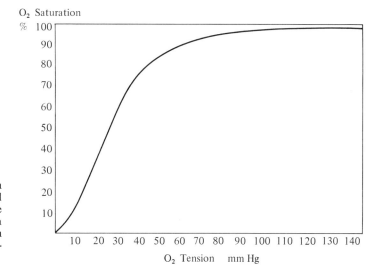

O$_2$ Saturation % 100

O$_2$ Tension   mm Hg

Figure 6–4. The oxyhemoglobin dissociation curve. This normal dissociation curve illustrates the relationship between oxygen saturation and oxygen tension for whole blood of normal hematocrit at a pH of 7.4 at 37°.

$$\text{Arterial } pCO_2 = K \frac{\text{Metabolic } CO_2 \text{ production } (\dot{V}CO_2)}{\text{Alveolar ventilation } (\dot{V}_A)}$$

Carbon dioxide readily diffuses across alveolar capillary membranes and normally is easily eliminated by the lungs. Under circumstances of increased $\dot{V}CO_2$ (e.g., fever or exercise), increased $\dot{V}_A$ maintains the arterial pCO_2 within a narrow normal range. When arterial pCO_2 is abnormal, $\dot{V}_A$ may be responsible (e.g., during ventilation of underperfused alveoli, if a compensatory increase in normally ventilated areas does not occur, or if total ventilation is decreased).

Estimates of pCO_2 based on clinical criteria alone are inaccurate (Mithoefer *et al.*, 1968). Accuracy is obtained when pCO_2 is measured in arterial blood. *Principle: Accurate measurements of blood gases are critical to proper therapy of many respiratory and cardiovascular diseases. Abnormalities must be suspected, measurements made, and therapy directed by the results of tests. Because disease states are dynamic in the critically ill patient, tests should be run at close intervals if they are to be maximally useful.*

Effect of Alveolar pO_2 on pCO_2

Alveolar gases include nitrogen, oxygen, carbon dioxide, and water vapor. The sum of their partial pressures is equal to atmospheric pressure. Since alveolar nitrogen varies little from that of inspired air and since water vapor pressure is constant, a rise in alveolar pCO_2 is accompanied by a fall in pO_2 and vice versa. For clinical purposes, an estimate of alveolar pO_2 may be made by the following equation (resting subject breathing room air at sea level) (McNicol and Campbell, 1965):

$$\text{Alveolar } pO_2 = 150 - 1.25 \, (\text{arterial } pCO_2)$$

When alveolar pO_2 has been estimated, the arterial pO_2 can be predicted by allowing for an alveolar-arterial oxygen difference, due to minor mismatching of ventilation and perfusion. The difference is likely to be at least 15 mm Hg in patients with chronic respiratory failure. While the patient is breathing room air, the degree of hypercapnea is limited by the maximum tolerable alveolar hypoxia (20 to 30 mm Hg). If the arterial pCO_2 rises to 85 mm Hg, the pO_2 will fall to approximately 30 mm Hg, as demonstrated by the following calculation:

$$\begin{aligned}\text{Alveolar } pO_2 &= 150 - 1.25 \, (85) \\ &= 150 - 106 \\ &= 44 \\ 44 - 15 &= 29 \text{ mm Hg}\end{aligned}$$

Thus, the upper limit of carbon dioxide tension compatible with maximal hypoxia is approximately 85 mm Hg when the patient breathes room air.

For comprehensive reviews of pulmonary physiology, the student is referred to authoritative textbooks of Comroe and Dejours (1965, 1966).

CATEGORIES OF DRUGS AND THERAPEUTIC PRINCIPLES

In approaching the patient with pulmonary disease, the therapist should first identify the specific pathogenic agent or process whenever possible, then select therapeutic agents that may specifically reverse the process. A large number of pathogens, including allergens, bacteria, fungi, and chemical irritants, may be countered directly and specifically. Unfortunately, much of pulmonary therapeutics is directed against diseases of obscure etiology and pathogenesis. However, the type and extent of the lesion can usually be assessed and objective measurements can be made of the functional disturbance. Thus, a setting is created for rational selection of therapeutic agents and assessment of the impact of therapeutic interventions.

Proper selection of a therapeutic agent requires a working knowledge of the pharmacology of the agent. Several categories of drugs are discussed in this chapter, including bronchodilators, mucolytic drugs, expectorants, and corticosteroids. Anticoagulants and their use in pulmonary embolism and antibiotics are discussed in Chapters 5 and 10, respectively.

Bronchodilators

Some causes of airway obstruction are related to contraction of bronchial smooth muscle. If administration of a bronchial smooth-muscle relaxant improves expiratory flow rate, muscular bronchoconstriction may be inferred. However, if the agent has no effect bronchoconstriction should not be excluded, and the drug may still be potentially efficacious (Sobol et al., 1970).

In asthma, chronic bronchitis, and emphysema, bronchial secretions and distortion of airways may narrow or completely obstruct the lumen of some bronchi. Aerosolized drugs may fail to reach the obstructed area where they are most needed, because delivery of the agents may depend upon ventilation of the obstructed area. Under such circumstances, vigorous attempts must be made to clear secretions. Occasionally, parenteral administration of the bronchodilators may be efficacious.

The size of aerosol droplet is important for the proper distribution of the drug in the airways (see Chapter 2). Particles larger than 20 μ fail to reach the terminal bronchioles. Particles smaller than 2 μ may fail to deposit in the primary bronchi, and particles less than 0.6 μ in diameter are not retained. Particle size is determined by the type of dispensing apparatus used, the drug used, its concentration, and the vehicle in which it is dispersed or dissolved. When an anticipated response is not achieved, adjustment of particle size may be beneficial.

The mainstays of bronchodilator therapy are sympathomimetic drugs (isoproterenol, epinephrine, ephedrine, etc.) and the theophylline compounds, all of which cause relaxation of bronchial smooth muscle (Aviado, 1970). When adrenergic stimulators are used, bronchial smooth muscle relaxation results from stimulation of beta-adrenergic receptors. Agents with alpha-stimulating properties (epinephrine, phenylephrine) may be of some benefit when combined with isoproterenol because they result in a slightly greater reduction in airway resistance. Such summation of pharmacologic effect is presumably due to (1) the relief of mucosal edema as

alpha stimulators constrict vessels supplying the mucosa, and (2) a prolongation of the pharmacologic effect of isoproterenol (due to its slower transmucosal absorption in the presence of epinephrine or phenylephrine). In patients with chronic airway obstruction, the duration and magnitude of the response of airway resistance to a standard dose of an aerosol or isoproterenol are significantly greater in combination with phenylephrine (Cohen and Hale, 1965).

Sympathomimetics exert many other effects if they are absorbed and enter the systemic circulation in sufficient amounts. Cardiovascular effects are most evident. The drugs increase the heart rate and force of contraction, and the patient may experience palpitations (see Chapter 5). Phenylephrine increases blood pressure, resulting in reflex slowing of heart rate. When conventional doses of isoproterenol and phenylephrine are combined, the increase in heart rate is not so great as when isoproterenol is used alone (Cohen and Hale, 1965).

Many variable factors may influence the response to aerosolized bronchodilators, including the pathogenesis of the obstruction, the uniformity in delivery of the agent to the airways, the presence or absence of tachyphylaxis to the agent(s), changes in systemic pH, and the presence of other drugs. Even when these factors are stable, individual response to aerosolized agents varies widely.

The therapist's use of aerosols is limited by the appearance of systemic effects of the drug (e.g., unpleasant symptoms and dangerous adverse effects, such as arrhythmias). He must estimate the assets and liabilities of his maneuvers. The estimate can be made by quantitating the changes in $FEV_1\%$ and relating this therapeutic effect to systemic effects (e.g., change in heart rate and blood pressure after the bronchodilator has been administered). In essence a clinical therapeutic index is established for the drug in the particular patient. If the heart rate and blood pressure have dramatically changed 10 minutes after an inhalation but the $FEV_1\%$ is stable, the drug is probably not useful at that time. Generally, if the $FEV_1\%$ is favorably changed by isoproterenol, the maximum allowable dose should be set by an increase in heart rate 10 to 15 beats per minute greater than the pretreatment rate.

The rate of disappearance of effect on the $FEV_1\%$ may be used as a guide to the necessary frequency of dose administration. Dose frequency varies between patients with the same disease, and even more between patients with different diseases. *Monitoring a therapeutic and potentially toxic drug effect is even more important as dose size and frequency increase or if an associated disease increases the likelihood of toxicity.*

The response of the airway (as reflected in the $FEV_1\%$) and heart rate to therapy may help in establishing a diagnosis. Various types of response and their diagnostic implications are listed in Table 6–3. Whatever the response, it provides information that is often helpful in defining pathophysiology and directing the therapist's attention to effective measures.

Additional pharmacologic effects of sympathomimetic drugs must be considered in special clinical settings. Hyperglycemia may complicate the management of the diabetic patient; anxiety and apprehension may be aggravated; gastric motility may be inhibited; micturition may be impeded; and increased metabolic rates, mobilization of free fatty acid, increased concentration of lactate in blood, increased respiratory rate, and elevated white-blood-cell count could confuse the physician in his interpretation of the patient's condition unless he knows that these changes can be produced by the drug. *Principle: When the full pharmacologic potential of a drug is understood, misinterpretation of tests or new events in the patient's course caused by drugs is minimized.*

Pressurized aerosols are convenient and often efficient dispensers of drugs to the bronchi. However, in England and Wales, mortality from asthma increased substantially between 1961 and 1966. Eighty-six per cent of deaths occurred in patients using pressurized dispensers; in 72% of those who died, the drug used was isoproterenol (Speizer *et al.*, 1968). Fifty-seven per cent of the deaths occurred within 2 hours of the onset of the attack, and all but 5% of the people who died were using an aerosol. These data were retrospectively gathered and have inherent limitations. How-

ever, it is possible that death was due to an arrhythmia induced by an overdose of isoproterenol. Since patients tend to use the aerosol repeatedly during an acute attack, and since this practice has the potential of producing life-threatening arrhythmias, the physician should set strict limits on the frequency of drug administration.

Despite the potential hazards associated with the use of sympathomimetic bronchodilators, they are nevertheless a very useful group of drugs that are important in the treatment of obstructive airway disease. The hazards of the use of these drugs are discussed to emphasize the necessity of measuring drug effects in order to maximize therapeutic effects without creating toxicity and to permit early recognition of toxicity.

Modification of the structure of isoproterenol may increase the ratio of respiratory to cardiovascular effects of the drug. Studies of orciproterenol and salbutamol (Choo-Kang *et al.*, 1969; Tattersfield and McNicol, 1969) suggest that these agents produce fewer chronotropic effects than does isoproterenol for any standard improvement in maximum expiratory flow rates. In addition, the duration of action of these congeners is longer than that of isoproterenol. These agents must be compared with isoproterenol in a full clinical trial to decide which has the most beneficial effects and the lowest toxicity.

Claims of efficacy for orally active bronchodilator preparations containing several agents at fixed dosages may be confusing. Many formulations contain (1) ephedrine, (2) a sedative (usually a barbiturate), and (3) a theophylline salt. In addition, they may contain expectorants (potassium iodide, glyceryl guaiacolate), antihistamines, aspirin, and vitamins (Table 6–4).

Table 6–3. MEASURED RESPONSES TO AN ISOPROTERENOL AEROSOL

FEV_1	PULSE RATE	POSSIBLE CAUSES OF RESPONSE
No change	Increases	Obstruction may not be due to bronchial muscle constriction or small-airway involvement Drug is not being delivered uniformly to the bronchial tree (obstructed areas do not receive it)
Increase	No change	Ideal response, aerosol is delivering drug to site of desired pharmacologic response. More drug may be given if greater relief of obstruction is desired
No change	No change	Inadequate dosage Patient is tachyphylactic Drug is inactive Patient is receiving a drug that blocks β receptors Systemic acidosis is impeding drug responsiveness
Decrease	No change	An unusual response *Measuring the response to the drug is important*

Table 6–4. COMPOSITION OF FREQUENTLY PRESCRIBED ASTHMALYTIC COMPOUNDS

TRADE NAME	MANUFACTURER	EPHEDRINE (mg)	BARBITURATE (mg)	THEOPHYLLINE (mg)	OTHER INGREDIENTS
Aiadrine	Table Rock or Merit	8	Seco 8	×	
Amesec	Lilly	25	Amo 25	130	
Amodrine	Searle	Race 25	Pheno 8	100	
Asminyl	Cole	30	Pheno 8	120	
Brondilate	Walker	15	Buta 20	×	Isoproterenol
Bronkotab	Breon	25	Pheno 8	100	Thenyldiamine + glyceryl guaiacolate
Dainite	Mallinckrodt	15	Pheno 15	200	With or without K
Deltasmyl	Roussel	15	Pheno 8	120	Prednisone
Ephedrine with Amytal	Lilly	25	Amo 50	×	
Ephedrine with Seconal	Lilly	25	Seco 50	×	
Ephoxamine	Unimed	Race 30	×	×	Phenyltoloxamine
Hyadrine	Searle	Race 25	×	150	Diphenhydramine
Luasmin	Cooper	30	Pheno 30	120	
Marax	Roerig	25	×	130	Hydroxyzine (Atarax)
Mudrane	Poythress	16	Pheno 20	120	K or glyceryl guaiacolate
Numa (prolonged action)	Cooper	50	Buta 25	225	
Quadrinal	Knoll	25	Pheno 25	120	K
Synate-M	Central	Race 25	Seco 45	165	K + niacinamide
Tedral	Warner	25	Pheno 8 or buta 25	125	With or without chlorpheniramine
Verequad	Knoll	25	Pheno 8	130	Glyceryl guaiacolate

* Modified from Harris, M. C., and Shure, N.: *Sensitivity Chest Diseases.* F. A. Davis Co., Philadelphia, 1964. Based on the Report of the Committee on Allergy, American College of Physicians, 1965.

The efficacy of each of the preparations can be attributed only to the ephedrine. The dosages of theophylline salts (100 to 200 mg) are probably inadequate to relax the bronchi (Report of the Committee on Allergy, 1965), but have been kept low to avoid gastric irritation. Initially, the sedative was added to reduce the hypertension, agitation, and sleeplessness caused by ephedrine. The fallacy of this reasoning is obvious: (1) the hypertensive effects of ephedrine are minimal during chronic or frequent use of the drug, as are the central-nervous-stimulating effects (Innes and Nickerson, 1965); (2) barbiturates do not depress the hypertensive effects of ephedrine; and (3) in patients with severe chronic obstructive airway disease, doses of barbiturates may depress ventilation through their action on the central nervous system and may produce life-threatening hypoventilation. Antihistamines are not useful during bronchoconstriction (Schiller, 1963) and may aggravate inspissation of secretions by their atropine-like effects. *Principle: Fixed-combination preparations are generally very difficult to use properly even when appropriate drugs are combined in average dosage. When inappropriate drugs are combined in inappropriate*

doses, drug interactions and adverse responses occur frequently (see Chapters 15 and 16). Logic condemns the routine use of preparations containing a number of drugs in fixed dosage.

The xanthines and catecholamines share many pharmacologic properties (Table 6–5) that may

Table 6–5. SIMILARITIES IN RESPONSE TO EPINEPHRINE AND AMINOPHYLLINE*

	EPINEPHRINE	AMINOPHYLLINE
Pulse rate	↑	0, ↑
Pulse pressure	↑	↑
Cardiac output	↑	↑
CNS stimulation	↑	↑
Bronchodilation	↑	↑
Blood glucose	↑	
Free fatty acid mobilization	↑	↑
Metabolic rate	↑	↑
Respiratory rate	↑	↑

* Modified from Ritchie, J. M.: Central nervous system stimulants. II. The Xanthines. In Goodman, W. S., and Gilman, A. (eds.): *The Pharmacological Basis of Therapeutics*, 4th ed. The Macmillan Co., New York, 1970.

be attributed to similar biochemical mechanisms (Sutherland *et al.*, 1968). The methyl xanthines inhibit phosphodiesterase, an enzyme that inactivates cyclic AMP. Beta-adrenergic drugs stimulate the formation of cyclic AMP by activation of adenyl cyclase. Both drugs tend to increase intracellular concentrations of cyclic AMP, which is thought to be the messenger that mediates bronchial smooth-muscle relaxation, increases myocardial inotropism and chronotropism, and produces the metabolic effects represented in Table 6–5 (see Chapters 5, 7, and 9).

Theophylline and aminophylline (which contains theophylline) are xanthines used in the treatment of obstructive airway disease. The effects of aminophylline on bronchial smooth muscle are similar to those produced by the adrenergic agents and presumably are related to the increase in cyclic AMP, as has been shown to occur in heart muscle and intestinal smooth muscle (Rall and West, 1963; Wilkenfield and Levy, 1969). The effects of aminophylline are not influenced by beta blocking agents; therefore, this drug may be useful in patients who develop bronchospasm while taking beta blocking agents. Theophylline and aminophylline can be administered orally; aminophylline may also be given intravenously or by rectal suppository. When given by the intravenous route, aminophylline must be diluted and delivered slowly, since rapid administration may produce serious arrhythmias and hypotension (Bresnick *et al.*, 1948) (see Chapter 5). Chronic administration by rectal suppository irritates the rectal mucosa and causes severe proctitis.

Mucolytic and Expectorant Drugs

The efficacy of mucolytic and expectorant agents is difficult to establish, because adequate tests of their effectiveness have been difficult to define, standardize, and validate. The quantity, viscosity, and stickiness of sputum are not easily measured, and the relevance of these qualities to a changing pathophysiologic process or a clinical response has not been defined (Forbes and Wise, 1957). Many reports have recorded subjective rather than objective evaluations of variables obtained from double-blind studies. For example, the inorganic iodides have been accepted for years on the basis of subjective reports. Like many other drugs enjoying traditional use, iodides should be subject to the same scientific inquiry as new drugs.

The pathophysiology of asthma, chronic bronchitis, bronchiectasis, and mucoviscidosis includes excessive production of secretions, increased viscosity and retention of sputum, and

the presence of infection, all of which aggravate airway obstruction. Sputum production can be limited by avoiding inhalation of irritants and properly treating infection. Increasing the water content of sputum and reducing its mucopolysaccharide and protein content may minimize the viscosity and stickiness of secretions, thereby facilitating their clearance from the bronchial tree.

The simplest means of increasing the water content of sputum is hydration of the patient. Within limits, hydration appears to be quite safe. Water intoxication and pulmonary edema must be prevented in susceptible patients with renal insufficiency, heart failure, adrenal or thyroid insufficiency, or potassium depletion. Water must be considered a drug, and objectives must be set before it is used. The response must be assessed and adverse reactions must be anticipated and prevented. A patient showing an optimal response to hydration has thin sputum that is easily raised and dilute urine (< 1.010 specific gravity). The vital capacity and maximum expiratory flow rate should be improved, and hyponatremia should not be present.

Several mucolytic, proteolytic, and nucleolytic drugs can decrease the viscosity of sputum. Potassium iodide increases the volume of aqueous secretions from bronchial glands, and at high concentrations induces enzymatic hydrolysis of protein (Lieberman and Kurnick, 1964). The expectorant action of iodides is dose related and closely parallels other effects of iodides, including rhinorrhea, skin rash, parotid and submaxillary pain and swelling, gastrointestinal distress, and fever. Of these effects, gastrointestinal irritation, anorexia, vomiting, and epigastric pain are the most frequent (seen in 11% of patients taking 5 to 7 g KI per day, and in 41% of patients taking 18 to 36 g KI per day [Bernecker, 1969]).

Iodide-induced hypothyroidism may develop insidiously, and substantially contributes to hypoventilation when it appears (Massumi and Winnacker, 1964). Fortunately, the incidence of iodide-induced goiter and hypothyroidism appears to be low (Bernecker, 1969). However, goiter may be seen in 30% of patients receiving iodopyrine, which contains both iodide and antipyrine (Begg and Hall, 1963). The inordinately high incidence of goiter in patients taking this preparation is attributed to the additive effects of iodide and the antithyroid effect of antipyrine (Pasternak *et al.*, 1969). The incidence of iodide-induced myxedema may rise when these agents are given to patients with thyroid diseases such as Hashimoto's thyroiditis, Graves's disease, or abnormalities in the biosynthesis of thyroid hormones (Falliers, 1960; Wolff, 1969).

Although a substantial number of patients appear to respond well to iodides, less toxic alternative drugs should be considered. Glyceryl guaiacolate may be a suitable substitute for iodides. The guaiacolates may induce an increased avidity of the sputum for water, but the biochemical mechanism by which they thin sputum and increase sputum volume has not been defined (Chodosh, 1964). Adverse effects are infrequent, subjective improvement has been verified using double-blind crossover studies, and sputum surface tension and viscosity are reduced in patients with chronic bronchitis (Chodosh, 1967). (The drug may interfere with the laboratory tests for carcinoid syndrome, producing false-positive tests for 5-hydroxy-indolacetic acid.) The mucolytic agent N-acetyl-L-cysteine (Mucomyst) is effective in thinning extremely viscid tracheobronchial secretions. *In vitro* it reduces viscosity of sputum, probably by sulfhydryl-disulfide interchange with mucoprotein. The sodium salt of the drug also reduces viscosity of deoxyribonucleic acid and hyaluronic acid (Sheffner, 1965). Its clinical usefulness has been limited because it is difficult to administer. The drug reacts with most metals, rubber, and, to some extent, oxygen. The most effective means of administration has been direct instillation in the tracheobronchial tree through a percutaneous catheter, tracheotomy, or bronchoscope. It is given in 2–5% aqueous solution to one side at a time. Twenty minutes later it is removed with postural drainage or bronchial lavage. It decreases the consistency of sputum to a much greater extent than does a saline control (Hirsh and Kory, 1967). However, the drug may increase bronchial constriction independent of its effect on sputum, particularly in patients with bronchial asthma (Bernstein and Ausdenmoore, 1964). This effect may lead to serious bronchial obstruction; therefore, this agent should not be used in asthmatic patients without concomitant bronchodilator treatment. The drug may also produce stomatitis, rhinorrhea, and hemoptysis.

At present, the use of N-acetyl-L-cysteine has been largely restricted to those nonasthmatic tracheobronchial diseases in which conventional modes of therapy have been ineffective and retention of viscous secretions aggravates a severe pathophysiologic state. The beneficial effects of this agent have been demonstrated in children with mucoviscidosis (Stamm and Docter, 1965). Even in these patients, proper postural drainage, adequate fluid intake, and encouragement of cough are more important, although only supportive, therapeutic measures.

Neglect of these routine, relatively simple, but critical maneuvers can minimize or cancel the major beneficial effects of the drug. When powerful drugs are used, there is a general tendency to neglect other more important "ancillary" therapeutic measures. This "pitfall" must be avoided.

Proteolytic enzymes are being tested to determine their efficacy and toxicity. However, when they are administered via aerosol, these enzymes generally produce an unacceptably high incidence of toxic reactions without evidence of sustained mucolytic activity.

The clinical pharmacology of mucolytic and expectorant drugs is not fully developed, nor has the ideal mucolytic and expectorant drug been identified. In lieu of a standardized, relevant, objective criterion of a drug's effectiveness, future studies must employ a combination of double-blind techniques for evaluation of subjective effects with objective measurements of changes in pulmonary function and the physical properties of sputum. These studies should be conducted over both brief and prolonged periods if the drug's effect on prognosis is to be adequately assessed (Medical Letter, 1970).

Corticosteroids

The use of corticosteroids in the treatment of respiratory diseases is based, for the most part, on the empiric observation that they have potent effects that may relieve obstructive airway disease in asthmatic patients and resolve some infiltrative or inflammatory processes in the lungs. The fundamental pharmacologic mechanisms of corticosteroid action in man have not been identified, although most therapists agree that the anti-inflammatory effect of these drugs accounts for most of their effectiveness. Corticosteroids also inhibit antibody production, reduce tissue sensitivity, and inhibit contraction of bronchial smooth muscle.

The effects of corticosteroids are only palliative. The drugs do not significantly interrupt the etiology or fundamental pathogenetic mechanisms of any respiratory disease.

Weighed against the potent anti-inflammatory effects of corticosteroids are the severe side effects that invariably accompany long-term use of these agents in pharmacologic doses. Once the drug is administered, it may be difficult or impossible to withdraw it. Its application must always be based on assessment of the risks in using the drug versus the likelihood of symptomatic control of a given disease process. The patient's degree of symptomatic disability, his limitation of function, the rapidity of progress of the disease, and his response to other forms of treatment must be considered in the decision to use corticosteroids (see Chapters 9 and 15). *Principle: Use of corticosteroids should be restricted to disabling or rapidly progressive disease that is unresponsive to conventional forms of treatment.*

How hazardous is corticosteroid therapy?

1. A single dose, even a large one, seldom results in a harmful effect.

2. Corticosteroids given for less than 2 weeks rarely produce harmful effects, unless the patient has unusual risk factors (e.g., an underlying psychosis, a peptic ulcer, hypertension, tuberculosis).

3. As the dose of drug exceeds the normal daily secretion rate, and the duration of treatment extends beyond two weeks, the incidence of disfiguring, disabling, and life-threatening side effects increases. Alternate-day therapy reduces but does not eliminate the side effects of corticosteroids; however, not all asthmatics can be controlled with this regimen (see Asthma, below).

4. The palliative anti-inflammatory, antipyretic, and mood-elevating properties of these drugs often give both the patient and the doctor a false impression that the disease process has been arrested. Objective measurements of response must supplement the patient's subjective impressions. In addition, the ability of the drug to mask symptoms of a superimposed illness must be appreciated.

5. Intercurrent illness in a patient taking low doses of corticosteroids, or exposure of the patient to any undue stress up to 1 year after the drug has been withdrawn, may precipitate adrenal insufficiency (Travis and Sayers, 1965).

The physician must use corticosteroids with flexible reticence. These drugs should not be used if therapy is likely to be chronic. If long-term therapy is unavoidable, the minimum effective dose should be established, and the need for the drug should be reassessed at frequent intervals. Objective measurements of pulmonary function provide a useful guide in determining the changes in the minimum effective dose.

Corticosteroids have been administered via aerosol in an attempt to favor the ratio of pulmonary to systemic effects of the drugs. Theoretically, systemic effects of these drugs could be minimized while achieving adequate concentrations of drug in the lungs. However, no clear advantage of this form of therapy has been established. Adrenal suppression and cushingoid features may appear in children after only four inhalations per day (Crepea, 1963). In addition, if absorption is unreliable or variable, the minimum effective therapeutic dose is difficult if not impossible to establish. The variability becomes particularly important if the adrenal gland has been suppressed and it is imperative that replacement be reliable. Failure to sustain pharmacologic levels of the drug because of variable use or absorption, a change in the technique of administration, or a change in the airways that impedes delivery of the drug carries the potential risk of precipitating adrenal insufficiency. There are no apparent advantages to the administration of corticosteroids by aerosol over more conventional routes, and there may be a considerable number of disadvantages.

CLINICAL THERAPY

This section illustrates the application of therapeutic principles in asthma, sarcoidosis, chronic bronchitis, and emphysema. These diseases were selected to illustrate principles of good clinical pharmacology of lung diseases outlined in the first part of this chapter. There is considerable information about the pathogenesis, pathophysiology, and abnormalities in pulmonary function in patients with asthma. Knowledge of this information affords an opportunity to use both specific and nonspecific therapeutic measures rationally. The cause of sarcoidosis is unknown, and treatment must take into account the variable course of this disease. Despite the variabilities, principles of therapeutics may still be rationally and successfully applied. The discussion of chronic bronchitis, emphysema, and respiratory failure is intended to illustrate further the approach to diseases of unknown origin.

Asthma

Bronchial asthma is a chronic disease characterized by episodic bronchial obstruction that is clinically manifested by wheezing, dyspnea, cough, and production of mucoid sputum. Asthma is classified into two types: extrinsic asthma, about which there is considerable information regarding immunologic and biochemical pathogenetic mechanisms; and intrinsic asthma, the causes of which are poorly understood. Extrinsic asthma (Figure 6–5) occurs in young (aged 5 to 35), genetically susceptible individuals who have become sensitized to one or more of a variety of antigens delivered transmucosally (Salvaggio *et al.*, 1964). The exposure gives rise to a reaginic (skin-sensitizing) antibody (IgE) that characterizes atopic disease. The IgE globulin becomes cell fixed and reacts with the antigen to produce a series of biochemical changes in cells, of which the mast cell seems to be the principal participant (see Chapters 9 and 15). This interaction results in the liberation of several substances that produce increased

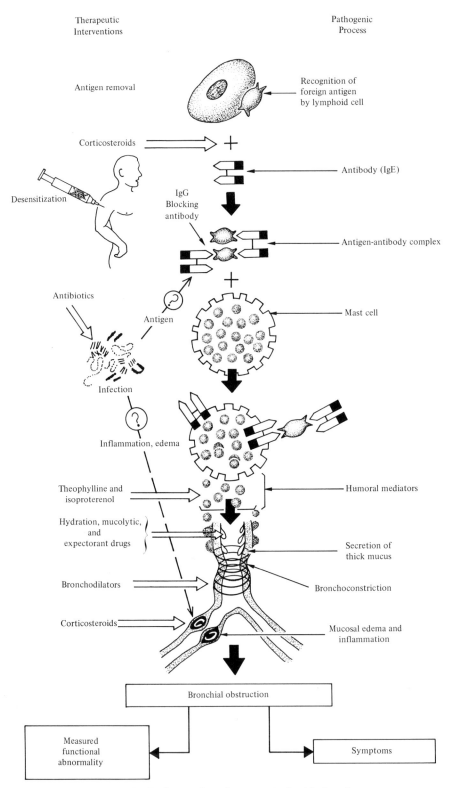

Therapeutic
Interventions

Pathogenic
Process

Antigen removal

Recognition of
foreign antigen
by lymphoid cell

Corticosteroids

Desensitization

IgG
Blocking
antibody

Antibody (IgE)

Antigen-antibody complex

Antibiotics

Antigen

Mast cell

Infection

Inflammation, edema

Theophylline and
isoproterenol

Humoral mediators

Hydration, mucolytic,
and
expectorant drugs

Secretion of
thick mucus

Bronchodilators

Bronchoconstriction

Corticosteroids

Mucosal edema and
inflammation

Bronchial obstruction

Measured
functional
abnormality

Symptoms

Figure 6–5. Pathogenesis and treatment of extrinsic asthma.

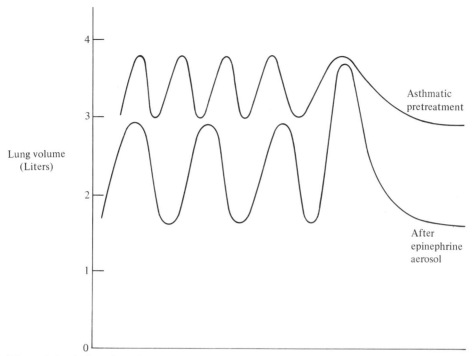

Figure 6–6. Asthmatic patient with markedly increased residual volume, small tidal volume, and vital capacity with delayed expiratory flow rates responding dramatically to aerosolized epinephrine. (Modified from Comroe, J. H.; Forster, R. E.; Dubois, A. B.; Briscoe, W. A.; and Carlsen, E.: *The Lung: Clinical Physiology and Pulmonary Function Tests*, 2nd ed. Year Book Medical Publishers, Inc., Chicago, 1962.)

capillary permeability (edema), hypersecretion by the mucous glands, contraction of bronchial smooth muscle, and responses in the bronchi and bronchioles typical of acute inflammation. Mast cells are rich in histamine, which is released on exposure to specific antigens (Schild *et al.*, 1951; Brocklehurst, 1956). Histamine is a potent constrictor of bronchial smooth muscle; it increases capillary permeability and causes bronchial glands to secrete excessive quantities of mucus. Patients with asthma are overly sensitive to the action of inhaled histamine (Curry and Lowell, 1948). Despite these observations, antihistaminic drugs have been ineffective in preventing asthmatic attacks or in reversing those already initiated (see Chapter 9).

As in other inflammatory diseases, additional chemical substances have been implicated as mediators of the asthmatic attack. Exact identification of these mediators and the extent of their contribution to the pathogenesis of asthma has not been accomplished. One such possible mediator deserves special mention. This substance is SRS-A (slow-reacting substance of anaphylaxis). A recent symposium (Pepys and Frankland, 1969) evaluated disodiumchromoglyc-ate, an inhibitor of SRS-A. The consensus of

investigators was that this new drug may be beneficial in allergic asthma, but even today the results must be considered preliminary (Mathison *et al.*, 1971). Whatever the active chemical mediators are, they contribute to the narrowing of airways and the obstruction of the flow of air. Infection may precipitate the process or may result from intrabronchial accumulation of mucus. Inspissated or stagnated mucus can aggravate the bronchoconstriction or even lead to complete obstruction of airways.

The functional abnormalities and clinical features of asthma usually are easily recognized and objectively documented by demonstration of prolonged expiration, reduced maximal expiratory flow rates, and a reduced vital capacity. The patient's symptoms and abnormalities of the spirographic tracing often rapidly and dramatically revert to normal during the administration of a bronchodilator (Figure 6–6). Responsiveness to bronchodilators is characteristic of asthma and helps to distinguish it from disease states with fixed obstruction of airways. Absence of responsiveness to drugs, however, does not differentiate between these alternative disease states (see Obstructive Airway Disease, page 264).

Testing of pulmonary function in the asthmatic patient during an acute attack demonstrates that the reduction in vital capacity is due to an increased residual volume, resulting from trapping of air. Although the total lung capacity is usually normal, distribution of inspired gas frequently is abnormal and, because poorly ventilated alveoli are perfused, arterial hypoxemia is nearly always present.

During chronic asthma and after prolonged and repeated attacks, the pattern of pulmonary function usually changes. Residual volume and functional residual capacity may increase, reflecting hyperinflation of the lung. This abnormality can persist for some time after relief of the obstruction. In addition, airway resistance and total lung capacity may increase between attacks and may be accompanied by reduced elastic recoil of the lung (Gold et al., 1967; Woolcock and Read, 1968). Maldistribution of inspired gas usually continues, but diffusion capacity remains normal (Bates, 1952) and pCO_2 values reflect the adequacy of alveolar ventilation. All these abnormalities may return to normal once the disease has been adequately controlled.

Early in the course of an attack of asthma, modest desaturation of arterial blood occurs as mismatching of ventilation to perfusion develops. Arterial pCO_2 tends to fall as ventilation increases in response to the hypoxia. Later, as the bronchospasm progresses, the pO_2 falls further and pCO_2 tends to return to normal. In severe status asthmaticus, the pO_2 may continue to fall and the pCO_2 may rise above normal. As the patient becomes exhausted from the increased work of breathing, these changes in gas content of blood indicate that alveolar hypoventilation may soon be life threatening. Thus, in the asthmatic patient with an acute attack, an increase of pCO_2 from 40 to 45 (a change that would seldom alarm the physician treating a patient with chronic bronchitis or emphysema) is an important finding requiring vigorous efforts to improve alveolar ventilation.

Specific Therapy for Extrinsic Asthma. The introduction of antigen via the respiratory tract initiates the asthmatic response in susceptible patients. If a history can be obtained that links exposure of the patient to pollens, animal danders, or components of the diet to asthmatic symptoms, the offending antigen may be accurately identified. If the suspected antigen produces an immediate reaction when injected into the skin, its removal from the patient's environment is logical and often efficacious.

When exposure of the patient to antigens cannot be effectively avoided, in selected cases desensitization may be attempted by multiple injections of small doses of aqueous extract of specific allergens, or by injections of emulsion containing the actual allergen (see Chapter 15).

"Desensitization" connotes the binding and removal of antibody with small amounts of antigen, theoretically lowering the allergic reactivity of the patient to involuntary exposure to antigen. Desensitization thus defined does not occur. Titers of skin-sensitizing antibody may actually rise after "desensitization," as does specific reactivity of the skin (Tuft and Heck, 1954; Sherman, 1957) and IgE concentrations in blood (Berg and Johansson, 1969). Despite this "paradoxical response," the constitutional symptoms may decrease and tolerance to repeated injections and spontaneous exposures to the allergen may increase. Recent evidence suggests that the mechanism for tolerance is related to production of neutralizing or blocking (IgG) antibodies (Lichtenstein and Norman, 1969) (see Chapter 15).

Although "desensitization" is widely used, its effectiveness in adult patients with asthma has not been documented. Studies in children show that despite considerable placebo effect in control groups (Frankland and Augustin, 1954; Feinberg, 1961), treated groups experience significant amelioration of asthmatic symptoms and a lower incidence of disease activity after the age of 16 (Johnstone and Dutton, 1968). However, desensitization therapy in adult asthmatic patients has not been studied as carefully as has the treatment of ragweed hay fever in children. Two promising developments in this area have been described (Lichtenstein et al., 1966): (1) an in vitro test, in which antigen causes the release of histamine from white blood cells of patients with allergic rhinitis, which closely parallels the clinical state of allergic rhinitis, (2) that the large doses of antigen used in this study reduced symptoms in children with allergic rhinitis more effectively than the smaller doses used by other investigators (Frankland and Lowell, 1967). Perhaps these results can be extrapolated to the desensitization of adult asthmatic patients; however, in vitro there are differences in cell reactions to antigen between children and adults (Sadan et al., 1968). Despite the lack of valid data, desensitization (a potentially dangerous form of therapy) is widely employed in the treatment of adult asthmatic patients. The "desensitization process" is laborious, painful, expensive, and subject to adverse reactions, including local swelling and erythema, urticaria, angioedema, asthmatic attacks, chills and fever, or even anaphylactic shock. It is far from an ideal form of therapy for asthma, and favorable results are not well documented. Desensitization should be reserved for the patient whose disease is substantially disabling and unresponsive to a well-tested vigorous therapeutic program found efficacious in most patients. *Principle: Popularity of a therapeutic maneuver does not establish its efficacy or safety or justify its use.*

Treatment of Intrinsic Asthma. Intrinsic asthma has many physiologic and pathologic abnormalities in common with extrinsic asthma but afflicts individuals of a different age group (younger than 5 and older than 35). Many of these patients have no previous history of atopy or response to skin test antigens that commonly produce reactions in atopic individuals. An immunologic mechanism for intrinsic asthma has not been demonstrated. Although the "specific" forms of therapy (antigen withdrawal and "desensitization") sometimes useful in extrinsic asthma are of no value in patients with intrinsic asthma, most drug therapy is directed toward reversal of selected abnormalities regardless of their etiology (e.g., bronchoconstriction, mucosal edema, and production of sputum). Many nonspecific forms of therapy (bronchodilators, mucolytic and expectorant agents, and corticosteroids) are useful in both types of asthma (Figure 6–5) (Quimby *et al.*, 1958).

In treating the asthmatic patient, the therapist must answer the following questions: (1) How can the knowledge of pathogenic, pathophysiologic, and pharmacologic information be integrated and used to establish effective therapeutic programs? (2) What is the role of pulmonary function testing in acute and long-term management? (3) Which therapeutic approach is used for which type of patient? (4) What governs the intensity of the therapeutic program? (5) What are the pitfalls and common errors that appear during management of the patient?

Asthma is a chronic disease with variable severity. Because the disease is chronic and the therapy palliative, the therapist is consulted for long periods. A good therapeutic regimen must be carefully planned and the benefit-to-risk ratio estimated for each decision.

Treatment of the Ambulatory Patient. In the patient with extrinsic asthma, the offending antigen should be identified and eliminated if possible. During the initial clinical evaluation, the physician should evaluate the degree of disability caused by the disease (which will influence the vigor of the therapeutic approach) and environmental, emotional, and other factors that might aggravate the disease. He must note the effectiveness of previous therapeutic programs. Acute flares of the disease may result from an infectious process in the bronchi, which can be very difficult to diagnose. Infection may be reflected in the texture, color, or cellular content of the sputum or in the patient's temperature,

differential white-blood-cell count, or chest x-ray. Often the only clue to infection is a change in the character of the sputum, especially if the patient is already taking anti-inflammatory drugs.

The rate of onset and the severity of the disease process should be estimated. The spirographic recording of vital capacity and maximum flow rates offers the means for objective appraisal of the severity of the disease and the frame of reference against which therapeutic interventions must be judged. If aerosolized catecholamines fail to alter the course of the disease, the obstruction is due to factors other than spasm of bronchial muscle, adequate amounts of the drug are not being delivered to the constricted bronchi, or the drug is ineffective because of systemic acidosis. If tenacious secretions have accumulated, they must be removed. If accumulation of sputum is not responsible for resistance to therapy, other causes of obstruction, such as acidosis, should be sought and treated (Table 6–3).

Once obstruction of bronchi has been reversed, a program that helps to minimize residual functional abnormality and to prevent recurrences without encountering undue drug toxicity must be fashioned. In most ambulatory patients, the treatment includes hydration, use of an aerosol and/or an orally active bronchodilator, and possibly an effective expectorant. Often patients require a custom-tailored dose of isoproterenol delivered by a DeVilbiss nebulizer at home, but use the more convenient proprietary aerosol preparations when away from home. Oral administration of theophylline or the use of suppositories of aminophylline should be considered to add to the effect of other measures. Given orally, theophylline produces more predictable concentrations in blood than when suppositories are used.

Changes in blood pressure, heart rate, and cardiac rhythm must be carefully and frequently observed to establish the maximal acceptable dose of bronchodilators. Measurement of pulmonary function and pulse rate before and 10 minutes after the initial dose of aerosol and at subsequent office visits is important in assessing the maintenance of a therapeutic effect.

The use of sedatives in asthmatic patients is controversial. The decision to use these drugs must weigh the emotional components that may contribute to the disease state and the effects of sedatives on depressing respiration. In general, sedatives should not be used in most patients with pulmonary disease (Catchlove and Kafer, 1971).

Many patients seek help only during acute

phases of an asthmatic attack and receive no preventive treatment between attacks. Typically, a patient appears in an emergency room with severe bronchospasm; his symptoms are relieved with a single subcutaneous dose of epinephrine or intramuscular epinephrine in oil. When he returns to the same environmental setting in which the attack was precipitated, another attack occurs. The patient may reappear in the emergency room many times before the short-comings of this form of treatment are realized. *Intercurrent treatment may forestall the occurrence of an asthmatic attack.* If an attempt is made to control the patient with a program progressing from hydration, oral ephedrine, or elixir of theophylline to an aerosol of isoproterenol with or without phenylephrine as needed, the exacerbations can often be prevented and the patient may experience little disability. If an acute severe attack occurs while the patient is taking a full therapeutic maintenance program, he should be hospitalized. The emergency room is a poor setting for the treatment of chronic or recurrent asthma attacks, except for the emergency care preliminary to hospitalization.

Care of the Hospitalized Asthmatic. When a patient's disease suddenly worsens, reasons for the change must be sought so that proper therapy may be instituted. The following questions should be asked: (1) Has infection developed? (2) Has the patient been taking the drugs as prescribed? (3) Have mucus plugs obstructed airways? (4) Has the patient suddenly and unwittingly exposed himself to a source of antigen? Infection should be suspected first, as it very often accounts for the exacerbation of symptoms.

Status asthmaticus (asthma refractory to conventional treatment) is usually life threatening; regardless of the precipitating event, vigorous therapy is necessary, including intravenous or oral replacement of fluids, a bronchodilator drug in dilute aerosol form delivered by an effective nebulizer, and an intermittent positive-pressure breathing apparatus and oxygen (if arterial pO_2 is too low) (Bocles, 1970).

When intravenous aminophylline is used, it should be diluted (1 to 2 mg/ml) and no more than 1 g should be given in the first 15 to 30 minutes. Subsequent doses can be chosen after the therapeutic and toxic effects of the first dose are determined. Xanthines and catecholamines may add to the effects of acidosis, hypoxia, and pulmonary hypertension in predisposing the severely ill patient to dangerous arrhythmias. Sodium bicarbonate may be helpful if acidosis is severe and not readily reversed by more specific therapy (e.g., administration of oxygen,

fluids, and drugs that support ventilation and cardiovascular function).

If the patient has developed severe symptoms but demonstrates no signs of extensive fatigue or severe hypoxia and hypercapnia, a trial of intensive therapy excluding corticosteroids should be initiated. If a favorable response does not promptly ensue, or if the disease progresses (as shown by deterioration of arterial blood gas measurements), corticosteroids should be added to the therapeutic program. If the patient continues to worsen, endotracheal intubation may be needed to control or assist ventilation. Ether or halothane anesthesia, bronchial lavage, and bronchoscopy for removal of bronchial plugs may be employed when severe bronchoconstriction is unresponsive to the above measures.

After airway obstruction is relieved, corticosteroids should be cautiously tapered until the minimum dose that effectively controls symptoms and bronchial obstruction is reached. The ultimate goal is maximum control of the disease without the use of corticosteroids. However, if careful attempts to wean the patient from the drug lead to recrudescence of signs and symptoms and impose disability, long-term corticosteroid therapy must be employed. Most patients respond to a low dose of 5 to 10 mg of prednisone per day; corticosteroid therapy given every other day is usually successful. As the dose of drug and the duration of treatment increase, or as dose intervals decrease, the incidence of adverse effects increases. When patients require prolonged therapy, the dose should be adjusted according to subjective appraisal of disability and objective appraisal of functional disturbance measured by changes in vital capacity and $FEV_1\%$. When the therapist is forced to use corticosteroids, he may have to settle for a dose that, in combination with other forms of treatment, prevents severe disability, even though some wheezing and abnormalities of $FEV_1\%$ persist.

A patient may remain resistant to all the above measures, even when 40 mg of prednisone are being administered daily. At this point the diagnosis should be questioned. Does the patient have periarteritis, Wegener's granulomatosis, or some other underlying disease? The therapist should also remember that variations exist between different asthmatic patients in the quantity and duration of pharmacologic effect of corticosteroids and, therefore, in their dose requirements for any standard effect of the drug (Walsh and Grant, 1966). Perhaps some variability between patients is accounted for by the inherent differences in their ability to metabolize corticosteroids. Patients who metabolize prednisone rapidly may be unresponsive to conventional doses (40 mg of prednisone per day), but may demonstrate beneficial effects without toxicity at doses considered very high for most individuals. In a study of small numbers of asthmatic patients (Dwyer *et al.*, 1967), very high doses of cortisol were necessary to achieve blood levels of 100 μg/100 ml, at which concentration a good therapeutic response was seen in all patients. Conversely, if the patient develops severe liver disease from any cause (e.g., cardiac cirrhosis associated with chronic failure of the right ventricle, alcoholic cirrhosis, or other disease processes), metabolism of corticosteroids may be considerably slowed, and both therapeutic and toxic effects may be seen at doses substantially lower than those required for the typical patient.

Dosage form and dose interval may be critical to effective therapy. Attempts have been made to manipulate doses of corticosteroids in order to favor the therapeutic-to-toxic ratio in asthmatic patients. Alternate-day therapy or other forms of interrupted therapy have been based on the theory that the effects of corticosteroids in relieving airway obstruction may be more prolonged than the effects that suppress the pituitary-adrenal axis. In selected patients such assumptions may be justified. Similarly, a wide dose interval might allow frequent periods free of the systemic effects of high concentrations of the drug; this might eliminate or reduce some of the disabling and disfiguring adverse effects of these agents (Harter *et al.*, 1963). Intermittent use of corticosteroids may be used only if the therapist takes into account the variable half-life of these drugs among individuals and between the various corticosteroid analogs. It would not be rational to use dexamethasone (duration of ACTH suppression, 2 3/4 days) every other day. The dose should be spaced as widely as symptoms and functional impairment permit; some patients may require daily therapy (Walsh and Grant, 1966).

If corticosteroids do not produce a noticeable therapeutic effect, the therapist must determine whether fluid retention, increased blood pressure, changes in electrolyte balance, hyperglycemia, and eosinopenia are present. If they are not, more drug may be required; if they are present, a different drug or re-evaluation of the diagnosis may be required. Each step in the treatment must be matched to the severity of the disease.

Sarcoidosis

The treatment of sarcoidosis challenges the therapist because (1) the etiology of the disease is unknown; (2) the disease runs a variable course with frequent spontaneous remissions; (3) there is poor correlation between radiologic findings, symptoms, and abnormalities of pulmonary function; and (4) the corticosteroids often used to treat the disease are toxic and their efficacy is open to question. In light of the obstacles to definitive therapy, what information can be used for rational and effective therapy? Understanding available data on the pathology and pathophysiology of sarcoid allows the therapist to make rational therapeutic choices and meaningful measurements useful in following the course of the disease and the effects of therapy.

The morphologic changes include multiple small noncaseating granulomata that are widely distributed throughout the lungs, lymphatics, and other tissues (Mayock *et al.*, 1963). The granulomata are consistent with inflammation, an observation that forms the basis for using anti-inflammatory agents to treat the disease. Although the lymphatic involvement may be most prominent (demonstrated by enlargement of the hilar lymph nodes), accompanying abnormalities of the parenchyma of the lung often can be detected by using tests of pulmonary function. Sometimes even when the appearance of the chest x-ray and pulmonary hemodynamics are normal (Coates and Comroe, 1951; Marshall *et al.*, 1958; Svanborg, 1961), small reductions in vital capacity, residual volume, and D_LCO may be present (Marshall *et al.*, 1958; Svanborg, 1961; Hamer, 1963). When mild parenchymal involvement is demonstrated by a chest x-ray, a somewhat variable pattern of pulmonary functional abnormalities is usually present. Lung volumes, compliance, and D_LCO are often reduced, and the D_LCO abnormality is accentuated during exercise. At this stage of the disease, arterial blood gas tensions at rest and hemodynamics during exercise may be normal, and wasted ventilation is not increased (Svanborg, 1961). Sometimes despite severe radiographic abnormalities, remarkably good pulmonary function may exist with only minor reductions in D_LCO. However, most patients with pulmonary fibrosis or long-standing infiltrative disease have severe functional abnormalities, with evidence of airway obstruction, hypoxia, and pulmonary hypertension. In the late stages of the disease, low pO_2 and low or normal pCO_2 are common findings.

The presence of extrapulmonary disease may influence therapeutic decisions. Involvement of the eye, central nervous system, or heart may constitute greater immediate risk to the patient than either the lung lesion or the adverse effects of corticosteroids. Ocular sarcoid may occur in as many as 25% of patients (Mayock *et al.*, 1963). Uveitis is the most common ocular manifestation of the disease and may lead to synechiae and secondary glaucoma. Involvement of the posterior chamber of the eye may also occur. Lesions in the nervous system, consisting of a wide variety of peripheral and central disturbances, occur in about 5% of patients (Mayock et al., 1963). Cardiac involvement may be secondary to advanced pulmonary disease (cor pulmonale), due to the pharmacologic effect of hypercalcemia on the heart or to direct involvement of the heart with granulomata, causing conduction disturbances, paroxysmal arrhythmias, heart failure, and sudden death (Porter, 1960). Elevation of serum calcium occurs in 15 to 20% of patients (Winnacker et al., 1968) and is in part due to increased sensitivity to vitamin D expressed by increased absorption of calcium (Bell et al., 1961).

These summary points are pertinent to the treatment of sarcoidosis: (1) The x-ray is inadequate to document the course of the disease and must be supplemented by tests of pulmonary function. (2) Careful attention must be paid to the possibility of hypercalcemia and to the function of the kidney, eye, nervous system, and heart. (3) Corticosteroids are the major empiric therapeutic tool in the treatment of sarcoidosis. They are used both for their anti-inflammatory effects and for their ability to reduce serum calcium concentrations (see Chapter 7). (4) The effectiveness of steroids in treating the pulmonary manifestations of the disease is debatable. Corticosteroids should be used only if they produce improvement in pulmonary function in the disabled patient, and not just to produce roentgenographic improvement in the lung. Although corticosteroids may cause functional improvement (Sharma et al., 1966), pulmonary function usually reverts to the pretreatment state after withdrawal of the drug (Sharma et al., 1966) and its use may be of little value (Young et al., 1970).

Several extrapulmonary and pulmonary manifestations of sarcoidosis require treatment with corticosteroids: (1) Corticosteroids should be employed to prevent the complications of uveitis. They can be used topically with little risk of systemic manifestations, although rises in intraocular pressure due to corticosteroids may occur. (2) Cutaneous sarcoid in areas of cosmetic importance should be treated with corticosteroids. Topical application may result in significant improvement with little risk of drug toxicity. However, corticosteroids can be absorbed from both normal and inflamed skin (especially when occlusive dressings are used). The total dose of drug and the surface area to which corticosteroids are applied determine whether systemic manifestations will appear

(Scoggins and Kliman, 1965). (3) Reversal of hypercalcemia may be life saving and is often dramatically facilitated by corticosteroids. Corticosteroid therapy of 1 to 2 weeks may be sufficient, if exposure to sunlight and dietary vitamin D are avoided. (4) Serious neurologic manifestations and disturbances of cardiac rhythm may require corticosteroid therapy. Although therapists often resort to the use of corticosteroids, there has been no clear demonstration of the efficacy of these drugs for neurologic complications of sarcoid (Porter, 1960). *Principle: When indications for therapy are not clearly defined, the decision to use any therapeutic agent must weigh the risk of the disease against the potential benefit and risk of therapy.*

Table 6–6. DRUGS USED TO TREAT SARCOIDOSIS IN THE PAST*

Cacodylate
Sodium morrhuate
Thorium X
Gold salts
Antilepral agents
Bismuth
Penealler
Sulfone derivatives and streptomycin
Chlortetracycline
Vitamin E
Vitamin C
Vitamin D
Mepacrine
Potassium para-aminobenzoate
Isoniazid
Chalmoogra oil
Chelating agents
Methotrexate
Chloroquine
Corticosteroids
Nitrogen mustard
Quinacrine
X-ray

* Wide spectrum of empirically chosen drugs employed in the treatment of sarcoidosis. Of special interest is the use of vitamin D (see text).

In the treatment of sarcoidosis, therapeutic trials have been initiated with many drugs chosen empirically. Table 6–6 provides a partial list of the agents reported. A list this long reflects poor understanding of the disease and failure to find a completely satisfactory therapeutic agent. Therapeutic efficacy has even been claimed for vitamin D. The testimonial account of remissions in cutaneous sarcoid with vitamin D therapy illustrates the dangers created when the acceptance of dogma is based on uncritical appraisal of uncontrolled reports. Subsequent information showed that vitamin D had falsely been given credit for a spontaneous remission of the skin lesions. However, vitamin D did produce hypercalcemia, leading to renal calculi, nephrocalcinosis, and renal failure (Ballard, 1960).

Chronic Bronchitis and Emphysema

There is some doubt that therapy for chronic bronchitis and emphysema influences longevity (McClement, 1965; Burrows and Earle, 1969; Emirgil et al., 1969). However, the quality if not the quantity of life may be favorably influenced by careful therapeutic intervention in these two disorders.

Management of the Ambulatory Patient. Advanced chronic bronchitis, characterized by dyspnea on mild exertion, cough with production of excessive amounts of sputum, and episodic exacerbations of both infection and respiratory failure, is successfully managed only when the numerous medical and community resources for its therapy are mobilized and integrated. The physician who enlists the patient in a program of (1) abstinence from smoking, (2) exercise, (3) accommodation to the home environment, (4) physical therapy aimed at facilitating sputum clearance, and (5) occupational rehabilitation in addition to pharmacologic treatment unquestionably helps the patient to improve his exercise tolerance, the quality of his life, and perhaps even some aspects of his pulmonary function (Figure 6–7) (Pierce et al., 1964; Woolf and Suero, 1969; Bass and Whitcomb, 1970; Petty et al., 1970).

Cessation of smoking may be much more important than any of the pharmacologic therapeutic measures. The physical therapist may help the patient by assisting him with postural drainage and chest percussion to facilitate clearing of secretions from the bronchial tree. In addition, the therapist may assist in a program of physical conditioning designed to improve the peripheral utilization of the limited oxygen supply. Administration of oxygen at low flow rates during exercise periods may permit activity and performance that would otherwise be impossible (Pierce et al., 1964; Petty and Finigan, 1968). *Principle: Although drugs may be the most convenient therapeutic tool, they may not be the safest, most efficacious, or most acceptable form of therapy.*

Treatment of Infections. The treatment or prevention of infections in the chronic bronchitic patient is designed to decrease the number of acute exacerbations of bronchitis that frequently cause prolonged morbidity and even death. The patient whose pO_2 is on the steep part of the oxygen-hemoglobin dissociation curve is in a precarious position; a minor infection may cause respiratory decompensation and inadequate oxygenation of peripheral tissues.

Several bacterial species and viral agents have been incriminated in the acute exacerbations of chronic bronchitis (see Chapter 10). These organisms include *Hemophilus influenzae, Diplococcus pneumoniae, Staphylococcus aureus,* species of *Klebsiella,* group A streptococci, the *Bacteroides* group, anaerobic streptococci, and many viral agents (Smith, 1930; Benstead, 1950; May, 1954; Carrilli et al., 1964; Storey et al., 1964; Ross, 1966). Regardless of the etiology of the infection, this is one of few instances in medicine in which the value of the prophylactic use of antibiotics has been confirmed (Francis et al., 1961, 1964; Report to the Medical Research Council, 1966). Tetracycline given daily reduces the patient's time out of work, his days of hospitalization, the number of febrile episodes, and his sputum volume. Ampicillin may have similar effectiveness, but penicillin, erythromycin, and sulfa drugs are not as useful (Francis et al., 1964). An alternative to prophylactic therapy is the use of antibiotics when an early but not fully developed infectious process is suspected. In such a program, the early treatment is initiated by the patient as soon as he (not the doctor) suspects infection of the respiratory tract; 1 to 2 g of tetracycline given daily for a week to 10 days, or ampicillin in equivalent dosage, is usually employed. Both regimens apparently meet therapeutic objectives.

Prophylactic antibiosis does not entail disruption of basic principles of therapeutics. In both prophylactic and early treatment, antibiotics are administered before attempts are made to identify the offending organism. In addition, the organism responsible for the infection may sometimes not be affected by the antibiotic chosen, and at times infection may not be present (Stone et al., 1953). If a gram stain of the sputum smear and culture of sputum impose little delay to the initiation of therapy there is an advantage in conducting these tests first. Then therapy may be begun and the results of the tests consulted for a proper choice of agents if the initial program fails. However, the prophylactic and early programs are suggested because rapid initiation of therapy is essential; infection is extremely detrimental to these patients, and it is caused in the overwhelming majority of patients by organisms predictably susceptible to tetracyclines (Stone et al., 1953). In addition, it is often difficult to isolate an organism from sputum (even by transtracheal aspiration) that can confidently be designated as the pathogen.

Treatment Aimed at Reversing the Pathophysiologic Abnormality. If expiratory flow

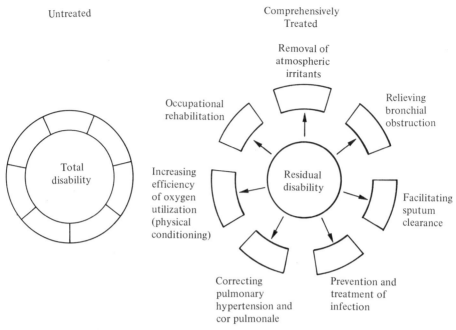

Figure 6–7. The impact of comprehensive therapy in chronic obstructive pulmonary disease.

rates increase when bronchodilators are given to patients with bronchitis, such therapy should be continued. If obstruction is persistent but the drugs demonstrate activity by affecting the cardiovascular system (pulse rate, blood pressure), the obstruction may not be due to bronchial muscle spasm. Likewise, the contribution of mucolytic and expectorant drugs must be individually assessed. In patients with emphysema, tissue destruction and consequent loss of elastic recoil may limit the improvement in expiratory flow rates regardless of the response of bronchial musculature.

Suppression of cough may be important in some patients. When the cough is frequent and in excess of its usefulness (nonproductive), it theoretically traumatizes the bronchial epithelium and causes persistent inflammation (Chodosh and Segal, 1964). It is not known whether the short- or long-term benefits of cough suppression outweigh its risks (depression of the respiratory center and pooling of uncleared secretions). If pCO_2 and $FEV_1\%$ can be measured frequently, symptomatic relief from frequent nonproductive cough by using codeine may be worth a therapeutic trial.

The use of corticosteroids to relieve bronchial edema, secretions, and spasm during chronic obstructive lung disease in adults has been extensively studied, but the efficacy of these drugs has not been established. Although some studies were controlled (Morgan and Rusche, 1964;

Klein et al., 1969), the double-blind method has not been employed and the duration of therapy has been inadequate to fully evaluate its effects. The results have not encouraged the use of steroids, except perhaps in patients with atopy (i.e., eosinophilia and immediate skin reactions to more than 50% of common antigens). These patients appear to represent intermediates between asthma and chronic bronchitis without atopy. Their disease has been labeled "asthmatic bronchitis" and may be responsive to steroids (Klein et al., 1969).

Most patients with chronic bronchitis have no history of atopy, no identifiable antigens, and no eosinophilia or immediate skin reactivity. They will probably not benefit from corticosteroids (Morgan and Rusche, 1964). Corticosteroids should not be used in most patients with bronchitis.

Physiologic disturbances other than airway obstruction may require therapy. Acid-base disturbance secondary to hypoventilation and retention of CO_2 occurs in association with cor pulmonale. Bicarbonate is retained by the kidney to compensate for the increased hydrogen ion load, and there are renal losses of chloride ion (see Chapter 3). The hydrogen ion load presented to the kidney induces ionic exchange for potassium with net loss of potassium. The signs and symptoms of right-heart failure may lead the well-meaning physician to employ kaluretic diuretics; this results in further total-body potassium depletion (with or without hypokalemia) and its attendant risks (Polak *et al.*, 1961; Murray, 1962).

The primary therapeutic approach to both cor pulmonale and respiratory acidosis should be directed at correction of the ventilatory defect. The hypoxemic patient with chronic bronchitis differs somewhat from the patient with emphysema who is not hypoxemic. In the patient with chronic bronchitis, any measures that reverse the hypoxemia also reduce pulmonary vascular resistance and the work load on the right ventricle, and thereby improve right or biventricular heart failure. Efforts to relieve bronchial obstruction, reduce or dispose of secretions, and improve ventilation have a salutary effect on cor pulmonale.

Increasing oxygen tension for prolonged periods may substantially lower pulmonary artery resistance and right ventricular afterload (Abraham *et al.*, 1968; Bedon *et al.*, 1970). Low-flow oxygen can be tried in patients who are undergoing graded exercise training. Oxygen is supplied by portable oxygen apparatus (Petty and Finigan, 1968; Neff and Petty, 1970). The salutary effects of chronic oxygen administration, especially on longevity, have not been established. Administration of oxygen may depress respiration in a patient with respiratory insufficiency and should be attempted only when the patient can be closely observed by skilled personnel.

The polycythemia accompanying chronic hypoxemia increases the viscosity of the blood, when hematocrits exceed 55 to 60%. An increased viscosity contributes to the resistance to flow through the pulmonary vascular bed and to congestive heart failure. Some therapists have suggested that chronic administration of oxygen at low flow rates may alleviate the polycythemia as well as the constriction of the pulmonary artery. Relief of polycythemia secondary to pulmonary disease by venesection or oxygen administration is probably worthwhile if cor pulmonale is present.

The usual patient with emphysema has less hypoxemia and a more fixed pulmonary vascular resistance than does the patient with "pure" chronic bronchitis. However, most of these patients have both chronic bronchitis and emphysema. In general, the salutary effects of oxygen are more pronounced in patients with predominant features of chronic bronchitis.

The value of digitalis in the treatment of cor pulmonale has been questioned. Responses to digitalis are not dramatic in patients with this disease. Digitalis may potentiate the arrhythmic potential of hypoxia, acid-base imbalance, and potassium deficit (see Chapter 5). Faced with a lessened likelihood of response to digitalis and an increased likelihood of adverse effects, the physician must exercise caution if he uses the drug. Despite these limitations, most investigators feel that the drug is useful if cautiously applied to patients with cor pulmonale (Oakley and Goodwin, 1967).

Left ventricular failure can be secondary to respiratory failure (Rao *et al.*, 1968). In such cases treatment of left ventricular failure is similar to its treatment in other cardiac diseases (see Chapter 5).

Treatment of Respiratory Failure. Usually rapid deterioration of a patient with chronic bronchitis is easily diagnosed. The patient is cyanotic, breathes laboriously through pursed lips, and employs accessory muscles of respiration with each breath; breath sounds are often inaudible. Signs of right ventricular heart failure may be present. Skillful therapy may reduce the mortality in this group of patients by 30 to 40%, restoring years of useful life (Sukumalchantra *et al.*, 1966).

The first steps in evaluating such a patient are to determine the pH, pCO_2, and pO_2 of arterial blood and to seek out any triggering factor that may have precipitated respiratory failure. If the function of the central nervous system or heart is compromised owing to low arterial pO_2, immediate attempts to increase pO_2 must be made. If the pO_2 is 30 mm Hg or less, the patient needs oxygen regardless of the state of cardiac or central nervous system function. Oxygen must be utilized like any drug and should be given only in the quantity sufficient to keep the pO_2 between 60 and 80 mm Hg, or to reverse the changes in cerebral or cardiac function. This can be accomplished by using a nasal catheter, mask, or mouthpiece. Another method of achieving controlled oxygen concentrations in inspired gas is to use a Venturi mask, which allows delivery of a predetermined oxygen concentration. These techniques minimize the production of coma (due to CO_2 narcosis) when oxygen is given to patients with respiratory failure (Campbell, 1967). Controlled oxygen therapy for respiratory failure requires constant supervision by a team of physicians and trained nursing staff. The response to O_2 should be evaluated in terms of the level of consciousness, the cardiac function, and the changes in measured pO_2 and pCO_2. Patients with cor pulmonale and heart failure that have been refractory to the usual therapeutic measures may dramatically respond to the improved pO_2.

As long as the pH is nearly normal, the pCO_2 should not be allowed to increase more than 10 to 15 mm Hg during therapy with oxygen. If the patient cannot be adequately oxygenated or if the pCO_2 rises dangerously (above 65 mm Hg), the patient's ventilation must be assisted or controlled. This usually requires endotracheal intubation. Following intubation, CO_2 may be eliminated too rapidly, producing a high concentration of bicarbonate in serum and a resultant alkalosis with hypokalemia. During this interval it is important to replace potassium and chloride simultaneously. Alkalosis and hypokalemia can be accompanied by cerebral vasoconstriction, reduced cerebral blood flow, coma, seizures, cardiac arrhythmias, and death (Robin, 1963; Kilburn, 1966). *Principle: "The longest way round is the shortest way home." The treatment should be no more intense than absolutely necessary to initiate improvement in the clinical and laboratory abnormalities.* No prizes are given to the physician who reduces the patient's pCO_2 to 40 mm Hg "first" at the expense of a seizure.

Chronic bronchitis and emphysema differ from asthma and sarcoidosis in that they more often run a relentlessly progressive course despite therapy. To equate this course with futility is, however, a grave error. The quality of life of these patients, regardless of the stage of their disease, can be favorably influenced by a rational therapeutic program, the sum total of which can significantly influence the patient's degree of disability (Figure 6-7).

REFERENCES

Abraham, A. S.; Cole, R. B.; and Bishop, J. M.: Reversal of pulmonary hypertension by prolonged oxygen administration to patients with chronic bronchitis. *Circ. Res.,* 23:147–57, 1968.

Acetylcysteine-respaire and mucomyst. *Med. Lett. Drugs Ther.,* 12:25–26, 1970.

Aviado, D.: Acute asthmatic action of sympathomimetics: a review of the literature on their bronchopulmonary effects. *J. Clin. Pharmacol.,* 10:217–21, 1970.

Ballard, H. S.: Irreversible renal failure following short term therapy in sarcoidosis. *Arch. Intern. Med. (Chicago),* 106:112–16, 1960.

Bass, H., and Whitcomb, E.: Exercise training: therapy for patients with chronic obstructive pulmonary disease. *Chest,* 57:116–21, 1970.

Bates, D. V.: Impairment of respiratory function in bronchial asthma. *Clin. Sci.,* 11:203–207, 1952.

Bates, D. V., and Christie, R. V.: *Respiratory Function in Disease.* W. B. Saunders Co., Philadelphia, 1964, pp. 46–47.

Bedon, G. A.; Block, A. J.; and Ball, W. C.: The 28% venturi mask in obstructive airway disease. *Arch. Intern. Med. (Chicago),* 125:106–13, 1970.

Begg, T. B., and Hall, R.: Iodide goiter and hypothyroidism. *Quart. J. Med.,* 32:351–62, 1963.

Bell, N. H.; Gill, J. R.; and Bartter, F. C.: Calcium metabolism in sarcoidosis. *Amer. Rev. Resp. Dis.,* 84:27–31, 1961.

Bendixen, H. H., and Laver, M. B.: Hypoxia in anesthesia: a review. *Clin. Pharmacol. Ther.,* 6:510–39, 1965.

Benstead, J. G.: The flora of 100 bronchial secretion, with particular reference to anaerobic cocci. *Lancet,* 1:206–208, 1950.

Berg, T., and Johansson, S. G. O.: IgE concentrations in children with atopic diseases. *Int. Arch. Allergy Appl. Immunol.,* 36:219–32, 1969.

Bernecker, C.: Intermittent therapy with potassium iodide in chronic obstructive disease of the airways. *Acta Allerg.,* 24:216–25, 1969.

Bernstein, I. L., and Ausdenmoore, R. W.: Iatrogenic bronchospasm occurring during clinical trials of a new mucolytic agent, acetylcysteine. *Dis. Chest,* 46:469–73, 1964.

Bocles, J. S.: Status asthmaticus. *Med. Clin. North Amer.,* 54:493–509, 1970.

Bresnick, E.; Woodard, W. K.; and Sageman, C. B.: Fatal reaction to intravenous administration of aminophyllin: report of 3 cases. *J.A.M.A.,* 136:397–98, 1948.

Brocklehurst, W. E.: A slow reacting substance in anaphylaxis—"SRS-A". In Wolstenholme, G. E. W., and O'Connor, C. M. (eds.): *Ciba Foundation Symposium jointly with the Physiological Society and the British Pharmacological Society on Histamine.* J. & A. Churchill, Ltd., London, 1956, pp. 175–79.

Burgess, J. H., and Bishop, J. M.: Pulmonary diffusing capacity and its subdivisions in polycythemia vera. *J. Clin. Invest.,* 42:997–1006, 1963.

Burrows, B., and Earle, R. H.: Course and prognosis of chronic obstructive lung disease. *New Eng. J. Med.,* 280:397–404, 1969.

Campbell, E. J. M.: The J. Burns Amberson Lecture. The management of acute respiratory failure in chronic bronchitis and emphysema. *Amer. Rev. Resp. Dis.,* 96:626–39, 1967.

Carrilli, A. D.; Gohd, R. S.; and Gordon, W.: A virologic study of chronic bronchitis. *New Eng. J. Med.,* 270:123–27, 1964.

Catchlove, R. H. F., and Kafer, E. R.: The effect of diazepam on the ventilatory response to carbon dioxide and on steady-state gas exchange. *Anesthesiology,* 34:9–13, 1971.

Chodosh, S.: Glyceryl guaiacolate: a controlled laboratory and clinical study. *Amer. Rev. Resp. Dis.,* 90:285–86, 1964.

———: Newer drugs in the treatment of chronic bronchitis. *Med. Clin. N. Amer.,* 51:1169–79, 1967.

Chodosh, S., and Segal, M. S.: Chronic bronchitis. *New Eng. J. Med.,* 270:894–97; 1057–59, 1964.

Choo-Kang, Y. F. J.; Simpson, W. T.; and Grant, I. W. B.: Controlled comparison of the bronchodilator effects of three β-adrenergic stimulant drugs administered by inhalation to patients with asthma. *Brit. Med. J.,* 2:287–89, 1969.

Coates, E. O., and Comroe, J. H., Jr.: Pulmonary function studies in sarcoidosis. *J. Clin. Invest.,* 30:848–52, 1951.

Cohen, A. A., and Hale, F. C.: Comparative effects of isoproterenol aerosols on airway resistance in obstructive pulmonary diseases. *Amer. J. Med. Sci.,* 249:309–15, 1965.

Comroe, J. H.: *Physiology of Respiration: An Introductory Text.* Year Book Medical Publishers, Chicago, 1965.

Comroe, J. H.; Forster, R. E.; Dubois, A. B.; Briscoe, W. A.; and Carlsen, E.: *The Lung: Clinical Physiology and Pulmonary Function Tests,* 2nd ed. Year Book Medical Publishers, Inc., Chicago, 1962.

Crepea, S. B.: Inhalation corticosteroids (dexamethasone PO_4) management of chronically asthmatic children. *J. Allergy,* 34:119–26, 1963.

Curry, J. J., and Lowell, F. C.: Measurement of vital capacity in asthmatic subjects receiving histamine and acetyl-beta-methyl choline. *J. Allergy,* 19:9–18, 1948.

Dejours, P.: *Respiration.* Oxford University Press, New York, 1966.

Duffell, G. M.; Marcus, J. H.; and Ingram, R. H.: Limitation of expiratory flow in chronic obstructive pulmonary disease. *Ann. Intern. Med.*, **72**:365–74, 1970.

Dwyer, J.; Lazarus, L.; and Hickie, J. B.: A study of cortisol metabolism in patients with chronic asthma. *Aust. Ann. Med.*, **16**:297–303, 1967.

Emergil, C.; Sobol, B. J.; Herbert, W. H.; and Trout, K. W.: Routine pulmonary function studies as a key to the status of the lesser circulation in chronic obstructive pulmonary disease. *Amer. J. Med.*, **50**:191–99, 1971.

Emirgil, C.; Sobol, B. J.; Norman, J.; Moskowitz, E.; Prakash, G.; and Wadhwani, B.: A study of the long-term effect of therapy in chronic obstructive pulmonary disease. *Amer. J. Med.*, **47**:367–77, 1969.

Falliers, C. J.: Goiter and thyroid dysfunction following the use of iodides in asthmatic children. *Amer. J. Dis. Child.*, **99**:428–36, 1960.

Feinberg, S. M.: Repository antigen therapy: its present status. *J. Allergy*, **32**:271–73, 1961.

Finley, T. N.; Swenson, E. W.; and Comroe, J. H.: The cause of arterial hypoxemia at rest in patients with "alveolar-capillary block syndrome." *J. Clin. Invest.*, **41**:618–22, 1962.

Forbes, J., and Wise, L.: Expectorants and sputum viscosity. *Lancet*, **2**:767–70, 1957.

Francis, R. S.; May, J. R.; and Spicer, C. C.: Chemotherapy of bronchitis: influence of penicillin and tetracycline administered daily, or intermittently for exacerbations. *Brit. Med. J.*, **2**:979–85, 1961.

———: Influence of daily penicillin, tetracycline, erythromycin and sulphamethoxypyridazine on exacerbations of bronchitis. *Brit. Med. J.*, **1**:728–32, 1964.

Frankland, A. W., and Augustin, R.: Prophylaxis of summer hay fever and asthma: a controlled trial comparing crude grass-pollen with the isolated main protein component. *Lancet*, **1**:1055–57, 1954.

Frankland, A. W., and Lowell, F. C.: Comparison of two dosages of ragweed extract in the treatment of pollinosis. *J.A.M.A.*, **201**:95–97, 1967.

Fry, D. L., and Hyatt, R. E.: Pulmonary mechanics: a unified analysis of the relationship between pressure, volume, and gas flow in the lungs of normal and diseased human subjects. *Amer. J. Med.*, **29**:672–89, 1960.

Gazioglu, K.; Condemi, J. J.; Hyde, R. W.; and Kaltreider, N. L.: Effect of isoproterenol on gas exchange during air and oxygen breathing in patients with asthma. *Amer. J. Med.*, **50**:185–90, 1971.

Gold, W. M., and Jennings, D. B.: Pulmonary function in patients with systemic lupus erythematosus. *Amer. Rev. Resp. Dis.*, **93**:556–67, 1966.

Gold, W. M.; Kaufman, H. S.; and Nadel, J. A.: Elastic recoil of the lung in chronic asthmatic patients before and after therapy. *J. Appl. Physiol.*, **23**:433–38, 1967.

Gracey, D. R.; Divertie, M. B.; and Brown, A. L.: Alveolar-capillary membrane in idiopathic interstitial pulmonary fibrosis: electron microscopic study of 14 cases. *Amer. Rev. Resp. Dis.*, **98**:16–21, 1968.

Hamer, N. A. J.: Changes in the components, of the diffusing capacity in pulmonary sarcoidosis. *Thorax*, **18**:275–87, 1963.

Harter, J. G.; Reddy, W. J.; and Thorn, G. W.: Studies on an intermittent corticosteroid dosage regimen. *New Eng. J. Med.*, **269**:591–96, 1963.

Hirsh, S. R., and Kory, R. C.: An evaluation of the effect of nebulized N-acetylcysteine on sputum consistency. *J. Allergy*, **39**:265–73, 1967.

Innes, I. R., and Nickerson, M.: Drugs acting on post-ganglionic adrenergic nerve endings and structures innervated by them (sympathomimetic drugs). In

Goodman, L. S., and Gilman, A. (eds.): *The Pharmacological Basis of Therapeutics*, 3rd ed. The Macmillan Co., New York, 1965, pp. 505–506.

Johnstone, D. E., and Dutton, A.: The value of hyposensitization therapy for bronchial asthma in children: a 14 year study. *Pediatrics*, **42**:793–802, 1968.

Kilburn, K. H.: Shock, seizures, and coma with alkalosis during mechanical ventilation. *Ann. Intern. Med.*, **65**:977–84, 1966.

Klein, R. C.; Salvaggio, J. E.; and Kundur, V. G.: The response of patients with "idiopathic" obstructive pulmonary disease and "allergic" obstructive bronchitis to prednisone. *Ann. Intern. Med.*, **71**:711–18, 1969.

Lichtenstein, L. M., and Norman, P. S.: Human allergic reactions. *Amer. J. Med.*, **46**:163–73, 1969.

Lichtenstein, L. M.; Norman, P. S.; Winkenwerder, W. L.; and Osler, A. G.: *In vitro* studies of human ragweed allergy: changes in cellular and humoral activity associated with specific desensitization. *J. Clin. Invest.*, **45**:1126–36, 1966.

Lieberman, J., and Kurnick, N. B.: The induction of proteolysis in purulent sputum by iodides. *J. Clin. Invest.*, **43**:1892–1904, 1964.

McClement, J. H.: The problem of chronic obstructive lung disease restated. In *Conference on Research in Emphysema: 8th Meeting in Aspen, Colorado, 1965: Management of Chronic Obstructive Lung Disease.* U.S. Department of Health, Education, and Welfare, Washington, D.C., 1965, pp. 1–6.

Macklem, P. T., and Mead, J.: Resistance of central and peripheral airways measured by a retrograde catheter. *J. Appl. Physiol.*, **22**:395–401, 1967.

McNicol, M. W., and Campbell, E. J.: Severity of respiratory failure. Arterial blood-gases in untreated patients. *Lancet*, **1**:336–38, 1965.

Marshall, R.; Smellie, H.; Maylis, J. H.; Hoyle, C.; and Bates, D. V.: Pulmonary function in sarcoidosis. *Thorax*, **13**:48–58, 1958.

Massumi, R. A., and Winnacker, J. L.: Severe depression of the respiratory center in myxedema. *Amer. J. Med.*, **36**:876–82, 1964.

Mathison, D. A.; Condemi, J. J.; Lovejoy, F. W.; and Vaughan, J. H.: Cromolyn treatment of asthma; trials in corticosteroid-dependent asthmatics. *J.A.M.A.*, **216**:1454–58, 1971.

May, J. R.: Pathogenic bacteria in chronic bronchitis. *Lancet*, **2**:839–42, 1954.

Mayock, R. L.; Bertrand, P.; Morrison, C. E.; and Scott, J. H.: Manifestations of sarcoidosis. *Amer. J. Med.*, **35**:67–89, 1963.

Mithoefer, J. C.; Bossman, O. G.; Thibeault, D. W.; and Mead, G. D.: The clinical estimation of alveolar ventilation. *Amer. Rev. Resp. Dis.*, **98**:868–71, 1968.

Morgan, W. K. C., and Rusche, E.: A controlled trial of the effect of steroids in obstructive airway disease. *Ann. Intern. Med.*, **61**:248–54, 1964.

Murray, J. F.: Carbon dioxide retention without acidosis: a common occurrence due to co-existing potassium depletion. *Amer. Rev. Resp. Dis.*, **86**:126, 1962.

Nadel, J. A.; Gold, W. M.; and Burgess, J. H.: Early diagnosis of chronic pulmonary vascular obstruction. *Amer. J. Med.*, **44**:16–25, 1968.

Naeye, R. L.: Pulmonary vascular lesions in systemic scleroderma. *Dis. Chest*, **44**:374–80, 1963.

Neff, T. A., and Petty, T. L.: Long-term continuous oxygen therapy in chronic airway obstruction. *Ann. Intern. Med.*, **72**:621–26, 1970.

Nunn, J. F.: *Applied Respiratory Physiology*. Butterworth & Co., Ltd., London, 1969, pp. 359–62.

Oakley, C. M., and Goodwin, J. F.: The current status of pulmonary embolism and pulmonary vascular disease in relation to pulmonary hypertension. *Progr. Cardiov. Dis.*, 9:495–521, 1967.

Palmer, K. N. V., and Diament, M. L.: Effect of aerosol isoprenaline on blood-gas tensions in severe bronchial asthma. *Lancet*, 2:1232–33, 1967.

Pasternak, D. P.; Socolow, E. L.; and Ingbar, S. H.: Synergistic interaction of phenazone and iodide on thyroid hormone biosynthesis in the rat. *Endocrinology*, 84:769–77, 1969.

Pepys, J., and Frankland, A. W.: *Disodiumchromoglycate in Allergic Disease*. Butterworth, London, 1969.

Petty, T. L.; Brink, G. A.; Miller, M. W.; and Corsello, P. R.: Objective functional improvement in chronic airway obstruction. *Chest*, 57:216–23, 1970.

Petty, T. L., and Finigan, M. M.: Clinical evaluation of prolonged ambulatory oxygen therapy in chronic airway obstruction. *Amer. J. Med.*, 45:242–52, 1968.

Pierce, A. K.; Taylor, H. F.; Archer, R. K.; and Miller, W. F.: Responses to exercise training in patients with emphysema. *Arch. Intern. Med. (Chicago)*, 113:28–36, 1964.

Polak, A.; Haynie, G. D.; Hays, R. M.; and Schwartz, W. B.: Effects of chronic hypercapnia on electrolyte and acid-base equilibrium. I. Adaptation. *J. Clin. Invest.*, 40:1223–37, 1961.

Porter, G. H.: Sarcoid heart disease. *New Eng. J. Med.*, 263:1350–57, 1960.

Quimby, C. W., Jr.; Aviado, D. M., Jr.; and Schmidt, C. F.: The effects of aminophylline and other xanthines on the pulmonary circulation. *J. Pharm. Exp. Ther.*, 122:396–405, 1958.

Rall, T. W., and West, T. C.: The potentiation of cardiac inotropic responses to norepinephrine by theophylline. *J. Pharm. Exp. Ther.*, 139:269–74, 1963.

Rao, S. B.; Cohn, K. E.; Eldridge, F. L.; and Hancock, E. W.: Left ventricular failure secondary to chronic pulmonary disease. *Amer. J. Med.*, 45:229–41, 1968.

Report of the Committee on Allergy, American College of Physicians: Asthmalytic and antihistamine compounds. *Dis. Chest*, 48:106–10, 1965.

Report to the Medical Research Council by their working party on trials of chemotherapy in early chronic bronchitis: value of chemoprophylaxis and chemotherapy in early chronic bronchitis. *Brit. Med. J.*, 2:1317–22, 1966.

Robin, E. D.: Abnormalities of acid-base regulation in chronic pulmonary disease, with special reference to hypercapnea and extracellular alkalosis. *New Eng. J. Med.*, 268:917–22, 1963.

Ross, C. A. C.: Infective agents and chronic bronchitis. *Thorax*, 21:461–66, 1966.

Sadan, N.; Rhyne, M. B.; Mellits, D. E.; Goldstein, E. O.; Levy, D. A.; and Lichtenstein, L. M.: A study of clinical and immunologic parameters in children receiving immunotherapy for ragweed hay fever. *J. Allergy*, 41:116–17, 1968.

Salvaggio, J. E.; Cavanaugh, J. J. A.; Lowell, F. C.; and Leskowitz, S. A.: A comparison of the immunologic responses of normal and atopic individuals to intranasally administered antigen. *J. Allergy*, 35:62–69, 1964.

Schepers, G. W. H.: Comparative vascular pathology of occupational chest diseases. *Arch. Indust. Health (Chicago)*, 12:7–25, 1955.

Schild, H. O.; Hawkins, D. F.; Mongar, J. L.; and Herxheimer, H.: Reaction of isolated human asthmatic lung and bronchial tissue to a specific antigen: histamine release and muscular contraction. *Lancet*, 2:376–82, 1951.

Schiller, I.: Bronchial asthma: views on therapy. *New Eng. J. Med.*, 269:94–97; 201–204, 1963.

Scoggins, R. B., and Kliman, B.: Percutaneous absorption of corticosteroids. *New Eng. J. Med.*, 273:831–40, 1965.

Severinghaus, J. W.: Personal communication, 1970.

Severinghaus, J. W., and Stupfel, M.: Alveolar dead space as an index of distribution of blood flow in pulmonary capillaries. *J. Appl. Phys.* 10:335–48, 1957.

Sharma, O. P.; Colp, C.; and Williams, M. H., Jr.: Course of pulmonary sarcoidosis with and without corticosteroid therapy as determined by pulmonary function studies. *Amer. J. Med.*, 41:541–51, 1966.

Sheffner, A. L.: Mucolytic activity mechanism of action and metabolism of acetyl cysteine. *Pharmakotherapeutica*, pp. 47–73, 1965.

Sherman, W. B.: Reaginic and blocking antibodies. *J. Allergy*, 28:62–75, 1957.

Smith, D. T.: Etiology of primary bronchiectasis. *Arch. Surg. (Chicago)*, 21:1173–87, 1930.

Smith, G. T.; Dammin, G. J.; and Dexter, L.: Postmortem arteriographic studies of the human lung in pulmonary embolization. *J.A.M.A.*, 188:143–51, 1964.

Sobol, B. J.; Emergil, C. E.; Wodhwani, B.; and Sowkor, L.: The response to bronchodilator in asthmatic subjects as assessed by pulmonary function tests. *J. Allergy*, 46:65–72, 1970.

Speizer, F. E.; Doll, R.; Heaf, P.; and Strangs, L. B.: Investigation into use of drugs preceding death from asthma. *Brit. Med. J.*, 1:339–43, 1968.

Stamm, S. J., and Docter, J.: Clinical evaluation of acetylcysteine as a mucolytic agent in cystic fibrosis. *Dis. Chest*, 47:414–20, 1965.

Stone, D. J.; Schwartz, A.; Newman, W.; Feltman, J. A.; and Lovelock, F. J.: Precipitation by pulmonary infection of acute anoxia, cardiac failure and respiratory acidosis in chronic pulmonary disease. *Amer. J. Med.*, 14:14–22, 1953.

Storey, P. B.; Morgan, W. K. C.; Diaz, A. J.; Klaff, J. L.; and Spicer, W. S.: Chronic obstructive airway disease: bacterial and cellular content of the sputum. *Amer. Rev. Resp. Dis.*, 80:730–35, 1964.

Sukumalchantra, Y.; Dinakara, P.; and Williams, M. H.: Prognosis of patients with chronic obstructive pulmonary disease after hospitalization for acute ventilatory failure: a three year followup study. *Amer. Rev. Resp. Dis.*, 93:215–22, 1966.

Sutherland, E. W.; Robison, G. A.; and Butcher, R. W.: Some aspects of the biological role of adenosine 3′,5′-monophosphate (cyclic AMP). *Circulation*, 37:279–306, 1968.

Svanborg, N. (ed.): Studies on cardiopulmonary function in sarcoidosis. *Acta Med. Scand.* (Suppl. 336), 1961.

Tattersfield, A. E., and McNicol, M. W.: Salbutamol and isoproterenol: a double-blind trial to compare bronchodilator and cardiovascular activity. *New Eng. J. Med.*, 281:1323–26, 1969.

Travis, R. H., and Sayers, G.: Adrenocorticotropic hormone; adrenocortical steroids and their synthetic analogs. In Goodman, L. S., and Gilman, A. (eds.): *The Pharmacological Basis of Therapeutics*. The Macmillan Co., New York, 1965, pp. 1608–48.

Tuft, L., and Heck, V. M.: Studies in sensitization as applied to skin test reactions. I. Do skin test reactions change? *J. Allergy*, 25:340–54, 1954.

Tuller, M. A., and Mehdi, F.: Compensatory hypoventilation and hypercapnia in primary metabolic alkalosis. Report of three cases. *Amer. J. Med.*, 50:281–90, 1971.

Walsh, S. D., and Grant, I. W. B.: Corticosteroids in treatment of chronic asthma. *Brit. Med. J.*, 2:796–802, 1966.

Wilkenfield, B. E., and Levy, B.: The effects of theophylline, diazoxide, and imidazole on isoproterenol-induced inhibition of the rabbit ileum. *J. Pharm. Exper. Ther.*, 169:61–67, 1969.

Winnacker, J. L.; Becker, K. L.; and Katz, S.: Endocrine aspects of sarcoidosis. *New Eng. J. Med.*, **278**: 427–34, 1968.

Wolff, J.: Iodide goiter and the pharmacologic effects of excess iodide. *Amer. J. Med.*, **47**:101–24, 1969.

Woolcock, A. J., and Read, J.: The static properties of the lungs in asthma. *Amer. Rev. Resp. Dis.*, **98**:788–94, 1968.

Woolf, C. R., and Suero, J. T.: Alterations in lung mechanics and gas exchange following training in chronic obstructive lung disease. *Dis. Chest*, **55**:37–44, 1969.

Young, R. L.; Harkleroad, L. E.; Lordon, R. E.; and Weg, J. G.: Pulmonary sarcoidosis: a prospective evaluation of glucocorticoid therapy. *Ann. Intern. Med.*, **73**:207–12, 1970.

Chapter 7

ENDOCRINE DISORDERS

Hibbard E. Williams and *Charles E. Becker*

The 1971 *Physicians' Desk Reference* lists over 500 hormonal preparations for use in man. This chapter does not describe the use of these preparations but rather outlines basic principles for hormonal and antihormonal therapy in the major endocrinopathies.

The agents used to treat endocrine disorders often are naturally occurring compounds. Many disorders are deficiency syndromes requiring only the simple replacement of the missing hormone. No controversy exists as to which hormone to replace, and replacement therapy gives some of the most effective and rewarding results in therapeutics. In few situations in therapeutics is there an opportunity to deal with such straightforward and simple principles. However, one need only mention the treatment of hyperthyroidism, the methods of controlling diabetes mellitus, or the use of "the pill" to raise the hackles of many an enthusiastic endocrinologist. This chapter includes discussions both of simple hormonal replacement therapy and of the more controversial methods of treatment.

CHARACTERISTICS OF THE ENDOCRINE SYSTEM

The most characteristic feature of the endocrine system is the ability of the glands of internal secretion to produce hormones essential for normal metabolic functions. The number of recognized hormones produced by endocrine tissues is small. The anterior pituitary hormones include growth hormone, adrenocorticotropin, melanocyte-stimulating hormone, thyrotropin, luteotropin or interstitial-cell-stimulating hormone, follicle-stimulating hormone, and prolactin. The neurohypophysis produces vasopressin and oxytocin, which are stored in the posterior pituitary. The three major hormones of the human thyroid include thyroxine, triiodothyronine, and thyrocalcitonin, whereas parathormone is the only hormone produced by the parathyroids. Several steroid hormones have been isolated from human adrenal venous blood, including the glucocorticoids, cortisol and corticosterone; a mineralocorticoid, aldosterone; an androgen, Δ4-androstenedione; an estrogen, estradiol; and the progestins, progesterone and pregnenolone. The pancreatic islets produce insulin (and proinsulin) and glucagon; the adrenal medulla, epinephrine and norepinephrine; and the testes, Δ4-androstenedione and testosterone. The human ovary produces three major estrogenic hormones (estriol, estradiol, and estrone), as well as testosterone, progesterone, and relaxin. The gastrointestinal tract hormones are not discussed in this chapter (see Chapter 4).

The hormones differ chemically and in their physiologic effect. Most hormones (e.g., ACTH, TSH, FSH, and MSH) are polypeptides, and many circulate in plasma bound to specific proteins. The steroid hormones are simpler chemicals composed of the cyclopentano-perhydro-phenanthrene ring with a myriad of side-chain substitutions and varying degrees of ring saturation, which account for their differing metabolic actions. Amino acids such as thyroxine and triiodothyronine are chemically the simplest of all. Beside variations in basic structure, hormones differ in their major roles—the "doers," which actually affect a number of metabolic processes, and the "controllers," which primarily control the secretion and production of other hormones.

Control of Hormone Production

The control of corticosteroid production is presented as a model for other control systems. Corticosteroid production requires a balance between hormones, feedback mechanisms, and releasing and inhibiting factors. Cortisol secretion by the adrenal cortex actually is controlled in the median eminence of the pituitary stalk, where the polypeptide corticotropin-releasing factor (CRF) is released into the hypophyseal portal system. CRF production increases when the concentration of glucocorticoids in plasma decreases. CRF then stimulates release of ACTH from its stores within the anterior pituitary. ACTH in turn stimulates the secretion of corticoids from the zona fasciculata of the adrenal cortex. As corticoid concentration in the blood rises, release of CRF is inhibited and, in turn, ACTH secretion diminishes. This fine homeostatic control or feedback mechanism results in the maintenance of necessary levels of corticoids for normal body function. Similar feedback mechanisms exist for the control of thyroid hormones, estrogens, and progesterone. In contrast to positive control, production of prolactin and melanocyte-stimulating hormone is normally rapid and requires inhibition rather than stimulation by hypothalamic factors. *Principle: Keep feedback mechanisms in mind when treating an endocrine disorder or using a hormone as a therapeutic tool, as therapeutic interventions undoubtedly affect these mechanisms.*

Mechanism of Action of Hormones

The complexity and variety of molecular mechanisms of action of hormones on target tissues are impressive and important to the therapist. Although they cannot be detailed in this book, they are summarized when appropriate. The complex effects of insulin are listed in part in Table 7–1; ACTH affects carbohydrate, lipid, and protein metabolism in the adrenal cortex (Forsham, 1968); TSH changes iodide transport, as well as other metabolic processes within the gland required for normal production of thyroid hormones (Ingbar and Woeber, 1968). Aldosterone and vasopressin affect sodium transport only after a number of metabolic processes, including increased RNA production and activation of an adenyl cyclase system, have been accomplished (Leaf and Coggins, 1968). *Principle: A similar clinical endocrinopathy may result from one of many abnormalities in a biochemical pathway. When hormones are used therapeutically, their effect or lack thereof may depend on the integrity of the potential pathways involved in their action. The rational use of hormones or of new drugs developed for treatment of endocrine disorders depends on a thorough knowledge of their biochemical effects.*

Table 7–1. METABOLIC EFFECTS OF INSULIN

STIMULATION OF	INHIBITION OF
Hexose transport	Glycogenolysis
Glycogen synthesis	Gluconeogenesis
Glycolysis	Lipolysis
Oxidative phosphorylation	Proteolysis
Lipogenesis	
Protein synthesis	
DNA and RNA synthesis	

Protein Binding of Hormones

Nearly all endocrine hormones are carried by specific transport proteins in the blood. They remain biologically inactive until they are transferred to peripheral effector sites. For example, cortisol is bound to a specific alpha-globulin (corticosteroid-binding globulin [CBG] or transcortin) with a molecular weight of approximately 52,000. The binding is specific, in that cortisol and progesterone are bound with high affinity, but aldosterone is bound only weakly. Ordinarily, saturation of CBG binding sites occurs at a plasma concentration of cortisol of approximately 20 to 30 $\mu g/100$ ml, and the physiologic effects of the hormone are not seen unless the concentrations exceed that value. However, plasma binding of cortisol depends on the concentrations of CBG and cortisol in the plasma. Each factor has several determinants. As CBG is produced by the liver, chronic liver disease may decrease CBG's production or catabolism, leading to unpredictable changes in plasma concentrations. Some changes in CBG or cortisol binding are predictable. Estrogens increase CBG formation, leading to increased concentrations in blood and increased binding capacity for cortisol; progesterone may displace cortisol from the CBG binding sites, resulting in increased concentrations of free cortisol in the plasma. Specific protein binding has been described for thyroxine, insulin, and some of the pituitary hormones. *Principle: When drugs or hormones are used in situations where concentrations of the active agent may be unpredictable or variable, objectives of therapy must be well defined and frequent measurements must be made of reliable variables affected by the drug. Only by setting clear goals and objectively assessing progress can the dose and dose interval be adjusted, efficacy assured, and toxicity avoided.*

Hormone Preparations and Their Practical Use

Unlike many other areas of therapeutics, the treatment of endocrinologic diseases is largely dependent on the use of hormone preparations derived from animal and human sources. The standardization of these preparations is often based on relatively nonspecific bioassay techniques. Therefore, potency of various preparations may vary from batch to batch, and instability of the active ingredients is often a problem. These factors must be considered in evaluating the effectiveness of all nonsynthetic hormone preparations. Fortunately the development of many synthetic hormones in the past decade has obviated many of these disadvantages.

Many polypeptide hormones that are derived from animal sources may be antigenic for man. This has led to the development of significant allergic reactions and sometimes to resistance to exogenous hormone action. An example of this problem is discussed in the section on pancreatic disorders. The practical use of many hormones is dependent on their ability to be absorbed and transported across cell membranes, a factor especially important in the use of polypeptide hormones. *Principle: The practical use of hormonal preparations must take into account the source, methods of production, stability, standardization procedures, and host reactions to the particular preparation.*

Diseases Caused by Excess Hormone Production

Hyperfunction of endocrine tissues is studied early by most students of medicine, perhaps because of the characteristic clinical picture presented by most patients with excessive production of a hormone. Thyrotoxicosis, acromegaly, Cushing's syndrome, and hyperparathyroidism are but a few of the endocrine hyperfunction states in which the physiology of hormone action can be correlated accurately with the clinical manifestations of the disease. Diagnosis of these disorders has been greatly simplified in the past decade by the development of highly sensitive and specific techniques for hormone assay in various fluids. This rapidly expanding area of research in clinical endocrinology should lead to the complete characterization of a patient's "hormone profile" by rapid examination of small samples of blood and urine. Diagnosis of an endocrine hyperfunction state may soon be greatly assisted by the autoanalyzer and computer, removing much of the excitement in diagnosis from this intriguing area of endocrinology. These aids will presumably be helpful in monitoring the response to therapy.

The causes of excessive hormone production by endocrine tissues are three: inflammatory disease, neoplastic disease, and hyperplasia. The least frequent of these mechanisms, inflammation, is exemplified by the rare appearance of symptoms of thyrotoxicosis in cases of thyroiditis. More commonly, inflammatory disease leads to endocrine hypofunction. Neoplastic involvement of the endocrine system is a common cause of hyperfunction. This may be benign (e.g., parathyroid adenoma) or malignant (e.g., adrenal-cell carcinoma). Hyperplasia as a cause of excessive hormone production is generally rarer than neoplasia and may be primary, as in some cases of thyrotoxicosis, or secondary, as in hyperparathyroidism secondary to chronic renal disease. Glandular hyperplasia may be due to excessive trophic hormone production, as in certain cases of Cushing's syndrome associated with adrenal hyperplasia, and treatment of this disorder may be directed toward the pituitary rather than toward the adrenals. Numerous syndromes of hormone excess may be seen in patients with nonendocrine malignant tumors; Cushing's syndrome is found in patients with oat-cell carcinoma of the lung due to excessive ACTH production by the undifferentiated tumor cells. Severe hypoglycemia may occur in patients with massive retroperitoneal sarcomas, in some cases owing to production by the tumor of an insulin-like substance. This group of paraendocrine syndromes associated with tumors of nonendocrine origin emphasizes the need to examine all patients with endocrine hyperfunction for nonendocrine as well as endocrine neoplasia. *Principle: Treatment of diseases caused by excess hormone production must be guided by a thorough understanding of the mechanisms involved in the overproduction of the particular hormone.*

Diseases Caused by Deficient Hormone Production

Endocrine deficiency states usually represent well-defined clinical entities. Diagnosis is based on the demonstration of specific hormone lack or on provocative tests used to stress the gland in question (e.g., the ACTH stimulation test). The causes of endocrine hypofunction are more numerous than the causes of hyperfunction. Hypothyroidism is seen in many cases of Hashimoto's thyroiditis, diabetes mellitus in chronic pancreatitis, and occasionally hypogonadism following mumps orchitis. The replacement of glandular tissue by either neoplastic or granulomatous tissue results in several endocrine deficiency states (e.g., hypopituitarism, due to sarcoidosis involving the pituitary, and adrenal insufficiency, resulting from tuberculosis or neoplastic involvement of the adrenals). Genetic defects may cause endocrine hypofunction, as evidenced by the enzyme deficiency states that produce goitrous cretinism, the adrenogenital syndrome, and the hypogonadal states produced by sex chromosome abnormalities. Since Albright recognized that pseudohypoparathyroidism represented target organ resistance to parathormone's activity, this mechanism of endocrine dysfunction has received wider study and confirmation. The number of "idiopathic" endocrine deficiency states emphasizes the need for continued study. The roles of autoimmunity, rapid hormone inactivation, excessive hormone binding to serum proteins, and production of biologically inactive (but immunologically active) hormones as mechanisms for endocrine deficiency syndromes require extensive investigation. *Principle: Although the treatment of endocrine hypofunction states may often be simple hormonal replacement, an understanding of the basic mechanism of the hypofunction may lead to more rational therapy directed toward the correction of the underlying pathogenetic abnormality.*

Drug-Induced Endocrine Abnormalities

Iatrogenic disorders are a growing fraction of the endocrinologist's practice. To a large extent the consultative function of the endocrinologist involves the evaluation and treatment of drug-induced endocrinopathies. Exogenously induced Cushing's syndrome is more frequently seen than the other causes of adrenal hyperfunction. The excessive and often unwarranted use of corticosteroids has done more to elucidate the importance of the pituitary-adrenal axis and its feedback mechanisms than many of the planned investigations of the past 20 years. The hypoglycemic states associated with sulfonylurea therapy have been useful in defining the mechanisms controlling insulin secretion and the importance of drug interactions in the therapy of endocrine disorders. Similarly, the hyperglycemia following therapy with thiazide diuretics has led to important studies of the prediabetic state, the role of cations in insulin secretion, and the peripheral actions of these drugs. In reviews of endocrine hyperfunction states, every differential diagnosis list includes iatrogenic causes: hypoglycemia, hyperthyroidism, Cushing's disease, gynecomastia, and hypervitaminosis D, to name but a few. *Principle: The frequent inappropriate use of therapeutic agents in the treatment of endocrine disorders has helped to advance knowledge of the mechanisms of hormone action and the control of endocrine function. Knowledge gained from such clinical models has been instrumental in the more rational use of these agents in the treatment of endocrine and nonendocrine abnormalities.*

CATEGORIES OF DRUGS AND THERAPEUTIC PRINCIPLES

By far the most important therapeutic role of the endocrinologist is the guidance of hormonal replacement therapy. For this to be accomplished successfully and accurately, a thorough understanding of the pathogenesis of the endocrine disorder and of the clinical pharmacology of the hormone is essential. This latter aspect includes pharmacokinetic as well as pharmacologic actions of the particular hormone. Treatment of the newly diagnosed diabetic patient must take into account the underlying mechanism of the hyperglycemia as well as the mechanism of action of the various hypoglycemic agents. The gastrointestinal absorption of thyroid hormone preparations is important in the therapy of myxedema. Estrogen therapy of the patient on corticosteroid replacement may affect plasma binding of cortisol and warrant adjustment of drug dosage. Problems of proper hormone replacement are discussed extensively in later sections of this chapter.

A second major role of the endocrinologist is the control of excessive hormone production in endocrine hyperfunction states. An example of drug therapy for hyperfunction of an endocrine gland is the use of the thioamide drugs (such as propylthiouracil) to control the clinical manifestations of hyperthyroidism. Despite the controversial aspects of this mode of long-term therapy, its use in the initial therapy of hyperthyroidism, often before or concurrent with other definitive measures, is well accepted. Most other drugs for the treatment of excessive hormone production have enjoyed little of the acceptance of the thioamide compounds. The alpha- and beta-adrenergic blocking drugs have been useful in the preoperative therapy of patients with pheochromocytoma. Alloxan, a specific poison of pancreatic islet cells, has been used, mostly unsuccessfully, in the treatment of islet-cell carcinomas. An analog of amphenone, o,p'-DDD, has been administered with varying success to patients with adrenal carcinomas. The use of peripheral antagonists to insulin, such as growth hormone, and the inhibition of insulin secretion by diazoxide have both proved useful in small numbers of patients with various hypoglycemic states. *Principle: Although generally less successful than simple hormonal replacement therapy, the use of drugs for the control of excessive hormone production is important in the treatment of certain endocrine hyperfunction states.*

A unique form of therapy for certain endocrine disorders is the stimulation of secretion of one hormone by the administration of its appropriate trophic hormone. The most widely used example of this form of therapy is the administration of ACTH to stimulate corticosteroid release from the adrenal cortex. Discussions of ACTH use are encountered frequently throughout this book, as this type of hormonal therapy is popular among gastroenterologists, neurologists, and hematologists. However, endocrinologists have utilized ACTH more as a diagnostic preparation than as a therapeutic tool. TSH and chorionic gonadotropin are additional trophic hormones useful in specific endocrinologic situations. In contrast to this mode of therapy, the recent application of estrogens and progestins as birth control preparations represents inhibition of trophic hormone release as a means of specific therapy. The opposite effect may be elicited by clomiphene. The use of thyroid hormones to diminish TSH secretion in thyroid cancer is an additional example of this type of therapy. *Principle: Knowledge of control mechanisms important for normal hormone secretion is essential for the rational use of trophic*

hormones or of agents that interfere with normal feedback mechanisms.

An important use of many of the hormones and drugs to be discussed in this chapter is in the diagnosis of endocrine dysfunction. A wide variety of stimulatory and inhibitory tests utilizing natural feedback mechanisms have been developed over the past 20 years. Of the pituitary hormones, both ACTH and TSH stimulation tests have been useful in separating primary from secondary hypofunction of the adrenal cortex and thyroid, respectively. The availability of purified gonadotropin preparations should allow the use of these hormones to test gonadal function. Chorionic gonadotropin administration forms the basis of a test for testicular Leydig-cell function. Tolbutamide is now widely used as a test for islet-cell function in the diagnosis of both diabetes and islet-cell adenomas.

An understanding of the adrenal-pituitary feedback mechanisms has led to the use of dexamethasone administration as a test for the suppressibility of ACTH release. Metyrapone, by inhibiting cortisol synthesis within the adrenal, leads to enhanced secretion of corticotropin-releasing factor (CRF), which in turn stimulates ACTH output from the anterior pituitary. Administration of triiodothyronine in large doses for several days leads to inhibition of pituitary TSH release and a consequent fall in thyroidal uptake of ^{131}I in normal patients. In thyrotoxicosis T_3 administration fails to reduce the increased ^{131}I uptake, synthesis, and release of thyroid hormone.

The effect of hormones on peripheral tissues has also been used to diagnose a variety of conditions. Glucagon administration leads to increased glycogenolysis, a prompt rise in blood glucose, and an increase in serum insulin levels by a direct effect on pancreatic islets. Failure of the blood glucose to rise after glucagon administration may be due to deficient hepatic glycogen stores or to a specific metabolic block in glycogenolysis, as occurs in the glycogen-storage diseases. Insulin-induced hypoglycemia is useful in studying growth hormone and ACTH secretion, gastric acid production, and the responsiveness of peripheral tissues to insulin. The response of the renal tubules to parathormone forms the basis for the differentiation of parathormone deficiency from tissue unresponsiveness to parathormone.

In the diagnosis of some thyroid hypofunction states the administration of potassium thiocyanate at the time of ^{131}I testing is a useful diagnostic tool. The thiocyanate ion, which competes with the trapping mechanism for iodine, displaces

[131]I from a gland previously labeled with [131]I. The amount of ^{131}I displaced depends on the utilization of the iodide. In the event of a metabolic block in organification of iodine, increased amounts of ^{131}I are displaced by the thiocyanate. *Principle: As with the therapeutic use of hormonal agents and other drugs in the treatment of endocrine abnormalities, an understanding of normal physiologic mechanisms of endocrine function has led to the wide applicability of these agents in the diagnosis of endocrine diseases.*

THE PANCREAS

Proper therapy of disorders of pancreatic islet-cell function relies on a thorough understanding of the hormones produced by these cells and of the factors controlling hormone synthesis and secretion.

Human pancreatic insulin is composed of two polypeptide chains bound by two disulfide bridges (Sanger, 1959). The A chain has 21 amino acids and an intrachain disulfide bridge between amino acids 6 and 11. The B chain is composed of 30 amino acids. Differences between mammalian species of insulin occur primarily at amino acids 8, 9, and 10 of the A chain and at amino acid 30 of the B chain. Pig insulin differs from human insulin only in the substitution of alanine for threonine in position 30 of the B chain (Smith, 1966).

Although the biologically active center of insulin is unknown, the area between amino acids 6 and 11, in the intrachain disulfide bridge area of the A chain, may be important in the binding of insulin to muscle and other tissues. The disulfide bridge must be intact for full biologic activity, as reduction of the disulfide groups inactivates insulin. Esterification of carboxyl groups and modification of the phenolic hydroxyl and imidazolyl groups also lead to loss of activity (Williams, 1968).

The antigenic determinants of insulin appear to be present in the A chain, particularly involving amino acids 8, 9, and 10 (Prout, 1963). Although amino acids 23 to 30 in the B chain are essential for full biologic activity, they are not necessary for antigenicity. Tertiary structure may also be important, since dealaninated pig insulin, which is identical to human insulin except for the absence of the final amino acid in the B chain, retains its antigenicity in man. Antigenicity is also dependent upon secondary structure and polymer formation.

Aggregation of insulin molecules in solution depends upon temperature, pH, and zinc content. Since extraction methods for insulin remove zinc, this ion must be added for crystallization of the hormone. Insulin, with an isoelectric point of 5.3, is relatively insoluble between pH 4 and 7. Below pH 3.5, molecules of insulin in heated solutions aggregate to form fibers, which are then stable at pH values from 0 to 10. Fibril formation is inhibited by disruption of the disulfide bridges.

The discovery of a precursor of insulin, known as proinsulin, in pancreatic preparations and blood has shed light on the early synthesis of the insulin molecule (Steiner et al., 1967). Proinsulin has a molecular weight of approximately 9000, and contains 104 amino acids in a single continuous polypeptide chain, connected by two disulfide bridges; it is now thought to be the precursor of the normal storage form of insulin (Frank and Veros, 1968). Islet cell granule formation follows proinsulin synthesis; a "C" peptide of 33 amino acids is split from the proinsulin molecule in granules ready for secretion (Steiner et al., 1967). Although the "C" peptide is biologically inactive, proinsulin demonstrates a biologic activity approximately one-tenth that of insulin in *in vitro* test systems (Steiner et al., 1968; Kitabchi, 1970). Although proinsulin is not normally secreted into the blood in significant quantities, numerous laboratories are now engaged in the assay of this less active form of insulin in various clinical states associated with glucose intolerance (Chance and Ellis, 1969; Fineberg and Merimee, 1970).

Factors affecting insulin secretion are listed in Table 7–2. The most important stimulus for insulin secretion appears to be increased blood concentrations of glucose (Grodsky and Bennett, 1966). This

Table 7–2. FACTORS AFFECTING INSULIN SECRETION

Stimulation
Glucose and other monosaccharides
Amino acids
Fatty acids
Ketones
Cations—Ca^{++}, Mg^{++}, K^+
Glucagon
Growth hormone
Placental lactogen
ACTH
Secretin
Gastrin
Pancreozymin
Sulfonylurea drugs
Isoproterenol
Phentolamine
Inhibition
2-Deoxyglucose
Insulin
Epinephrine
Norepinephrine
Diazoxide

hexose causes immediate release of stored insulin within seconds after intravenous administration, and *in vitro* studies show that release of insulin ceases within 1 minute after glucose perfusion of the isolated pancreas is discontinued. Glucose also causes an increase in the synthesis of pancreatic insulin (Jarrett et al., 1967). In addition to glucose, several other sugars are capable of increasing insulin secretion, including fructose, galactose, ribose, and mannose, whereas 2-deoxyglucose and D-mannoheptulose both decrease insulin secretion (Haist,

1965). Stimulation of insulin release by fructose cannot be demonstrated in patients with hereditary fructose intolerance, suggesting that conversion of fructose to glucose or its glycolytic intermediates is necessary for this action of fructose (Frohman, 1969). On the other hand, fructose stimulates insulin secretion in patients with glucose-6-phosphatase deficiency, suggesting that glycolytic intermediates are more important than glucose itself in stimulating release of insulin (Hug and Schubert, 1967).

Insulin secretion is also stimulated by protein ingestion and administration of essential amino acids (Floyd et al., 1966). All the essential amino acids are capable of this stimulatory effect, although arginine is the most potent. The mechanism of stimulation is not entirely known, but, in general, amino-acid-stimulated insulin secretion is not suppressed by inhibitors of glucose-stimulated insulin release (e.g., epinephrine) (Rabinowitz et al., 1966). Leucine acts differently in this regard; its stimulatory effect appears to be similar to that of glucose, being enhanced by sulfonylurea therapy and decreased by inhibitors of glucose-mediated insulin release (Fajans et al., 1967). Amino acid infusion tests have been utilized to elicit hypoglycemic reactions as a diagnostic maneuver in islet-cell tumors and infantile hypoglycemic states.

Both long- and short-chain fatty acids, as well as ketone bodies, are capable of stimulating insulin release in experimental conditions (Linscheer et al., 1967; Manns and Boda, 1967). Although the increased release of insulin in response to long-chain fatty acids has been suggested as a mechanism by which insulin controls the rate of lipolysis, little is known about the physiologic role of these acids in insulin secretion. Hyperlipidemic states are usually associated with glucose intolerance, possibly by means of peripheral antagonism of insulin's effects by lipids.

Certain cations, particularly calcium, magnesium, and potassium, may play an important role in the normal release of insulin in response to glucose administration (Milner and Hales, 1968). The glucose intolerance sometimes found in potassium-depleted patients may be secondary to this mechanism. In addition, sodium is necessary for insulin release in response to glucose and other stimuli.

Central nervous system control of insulin secretion has been studied for many years with few conclusive results (Frohman et al., 1966, 1967a). In the dog, insulin secretion is increased by vagal stimulation, an effect that can be blocked by atropine. Insulin concentration in plasma is also elevated after destruction of the ventromedial nucleus of the hypothalamus in weanling rats (Frohman and Bernardis, 1968). However, the transplanted, denervated pancreas is capable of insulin secretion (Frohman, 1967a). The physiologic role of the central nervous system in insulin secretion is not known.

Glucagon stimulation of insulin secretion is independent of its hyperglycemic action, since it occurs in patients with glucose-6-phosphatase deficiency who do not have a hyperglycemic response following glucagon administration (Samols et al.,

1965; Crockford et al., 1966). The stimulatory effect of glucagon on insulin secretion may be mediated by stimulation of the adenyl cyclase system, leading to increased levels of adenosine 3′,5′-monophosphate (cyclic AMP). Since conditions that favor insulin secretion inhibit glucagon secretion, the physiologic importance of glucagon-stimulated insulin release has been questioned. Catecholamines may also regulate insulin secretion (Porte et al., 1966; Porte, 1967). Epinephrine and norepinephrine inhibit insulin release from the pancreas, whereas isoproterenol stimulates its release. The increase in insulin secretion following alpha-receptor blockade with phentolamine, and the inhibition of isoproterenol-stimulated insulin release with the beta blocker propranolol, has suggested that alpha receptors are inhibitory for insulin release and beta receptors are stimulatory. Direct inhibition of insulin secretion in vitro has also been demonstrated for epinephrine and norepinephrine (Malaisse et al., 1967). Although the physiologic importance of these effects is not entirely known, under normal conditions the inhibitory alpha effect appears to predominate. Chemical diabetes is a regular finding in patients with a pheochromocytoma.

Growth hormone appears to enhance normal insulin secretion in response to glucose, although no direct stimulatory effect of growth hormone on insulin secretion can be demonstrated (Frohman, 1969). This may be important in growth-hormone deficiency, since in this condition the decreased insulin release in response to glucose can be corrected within minutes by growth hormone administration (Frohman et al., 1967b). Growth hormone has a diabetogenic action, causing hyperglycemia, and hypoglycemia occurs occasionally in its absence. In some cases of growth hormone deficiency, relative insulinopenia following a glucose load has been observed (Rabinowitz et al., 1968). Human placental lactogen may have an effect similar to that of growth hormone (Beck and Daughaday, 1967). ACTH stimulation of insulin secretion may be mediated by the adenyl cyclase system, but further studies are necessary to document this (Lebovitz and Pooler, 1967). The effects of oxytocin, vasopressin, and angiotensin in altering insulin secretion may represent effects on pancreatic blood flow (Kaneto et al., 1967). Oral contraceptive agents increase insulin secretion in response to intravenous glucose without altering the rate of glucose disappearance (Spellacy et al., 1967). Effects of estrogens on growth-hormone secretion make evaluation of these findings difficult.

The greater output of insulin in response to oral administration of glucose, compared to intravenous glucose administration, has suggested a role for gastrointestinal hormones in the control of insulin secretion. Secretin, pancreozymin, gastrin, and intestinal glucagon all stimulate pancreatic insulin release (Dupre et al., 1966; Meade et al., 1967; Unger et al., 1967; Mahler and Weisberg, 1968). Although secretin administration can affect insulin secretion, the observation that intraduodenal administration of acid, a potent stimulus for release of secretin, does not stimulate insulin release has raised questions about the physiologic importance of these studies (McIntyre *et al.*, 1965). Further study of the effects of these intestinal factors is necessary before their physiologic role can be assessed.

Hormonal effects on insulin secretion are numerous but difficult to evaluate for clinical relevance because of the pharmacologic doses used in many of the studies. As with other stimuli of insulin secretion, the importance of hormones in the normal physiologic control of this process cannot be completely determined at the present time. A therapeutic approach to any state related to abnormal glucose tolerance must consider possible abnormalities in any of the control mechanisms. Therapy is unjustified until these factors have been assessed.

The rational therapy of clinical states associated with disorders of carbohydrate tolerance is also dependent on an understanding of those factors that affect the peripheral action of insulin. Perhaps the most important inhibitors of peripheral insulin action are those humoral factors which also affect the secretion of insulin. Many of these hormones have dual effects on insulin action, which in some cases potentiate and in some antagonize one another. Glucagon stimulates glycogenolysis and lipolysis; the latter effect antagonizes insulin's action on glucose uptake in muscle. Epinephrine, however, has actions similar to glucagon on glycogenolysis and lipolysis, but unlike glucagon it inhibits insulin secretion from the pancreas. The net effect of glucocorticoids on glucose tolerance is complicated by the numerous metabolic effects of these hormones, particularly an increase in gluconeogenesis, ketogenesis, and lipolysis, and a decrease in peripheral glucose utilization. In clinical states associated with excessive endogenous glucocorticoid synthesis or with exogenous administration of glucocorticoids, glucose intolerance is worsened.

Although all the pituitary hormones affect carbohydrate tolerance in man, the most potent in this regard are growth hormone and ACTH. Their effect on glucose tolerance is complex and is related to the many metabolic factors altered by these hormones. Growth hormone stimulates lipolysis, leading to an increase in serum free fatty acids and subsequent inhibition of glucose uptake, particularly in muscle (Williams, 1968). In addition, growth hormone increases gluconeogenesis and protein synthesis, the latter effect being considerably greater in the presence of insulin. ACTH is lipolytic and ketogenic and increases insulin secretion (Lebovitz and Pooler, 1967). Although the pituitary hormones can individually affect glucose tolerance, their combined effects are usually additive. Thyroxine increases gluconeogenesis, proteolysis, glycogenolysis, and glucose uptake in peripheral tissues (Frohman, 1969). The net effect of these changes is usually diabetogenic. Oxytocin stimulates lipogenesis and increases glucose utilization (Williams, 1968).

In addition to these humoral agents, there are a number of nonhormonal insulin antagonists. Vallance-Owen demonstrated a substance capable of antagonizing insulin action on rat diaphragm in the serum of normals and diabetics (Vallance-Owen, 1965). The substance responsible for this antagonism migrated with the albumin peak during serum electrophoresis and was named synalbumin. An increased amount of synalbumin was found in most diabetic subjects and in a large number of clinically nondiabetic relatives of diabetics, suggesting that the excessive synalbumin synthesis was inherited as an autosomal dominant trait. More recent evidence suggests that synalbumin may be the B chain of insulin complexed with albumin (Fenichel *et al.*, 1966). Other investigators have both confirmed and denied this hypothesis. The demonstration that the Visking dialysis tubing used in the original studies contains a substance that antagonizes insulin and combines with albumin has raised questions about the validity of the original observations (Ensinck *et al.*, 1967). More evaluation of this subject is necessary before synalbumin's physiologic and pharmacologic role in diabetes can be determined.

Additional antagonists of insulin have been found in the serum of certain diabetics. Field and co-workers described a protein antagonist of insulin in some patients with diabetic ketoacidosis that disappeared slowly following treatment of the ketoacidotic state (Field and Stetten, 1956). Similar antagonists have been described in diabetics with severe infection and in acromegalic patients with glucose intolerance. The clinical importance of these antagonists has not been fully defined.

The single most widely studied factor affecting peripheral action is insulin antibodies (Shipp *et al.*, 1965). Circulating antibodies to exogenous insulin can be demonstrated in all diabetic subjects who have received therapy with any preparation of insulin for more than a few weeks (Berson and Yalow, 1966). Although such antibodies are capable of binding to circulating insulin, they may not reduce the biologic effectiveness of the endogenous hormone (Berson and Yalow, 1964). The only clinical situation in which insulin antibodies are significantly important is the syndrome of chronic insulin resistance. In this situation, high titers of neutralizing antibodies to insulin may result in a tremendous insulin requirement. As these antibodies appear to be species specific, treatment of these patients with pork or fish insulin, rather than beef insulin, may effectively reduce the insulin requirement (Akre *et al.*, 1964). Corticosteroid therapy has also been effective in some patients with chronic insulin resistance (Shipp *et al.*, 1965), although the capacity of serum globulins to bind insulin may not be affected by this treatment. The exact mechanism whereby corticosteroids are effective in this circumstance is not understood. Although many attempts have been made to implicate insulin antibodies in the etiology of the diabetic state, there appears to be no conclusive evidence to support a causal relationship of these antibodies to the genesis of diabetes mellitus.

Other factors may affect peripheral insulin action. Severe acidosis (arterial blood pH values of 7.1 or less) may interfere with insulin activity. Excessive serum osmolality can increase glucose uptake and oxidation and stimulate lipogenesis in adipose tissue (Kuzuya *et al.*, 1965). Certain cations, particularly Na^+, K^+, Ca^{++}, and Zn^{++}, may affect insulin activity under certain experimental conditions (Grodsky and Bennett, 1966). Although the exact role of these factors in alterations of glucose tolerance in normal and diabetic subjects is not fully understood, the limited information available should be borne in mind in treatment of diabetes mellitus. Failure of the patient to respond in the predicted manner may indicate the presence of another abnormality.

Treatment of Diabetes Mellitus

Although the dietary treatment of diabetes mellitus will not be discussed in detail, certain basic principles of dietary management deserve comment (Hamwi, 1964). Calorie intake should be tailored to the needs of the individual who should maintain a normal body weight. This is particularly important in young diabetics and diabetic women during pregnancy. The obese diabetic should be given a diet to allow significant weight loss. In some mildly obese diabetics, weight reduction is often associated with improvement in glucose tolerance sufficient to obviate the need for insulin therapy. In general, small feedings given frequently throughout the day are preferable to large feedings, to avoid wide "swings" in blood sugar. This may be particularly useful in the brittle juvenile diabetic. Some investigators have recommended that carbohydrate be supplied chiefly as large polymers such as starch rather than as monosaccharides or disaccharides, or that a large proportion of the diet be in the form of protein. In each instance, smaller swings in the glucose concentration in blood result. Because attempts to restrict rigidly the amount of carbohydrate in the diet often result in diets unnecessarily high in fat, strict limitations of carbohydrate intake should probably be avoided. *The most important therapeutic principle should be to maintain an ideal body weight while attempting to control large variations in the glucose concentration in blood.*

Insulin Therapy. Insulin preparations generally used in the United States are outlined in Table 7–3. The major differences among these preparations relate to their length of action, the pH of the buffer used, and the presence of binding proteins that affect their duration of action (Peck, 1964). Crystalline zinc insulin is a clear solution that may be mixed with most other preparations. NPH and lente preparations should not be mixed, because the phosphate buffer of the NPH solution disrupts the solubilities of the lente crystals in acetate buffer (Peck, 1964). Note that the duration of action of ultralente and PZI insulin is greater than 36 hours, which makes utilization of these preparations more difficult on a once-a-day schedule. The most useful and popular preparations for single daily therapy are NPH and lente insulins. Since lente insulin contains no exogenous binding protein and may therefore be less allergic than NPH, some physicians prefer this preparation to NPH. There is, however, no evidence that the biologic effects of these preparations or their long-term effects on blood sugar are significantly different.

Intermediate-acting insulin is usually administered once daily, 1/2 hour before breakfast (Ricketts, 1964). The dose is determined by the presence or absence of symptoms of hyperglycemia or hypoglycemia, and by the results of urine and blood tests for glucose. Some physicians prefer the use of crystalline insulin given two to four times per day, usually before meals (Oakley, 1968). This dosage schedule has obvious disadvantages: frequent injections are needed, and there is greater likelihood of hypoglycemic reactions and of wide "swings" in the concentration of glucose in blood during the day. For these reasons crystalline insulin therapy is usually reserved for cooperative, intelligent patients who are willing to administer frequent injections and who can be followed closely and conveniently. Proponents of the multiple-daily-dose schedule of treatment emphasize its physiologic advantages as compared with single-daily-dose schedules. Since glucose concentrations in blood fluctuate normally between fasting and postprandial states, frequent doses of crystalline insulin produce a blood sugar response closer to the normal subject's than does single-dose therapy (although admittedly at higher blood sugar concentrations, and with wider "swings"). No convincing evidence demonstrates that any particular dose regimen is likely to prevent the long-term complications of diabetes. In the absence of unequivocal demonstration of superiority of a single preparation or dosage schedule for the insulins, the physician may select the drug form, degree of control, and dosage schedule felt to be optimal for the individual patient. This selection may take into consideration the patient's ability to cooperate, his age (juvenile diabetics being "brittle"; old patients tolerating hypoglycemia poorly), and other factors outlined below.

Because insulin therapy alone cannot prevent the progress of atherosclerosis or other vascular complications of diabetes, realistic objectives should be set for its use. Most important, the therapist should avoid detrimental hypoglycemic episodes. Positive overall objectives for the use of insulin are to protect the patient from ketoacidosis and to allow him to live as normal

Table 7–3. MAJOR INSULIN PREPARATIONS

TYPE	BUFFER	pH	MAXIMUM ACTION IN HOURS	DURATION OF ACTION IN HOURS
Rapid acting				
Crystalline zinc	None	2.5–3.5	4–6	6–8
Semilente	Acetate	7.1–7.5	4–6	12–16
Intermediate acting				
NPH	Phosphate	7.1–7.4	8–12	18–24
Globin	None	3.4–3.8	6–10	12–18
Lente	Acetate	7.1–7.5	8–12	18–24
Long acting				
Protamine zinc	Phosphate	7.1–7.4	14–20	24–36
Ultralente	Acetate	7.1–7.5	16–18	30–36

a life as possible. When the therapist concentrates on narrow and precise management of the glucose concentrations in blood, he often is only treating himself and making the patient's life miserable. Above all, the therapist must not inadvertently complicate the disease course by unnecessarily introducing drugs that make management impossible, or mistake sudden unmanageable swings in blood glucose concentrations as disease induced when additional drugs are responsible for the problem.

Indications for Insulin Therapy. Insulin is required for the treatment of most juvenile diabetics to prevent ketosis, maintain the patient free of symptoms, help maintain ideal body weight, and assist in the prevention of certain complications, particularly infections of the skin, vagina, and urinary tract. For example, the incidence of urinary tract infections in diabetic subjects is directly related to the amount of glucose excreted in the urine per 24 hours (Cahill, 1966). Similar relationships for skin and vaginal infections have been claimed (Cahill, 1966). Insulin is also useful in the control of symptoms in patients with diabetes secondary to pancreatectomy and chronic pancreatitis, and in some maturity-onset diabetics who fail to respond to oral hypoglycemic therapy.

The prevention of other complications of diabetes by insulin therapy has been argued since the advent of this method of treatment. Although a number of studies have suggested that rigid control of the blood glucose concentration forestalls the onset of vascular complications, most were inappropriately controlled and inadequately designed. At the present time "there is as yet no scientifically acceptable evidence that any particular form of treatment is better than any other" for the prevention of these complications (Bondy, 1966). The papers of Marble, Bondy, and Cahill provide an excellent discussion of this topic (Bondy, 1966; Cahill, 1966; Marble, 1966).

Special Problems in the Treatment of Diabetes. BRITTLE DIABETES. "Brittle" diabetes refers to the wide variations in blood glucose concentration seen in some juvenile diabetics treated with insulin (Knowles, 1964). These patients often are precariously balanced between severe hypoglycemic reactions and episodes of ketoacidosis. The cause of this variation is generally unknown, but changes in diet and exercise, inaccuracies in insulin administration (sometimes because the patient is blind), mild infections, and emotional factors have been incriminated. Changes in the concentration of circulating insulin antibodies have also been suspected. Of these factors occult infection is the most common, and careful examination for occult infections, such as sinusitis, osteomyelitis, and prostatitis, is necessary in all patients with apparent insulin resistance.

The treatment of the brittle diabetic is difficult and frustrating because of the uncertainties of causal factors. A number of treatment programs have met with some success in individual patients. Attempts should be made to control physical activity and diet. The use of frequent small feedings throughout the day and evening is particularly useful in this circumstance. Single-dose insulin therapy is usually more difficult to use in these patients than is some form of divided-dose therapy. Three types of divided-dose therapy have been employed:

1. Frequent injections of crystalline insulin usually given 1/2 hour before each meal, the dose being dependent on the amount of glucose in urine. This concentration is best determined by emptying the bladder 1 hour before the dose, then testing the urine collected in the subsequent 1/2 hour ("true spot" specimens). With

this "rainbow" type of schedule a predetermined number of units of insulin is administered for each degree (1+ to 4+) of glycosuria. Further dose modifications may be linked to the presence or absence of urinary ketone bodies in the specimen. The amount prescribed for an individual patient depends on his prior needs and on complicating features such as diet or infection. An average "rainbow" insulin dose schedule would be: urine glucose 0 to 1+, no insulin; urine glucose 2+, 5 units; 3+, 10 units; 4+, 20 units; if ketones present, add 5 units to dose. The range of insulin requirements is quite wide in individual patients; this schedule is an example, not a rule, for use of the "rainbow" method.

2. Combinations of intermediate- and short-acting insulin. Part of the daily insulin requirement is administered as an intermediate-acting preparation and additional doses of short-acting preparations are added, depending on results of urine tests.

3. Split dosage of intermediate-acting insulin providing approximately two-thirds of the daily requirement in the morning and one-third in the early evening, usually just before supper. This form of therapy requires precautions against early-morning hypoglycemia, usually by ingesting late-evening snacks containing protein or large-polymer polysaccharides.

None of these forms of therapy is universally successful in the brittle diabetic subject, and careful trial and error is usually necessary to determine the most acceptable method.

The patient whose insulin requirement appears to be steadily increasing without obtaining successful control may exhibit the Somogyi effect (Perkoff and Tyler, 1954). In some juvenile diabetic subjects, when single morning urine tests are utilized to guide insulin dosage, increasing the dose of insulin often is used to "cover" persistently positive urine tests for glucose. In some of these patients, unnoticed hypoglycemic reactions may occur during the early morning or late evening, leading to excessive catecholamine release in response to the hypoglycemia. This in turn leads to a subsequent hyperglycemia and positive urine glucose tests, particularly in the early morning. In these patients, less insulin rather than more insulin is required to avoid the hypoglycemic reactions and the associated hyperglycemia. Careful questioning of patients for subtle symptoms of hypoglycemia (morning headache, night sweats, paresthesias, frequent nightmares) and frequent blood glucose determinations (sometimes during the evening hours) are important in determining the presence of the Somogyi effect.

DIABETIC KETOACIDOSIS. Space does not permit a complete analysis of the complex metabolic alterations that occur in this condition. Interested readers are referred to several recent reviews (Sheldon and Pyke, 1968; Williams, 1968; Kiraly et al., 1970). Certain aspects of the initial therapy of ketoacidosis deserve comment and illustrate principles of therapeutics:

1. Insulin therapy. Patients with diabetic ketoacidosis have an absolute deficiency of insulin, as well as some resistance to the peripheral actions of insulin caused by a number of factors. Insulin requirements in the first 12 to 24 hours of treatment frequently reach 500 to 1000 units. In most patients who have previously received insulin treatment, some degree of insulin binding to neutralizing antibody can be anticipated. This leads to some resistance to insulin in the early phases of treatment and may be followed several days later by hypoglycemic reactions thought to be due to release of insulin from antibody. Direct proof for this mechanism is lacking.

Patients with diabetic ketoacidosis usually require much more insulin than patients with hyperosmolar, nonketotic, diabetic coma (Williams, 1968). The frequency and size of individual doses of insulin must be related not only to the blood glucose concentration but also to serial dilutions of the patient's serum for ketone bodies. If ketones are present at serum dilutions of 1:8 to 1:16, a large insulin dose is necessary. As serum ketone concentrations diminish, the dose of insulin is reduced. Intravenous insulin is given every 1 to 2 hours, depending on the urgency of the clinical situation. Further details of management are included in the programmed case in Unit IV.

Only intravenous crystalline insulin should be used in the treatment of ketoacidosis. Because of the ability of insulin to bind nonspecifically to glass surfaces (Williams, 1968), glass bottles should not be used for intravenous administration of insulin. *Principle: Hypotension is often associated with ketoacidosis. The variability in absorption from subcutaneous sites in patients may be related to the circulatory instability and to unstable, unpredictable perfusion of the subcutaneous tissue. Therefore, this site of administration is undesirable.*

2. Intravenous fluids. Hyperosmolality and sodium depletion complicate most cases of ketoacidosis; hypotonic fluids are usually required, particularly hypotonic saline. Large amounts of fluid are necessary in the first 24 hours of treatment, and fluid deficits may be as high as 6000 ml (Kiraly et al., 1970). With the associated osmotic diuresis that occurs during much of the early period of treatment, as much as 10 to 12 liters of fluid are sometimes necessary

to re-establish fluid balance. In some instances, if the fluids are rapidly administered, rapid reversal of the hyperosmolality in the serum may be accomplished. However, the intracellular osmolality, particularly in the central nervous system, may not be corrected so quickly, and large shifts of water from the extracellular to the intracellular space may occur after the first several hours of fluid therapy, leading to worsening of central nervous system function. Indeed, death secondary to cerebral edema has been documented in some patients with hyperosmolar coma (Williams, 1968). For this reason the hyperosmolality should not be corrected too rapidly.

3. Alkali therapy. Although arterial blood pH values as low as 7.1 to 7.0 may interfere with the peripheral action of insulin (Rogers, 1958), rapid correction of the acidosis with alkali therapy may be dangerous for the same reasons as those applying to rapid correction of acidosis in uremia (see Chapter 3). Rapid alkalinization leads to movement of potassium into cells, resulting in a rapid fall in serum potassium concentrations. Very rapid decreases in serum potassium concentration in the diabetic may be difficult to correct with intravenous administration of potassium, and under these circumstances severe cardiac effects may result. Therefore, alkali therapy in ketoacidosis must be utilized extremely carefully with frequent monitoring of the electrocardiogram and measurements of the serum potassium concentration. Correction of extracellular acidosis with bicarbonate therapy does not assure simultaneous amelioration of central nervous system acidosis. Extracellular pH, bicarbonate, and pCO_2 are quickly increased after intravenous bicarbonate therapy; equilibration of blood and cerebrospinal fluid pCO_2 is rapid, but cerebrospinal fluid bicarbonate increases slowly, allowing continued or even temporarily worsened cerebrospinal fluid acidosis (Posner and Plum, 1967). Correction of acidosis should be gradual and incomplete, as correction of the ketoacidosis with insulin will eventually lead to the metabolic generation of base from betahydroxybutyrate, acetoacetate, and the like. Overly zealous correction may lead to the later appearance of a metabolic and respiratory alkalosis. If alkali therapy is to be used, sodium bicarbonate is preferable to sodium lactate because of the occasional appearance of lactic acidosis in some patients with diabetic ketoacidosis (see Chapter 3).

4. Potassium therapy. A significant fall in the serum potassium concentration attends insulin therapy in all patients with ketoacidosis (Kiraly et al., 1970). Additional potassium supplementation by the intravenous route is necessary in the treatment of nearly all patients with this syndrome. Despite elevated serum concentrations of potassium at the onset of treatment, large total-body deficits of potassium are present, often requiring administration of 200 to 400 mEq or more of potassium for balance to be re-established. The amount of potassium needed for replacement therapy and its rate of replacement are influenced by multiple determinants, such as the initial degree of depletion, effect of correction of acidosis, direct effect of insulin on cellular uptake of potassium, presence or absence of tissue hypoperfusion, continuing loss rates of potassium in the urine due to dehydration and osmotic diuresis, and the patient's renal function. In such a complex situation, the best guide to therapy is the patient's response, not some rigid estimate derived from a formula or from the patient population experience. Frequent measurements of the serum potassium concentration and its physiologic effect (electrocardiogram) for signs of hypokalemia or hyperkalemia are necessary in the early treatment of ketoacidosis.

5. Carbohydrate needs. Most patients with ketoacidosis have moderate-to-severe depletion of carbohydrate stores. Once ketoacidosis is corrected, additional carbohydrate is necessary, usually in the form of glucose. Intravenous glucose therapy can safely be administered in these patients once the blood glucose concentration is less than 300 mg/100 ml.

INSULIN RESISTANCE. The syndrome of insulin resistance may be either acute or chronic. The acute form is related to complications such as infection and other inflammatory diseases that temporarily raise the daily requirement for insulin. Adjustment of insulin dosage and proper treatment of the complications are usually sufficient to control this problem.

In contrast, chronic insulin resistance refers to the persistent requirement for more than 200 units of insulin per day. This clinical condition is usually related to the presence of large amounts of neutralizing anti-insulin antibodies. Two general approaches to the treatment of this problem have been attempted, each with some success:

1. Use of insulin that is not neutralized by antibodies to the usual beef-pork insulin mixtures. Since antibodies appear to be directed primarily against beef insulin, substitution of pure pork insulin is helpful in some instances (Forsham, 1964). Pork insulin in which the terminal amino acid in the B chain has been removed is termed "dealaninated insulin." It has the same amino acid sequence as human insulin, lacking the terminal threonine in the B

chain. Unfortunately, this form of insulin has not been more effective in this syndrome than ordinary pork insulin (Boshell *et al.*, 1964). Sulfated insulin and fish insulin have been used successfully in some patients (Little and Arnott, 1966). Other unusual insulins, such as whale or turtle insulin, have not generally been effective.

In some patients with maturity-onset diabetes who develop chronic insulin resistance, addition of an oral sulfonylurea has been useful in stimulating release of endogenous pancreatic insulin that may not be neutralized by antibodies to beef insulin (Segre, 1962). This form of therapy cannot be used in juvenile diabetic subjects who show no response to sulfonylurea therapy.

2. Use of corticosteroids. The exact mechanism by which this therapy is effective in chronic insulin resistance is not known. Nonetheless, it is probably the most consistently effective treatment when insulin resistance is caused by excessive neutralizing antibodies to insulin (Kantor and Berkman, 1967). Relatively small doses of corticosteroids (20 to 40 mg of prednisone) are necessary to reduce the insulin requirement, but treatment is often required for several months (Bondy, 1966). When corticosteroid therapy is effective, severe hypoglycemia may initially result, as large amounts of circulating insulin previously bound to antibody become biologically active (Bondy, 1966).

HYPOGLYCEMIC REACTIONS IN THE DIABETIC. All diabetics taking insulin must be warned of the symptoms of hypoglycemia. The symptoms vary with the preparation used. When intermediate-acting insulin preparations are used, hypoglycemia develops relatively slowly; mild central nervous system symptoms predominate and may not be recognized as hypoglycemia. Rapid-acting insulin preparations produce symptoms referable to sympathetic discharge. Hypoglycemia occurring at night may go unnoticed by the patient and may be accompanied only by abnormalities in the sleep pattern: frequent nightmares, night sweats, morning headache, and enuresis in children.

The most effective and appropriate therapy for hypoglycemic reactions is the intravenous administration of glucose. Since the glucose is often utilized very rapidly, treatment should be followed by additional dietary carbohydrates and protein over the next few hours. Oral glucose administration during an acute hypoglycemic episode is less reliable, because gastric emptying and absorption may be inadequate as a result of autonomic dysfunction in the hypoglycemic period. Intramuscular glucagon may be helpful, particularly when intravenous therapy is difficult, but glucagon therapy has two disadvantages: (1) The immediate effect of

glucagon on raising the blood glucose level depends on adequate stores of liver glycogen. In some diabetic subjects with hypoglycemic episodes, hepatic glycogen is insufficient. (2) Glucagon stimulates insulin release from the pancreatic islets (Samols *et al.*, 1965). In patients with maturity-onset diabetes with some remaining islet-cell function, this effect of glucagon may be disadvantageous. ***Principle: Glucose therapy is the treatment of choice for hypoglycemic reactions in the diabetic and may necessarily be prolonged depending upon the severity of the reaction, the time of onset in relation to the dose of insulin, and the type of insulin used.***

Oral Hypoglycemic Therapy of Diabetes: The Sulfonylureas. Since the development of these drugs following the work of Janbon in 1942 (Janbon *et al.*, 1942), many diabetics have been treated for over 14 years. The sulfonylureas have provided convenient therapy for many symptomatic maturity-onset diabetic subjects. They also illustrate how basic pharmacologic features can be related to their clinical usefulness in controlling the concentration of blood glucose.

Pharmacology of the Sulfonylureas. The formulas for the useful sulfonylurea drugs are shown in Figure 7–1. The biologically active portion of the molecule is evident in each. Alterations in both end groupings have modified the metabolism and duration of action of these drugs (Seidensticker and Hamwi, 1967). Tolbutamide (Orinase), the first practical and most commonly used sulfonylurea, is well absorbed from the gastrointestinal tract and has a half-life of about 4 to 5 hours. It is metabolized in the liver to carboxytolbutamide, which is inactive as a hypoglycemic compound. Both the metabolite and the unmetabolized drug are excreted in the urine. Protein binding of tolbutamide does occur, but the exact percentage of circulating tolbutamide bound or the affinity of protein for the drug is not well known. The duration of action of tolbutamide is approximately 6 to 12 hours.

Chlorpropamide, the first long-acting sulfonylurea, is well absorbed from the gastrointestinal tract and has a half-life of 18 hours and a duration of action of more than 36 hours. The drug apparently is not metabolized, and virtually all of an administered dose can be recovered unchanged from the urine (Seidensticker and Hamwi, 1967). Acetohexamide has an intermediate duration of action (12 to 24 hours) and a half-life of 5 to 8 hours. The duration of action is related to the unique metabolism of acetohexamide: the drug is normally reduced in the liver to hydroxyhexamide, which has the same hypoglycemic properties as the parent drug. Both metabolite and drug are excreted in the

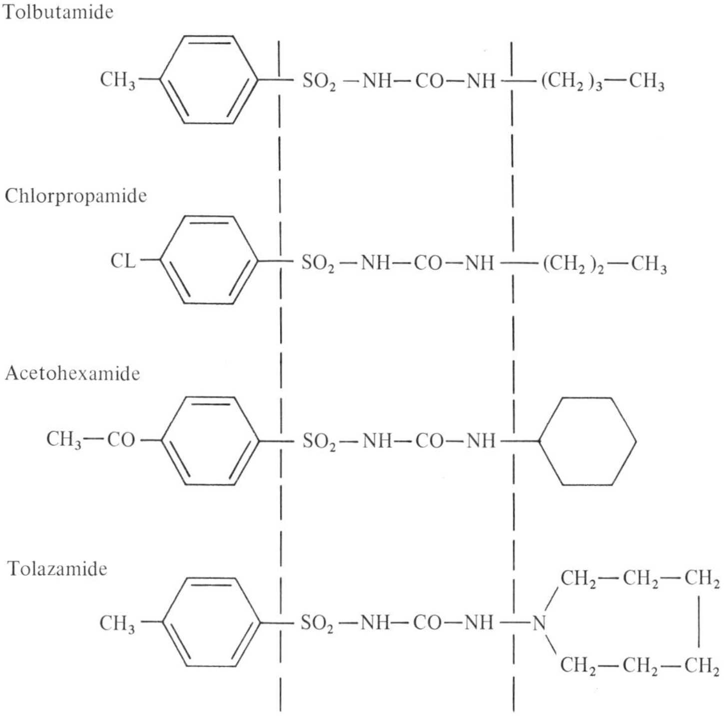

Tolbutamide

$$CH_3 \!-\! \bigcirc \!-\! SO_2 \!-\! NH \!-\! CO \!-\! NH \!-\! (CH_2)_3 \!-\! CH_3$$

Chlorpropamide

$$CL \!-\! \bigcirc \!-\! SO_2 \!-\! NH \!-\! CO \!-\! NH \!-\! (CH_2)_2 \!-\! CH_3$$

Acetohexamide

$$CH_3 \!-\! CO \!-\! \bigcirc \!-\! SO_2 \!-\! NH \!-\! CO \!-\! NH \!-\! \bigcirc$$

Tolazamide

$$CH_3 \!-\! \bigcirc \!-\! SO_2 \!-\! NH \!-\! CO \!-\! NH \!-\! N \begin{array}{c} CH_2 \!-\! CH_2 \!-\! CH_2 \\ \diagup \\ \diagdown \\ CH_2 \!-\! CH_2 \!-\! CH_2 \end{array}$$

Figure 7–1. Major sulfonylurea drugs.

urine. About 10% of the drug is excreted in the bile. In addition to its hypoglycemic properties, acetohexamide is uricosuric in doses usually utilized for treatment of diabetes. Tolazamide, one of the newest intermediate-acting drugs, has a half-life similar to that of acetohexamide. Its metabolism is not well studied, but there appear to be several metabolites of the drug recovered in the urine, some of which have hypoglycemic properties (Comment, 1966). During the diabetic state, especially in the older patients who are most likely to be given these drugs, liver or renal failure may occur. Under such circumstances one preparation may be most desirable in one instance but contraindicated in another. When would any or all preparations of the sulfonylureas be contraindicated or used with a modified dosage schedule owing to factors unrelated to blood glucose concentrations? There are a number of sulfonylurea compounds, and a tendency in medicine is to "learn how to use one preparation" successfully. However, different clinical settings require different preparations, and probably in few other areas of therapeutics is a knowledge of the chemical differences in drug preparations so potentially helpful.

The major mechanism of action of all sulfonylureas is stimulation of pancreatic insulin secretion. Therefore, some functional islet-cell tissue is necessary in patients receiving these drugs. The effect of sulfonylureas on pancreatic insulin release is prompt, occurring within minutes of intravenous administration in man (Perley and Kipnis, 1966). A number of other effects of the sulfonylureas have been described (Davidoff, 1968). *In vivo* and *in vitro* studies have suggested some peripheral augmentation of insulin action, particularly in muscle. An effect of the sulfonylureas to decrease hepatic glucose output has been suggested by studies that have demonstrated decreased hepatic gluconeogenesis and glycogenolysis in the presence of these compounds. The clinical relevance of the ability of the sulfonylureas to decrease the degradation of insulin by insulinase and to decrease insulin binding to circulating proteins is difficult to evaluate because large doses were used in these studies (Hasselblatt, 1963). Although a number of the extrapancreatic effects of sulfonylureas may be important under selected conditions, the single most important mechanism of action of the sulfonylureas is their effect on release of pancreatic insulin.

Clinical Usefulness of the Sulfonylureas. Sulfonylurea therapy is most useful in the treatment of symptomatic maturity-onset diabetics in whom some beta-cell function is preserved. Sulfonylureas should not be employed as primary treatment in juvenile diabetics, in individuals who have diabetes secondary to pancreatectomy or chronic pancreatitis, or in maturity-onset diabetics who are asymptomatic. The overall success of sulfonylurea therapy in patients with symptomatic maturity-onset diabetes in terms of control of symptoms and control of the blood glucose level is estimated at 65 to 70% (Balodimos *et al.*, 1966). About 10 to 15% of patients are secondary failures; that is, response fails after 3 to 6 months of good control. The reasons for both primary and secondary failures are unknown, but in some instances failure may represent easing of dietary restrictions owing to reliance on expected drug effectiveness and inadequate or inaccurate drug ingestion by the patient. These factors do not entirely explain the cause of secondary failures, and further studies are necessary to investigate the phenomenon.

The long-term effects of the oral sulfonylurea drugs are not known. As with insulin, there is no evidence that chronic sulfonylurea therapy has any effect on the appearance or progression of the vascular complications of diabetes. Most investigators prefer insulin therapy to sulfonylurea therapy during severe infections in patients with maturity-onset diabetes. Sulfonylureas are not used to treat diabetic ketoacidosis.

Treatment of mild diabetes mellitus or prediabetes with sulfonylurea drugs for periods of 1 to 2 years may lead to an improvement in glucose tolerance (Fajans and Conn, 1962; Sheldon *et al.*, 1966; Reaven and Dray, 1967). These studies have been supported by animal studies that demonstrate a decreased incidence of diabetes in partly pancreatectomized animals treated with a high-carbohydrate intake and sulfonylureas, when compared with animals receiving only the high-carbohydrate intake (Williams, 1968). Some caution must be used in interpreting the studies in man. Since glucose tolerance may vary from day to day in mild diabetics and prediabetics, appropriate rigidly controlled studies on large populations of patients must be included in any evaluation of a drug's effect on glucose tolerance. Extensive controlled studies indicate that in asymptomatic patients who have recently developed maturity-onset diabetes, the long-term effects of sulfonylurea drugs on forestalling symptomatic disease are unimpressive. In fact the drugs may be much less effective than insulin and considerably more toxic than either insulin or no drug at all. Because hepatic metabolism plays an important role in the elimination of tolbutamide, this drug should be administered cautiously to patients with severe chronic liver disease. The importance of renal excretion in the elimination of all sulfonylureas makes their use in patients with

significant renal insufficiency dangerous, although tolbutamide may be the safest in this clinical situation. Owing to its uricosuric effect, acetohexamide may be the drug of choice in the symptomatic maturity-onset diabetic with gout.

Recently the results of the University Group Diabetes Program (Comment, 1970) have raised some rather serious questions concerning the safety of oral sulfonylurea drugs. In this multi-institutional, prospective, controlled study, a significantly increased mortality from cardiovascular causes was found in 204 tolbutamide (1.5 g per day)-treated patients when compared with 205 placebo-treated diabetics. At the end of the eighth year of follow-up, the cardiovascular mortality rate was 75% higher in the tolbutamide treatment group than in the placebo-treated patients. Although a number of criticisms have been offered concerning the experimental design of this study (Feinstein, 1971), it has raised serious doubts about the use of oral sulfonylurea agents in the routine treatment of maturity-onset diabetes. As a result of this study, on October 30, 1970, the Food and Drug Administration made the following recommendation: "...the use of Orinase (tolbutamide) and other sulfonylurea type agents, Dymelor (acetohexamide), Diabinese (chlorpropamide), Tolinase (tolazamide), should be limited to those patients with symptomatic adult-onset nonketotic diabetes mellitus which cannot be adequately controlled by diet or weight loss alone and in whom the addition of insulin is impractical or unacceptable" (Comment, 1970).

Evaluation of this important study must take into account other conflicting data. In Keen's study (Keen, 1970) of 248 borderline diabetics, one half of whom were treated with tolbutamide and one half with placebo, a significantly lower percentage of arterial events (myocardial infarction, angina pectoris, stroke and intermittent claudication) was found in the tolbutamide-treated group than in the placebo group, despite no significant differences in blood sugar. This study, which suggests a protective effect of tolbutamide in regard to arterial disease, together with the UGDP study, emphasizes the need for continued evaluation of the usefulness and safety of the oral hypoglycemic agents.

Toxicity of the Sulfonylureas. The major toxic manifestations of these drugs are similar, with insignificant differences in the incidence of particular side effects. The overall incidence of toxic reactions to sulfonylurea compounds is approximately 3 to 5%, mostly consisting of mild gastrointestinal reactions or mild skin rashes. Severe toxicity is seen in less than 1% of patients. Such reactions include hepatic toxicity, bone marrow toxicity, and prolonged hypoglycemic reactions. Cholestatic jaundice has been seen in a small number of patients given oral sulfonylurea therapy, particularly chlorprop-amide. The liver damage appears to be revers-ible in most instances following discontinuation of the drug. Therefore, liver function should be frequently tested in patients on sulfonylurea therapy. Rare instances of hematologic reactions, including leukopenia (apparently the most common hematologic side effect), thrombocyto-penia, and hemolytic anemia, have been reported in patients taking sulfonylureas. Corticosteroid therapy has sometimes been used to reverse these abnormalities.

The most common and life-threatening toxic effect of the sulfonylureas is prolonged hypo-glycemia, sometimes persisting for several days after drug therapy is stopped and requiring continuous intravenous glucose administration. This problem has been noted most often in patients with some degree of renal insufficiency. In such patients markedly elevated concentra-tions of the drug in blood are probably related to the inability to eliminate the drug or its metabolites from the body by the normal renal mechanisms. These clinical observations should emphasize the danger of using these drugs in any patient with significant renal insufficiency. Because of its hepatic metabolism, tolbutamide may be the least likely to produce hypoglycemia in the patient with renal disease. For the same reason tolbutamide is much *more* likely to produce prolonged hypoglycemia in the patient with severe hepatic disease than are the other sulfonylureas. Prolonged hypoglycemia has also been seen more commonly in elderly, debilitated, or cachectic patients treated with these drugs. Since islet-cell adenomata have appeared in patients with a previous history of diabetes mellitus, prolonged hypoglycemic reactions to sulfonylureas may herald this diagnosis. The relatively high mortality rate seen in asympto-matic patients taking selected oral hypoglycemic agents has not been explained. Until these drugs are proved to be efficacious for long-term control of hyperglycemia or to prevent complications in the diabetic patient, they should not be used in the asymptomatic patient. If they are used, extreme caution should be exercised. The inter-ested student is directed to the following refer-ences related to the use and dangers of oral hypo-glycemic agents. He will certainly be impressed by the data leading to therapeutic decisions in transition. *Principle: No drug should be used unless there are very well-established objectives for giving the drug, and the risks of drug use are clear and are balanced in the overall therapeutic decision* (Comment, 1970; Keen, 1970; Feinstein, 1971).

Prolonged hypoglycemia has developed in a number of patients treated with tolbutamide following administration of another drug. These represent some of the classic examples of drug interactions in man. Evidence suggests that sulfonamides, phenylbutazone, and bishydroxy-coumarin may competitively interfere with tolbutamide metabolism in the liver, leading to elevated concentration of the drug in blood and to severe hypoglycemia (Field *et al.*, 1967; Solomon and Schrogie, 1967). Acetylsalicylic acid may displace tolbutamide from binding sites on serum proteins, freeing the drug and producing severe hypoglycemia. Monoamine oxidase inhibitors and propranolol have preci-pitated severe hypoglycemia in patients taking sulfonylureas, by mechanisms almost surely dependent in part on the adrenergic blocking qualities of each of the agents.

Interactions resulting in potentiation of the effects of other drugs are also important. Tolbutamide therapy may make patients more sensitive to the anticoagulant effects of bis-hydroxycoumarin and to the intoxicating effects of alcohol (Larsen and Madsen, 1962). The latter is apparently related to interference with alcohol metabolism by the sulfonylureas.

A few patients have developed severe hypo-glycemia with the initial dose of tolbutamide (Bird and Schwalbe, 1965). Elevated concentra-tion of the drug and decreased concentrations of the major metabolite of tolbutamide have been found in these patients, suggesting that they may lack the enzyme responsible for the oxidation of tolbutamide in the liver. Further work will be required before factors predisposing to this effect can be defined.

Phenethyl Diguanide. A nonsulfonylurea oral hypoglycemic agent, phenethyl diguanide or phenformin, has been utilized in the treatment of diabetes mellitus for several years. It is well absorbed from the gastrointestinal tract and for the most part is not metabolized. Only one third of the drug is hydroxylated in the para position of the phenyl ring. Both parent drug and meta-bolite are rapidly excreted in the urine, with an estimated half-life of the drug of approximately 3 hours. Because of its short half-life, the drug is usually administered in a "timed-disintegra-tion" form.

The mechanism of the hypoglycemic action of phenformin continues to be debated. Early studies demonstrated interference with oxidative phosphorylation (Falcone *et al.*, 1962). Thus in peripheral tissues, a secondary increase in the uptake of glucose and in oxidation by anaerobic glycolysis leads to decreased concentration of glucose in blood. However, the dose of drug necessary to show this effect was greater than the usual pharmacologic doses effective in diabetic man. Therefore, additional sites of action of the drug have been proposed. Inhibition of hepatic gluconeogenesis (Meyer *et al.*, 1967) and release of glucose have been demonstrated in laboratory animals, but studies in man have shown that phenformin accelerates the turnover of glucose in nondiabetic subjects (Searle *et al.*, 1966). This increased turnover may be due both to increased hepatic glucose output and to increased peripheral utilization of glucose, the balancing of the two effects accounting for the inability to demonstrate hypoglycemia in most nondiabetic subjects given phenformin. Phenformin has no immediate effect on the release of pancreatic insulin or the disposition of circulating insulin (serum insulin levels do not rise after administration of this drug in man).

The clinical uses of phenformin are not so clearly defined as are those of the sulfonylurea drugs. The following uses of the drug have been recommended:

1. Primary therapy of maturity-onset diabetes, particularly in obese subjects. Since this drug does not increase serum insulin levels, the lipogenic effect of insulin can be avoided, which might be advantageous in the obese diabetic. Although some obese patients treated with phenformin lose weight, this result could be due to the anorexia sometimes produced by this drug.

During chronic ingestion of phenformin, maturity-onset diabetics have shown blunting of the peak plasma insulin concentrations after a glucose load. The clinical relevance of these findings is elusive, since it is not known whether the lower insulin concentrations constitute an advantage or a disadvantage in treatment of the disease. Phenformin therapy does not appear to have a definite advantageous effect in the long-term treatment of maturity-onset diabetes.

2. Combined therapy with sulfonylurea drugs. Since phenformin and the sulfonylureas have different mechanisms of action, their effects on blood sugar may be separate and additive. Clinical studies have indicated the usefulness of combined therapy with phenformin and sulfonylureas in some patients who represent secondary failures to sulfonylurea therapy alone. Most patients with this syndrome, however, eventually require insulin therapy. *Principle: In general there is little reason for combination therapy when both drugs or all drugs have similar mechanisms of action, unless the nontherapeutic or unwanted effects of one agent prevent the maximum possible therapeutic effect. A combination of drugs is most useful when agents of different chemical composition and different major mechanism of action can accomplish the same end result and when the maximum effect of one agent is insufficient* (see Chapters 3 and 5).

3. Control of the brittle diabetic. Although phenformin has been recommended in brittle diabetes, there is little evidence that the drug is truly beneficial. Because of the toxicity of the drug, many physicians are hesitant to use phenformin in the juvenile diabetic.

Toxic side effects occur more frequently during phenformin therapy than during sulfonylurea therapy. The most common problems are anorexia, nausea, vomiting, and diarrhea. The intestinal symptoms are much less common than with the sulfonylureas. Prolonged hypoglycemic reactions have been seen, mostly in patients with renal insufficiency. The toxic manifestation receiving the greatest attention is lactic acidosis, which has been reported in several patients taking this drug (Williams, 1969). Because lactic acidosis occurs more frequently in diabetics than in the normal population, the exact relationship of phenformin to this syndrome is uncertain. Lactate accumulation and subsequent acidosis might be expected during the use of phenformin because of its ability to inhibit oxidative phosphorylation. Nearly all patients with lactic acidosis associated with phenformin therapy have had significant renal insufficiency. At the present time, although an exact causal relationship between phenformin and the syndrome of lactic acidosis cannot be established unequivocally, it seems inadvisable to use this drug in patients with renal insufficiency or with other conditions that might predispose to anoxemia and lactate accumulation. *Principle: The knowledge of the chemistry of a drug, its metabolism, and its pharmacokinetics may help in determining (1) proper choice between drugs in different clinical situations associated with the same disease, (2) proper combinations of drugs ostensibly used to obtain the same therapeutic end point, and (3) some of the reasons for extension of toxicity beyond the ordinary half-life of the drug* (see Chapters 2 and 15).

Treatment of the Hypoglycemic State

The causes of hypoglycemia are multiple, involving many different pathogenetic mechanisms (Table 7–4). In many of these conditions only dietary manipulation may be required. This is particularly true with the various causes of reactive hypoglycemia and in some of the inborn errors of metabolism associated with hypoglycemia. The treatment of insulin reactions has already been discussed. Another of the most serious causes of hypoglycemia is islet-cell adenoma or carcinoma. In this disorder as well as in some of the severe forms of hypoglycemia in childhood, drug therapy has been necessary to maintain normal glucose concentrations in blood. A number of drugs have been tried in these situations, including corticosteroids, catecholamines, glucagon, growth hormone, streptozotocin, and diazoxide (Williams, 1968). Corticosteroids, although effective in raising the concentration of glucose in blood, are usually not warranted because of the serious side effects that occur after long-term therapy. Various short- and long-acting catecholamine preparations have been tried for a number of years, but their effect on the sugar content of blood is often associated with symptoms of excessive sympathetic activity. Long-acting glucagon preparations (zinc, oil, or gel) can maintain a normal glucose concentration in these patients for periods of 8 to 12 hours and have been used particularly at night or during other long periods of fasting (Roth *et al.*, 1966). Because these drugs also stimulate insulin release, objection has been raised to their use during insulinogenic hypoglycemia. Growth hormone, although very effective in raising glucose concentrations in blood, is impractical at the present time because expensively large amounts (2 to 5 mg per day) are necessary to maintain the effect.

Table 7–4. CAUSES OF HYPOGLYCEMIA

Insulinogenic hypoglycemia
  Islet-cell adenoma
  Reactive hypoglycemia
  Prediabetes
  Drugs
  Leucine-sensitive hypoglycemia
  CNS disease
Insulinopenic hypoglycemia
  Nonpancreatic tumors
  Inborn errors of metabolism
  Hepatic disease
  Alcohol hypoglycemia
Increased sensitivity to insulin
  Endocrine disorders
Artifactual hypoglycemia

Perhaps the most useful agent in the treatment of chronic hypoglycemia is an antihypertensive, nondiuretic thiazide analog, diazoxide (Field *et al.*, 1968; Marks and Samols, 1968). This drug has been extensively used in patients with severe hypoglycemia of various etiologies, including infantile hypoglycemia (Drash *et al.*, 1968), glycogen-storage disease (Drash *et al.*, 1968), islet-cell carcinoma (Field *et al.*, 1968), retroperitoneal sarcomas (Tucker *et al.*, 1968), and leucine-sensitive hypoglycemia (Green and Berger, 1968). The drug appears to inhibit insulin release from islet-cell tissue (Graber *et al.*, 1968; Porte, 1968). Direct effects of diazoxide on hepatic glycogenolysis and catecholamine

release may be additional modes of action but are less well delineated. Synergism with other thiazides may be utilized to keep drug dosage low. Toxic manifestations of the drug include hypertrichosis, hyperuricemia, edema, and excessive hyperglycemia. Although long-term studies are not available, diazoxide appears to be the drug of choice for treatment of severe, chronic hypoglycemic states in both children and adults. The use of diazoxide in the treatment of hypertension is discussed in Chapter 5.

THE THYROID

The major function of the thyroid gland is to synthesize, store, and secrete two hormonally active iodinated amino acids, L-thyroxine (T_4) and L-triiodothyronine (T_3), which are necessary for body metabolism, development, and growth. One determinant of the rate of formation of thyroid hormone is the availability of sufficient quantities of iodine. Normally, iodine is efficiently absorbed from the gastrointestinal tract, is largely confined to the extracellular space, and is cleared primarily by the kidney and thyroid gland (Figure 7–2). The renal tubules passively reabsorb iodide, and major changes in iodide clearance are usually dependent upon changes in the glomerular filtration rate (Ingbar and Woeber, 1968). In patients with the nephrotic syndrome, T_4 is inappropriately excreted, bound to its transport protein. Other valuable iodinated derivatives may be lost in the urine in patients with the rare familial enzyme deficiency of iodotyrosine dehalogenase or may be lost in the stool when gastrointestinal absorption is impaired or when they are bound to certain nonabsorbable dietary constituents such as soybeans and walnuts (Ingbar and Woeber, 1968).

The thyroid gland actively extracts iodide from the plasma, the intrathyroidal iodide concentration being greater than that in the extracellular fluid. The iodide-trapping mechanism is energy dependent and is inhibited by anoxia, by inhibitors of oxidative metabolism (cyanide and fluoride), and by agents known to uncouple oxidative phosphorylation, such as 2,4-dinitrophenol and bishydroxycoumarin (Ingbar and Woeber, 1968). The iodide-trapping mechanism can also be inhibited by certain monovalent anions, which act as competitive inhibitors owing to the similarity of their atomic diameters. Those most frequently used in therapy are perchlorate and thiocyanate. Features that limit their effectiveness include their high solubility in water, their rapid excretion from the body, and extrathyroidal effects such as aplastic anemia. ***Principle: Even if drugs are efficacious, they may be impractical, and the choice between agents may be independent of their proven primary pharmacologic effects.***

By virtue of their competitive effects on iodide trapping, thiocyanate and perchlorate can be used as diagnostic tools. The perchlorate discharge test has been of value in the diagnosis of an absolute or relative defect in thyroid hormone biosynthesis when the defect lies in the ability of the thyroid to carry out organic iodination. Since iodide transport is

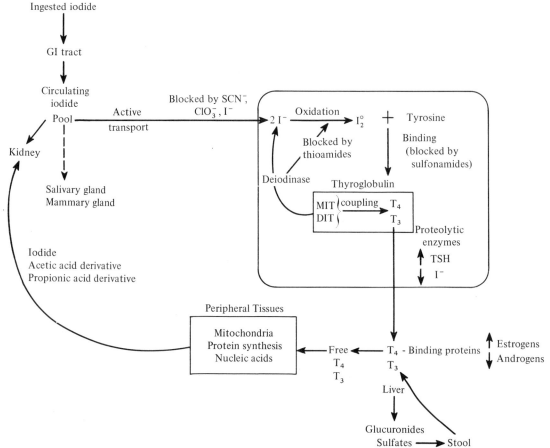

Figure 7–2. Schema of iodide metabolism. *SCN*, thiocyanate; *ClO₃*, perchlorate; *MIT*, monoiodotyrosine; *DIT*, diiodotyrosine; *TSH*, thyroid-stimulating hormone; T_3, triiodothyronine; T_4, *L*-thyroxine.

normal, the initial thyroid uptake of radioactive iodine is normal or high. When perchlorate is given, this anion discharges the iodine, since the labeled iodine does not bind organically to the tyrosine molecules to form iodotyrosines. Normally the organic binding of iodine to tyrosine occurs sufficiently rapidly that perchlorate discharges only small amounts of labeled iodine.

The thyroidal iodide transport mechanism is directly influenced by the hypothalamic-pituitary axis through secretion of thyrotropin-releasing factor (TRF) and thyroid-stimulating hormone or thyrotropin (TSH). TRF, which has been isolated from the human hypothalamus, influences thyrotropin release from the pituitary (Schally *et al.*, 1967). Both TRF and TSH participate in a negative feedback mechanism; their release is diminished by free thyroid hormones in the blood. When TSH is given intravenously to mice pretreated with ¹³¹I, it causes release of radioactive iodine from the thyroid gland. A peak of radioactive iodide appears in the blood usually at 2 hours and falls by 24 hours. Long-acting thyroid stimulator (LATS) is a 7S gamma globulin

found in some patients with hyperthyroidism and in most patients with pretibial myxedema. LATS causes delayed release of iodine from the prelabeled gland, the peak appearing in 8 to 16 hours. The longer duration of thyroid stimulation by LATS is apparently due to its longer biologic half-life compared with TSH. The concentration of LATS in serum does not correlate with the severity of hyperthyroidism and may remain elevated long after hyperthyroidism is treated.

Although TSH seems to be the major regulatory hormone for thyroid function, intrinsic thyroid autoregulation is also important. High concentrations of intrathyroidal iodide decrease the rate of utilization of thyroidal iodine (Braverman and Ingbar, 1963). Studies utilizing radioimmunoassay of TSH have aided understanding of the TSH control mechanism (Odell *et al.*, 1967). Tests of TSH reserve are not generally available, since even large doses of antithyroid drugs do not usually increase the concentration of TSH in plasma. Recently a test of TSH reserve has been proposed that depends on changes in the absolute thyroidal iodide uptake and in plasma inorganic iodide (indirect evidence of TSH effect) after 7 days of carbimazole therapy (Jensen, 1969). Glucocorticoids decrease TSH concentration in plasma within 8 hours of their administration; there is a significant increase in the concentrations of TSH above control levels in both normal and hypothyroid patients when the steroid is withdrawn (Wilber and Utiger, 1969). This "rebound" in TSH production or release may provide a method for testing TSH reserve and suggests that glucocorticoids play a significant role in normal regulation of TSH release (Nicoloff et al., 1969). *Principle: Pharmacologic manipulation of a control mechanism may aid in both diagnosis and therapy of disease. When careful observations are made of the effects of the manipulation, information concerning normal physiologic mechanisms can be obtained.*

Iodide within the thyroid cell undergoes a series of complex reactions leading to its incorporation into active thyroid hormones. The reactions include oxidation of iodide, organic binding, and coupling of iodotyrosines to yield active iodothyronines. These are stored as part of a large molecule (thyroglobulin) in the thyroid follicles (Figure 7–2). Because thyroglobulin is too large to be transported across the thyroid acinar cell wall, the active iodothyronines (T_3 and T_4) are released from thyroglobulin by proteolytic enzymes and transported into the circulation. The storage of relatively large amounts of active thyroid hormone in thyroglobulin protects against sudden deficiency.

The total daily turnover or disposition of T_4 is approximately 85 μg, with a serum concentration of 7.5 μg/100 ml, a half-time in the serum of 7.6 days, a volume of distribution of 12 liters, and a fractional daily turnover of 9% (Green, 1968). It has been estimated in a less precise fashion that the daily turnover rate of T_3 is approximately 37 μg, with a serum concentration of 0.3 μg/100 ml, a half-time in the serum of 1.4 days, a volume of distribution of 25 liters, and a fractional daily turnover of 50% (Green, 1968).

T_4 is bound to specific plasma proteins. Thyroxine-binding globulin (TBG) is a glycoprotein that has high affinity for T_4; thyroxine-binding prealbumin has a weaker affinity for T_4. As a result of protein binding, only a small fraction of T_4 circulates freely in the plasma. T_3 is also bound to TBG, but less firmly than is T_4. This weaker binding affinity may explain the more rapid turnover of T_3.

Many drugs can alter the concentration of thyroid-binding proteins in plasma, thereby affecting thyroid function tests that measure bound T_4. However, under these circumstances the concentration of free T_3 and T_4 usually remains normal and there is no change in body metabolism. The most commonly used drugs that increase binding proteins are estrogenic hormones, especially the oral contraceptives. Clinical situations associated with increased hormonal binding include pregnancy, genetically induced increases in thyroid-binding proteins, acute intermittent porphyria, feminizing tumors, and acute liver disease (Ingbar and Woeber, 1968). Drugs that decrease the plasma concentration of binding proteins include anabolic steroids and glucocorticoids. Genetic abnormalities, nephrosis, chronic liver disease, and dysproteinemias are also associated with decreased concentrations of thyroid-binding proteins in blood. Salicylates and aminosalicylic acid (para-aminosalicylic acid, PAS) compete for binding sites on thyroid-binding proteins and decrease binding of T_4 to thyroid-binding prealbumin without affecting the concentration of the protein. Compounds such as triparanol, o,p'-DDD, amphenone B, 2,4-dinitrophenol, bishydroxycoumarin, and diphenylhydantoin are structurally similar to active thyroid hormones and may displace T_4 from binding proteins (Astwood, 1965).

The T_4-binding capacity of TBG affects the distribution of T_4 (whether endogenous or exogenous) within the body and the rate of disappearance from the plasma of T_3 and T_4. When estrogens increase TBG, they reduce the hepatic incorporation, hepatic volume of distribution, and hepatic clearance of T_3 and T_4 without altering extrahepatic functions of the hormone (Musa et al., 1969). Glucocorticoids affect the hepatic uptake of thyroid hormones independent of their ability to decrease the synthesis of thyroid-binding proteins (Kumar et al., 1968). Large doses of glucocorticoids may precipitate thyrotoxicosis in a patient on a fixed intake of T_3 by increasing the availability of free hormone in the plasma owing to an acute fall in the blood concentration of TBG (Greenspan, 1969). *Principle: The use of a laboratory test for the detection of disease or the determination of drug dosage requires a thorough knowledge of the factors that can alter the results of the specific test.*

It is not known whether T_3 is formed from T_4, although recent studies suggest that deiodination of T_4 to yield T_3 is a prominent pathway of T_4 metabolism (Braverman et al., 1969).

The primary pathway of thyroid hormone degradation is conjugation to glucuronic and sulfuric acids through the phenolic hydroxy groups (Astwood, 1965). After conjugation in the liver, the products are excreted in the bile and partially reabsorbed. Many tissues deiodinate T_3 and T_4 to iodide and acetic and propionic acid derivatives that are excreted in the urine. There are several known inhibitors of thyroid hormone deiodination (thiouracil, serotonin, 3,3',5-triiodothyronine) (Ingbar and Woeber, 1968), but their exact physiologic significance is unknown. The rate of degradation of thyroid hormones is greatly influenced by the status of thyroid and hepatic function. This must be kept in mind during the management of patients who require thyroid hormones.

The action of thyroid hormones on peripheral tissues is complex, and no unified concept of their action is well accepted. Most attention has been directed to the ability of thyroid hormone to uncouple oxidative phosphorylation, alter mitochondrial histology, and affect protein synthesis or nucleic acid metabolism. Many analogs of thyroid hormones have been synthesized in an attempt to develop active competitive inhibitors of the peripheral effects of thyroid hormone, but no clinically useful analog is available.

Drugs Affecting Thyroid Function Tests

Tests of thyroid function mainly involve the measurement of bound thyroid hormones in blood or of the thyroidal accumulation of radioiodine (^{131}I). Although free unbound thyroid hormones have been measured by gas-liquid chromatography (Hollander et al., 1969), most methods for determination of these hormones measure bound hormones or bound iodinated proteins and are thereby influenced by contamination with organic or inorganic iodide, by release of hormonal precursors, or by changes in thyroid-binding proteins. The protein-bound iodine test quantitates the iodide after precipitation and washing of the plasma proteins. A useful variation of the PBI is the butanol-extractable iodine test (BEI), which measures only T_4 and usually has a value 20% less than that of the PBI. The BEI does not measure biologically inactive iodoproteins, which are frequently increased in Hashimoto's thyroiditis. Unfortunately, most iodinated dyes that increase the PBI are extractable into butanol and cannot be distinguished by this test.

The most reliable commercially available method for measuring T_4 is the binding displacement method (Murphy and Pattee, 1964). X-ray contrast media are measured by the PBI and the BEI, but do not interfere with the Murphy-Pattee method. Dyes excreted in the bile undergo enterohepatic recirculation and may remain in the body for long periods. Iophenoxic acid (Teridax) is tightly bound to protein, sometimes remaining for several years, and crosses the placenta, increasing the fetal PBI (Shapiro and Man, 1960). The PBI may be artificially lowered by heavy metals, especially mercurial diuretics (a transient effect) and gold salts (a more prolonged effect), which interfere with the colorimetric reaction for iodide used in the determination of the PBI (Fisher et al., 1965). Any inorganic iodide may increase the PBI. Cleansing the venipuncture site with an iodide-containing antiseptic may spuriously raise the PBI. A thorough review calls attention to the increase in the PBI by iodide contamination by some proprietary preparations such as vaginal and rectal suppositories, tincture of iodine, cough medications, suntan lotions, nail hardeners, antidandruff medications, toothpaste, vitamin and mineral preparations, cod-liver oil, cosmetics, and even iodized salt (Davis, 1966). Some preparations of bromsulfophthalein (BSP) and barium sulfate may contain excess iodide. Recently, tubing used for intravenous therapy was found to be contaminated with iodine, causing an increase in the PBI concentration in several patients (Simbari and Houghton, 1969).

Several in vitro tests have been developed to measure free thyroid hormone present in the plasma. These in vitro uptake tests are based on the principle that exogenous free thyroid hormone competes with binding sites on the patient's own thyroid-binding proteins in plasma and with nonspecific binding sites on an inert particle or erythrocyte. Tracer amounts of isotopic thyroid hormone (T_3) are added to the patient's plasma in the presence of a resin or erythrocytes. The particles are separated and the ratio of isotope bound to the resin and that bound to the patient's plasma proteins is determined. In hyperthyroidism, binding sites on the patient's plasma proteins are saturated, more isotope binds to the resin particles, and the in vitro resin uptake of isotope is elevated. In the hypothyroid state, a low resin uptake is seen because the large number of available binding sites on the patient's plasma proteins selectively bind the isotope, leaving less available for binding to resin. During oral contraceptive therapy or pregnancy, increased binding proteins result in low resin uptakes, even though the PBI may be high. This test is of great value in the difficult diagnosis of hyperthyroidism in pregnancy. In the nephrotic syndrome, excessive urinary loss of T_4 bound to its transport proteins leads to an increase in the resin uptake. Erythrocytes appear to be less accurate than resin as a binding agent, because the red-cell uptake may be influenced by nonthyroidal illnesses such as liver disease, cancer, and respiratory failure, and even by bishydroxycoumarin therapy (Ingbar and Woeber, 1968). By multiplying the free thyroxine value (normal 3 to 7 μg/100 ml) (Murphy-Pattee method) by the T_3 resin uptake (normal 25 to 35%), a clinically useful free thyroxine index can be calculated, with normal values between 0.75 and 2.5. Thus patients on oral contraceptives have a high free thyroxine and a low T_3 resin, giving a normal free thyroxine index, whereas a hyperthyroid pregnant patient has an increased free thyroxine as well as an increased T_3 resin, giving an increased free thyroxine index (Greenspan, 1970).

Certain drugs affect thyroidal accumulation of radioiodine. Drugs containing iodine (organic, inorganic, or elemental) increase the iodide pool size and decrease the radioactive iodine uptake by "diluting" the tracer dose. Drugs that decrease the glomerular filtration rate or contribute to renal insufficiency increase the concentrations of plasma inorganic iodide and depress thyroidal uptake of iodide (Becker et al., 1969). Prolonged use of diets severely restricted in sodium may result in iodide deficiency and may lead to an increase in the ^{131}I uptake. Despite these limitations, the 24-hour ^{131}I uptake appears to be the most reliable test of thyroid function in uremic patients and in patients undergoing intermittent hemodialysis (Bailey et al., 1967). Some drugs affect the ^{131}I uptake directly. Thyroid hormones decrease ^{131}I uptake by suppressing pituitary TSH. Resorcinol may cause myxedema by decreasing iodine uptake (Bull and Fraser, 1950). In large doses both salicylates and phenylbutazone decrease the ^{131}I uptake (Myhill and Hales, 1963). Lithium and imipramine cause goiter in some psychiatric patients, although changes in thyroid function have been inconsistent (Fieve and Platman, 1969). The sulfonylureas may decrease the ^{131}I uptake by a direct antithyroid effect, but this has been disputed (Hunton et al., 1965; Burke et al., 1967).

Treatment of Hypothyroidism

Treatment of hypothyroidism in adults is specific, inexpensive, relatively nontoxic, dramatic for the patient, and satisfying for the physician. Four types of thyroid hormone replacement therapy are available (Table 7–5).

Historically, the standard treatment of hypothyroidism was administration of desiccated thyroid U.S.P. This powder, derived from dried, defatted animal thyroid glands, is standardized only by its content of organic iodide (0.17 to 0.23%). Preparations of similar iodide content may vary markedly in their biological activity owing to variation in T_3 and T_4 content. The extract is unstable, with loss of activity on storage in air. The theoretic and practical disadvantages to the use of desiccated thyroid have led to its recent removal from U.S.P. preparations.

Thyroglobulin extract (Proloid) is partly purified, denatured thyroglobulin that is standardized by organic iodide content and by bioassay to give a T_4/T_3 ratio of 2.5/1. Since desiccated thyroid and Proloid contain both T_3 and T_4, the PBI should be maintained within normal limits during full replacement therapy as long as these preparations do not contain excess T_3.

Because of the advantages of using a pure chemical, many physicians prefer levothyroxine sodium (T_4) or liothyronine sodium (T_3). Major differences exist between T_3 and T_4 therapy. T_3 is efficiently absorbed from the gastrointestinal tract, has a rapid turnover, quickly corrects the hypothyroid state, and allows rapid return to a hypothyroid state if therapy is discontinued. In contrast, T_4 is variably absorbed, is firmly bound to protein, and turns over more slowly than T_3. The PBI in a patient made euthyroid with T_3 is usually 1 to 2 $\mu g/100$ ml, since T_3 is more potent than T_4, contains less iodine, and is less firmly protein bound. The effectiveness of T_3 therapy is best assessed by changes in clinical symptoms and by a decrease in the concentration of cholesterol in serum. When the patient is rendered euthyroid by T_4, the PBI is higher than in normals,

usually 6 to 10 $\mu g/100$ ml. The elevation in PBI is due to the fact that the normal thyroid produces both T_3 and T_4, resulting in a PBI of 4 to 8 $\mu g/100$ ml. Both hormones have biologic activity, but only T_4 is measured by the PBI. A "new" synthetic thyroid hormone combination of T_3 and T_4 has been described that produces normal PBI measurements when the patient is euthyroid (Selenkow and Wool, 1967). Use of the "new" drug may be reassuring to the physician who relies on laboratory confirmation of the euthyroid state, but it has no pharmacologic advantage over therapy with either T_3 or T_4, which can reverse all the known abnormalities of the thyroid deficiency. *Principle: Before using a "new" preparation, study its merits. Unless the drug has clear advantages that are related to effects on the disease state and not to effects on the physician, the new preparation may not be preferable. The experience and data derived from drugs used over long periods are often invaluable and should not be abandoned without good reason and clear advantages for the patient.*

The rapid disappearance of T_3 might suggest its usefulness in the treatment of a hypothyroid patient with cardiac disease. Presumably, if cardiac toxicity occurs, the drug and its effects will disappear more rapidly than would T_4. However, many observers are convinced that T_3 is more likely than T_4 to cause untoward cardiac effects by inducing abrupt changes in metabolic demands (Green, 1968).

Since rapid reversal of the hypothyroid state is rarely necessary, most physicians prefer T_4 therapy for hypothyroidism. The effects of T_4 may be produced rapidly as long as doses sufficient to overcome binding to proteins are administered (Holvey *et al.*, 1964). A single weekly dose of T_4 (2.0 mg) may maintain the hypothyroid patient in a euthyroid state, as evidenced by adequate suppression of thyroidal ^{131}I uptake and by normal cholesterol levels. Despite the administration of a single large

Table 7–5. TYPES OF THYROID REPLACEMENT THERAPY

	COMPOSITION	APPROX. EQUIV. DOSE	DAILY DOSE	METHOD OF STANDARD- IZATION	EFFECT ON PBI
Desiccated thyroid	Animal T_3, T_4	60 mg	120–180 mg	Organic iodide content 0.17–0.23%	Normal 4–8 $\mu g/100$ ml
Thyroglobulin (Proloid)	Animal T_3, T_4	60 mg	120–180 mg	Iodide content and bioassay	Normal 4–8 $\mu g/100$ ml
Sodium levothyroxine (Synthroid)	Synthetic T_4	0.1 mg	0.2–0.3 mg	Sodium salt of natural isomer	6–10 $\mu g/100$ ml
Sodium liothyronine (Cytomel)	Synthetic T_3	25 μg	50–75 μg	Sodium salt of natural isomer	1–2 $\mu g/100$ ml

dose of T_4, no adverse cardiovascular effects were observed in the patients studied (Bernstein and Robbins, 1969). If such a large dose of thyroxine were administered to euthyroid patients in whom most of the thyroxine binding sites were saturated, more free hormone might be available and adverse cardiovascular effects might appear.

Thyroid replacement therapy, guided by assessments of the clinical state and by measurements of the PBI, is generally indicated in documented thyroid hormone deficiency. T_4 can be used regardless of the cause of the hypothyroidism (including simple or nontoxic goiter, chronic thyroiditis, use of complete blocking doses of antithyroid drugs, thyroid cancer, and use of ^{131}I therapy). An excellent review provides further information on clinical thyroid problems (Ingbar and Woeber, 1968).

Full-replacement therapy in myxedema is usually not difficult to achieve, although the broad range of normal thyroid function makes serial PBI determinations necessary. As long as the drug is of uniform potency, 90 to 180 mg of desiccated thyroid per day will usually produce euthyroidism. The advantage of using synthetic and well-standardized preparations is emphasized. Orally, 0.1 mg of T_4 is equivalent to approximately 60 mg of desiccated thyroid; the replacement dose of T_4 is 0.15 to 0.3 mg per day. A T_3 dose of 25 to 40 μg is equivalent to approximately 60 mg of desiccated thyroid, and the replacement dose is usually 50 to 100 μg per day (Green, 1968). The dose may vary with body weight and is conventionally lower in the older patient who has cardiac disease. The therapeutic response can be judged by reversal of skin changes, improvement in delayed relaxation of deep-tendon reflexes, increase in body temperature, rise in pulse, fall in the plasma cholesterol, and changes in the serum PBI.

In two clinical situations, therapy is less than satisfactory: myxedema with coma and cretinism.

The management of severe hypothyroidism and coma is complex and difficult (Catz and Russell, 1961). The factors that may contribute to coma during severe hypothyroidism are carbon dioxide retention, fluid and electrolyte disturbances, marked hypothermia, or a combination of these factors. In addition to replacement of thyroid hormone, attention should be directed toward treating associated illness such as infection, gastrointestinal bleeding, paralytic ileus, congestive heart failure, inappropriate ADH secretion, hypoglycemia, or respiratory acidosis. These complications of hypothyroidism often are not recognized unless they are carefully sought. Sometimes the major clinical features of

a primary disease, and the opportunity to reverse them with specific therapy, may so consume a physician's interest and attention that complicating features are ignored or remain undiscovered for prolonged and sometimes critical periods. This may occur despite the knowledge and observation that the complications can be fatal and can be as readily and specifically reversed as the primary disease.

The dose and type of thyroid replacement in severe myxedema coma are controversial. Based on calculations of the estimated depletion of the extrathyroidal hormone pool and of the diminished fractional turnover rate, an intravenous dose of 500 μg of L-thyroxine, followed by 50 μg of oral L-thyroxine daily to restore the euthyroid state gradually, was suggested (Holvey et al., 1964). In contrast, both oral and intravenous triiodothyronine in small doses have been successful. Because of the difficulty in excluding associated adrenal insufficiency in myxedema, corticosteroids are generally recommended in coma, although their efficacy has not been fully documented. Sedation should be avoided because it can accentuate respiratory depression. Overhydration is a risk, as water excretion is impaired in the hypothyroid state; dilutional hyponatremia can be severe (Goldberg and Reivish, 1962). Rapid reversal of the associated hypothermia may be dangerous because of the redistribution of blood away from vital tissues to tissues such as skin.

Most drugs given to a patient with hypothyroidism have a markedly prolonged effect because of decreased glomerular filtration and delayed hepatic metabolism. Drug absorption from gut or even from intramuscular injections may be compromised. *Principle: Although reversal of the primary disease is the major consideration of therapy, ancillary measures should be evaluated for potentially detrimental effects.*

Cretinism is often not detected at birth. It is usually recognized at age 3 to 6 months, when bone and growth retardation is severe. If therapy is begun soon after birth, normal mental and physical function may develop; mental impairment is never fully recovered if therapy is delayed. Hypothyroid infants require relatively larger doses of thyroid hormone replacement therapy than do adults. Initial administration of 25 μg of L-thyroxine daily, with an increase in the daily dose of 25 μg each week until a dose of 100 μg is reached after 3 to 4 weeks, has been recommended (Ingbar and Woeber, 1968). The PBI should be maintained at 8 to 10 μg/100 ml, but if normal intellectual function does not develop, higher doses should be tried.

Thyroid hormone therapy has often been used to treat a wide variety of illnesses unassociated with hypothyroidism, such as obesity, hyper-cholesterolemia, habitual abortions, and infertility. The efficacy of this therapy is doubtful unless hypothyroidism exists. Since the symptoms of hypothyroidism are nonspecific, empiric therapy without documentation of depressed thyroid function may obscure a primary disease responsible for the symptoms. *Principle: Whenever possible, a proper and reliable diagnosis should be established before therapy is instituted. This requirement prevents toxicity of a drug used irrationally and often leads to appropriate diagnosis and therapy.*

Treatment of Hyperthyroidism

The etiology of hyperthyroidism is uncertain. Therapy for the severe metabolic derangement of thyrotoxicosis is directed toward interference with the synthesis, release, or peripheral effects of thyroid hormones. Lack of firm agreement concerning the relative benefits of each of these forms of therapy reflects the problems encountered in the treatment of some patients with hyperthyroidism and the observation that no one method is clearly more efficacious than the others.

Iodide is the oldest therapeutic agent for hyperthyroidism. The clinical response of the thyrotoxic patient is often rapid and dramatic. The effects may be discernible in 24 hours, and the maximal effects occur in approximately 2 weeks. The vascularity of the thyroid gland is greatly reduced, and the gland becomes small and firm. Unfortunately, iodide therapy usually does not completely control the disease and hyperthyroidism may return in a more fulminant form if the iodide is discontinued suddenly or if doses are omitted. Some normal patients, when treated with large doses of saturated solutions of potassium iodide for long periods, may develop goiter and hypothyroidism, without previous evidence of hyperthyroidism (Cerletty and Engbring, 1969). Treatment of chronic bronchitis with saturated solutions of potassium iodide as an expectorant may cause hypothyroidism (see Chapter 6).

Although large doses of iodide can induce an abrupt decrease in organic binding of iodide by the thyroid, this effect is apparently transient. The major action of iodide is to inhibit release of active hormones (Ingbar and Woeber, 1968). When large doses of iodide are administered prior to thioamide therapy, the organic iodide stores within the gland increase, retarding the clinical response to antithyroid drugs. In addition, the high plasma iodide concentration lowers the thyroidal ^{131}I uptake and increases the total dose of radiation necessary to affect the gland. *Principle: Careful consideration allows choice of a nonconflicting sequence of drugs when it is likely that more than one drug will be necessary to manage a disease state.*

Iodide therapy is indicated when a rapid clinical response is necessary (e.g., when treating thyroid storm, acute hyperthyroidism occurring during or after thyroid gland surgery, and severe cardiac disease associated with or precipitated by hyperthyroidism). The exact dosage and form in which iodide is administered bear little relationship to the inhibition of release of thyroid hormones, provided not less than 6 mg is given daily. Ten drops of Lugol's solution are usually given three times a day, providing almost 40 times the necessary dose. The large dose is given to preclude a "breakthrough" of thyroid function. The dose interval is important because the drug has a short half-life. If iodide is not given every 8 hours, periods of escape from thyroid suppression may lead to the clinical interpretation of an inadequate drug response. On the other hand, excesses of iodide lead to adverse reactions and also interfere with the ability to follow the PBI and the ^{131}I uptake as parameters of the therapeutic response. During the use of iodide, the "true T_4" and T_3 resin uptake tests are still valid measurements of thyroid function.

Side effects of iodide include sialadenitis, which may respond to a decrease in dose. Other side effects such as drug fever, skin rash or lesions resembling periarteritis nodosa, and thrombotic thrombocytopenic purpura require that iodide be discontinued.

A group of monovalent anions, including thiocyanate and perchlorate, inhibits thyroid function by competitive inhibition of the active iodide-concentrating system, eventually leading to goiter formation. The inhibition may be overcome by increasing iodide intake. Despite their antithyroid efficacy, both drugs have been abandoned owing to their severe toxic effects on bone marrow.

The major drugs used in the therapy of hyperthyroidism are the thioamides, propylthiouracil, and methimazole (Tapazole) (Figure 7–3). In earlier studies the mechanism of action of these drugs was thought to involve only inhibition of the oxidation of iodide to iodine. However, their action is more complex, involving effects on organic binding and coupling. These effects may help to explain why the early ^{131}I uptake may remain elevated in the hyperthyroid patient even though euthyroidism is approached.

Studies on the pharmacokinetics of these drugs have been hampered by inability to measure these compounds directly. Although most studies indicate rapid metabolism, rapid

Thioamides

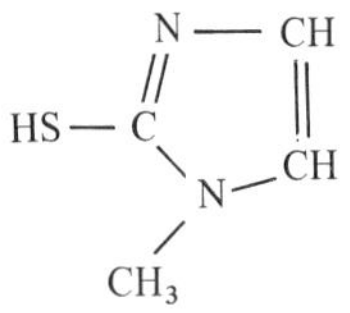

Methimazole 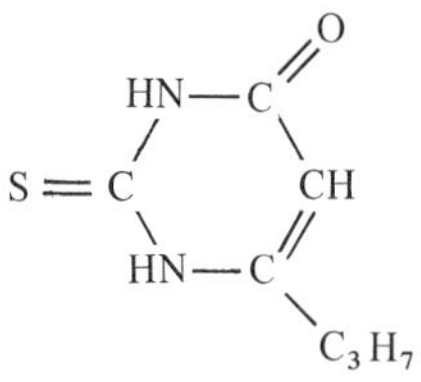   Propylthiouracil

Amino Heterocyclic Compounds and Substituted Phenols

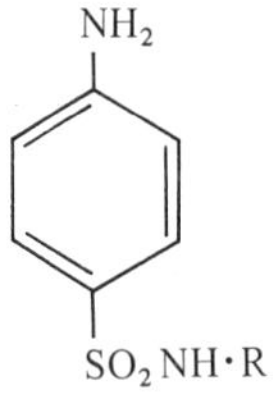

Sulfonamides 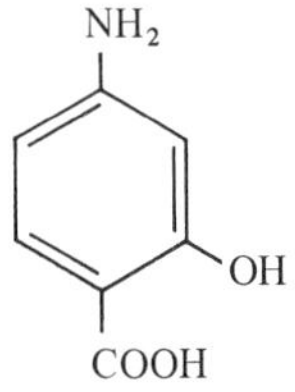   p-Aminosalicylic Acid 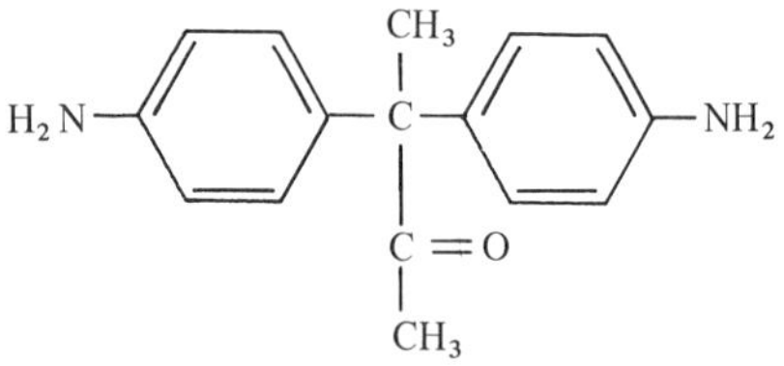   Amphenone B

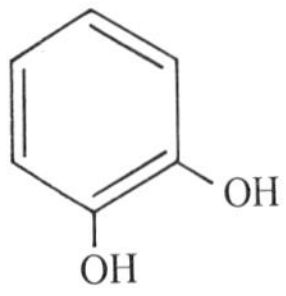

Resorcinol

Figure 7–3. Drugs with antithyroid action.

absorption (20 to 30 minutes), and a brief duration of action (usually 2 to 3 hours) (Maloof and Soodak, 1963), treatment of hyperthyroid patients with a single daily dose of propylthiouracil has been accomplished (Greer *et al.*, 1965). The thioamides cross the placental barrier and are excreted in the breast milk; they can suppress thyroid function in the fetus or neonate.

The clinical response to these drugs is delayed for approximately 1 to 2 weeks, since the thioamides do not affect the release of thyroid hormones, as does iodide. The rapidity of the response probably depends upon the completeness of the blockade of thyroid hormone synthesis, the quantity of preformed hormone in the gland, and the peripheral rate of turnover of the thyroid hormones. The decrease in size of the thyroid gland during treatment is a good index of drug efficacy. Late enlargement of the gland, while the patient takes effective blocking doses of these drugs, suggests an increase in pituitary TSH that can be suppressed by replacement doses of T_4. Combination therapy of thioamide and T_4 has proved successful and averts hypothyroidism (Howard, 1967).

How long should antithyroid drug therapy be maintained? Because hyperthyroidism is a disease with exacerbations and remissions, medical therapy may not be needed on a continuous basis. However, in view of the severity of the disease, the complete natural course of the illness cannot be studied without drug or palliative therapy. In practice, thioamide therapy is usually continued until the patient has been euthyroid for 6 to 12 months. A T_3 suppression test is then performed while the patient remains on therapy. If the early ^{131}I uptake is suppressed by T_3, indicating a physiologic pituitary-thyroid response, drugs are withdrawn. The likelihood of permanent remission is approximately 50 to 60% (Reveno and Rosenbaum,

1964). If another course of medical therapy is needed, improvement and remission may be expected in another 10 to 20%. Prognostic signs for predicting a poor response to drug therapy include a very large goiter, severe cardiovascular and ocular manifestations of hyperthyroidism at the onset of the disease, and lack of response to the T_3 suppression after an adequate course of drug therapy.

The relative toxicities of the antithyroid drugs have been compared (Trotter, 1962). The overall risk of thioamide drug therapy is small. The most common untoward reaction is skin rash, which may disappear even if the therapy is continued. The most serious side effects are agranulocytosis and bone marrow aplasia, which usually improve when therapy is discontinued (Martelo et al., 1967). The fact that mild granulocytopenia may occur as a result of hyperthyroidism makes evaluation of small changes in the leukocyte count difficult in the patient taking these drugs. Since serial white-blood-cell counts in all hyperthyroid patients on thioamide therapy are not generally helpful, it is recommended that any sore throat or fever be quickly evaluated by the physician and that any fall in the leukocyte count be carefully followed. If a drug reaction occurs with propylthiouracil or methimazole, the alternate drug may be tried. If a similar reaction occurs, surgery or ^{131}I therapy must be considered.

Surgery for Hyperthyroidism. Prior to 1950, surgical therapy was performed in almost all thyrotoxic patients, in spite of the risk of thyroid storm, sudden death, and the other complications of surgery. With the advent of effective antithyroid drugs and careful iodide therapy, surgery was made safer, but patients referred for surgery were often sicker than those treated by drugs alone and reported complication rates remained high, perhaps artificially so. One of the most thorough series reviewed approximately 4000 patients treated surgically for hyperthyroidism (Hershman, 1966). The study found a mortality rate from surgery of 0 to 3%, recurrence or persistence of hyperthyroidism of 1 to 18%, vocal cord paralysis of 0 to 4%, and permanent hypothyroidism of 4 to 30%. As more patients are followed for longer periods, the incidence of permanent hypothyroidism after surgery approaches that following ^{131}I therapy (Nofal et al., 1966; Werner, 1967b). Although the risk of recurrent hyperthyroidism after surgery is less than 10%, the added risk of surgical complications makes this form of "definitive therapy" less than ideal. The argument that a very small percentage of patients with diffuse toxic goiter may have microscopic papillary carcinoma does not seem sufficient to warrant the surgical risk. The development of thyroid cancer after ^{131}I therapy does not prove that the cancer results from the therapy, since it may occur independent of ^{131}I therapy. Because the hyperthyroid state must be controlled before surgery is performed, surgery is not the initial therapy of choice in the acutely ill hyperthyroid patient.

"RAI Therapy." Radioactive iodine therapy was first used by Hertz and Roberts in 1942. Like stable iodine, radioactive iodine is concentrated in the thyroid gland and selectively irradiates the thyroid, sparing other vital organs. The fear of the increased risk of thyroid cancer has not been verified (Saenger et al., 1968). Radioactive iodine has many advantages in the therapy of hyperthyroidism. It is inexpensive, relatively safe, and easy to administer; has few immediate complications; and slowly reverses the hyperthyroid state. Commonly recognized disadvantages of this therapy include its delayed action, production of radiation thyroiditis, difficulty in establishing a safe but effective dose, questionable safety in young patients and during pregnancy, and the uncertainty as to the induction of genetic abnormalities. Recently, much emphasis has been placed on the high incidence of latent hypothyroidism and on the possible persistent chromosomal aberrations following ^{131}I therapy. *Principle: The physician must be prepared to assess the long-range effects of therapy as well as initial results. Data on prolonged and subtle effects of therapy are much more difficult to record than are acute cause-and-effect events. However, such data may be most critical in establishing a risk-benefit ratio for the therapy and, therefore, in establishing a logical choice between modes with differing acute effects.*

The incidence of hypothyroidism among 848 hyperthyroid patients treated with ^{131}I therapy and 121 patients treated with surgery has been compared (Nofal et al., 1966). At least 15% of those treated with ^{131}I therapy (in a dose of approximately 180 μc/g of thyroid) developed hypothyroidism with a cumulative increase of approximately 3% per year. In the surgically treated group, approximately 2% per year developed hypothyroidism. Other authors have also noted the disturbing increase of latent hypothyroidism after ^{131}I therapy. Therefore, smaller doses, usually one half the originally prescribed dose (i.e., 70 to 90 μc/g of thyroid), have recently been employed with good clinical success and with an apparent decrease in the incidence of permanent hypothyroidism (Hagen et al., 1967). Few data are available at present on the natural history of untreated hyperthyroidism. Perhaps a significant percentage of untreated hyperthyroid patients also would develop hypothyroidism.

Consistent chromosomal aberrations in peripheral leukocytes were reported in five hyperthyroid patients who received ^{131}I therapy (Cantolino et al., 1966). The clear-cut difference reported between the normal control population and patients receiving ^{131}I therapy is striking. Since no chromosomal abnormality is desirable, ^{131}I therapy may be potentially hazardous; further study is needed to establish the relative risk of all types of antithyroid therapy.

A comparison of 22,000 hyperthyroid patients receiving ^{131}I treatment with 14,000 patients treated without ^{131}I found the incidence of leukemia to be similar in the two groups, although hyperthyroid patients as a group may have a somewhat greater risk of leukemia independent of therapy (Saenger et al., 1968). [125]I therapy has been used to treat the hyperthyroidism more rapidly, with less damage to the entire thyroid, in hopes of inducing fewer instances of late latent hypothyroidism (Grieg et al., 1969). With this treatment, the lower energy of radiation emitted by the isotope may less severely damage the thyroid cell nuclei and the thyroid stroma.

Adrenergic Receptor Blockade Therapy. Various antagonists of the sympathetic nervous system have been used to control the sympathetically mediated manifestations of hyperthyroidism (Das and Krieger, 1969; Stout et al., 1969). Since these drugs do not affect the PBI or the ^{131}I uptake, they are thought to act solely by blocking the peripheral actions of circulating catecholamines. They are not primary therapeutic measures for hyperthyroidism. Hyperthyroid patients show increased responsiveness to adrenergic stimulation; reserpine and guanethidine (both catecholamine depletors) have been used to decrease some of the cardiovascular manifestations of the disease (Canary et al., 1957). The true efficacy of these drugs is difficult to evaluate, as antithyroid drug therapy was given simultaneously; improvement could have been due in part to control of the thyrotoxicosis. Seventy-five thyrotoxic patients were successfully treated with the beta-blocking drug propranolol, the therapeutic end points being a slowing of pulse and improvement of symptoms (Vinik et al., 1968). Other investigators have been less successful with beta blockade, but this may be partly related to the earlier use of pronethalol, which unlike propranolol has intrinsic sympathomimetic activity. Although propranolol creates sympathetic blockade in hyperthyroid patients, myocardial function may continue to be abnormal. The possibilities of being able to prepare patients for surgery more

rapidly and of being able to control symptoms by immediate nonspecific therapy, while waiting for results of laboratory tests, are important clinical considerations. Alpha blockade with phenoxybenzamine HCl, in combination with beta blockade with propranolol, has also been advocated to reverse the cardiac manifestations of the hyperthyroid state rapidly (Stout et al., 1969). Before undertaking this potentially dangerous therapy, the physician must weigh the risks of increased heart failure and worsened asthma and the known improvement with established forms of therapy with the benefits of slowed pulse, decreased oxygen consumption, decreased Achilles reflex time, and decreased symptoms. Further evaluation of the effect of sympathetic blockade on metabolic functions in peripheral tissues must be completed before these drugs can be strongly recommended in the treatment of hyperthyroidism. *Principle: The advantages of a drug compared to a standard therapy, or a low risk-benefit estimate of a drug during its early evaluation, often are not considered in the zealous attempt to establish drug efficacy. Unless the risk-benefit ratio is compared to that of standard therapy, a drug cannot be established as desirable.* Such comparisons using antiadrenergic or adrenergic blocking agents have not been made. Therefore, data on the management of thyroid storm with reserpine may be valid but are uninterpretable in terms of establishing the drug's role (see Chapter 1).

Special Pharmacologic Problems in Thyroid Storm. Thyroid storm is frequently, although not invariably, abrupt in onset, occurring in the partly treated thyrotoxic patient (Ingbar, 1966). This serious complication of thyrotoxicosis is often precipitated by severe infection, surgery, diabetic ketoacidosis, or complications of pregnancy. General medical supportive measures include correction of hyperthermia, adequate hydration, a diet high in calories and vitamins, sedatives, and frequent observation in quiet surroundings.

The major therapeutic goals are the rapid interruption of synthesis, blockage of release, and antagonism of the peripheral actions of thyroid hormones. Large doses of antithyroid drugs (900 to 1200 mg of propylthiouracil a day) are usually begun to help prevent storage of iodine. The antithyroid drugs must be given by mouth or by nasogastric tube, since parenteral therapy is generally unavailable. In extreme emergency, methimazole may be prepared in solution for intravenous use and may be given in doses of approximately 20 mg every 4 hours. Iodide rapidly blocks hormonal release and should be given either orally as Lugol's solution (30 drops in divided doses every 8 hours) or intravenously as sodium iodide (1 to 2 g). If severe cardiac manifestations (other than congestive heart failure) are present, beta blockade with propranolol may be undertaken with approximately 2 mg of propranolol intravenously or 20 mg by mouth every 4 hours (Das and Krieger, 1969). Treatment of arrhythmias and congestive heart failure in patients with thyroid storm may be exceedingly difficult until the hyperthyroidism is controlled. Large doses of digitalis are generally ineffective, and digitalis toxicity may occur as the hyperthyroidism is controlled. Often the patient is too ill to await laboratory confirmation of thyroid storm, and therapy must be started after appropriate studies have been conducted. Although adrenocortical insufficiency is poorly documented in this condition, glucocorticoid therapy during the acute phase of the illness may increase survival (Waldstein et al., 1960). Attempts to lower circulatory levels of thyroxine acutely by blood exchange and plasmapheresis have been successful (Ashkar et al., 1970).

Thyrotoxicosis During Pregnancy. Thyrotoxicosis during pregnancy is one of the most disputed and difficult therapeutic problems in the management of hyperthyroidism. Since hyperthyroidism and pregnancy have many features in common and diagnostic radioactive iodine studies are generally not used during pregnancy, the laboratory confirmation of hyperthyroidism is often difficult. Although the absolute level of the PBI, the high T_3 resin uptake, and the decrease in the PBI with large doses of T_3 may be helpful, the absolute diagnosis often remains in doubt (Kaori and Itelson, 1969). The oral tyrosine tolerance test may be especially helpful in diagnosing hyperthyroidism during pregnancy (Rivlin et al., 1965).

Another difficulty in the management of this type of hyperthyroidism results from the lack of understanding of the kinetics of placental transfer of thyroid hormones. Although TSH does not cross the placenta, antithyroid drugs readily enter the fetal circulation and may induce hypothyroidism in the fetus. It is unknown whether fetal requirements for thyroid hormones are met largely by secretion of the fetal or of the maternal thyroid (Werner, 1967a).

If hyperthyroidism is mild, therapy may be delayed, provided frequent clinical observations are made to ensure detection of any rapid worsening of the hyperthyroid state. Surgical thyroidectomy for the ill pregnant patient with hyperthyroidism has the distinct advantage of avoiding drug effects on the fetal thyroid. Since the exact adjustment of antithyroid drug dosage to ensure adequate control of hyperthyroidism and yet preserve fetal thyroid function is difficult, elective thyroidectomy at the end of the first trimester of pregnancy may be the best therapy. The dose of T_3 necessary to suppress the pituitary-thyroid axis of the pregnant patient may be greater than normal, and large doses of T_3 (300 μg) may cross the placenta and preserve fetal thyroid function during antithyroid drug therapy (Raiti et al., 1967). Since thyroid hormones may not completely counteract the block induced by antithyroid drugs, and since fetal hypothyroidism might lead to severe central nervous system damage, the most reasonable approach would seem to be surgery at the end of the first trimester or careful adjustment of antithyroid drug dosage to the minimum required for borderline control of thyroid function. Because antithyroid drugs can enter the mother's milk, breast feeding should be avoided. Iodide therapy should not be utilized because of the likelihood of inducing iodide goiter in the fetus. In the third trimester of pregnancy, propylthiouracil in doses of 100 mg or less every 6 hours, or methimazole in doses of 10 mg or less every 6 hours, may be used to sustain the mother through parturition, after which a definitive therapeutic decision can be made. The incidence of fetal thyroid blockade decreases as the dose of antithyroid drugs decreases.

Juvenile Hyperthyroidism. Although juvenile hyperthyroidism is rare, it is of special interest because of the difficulties encountered in its treatment. Therapy with radioactive iodine is often avoided because of the dangers of possible genetic damage, fear of inducing thyroid cancer or other malignancy, and the high incidence of late hypothyroidism. Antithyroid drug therapy plus supplemental T_4 is efficacious and will prevent even mild hypothyroidism, although frequent relapses, lack of apparent response to therapy, drug toxicity, and failure of the patient to cooperate may make surgery necessary. Subtotal thyroidectomy was considered to be the treatment of choice after experience with 253 hyperthyroid children less than 15 years old (Hayles and Chaves-Carballo, 1965). Similarly, surgery was concluded to be the therapy of choice after a review of 45 hyperthyroid children under the age of 16 (Kogut et al., 1965). Despite these reports, in view of the rising incidence of latent hypothyroidism after extensive surgery, the exacerbations of hyperthyroidism if surgery is not extensive enough, the operative risks of hypoparathyroidism and damage to the recurrent laryngeal nerves, and the surgical mortality, an adequate trial of the antithyroid drugs should be considered prior to surgical therapy. *Principle: When young people are considered for therapy, a relatively effective, safe, and* *specific drug may be elected because it is associated with the fewest long-term detrimental effects. This consideration is particularly germane for an intermittent disease in which there is a reasonable chance of inducing a prolonged remission.*

Infiltrative Ophthalmopathy and Pretibial Myxedema. Infiltrative ophthalmopathy may be an extremely severe complication of thyroid disease. In its most severe form, it may be very resistant to therapy and may cause loss of vision. The natural history of exophthalmos is quite variable and may include exacerbations and remissions that are apparently unrelated to the degree of thyroid dysfunction. The only accepted relation of thyroid function and exophthalmos is worsening of the ophthalmopathy if hypothyroidism supervenes rapidly. For mild cases, local measures such as dark glasses, diuretics, elevation of the head of the bed, local lubricants, and patching of the eyes at night help prevent corneal breakdown and serious eye damage. Fortunately, the ophthalmopathy most often is not progressive; conservative and palliative therapy is adequate until a spontaneous remission occurs.

In the severe form, several modes of therapy have been suggested. Massive doses of corticosteroids (120 to 140 mg of prednisone each day) may be of value (Werner, 1966). This dose can be tapered, once remission is induced, to one that controls progression and maintains remission with a minimum of side effects. Steroid therapy in the absence of thyroid disease has been associated with development of marked exophthalmos and has also caused an increase in intraocular pressure, precipitating glaucoma.

Large doses of radioactive iodine after aggressive surgical thyroidectomy have been advocated (Bauer and Catz, 1966). These investigators treated 126 patients with Graves's disease and 8 patients with pretibial myxedema with this program. Improvement in proptosis, ophthalmopathy, and pretibial myxedema occurred in 129 patients (Catz, 1967). Other investigators have not been as successful with this approach and feel that total thyroidectomy has no value in the therapy of the active eye changes of Graves's disease (Werner *et al.*, 1967).

X-ray therapy to the orbit and total hypophysectomy, although not well studied, have also been suggested. If steroid therapy does not control the disease and if visual acuity is compromised, surgical closure of the lids and surgical orbital decompression should be undertaken. The natural history of infiltrative exophthalmos often includes spontaneous stabilization, but it may leave residual muscle damage. Surgical correction of the diplopia and the stare may be successful.

In some patients with Graves's disease a violaceous, elevated induration appears on the pretibial area and on the dorsum of the feet. This unusual manifestation of Graves's disease, termed pretibial myxedema, is always associated with a high serum titer of LATS. Therapy of this lesion was generally unsuccessful until corticosteroids were shown to decrease the circulating levels of LATS and to improve the skin lesions (Benoit and Greenspan, 1967). Striking remissions with local steroid creams (0.2% fluocinolone acetonide) under occlusive dressings have been demonstrated with a low frequency of undesirable steroid side effects (Kriss *et al.*, 1967).

Principle: When possible therapies are diverse and clinical data are conflicting, the therapist must look for strengths and weaknesses in the data in order to make his own decision: (1) The conclusions related to results or to comparisons of results may be invalid by virtue of patient selection or improper design (see Chapter 1). (2) The drugs may all be relatively ineffective (particularly with a disease whose natural history is either unknown or notoriously variable) or may not have been used in a manner that can establish their effect. (3) The pathogenesis of the disease may be so poorly understood that all therapy must be considered palliative, and heroic doses or irreversible measures should be approached with caution. (4) If alternative 3 applies (as with exophthalmos and perhaps with pretibial myxedema) the physician can recognize that his therapy is empiric and palliative, use the therapy, but remain open to valid studies suggesting unconventional approaches. If the disease is uncommon, the patient may be referred to therapists skilled in the special care of such patients. Often a carefully selected referral may be a valuable therapeutic maneuver.

Management of Thyroiditis

The diagnosis of Hashimoto's thyroiditis is indicated by the presence of an enlarged thyroid, a high titer of thyroid antibodies, association with other diseases presumed to have an "autoimmune etiology," evidence of iodoprotein production (an unusually large difference between the PBI and BEI or true T_4), decreased responsiveness to TSH, and a rapid decrease in the size of the goiter following corticosteroid therapy. Although most patients need no therapy, thyroid hormone and corticosteroids are indicated if the goiter is exceedingly large, leading to compression symptoms, or if there is severe local pain. Steroid therapy dramatically decreases the signs and symptoms of the disease, diminishes the thyroid antibody titer, and may return thyroid function tests to normal (except for the ^{131}I uptake) (Blizzard *et al.*, 1962).

However, once the steroid therapy is discontinued, the signs and symptoms recur and long-term thyroid hormone therapy may be required to suppress the gland's activity. In many patients, no therapy is needed, but each patient must be watched for clinical signs and laboratory evidence.

A major problem in the management of Hashimoto's thyroiditis is its differentiation from thyroid cancer. A rapid increase in size and rock-hard texture of the thyroid gland, increased size of regional lymph nodes, hoarseness, lack of laboratory evidence for thyroiditis (increased thyroid antibodies or increased iodoprotein), and absence of a decrease in the size of the gland with steroid therapy or thyroid hormone therapy may all suggest thyroid cancer. If the diagnosis is uncertain, open surgical biopsy is indicated; needle biopsy is probably not a reliable means for excluding the presence of cancer (Colcock and Pena, 1968).

Three other distinct types of thyroiditis deserve brief mention. Pyogenic thyroiditis, a severe but uncommon infection of the thyroid gland caused by bacteria, usually responds to appropriate antibiotics. Subacute thyroiditis apparently is a viral infection of the thyroid occurring frequently in middle-aged females, often misdiagnosed as pharyngitis. It differs from Hashimoto's thyroiditis in that there is no apparent association with autoimmune diseases, and it often subsides in a few months leaving a histologically normal thyroid, only rarely ending in hypothyroidism. A very rare type of thyroiditis is Riedel's thyroiditis, characterized by extensive fibrosis of the thyroid with involvement of mediastinal structures and retriperitoneal areas. The characteristic feature of the disease is a rock-hard thyroid gland, often confused with thyroid cancer. Therapy with thyroid hormone reverses associated hypothyroidism, but the gland rarely decreases in size and biopsy is often necessary to eliminate the possibility of cancer. The basis for the use of corticosteroids in thyroiditis is twofold. The primary disease has all the characteristics of an active inflammatory process; nonspecific suppression of its acute manifestations occurs (see Chapter 9). In addition, the response to the drug can be used as a diagnostic tool. *Principle: When a response to a drug has been well characterized, the changes it produces in the character of a disease can be used to establish the diagnosis with confidence when the response is favorable, or to indicate the need for further research for the proper diagnosis when the response is "poor" or unexpected.*

Management of Thyroid Cancer

The management of thyroid cancer is extremely complex. Literature reviewing the subject is controversial, owing to uncertain pathological diagnostic criteria, variation in the clinical course, uncertainty as to the natural history of the disease, inadequate follow-up studies, and bias in patient selection. The management and evaluation of thyroid cancer represent a problem in approaching a patient with a nodular thyroid gland, which has been excellently reviewed (Ingbar and Woeber, 1968).

The Thyroid Clinic at the University of California in San Francisco, under the direction of Dr. Francis S. Greenspan, has evaluated some 90 patients with nodular thyroid glands during the past 5 years. Those patients considered to be at high risk of thyroid cancer were young children and young adult males with previous x-ray therapy to the head or neck, recent hoarseness, a solitary firm dominant nodule that did not concentrate ^{131}I, cervical lymphadenopathy, diffuse calcification within a nodule, or failure of the gland to regress in size or an increase in gland growth when the patient was taking 0.3 mg T_4 per day. Of the 90 patients, 21, judged to be at high risk of thyroid cancer, had surgical biopsies of the thyroid; 14 of these patients had thyroid cancer. Those patients considered to be at low risk had a family history of goiter, a diffuse multinodular goiter, soft nodules that concentrated ^{131}I, very high antithyroid antibody titers, shell-like calcifications of the nodules, and definite regression in gland size during T_4 therapy. Of the 90 patients 69 were judged to be at low risk; 16 of these eventually had a surgical biopsy and only 2 proved to have thyroid cancer.

It is exceedingly difficult to evaluate any form of therapy when dealing with a cancer that grows as slowly as does well-differentiated cancer of the thyroid. Two major factors determine the prognosis of thyroid cancer: the cell type and the extent of the disease. Approximately 60% of thyroid cancer is papillary, 20% follicular, 10% solid with amyloid stroma, and 10% anaplastic (Winship, 1967).

If a well-differentiated thyroid cancer is found at surgery, a total thyroidectomy is usually recommended, with removal of those regional lymph nodes that are clinically enlarged. Some therapists advocate only lobectomy and neck dissection to decrease the risk of hypoparathyroidism, since development of thyroid cancer in the contralateral lobe is rare. However, intraglandular spread of papillary cancer may be demonstrated in serially sectioned thyroid glands (Winship, 1967). A postoperative whole-body radioactive iodine uptake and scan, as well as determination of urinary radioactivity, should be utilized to quantitate the degree of metastatic follicular elements remaining. This procedure may be of value in patient follow-up.

Radioactive iodine is not always effective in treating metastatic thyroid cancer, since only a small portion of the tumor may contain follicular elements capable of trapping radioactive iodine. Several methods have been used to augment radioactive iodine uptake by the tumor, including discontinuation of thyroid replacement therapy to induce hypothyroidism, administration of exogenous TSH, and the induction of iodine depletion with a low-iodine diet, mannitol diuresis, or diuretic therapy (Hamburger and Desai, 1966). Despite these measures, ^{131}I uptake by the tumor is generally slight and the doses of radioactive iodine needed are very high, often leading to severe radiation damage to the lungs and bone marrow.

Long-term thyroid hormone therapy to reduce TSH levels and prevent TSH stimulation of tumor growth is strongly recommended. The less differentiated cancers are much more malignant and less responsive to any form of therapy. Occasionally a syndrome of hyperthyroidism due to functioning metastasis from thyroid cancer may occur. Usually this arises in well-differentiated cancer, with a long latent period before the onset of the clinical hyperthyroidism. The metastases are most often found in the bones and lung (Federman, 1964). These patients should be treated with large doses of radioactive iodine followed by antithyroid drugs to destroy the metastases and to control the acute symptomatology. *Principle: Although the treatment of thyroid cancer may be too vigorous with some lesions, effective care of the severe forms becomes effective only after factors controlling thyroid function are appreciated and applied in a rational manner.*

THE PITUITARY

The pituitary gland consists of the anterior, posterior, and intermediate lobes, which differ from each other functionally, embryologically, and histologically. The anterior lobe has a richly vascular portal system draining the hypothalamus and is under the direct influence of hypothalamic releasing factors to secrete growth hormone (GH) adrenocorticotropin (ACTH), thyrotropin (TSH), follicle-stimulating hormone (FSH), luteinizing hormone (LH), and prolactin. Secretion of these hormones is controlled by feedback mechanisms dependent on the concentration of the end-organ hormones in the blood. Most feedback mechanisms are thought to function by decreasing secretion of hypothalamic releasing factors.

The intermediate lobe of the pituitary produces two polypeptide hormones, alpha and beta melanocyte-stimulating hormones (MSH), which increase skin pigmentation. The posterior lobe is directly connected with the hypothalamus through numerous nerve fibers and stores vasopressin and oxytocin, which are synthesized in the supraoptic and paraventricular nuclei of the hypothalamus.

Most cases of hypopituitarism involve the sequential loss of GH, gonadotropins, ACTH, and TSH (Rabkin and Frantz, 1966). Deficiency of growth hormone can most accurately be detected by the failure of insulin-induced hypoglycemia to increase the plasma growth hormone concentration. Loss of gonadotropin function can be assessed by the failure of clomiphene citrate to increase pituitary gonadotropins. The diagnosis of ACTH deficiency can be established by failure of metyrapone or vasopressin to stimulate ACTH release. An adequate TSH reserve is implied by an increase in plasma TSH following administration of antithyroid drugs (Studer et al., 1964), or by a rise in thyroidal ^{131}I uptake after cessation of TSH suppression with triiodothyronine (Stein and Nicoloff, 1969). TSH can also be directly measured (Mayberry et al., 1971; Hershman and Pittman, 1971; Editorial, 1971).

Recent purification and synthesis of the hypothalamic releasing factors have led to the discovery that thyrotropin-releasing factor may be a single tripeptide containing glutamic acid, histidine, and proline. Administration of the synthetic tripeptide to animals led to a rapid rise in circulating TSH level (Bowers et al., 1969). Future study may allow application of this technique to the other pituitary trophic hormones and may lead to the accurate and rapid diagnosis of pituitary dysfunction in man. *Principle: In a system of interrelating controls, therapeutic agents can be used as diagnostic tools. Pharmacologic principles apply, but the objectives of "therapy" in this circumstance are already explicitly quantitated, the dose of the drug is specified, and the drug is administered to determine whether the individual's response falls within preset limits. When the diagnosis has been established, the test drug often becomes a therapeutic agent. The only preset goal is the desired response; the dosage selected is an amount adequate to meet the predetermined goal.*

Treatment of Pituitary Hypofunction

Panhypopituitarism may be caused by postpartum pituitary necrosis, irradiation or surgical ablation, tumors (either primary or metastatic), infarction of pituitary tumors, or several granulomatous "storage" diseases. The clinical manifestations include wrinkled skin, pallor out of proportion to a mild anemia, loss of axillary and pubic hair, amenorrhea and loss of libido, breast atrophy in females, myxedema facies, signs of hypothyroidism, low blood pressure, hypoglycemia, and a variable degree of inanition, but not emaciation to a degree suggesting starvation. Specific radioimmunoassays for each of the pituitary trophic hormones have allowed the recognition of specific isolated deficiencies of the anterior pituitary hormones GH, ACTH, TSH, and gonadotropins (Odell, 1966). Isolated iatrogenic hypopituitarism also may occur following long-term, high-dose corticosteroid hormone therapy. Alternate-day corticosteroid therapy may also alter the functional capacity of the hypothalamic pituitary axis, but growth hormone release is apparently preserved with either form of steroid therapy (Martin *et al.*, 1968).

Anorexia nervosa may be difficult to distinguish from panhypopituitarism. In patients with anorexia nervosa, the psychiatric history, extreme inanition, alert mental status, presence of axillary and pubic hair, and borderline tests of adrenal, thyroid, and gonadal function may help to establish the diagnosis. The concentration of growth hormone in serum is strikingly increased during starvation; assessment of this hormone probably is the most sensitive method to differentiate patients with anorexia nervosa from those with hypopituitarism (Roth *et al.*, 1967).

Although theoretically attractive, the use of pituitary or placental hormones for treatment of panhypopituitarism is impractical, because the preparations are impure and expensive, rapidly provoke antibody production, and must be administered parenterally. Potent and effective hormones (corticosteroids, thyroid hormones, and androgens or estrogens) usually are employed in replacement therapy. Exceptions to this general rule will be cited.

Corticosteroid therapy is essential in the treatment of panhypopituitarism. Cortisone acetate in doses of about 25 mg daily is usually sufficient. Some investigators recommend divided doses of 15 mg in the morning and 10 mg at night, in consideration of the drug's metabolism and the normal diurnal secretion pattern of the hormone. Specific mineralocorticoid therapy may not be required if adequate salt intake is maintained, since aldosterone secretion is usually normal in patients with hypopituitarism, although an occasional patient may not increase aldosterone secretion normally in response to sodium restriction. The daily dose of cortisone acetate or of its equivalent must be tailored to the individual patient.

The correction of thyroid hormone insufficiency can best be achieved by slowly increasing the dose of L-thyroxine from 0.05 mg daily to the normal maintenance dose of 0.2 to 0.3 mg daily. Rapid reversal of the hypothyroid state with triiodothyronine may prove hazardous if it stimulates metabolism and demand for cardiac output prior to its full cardiotonic effects. When both thyroid and adrenal insufficiency are documented, adequate corticosteroid therapy should be administered before correction of the hypothyroid state. If thyroid replacement is given first, precipitation of adrenal insufficiency occasionally results, presumably because of the ability of thyroid hormone to increase the rate of metabolism of corticosteroids.

In men, oral or parenteral administration of androgens will improve well-being, strength, and libido. Estrogen therapy in women will reverse the genital atrophy, symptoms of osteoporosis, and skin changes of panhypopituitarism. Although most adult patients with panhypopituitarism do not require pituitary gonadotropins, these hormones must be administered to normalize gametocyte function if conception is desired. Clomiphene citrate therapy is of no value in panhypopituitarism because the drug induces ovulation by releasing pituitary gonadotropins. This represents a clear instance in which knowledge of the mechanism of action of a drug is mandatory before it can be used rationally.

When hypopituitarism occurs before puberty, special therapeutic problems arise, since the combined deficiencies of growth hormone, sex hormones, and thyroid hormone cause severe proportional dwarfism. This abnormality must be treated with both replacement hormones and parenteral growth hormone. Although preparations of growth hormone are not commercially available, small quantities can be obtained for clinical investigation. Patients with isolated growth hormone deficiency or prepubertal panhypopituitarism respond well to parenteral growth hormone if the other hormones are present in normal quantities.

Without the delicate control provided by normal hypothalamic–pituitary–target organ function, the patient given replacement hormonal therapy may need to alter his therapy, especially corticosteroids, to meet the increased requirements of trauma, infection, surgery, or pregnancy. Side effects of replacement therapy must be carefully assessed. Mild hyperadrenocorticism can frequently occur unless criteria such as changes in body weight, blood pressure, and white-blood-cell count are frequently measured and limits of these changes are preset as guides to therapy. Diabetic patients become sensitive to insulin when they undergo pituitary ablation as treatment for fulminant diabetic retinopathy.

Summary Principles: (1) The simple absence of a hormone does not mean that it should necessarily be replaced, unless there is specific therapeutic intent. (2) When the physiologic effects of several substances are interrelated, it may be necessary to replace all before the pharmacologic effects of any one are fully expressed. (3) As hormones may be considered monitors of the milieu intérieur, *the effects of one may balance or modulate the effects of others (e.g., the effects of corticosteroids, growth hormone, catecholamines, and insulin on glucose concentrations in blood). When several but not all hormones are absent and their balanced effect is critical for a vital function (e.g., blood glucose concentration), administration of exogenous hormone must be carefully planned and frequently assessed.*

Treatment of Pituitary Hyperfunction

Hyperfunction of the acidophilic cells of the pituitary results in the well-recognized syndromes of acromegaly and prepubertal gigantism. Acidophilic adenomatas are usually large enough to erode and enlarge the walls of the sella turcica, resulting in an abnormal skull x-ray (especially if sellar volumes are calculated from tomograms of the sella turcica). Tumor growth has a variable effect on the production of the other pituitary hormones, and hypogonadism, hypoadrenalism, and hypothyroidism may complicate the condition, each requiring treatment. The clinical diagnosis of acromegaly can be confirmed by the demonstration of excessive circulating growth hormone in the fasting state that is not suppressed by glucose administration (Roth *et al.*, 1967).

Basophilic adenomata are small pituitary tumors that do not usually erode the sella turcica and are associated with Cushing's syndrome. Many instances of the syndrome have been described without evidence of a pituitary tumor (see Treatment of Cushing's Syndrome, page 329).

After bilateral adrenalectomy, some patients develop a marked increase in skin pigmentation and progressive enlargement of the sella turcica (Nelson *et al.*, 1960). As these pituitary tumors enlarge they may impair visual acuity. Following bilateral adrenalectomy, frequent x-ray examination of the skull should aid in the identification of this pituitary tumor before loss of other pituitary hormones or decreased visual acuity occurs.

Although the radioimmunoassay of growth hormone is of value in the *diagnosis* of acromegaly, its major use has been to assess therapeutic progress and to indicate the required intensity and duration of *therapy* in acromegaly. In the past, irradiation of the pituitary has been the treatment of choice for acromegaly, in the absence of significant parasellar extension of the tumor. Although the disease may be slowed by radiation, circulating concentrations of growth hormone generally remain elevated. Therefore, more aggressive measures have been undertaken, including cryosurgery (Rand, 1966), stereotactic implantation of yttrium or iridium (Jadresic and Poblete, 1967), proton beam radiotherapy (Kjellberg *et al.*, 1968), and surgical hypophysectomy. These specialized procedures are available only at certain medical centers. Acute visual loss and disturbance of extraocular muscle function are the primary indications for immediate surgical

removal of the tumor. If there is significant parasellar extension, as demonstrated by encephalography or angiography, surgical hypophysectomy may be the most effective form of therapy. Regardless of the type of therapy in acromegaly, restoration of a normal growth hormone concentration is often followed by rapid regression of the soft-tissue involvement, improved glucose tolerance, and loss of symptoms of fatigue, headache, and arthritis.

Because of a relative resistance to insulin, the glucose intolerance associated with acromegaly may be difficult to manage with oral hypoglycemic agents or even with insulin. Transient improvement in carbohydrate tolerance has been reported in some acromegalic patients treated with estrogens (Mintz *et al.*, 1967). Recently, progestins have been used to treat acromegaly (Lawrence, 1969). Medroxyprogesterone acetate caused a striking diminution in blood growth hormone concentration, along with some symptomatic and cosmetic benefit. Further study is needed to clarify the role of each of these modalities of therapy.

At the time of diagnosis or following aggressive therapy of a pituitary tumor, relative or absolute deficiency of ACTH, TSH, or gonadotropins may develop. It is important to suspect these deficiencies and to treat them when they are documented.

Treatment of Posterior Pituitary Disease

Diabetes insipidus is a relatively rare disease resulting from complete or partial loss of the posterior pituitary hormone, arginine vasopressin, or, in some cases, from failure of end-organ response to the hormone. Vasopressin is produced in nerve cells of the hypothalamus and is stored in the posterior pituitary. Its release is controlled primarily by osmoreceptors. Dehydration and hyperosmolarity increase rates of hormone release. Emotional and physical stress, as well as some drugs (e.g., morphine and nicotine), can also discharge vasopressin, whereas alcohol inhibits its release. Destruction of the hypothalamus or the posterior pituitary by infection, neoplasia, or trauma leads to marked polyuria and polydipsia. Fluid loss may reach distressing proportions (sometimes exceeding 10 liters in 24 hours). The specific gravity of the urine is usually less than 1.004. If an adequate thirst mechanism is present, and the patient has access to fluid, physiologic balance can be maintained by increasing oral intake. If the patient becomes unconscious because of surgery or trauma, severe dehydration may ensue. Careful records of intake, output, and body weight are critical in managing these patients.

The differential diagnosis of diabetes insipidus must include persistent excessive water intake and either renal unresponsiveness to adequate amounts of vasopressin or inadequate secretion of vasopressin. These conditions can usually be distinguished by demonstrating unresponsiveness of the ADH release mechanism to hypertonic saline infusions or to dehydration. The creatinine clearance must remain stable during these maneuvers, as acute decreases in glomerular filtration rate may result in an increase in urine osmolality. Dehydration in a patient with diabetes insipidus may be exceedingly dangerous, and careful measurements of body weight and cardiovascular signs must be made to avoid severe hypovolemia. Pharmacologic means of releasing ADH with nicotine have produced variable responses. If the ADH release mechanisms are thought to be impaired, normal renal responsiveness to exogenous hormone (aqueous vasopressin or pitressin tannate in oil) must be demonstrated. These tests usually distinguish renal unresponsiveness and inadequate vasopressin secretion, but persistent excessive water intake may be difficult to exclude without overt evidence of severe psychiatric disease (Leaf and Coggins, 1968).

Some patients with mild diabetes insipidus can be treated with fluid alone. The most valuable replacement therapy of vasopressin deficiency is pitressin tannate in oil, administered intramuscularly every 24 to 72 hours. In this dosage form, the antidiuretic action is prolonged. The preparation is supplied in vials that must be warmed and shaken vigorously to ensure adequate dispersion of the hormone. To avoid water intoxication, intramuscular vasopressin should be administered only after the therapeutic effect of the previous dose has disappeared, and the patient should regulate fluid intake based on urine volume. Following head trauma or neurosurgical procedures, transient diabetes insipidus may occur. Since this complication may disappear spontaneously, medication should be periodically withdrawn before a diagnosis of permanent diabetes insipidus is made. After prolonged excessive intake of water, in either psychogenic or true diabetes insipidus, the initial response to maximal doses of ADH is blunted, possibly because the tonicity of the renal medullary interstitium is decreased. With correction of the polydipsia, sensitivity to ADH is restored and dose requirements diminish.

Vasopressin may be given intramuscularly in aqueous form, but its short duration of action makes it clinically undesirable except as a diagnostic test or in treating patients for short periods. Because the drug has a half-life of only 20 minutes when administered intravenously, this route of administration is not recommended for treatment of diabetes insipidus. Vasopressin can be given as a nasal snuff. Local irritation to the nasal mucosa and uncertain absorption limit the usefulness of this dosage form. Since these preparations are of animal origin, allergic reactions to them are common. A synthetic substitute, lysine-8-vasopressin, administered as a nasal spray every 8 hours, is generally free of allergic reactions and offers promise as a more ideal replacement therapy (Rallison and Tyler, 1967; Mimica et al., 1968).

Vasopressin is a powerful constrictor of smooth muscle, causing severe vasoconstriction in both peripheral and visceral blood vessels. This effect on visceral blood flow has led to the use of vasopressin as a temporary means of decreasing bleeding in the gastrointestinal tract, especially from esophageal varices (see Chapter 4).

The ability of vasopressin to release ACTH and other pituitary hormones has led to its use as a diagnostic tool in assessing pituitary function (Tucci et al., 1968), but the large doses of vasopressin required cause vasoconstriction, an increase in blood pressure, and abdominal cramps. These tests should not be performed in patients with known coronary artery disease, as they may precipitate severe angina or myocardial infarction. An electrocardiographic monitor should be available during these tests.

In addition to specific hormonal replacement therapy, diuretic therapy and salt restriction may reduce polyuria in these patients, decreasing urine volumes by one-half to one-third. This antidiuresis has been observed with several diuretic agents and appears to be related to sodium depletion; it can be overcome with salt loading and may be maintained in the salt-depleted patient on a low-salt diet after diuretic therapy has been discontinued. An increased fractional absorption of water in the proximal tubule, with delivery of less water to the distal segment, accounts for the antidiuresis. Whether this phenomenon is related to reduced glomerular filtration rate, intrarenal vascular changes, or increased renin and angiotensin production has not been decided conclusively (Brown et al., 1969). Recently the sulfonylurea, chlorpropamide, has been shown to diminish polyuria in these patients. The exact mode of action is not certain (Arduino et al., 1966), although chlorpropamide and vasopressin may share a common site of action on the renal tubule (Ingelfinger and Hays, 1969). *Principle: Changing the dosage form of a single chemical may provide wide latitude in its effectiveness in a variety of clinical settings. An understanding of renal physiologic mechanisms may allow the paradoxical use of a diuretic to elicit an antidiuretic response!*

Prolonged exposure of normal subjects on a normal fluid intake to excessive amounts of vasopressin leads to a state of hyponatremia with a normal glomerular filtration rate and sodium wasting in the urine, but no edema or dehydration. A similar constellation of findings, referred to as the inappropriate ADH syndrome, occurs in a variety of conditions associated with pulmonary and cerebral disease states (Bartter and Schwartz, 1967). The typical features of the syndrome include hyponatremia with continued renal excretion of sodium, urine osmolality greater than that appropriate to the tonicity of the plasma, correction of the hyponatremia by fluid restriction, and absence of clinical evidence of volume depletion, edema, or renal or adrenal impairment. An ADH-like material may be produced by certain nonpituitary tumors or may originate from the hypothalamic-pituitary region under nonphysiologic conditions (Ivy, 1968). Chlorpropamide has an ADH-like action in both normal subjects and patients with diabetes insipidus (Arduino *et al.,* 1966). A syndrome resembling inappropriate secretion of ADH was described in a patient receiving chlorpropamide. The syndrome abated when the drug was stopped and reappeared when the therapy was resumed on three separate occasions (Fine and Shedrovilzky, 1970).

THE ADRENAL CORTEX

Since the classic descriptions of adrenal insufficiency by Addison and Brown-Séquard over a century ago, our knowledge of the physiologic functions of the adrenal cortex has remarkably increased. The adrenals secrete a number of steroidal hormones that have important effects on a variety of metabolic processes in nearly every organ of the body. The hormones include progesterone, corticosteroids (corticosterone and cortisol), aldosterone, androgens (androstenedione and testosterone), and estrogen (estradiol). Aldosterone production occurs in the zona glomerulosa of the cortex; the remaining hormones are synthesized in the zona fasciculata and zona reticularis.

The synthesis of the adrenal steroids occurs through a number of metabolic steps beginning with cholesterol, the major precursor of all steroid hormones (Figure 7–4). Although cholesterol can be synthesized from precursors by the adrenal cortex, free plasma cholesterol appears to be utilized preferentially for adrenal steroidal biosynthesis. The next series of reactions, often referred to as the desmolase reactions, leads to cleavage of the cholesterol side chain, resulting in the formation of a 21-carbon steroid, Δ5-pregnenolone. This compound

can then undergo a number of hydroxylations, primarily on carbons 11, 17, and 21. The intracellular site of hydroxylation is not entirely clear, but both microsomes and mitochondria appear to be involved. During this sequence of reactions, either before or after hydroxylation, oxidation of the 3β-hydroxyl group occurs, with a shift in the double bond of the β ring from the 5-6 to the 4-5 position, followed by conversion to aldosterone by formation of the hemiacetal ring. The androgens of the adrenal cortex are apparently synthesized by cleavage of the C-20,21 side chain of 17-hydroxypregnenolone and 17-hydroxyprogesterone and subsequent reduction to the 17-ketones; estrogens are probably derived from testosterone by mechanisms similar to those described in the gonads.

Several hereditarily determined enzyme deficiencies in adrenal steroid biosynthesis, known collectively as the adrenogenital syndrome, lead to various degrees of virilization. The basic defect in these syndromes is deficient synthesis of cortisol resulting in increased release of ACTH, leading in turn to excessive production of androgenically active steroids. Certain complications (hypertension or salt loss) may accompany the fundamental defect, depending on the location of the enzymatic block. Female patients with the syndrome are often recognized at birth owing to masculinization of the external genitalia, whereas male patients are usually not discovered until later in infancy or early childhood (Bongiovanni and Root, 1963).

The most common form of this disorder is a partial or complete salt-losing syndrome secondary to a relative deficiency of a C-21 hydroxylating enzyme, which leads to a decreased formation of 11-desoxycortisol and 11-desoxycorticosterone. Most often this block is only partial, such that sufficient amounts of cortisol and aldosterone are produced to prevent dramatic adrenal insufficiency and sodium loss. A defect in the C-11 hydroxylating enzyme system results in an increase in 11-desoxycortisol and 11-desoxycorticosterone. The latter has potent mineralocorticoid effects, leading to hypertension. Metyrapone inhibition of C-11 hydroxylation followed by a fall in plasma cortisol and increase in plasma ACTH forms the basis of an important test of pituitary function (Figure 7–4).

A rare enzymatic defect in steroid biosynthesis involving the side-chain cleavage of cholesterol results in large, lipid-laden adrenals, inhibition of adrenal steroidogenesis, and death in early infancy. Aminoglutethimide (Elipten), initially marketed as an anticonvulsant, produces adrenal insufficiency by inhibition of side-chain cleavage of cholesterol. The therapeutic benefits of such a blocking drug to patients with adrenal carcinoma are under investigation.

The absence of an adrenal 17-hydroxylase enzyme has recently been documented (Biglieri *et al.,* 1966; Goldsmith *et al.,* 1967). In the presence of this enzyme deficiency, cortisol formation is inhibited, but corticosterone, a potent mineralocorticoid, is produced in excess, resulting in hypertension. This syndrome is similar to the 11-hydroxylase deficiency in which hypertension is caused by an increase in

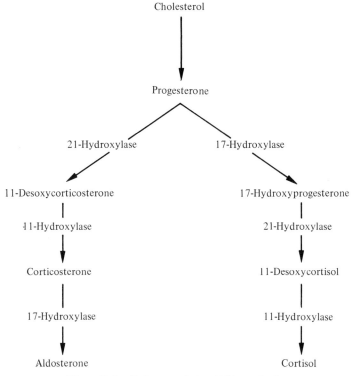

Cholesterol

Progesterone

21-Hydroxylase   17-Hydroxylase

11-Desoxycorticosterone   17-Hydroxyprogesterone

11-Hydroxylase   21-Hydroxylase

Corticosterone   11-Desoxycortisol

17-Hydroxylase   11-Hydroxylase

Aldosterone   Cortisol

Figure 7–4. Pathways of steroid biosynthesis.

desoxycorticosterone. Both forms of hypertension can be treated effectively by correcting the relative deficiency of cortisol.

The metabolism of steroid hormones occurs chiefly in the liver by several pathways, including reduction, hydroxylation, cleavage of the side chain, and esterification. The first mechanism results in reduction of the C-4-5 double bond of the A ring and reduction of the 3-ketone group. In hypothyroidism reduction of the 3-ketone group may occur in the absence of reduction of the A ring. Little is known about the importance of C-20,21 side-chain cleavage in the liver, but hydroxylation of cortisol in the 6 position increases water solubility of cortisol, facilitating its renal excretion. Increased excretion of 6-hydroxycortisol has been reported in newborn infants and in patients with Cushing's syndrome, chronic liver disease, hyperestrogenism after certain drug therapy that causes microsomal enzyme induction, and advanced cancer. This finding may be related in some patients to an inability to reduce the A ring of cortisol. The majority of the steroid hormones undergo esterification in the liver to water-soluble sulfates and glucuronides. Sulfation occurs through a soluble sulfotransferase, which utilizes 3'-phosphoadenosine-5'-phosphosulfate as the donor. Glucuronide formation is controlled by the enzyme glucuronyl transferase. *Principle: This brief review of the biosynthesis and metabolism of steroid hormones stresses the complexity of biotransformation, the chemical similarity between hormones with widely divergent physiologic and pharmacologic potential, and the fact that abnormalities in synthesis (genetically inherited or metyrapone induced) could simultaneously produce excesses of one hormone and deficiencies of another, which may require specific therapeutic intervention.*

The major factor contolling the biosynthesis of corticosterone and cortisol is ACTH. The primary site of action of this pituitary hormone is not entirely clear. ACTH activates adrenal adenyl cyclase activity, increasing cyclic AMP generation from ATP. Cyclic AMP may in turn increase membrane permeability to cholesterol. At high concentrations of ACTH, increased synthesis of a specific highly labile protein occurs under the stimulus of cyclic AMP. This protein may stimulate the desmolase reaction, facilitating utilization of cholesterol in the steroid synthetic pathway. ACTH may also increase the transfer of stored cholesterol from adrenal cellular liposomes, making more free cholesterol available for steroid biosynthesis. ACTH reduces the amount of adrenal ascorbic acid and liberates free fatty acids from adipose tissue. *Principle: When using ACTH or any drug, remember both the primary and the secondary effects (often called side effects) of the drug. Both are part of the pharmacologic effects of the drug and usually cannot be separated unless the dose response for each effect is different. This principle emphasizes the necessity to carefully establish the choice of dose and dose interval for any given therapeutic effect* (see Chapter 15).

ACTH production is directly influenced by the hypothalamus. A specific hypothalamic polypeptide, corticotropin-releasing factor (CRF), is secreted into the pituitary portal system and stimulates both the release and the production of ACTH in the anterior pituitary. The daily fluctuations (diurnal variation) in ACTH output by the pituitary appear to be related to variations in the output of hypothalamic CRF.

A number of factors affect the hypothalamic production of CRF and therefore the release of ACTH. A daily diurnal rhythmicity in pituitary production of ACTH results in peak levels in the serum just prior to awakening, the lowest levels being reached during the early part of sleep. A rhythmic daily pattern of growth hormone has also been detected (Quabbe et al., 1966), which is greatly influenced by sleep patterns (Honda et al., 1969). The ACTH pattern can be altered by disrupting the normal sleep pattern for several days and disappears in patients with Cushing's syndrome. The diurnal rhythmicity of ACTH release is not related to the concentration of circulating corticosteroids, since it persists in patients with bilateral adrenalectomy who are given exogenous steroid replacement. Adrenal steroids do, however, affect CRF and ACTH production, elevated concentrations in blood causing indirect depletion of pituitary ACTH. The release of ACTH is increased by a number of other stimuli, including psychologic stress, trauma, surgery, hyperthermia, exposure to cold, hypotension, hypovolemia, hypoglycemia, acute hemorrhage, anoxia, and increased secretion of epinephrine and vasopressin. In many of these situations, the increase in ACTH can be blocked by administration of exogenous corticosteroids. ACTH release can occasionally "break through" suppression by exogenous corticosteroids. Several drugs, including reserpine, diphenylhydantoin, and the phenothiazines, can interfere with the release of ACTH in response to trauma. *Principle: The diurnal variation of corticosteroid release and the feedback effects of corticosteroids on ACTH release and on ACTH stores should be kept in mind when considering the pharmacologic use of corticosteroids. Replacement of steroids should closely simulate the physiologic pattern of release.* Not only dose but also dosage form and interval between doses should be considered. Pathologic stress stimulates endogenous corticosteroid secretion. During stress, an amount of corticosteroids equal to that produced during maximal endogenous secretion may be required.

The accuracy of estimation of steroid secretory rates in man is largely dependent on the methods utilized. In normal subjects, the secretion of cortisol has been estimated by isotope dilution methods to be 14 to 23 mg per 24 hours. In the morning, approximately 600 μg per hour of cortisol are secreted. Normal corticosterone secretory rates have been estimated at 2.0 mg per 24 hours. Following administration of ACTH cortisol secretion increases to approximately 250 mg per 24 hours and corticosterone to 40 mg per 24 hours. The volume of distribution of cortisol is about 10 liters; the half-life in plasma is about 80 minutes after tracer doses and 120 minutes after larger doses. Factors decreasing the rate of removal of cortisol from the plasma include chronic liver disease, chronic renal failure, and hypothyroidism. Hyperthyroidism and drugs that stimulate hepatic microsomal enzymes increase the rate of removal of cortisol from plasma.

In plasma, cortisol is normally bound to an alpha-globulin (corticosteroid-binding globulin, CBG) that is synthesized in the liver. This specific globulin has a high affinity for cortisol. When all binding sites are occupied, cortisol adheres weakly to albumin. Aldosterone is chiefly bound to albumin and has only a weak affinity for CBG (Forsham, 1968). Approximately 90% of cortisol circulates in the bound form and only 10% in the free (active) fraction. At plasma concentrations of cortisol exceeding the binding capacity of CBG, free urinary cortisol increases, serving as a sensitive index of adrenal hyperfunction. Unfortunately, the assay procedure for free urinary cortisol is technically difficult and not generally available. The conjugated metabolites of cortisol are water soluble and do not bind to carrier proteins. CBG is increased by estrogen therapy and pregnancy and diminished by chronic liver disease or nephrosis. These changes in CBG do not lead to clinical manifestations of cortisol excess or deficiency, since the same amount of active free hormone is still available to the tissues (only free cortisol inhibits the hypothalamus-pituitary feedback mechanism). This carrier-protein binding mechanism protects cortisol from rapid inactivation in the liver and may allow a large peripheral store of readily available hormone for emergency use.

The corticosteroids have many vital biochemical and physiologic actions that have important pharmacologic implications. Depending on the dose and on the tissue affected, corticosteroids may act directly or may affect the actions of other hormones (e.g., catecholamines) in a permissive way.

The corticosteroids affect the skeletal system by blocking the effects of growth hormone on bone, by antagonizing the effects of vitamin D, and by inhibiting protein synthesis necessary for bone matrix development. They have profound effects on carbohydrate and fat metabolism, increasing gluconeogenesis, producing glucose intolerance, and causing hyperlipidemia. Corticosteroids affect nervous system function by altering nerve conduction and may produce changes in personality. They affect the gastrointestinal system by altering gastric mucus and increasing gastric acid production. Administration of corticosteroids may result in polycythemia, thrombocytosis, and leukocytosis with an increase in total granulocytes but a decrease in lymphocytes and eosinophils. Cortisol is essential for the normal excretion of a water load by the kidneys. The complex effects of mineralocorticoids on electrolyte excretion are described in detail in Chapter 3. The vascular compartment is expanded by the mineralocorticoid effect of corticosteroids, and cortisol may play a permissive role in catecholamine effects on peripheral vasculature, but this has been disputed (Verrier et al., 1969). Corticosteroids have anti-inflammatory properties that alter the normal responses of connective tissues to injury. This effect, combined with the lysis of lympho-cytes, reduces antibody production and impairs immune responses.

Many of the diverse biologic actions of the corticosteroids can be measured quantitatively in animals; these form the basis for potency estimates that may be applicable pharmacologically in humans. Those steroidal functions most often tested by bioassay are anti-inflammatory activity, ACTH suppression, actions to increase gluconeogenesis, thymolytic and eosinopenic responses, ulcerogenic activity, sodium retention, potassium wasting, and effects on calcium and phosphorus metabolism (Steelman and Hirschmann, 1967). Unfortunately the estimation of anti-inflammatory activity is difficult; full appreciation of this therapeutic effect requires a more precise understanding of the process of inflammation.

Alterations in the structure of the corticosteroids (Figure 7–5) may greatly affect the rate of metabolism of the hormones. For example, when a double bond is added to the basic cortisol structure (e.g., dexamethasone), the half-life is prolonged since the rate of liver inactivation is decreased. The increases in biologic half-life of corticosteroid preparations

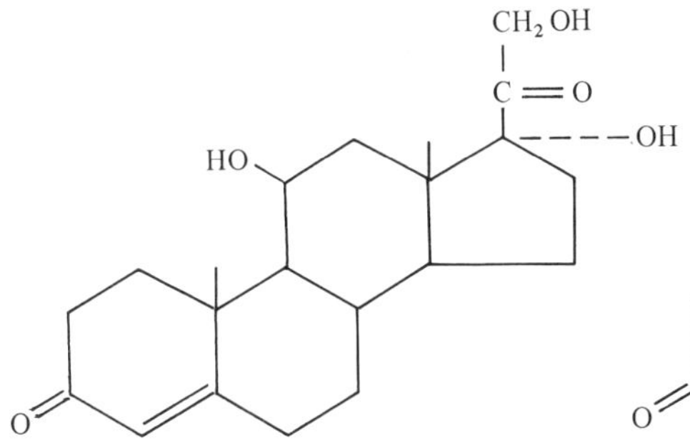

Cortisol (hydrocortisone)

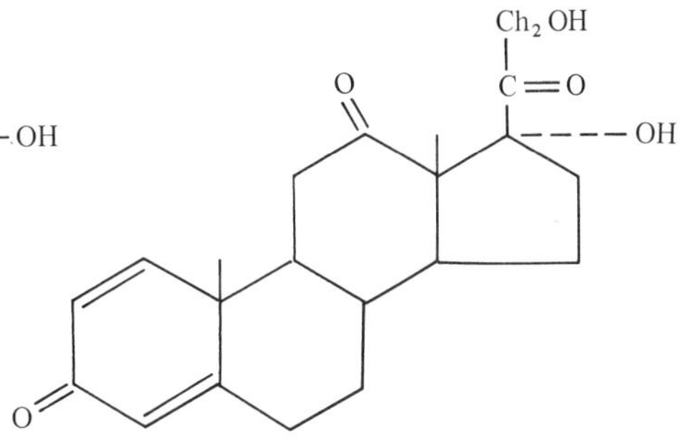

Prednisone

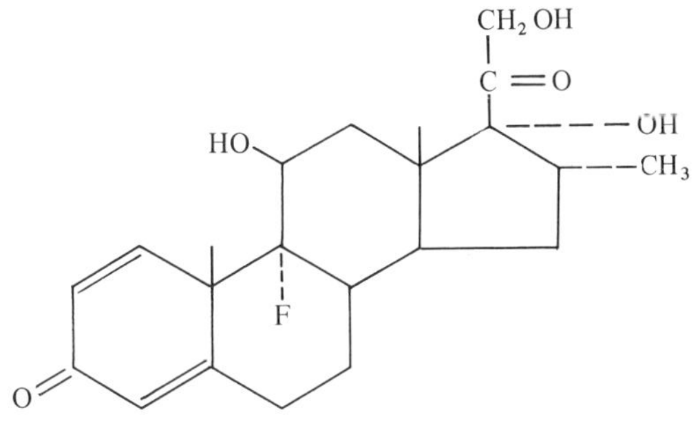

Dexamethasone

Figure 7–5. Structures of some commonly used steroid preparations.

Table 7–6. COMPARISONS OF SEVERAL NATURAL AND SYNTHETIC CORTICOSTEROID PREPARATIONS

COMPOUND	NONPROPRIETARY NAME	EQUIV. ORAL DOSE (mg)	ANTI-INFLAM-MATORY POTENCY	RELATIVE SALT-RETAINING POTENCY
Hydrocortisone	Cortisol	20	1	+ +
Cortisone	Cortisone	25	0.7	+ +
1-Dehydrohydrocortisone	Prednisolone	5	4	+
1-Dehydrocortisone	Prednisone	5	3.9	+
6α-Methylprednisolone	Methylprednisolone	4	5	0
6α-Fluoro-16α-methylprednisolone	Paramethasone	2	11	0
16α-Hydroxy-9α-fluoroprednisolone	Triamcinolone	4	4	0
16β-Methyl-9α-fluoroprednisolone	Betamethasone	0.6	26	0
16α-Methyl-9α-fluoroprednisolone	Dexamethasone	0.75	30	0
9α-Fluorohydrocortisone	Fluorocortisone	0.1	15	+ + + +

following alterations in structure are: cortisone, 30 minutes; prednisone, 60 minutes; corticosterone, 70 minutes; cortisol, 90 minutes; prednisolone, 200 minutes; and dexamethasone, 200 minutes (Forsham, 1968).

Many attempts have been made to alter the corticosteroid molecule to obtain the most desirable clinical effects with the least undesired effects. The 9α-halogenated steroids have proved to be more potent anti-inflammatory agents than cortisol, but produce excessive sodium retention; 9α-fluorohydrocortisone is a potent mineralocorticoid used in the treatment of adrenal insufficiency. With the introduction of the C-1,2 double bond (e.g., prednisolone) a preparation with marked anti-inflammatory activity and less sodium retention than cortisol has been obtained. Some methylated and hydroxylated corticosteroids have been synthesized and tested clinically, but further study is needed to define their structure-activity relationships. Knowledge of the method of administration and of the basic steroidal structure can be utilized to tailor therapy to specific needs. Triamcinolone is useful for topical administration because of its relatively poor absorption from skin. Cortisol acetate and methylprednisolone, when given intramuscularly, have a slower absorption and more prolonged effects than does cortisol or prednisolone. *Principle: Learning to use only a single preparation would limit the therapist's flexibility in use of the steroids for different purposes.*

The relative potencies of the major synthetic anti-inflammatory adrenal steroids and mineralocorticoids available in the United States are listed in Table 7–6.

Treatment of Adrenal Insufficiency

Deficiency of adrenal corticosteroid hormones may be primarily due to destructive lesions of the adrenal, including chronic infections such as tuberculosis or other granulomatous diseases, malignant disease, and massive hemorrhage, and secondarily to a deficiency of ACTH production by the pituitary. Idiopathic atrophy of the adrenal gland is the most frequent cause of Addison's disease (Eisenstein, 1968). There is abundant evidence that autoimmunity may cause this type of adrenal insufficiency. Idiopathic atrophy of the adrenal is occasionally associated with other endocrine disturbances, especially thyroid disease, diabetes mellitus, hypoparathyroidism, and pernicious anemia (Eisenstein, 1968). Deficiency of glucocorticoids is suggested by weakness and fatigue, nausea and vomiting, dehydration, hypotension, muscle cramps, hyponatremia, and low 17-hydroxycorticoids that do not rise following ACTH stimulation. Increased skin pigmentation may result from high ACTH concentrations. Loss of adrenal androgen is indicated by low urinary 17-ketosteroids and by loss of pubic hair and libido. Aldosterone deficiency is suggested by hypotension, low urinary aldosterone levels that do not increase after salt deprivation, and a serum Na^+/K^+ ratio of less than 30 (Frawley, 1967).

Glucocorticoid deficiency is generally treated by daily oral administration of 20 to 30 mg of hydrocortisone or its equivalent. Divided doses are given to mimic the normal diurnal variation (i.e., two thirds of the daily dose with the morning meal and one third with the evening meal). Clinical guidelines to the appropriate dose include improved strength, freedom from gastrointestinal complaints, increased white-blood-cell count with a decreased percentage of lymphocytes, normalization of electrolytes, decreased postural hypotension, and decreased skin pigmentation. Side effects warranting a decrease in dose include excessive weight gain, ravenous appetite, severe insomnia, or psychosis.

If the adrenal is entirely destroyed, mineralocorticoid therapy as well as glucocorticoid hormonal therapy may be required. If adrenal insufficiency is secondary to pituitary disease, retention of mineralocorticoid function may occur. During acute illness or surgery the glucocorticoid dosage must be increased to prevent adrenal crisis. In addition to intravenous cortisol, therapy requires adequate volume replacement with saline or whole blood, treatment of the underlying precipitating event (usually infection), and control of associated hypoglycemia with intravenous dextrose. Since the half-life of cortisol is only 90 minutes, therapy must be given every 4 to 6 hours to ensure complete and continuous therapeutic effects. Each patient with adrenocortical insufficiency should carry identification stating the need for additional glucocorticoid therapy in the event of acute illness. *Principle: The danger of stating that a given dose of a drug should be used to manage a specific state in all patients is illustrated by the use of corticosteroids in the treatment of Addison's disease. The objectives of therapy should be explicit and repeatedly evaluated. The potential variables influencing dose requirements (body size, adiposity, hepatic and thyroid function, or stress) must be considered to avoid arbitrary or irrational drug administration.*

Mineralocorticoid need is best met with the potent sodium-retaining hormone 9α-fluorocortisol since aldosterone is relatively inactive by mouth. Guidelines for this therapy include stabilization of body weight, normalization of urinary and plasma sodium and potassium, and improved blood pressure. Side effects include excessive weight gain, edema, hypertension, potassium loss, and congestive heart failure due to sodium retention.

Treatment of Cushing's Syndrome

Treatment of Cushing's syndrome requires an accurate diagnosis of the underlying disorder. The diagnosis can usually be established by the demonstration of an increased amount of Porter-Silber chromogen (17-hydroxysteroids) in the urine, loss of the normal diurnal variation of plasma cortisol, failure of the adrenal-pituitary axis to be suppressed following dexamethasone administration, or increased free cortisol in the urine (Liddle, 1967; O'Neal, 1968; Sawin *et al.*, 1968) (Table 7–7). The most frequent cause of spontaneous Cushing's syndrome is bilateral adrenal hyperplasia associated with increased concentration of plasma ACTH but without an obvious pituitary tumor. An increasing number of nonendocrine tumors associated with production of an ACTH-like polypeptide are now recognized by their ful-

minant course, pronounced hypokalemic alkalosis, and resistance to stimulation with ACTH or to suppression with large doses of dexamethasone (Nichols *et al.*, 1968). A relatively small number of cases of Cushing's syndrome are due to benign or malignant tumors of the adrenal.

Surgical excision is usually the most effective form of therapy for tumors of the adrenal. Treatment of patients with both inoperable functioning and nonfunctioning adrenal carcinomas may be achieved with the use of a congener of DDT called o,p'-DDD. The exact mechanism of action of this drug is not known, but its usefulness was initially suggested by the observation that dogs treated with DDD develop atrophy and necrosis of the adrenal cortex (Hutter and Kayhoe, 1966). The usefulness of this drug is limited by tumor unresponsiveness, gastrointestinal side effects, mental depression, and somnolence (Netto *et al.*, 1963; O'Neal, 1968). Only one-third of patients treated with this drug have objective tumor regression (Hutter and Kayhoe, 1966). Aminoglutethimide (Elipten) therapy has also been associated with transient improvement in some patients with Cushing's syndrome due to metastatic adrenal cancer (Schteingart *et al.*, 1966). Although initially introduced as an anticonvulsant, this drug was found to have toxic effects for both the adrenal and thyroid. The inhibition of adrenal steroidogenesis probably occurs at a step early in the steroid biosynthetic pathway involving the desmolase side-chain cleavage of cholesterol (Cash *et al.*, 1967).

Many drugs affect hepatic enzyme systems, thereby altering both normal metabolic processes and the metabolism of the administered drug. Several structurally unrelated drugs and insecticides that stimulate drug-metabolizing enzyme activity also stimulate steroid hydroxylase activity. In man, treatment of patients with phenobarbital, diphenylhydantoin, and phenylbutazone markedly stimulates the metabolism of cortisol to 6β-hydroxycortisol (Conney, 1969). The full clinical importance of these drug interactions requires further study.

If bilateral adrenal hyperplasia is associated with increased production of pituitary ACTH, pituitary irradiation may be of value (Heuschele and Lampe, 1967). Unless the physician is certain that the patient does not have an adrenal neoplasm as the cause of the Cushing's syndrome, adrenal exploration is indicated (Egdahl, 1968). If adrenocortical hyperfunction is caused by a nonendocrine tumor, treatment depends upon the primary tumor. If the primary tumor is slowly progressive and the symptoms of excess cortisol production are severe, total adrenalectomy may be indicated. Occasionally

Table 7-7. ADRENAL-PITUITARY FUNCTION STUDIES IN THE DIAGNOSIS OF CUSHING'S SYNDROME*

TEST	NORMAL	BILATERAL HYPERPLASIA	ADENOMA	ADRENAL CARCINOMA	ECTOPIC ACTH SYNDROME
Baseline urinary					
17OH	10 mg/24 hr	>2X ↑	>3X ↑	>5X ↑	>6X ↑
17KS	12 mg/24 hr	>2X ↑	>3X ↑	>10X ↑	>12X ↑
Rhythmic plasma F	+	−	−	−	−
Plasma ACTH	Normal	High	Low	Low	High
ACTH stimulation	↑ ↑ ↑ ↑	↑ ↑	↑	±	±
Dexamethasone suppression					
2 mg/day	↓ ↓	↓	−	−	−
8 mg/day	↓ ↓ ↓	↓ ↓	↓	−	−
Metyrapone	↑ ↑ ↑ ↑	↑ ↑	−	−	±

* Direction of arrows indicates net increase or decrease; relative magnitude of change is indicated by number of arrows.

patients with the ectopic ACTH syndrome may respond to metyrapone (Coll et al., 1968) or Elipten (Gorden et al., 1968).

Regardless of the cause of Cushing's syndrome, patients undergoing bilateral adrenal resection must be given additional corticosteroids to prevent a precipitous fall in the concentration of plasma cortisol. If a unilateral adrenalectomy is done for adenoma or carcinoma, the contralateral gland is atrophic and exogenous corticosteroids are similarly required. After adrenalectomy, patients may develop a progressive increase in skin pigmentation and an increase in the size of the sella turcica secondary to a pituitary adenoma. If ocular abnormalities result, hypophysectomy is indicated. In most cases, serial x-rays of the skull reveal a gradual increase in the size of the sella turcica, and pituitary radiation therapy may prevent rapid progression (Nelson et al., 1960). *Principle: Successful therapy of an endocrine abnormality usually involves nearly continuous observations of the patient and extraordinary commitment by the therapist. He must be able to predict the complex consequences of intervention with the control mechanisms of hormone synthesis, release, or metabolism. By virtue of the therapy he undertakes, he often trades one disease for another.*

Therapy of diseases of the adrenal medulla and of primary hyperaldosteronism is discussed in Chapter 5.

Treatment of Nonadrenal Disorders with Corticosteroids

The glucocorticoids have been extensively used to treat diseases in which there is no known disturbance of adrenal function, specifically, allergic reactions, inflammatory disease, disease associated with "autoimmunity," "immunosuppression" during transplantation, and certain

malignancies. The benefits of this therapy must be evaluated in each patient by serial observations of the course of the disease, and the observed therapeutic benefits must be weighed against the serious side effects of the treatment. The major principle in using this therapy safely is to administer the smallest possible dose for the shortest period of time necessary to obtain the desired result. For example, if a patient with nephrotic syndrome is responsive to glucocorticoid therapy, it is often most convenient to start with a dose that produces a fall in urinary protein and a rise in serum albumin. Once the desired therapeutic goal is achieved, the dose must be decreased to the point where the therapeutic benefit is maintained. Some diseases respond best to small doses given frequently; others respond to doses given every other day or perhaps administered locally (Harter et al., 1963). Even a slight excess of corticosteroid given for prolonged periods will induce Cushing's syndrome. *Therapy must be individualized to the patient's observed response to the drug.*

The anti-inflammatory effect of corticosteroids represents one of the most useful pharmacologic properties in the treatment of diseases with no apparent adrenal defect. Steroids inhibit exudation and local cellular response to injury, delay fibroblast formation, and stabilize lysosomal membranes. By lysing plasma cells and lymphocytes, they help impair the immune responses that may accentuate and perpetuate inflammation. They are not, however, a panacea for inflammatory disorders. They control the manifestations of inflammation rather than the underlying process of tissue destruction and fibrosis, as in rheumatoid arthritis, where progressive joint destruction occurs despite their use.

Consideration of the nature of the disease and

of the inflammatory stimulus is essential. For example, an acute reaction to a bee sting may require a large dose of rapid-acting steroid that should be continued only until the inflammatory stimulus is dissipated. In ulcerative colitis or lupus erythematosus, where the exact inflammatory stimulus is not defined, moderate doses may be required for prolonged periods to suppress the symptoms, if not to reverse the permanent injury, that result from chronic, low-grade inflammation. In chronic inflammatory disorders, periods of drug withdrawal are indicated because the diseases are characterized by intermittent remissions, and unnecessary exposure of the patient to the drug is undesirable.

A major complication of corticosteroid therapy is interference with the normal pituitary-adrenal feedback mechanism. When glucocorticoids are administered, even in large doses for short periods (3 to 4 weeks), serious side effects are unusual and adrenal suppression is rare (Danowski et al., 1964). The degree of adrenal suppression is primarily a function of the length of time that suppressing doses are given. Once the pituitary-adrenal axis is suppressed, recovery follows a definite pattern requiring at least several months for completion (Graber et al., 1965). After steroid therapy is discontinued, initial plasma concentrations of both ACTH and corticosteroid are low. After a period of up to 6 months, ACTH concentrations gradually increase until supernormal concentrations are reached. Supernormal plasma ACTH concentrations persist for several months before normal adrenal responsiveness is recovered. Because of this delay in adrenal response to increased plasma concentrations of endogenous ACTH, some authors have advocated administration of ACTH to activate the adrenal cortex before final withdrawal of corticosteroids (Thorn, 1966). Despite interference with normal pituitary-adrenal function following steroid therapy, the subnormal corticosteroid and ACTH secretion still follows a definite diurnal pattern.

ACTH, rather than corticosteroids, has been advocated for the treatment of certain neuromuscular illnesses, since ACTH stimulates both adrenal androgens and adrenal corticosteroids. Adrenal androgens may diminish somewhat the catabolism and myopathy that result from corticosteroid therapy. Unfortunately, the problems of parenteral injections, and the salt and water retention associated with ACTH therapy, have limited its use.

The method of administration of steroid therapy may greatly influence the incidence of side effects and the degree of pituitary adrenal suppression. If the disease process can be controlled by therapy given once daily, as judged by the measurements for disease activity chosen to reflect changes in the course of the illness, therapy should be administered between 8 and 9 A.M. to prevent interference with maximal release of ACTH in the evening. In some illnesses, such as nephrosis and systemic lupus erythematosus, therapeutic doses administered every other day or three times a week may control the disease and at the same time lessen the degree of ACTH suppression (Harter et al., 1963; Ackerman and Nolan, 1968; Martin et al., 1968). These treatment programs do not, however, entirely prevent the side effects of long-term corticosteroid therapy.

Several programs for steroid withdrawal have been suggested, with subsequent assessment of pituitary-adrenal responsiveness to ACTH and metyrapone stimulation tests. These tests may be of value in demonstrating relative pituitary or adrenal unresponsiveness despite apparently normal function under basal conditions (Thorn, 1966). Failure of urinary 17-hydroxycorticoids to increase following stimulation by ACTH indicates unresponsive adrenal glands. Having demonstrated intact adrenal function, lack of increase of urinary 17-hydroxycorticoids following metyrapone's inhibition of the conversion of 11-desoxycortisol to cortisol indicates pituitary failure (11-desoxycortisol does not inhibit ACTH release; the decrease in free cortisol stimulates a normal pituitary to secrete ACTH, which increases urinary Porter-Silber chromogens [17-hydroxycorticoids]). Normal tests in a basal condition may not accurately assess the reserve of the pituitary-adrenal axis under the stress of associated illness. A patient previously treated with corticosteroids should carry identification indicating possible relative adrenal insufficiency and should be treated with corticosteroids at times of severe stress, trauma, or surgery. Because of the prolonged adrenal and pituitary suppression following chronic corticosteroid therapy, this precaution must be taken for as long as 1 year following cessation of therapy.

Most patients treated with corticosteroids in pharmacologic doses develop iatrogenic Cushing's syndrome, characterized by facial rounding, truncal obesity, acne, easy bruisability, thinning of the skin, striae, and poor wound healing. The rate of development and severity of these side effects are generally dose related. Other more serious side effects include weight gain with sodium retention, hypertension, osteoporosis, gastrointestinal bleeding, potassium wasting, psychosis, superinfection or reactivation of latent infections, growth retardation, carbohydrate intolerance, increased intraocular pressure (most pronounced with local steroid application), myopathy, posterior subcapsular cataracts, pseudotumor cerebri, pancreatitis, fatty liver with or without fat emboli, and aseptic bone necrosis. *Principle: Although corticosteroids are very useful pharmacologic agents, their use is probably greater than would be suggested by their proven efficacy.* The therapist should carefully examine the data upon which a recommendation for the use of corticosteroids is based. When conclusions are tenuous (e.g., during endotoxemia in man), their use should be restricted or therapeutic objectives clearly defined and assessed in relation to the drug's effect.

Certain adjuvants to steroid therapy have been used to help diminish some of the undesirable side effects. These adjuvants generally include sodium restriction and diuretic therapy if edema worsens, and potassium supplementation and oral hypoglycemics or insulin if carbohydrate tolerance worsens and if symptoms of hyperglycemia occur. High calcium and protein intake in addition to regular physical activity has been advocated to help lessen osteoporosis, but this therapy has not been proved effective; the increased calcium intake may enhance the hypercalcuria associated with high-dose corticosteroid therapy and may predispose to renal calculi. No well-controlled studies have shown the efficacy of antacid therapy in protecting against ulcers resulting from changes in gastric secretion due to steroid therapy. Superinfection or reactivation of latent infections such as tuberculosis must be treated. A skin test for tuberculosis should be done before corticosteroids are administered. Intermittent therapy with corticosteroids given 3 to 5 days a week, or large doses given every other day, may provide satisfactory therapy for some diseases. Such treatment programs apparently diminish the incidence of undesirable steroid side effects and cause less hypothalamic-pituitary suppression (Harter et al., 1963; Thorn, 1966; Ackerman and Nolan, 1968). Although apparent side effects are less severe and pituitary function is less suppressed with intermittent steroid therapy, relative adrenal insufficiency can occur; such patients should be given supplemental steroid therapy in times of increased stress.

THE PARATHYROIDS AND METABOLIC BONE DISEASE

A discussion of the treatment of disorders of parathyroid function involves a consideration of the factors that control calcium homeostasis. These include (1) three important humoral factors, vitamin D, parathormone, and thyrocalcitonin; (2) to a lesser extent, growth hormone, gonadal hormones, thyroxine, glucocorticoids,

and pancreatic hormones; and (3) nonhormonal dietary factors such as inorganic phosphate and citrate.

The calcium content of the normal adult is about 1000 to 1200 g, of which over 99% is in bone as hydroxyapatite (Rasmussen, 1968). Of the 1 g of calcium in the extracellular fluids, 54% is ultrafilterable (ionized) and 46% is bound to albumin. About 15% of the ionized calcium is normally complexed to various anions, particularly to phosphate and citrate. The concentration of ionized calcium in blood is the major factor responsible for the physiologic effects of calcium and for the regulation of the feedback system that controls calcium balance, but most laboratories report the total concentration of calcium in serum without regard to the ionized fraction. A given elevation in serum calcium in patients with hypoalbuminemia is potentially of graver consequence than in patients with normal albumin, since each gram of serum albumin binds about 0.8 mEq of calcium ion. Control of calcium homeostasis has been discussed extensively in a recent excellent review (Kleeman et al., 1971).

Humoral Factors and Calcium Homeostasis

Vitamin D_3 is a natural vitamin found in fish oils. It is absorbed from the distal portion of the ileum, transported in the serum bound to protein, and delivered to the liver, then to bone, kidney, and intestine. Recent evidence suggests that the vitamin is converted in several tissues to a metabolically active form, probably the 25-hydroxylated derivative (Blunt et al., 1968; Hallick and DeLuca, 1969; Horsting and DeLuca, 1969). The major site of action of D vitamin is the gastrointestinal tract (Schachter, 1963), where it increases the permeability of the entire small bowel to calcium, stimulates the synthesis of a specific calcium-binding protein in the gastrointestinal mucosal cells (Wasserman et al., 1968; Wasserman and Taylor, 1968), and may stimulate a separate energy-linked transport system of calcium found in the duodenum and upper jejunum (Rasmussen, 1968). Physiologic doses of vitamin D also play an ill-defined permissive role in the action of parathormone on bone. Even in the absence of parathormone, pharmacologic doses of vitamin D enhance bone resorption (Rasmussen, 1968). The vitamin does not appear to have important direct effects on the kidney.

Preparations of bovine parathormone have allowed study of parathormone's structure and activity (Potts and Deftos, 1969). The hormone appears to be a polypeptide consisting of a single chain of 83 amino acids. The biologic and antigenic sites of the molecule appear to reside in the 35 amino acids at the amino terminal end of the molecule. Isolation of parathormone has led to development of radioimmunoassay techniques which permit accurate determination of hormone concentrations in serum during various disease states in man. These include hyperparathyroidism (Reiss and Canterbury, 1969), pseudo-hypoparathyroidism (Lee *et al.*, 1968), and chronic renal failure (Reiss *et al.*, 1969).

The major effects of parathormone are on calcium transport in the bone, kidney, and gut. In bone, parathormone stimulates adenyl cyclase and rapidly promotes osteocytic osteolysis, leading to an increased release of calcium from bone (Aurbach and Potts, 1964; Talmage, 1967). In addition, the hormone has a slower but more prolonged effect on bone remodeling. In the kidney, parathormone inhibits the tubular resorption of phosphate, an effect that is also mediated by the activation of renal adenyl cyclase (Aurbach and Potts, 1964). Increased renal excretion of cyclic AMP precedes the phosphaturic effect of parathormone (Chase *et al.*, 1968). In addition to its effects on phosphate clearance, parathormone decreases the renal clearance of calcium. This may explain the relatively low incidence of hypercalcuria in hyperparathyroidism despite the presence of hypercalcemia. Parathormone has no apparent direct action on intestinal calcium transport (Potts and Deftos, 1969).

Recently, thyrocalcitonin has been implicated in calcium homeostasis. This relatively small polypeptide, produced by the parafollicular cells of the thyroid, reduces serum concentrations of calcium, apparently by inhibiting bone resorption without changing renal or gastrointestinal transport of calcium. The basic mechanism of action of thyrocalcitonin on bone has not been delineated, but effects on adenyl cyclase do not appear to be involved.

The major factor controlling the secretion of parathormone and of thyrocalcitonin is the concentration of ionized calcium in the blood perfusing the thyroid and parathyroid glands (Sherwood *et al.*, 1966). When calcium concentration increases, parathormone secretion decreases and thyrocalcitonin increases. Conversely, decreases in calcium concentrations in blood lead to an increase in parathormone and a decrease in thyrocalcitonin release (Deftos *et al.*, 1968). The rather small stores of parathormone in the parathyroid gland require increased biosynthesis of the hormone after relatively short periods of hypocalcemia. In contrast, thyrocalcitonin stores are generally large and can be released for several hours without need for hormone synthesis. Estimates of daily parathormone production in man vary between 400 μg and 2 mg (Potts and Deftos, 1969).

Growth hormone increases the rate of bone formation, reduces the renal excretion of phosphate, and increases the renal excretion of calcium (Rasmussen, 1968). Gonadal hormones are important in normal bone maturation and promote retention of phosphate, calcium, and nitrogen, although there is no evidence that these hormones directly affect mineral transport. Thyroxine and triiodothyronine appear to increase the responsiveness of osteolytic cells to parathormone and may have a direct effect on bone resorption. Mild hypercalcemia is occasionally seen in thyrotoxicosis.

The glucocorticoid hormones have complex actions on calcium homeostasis (Epstein, 1968). These hormones are catabolic and cause a decrease in the biosynthesis of collagen in bone. In addition, corticosteroids indirectly increase bone resorption because they antagonize the effect of vitamin D on the gut transport of both calcium and phosphate, leading to decreased absorption of both elements (Avioli *et al.*, 1968). When hypocalcemia develops, parathormone secretion is stimulated. Corticosteroids may also block the effect of vitamin D on bone. Chronic excesses of endogenous or exogenous adrenal hormones result in profound osteoporosis. Interestingly, patients with Addison's disease may have hypercalcemia, possibly related to sodium depletion, which may cause an increase in protein-bound calcium (Walser *et al.*, 1963).

Inorganic pyrophosphate inhibits precipitation of calcium and phosphate from metastable solutions and may prevent the formation and dissolution of hydroxyapatite (Fleisch *et al.*, 1966). Administration of inorganic phosphate in man leads to a decrease in urinary calcium, which has been attributed to a reduced filtered load of calcium secondary to increased deposition of calcium and phosphate in tissues. Phosphate administration also increases the urinary excretion of pyrophosphate, possibly accounting for the ability of phosphate to prevent stone formation in states associated with nephrolithiasis. *Principle: Therapeutic manipulation of ionized calcium concentrations in serum requires knowledge of the complex factors responsible for its homeostasis.*

Treatment of Disorders of Parathyroid Function

Hyperparathyroidism. The excessive production of parathyroid hormone results from hyperplasia, adenoma, or carcinoma of the parathyroid glands, or from aberrant production of parathormone by some malignancies of non-parathyroid tissue. Regardless of the pathologic process, the clinical manifestations of hyperparathyroidism are primarily related to hypercalcemia and hypercalcuria induced by excessive production of this hormone. The symptoms include polyuria and polydipsia, obstipation, disorders of mentation, disorders of cardiac rhythm, symptoms secondary to renal calculi, and bone pain. Diagnosis is based on the accurate demonstration of hypercalcemia and hypophosphatemia, usually with depression of the tubular resorption of phosphate (Strott and Nugent, 1968), demonstration of subperiosteal bone resorption, and, in most cases, failure of corticosteroid therapy to lower the concentration of calcium in serum (Gleason and Protchen, 1967). Sensitive immunoassay techniques for measuring serum concentrations of parathyroid hormone have demonstrated autonomy of hormone secretion in hyperparathyroidism (Potts *et al.*, 1967; Potts and Deftos, 1969) and should permit more accurate diagnosis of this endocrinopathy.

The therapy of hyperparathyroidism is primarily surgical. Removal of a parathyroid adenoma or of hyperplastic parathyroid glands is usually indicated once the diagnosis of hyperparathyroidism is established. In those patients with extraparathyroid tumors associated with excessive parathormone secretion, surgical removal of the tumor usually relieves the manifestations of hyperparathyroidism. If metastatic disease precludes the surgical removal of such tumors, chemotherapeutic agents appropriate for controlling the tumor may be effective in some instances, without other medical therapy of hypercalcemia. However, when widely metastatic carcinoma of the parathyroids or of extraparathyroid tissue results in hypercalcemia, chronic medical therapy of the hypercalcemia is indicated (Goldsmith and Ingbar, 1966).

The most acute and life-threatening problem in hyperparathyroidism is hypercalcemic crisis. In this situation, the management of hypercalcemia must be vigorous, rapid, and based on several pharmacologic principles. Large amounts of fluid increase calcium clearance by the kidneys, thereby reducing concentrations of calcium in serum. Intravenous infusions of saline increase renal clearance of calcium by mechanisms discussed below. Although administration of the chelating agent ethylenediaminetetraacetic acid is theoretically attractive because it rapidly lowers the serum calcium concentration, excretion of calcium-EDTA complexes may cause severe renal damage (Kennedy et al., 1953; Goldsmith and Ingbar, 1966).

Administration of salts of inorganic phosphate has been advocated for the treatment of hypercalcemia (Goldsmith and Ingbar, 1966). The hypocalcemic effect of phosphate is prompt, often occurring within hours of intravenous administration. Intravenous administration of 1 liter of an 0.1 M solution of disodium phosphate and monopotassium phosphate over 6 to 8 hours may lead to normocalcemia for 24 to 72 hours. Daily oral therapy with 1 to 3 g of phosphate given as the disodium or dipotassium salt has also been effective in maintaining eucalcemia for several days, weeks, and even years (Goldsmith and Ingbar, 1966). During either oral or intravenous phosphate therapy, careful and frequent measurements of serum calcium are essential. It may be necessary to monitor the electrocardiogram to prevent the appearance of hypocalcemia (prolonged Q-T interval) if parenteral therapy is undertaken.

The major disadvantage of phosphate therapy during hypercalcemic states appears to be related to its presumed mechanism of action. Widespread metastatic calcification, particularly in the kidney and blood vessels, has been reported (Shackney and Hasson, 1967; Spaulding and Walser, 1968). During renal disease, phosphate concentrations in serum are high and the likelihood of metastatic calcification during phosphate administration is increased. Phosphate therapy should be avoided in the treatment of hypercalcemia in patients with this disorder. A side effect of oral phosphate therapy is diarrhea, which may become very important if dehydration is already present (Potts and Deftos, 1969).

Other agents have been employed in the treatment of hypercalcemia, including salts of sulfate and citrate, corticosteroids, dialysis, oral cellulose phosphate to interfere with gastrointestinal absorption of calcium, and thyrocalcitonin (Pak et al., 1968). Sodium sulfate and sodium citrate both lower calcium concentrations in serum by increasing the urinary excretion of calcium (Kennedy et al., 1953; Kenny and Holliday, 1964). When these preparations are used, the rate of fall of serum concentrations of calcium appears to be slower than with phosphate therapy, and sometimes 72 hours of treatment are required to obtain eucalcemia. Because the effect of sulfate and citrate salts is dependent on the increased renal excretion of calcium, their effectiveness in patients with renal insufficiency or congestive heart failure is limited. These agents are preferable to phosphate because they do not induce metastatic calcification, but severe hypernatremia may occur.

Recently eight patients with hypercalcemia were treated with large doses of furosemide intravenously and careful fluid replacement to prevent contraction of blood volume (Suki et al., 1970). Significant reductions of serum calcium secondary to increased urinary losses of calcium were observed in six of the patients. This form of therapy may prove to be a safe and effective means for the in-hospital treatment of severe hypercalcemia, but more clinical experience is needed.

Because the hypercalcemia of hyperparathyroidism appears to be resistant to the hypocalcemic effects of corticosteroids, this form of therapy in patients with hyperparathyroidism is usually not efficacious. Corticosteroid therapy can lower the concentration of calcium in serum when the hypercalcemia is secondary to vitamin D intoxication, sarcoidosis, or certain malignant tumors. Thyrocalcitonin has obvious theoretic advantages in the treatment of hypercalcemia, but available preparations are antigenic and clinical experience with this hormone is scant (Potts and Deftos, 1969). The use of the more potent salmon calcitonin in states associated with increased bone resorption has been encouraging (Neer et al., 1970; Potts, 1970).

A secondary problem seen in hyperparathyroidism and in other hypercalcemic states associated with hypercalcuria is the formation of renal calculi. The most important therapeutic maneuver in this circumstance is removal of the cause of hypercalcuria. If definitive cure cannot be accomplished, other methods of treatment are available. As with any disorder associated with renal stones, increased fluid intake reduces the concentration of urinary crystalloids. Therapy with inorganic phosphate lowers urine calcium excretion and increases the excretion of pyrophosphate (Howard and Thomas, 1968). However, the danger of inducing metastatic calcification with phosphate therapy has limited its usefulness in any hypercalcuric state. Citrate, like pyrophosphate, inhibits calcium phosphate precipitation from supersaturated solutions and has been used in the treatment of both hypercalcemia and recurrent calcium-containing renal stone disease (Howard and Thomas, 1968). *Principle: A drug may be both efficacious and dangerous to use. If the therapeutic index is narrow, assessment of progress and of possible developing toxicity must be made frequently.* In the case of renal stone disease, this assessment must rely both on sensitive indices (urinary content of calcium) and on more definitive but insensitive measurements (radiographic changes in the kidneys).

Because of the recently observed increase in calcium clearance following increases in sodium clearance in man, maneuvers that lead to depletion of total-body sodium have been used in the treatment of stone disease secondary to idiopathic hypercalcuria with normocalcemia (Epstein, 1968). Thiazide diuretics, by their ability to increase renal sodium clearance and deplete total-body sodium, lead to a decrease in urine calcium excretion (Nassim and Higgins, 1965). Long-term studies are needed to determine whether chronic thiazide therapy of renal stone formation produces unwanted effects, (e.g., hyperuricemia, hypokalemia, or glucose intolerance).

Hypoparathyroidism. Hypoparathyroidism may result from loss of parathyroid tissue secondary either to total thyroidectomy or to interruption of the vascular supply of the glands during thyroid surgery. Idiopathic hypoparathyroidism involves nearly total atrophy of the parathyroids by pathogenetic mechanisms that are not well understood. The disorder often is associated with monilial skin infections, Hashimoto's thyroiditis, pernicious anemia, Addison's disease, and circulating antibodies to adrenal, thyroid, and parathyroid tissue and to gastric mucosa. The immunologic abnormalities are often present in several family members, suggesting an autoimmune etiology for idiopathic hypoparathyroidism. The disorder pseudohypoparathyroidism represents an end-organ unresponsiveness to parathyroid hormone in which serum concentrations of parathormone are actually elevated (Potts and Deftos, 1969). Although the mechanism of relative unresponsiveness of kidney and bone to parathyroid hormone is not known, studies have demonstrated a failure in the rise of urinary cyclic AMP in response to parathyroid hormone administration in patients with pseudohypoparathyroidism (Chase et al., 1968).

The clinical manifestations of hypoparathyroidism are related primarily to hypocalcemia and to resultant increases in neuromuscular irritability. Symptoms include tetany, seizures, paresthesias, muscle cramps, and personality changes. Signs include cataracts, soft-tissue calcification, arrhythmias, electrocardiogram changes, and skin changes. The diagnosis is confirmed by persistent hypocalcemia and hyperphosphatemia in patients with normal renal function. A somewhat similar constellation of symptoms may follow parathyroid surgery for hyperparathyroidism despite normalization of serum calcium and may be related to magnesium deficiency. Ultimately the diagnosis can be made by measurement of parathormone concentration in serum, which should be low during hypoparathyroidism and elevated during pseudohypoparathyroidism (Potts and Deftos, 1969). In patients with pseudohypoparathyroidism, a number of characteristic developmental skeletal abnormalities also occur (Aurbach and Potts, 1964).

The therapy of hypoparathyroidism depends to a large extent on the careful and appropriate use of calcium and vitamin D. During acute hypocalcemic states, particularly those following thyroid surgery, intravenous calcium administration is usually indicated and should be maintained for several hours. Careful and frequent measurements of serum calcium and evaluation of the Q-T interval by electrocardiography are essential when administering intravenous calcium.

An understanding of the pharmacology of vitamin D preparations is necessary for the rational use of these drugs in patients with chronic hypocalcemia. The major vitamin D preparations include vitamin D_2 (calciferol or ergocalciferol), vitamin D_3 (activated 7-dehydrocholesterol or cholecalciferol), and the synthetic preparation dihydrotachysterol. The relative potency of these preparations has been studied in both animals and man. In the hypoparathyroid, vitamin-D-deficient rat, dihydrotachysterol is approximately ten times as effective as ergocalciferol in restoring normal blood concentrations of calcium (Harrison et al., 1968). In hypoparathyroid man, dihydrotachysterol seems to have an equivalent increased potency over ergocalciferol (Harrison *et al.*, 1967). Both the onset of action and the length of action of crystalline dihydrotachysterol appear to be shorter in comparison with ergocalciferol (Harrison *et al.*, 1967). The active metabolite of cholecalciferol, 25-hydroxycholecalciferol, has a shorter biologic half-life than the parent compound (DeLuca, 1969).

During chronic hypoparathyroidism, the major goal of therapy is the maintenance of serum concentrations of calcium sufficiently close to normal to eliminate the neuromuscular symptoms of hypocalcemia. Because of the dangers of hypercalcemia and the difficulty in regulating serum calcium concentrations in hypoparathyroid subjects, many therapists favor the maintenance of slightly low or low normal concentrations of serum calcium. Regardless of the therapy chosen, serum calcium concentrations must be measured frequently and drug dosage must be adjusted according to the results of these measurements.

Most of the clinical manifestations of hypoparathyroidism can be controlled with vitamin D in doses of 50,000 to 100,000 units per day (Potts and Deftos, 1969). The onset of action of ergocalciferol and cholecalciferol is slow, and several days or even weeks must elapse before the full effects of a single regimen can be determined or changes in the dose evaluated. Thus, considerable time periods may be required for adjustment of dose or, more important, for reversal of any toxicity that may have been caused by an improper dose. The more rapidly acting crystalline dihydrotachysterol, which also has a shorter duration of action, has obvious advantages in the treatment of hypoparathyroidism (Harrison *et al.*, 1967) (see Chapter 2). At present, the great expense of this preparation has limited its application. The usual daily dose of dihydrotachysterol is 1 to 1.5 mg. Although all vitamin D preparations are effective in maintaining patients free of hypocalcemic neuromuscular symptoms, some of the features of this disease, particularly cataracts, may progress despite adequate control of serum calcium. *Principle: If all signs or symptoms do not disappear when the patient is receiving what is considered adequate and specific therapy, re-examination of the pathogenesis of the disease and a search for more appropriate drugs are indicated.*

The major complications of vitamin D therapy are hypercalcemia and soft-tissue deposition of calcium, particularly in the kidneys. Such deposition can be prevented only by careful regulation of serum calcium concentrations. Determinations of urinary calcium concentration, particularly qualitative measurements such as the Sulkowitch test, do not accurately enough assess for hypercalcemia to permit their substitution for serum calcium determinations. Factors affecting an individual's response to vitamin D may vary, and some patients may develop hypercalcemia while taking relatively modest doses of vitamin D. For example, magnesium deficiency reduces the physiologic response to vitamin D, and administration of magnesium to some patients with hypoparathyroidism leads to an improved reponse to vitamin D (Welt and Gitelman, 1965; Harrison *et al.*, 1967). If vitamin D intoxication does occur in hypoparathyroid patients, saline infusions and corticosteroid therapy may reverse the hypercalcemia. Such therapy may have to be continued for several days or weeks because of the long biologic half-life of most vitamin D preparations.

Many patients with hypoparathyroidism do not require additional calcium supplements. Indeed, because of the dangers of hypercalcemia, calcium supplements must always be given with caution. When calcium supplementation is required, careful monitoring of changes in serum calcium concentration is necessary to evaluate drug dosage.

Treatment of Metabolic Disorders of Bone

Osteoporosis. This common disorder of bone, seen most frequently in elderly females, is characterized by a progressive decrease in total bone mass (Lutwak and Whedon, 1963). This leads to gradual thinning of cortical bone, resulting in bone pain, compression fractures of the spine, loss of height, and increased frequency of long-bone fractures. The underlying pathogenetic mechanisms are, for the most part, poorly understood, and progress in both diagnosis and therapy has been hampered because accurate methods for the determination of bone formation and resorption are not universally available. Recent microradiographic and calcium kinetic studies have suggested that bone formation is normal and that bone resorption may exceed formation in this disorder (Klein *et al.*, 1964; Avioli *et al.*, 1965; Jowsey, 1966; Neer *et al.*, 1966; Lukert *et al.*, 1967). On the other hand, morphometric methods utilizing tetracycline as a measure of appositional rates have indicated some impairment of bone formation. The chemical and crystalline structure of osteoporotic bone is considered normal (Urist, 1960). It has not been possible to incriminate fluoride deficiency, abnormalities in parathormone or thyrocalcitonin secretion, immobilization, corticosteroid hormone excess, or other hormonal changes as primary factors in the etiology of idiopathic osteoporosis (Potts and Deftos, 1969). However, each of these factors may at times be associated with changes in bone formation and absorption.

Secondary osteoporosis has been encountered in a number of endocrinopathic states, including Cushing's syndrome, hyperthyroidism, acromegaly, hyperparathyroidism, and diabetes mellitus. In addition, osteoporosis may occur during immobilization, particularly at times of active bone growth, following administration of large doses of heparin for long periods, and in a number of rare "storage diseases" such as Gaucher's disease and glycogen storage disease. As with idiopathic osteoporosis, the molecular mechanism for secondary osteoporosis is generally poorly defined. Accurate treatment of osteoporosis has been hampered by a lack of understanding of basic pathogenetic mechanisms and by inaccurate methods for evaluation of therapeutic effects.

The ideal treatment of osteoporosis should include control of symptoms, improvement in the radiographic appearance of bone, and evidence for correction of defects in either bone formation or resorption, A number of therapeutic approaches, such as high-protein and high-calcium intake, vitamin C and D supplementation, and androgen therapy, have been successful in controlling symptoms, but evidence for improvement in bone structure is generally lacking.

Estrogen therapy has been the most widely used and accepted form of treatment for idiopathic osteoporosis. Although definite symptomatic benefit occurs, there is little evidence for sustained remineralization of osteoporotic bone during long-term estrogen treatment (Potts and Deftos, 1969). Estrogen therapy does lead to short-term increases in calcium balance, but this does not persist with continued therapy (Urist, 1960; Lutwak and Whedon, 1963). However, densimetric studies have demonstrated that estrogen therapy significantly retards loss of bone substance in postmenopausal women (Meema and Meema, 1968). In addition, although estrogens may produce a decrease in bone resorption, this effect unfortunately appears to be diminished by an eventual slowing of bone formation. Despite these considerations, the use of estrogens in the postmenopausal female with osteoporosis is probably the single most beneficial treatment presently available (Gordan, 1971). Supportive therapy with analgesics, adequate nutrition and calcium intake, avoidance of vitamin deficiency, and a program of regular (but not strenuous) exercise may be important in preventing aggravation of the osteoporotic process. Treatment of the primary disease process is essential for arresting the osteoporosis secondary to endocrinopathic states.

Three new experimental approaches to the treatment of osteoporosis deserve brief comment. A high-phosphate intake may lead to increased deposition of bone mineral, but toxicity related to calcium phosphate deposition in other soft tissues must be evaluated more carefully before this therapy can be recommended for osteoporosis. A high-fluoride intake may increase bone density in osteoporosis, but gastrointestinal toxicity at high fluoride levels has limited its usefulness (Rich et al., 1964; Cohen and Gardner, 1966; Schenk et al., 1970). Thyrocalcitonin has been suggested as a useful agent in this disorder because of its ability to inhibit bone resorption. As with estrogen therapy, an eventual slowing of bone formation with thyrocalcitonin therapy might be expected (Martin and Melick, 1969; Potts and Deftos, 1969). These approaches, either singly or in combination, may contribute to the more rational therapy of osteoporosis in the future.

Osteomalacia. Osteomalacia, a bone disorder associated with multiple causal factors, is characterized by defective mineralization of bone matrix. The clinical manifestations are related to the age of onset. In children, growth retardation, abnormalities of the skull and pelvis, and incomplete fractures are the most common problems. In adults, skeletal deformities are rarer, and bone pain and proximal muscle weakness predominate. Radiographic findings show evidence of generalized demineralization and zones of rarefaction, termed Looser's zones (Looser, 1908). Laboratory findings generally include hypophosphatemia, increased serum alkaline phosphatase activity, and sometimes modest hypocalcemia. This picture of osteomalacia is seen in a number of clinical syndromes, including chronic renal disease, vitamin D deficiency, malabsorption states, renal tubular disorders, hypophosphatasia, and so-called phosphate diabetes.

The underlying molecular mechanism for the mineralization abnormality in osteomalacia is not entirely known. Hypophosphatemia, regardless of the cause, appears to be the single most important pathogenetic mechanism. Although it has been speculated that the role of hypophosphatemia in osteomalacia is related to a decrease in the $Ca \times PO_4 =$ solubility product, the finding of osteomalacia in patients with normal solubility products has raised some question about this simplified view. Although osteomalacia has been observed in patients with normal concentrations of serum phosphate, beneficial effects have been seen following vitamin D therapy in the absence of phosphate treatment. Evidence suggests some impairment in vitamin D metabolism in certain disorders associated with osteomalacia (Avioli et al.,

1966). Investigations of the basic pathogenetic mechanisms of bone demineralization in osteomalacia may define the role of such factors as parathormone and vitamin D metabolism and their action on bone in this disorder.

The therapy of osteomalacia is dependent on an understanding of the primary cause of the bone disease. In rickets or vitamin D deficiency, replacement of adequate amounts of vitamin D (usually 5000 units per day) is curative (Arnstein et al., 1967). Because of the rather rapid effects of vitamin D in this condition, initial therapy should also include calcium and phosphate supplementation to avoid hypocalcemia and hypophosphatemia as remineralization occurs. In malabsorptive states that are not amenable to reversal, modest parenteral doses of vitamin D (10,000 units per day) usually suffice.

The treatment of osteomalacia associated with various renal diseases is more complex and difficult. In renal tubular acidosis, reversal of the acidosis with sodium bicarbonate therapy may be sufficient to reverse the osteomalacia (Greenberg et al., 1966). In the Fanconi syndrome, in addition to correction of acidosis, phosphate therapy may be necessary because of the severe hypophosphatemia seen in this condition (Wilson and Yendt, 1963). If phosphate therapy is ineffective, large doses of vitamin D (50,000 to 100,000 units per day) may be required. In the syndrome of phosphate diabetes secondary to a defect in the metabolism of vitamin D, administration of the active metabolite, 25-hydroxycholecalciferol, is indicated (Avioli et al., 1966). When the disease appears to be due to a true renal phosphate leak, as opposed to abnormal vitamin D metabolism, phosphate supplementation is the therapy of choice (Nagant de Deuxchaisnes and Krane, 1967).

The recent demonstration of a defect in the conversion of vitamin D to its active metabolite in chronic renal disease has suggested that therapy with 25-hydroxycholecalciferol may be useful for the osteomalacia of this condition (DeLuca et al., 1967; Potts and Deftos, 1969). No long-term trials have as yet been reported. For this reason, most physicians dealing with chronic renal disease recommend large doses of vitamin D, usually 50,000 to 500,000 units per day (Stanbury, 1966). The danger of producing significant hypercalcemia with these doses cannot be overemphasized; blood concentrations of calcium must be frequently measured in all patients receiving large doses of vitamin D. When secondary or tertiary hyperparathyroidism appears in patients with chronic renal disease, subtotal parathyroidectomy may be required. A more complete discussion of this problem is included in Chapter 3.

Paget's Disease of Bone. This common bone disease, of unknown etiology, represents a disorder of bone remodeling. The axial skeleton is the most common site of involvement, and major clinical manifestations include bone pain, deformities, and fractures. Sarcomatous degeneration and a form of high-output congestive heart failure may occur when extensive skeletal involvement is present. The major pathologic process appears to be an increase in bone resorption followed by replacement with irregular, disordered new bone that apparently does not undergo normal remodeling (Nagant de Deuxchaisnes and Krane, 1964). Calcium kinetic studies have demonstrated a bone turnover rate of 10 to 20 times normal (Harris and Krane, 1968). Other laboratory findings in Paget's disease include elevation in the serum alkaline phosphatase activity, increased urinary hydroxyproline excretion, and excretion in the urine of a high-molecular-weight protein containing hydroxyproline (Krane et al., 1967). Despite these findings the underlying pathogenetic mechanisms of the disease are unknown.

Because of insufficient knowledge concerning the pathogenesis of Paget's disease, treatment programs have generally been inadequate. Attempts to interfere with the initial process of bone resorption have been partly successful. Both salicylates and corticosteroids in very large doses may decrease bone turnover and interfere with bone resorption, but this has been accomplished only at the expense of severe toxicity (Henneman et al., 1963). In addition, compounds that slow bone resorption may lead to a compensatory slowing of bone formation, an effect that could be potentially harmful. For these reasons long-term, high-dose salicylate or corticosteroid therapy is far from ideal.

Estrogen therapy in women with Paget's disease and androgen therapy in men may decrease both the urinary calcium excretion and the serum alkaline phosphatase levels (Gordan, 1971). However, it has not been demonstrated that the course of the disease has been altered by this therapy.

Symptomatic improvement and increases in calcium balance following sodium fluoride therapy have been reported in small numbers of patients with Paget's disease (Purvis, 1962; Rich et al., 1964; Avioli and Berman, 1968), but no long-term evaluation of large numbers of patients has appeared. The successful use of mithramycin in two patients with Paget's disease to decrease bone accretion rates and to improve symptoms should lead to further study of this approach (Ryan et al., 1969).

The use of intramuscular thyrocalcitonin was initially successful in patients with Paget's disease

(Bijvoet *et al.*, 1968; Potts and Deftos, 1969). The administration of 8 to 32 units of thyrocalcitonin per kilogram per day led to a marked reduction in bone resorption, accompanied by a marked fall in urinary hydroxyproline excretion and in serum alkaline phosphatase levels. This form of therapy avoids much of the toxicity experienced with other modes of treatment, but effects of thyrocalcitonin on bone formation have not been determined. The results of long-term therapy of Paget's disease with thyrocalcitonin must be evaluated before this approach can be recommended.

THE GONADS

The Ovary

The release of ova and female hormones is mediated by the pituitary gonadotropins, the latter being influenced by the hypothalamus and higher brain centers. At puberty, the ovary begins its cyclic function. At the beginning of each cycle, ovarian follicles develop in response to follicle-stimulating hormone (FSH). Luteinizing hormone (LH) causes ovulation of the follicle that has matured under the influence of FSH. As the follicle develops, it secretes estrogens, probably independent of FSH, but requiring small amounts of LH (Lloyd, 1968). At the time of peak LH release by the pituitary, synthesis of the other major female sex hormone, progesterone, begins. After ovulation, the ruptured follicle cavity fills with blood and forms the corpus luteum, which produces estrogens and progesterone. If the released ovum is fertilized, the chorion of the placenta produces chorionic gonadotropin, which maintains the corpus luteum. If the ovum is not fertilized, the corpus luteum degenerates and the content of estrogens and progesterone falls precipitously, causing shedding of the lining of the endometrium (menstruation).

The synthesis and release of LH and FSH by the pituitary are regulated by centers in the hypothalamus, where their individual releasing factors have been identified in humans (Schally *et al.*, 1967). It is likely, although not proven in humans, that estrogens and androgens inhibit the secretion of hypothalamic releasing factors (Swerdloff and Odell, 1968).

Estrogens. Four major estrogenic steroids have been isolated from human ovarian tissue or urine: alpha and beta estradiol, estrone, and estriol. All are C18 steroids in contrast to the androgenic C19 steroids (Figures 7–6 and 7–7). In addition to the naturally occurring estrogenic steroids a number of potent, nonsteroidal estrogens have been synthesized. Naturally occurring estrogens have an aromatic A ring and do not have methyl groups at position 10. Beta-estradiol appears to be the major secretory product of the ovary, whereas α-estradiol, estrone, and estriol are metabolic products of β-estradiol. The ovary usually is the principal site of estrogen synthesis, smaller quantities being synthesized by the adrenals, but during pregnancy large amounts of estrogen are synthesized by the placenta.

The naturally occurring estrogens are most effective when administered parenterally, thereby bypassing early metabolism by the liver. Synthetic estrogens (ethinyl estradiol and stilbestrol) are active orally because they are resistant to inactivation by the liver (Astwood, 1965). Ethinyl estradiol has approximately ten times the biologic activity of estrone (White *et al.*, 1968). Both synthetic compounds are used clinically as replacement therapy during menopause since they are more slowly degraded, making oral therapy feasible. *Principle: Congeners are designed for several purposes: (1) to select out or eliminate a given pharmacologic property of the drug, (2) to develop more potent agents, (3) to develop pharmacologic antagonists of the parent compound, and (4) to alter the pharmacokinetics of the drug so that it can be used more conveniently. Often detailed information on a drug's polarity, pK_a, and metabolism is necessary before a proper congener can be synthesized.*

The synthesis of estrogens occurs primarily in the ovary and adrenal glands, but synthesis by "nonhormonal" tissues has also been demonstrated. Within the ovary, estrogen synthesis occurs within the follicle; androgens are synthesized by stromal tissues, and the corpus luteum produces progestogens. Estimated production rates of estrone and estradiol in the normal female are approximately 0.1 to 0.5 mg per 24 hours.

Naturally occurring estrogens are conjugated rapidly by the liver and are excreted in the urine as water-soluble sulfates and glucuronides. In this soluble form estrogens are acidic and fully ionized at physiologic pH, a property that limits their entry into cells and favors excretion by the kidney. Renal tubular reabsorption of estrogens is minimal. Estrogens circulate in the blood loosely associated with serum proteins.

Although the biochemical mode of action of estrogenic hormones is unknown, numerous physiologic actions have been documented. Estrogens increase the size of the uterus by increasing mitotic activity in the myometrium and endometrium, and affect endometrial water, protein, and nucleotide content, and endometrial enzyme activity. They cause thickening of the vaginal mucosa and cornification of vaginal epithelium, increase cervical mucus secretion, and stimulate growth of the breast. In addition, estrogens increase the thickness and water content of the skin, delay the rate of epiphyseal bone growth during adolescence, and are anabolic for the secondary sex organs.

The estrogens are vitally important in normal female development. Most therapeutic uses of estrogens can be regarded as pharmacologic extensions of normal physiologic mechanisms, or as replacement of inadequate production. Estrogen therapy is effective in disease states where estrogen deficiency appears to play a pathogenetic role (e.g., menopause, senile vaginitis, and failure of ovarian development as in gonadal dysgenesis) and in relieving the symptoms of senile osteoporosis when calcium intake and gastrointestinal absorption are normal. In addition, estrogen therapy may be useful for hormone replacement in patients with pituitary

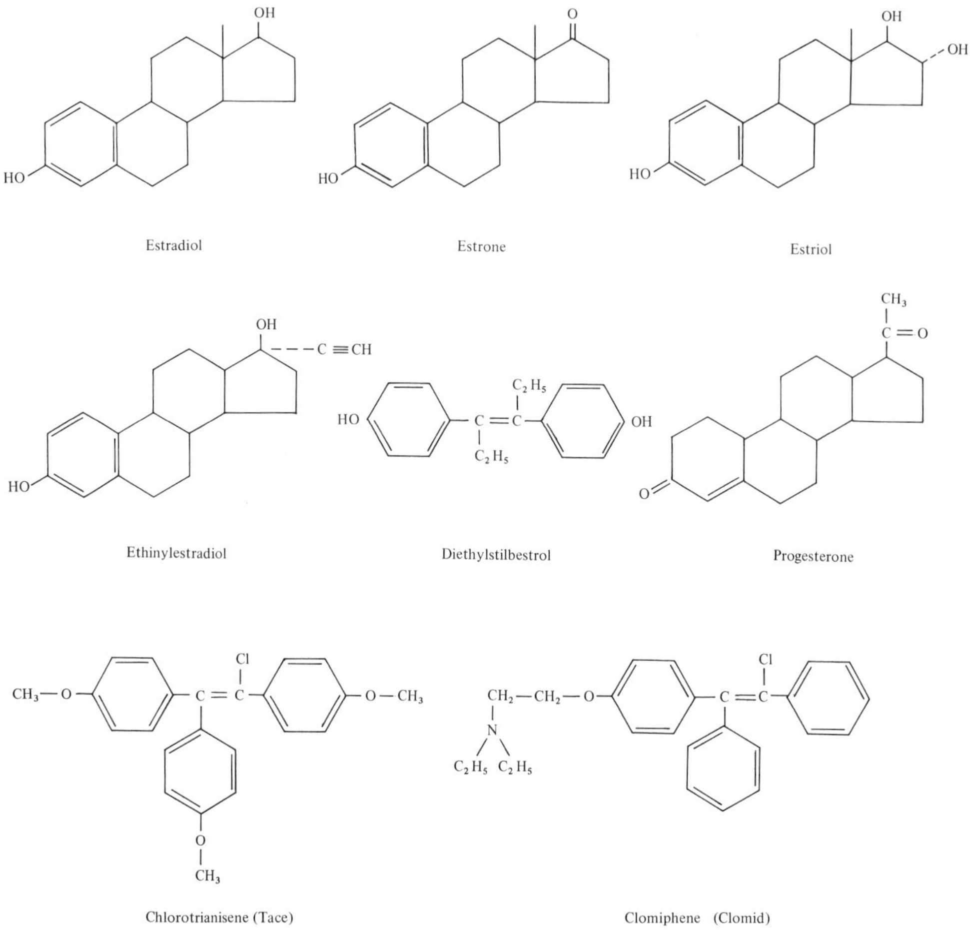

Figure 7–6. Estrogenic steroids.

failure, for suppression of lactation in the postpartum patient, and for suppression of bleeding from ectopic endometrial tissue in some patients with endometriosis. Cyclic administration of estrogens has been effective in instituting spontaneous menstruation in some patients with primary amenorrhea and in controlling dysfunctional uterine bleeding, particularly at the time of menopause. In the latter situation, progestational therapy for the last 7 days of each cycle of estrogen is required in order to produce complete desquamation of the endometrium. Continuous exposure of the endometrium to estrogens leads to abnormal hyperplasia and to abnormal vaginal bleeding. However, when estrogen and progesterone therapy is carefully adjusted, dysfunctional uterine bleeding and dysmenorrheic syndromes can be successfully managed.

In doses used clinically, estrogens have important effects on liver-cell function. Estrogens impair sulfobromophthalein (BSP) excretion, independent of its conjugation process (Gallagher et al., 1966), and enhance the synthesis of porphyrins, certain binding proteins (thyroxine-binding globulin, corticosteroid-binding globulin, and ceruloplasmin), and certain blood-clotting factors. Oral contraceptives containing estrogen increase plasma triglycerides by impairing lipolytic activity and removal of triglycerides from plasma (Gershberg et al., 1968).

Induction of Ovulation. The discovery of an important estrogenic analog, clomiphene citrate, illustrates important principles in creative pharmacology. During attempts to discover anti-fertility drugs, a compound was synthesized that was closely related to a long-acting estrogen, chlorotrianisene (Tace), and to the dangerous inhibitor of cholesterol synthesis, MER-29 (Triparanol). Not surprisingly, the newly synthesized compound proved to be a weak estrogen that blocked the action of more potent estrogens and apparently occupied the hypothalamic binding sites for estrogen (Igarashi et al., 1967). The clinical importance of this pharmacologic

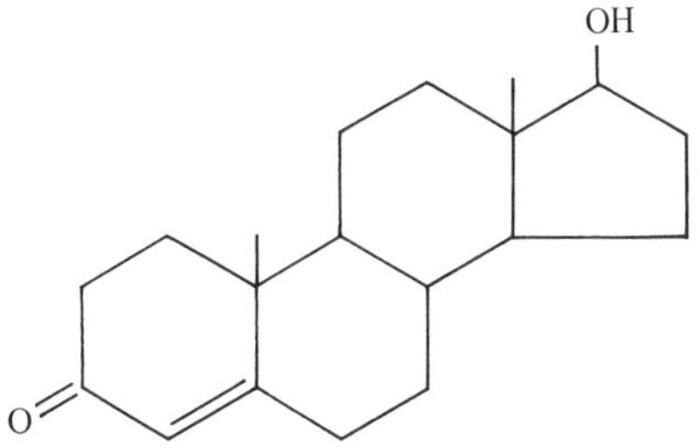

Figure 7–7. Androgenic steroids.

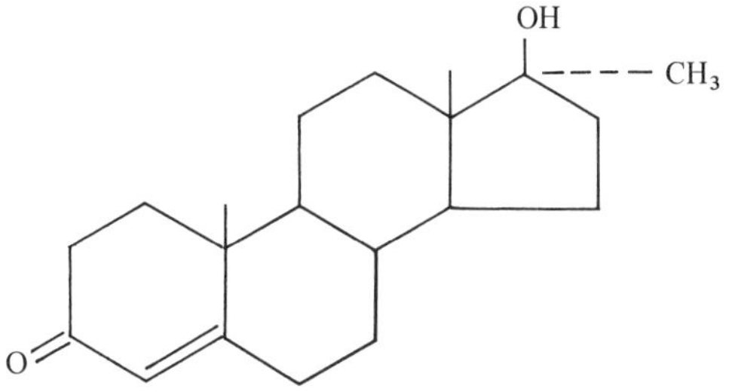

blockade involved not the antagonism of the peripheral effects of estrogen, but rather the subsequent discharge by the pituitary of large amounts of gonadotropins in response to the "apparent" decrease in circulating estrogen. Therefore, the drug has been used as a diagnostic tool to test pituitary function (Bardin *et al.*, 1967), and as a therapeutic agent in the treatment of disorders of ovulation when pituitary gonadotropins are releasable and when the ovary is capable of responding to large increases in the serum concentration of gonadotropins. Ovarian enlargement and multiple births have been the major side effects of clomiphene therapy, but these have been minimized, without compromising the therapeutic effects, by giving shorter courses and smaller doses of the drug.

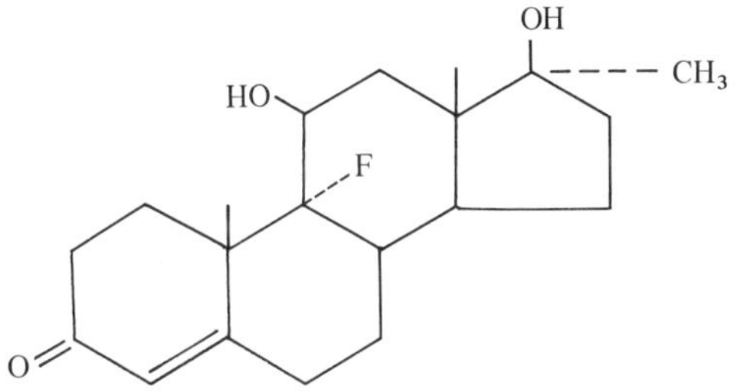

If central deficiency of gonadotropins (pituitary or hypothalamic) is present, preparations of human menopausal gonadotropin (HMG) having FSH activity may be utilized. HMG may be administered sequentially with HCG to induce ovulation in anovulatory patients (Taymor *et al.*, 1966). Therapy with HMG and HCG has been successful in patients with primary pituitary disease and gonadotropin deficiency.

Progestins. Progesterone is synthesized by

the corpus luteum (in the second half of the menstrual cycle), the placenta, and the adrenal. Physiologically, progesterone acts on the endometrium previously prepared by estrogen, inducing the mucus secretion necessary for implantation of the ovum. If pregnancy ensues, continued secretion of progesterone is essential for its completion. If pregnancy does not occur, progesterone secretion abruptly ceases at the end of the menstrual cycle. The decreasing concentration of circulatory progesterone appears to be the major determinant of the onset of menstruation. Progesterone is the precursor of estrogens, androgens, and some adrenal corticosteroids. It contributes to growth of the breasts and in large doses promotes retention of salt and water.

After oral or parenteral administration, progesterone is rapidly absorbed from the small intestine. Its half-life is short, and metabolism in the liver, largely to pregnanediol, is rapid (Little *et al.*, 1966). Pregnanediol is then conjugated with glucuronic acid. The urinary assay for pregnanediol serves as a useful but only approximate index of progesterone production.

Progesterone has been effectively used in combination with estrogens in oral contraceptive drugs and in the treatment of both dysfunctional uterine bleeding and dysmenorrhea. Progesterone has also been used empirically in the therapy of diseases of diverse pathogenesis, such as acromegaly (Lawrence, 1969), breast cancer (Muggia et al., 1968), alveolar hypoventilation associated with obesity (Lyons and Huang, 1968), type IV hyperlipoproteinemia (Glueck et al., 1969), and habitual and threatened abortions. Some uses of progesterone may be hazardous (e.g., in pregnant patients with habitual or threatened abortions). In these circumstances drug efficacy is uncertain and therapy may cause masculinization of a female fetus. *Principle: Although the rationale may be elusive, empiric therapy is justified when controlled studies prove its efficacy and safety.*

As with many other hormones, progesterone can be used as a diagnostic agent. Response to progesterone is a valuable test of the presence of estrogenic stimulation of the uterus. If there is no withdrawal bleeding of the estrogen-primed endometrium after 5 to 7 days of progesterone administration in a female with recent amenorrhea, a presumptive diagnosis of pregnancy can be made.

Oral Contraceptives. Oral contraceptives have been used for approximately 15 years by millions of women who have found these drugs a welcome approach to family planning. Increased experience with the application of these drugs has indicated the need for more caution in their use. *Principle: The therapeutic and toxic potentials of a new drug are seldom fully realized at the time that the drug is initially marketed.* The physician faces many important responsibilities when he considers the use of a new drug. If a drug is chosen because of its clear superiority to others used for the same purpose, the therapist must carefully observe its desirable and toxic effects, because pretesting (as defined by the FDA) often does not include adequate numbers of subjects, their variable physiologic states, or the duration of drug administration in all the clinical circumstances for which it is prescribed. Drug effects or drug interactions often become apparent first to the practicing physician. Unless he is critical and observant he may delay their discovery or may be unwilling to accept warnings about drug toxicity that "in his experience does not occur." The use of oral contraceptives illustrates the above principle.

There are three types of oral contraceptive treatment programs: (1) combination estrogen and progesterone therapy, (2) sequential therapy with estrogen followed by progesterone, and (3) continuous progesterone therapy. Despite the widespread use of these drugs, little is known about their metabolism or their mechanisms of action. The combination and sequential agents inhibit ovulation and alter cervical mucus; the progestins alone do not inhibit ovulation but presumably alter cervical mucus to make conception less likely. Radioimmunoassay of FSH and LH has demonstrated inhibition of FSH and of the midcycle LH peak by combination therapy, and occasional stimulation rather than inhibition of LH by sequential therapy. The difference in alteration of gonadotropin concentrations in serum may explain why sequential therapy is slightly less successful than combination therapy (Swerdloff and Odell, 1969). Regardless of which type of oral contraceptive is used, the failure rate is less than 1%, provided the therapy is taken as directed.

Side effects of these drugs usually represent only exaggerated physiologic responses to estrogens and progestins. The minor side effects of nausea, depression, headache, breakthrough bleeding, and edema are related to the estrogen content and usually can be controlled by altering the dose of estrogen or by changing the type of oral contraceptive. Despite the large-scale use of these drugs, some patients do reject them because of edema and nausea.

Because of the effects of estrogens on serum-binding proteins, oral contraceptive therapy makes assessment of thyroid, pituitary, and adrenal function more difficult. An increase in serum thyroxine-binding globulin concentration leads to increases in PBI and total serum thyroxine. This increase is related to the dose of estrogen, making evaluation of normal limits for each test somewhat difficult. The resin or particle uptake tests are also affected by estrogens, but in a reciprocal manner to the PBI. The thyroidal uptake of ^{131}I and the T_3 suppression test are unaffected by oral contraceptives. An increase in plasma transcortin concentration induced by estrogen leads to elevated plasma cortisol levels. Dexamethasone suppression and ACTH stimulation tests are usually normal and useful in excluding Cushing's syndrome or adrenal insufficiency. Metyrapone stimulation may be impaired (Leach and Margulis, 1965).

In addition to these changes in serum proteins, other abnormal laboratory tests have been related to oral contraceptives. An increase in serum transferrin concentration leads to elevations in both serum iron-binding and total iron-binding capacity. Plasminogen and alpha$_1$ antitrypsin levels decrease and serum cholinesterase and haptoglobins decrease as a result of oral contraceptive therapy (Elgee, 1970). Positive LE-cell preparations have also been noted in association with oral contraceptive use (Elgee, 1970).

The most serious disorders apparently associated with oral contraceptive therapy are vascular abnormalities, including thrombophlebitis and pulmonary embolism. Studies in Great Britain have shown a two- to threefold increased risk of thromboembolic disease in patients taking oral contraceptive therapy (Vessey and Doll, 1969). These studies have emphasized the definite association of oral contraceptives with superficial thrombophlebitis, deep-vein thrombosis, cerebral thrombosis, and pulmonary embolism. Studies in the United States conducted by the Food and Drug Administration have shown less striking increases in this severe complication. Patients with blood types A, AB, or B may be predisposed to the vascular abnormality (Jick et al., 1969; Talbot et al., 1970; Bates, 1971). Other vascular syndromes apparently associated with oral contraceptive therapy include pulmonary emboli in patients with hemoglobinopathies (Haynes and Dunn, 1967), increased blood pressure (Weinberger et al., 1969; Crane et al., 1971), midgut bowel infarction (Brennan et al., 1968), hepatic vein thrombosis (Sterup and Mosbech, 1967; Hoyumpa et al., 1971), various neuro-ophthalmic syndromes (Salmon et al., 1968), increased incidence of migraine headaches and other cerebrovascular complications (Editorial, 1969; Masi et al., 1970), and accelerated pulmonary vascular obstruction in patients with congenital heart lesions (Oakley and Somerville, 1968) and even myocardial infarction (Dear and Jones, 1971). Venous and arterial retinal thromboses have been suspected as a complication of oral contraceptive therapy. These possible side effects have raised concern about the administration of these drugs to patients with migraine, hemoglobinopathies, epilepsy, or hypertension and have suggested preclusion of their use in patients with a previous history of thromboembolic vascular disease. At this time, even a slight risk of severe complications should warrant caution in the use of oral contraceptives.

In some circumstances, when patients are unable to understand or afford other effective contraceptive measures, the physician can justly resort to the use of oral contraceptives. In addition, the natural risks of pregnancy in parts of India, South America, and Mexico are much more substantial than the risks of oral contraceptive therapy. In the majority of educated patients in the United States, the hazards of oral contraceptive therapy are probably too great to allow free prescription of the drugs each time a patient seeks advice about contraception. Before the drugs are recommended, each patient should be evaluated in terms of the socioeconomic consequences of pregnancy, ability (mental or physical) to use other contraceptive devices, and possible factors predisposing to vascular and other complications.

Because of the serious thromboembolic complications of oral contraceptive therapy, many studies have been undertaken to investigate its effect on clotting factors. Increased synthesis of clotting factors, similar to that seen during pregnancy, has been reported with oral contraceptive therapy. Larger doses of oral anticoagulants are required to adequately anticoagulate patients taking oral contraceptives than are required in a control population or in the same individuals after discontinuation of the drug (Schrogie et al., 1967). An increase in platelet sensitivity to adenosine diphosphate has also been reported (Caspary and Peberdy, 1965). Most studies in patients taking oral contraceptives have demonstrated normal bleeding and clotting times; a definite diagnosis of hypercoagulability related to drug administration is difficult to establish. Extreme caution is justified, however, in all patients who previously have demonstrated clotting abnormalities, predisposition to thrombophlebitis, or pulmonary emboli.

Other potentially serious side effects of oral contraceptive therapy include drug-induced changes in carbohydrate and lipid metabolism. Glucose tolerance decreases during use of oral contraceptives, especially when patients have a family history of diabetes mellitus. Although the exact mechanisms for changes in glucose tolerance are unclear, human growth hormone is released by estrogens (Yen and Vela, 1968) and may contribute to the phenomenon. Most subjects taking oral contraceptives show a substantial increase in plasma insulin levels, suggesting that deterioration in glucose tolerance is most likely related to increased peripheral resistance to insulin. Deterioration in the cortisone glucose tolerance test following oral contraceptive therapy has also been noted. Despite the reversibility of glucose intolerance after contraceptive therapy is withdrawn, the potential danger of long-term oral contraceptive therapy in patients with prediabetes or latent diabetes is uncertain (Szabo et al., 1970).

Estrogens have important effects on plasma proteins that bind triglycerides and cholesterol. Marked elevations in low-density and very-low-density lipoproteins and small increases in cholesterol have been reported. Increased concentrations of plasma triglycerides have been described in some subjects taking oral contraceptives. The mechanism of the increased triglyceride concentration may be related to a decrease in postheparin lipolytic activity and to impaired removal of triglyceride from the blood (Hazzard et al., 1969). The full significance or consequences of these changes in plasma lipids cannot be assessed at present, and long-term prospective studies will be required to evaluate the possible dangers of these abnormalities.

Cholestatic jaundice has been described in some patients on oral contraceptive therapy, especially those patients with a history of cholestatic jaundice during pregnancy (Hartley et al., 1969). A previous history of jaundice during the third trimester of pregnancy contraindicates the use of these drugs. Increased BSP retention is common with oral contraceptive therapy. Several studies from the United States and elsewhere report a varying incidence of abnormal BSP retention from 19 to 48% in women taking oral contraceptives (Elgee, 1970). Alkaline phosphatase elevations have been seen in only 2% of these subjects. If other liver function studies are abnormal and BSP secretion is increased, therapy should be discontinued (Ockner and Davidson, 1967).

Significant hypertension has been seen in a small number of patients on oral contraceptive therapy, although overall estimates of blood pressure show only a small increase in mean systolic and diastolic pressures. In a small number of patients with significant hypertension, cessation of drug therapy led to a fall in blood pressure with a subsequent rise when therapy was resumed. Both plasma renin and aldosterone levels have been shown to increase with oral contraceptive therapy. Although long-term evaluation has not been reported, it would seem advisable to discontinue oral contraceptive therapy in any woman who develops significant hypertension and to avoid use of these drugs in women with established hypertensive disease.

Oral contraceptives block the gastrointestinal conversion of polyglutamic folic acid to monoglutamic folic acid and may cause a folic acid deficiency that can be corrected with oral monoglutamic folic acid (Streiff, 1969).

Questions have been raised concerning the risk of cancer of the breast, endometrium, and cervix in completely normal, healthy females taking birth control "pills" for long periods (Hertz, 1968). Atypical endocervical hyperplasia and adenomatous hyperplasia of the uterine cervix have been noted in patients receiving oral contraceptives. The incidence of vulvovaginal moniliasis is also increased. More study is required, and any risk must be balanced against the need for this particular type of contraception. Based on the information available, many investigators feel that congestive heart failure, uterine myomata, liver disease, diabetes mellitus, lactation, cancer, migraine, or history of thromboembolic vascular disease are relative or absolute contraindications to the use of oral contraceptive therapy.

The Testis

The testis, like the ovary, has at least two important functions: production of gametes and synthesis of sex hormones. The seminiferous tubules of the testis are influenced by FSH and are responsible for the production of gametes. The Leydig cells are influenced by LH gonadotropin and are responsible for the synthesis of androgens. Estrogens have been isolated from the testis and androgens from ovarian tissue. The common embryologic origin of the testis and ovary may explain the production of male and female sex hormones by both organs.

The major androgenic hormone in man is testosterone (Figure 7–7). Androgen biosynthesis can occur from acetate or cholesterol, with the rate-limiting step apparently at the 20α-hydroxylation of cholesterol, a reaction under the influence of LH (White et al., 1968). Androgens also can be formed in peripheral tissue (liver, adrenal cortex, prostate gland, and skeletal muscle) by removal of the two-carbon side chains from circulating adrenal corticosteroids (Rivarola et al., 1966). Under normal circumstances these peripheral sites contribute less than 5% of the total testosterone pool (Lipsett et al., 1968). In addition to testosterone, two other androgens are secreted by the testes, dehydroepiandrosterone and $\Delta 4$-androstenedione. In man, under basal conditions, the testosterone production rate is approximately 6.0 mg per day and the plasma testosterone concentration approximately 0.5 μg/100 ml (Coppage and Cooner, 1965). In normal females the testosterone production rate is approximately 0.23 mg per day. In some hirsute females or in patients with polycystic ovary disease, testosterone production may be increased. In these patients the blood androgen concentration can be decreased by glucocorticoid therapy (Bardin et al., 1968). These problems and other disorders of androgen metabolism have recently been reviewed (Lipsett et al., 1968). Some of the circulating testosterone is bound to a specific protein and carried to the liver where biotransformation occurs. In the liver reduction of the double bond and keto groups of ring A occurs, followed by conjugation with glucuronic and sulfuric acid; the conjugates are then excreted in the urine. Since each of the many urinary metabolites of androgens has a ketone group at the 17 position, the urinary 17-ketosteroid determination is a relative index of the production of androgens. It should be emphasized that testosterone itself is not a 17-ketosteroid, and that not all 17-ketosteroids, such as etiocholanolone, have androgenic activity. These 17-ketosteroids derived from the adrenal cortex generally have a hydroxyl or keto group at the C_{11} position and are called 11-oxy,17-ketosteroids. Their concentration in urine may be an indicator of the secretion of testicular versus adrenal androgens.

With the onset of puberty in the male, testosterone secretion is responsible for a number of physiologic changes, including increase in genital size, changes in hair growth, increase in height, enlargement of the prostate and seminal vesicles, lowering of the voice, and changes in the psyche. Many of the growth changes that occur at this time are related to the potent anabolic effects of testosterone, as manifested by retention of nitrogen owing both to increased protein synthesis and to decreased amino acid catabolism, and by retention of potassium, calcium, and phosphorus.

The major use of testosterone is for replacement therapy in hypogonadal states where the Leydig cells are irreversibly damaged. Testosterone therapy is indicated in Klinefelter's syndrome, Reifenstein's syndrome, testicular agenesis, or adult Leydig-cell failure. Androgen therapy is useful in postpubertal pituitary failure, since response to stimulation with chorionic gonadotropin usually is poor. When chorionic gonadotropic therapy is impractical, androgen replacement therapy may also be effective in some patients with hypogonadotropic eunuchoidism.

The preparations of androgens currently available for replacement therapy are shown in Figure 7–7. Conjugated testosterone preparations are generally given by the intramuscular route and are more effective than oral preparations, because (like estrogens) they are rapidly metabolized after absorption from the gut. Methyltestosterone and fluoxymesterone, although less potent than conjugated testosterone preparations, are protected from metabolism by the liver, and therefore are effective when given by the oral route.

Androgens producing a maximal anabolic effect with minimal virilizing properties have been developed. Most so-called anabolic steroids, when given in doses sufficient to cause unequivocal anabolic effects, also have rather severe virilizing side effects. When oral therapy with methyltestosterone or fluoxymesterone or parenteral therapy with testosterone propionate is used in the treatment of androgen deficiency with delayed maturation, larger doses are required or full virilization may not be achieved. Androgens should be given cautiously prior to puberty, since therapy will enhance closure of the epiphyses.

Androgen replacement therapy has been shown to improve calcium balance in men with senile osteoporosis (Henneman and Wallach, 1957), but the evidence that androgen therapy improves other types of osteoporosis is much less convincing. Testosterone propionate therapy has been shown to have a beneficial effect in some women with advanced breast cancer (Goldenberg, 1964); however, the therapeutic benefits are often outweighed by the side effects of intense virilization. The prognosis of aplastic anemia has been improved with the introduction of testosterone therapy (Shahidi and Diamond, 1961). Other anabolic steroids have been used with striking clinical remission of congenital and

acquired aplastic anemia. Oral therapy with the anabolic hormones oxymetholone, methalone, dromostanolone propionate, and methenolone enanthate has been associated with clinical remissions in 70% of those cases of aplastic anemia treated for more than 2 months (Sanchez-Medal *et al.*, 1969).

An important side effect of these drugs is the production of hepatic abnormalities. A 3-ketone group in the drug's structure predisposes to a greater degree of BSP retention than does a 3-hydroxyl group; alteration of the C_{17} side chains also alters the incidence of abnormal BSP retention. These alterations of laboratory tests are directly related to the structure and dose (de Lorimer *et al.*, 1965). Clinically the hepatic abnormalities present as cholestatic hepatitis with jaundice. Other side effects of androgen therapy include virilization in females and sodium retention. *Principle: When possible, advantage should be taken of the structure-activity relationship. If several different structures produce the same therapeutic effect but have different propensities toward toxic effects, the latter may determine drug choice.*

Human chorionic gonadotropin (HCG), an extract from urine of pregnant women, possesses mainly LH activity and has been used in the treatment of certain hypogonadotropic states associated with hypogonadism. In patients with hypogonadotropic eunuchoidism, intramuscular administration of HCG three times weekly for 6 to 9 months may initiate spermatogenesis and pubertal changes. Human menopausal gonadotropin, an extract from urine of postmenopausal women, possesses both FSH and LH activity and has been used in the treatment of hypogonadotropic eunuchs, but present studies do not allow estimation of its usefulness. Similarly, clomiphene citrate, an ovulatory stimulant, has been inadequately studied in patients with hypogonadotropism.

A new contraceptive, WIN-17757, a 2,3-isoxazol derivative of 17-alpha-ethinyl testosterone, has been found to decrease pituitary gonadotropins and inhibit testicular function in males and may prove to be a useful male contraceptive agent (Sherins *et al.*, 1969).

Therapy with the testosterone drugs appears to have great commercial appeal. Methyltestosterone, for example, is offered in combination with other hormones, vitamins, or "tonics" in no less than 45 fixed-dose combination tablets (Wilson and Jones, 1968). One such combination pill contains 11 vitamins, iron, what is described as the active ingredient of rutin, betaine, methamphetamine, piperazine estrone sulfate, and methyltestosterone. Surely very few patients need so many drugs simultaneously, and the use of such preparations is strongly condemned.

With regard to other hormonal preparations, data for 1966 indicate that about 11% of patients aged 65 or over are given prescriptions for some form of sex steroid hormone, at an annual cost of $9,507,000. These figures do not include the sex hormones included in "tonic" preparations (Task Force on Prescription Drugs, 1968). An optimist might conclude that senile osteoporosis was responsible for this high prescription rate; a pessimist might fear that the drugs were being offered as general anabolic agents, the quality of the evidence justifying this use being generally poor. *Principle: A variety of clinical entities that are characterized by deficiency of sex steroid hormones or that are amenable to nonsex-related effects of the hormones are gratifyingly responsive to hormonal therapy. The use of these drugs in other clinical settings to achieve a "tonic" or "anabolic" effect is highly questionable.*

REFERENCES

Ackerman, G. L., and Nolan, C. M.: Adrenocortical responsiveness after alternate day corticosteroid therapy. *New Eng. J. Med.*, 278:405–409, 1968.

Akre, P. R.; Kirtley, W. R.; and Galloway, J. A.: Comparative hypoglycemic response of diabetic subjects to human insulin or structurally similar insulins of animal source. *Diabetes*, 13:135–43, 1964.

Arduino, F.; Ferraz, F. P. J.; and Rodrigues, J.: Antidiuretic action of chlorpropamide in idiopathic diabetes insipidus. *J. Clin. Endocr.*, 26:1305–28, 1966.

Arnstein, A. R.; Frame, B.; and Frost, H. M.: Recent progress in osteomalacia and rickets. *Ann. Intern. Med.*, 67:1296–1330, 1967.

Ashkar, F. S.; Katims, R. B.; Smook, W. M., III; and Gibson, A. J.: Thyroid storm treatment with blood exchange and plasmapheresis. *J.A.M.A.*, 214:1275–79, 1970.

Astwood, E. B.: Thyroid and antithyroid drugs. In Goodman, L. S., and Gilman, A. (eds.): *The Pharmacological Basis of Therapeutics*, 3rd ed. The Macmillan Co., New York, 1965, pp. 1466–1503.

———: Estrogens and progestins. *Ibid.*, pp. 1540–65.

Aurbach, G. D., and Potts, J. T., Jr.: The parathyroids. *Advance Metab. Dis.*, 1:45–93, 1964.

Avioli, L. V., and Berman, M.: Role of magnesium metabolism and the effects of fluoride therapy in Paget's disease of bone. *J. Clin. Endocr.*, 28:700–10, 1968.

Avioli, L. V.; Birge, S. J.; and Lee, S. W.: Effects of prednisone on vitamin D metabolism in man. *J. Clin. Endocr.*, 28:1341–46, 1968.

Avioli, L. V.; McDonald, J. E.; and Lee, S. W.: The influence of age on the intestinal absorption of ^{47}Ca in women and its relation to ^{47}Ca absorption in postmenopausal osteoporosis. *J. Clin. Invest.*, 44:1960–67, 1965.

Avioli, L. V.; McDonald, J. E.; and Williams, T. F.: Abnormal metabolism of vitamin D_3 in vitamin D-resistant rickets and familial hypophosphatemia. *J. Clin. Invest.*, 45:982–83, 1966.

Bailey, G. L.; Hampers, C. L.; and Merrill, J. P.: Thyroid function in chronic renal failure. *Clin. Res.*, 15:351, 1967.

Balodimos, M. C.; Camerini-Davalos, R. A.; and Marble, A.: Nine years' experience with tolbutamide in the treatment of diabetes. *Metabolism*, 15:957–70, 1966.

Bardin, C. W.; Hembree, W. C.; and Lipsett, M. B.: Suppression of testosterone and androstenedione production rates with dexamethasone in women with idiopathic hirsutism and polycystic ovaries. *J. Clin. Endocr.*, 28:1300–1306, 1968.

Bardin, C. W.; Ross, G. T.; and Lipsett, M. B.: Site of action of clomiphene citrate in men: a study of the pituitary Leydig cell axis. *J. Clin. Endocr.*, 27:1558–64, 1967.

Bartter, F. C., and Schwartz, W. B.: The syndrome of inappropriate secretion of antidiuretic hormone. *Amer. J. Med.*, 42:780–806, 1967.

Bates, M. M.: Venous thromboembolic disease and ABO blood type. *Lancet*, 1:239, 1971.

Bauer, F. K., and Catz, B.: Radioactive iodine therapy in progressive malignant exophthalmos. *Acta Endocr.*, 51:15–22, 1966.

Beck, P., and Daughaday, H. W.: Human placental lactogen: studies of its acute metabolic effects and disposition in normal man. *J. Clin. Invest.*, 46:103–10, 1967.

Beckers, C.; Strihou, C.; Coche, E.; Troch, R.; and Malvaux, P.: Iodine metabolism in severe renal insufficiency. *J. Clin. Endocr.*, 29:293–96, 1969.

Benoit, F. L., and Greenspan, F. S.: Corticoid therapy for pretibial myxedema. *Ann. Intern. Med.*, 66:711–20, 1967.

Bernstein, R. S., and Robbins, J.: Intermittent therapy with L-thyroxine. *New Eng. J. Med.*, 281:1444–48, 1969.

Berson, S. A., and Yalow, R. S.: The present status of insulin antagonists in plasma: October 1963. *Diabetes*, 13:247–59, 1964.

———: Insulin in blood and insulin antibodies. *Amer. J. Med.*, 40:676–90, 1966.

Biglieri, E. G.; Herron, M. A.; and Brust, N.: 17-Hydroxylation deficiency in man. *J. Clin. Invest.*, 45:1946–54, 1966.

Bijvoet, O. L. M.; Veer, J.; and Jansen, A. P.: Effects of calcitonin on patients with Paget's disease, thyrotoxicosis or hypercalcemia. *Lancet*, 1:876–81, 1968.

Bird, E. D., and Schwalbe, F. C., Jr.: Prolonged hypoglycemia secondary to tolbutamide. *Ann. Intern. Med.*, 62:110–12, 1965.

Blizzard, R. M.; Hung, W.; Chandler, R. W.; Aceto, T.; Kyle, M.; and Winship, T.: Hashimoto's thyroiditis: clinical and laboratory response to prolonged cortisone therapy. *New Eng. J. Med.*, 267:1015–20, 1962.

Blunt, J. W.; DeLuca, H. F.; and Schnoes, H. K.: 25-Hydroxycholecalciferol: a biologically active metabolite of vitamin D_3. *Biochemistry*, 7:3317–22, 1968.

Bondy, P. K.: Therapeutic considerations in diabetes mellitus. In Ingelfinger, F. J.; Relman, A. S.; and Finland, M. (eds.): *Controversy in Internal Medicine*. W. B. Saunders Co., Philadelphia, 1966, pp. 499–502.

Bongiovanni, A. M., and Root, A. W.: The adrenogenital syndrome. *New Eng. J. Med.*, 268:1283–88, 1342–51, 1391–99, 1963.

Boshell, B. R.; Barrett, J. C.; Wilensky, A. S.; and Patton, T. B.: Insulin resistance: response to insulin from various animal sources, including human. *Diabetes*, 13:144–52, 1964.

Bowers, C. Y.; Schally, A. V.; Enzmann, F.; Boler, J.; and Folkers, K.: Discovery of hormonal activity of synthetic tripeptides structurally related to thyrotropic releasing hormone. In *Program of the 45th Meeting, American Thyroid Association, Inc., Chicago, November, 1969*, p. 15.

Braverman, L. E., and Ingbar, S. H.: Changes in thyroidal function during adaptation to large doses of iodide. *J. Clin. Invest.*, 42:1216–31, 1963.

Braverman, L. E.; Ingbar, S. H.; and Sterling, K.: Conversion of thyroxine (T4) *in vivo* to triiodothyronine (T3). *Endocr. Soc.*, June, 1969, p. 68.

Brennan, M. F.; Clarke, A. M.; and MacBeth, W. A.: Infarction of the midgut associated with oral contraceptives. *New Eng. J. Med.*, **279**:1213–14, 1968.

Brown, J. J.; Chinn, R. H.; Lever, A. F.; and Robertson, J. I. S.: Renin and angiotensin as a mechanism of diuretic-induced antidiuresis in diabetes insipidus. *Lancet*, **1**:237–39, 1969.

Bull, G. M., and Fraser, R.: Myxedema from resorcinol ointment applied to leg ulcers. *Lancet*, **1**:851–55, 1950.

Burke, G.; Silverstein, G. E.; and Sorkin, A. I.: Effect of long-term sulfonylurea therapy on thyroid function in man. *Metabolism*, **16**:651–57, 1967.

Cahill, G. F., Jr.: Some thoughts concerning the treatment of diabetes mellitus. In Ingelfinger, F. J.; Relman, A. S.; and Finland, M. (eds.): *Controversy in Internal Medicine.* W. B. Saunders Co., Philadelphia, 1966, pp. 503–14.

Canary, J. J.; Schaaf, M.; Duffy, B. J.; and Kyle, L. H.: Effects of oral and intramuscular administration of reserpine in thyrotoxicosis. *New Eng. J. Med.*, **257**:435–42, 1957.

Cantolino, S. J.; Schmickel, R. D.; Ball, M.; and Cisar, C. F.: Persistent chromosomal aberrations following radioiodine therapy for thyrotoxicosis. *New Eng. J. Med.*, **275**:739–45, 1966.

Cash, R.; Brough, A. J.; Cohen, M. N. P.; and Satoh, P. S.: Aminoglutethimide (Elipten—Ciba) as an inhibitor of adrenal steroidogenesis: mechanism of action and therapeutic trial. *J. Clin. Endocr.*, **27**:1239–48, 1967.

Caspary, E. A., and Peberdy, M.: Oral contraception and blood platelet adhesiveness. *Lancet*, **1**:1142, 1965.

Catz, B.: Remnant thyroid tissue. *New Eng. J. Med.*, **276**:985–86, 1967.

Catz, B., and Russell, S.: Myxedema, shock and coma. *Arch. Intern. Med. (Chicago)*, **108**:407–17, 1961.

Cerletty, J. M., and Engbring, N. H.: Iodide-induced hypothyroidism. *Endocr. Soc.*, June, 1969, p. 129.

Chance, R. E., and Ellis, R. M.: Proinsulin: single-chain precursor of insulin. *Arch. Intern. Med. (Chicago)*, **123**:229–36, 1969.

Chase, L. R.; Melson, G. L.; and Aurbach, G. D.: Metabolic abnormality in pseudohypoparathyroidism: defective renal excretion of cyclic 3′5′-AMP in response to parathyroid hormone. *J. Clin. Invest.*, **47**:18a, 1968.

Cohen, P., and Gardner, F. H.: Induction of skeletal flurosis in two common demineralizing disorders. *J.A.M.A.*, **195**:962–63, 1966.

Colcock, B. P., and Pena, O.: Diagnosis and treatment of thyroiditis. *Postgrad. Med.*, **44**:83–86, 1968.

Coll, R.; Horner, I.; Kralem, Z.; and Gafni, J.: Successful metyrapone therapy of ectopic ACTH syndrome. *Arch. Intern. Med. (Chicago)*, **121**:549–53, 1968.

Comment: A new oral hypoglycemic agent: tolazamide (Tolinase). *J.A.M.A.*, **198**:308–309, 1966.

Comment: The University Group Diabetes Program. A study of the effects of hypoglycemic agents on vascular complications in patients with adult-onset diabetes. *Diabetes*, **19** (Suppl. 2):747–830, 1970.

Conney, A. H.: Drug metabolism and therapeutics. *New Eng. J. Med.*, **280**:653–60, 1969.

Coppage, W. S., and Cooner, A. E.: Testosterone in human plasma. *New Eng. J. Med.*, **273**:902–907, 1965.

Crane, M. G.; Harris, J. J.; and Winsor, W.: Hypertension, oral contraceptive agents, and conjugated estrogens. *Ann. Intern. Med.*, **74**:13–21, 1971.

Crockford, P. M.; Porte, D., Jr.; Wood, F. C., Jr.; and Williams, R. H.: Effect of glucagon on serum insulin, plasma glucose, and free fatty acids in man. *Metabolism*, **15**:114–22, 1966.

Danowski, T. S.; Bonessi, J. V.; Sabeh, G.; Sutton, R. D.;

Webster, M. W.; and Sarver, M. E.: Probabilities of pituitary-adrenal responsiveness after steroid therapy. *Ann. Intern. Med.*, **61**:11–26, 1964.

Das, G., and Krieger, M.: Treatment of thyrotoxic storm with intravenous administration of propranolol. *Ann. Intern. Med.*, **70**:985–88, 1969.

Davidoff, F. F.: Oral hypoglycemic agents and the mechanism of diabetes mellitus. *New Eng. J. Med.*, **278**:148–55, 1968.

Davis, P. J.: Factors affecting the determination of the serum protein-bound iodine. *Amer. J. Med.*, **40**:918–40, 1966.

Dear, H. D., and Jones, W. B.: Myocardial infarction associated with the use of oral contraceptives. *Ann. Intern. Med.*, **74**:236–39, 1971.

Deftos, L. J.; Lee, M. R.; and Potts, J. T., Jr.: A radioimmunoassay for thyrocalcitonin. *Proc. Nat. Acad. Sci.*, **60**:293–99, 1968.

de Lorimer, A. A.; Gordan, G. S.; Lowe, R. C.; and Carbone, J. V.: Methyltestosterone, related steroids, and liver functions. *Arch. Intern. Med. (Chicago)*, **116**:289–94, 1965.

DeLuca, H. F.: Recent advances in the metabolism and function of vitamin D. *Fed. Proc.*, **28**:1678–89, 1969.

DeLuca, H. F.; Lund, J.; Rosenbloom, A.; and Lobeck, C. C.: Metabolism of tritiated vitamin D_3 in familial vitamin D-resistant rickets with hypophosphatemia. *J. Pediat.*, **70**:828–32, 1967.

Drash, A.; Kenny, F.; Field, J.; Blizzard, R.; Langs, H.; and Wolff, F.: The therapeutic application of diazoxide in pediatric hypoglycemic states. *Ann. N.Y. Acad. Sci.*, **150**:337–55, 1968.

Dupre, J.; Rojas, L.; White, J. J.; Unger, R. H.; and Beck, J. C.: Effects of secretin on insulin and glucagon in portal and peripheral blood in man. *Lancet*, **2**:26–27, 1966.

Editorial: Strokes and the pill. *Brit. Med. J.*, **1**:733, 1969.

Editorial: Thyrotrophin radioimmunoassay: another test of thyroid function. *Ann. Intern. Med.*, **74**:627–30, 1971.

Egdahl, R. H.: Surgery of the adrenal gland. *New Eng. J. Med.*, **278**:939–49, 1968.

Eisenstein, A. B.: Addison's disease: etiology and relationship to other endocrine disorders. *Med. Clin. N. Amer.*, **52**:327–38, 1968.

Elgee, N. J.: Medical aspects of oral contraceptives. *Ann. Intern. Med.*, **72**:409–18, 1970.

Ensinck, J. W.; Proffenbarger, P. L.; Hogan, R. A.; and Williams, R. H.: Studies of insulin antagonists. I. An artifactual antagonist to insulin and plasma nonsuppressible insulin-like activity occurring in preparations of "albumin." *Diabetes*, **16**:289–301, 1967.

Epstein, F. H.: Calcium and the kidney. *Amer. J. Med.*, **45**:700–14, 1968.

Fajans, S. S., and Conn, J. W.: The use of tolbutamide in the treatment of young people with mild diabetes mellitus: a progress report. *Diabetes*, **11**(Suppl):123–26, 1962.

Fajans, S. S.; Floyd, J. C., Jr.; Knopf, R. F.; Guntsche, E. M.; Rull, J. A.; Thiffault, C. A.; and Conn, J. W.: A difference in mechanism by which leucine and other amino acids induce insulin release. *J. Clin. Endocr.*, **27**:1600–1606, 1967.

Falcone, A. B.; Mao, R. L.; and Shrago, E.: A study of the action of hypoglycemia-producing biguanide and sulfonylurea compounds on oxidative phosphorylation. *J. Biol. Chem.*, **237**:904–909, 1962.

Federman, D. D.: Hyperthyroidism due to functioning metastatic carcinoma of the thyroid. *Medicine*, **43**:267–74, 1964.

Feinstein, A. R.: Commentary. Clinical biostatistics. VIII. An analytic appraisal of the University Group

Diabetes Program (UGDP) study. *Clin. Pharmacol. Ther.*, **12**:167–91, 1971.

Fenichel, R. L.; Bechmann, W. H.; and Alburn, H. E.: Inhibition of insulin activity in mitochondrial systems and in normal rats by reduced insulin B chain-albumin complex. *Biochemistry*, **5**:461–66, 1966.

Field, J. B.; Boyle, C.; Remer, A.; and Drapanas, T.: Clinical and physiologic studies using diazoxide in the treatment of hypoglycemia. *Ann. N.Y. Acad. Sci.*, **150**:415–28, 1968.

Field, J. B.; Ohta, M.; Boyle, C.; and Remer, A.: Potentiation of acetohexamide hypoglycemia by phenylbutazone. *New Eng. J. Med.*, **277**:889–94, 1967.

Field, J. B., and Stetten, DeW., Jr.: Humoral insulin antagonism associated with diabetic acidosis. *Amer. J. Med.*, **21**:339–43, 1956.

Fieve, R. R., and Platman, S. R.: Follow-up studies of lithium and thyroid function in manic-depressive illness. *Amer. J. Psychiat.*, **125**:1443–45, 1969.

Fine, D., and Shedrovilzky, H.: Hyonatremia due to chlorpropamide: a syndrome resembling inappropriate secretion of antidiuretic hormone. *Ann. Intern. Med.*, **72**:83–87, 1970.

Fineberg, S. E., and Merimee, T. J.: Proinsulin: metabolic effects in the human forearm. *Science*, **167**:998–99, 1970.

Fisher, A. B.; Levy, R. P.; and Price, W.: Gold—an occult cause of low serum protein-bound iodine. *New Eng. J. Med.*, **273**:812–13, 1965.

Fleisch, H.; Russell, R. G. G.; and Straumann, F.: Effect of pyrophosphate on hydroxyapatite and its implications in calcium homeostasis. *Nature*, **212**:901–903, 1966.

Floyd, J. C., Jr.; Fajans, S. S.; Conn, J. W.; Knopf, R. F.; and Rull, J.: Stimulation of insulin secretion by amino acids. *J. Clin. Invest.*, **45**:1487–1502, 1966.

Forsham, P. H.: Therapy: insulin resistance. In Danowski, T. S. (ed.): *Diabetes Mellitus: Diagnosis and Treatment.* American Diabetes Association, Inc., New York, 1964, pp. 113–17.

———: The adrenal cortex. In Williams, R. H. (ed.): *Textbook of Endocrinology*, 4th ed. W. B. Saunders Co., Philadelphia, 1968, pp. 287–379.

Frank, B. H., and Veros, A. J.: Physical studies on proinsulin: molecular weight, association behavior and spectral studies. *Fed. Proc.*, **27**:392, 1968.

Frawley, T. F.: Adrenal cortical insufficiency. In Eisenstein, A. B. (ed.): *The Adrenal Cortex.* Little, Brown & Co., Boston, 1967, pp. 439–521.

Frohman, L. A.: The endocrine function of the pancreas. *Ann. Rev. Physiol.*, **31**:353–82, 1969.

Frohman, L. A., and Bernardis, L. L.: Growth hormone and insulin levels in weanling rats with ventromedial hypothalamic lesions. *Endocrinology*, **82**:1125–32, 1968.

Frohman, L. A.; Ezdinli, E. Z.; and Javid, R.: Effect of vagal stimulation on insulin secretion. *Diabetes*, **15**:522, 1966.

———: Effect of vagotomy and vagal stimulation on insulin secretion. *Ibid*, **16**:443–48, 1967a.

Frohman, L. A.; MacGillivray, M. H.; and Aceto, T., Jr.: Acute effects of human growth hormone on insulin secretion and glucose utilization in normal and growth hormone deficient subjects. *J. Clin. Endocr.*, **27**:561–67, 1967b.

Gallagher, T. F., Jr.; Mueller, M. N.; and Kappas, A.: Estrogen pharmacology. IV. Studies on the structural basis for estrogen-induced impairment of liver function. *Medicine*, **45**:471–79, 1966.

Gershberg, H.; Hulse, M.; and Javier, Z.: Hypertriglyceridemia during treatment with estrogens and oral contraceptives. *Obstet. Gynec.*, **31**:186–89, 1968.

Gleason, D. C., and Protchen, E. J.: The diagnosis of hyperparathyroidism. *Radiol. Clin. N. Amer.*, **5**:277–87, 1967.

Glueck, C. J.; Brown, W. V.; Levy, R. I.; Greten, H.; and Fredrickson, D. S.: Amelioration of hypertriglyceridemia by progestational drugs in familial type V hyperlipoproteinemia. *Clin. Res.*, **17**:284, 1969.

Goldberg, M., and Reivish, M.: Studies on the mechanism of hyponatremia and impaired water excretion in myxedema. *Ann. Intern. Med.*, **56**:120–30, 1962.

Goldenberg, I. S.: Testosterone propionate therapy in breast cancer. *J.A.M.A.*, **188**:1069–72, 1964.

Goldsmith, O.; Solomon, D. H.; and Horton, R.: Hypogonadism and mineralocorticoid excess: the 17-hydroxylase deficiency syndrome. *New Eng. J. Med.*, **277**:673–77, 1967.

Goldsmith, R. S., and Ingbar, S. H.: Inorganic phosphate treatment of hypercalcemia of diverse etiologies. *New Eng. J. Med.*, **274**:1–7, 1966.

Gordan, G. S.: Recent progress in calcium metabolism: clinical application. *Calif. Med.*, **114**:28–43, 1971.

Gorden, P.; Becker, C. E.; Levey, G. S.; and Roth, J.: Efficacy of amino-glutethimide in the ectopic ACTH syndrome. *J. Clin. Endocr.*, **28**:921–23, 1968.

Graber, A. L.; Ney, R. L.; Nicholson, W. E.; Island, D. P.; and Liddle, G. W.: Natural history of pituitary-adrenal recovery following long-term suppression with corticosteroids. *J. Clin. Endocr.*, **25**:11–16, 1965.

Graber, A. L.; Porte, D., Jr.; and Williams, R. H.: Clinical use of diazoxide and studies of the mechanism of its hyperglycemic effects in man. *Ann. N.Y. Acad. Sci.*, **150**:303–308, 1968.

Green, O. C., and Berger, S.: The clinical use of diazoxide in leucine-sensitive hypoglycemia. *Ann. N.Y. Acad. Sci.*, **150**:356–66, 1968.

Green, W. L.: Guidelines for the treatment of myxedema. *Med. Clin. N. Amer.*, **52**:431–50, 1968.

Greenberg, A. J.; McNamara, H.; and McCrory, W. W.: Metabolic balance studies in primary renal tubular acidosis: effects of acidosis on external calcium and phosphorus balances. *J. Pediat.*, **69**:610–18, 1966.

Greenspan, F.: Personal communication, 1969.

———: Thyrotoxicosis in pregnancy. *Calif. Med.*, **112**:41–46, 1970.

Greer, M. A.; Meihoff, W. C.; and Studer, H.: Treatment of hyperthyroidism with a single daily dose of propylthiouracil. *New Eng. J. Med.*, **272**:888–91, 1965.

Grieg, W. R.; Smith, J. F.; Gillespie, F. C.; Thomson, J. A.; and McGirr, E. M.: Iodine-125 treatment for thyrotoxicosis. *Lancet*, **1**:755–57, 1969.

Grodsky, G. M., and Bennett, L. L.: Effect of glucose "pulse," glucagon, and the cations Ca^{++}, Mg^{++}, and K^+ on insulin secretion *in vitro. J. Clin. Invest.*, **45**:1018, 1966.

Hagen, G. A.; Ouellette, R. P.; and Chapman, E. M.: Comparison of high and low dosage levels of ^{131}I in the treatment of thyrotoxicosis. *New Eng. J. Med.*, **277**:559–62, 1967.

Haist, R. E.: Effects of changes in stimulation on the structure and function of islet cells. In Leibel, B. S., and Wrenshall, G. A. (eds.): *On the Nature and Treatment of Diabetes.* Excerpta Medica International Congress Series #84. Excerpta Medica Foundation, New York, 1965, pp. 12–30.

Hallick, R. B., and DeLuca, H. F.: Stimulation of the template activity of rat intestinal mucosa chromatin by vitamin D_3. *Fed. Proc.*, **28**:759, 1969.

Hamburger, J. I., and Desai, P.: Mannitol augmentation of I^{131} uptake in the treatment of thyroid carcinoma. *Metabolism*, **15**:1055–58, 1966.

Hamwi, G. J.: Therapy: changing dietary concepts. In Danowski, T. S. (ed.): *Diabetes Mellitus: Diagnosis and Treatment.* American Diabetes Association, Inc., New York, 1964, pp. 73–78.

Harris, E. D., Jr., and Krane, S. M.: Paget's disease of bone. *Bull. Rheum. Dis.*, **18**:506–11, 1968.

Harrison, H. E.; Harrison, H. C.; and Lifshitz, F.: Interrelation of vitamin D and parathyroid hormone: the responses of vitamin D-depleted and of thyroparathyroidectomized rates to ergocalciferol and dihydrotachysterol. In Talmage, R. V., and Belanger, L. F. (eds.): *Parathyroid Hormone and Thyrocalcitonin (Calcitonin)*, Excerpta Medica International Congress Series #159. Excerpta Medica Foundation, New York, 1968, pp. 455–62.

Harrison, H. E.; Lifshitz, F.; and Blizzard, R. M.: Comparison between crystalline dihydrotachysterol and calciferol in patients requiring pharmacologic vitamin D therapy. *New Eng. J. Med.*, **276**:894–900, 1967.

Harter, J. G.; Reddy, W. J.; and Thorn, G. W.: Studies on an intermittent corticosteroid dosage regimen. *New Eng. J. Med.*, **269**:591–96, 1963.

Hartley, R. A.; Boitnott, J. K.; and Iber, F. L.: The liver and oral contraceptives. *Johns Hopkins Med. J.*, **124**:112–18, 1969.

Hasselblatt, A.: Liberation of insulin bound to serum protein by tolbutamide. *Metabolism*, **12**:302–10, 1963.

Hayles, A. B., and Chaves-Carballo, E.: Exophthalmic goiter in children. *Mayo Clin. Proc.*, **40**:889–94, 1965.

Haynes, R. L., and Dunn, J. M.: Oral contraceptives, thrombosis and sickle cell hemoglobinopathies. *J.A.M.A.*, **200**:994–96, 1967.

Hazzard, W. R.; Spiger, M. J.; Bagdade, J. D.; and Bierman, E. L.: Studies on the mechanism of increased plasma triglyceride levels induced by oral contraceptives. *New Eng. J. Med.*, **280**:471–74, 1969.

Henneman, P. H.; Dull, T. A.; Avioli, L. V.; Bastomsky, C. H.; and Lynch, T. N.: Effects of aspirin and corticosteroids on Paget's disease of bone. *Trans. Coll. Physicians Phila.*, **31**:10–25, 1963.

Henneman, P. H., and Wallach, S.: A review of the prolonged use of estrogens and androgens in postmenopausal and senile osteoporosis. *Arch. Intern. Med. (Chicago)*, **100**:715–23, 1957.

Hershman, J. M.: The treatment of hyperthyroidism. *Ann. Intern. Med.*, **64**:1306–14, 1966.

Hershman, J. M., and Pittman, A., Jr.: Utility of the radioimmunoassay of serum thyrotrophin in man. *Ann. Intern. Med.*, **74**:481–90, 1971.

Hertz, R.: Experimental and clinical aspects of the carcinogenic potential of steroid contraceptives. *Int. J. Fert.*, **13**:273–86, 1968.

Heuschele, R., and Lampe, I.: Pituitary irradiation for Cushing's syndrome. *Radiol. Clin. Biol.*, **36**:27–31, 1967.

Hollander, C. S.; Nihei, N.; and Burday, S. Z.: Abnormalities of T3 secretion in man: clinical and pathophysiological observations utilizing gas chromatographic techniques. *Clin. Res.*, **17**:286, 1969.

Holvey, D. N.; Goodner, C. J.; Nicoloff, J. T.; and Dowling, J. T.: Treatment of myxedema coma with intravenous thyroxine. *Arch. Intern. Med. (Chicago)*, **113**:89–96, 1964.

Honda, Y.; Takahashi, K.; Takahasi, S.; Azumi, K.; Irie, M.; Sakumura, M.; Tsushima, T.; and Shizume, K.: Growth hormone secretion during nocturnal sleep in normal subjects. *J. Clin. Endocr.*, **29**:20–29, 1969.

Horsting, M., and DeLuca, H. F.: Enzymatic conversion of cholecalciferol to 25-hydroxycholecalciferol. *Fed. Proc.*, **28**:351, 1969.

Howard, J. E.: Treatment of thyrotoxicosis. *J.A.M.A.*, **202**:706–709, 1967.

Howard, J. E., and Thomas, W. C., Jr.: Control of crystallization in urine. *Amer. J. Med.*, **45**:693–99, 1968.

Hoyumpa, A. M.; Schif, F. L.; and Helfman, E. L.: Budd-Chiari syndrome in women taking oral contraceptives. *Ann. Intern. Med.*, **50**:137–40, 1971.

Hug, G., and Schubert, W. K.: Serum insulin in type I glycogenosis: effect of galactose or fructose administration. *Diabetes*, **16**:791–95, 1967.

Hunton, R. B.; Wells, M. V.; and Skipper, E. W.: Hypothyroidism in diabetes treated with sulphonylurea. *Lancet*, **2**:449–51, 1965.

Hutter, A. M., and Kayhoe, D. E.: Adrenal cortical carcinoma: results of treatment with O,p'-DDD in 138 patients. *Amer. J. Med.*, **41**:581–92, 1966.

Igarashi, M.; Ibuki, Y.; Kubo, H.; Kamioka, J.; Yokota, N.; Ebara, Y.; and Matsumoto, S.: Mode and site of action of clomiphene. *Amer. J. Obstet. Gynec.*, **97**:120–23, 1967.

Ingbar, S. H.: Thyrotoxic storm. *New Eng. J. Med.*, **274**:1252–54, 1966.

Ingbar, S. H., and Woeber, K. A.: The thyroid gland. In Williams, R. H. (ed.): *Textbook of Endocrinology*, 4th ed. W. B. Saunders Co., Philadelphia, 1968, pp. 105–286.

Ingelfinger, J. R., and Hays, R. M.: Evidence that chlorpropamide and vasopressin share a common site of action. *J. Clin. Endocr.*, **29**:738–40, 1969.

Ivy, H. K.: The syndrome of inappropriate secretion of antidiuretic hormone. *Med. Clin. N. Amer.*, **52**:817–26, 1968.

Jadresic, A., and Poblete, M.: Stereotaxic pituitary implantation of yttrium-90 and iridium-192 for acromegaly. *J. Clin. Endocr.*, **27**:1503–1507, 1967.

Janbon, M.; Chaptal, J.; Vedel, A.; and Schaap, J.: Accidents hypoglycemiques graves par un sulfamidothiazol (le V.K. 57 ou 2254 RP). *Montpellier Med.*, **21–22**:441–44, 1942.

Jarrett, R. J.; Keen, H.; and Track, N.: Glucose and RNA synthesis in mammalian islets of Langerhans. *Nature*, **213**:634–35, 1967.

Jensen, S. E.: A new way of measuring thyrotropin (TSH) reserve. *J. Clin. Endocr.*, **29**:409–11, 1969.

Jick, H.; Westerholm, B.; Vessey, M. P.; Lewis, G. P.; Slone, D.; Inman, W. H.; Shapiro, S.; and Worcester, J.: Venous thromboembolic disease and ABO blood type. *Lancet*, **1**:539–42, 1969.

Jowsey, J.: Quantitative microradiography: a new approach in the evaluation of metabolic bone disease. *Amer. J. Med.*, **40**:485–91, 1966.

Kaneto, A.; Kosaka, K.; and Nakao, K.: Effects of the neurohypophysial hormones on insulin secretion. *Endocrinology*, **81**:783–90, 1967.

Kantor, F. S., and Berkman, P. M.: Steroid amelioration of immunogenic insulin-resistant diabetes: a proposed mechanism. *Yale J. Biol. Med.*, **40**:46–56, 1967.

Kaori, M., and Itelson, I.: Management of thyrotoxicosis in pregnancy: value of serial protein-bound iodine and Hamolski tests. *Israel J. Med. Sci.*, **5**:43–48, 1969.

Keen, H.: Minimal diabetes and arterial disease: prevalence and the effect of treatment. In Camerini Davalos, R. A., and Cole, H. S. (eds.): *Early Diabetes. Advances in Metabolic Disorders.* Academic Press, Suppl. 1, 1970, pp. 437–42.

Kennedy, B. J.; Tibbetts, D. M.; Nathanson, I. T.; and Aub, J. C.: Hypercalcemia, a complication of hormone therapy of advanced breast cancer. *Cancer Res.*, **13**:445–59, 1953.

Kenny, F. M., and Holliday, M. A.: Hypoparathyroidism, moniliasis, Addison's and Hashimoto's diseases. *New Eng. J. Med.*, **271**:708–13, 1964.

Kiraly, J.; Becker, C.; and Williams, H.: Diabetic ketoacidosis. *Calif. Med.*, **112**:1–9, 1970.

Kitabchi, A. E.: The biological and immunological properties of pork and beef insulin, proinsulin and connecting peptides. *J. Clin. Invest.*, **49**:979–87, 1970.

Kjellberg, R. N.; Shintani, A.; Frantz, A. G.; and Kliman, B.: Proton-beam therapy in acromegaly. *New Eng. J. Med.*, **278**:689–95, 1968.

Kleeman, C. R.; Massry, S. G.; and Coburn, J. W.: The clinical physiology of calcium homeostasis, parathyroid hormone and calcitonin, Parts I and II. *Calif. Med.*, **114**:16–43 (Mar.), 19–30 (Apr.), 1971.

Klein, L.; Lafferty, F. W.; Pearson, O. H.; and Curtiss, P. H., Jr.: Correlation of urinary hydroxyproline, serum alkaline phosphatase and skeletal calcium turnover. *Metabolism*, **13**:272–84, 1964.

Knowles, H. C., Jr.: Therapy: brittle diabetes. In Danowski, T. S. (ed.): *Diabetes Mellitus: Diagnosis and Treatment*. American Diabetes Association, Inc., New York, 1964, pp. 109–11.

Kogut, M. D.; Kaplan, S. A.; Collipp, P. J.; Tiamsic, T.; and Boyle, D.: Treatment of hyperthyroidism in children: analysis of 45 patients. *New Eng. J. Med.*, **272**:217–21, 1965.

Krane, S. M.; Munoz, A. J.; and Harris, E. D., Jr.: Collagen-like fragments: excretion in urine of patients with Paget's disease of bone. *Science*, **157**:713–16, 1967.

Kriss, J. P.; Pleshakov, V.; Rosenblum, A.; and Sharp, G.: Therapy with occlusive dressings of pretibial myxedema with fluocinolone acetonide. *J. Clin. Endocr.*, **27**:595–604, 1967.

Kumar, R. S.; Musa, B. U.; Appleton, W. G.; and Dowling, J. T.: Effect of prednisone on thyroxine distribution. *J. Clin. Endocr.*, **28**:1335–40, 1968.

Kuzuya, T.; Samols, E.; and Williams, R. H.: Stimulation by hyperosmolarity of glucose metabolism in rat adipose tissue and diaphragm *in vitro*. *J. Biol. Chem.*, **240**:2277–83, 1965.

Larsen, J. A., and Madsen, J.: Inhibition of ethanol metabolism by oral antidiabetics. *Proc. Soc. Exp. Biol. Med.*, **109**:120–22, 1962.

Lawrence, A. M.: Medical treatment of acromegaly with progestins. *Clin. Res.*, **17**:289, 1969.

Leach, R. B., and Margulis, R. R.: Inhibition of adrenocortical responsiveness during progestin therapy. *Amer. J. Obstet. Gynec.*, **92**:176–85, 1965.

Leaf, A., and Coggins, C. H.: The neurohypophysis. In Williams, R. H. (ed.): *Textbook of Endocrinology*, 4th ed. W. B. Saunders Co., Philadelphia, 1968, pp. 85–103.

Lebovitz, H. E., and Pooler, K.: Puromycin potentiation of corticotropin-induced insulin release. *Endocrinology*, **80**:656–62, 1967.

Lee, J. B.; Tashjian, A. H., Jr.; and Streeto, J. M.: Familial pseudohypoparathyroidism: role of parathyroid hormone and thyrocalcitonin. *New Eng. J. Med.*, **279**:1179–84, 1968.

Liddle, G. W.: Cushing's syndrome. In Eisenstein, A. B. (ed.): *The Adrenal Cortex*. Little, Brown & Co., Boston, 1967, pp. 523–51.

Linscheer, W. G.; Slone, D.; and Chalmers, T. C.: Effects of octanoic acid on serum levels of free fatty acids, insulin, and glucose in patients with cirrhosis and in healthy subjects. *Lancet*, **1**:593–97, 1967.

Lipsett, M. B.; Migeon, C. J.; Kirschner, M. A.; and Bardin, C. W.: Physiologic basis of disorders of androgen metabolism. *Ann. Intern. Med.*, **68**:1327–44, 1968.

Little, B.; Tait, J. F.; Tait, A. S.; and Erlenmeyer, F.: The metabolic clearance rate of progesterone in males and ovariectomized females. *J. Clin. Invest.*, **45**:901–12, 1966.

Little, J. A., and Arnott, J. H.: Sulfated insulin in mild, moderate, severe and insulin-resistant diabetes mellitus. *Diabetes*, **15**:457–65, 1966.

Lloyd, C. W.: The ovaries. In Williams, R. H. (ed.): *Textbook of Endocrinology*, 4th ed. W. B. Saunders Co., Philadelphia, 1968, pp. 459–536.

Looser, E.: Uber Spätrachitis und die Beziehungen zwischen Rachitis und Osteomalacia. *Mitt. Grenzgeb. Med. Chir.*, **18**:678–744, 1908.

Lukert, B. P.; Bolinger, R. E.; and Meek, J. C.: Acute effect of fluoride on ^{45}calcium dynamics in osteoporosis. *J. Clin. Endocr.*, **27**:828–35, 1967.

Lutwak, L., and Whedon, G. D.: Osteoporosis. *DM*, April, 1963, pp. 1–39.

Lyons, H. A., and Huang, C. T.: Therapeutic use of progesterone in alveolar hypoventilation associated with obesity. *Amer. J. Med.*, **44**:881–88, 1968.

McIntyre, N.; Holdsworth, C. D.; and Turner, D. S.: Intestinal factors in the control of insulin secretion. *J. Clin. Endocr.*, **25**:1317–24, 1965.

Mahler, R. J., and Weisberg, H.: Failure of endogenous stimulation of secretin and pancreozymin release to influence serum insulin. *Lancet*, **1**:448–51, 1968.

Malaisse, W.; Malaisse-Lagae, F.; Wright, P. H.; and Ashmore, J.: Effects of adrenergic and cholinergic agents upon insulin secretion *in vitro*. *Endocrinology*, **80**:975–78, 1967.

Maloof, F., and Soodak, M.: Intermediary metabolism of thyroid tissue and the action of drugs. *Pharmacol. Rev.*, **15**:43–95, 1963.

Manns, J. G., and Boda, J. M.: Insulin release by acetate, propionate, butyrate, and glucose in lambs and adult sheep. *Amer. J. Physiol.*, **212**:747–55, 1967.

Marble, A.: Control of diabetes lessens or postpones vascular complications. In Ingelfinger, F. J.; Relman, A. S.; and Finland, M. (eds.): *Controversy in Internal Medicine*. W. B. Saunders Co., Philadelphia, 1966, pp. 491–98.

Marks, V., and Samols, E.: Diazoxide therapy of intractable hypoglycemia. *Ann. N.Y. Acad. Sci.*, **150**:442–54, 1968.

Martelo, O. J.; Katims, R. B.; and Yunis, A. A.: Bone marrow aplasia following propylthiouracil therapy. *Arch. Intern. Med. (Chicago)*, **120**:587–90, 1967.

Martin, M. M.; Gaboardi, F.; Podolsky, S.; Raiti, S.; and Calcagno, P. L.: Intermittent steroid therapy: its effect on hypothalamic-pituitary-adrenal function and the response of plasma growth hormone and insulin to stimulation. *New Eng. J. Med.*, **279**:273–78, 1968.

Martin, T. J., and Melick, R. A.: The acute effects of porcine calcitonin in man. *Australas. Ann. Med.*, **18**:258–63, 1969.

Masi, A. T., and Dugdale, M.: Cerebrovascular diseases associated with the use of oral contraceptives. *Ann. Intern. Med.*, **72**:111–21, 1970.

Mayberry, W. E.; Gharib, H.; Bilstad, J. M.; and Sizemore, G. W.: Radioimmunoassay for human thyrotrophin: clinical value in patients with normal and abnormal thyroid function. *Ann. Intern. Med.*, **74**:471–80, 1971.

Meade, R. C.; Kneubuhler, H. A.; Schulte, W. J.; and Barboriak, J. J.: Stimulation of insulin secretion by pancreozymin. *Diabetes*, **16**:141–44, 1967.

Meema, H. E., and Meema, S.: Prevention of postmenopausal osteoporosis by hormone treatment of the menopause. *Canad. Med. Assoc. J.*, **99**:248–51, 1968.

Meyer, F.; Ipaktchi, M.; and Clauser, H.: Specific inhibition of gluconeogenesis by biguanides. *Nature*, **213**:203–204, 1967.

Milner, R. D. G., and Hales, C. N.: Cations and the secretion of insulin. *Biochim. Biophys. Acta*, **150**:165–67, 1968.

Mimica, N.; Wegienka, L. C.; and Forsham, P. H.: Lypressin nasal spray. *J.A.M.A.*, **203**:802–803, 1968.

Mintz, D. H.; Finster, J. L.; and Josimovich, J. B.: Effect of estrogen therapy on carbohydrate metabolism in acromegaly. *J. Clin. Endocr.*, **27**:1321–27, 1967.

Muggia, F. M.; Cassileth, P. A.; Ochoa, M.; Flatow,

F. A.; Gellhorn, A.; and Hyman, G. A.: Treatment of breast cancer with medroxyprogesterone acetate. *Ann. Intern. Med.*, 68:328–37, 1968.

Murphy, B. E., and Pattee, C. J. R.: Determination of thyroxine utilizing the property of protein-binding. *J. Clin. Endocr.*, 24:187–96, 1964.

Musa, B. U.; Kumar, R. S.; and Dowling, J. T.: Role of thyroxine-binding globulin in the early distribution of thyroxine and triiodothyronine. *J. Clin. Endocr.*, 29:667–74, 1969.

Myhill, J., and Hales, I. B.: Salicylate action and thyroidal autonomy in hyperthyroidism. *Lancet*, 1:802–805, 1963.

Nagant de Deuxchaisnes, C., and Krane, S. M.: Paget's disease of bone: clinical and metabolic observations. *Medicine*, 43:233–66, 1964.

———: The treatment of adult phosphate diabetes and Fanconi syndrome with neutral sodium phosphate. *Amer. J. Med.*, 43:508–43, 1967.

Nassim, J. R., and Higgins, B. A.: Control of idiopathic hypercalciuria. *Brit. Med. J.*, 1:675–81, 1965.

Neer, R. M.; Parson, J. A.; and Kraue, S. M.: Pharmacology of calcitonin, human studies. In Taylor, S. (ed.): *Calcitonin, Proc. 2nd Intern. Symposium.* Springer Verlag, Inc., New York, 1970, pp. 547–54.

Neer, R. M.; Zipkin, I.; Carbone, P. P.; and Rosenberg, L. E.: Effect of sodium fluoride therapy on calcium metabolism in multiple myeloma. *J. Clin. Endocr.*, 26:1059–68, 1966.

Nelson, D. H.; Meakin, J. W.; and Thorn, G. W.: ACTH-producing pituitary tumors following adrenalectomy for Cushing's syndrome. *Ann. Intern. Med.*, 52:560–69, 1960.

Netto, A. S. C.; Wajchenberg, B. L.; Ravaglia, C.; Pereira, V. G.; Shnaider, J.; Pupo, A. A.; and Cintra, A. B.: Treatment of adrenocortical cancer with O,p'-DDD. *Ann. Intern. Med.*, 59:74–78, 1963.

Nichols, T.; Nugent, C. A.; and Tyler, F. H.: Steroid laboratory tests in the diagnosis of Cushing's syndrome. *Amer. J. Med.*, 45:116–28, 1968.

Nicoloff, J. T.; Fisher, D. A.; and Appleman, M. D.: Glucocorticoid (G) regulation of thyroidal release (TR). *Endocr. Soc.*, June, 1969, p. 72.

Nofal, M. M.; Beierwaltes, W. H.; and Patno, M. E.: Treatment of hyperthyroidism with sodium iodide I¹³¹: a sixteen-year experience. *J.A.M.A.*, 197:605–10, 1966.

Oakley, C., and Somerville, J.: Oral contraceptives and progressive pulmonary vascular disease. *Lancet*, 1:890–92, 1968.

Oakley, W. G.: Treatment: management. In Oakley, W. G.; Pyke, D. A.; and Taylor, K. W. (eds.): *Clinical Diabetes and Its Biochemical Basis.* Blackwell Scientific Publications, Oxford, England, 1968, pp. 358–93.

Ockner, R. K., and Davidson, C. S.: Hepatic effects of oral contraceptives. *New Eng. J. Med.*, 276:331–34, 1967.

Odell, W. D.: Isolated deficiencies of anterior pituitary hormones: symptoms and diagnosis. *J.A.M.A.*, 197:1006–16, 1966.

Odell, W. D.; Utiger, R. D.; Wilber, J. F.; and Condliffe, P. G.: Estimation of the secretion rate of thyrotropin in man. *J. Clin. Invest.*, 46:953–59, 1967.

O'Neal, L. W.: Correlation between clinical pattern and pathological findings in Cushing's syndrome. *Med. Clin. N. Amer.*, 52:313–26, 1968.

Pak, C. Y. C.; Wontsman, J.; Beunett, J. E.; and Delea, C. S.: Control of hypercalcemia with cellulose phosphate. *J. Clin. Endocr.*, 28:1829–32, 1968.

Peck, F. B., Sr.: Therapy: insulin types. In Danowski, T. S. (ed.): *Diabetes Mellitus: Diagnosis and Treatment.* American Diabetes Association, Inc., New York, 1964, pp. 83–86.

Perkoff, G. T., and Tyler, F. H.: Paradoxical hyperglycemia in diabetic patients treated with insulin. *Metabolism*, 3:110–17, 1954.

Perley, M., and Kipnis, D. M.: Plasma insulin response to glucose and tolbutamide of normal weight and obese diabetic and nondiabetic subjects. *Diabetes*, 15:867–74, 1966.

Porte, D.: Beta adrenergic stimulation of insulin release in man. *Diabetes*, 16:150–55, 1967.

———: Inhibition of insulin release by diazoxide and its relation to catecholamine effects in man. *Ann. N.Y. Acad. Sci.*, 150:281–91, 1968.

Porte, D., Jr.; Graber, A. L.; Kuzuya, T.; and Williams, R. H.: The effect of epinephrine on immunoreactive insulin levels in man. *J. Clin. Invest.*, 45:228–36, 1966.

Posner, J. B., and Plum, F.: Spinal-fluid pH and neurologic symptoms in systemic acidosis. *New Eng. J. Med.*, 277:605–13, 1967.

Potts, J. T., Jr.: Recent advances in thyrocalcitonin research. *Fed. Proc.*, 29:1200–1208, 1970.

Potts, J. T., Jr., and Deftos, L. J.: Parathyroid hormone, thyrocalcitonin, vitamin D, bone and bone mineral metabolism. In Bondy, P. K., and Rosenberg, L. E. (eds.): *Duncan's Diseases of Metabolism: Endocrinology and Nutrition.* W. B. Saunders Co., Philadelphia, 1969, pp. 904–1082.

Potts, J. T., Jr.; Deftos, L. J.; Burke, R. M.; Sherwood, L. M.; and Aurbach, G. D.: Radioimmunoassay of parathyroid hormone: studies of the control of secretion of the hormone and parathyroid function in clinical disorders. In Hayes, R. L.; Goswitz, F. A.; and Murphy, B. E. (eds.): *Radioisotopes in Medicine: In Vitro Studies.* U.S. Atomic Energy Commission, Oak Ridge, 1967, pp. 207–29.

Prout, T. E.: The chemical structure of insulin in relation to biological activity and to antigenicity. *Metabolism*, 12:673–86, 1963.

Purvis, M. J.: Some effects of administering sodium fluoride to patients with Paget's disease. *Lancet*, 2:1188–89, 1962.

Quabbe, H.; Schilling, E.; and Helge, H.: Pattern of growth hormone secretion during a 24-hour fast in normal adults. *J. Clin. Endocr.*, 26:1173–77, 1966.

Rabinowitz, D.; Merimee, T. J.; Burgess, J. A.; and Riggs, L.: Growth hormone and insulin release after arginine: indifference to hyperglycemia and epinephrine. *J. Clin. Endocr.*, 26:1170–72, 1966.

Rabinowitz, D.; Merimee, T. J.; Rimoin, D. L.; Hall, J. G.; and McKusick, V. A.: Peripheral subresponsiveness to human growth hormone in a proportionate dwarf. *J. Clin. Invest.*, 47:82a, 1968.

Rabkin, M. T., and Frantz, A. G.: Hypopituitarism: a study of growth hormone and other endocrine functions. *Ann. Intern. Med.*, 64:1197–1207, 1966.

Raiti, S.; Holzman, G. B.; Scott, R. L.; and Blizzard, R. M.: Evidence for the placental transfer of triiodothyronine in human beings. *New Eng. J. Med.*, 277:456–59, 1967.

Rallison, M. L., and Tyler, F. H.: Treatment of diabetes insipidus in children with lysine-8-vasopressin. *J. Pediat.*, 70:122–25, 1967.

Rand, R. W.: Cryosurgery of the pituitary in acromegaly. *Ann. Surg.*, 164:587–92, 1966.

Rasmussen, H.: The parathyroids. In Williams, R. H. (ed.): *Textbook of Endocrinology*, 4th ed. W. B. Saunders Co., Philadelphia, 1968, pp. 847–965.

Reaven, G., and Dray, J.: Effect of chlorpropamide on serum glucose and immunoreactive insulin concentrations in patients with maturity-onset diabetes mellitus. *Diabetes*, 16:487–92, 1967.

Reiss, E., and Canterbury, J. M.: Primary hyperparathyroidism: application of radioimmunoassay to differentiation of adenoma and hyperplasia and to the pre-operative localization of hyperfunctioning para-thyroid gland. *New Eng. J. Med.*, **280**:1381–85, 1969.

Reiss, E.; Canterbury, J. M.; and Kanter, A.: Circulating parathyroid hormone concentration in chronic renal insufficiency. *Arch. Intern. Med. (Chicago)*, **124**:417–21, 1969.

Reveno, W. S., and Rosenbaum, H.: Observations on the use of the antithyroid drugs. *Ann. Intern. Med.*, **60**:982–89, 1964.

Rich, C.; Censinck, J.; and Ivanovich, P.: The effects of sodium fluoride on calcium metabolism of subjects with metabolic bone disease. *J. Clin. Invest.*, **43**:545–56, 1964.

Ricketts, H. T.: Therapy: insulin prescription. In Danowski, T. S. (ed.): *Diabetes Mellitus: Diagnosis and Treatment*. American Diabetes Association, Inc., New York, 1964, pp. 87–89.

Rivarola, M. A.; Saez, J. M.; Meyer, W. J.; Jenkins, M. E.; and Migeon, C. J.: Metabolic clearance rate and blood production rate of testosterone and androst-4-ene-3, 17-dione under basal conditions, ACTH and HCG stimulation: comparison with urinary production rate of testosterone. *J. Clin. Endocr.*, **26**:1208–18, 1966.

Rivlin, R. S.; Melmon, K. L.; and Sjoerdsma, A.: An oral tyrosine tolerance test in thyrotoxicosis and myxedema. *New Eng. J. Med.*, **272**:1143–48, 1965.

Rogers, T. A.: Inhibition of glucose uptake by acidosis *in vitro*. *Proc. Soc. Exp. Biol. Med.*, **97**:646–47, 1958.

Roth, H.; Thier, S.; and Segal, S.: Zinc glucagon in the management of refractory hypoglycemia due to insulin-producing tumors. *New Eng. J. Med.*, **274**:493–97, 1966.

Roth, J.; Glick, S. M.; Cuatrecasas, P.; and Hollander, C. S.: Acromegaly and other disorders of growth hormone secretion. *Ann. Intern. Med.*, **66**:760–88, 1967.

Ryan, W. G.; Schwartz, T. B.; and Perlia, C. P.: Effects of mithramycrin on Paget's disease of bone. *Ann. Intern. Med.*, **70**:549–57, 1969.

Saenger, E. L.; Thoma, G. E.; and Tompkins, E. A.: Incidence of leukemia following treatment of hyperthyroidism. *J.A.M.A.*, **205**:855–62, 1968.

Salmon, M. L.; Winkelman, J. Z.; and Gay, A. J.: Neuro-ophthalmic sequelae in users of oral contraceptives. *J.A.M.A.*, **206**:85–91, 1968.

Samols, E.; Marri, G.; and Marks, V.: Promotion of insulin secretion by glucagon. *Lancet*, **2**:415–16, 1965.

Sanchez-Medal, L.; Gomez-Leal, A.; Duarte, L.; and Rico, M. G.: Anabolic androgenic steroids in the treatment of acquired aplastic anemia. *Blood*, **34**:283–300, 1969.

Sanger, F.: Chemistry of insulin: determination of the structure of insulin opens the way to greater understanding of life processes. *Science*, **129**:1340–44, 1959.

Sawin, C. T.; Bray, G. A.; and Idelson, B. A.: Overnight suppression test with dexamethasone in Cushing's syndrome. *J. Clin. Endocr.*, **28**:422–24, 1968.

Schachter, D.: Vitamin D and the active transport of calcium by the small intestine. In Wasserman, R. H. (ed.): *The Transfer of Calcium and Strontium across Biological Membranes*. Academic Press, Inc., New York, 1963, pp. 197–210.

Schally, A. V.; Muller, E. E.; Arimura, A.; Bowers, C. Y.; Saito, T.; Redding, T. W.; Sawano, S.; and Pozzolato, P.: Releasing factors in human hypothalamic and neurohypophysial extracts. *J. Clin. Endocr.*, **27**:755–62, 1967.

Schenk, R. K.; Merz, W. A.; and Reutter, F. W.: Fluoride in osteoporosis. In *Fluoride in Medicine*. Hans Huber Publishers, Bern, 1970, pp. 153–68.

Schrogie, J. J.; Solomon, H. M.; and Zieve, P. D.: Effect of oral contraceptives on vitamin K-dependent clotting activity. *Clin. Pharmacol. Ther.*, **8**:670–75, 1967.

Schteingart, D. E.; Cash, R.; and Conn, J. W.: Aminoglutethimide and metastatic adrenal cancer. *J.A.M.A.*, **198**:1007–10, 1966.

Searle, G. L.; Schilling, S.; Porte, D.; Barbaccia, J.; deGrazia, J.; and Cavalieri, R. R.: Body glucose kinetics in nondiabetic human subjects after phenethyldiguanide. *Diabetes*, **15**:173–78, 1966.

Segre, E. J.: Diabetes mellitus with insulin resistance: report of a case successfully treated with tolbutamide. *Metabolism*, **11**:562–65, 1962.

Seidensticker, J. F., and Hamwi, G. J.: Oral hypoglycemic agents. *Geriatrics*, **22**:112–24, May, 1967.

Selenkow, H. A., and Wool, M. S.: A new synthetic thyroid hormone combination for clinical therapy. *Ann. Intern. Med.*, **67**:90–99, 1967.

Shackney, S., and Hasson, J.: Precipitous fall in serum calcium, hypotension, and acute renal failure after intravenous phosphate therapy for hypercalcemia: report of 2 cases. *Ann. Intern. Med.*, **66**:906–16, 1967.

Shahidi, N. T., and Diamond, L. K.: Testosterone induced remission in aplastic anemia of both acquired and congenital types. *New Eng. J. Med.*, **264**:953–67, 1961.

Shapiro, R., and Man, E. B.: Iophenoxic acid and serum-bound iodine value. *J.A.M.A.*, **173**:1352, 1960.

Sheldon, J., and Pyke, D. A.: Severe diabetic ketosis: precoma and coma. In Oakley, W. G.; Pyke, D. A.; and Taylor, K. W. (eds.): *Clinical Diabetes and Its Biochemical Basis*. Blackwell Scientific Publications, Oxford, England, 1968, pp. 420–55.

Sheldon, J.; Taylor, K. W.; and Anderson, J.: The effects of long-term acetohexamide treatment on pancreatic islet-cell function in maturity-onset diabetes. *Metabolism*, **15**:874–83, 1966.

Sherins, R. J.; Gandy, H. M.; and Paulson, C. A.: Depression of gonadotropin secretion and testicular function by a new steroidal compound WIN 17757. *Clin. Res.*, **17**:110, 1969.

Sherwood, L. M.; Potts, J. T., Jr.; Care, A. D.; Mayer, G. P.; and Aurbach, G. D.: Evaluation by radioimmunoassay of factors controlling the secretion of parathyroid hormone. *Nature*, **209**:52–55, 1966.

Shipp, J. C.; Cunningham, R. W.; Russell, R. O.; and Marble, A.: Insulin resistance: clinical features, natural course, and effects of adrenal steroid treatment. *Medicine*, **44**:165–86, 1965.

Simbari, R. D., and Houghton, E.: Distortion of PBI determination during coronary care. *Arch. Intern. Med. (Chicago)*, **123**:597, 1969.

Smith, L. F.: Species variation in the amino acid sequence of insulin. *Amer. J. Med.*, **40**:662–66, 1966.

Solomon, H. M., and Schrogie, J. J.: Effect of phenyramidol and bishydroxycoumarin on the metabolism of tolbutamide in human subjects. *Metabolism*, **16**:1029–33, 1967.

Spaulding, S. W., and Walser, M.: Oral phosphate therapy in experimental hypercalcemia. *Clin. Res.*, **16**:555, 1968.

Spellacy, W. N.; Carlson, K. L.; and Birk, S. A.: Carbohydrate metabolic studies after six cycles of combined type oral contraceptive tablets: measurement of plasma insulin and blood glucose levels. *Diabetes*, **16**:590–94, 1967.

Stanbury, S. W.: The treatment of renal osteodystrophy. *Ann. Intern. Med.*, **65**:1133–38, 1966.

Steelman, S. L., and Hirschmann, R.: Synthetic analogs of the adrenal cortical steroids. In Eisenstein, A. B. (ed.): *The Adrenal Cortex*. Little, Brown & Co., Boston, 1967, pp. 345–83.

Stein, R. B., and Nicoloff, J. T.: Triiodothyronine (T3) withdrawal test: a measure of the adequacy of TSH and thyroid reserve. In *Program of the 45th Meeting*,

American Thyroid Association, Inc., Chicago, November, 1969, p. 96.

Steiner, D. F.; Cunningham, D.; Spigelman, L.; and Aten, B.: Insulin biosynthesis: evidence for a precursor. *Science*, 157:697–700, 1967.

Steiner, D. F.; Hallund, O.; Rubenstein, A.; Cho, S.; and Bayliss, C.: Isolation and properties of proinsulin, intermediate forms, and other minor components from crystalline bovine insulin. *Diabetes*, 17: 725–36, 1968.

Sterup, K., and Mosbech, J.: Budd-Chiari syndrome after taking oral contraceptives. *Brit. Med. J.*, 4:660, 1967.

Stout, B. D.; Siener, L.; and Cox, J. W.: Combined alpha and beta sympathetic blockade in hyperthyroidism. *Ann. Intern. Med.*, 70:963–70, 1969.

Streiff, R. R.: Malabsorption of polyglutamic folic acid secondary to oral contraceptives. *Clin. Res.*, 17:345, 1969.

Strott, C. A., and Nugent, C. A.: Laboratory tests in the diagnosis of hyperparathyroidism in hypercalcemic patients. *Ann. Intern. Med.*, 68:188–202, 1968.

Studer, H.; Wyss, F.; and Jff, H. W.: A TSH reserve test for detection of mild secondary hypothyroidism. *J. Clin. Endocr.*, 24:965–75, 1964.

Suki, W. N.; Yium, J. J.; Von Minden, M.; Saller-Hebert, C.; Eknoyan, G.; and Martinez-Maldonado, M.: Acute treatment of hypercalcemia with furosemide. *New Eng. J. Med.*, 283:836–40, 1970.

Swerdloff, R. S., and Odell, W. D.: Gonadotropins: present concepts in the human. *Calif. Med.*, 109:467–85, 1968.

———: Serum luteinizing and follicle stimulating hormone levels during sequential and nonsequential contraceptive treatment of eugonadal women. *J. Clin. Endocr.*, 29:157–63, 1969.

Szabo, A. J.; Cole, H. S.; and Grimaldi, R. D.: Glucose tolerance in gestational diabetic women during and after treatment with a combination-type oral contraceptive. *New Eng. J. Med.*, 282:646–49, 1970.

Talbot, S.; Ryrie, D.; Wakley, E. J.; and Langman, M. J. S.: ABO blood-groups and venous thromboembolic disease. *Lancet*, 1:1257–59, 1970.

Talmage, R. V.: A study of the effect of parathyroid hormone on bone remodeling and on calcium homeostasis. *Clin. Orthopaed.*, 54:163–73, 1967.

Task Force on Prescription Drugs: *Background Papers: The Drug Users*. U.S. Dept. of Health, Education, and Welfare, Washington, D.C., 1968, p. 89.

Taymor, M. L.; Sturgis, S. H.; Lieberman, B. L.; and Goldstein, D. P.: Induction of ovulation with human postmenopausal gonadotropins. *Fertil. Steril.*, 17:731–35, 1966.

Thorn, G. W.: Clinical considerations in the use of corticosteroids. *New Eng. J. Med.*, 274:775–81, 1966.

Trotter, W. R.: The relative toxicity of antithyroid drugs. *J. New Drugs*, 2:333–43, 1962.

Tucci, J. R.; Espiner, E. A.; Jagger, P. I.; Lauler, D. P.; and Thorn, G. W.: Vasopressin in the evaluation of pituitary-adrenal function. *Ann. Intern. Med.*, 69:191–202, 1968.

Tucker, W. R.; Ryan, W. G.; Martin, B. F.; and Schwartz, T. B.: Studies in a patient with retroperitoneal sarcoma associated with severe hypoglycemia. *Ann. N. Y. Acad. Sci.*, 150:395–405, 1968.

Unger, R. H.; Ketterer, H.; Dupre, J.; and Eisentraut, A. M.: The effects of secretin, pancreozymin, and gastrin on insulin and glucagon secretion in anesthetized dogs. *J. Clin. Invest.*, 46:630–45, 1967.

Urist, M. R.: Observations bearing on the problem of osteoporosis. In Rodahl, K.; Nicholson, J. T.; and Brown, E. M. (eds.): *Bone as a Tissue.* McGraw-Hill Book Co., New York, 1960, pp. 18–45.

Vallance-Owen, J. Insulin antagonists. In Leibel, B. S., and Wrenshall, G. A. (eds.): *On the Nature and Treatment of Diabetes*, Excerpta Medica International Congress Series #84. Excerpta Medica Foundation, New York, 1965, pp. 340–53.

Verrier, R. L.; O'Neill, T. J.; and Lefer, A. M.: Functional capacity of resistance and capacitance vessels in adrenal insufficiency. *Amer. J. Physiol.*, 217:341–47, 1969.

Vessey, M. P., and Doll, R.: Investigation of relation between use of oral contraceptives and thromboembolic disease. *Brit. Med. J.*, 2:651–57, 1969.

Vinik, A. I.; Pimstone, B. L.; and Hoffenberg, R.: Sympathetic nervous system blocking in hyperthyroidism. *J. Clin. Endocr.*, 28:725–27, 1968.

Waldstein, S. S.; Slodki, S. J.; Kaganiec, G. I.; and Bronsky, D.: A clinical study of thyroid storm. *Ann. Intern. Med.*, 52:626–42, 1960.

Walser, M.; Robinson, B. H.; and Duckett, J. W., Jr.: The hypercalcemia of adrenal insufficiency. *J. Clin. Invest.*, 42:456–65, 1963.

Wasserman, R. H.; Corradino, R. A.; and Taylor, A. N.: Vitamin D-dependent calcium-binding protein: purification and some properties. *J. Biol. Chem.*, 243:3978–86, 1968.

Wasserman, R. H., and Taylor, A. N.: Vitamin D-dependent calcium-binding protein: response to some physiological and nutritional variables. *J. Biol. Chem.*, 243:3987–93, 1968.

Weinberger, M. H.; Collins, R. D.; Dowdy, A. J.; Nokes, G. W.; and Luetscher, J. A.: Hypertension induced by oral contraceptives containing estrogen and gestagen. *Ann. Intern. Med.*, 71:891–902, 1969.

Welt, L. G., and Gitelman, H.: Disorders of magnesium metabolism. *DM*, May, 1965, pp. 1–31.

Werner, S. C.: Prednisone in emergency treatment of malignant exophthalmos. *Lancet*, 1:1004–1007, 1966.

———: Two panel discussions on hyperthyroidism. I. Hyperthyroidism in the pregnant woman and the neonate. *J. Clin. Endocr.*, 27:1637–54, 1967a.

———: Two panel discussions on hyperthyroidism. II. Etiology and treatment of hyperthyroidism in the adult. *Ibid.*, 27:1763–77, 1967b.

Werner, S. C.; Feind, C. R.; and Aida, M.: Remnant thyroid tissue. *New Eng. J. Med.*, 276:986, 1967.

White, A.; Handler, P.; and Smith, E. L. (eds.): *The Principles of Biochemistry*, 4th ed. McGraw-Hill Book Co., New York, 1968.

Wilber, J. F., and Utiger, R. D.: The effect of glucocorticoids on thyrotropin (TSH) secretion. *Clin. Res.*, 17:295, 1969.

Williams, H. E.: Lactic acidosis. *Calif. Med.*, 110:330–36, 1969.

Williams, R. H.: The pancreas. In Williams, R. H. (ed.): *Textbook of Endocrinology*, 4th ed. W. B. Saunders Co., Philadelphia, 1968, pp. 613–802.

Wilson, C. O., and Jones, T. E.: *American Drug Index 1968.* J. B. Lippincott Co., Philadelphia, 1968.

Wilson, D. R., and Yendt, E. R.: Treatment of the adult Fanconi syndrome with oral phosphate supplements and alkali: report of two cases associated with nephrolithiasis. *Amer. J. Med.*, 35:487–511, 1963.

Winship, T.: Management of patients with cancer of the thyroid. *Cancer*, 20:1815–18, 1967.

Yen, S. S., and Vela, P.: Effects of contraceptive steroids on carbohydrate metabolism. *J. Clin. Endocr.*, 28:1564–70, 1968.

Chapter 8

HEMATOPOIETIC DISORDERS

John C. Marsh and *Joseph R. Bertino*

CHARACTERISTICS AND GENERAL CONSIDERATIONS

Correct diagnosis of hematologic disorders is imperative for rational treatment. Thorough evaluation is extremely important, as a disorder of the blood may manifest an underlying disease. For example, iron-deficiency anemia may be due to blood loss from an adenocarcinoma of the colon, and normocytic anemia may be secondary to severe renal disease. Simply treating the anemia without a thorough search for an underlying disorder may be disastrous.

The evaluation of a patient with a blood disorder should include calculation of red-cell indices and a reticulocyte count, in addition to enumeration of the formed elements. A careful examination of the blood smear is an essential part of the evaluation of every patient.

Principle: The use of "shotgun" hematinics has no place in clinical medicine. Specific replacement therapy is cheaper, confirms the diagnosis when successful, and, if not successful, suggests a mistaken diagnosis or other complicating factors. This chapter discusses specific treatment of the pathophysiologic processes in blood disorders.

Normal Erythropoiesis

Erythrocyte Physiology. The major function of the red cell, the transport of oxygen from lungs to tissues, is accomplished by the complexing of oxygen with hemoglobin, the principal protein of the erythrocyte. The efficiency of the transport process is reflected by the hemoglobin-oxygen dissociation curve, which is determined by the molecular configuration of hemoglobin and by the level of intracellular phosphates, the most important of which is 2,3-diphosphoglycerate (DPG). In conditions characterized by hypoxemia (anemia, pulmonary disease, high altitude) the level of red-cell DPG increases, resulting in an increased release of oxygen to the tissues (Benesch, 1969). Red cells are broken down at the end of their 120-day life-span by the reticuloendothelial system. The cleavage of the protoporphyrin ring of hemoglobin, and further separation of globin and iron from this ring, result in the formation of bilirubin (Figure 8–1). This pigment is bound to albumin and transported to the liver, where it is converted to the glucuronide and excreted in bile. The unconjugated bilirubin is measured as "indirect" in the van den Bergh reaction and, when elevated, gives a rough estimate of the degree of red-cell breakdown. The glucuronide is measured as the "direct" reacting pigment. The conjugated form is further broken down by bacteria in the intestine to a series of compounds collectively known as urobilinogens. These may be measured in the stool, and, to a lesser degree, in the urine, where they appear owing to colonic reabsorption and excretion by the kidney. Although other sources contribute to the pool of urobilinogens (Levitt *et al.*, 1968; Robinson, 1968), and although the correlation with hemoglobin breakdown is only approximate, measurements of these pigments may be helpful in diagnosing increased red-cell destruction. A more accurate

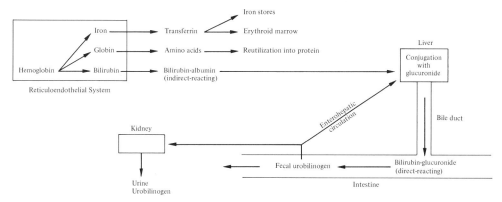

Figure 8–1. Hemoglobin catabolism and bilirubin metabolism.

estimate of the rate of destruction may be obtained by measuring the rate of disappearance of red cells labeled with radioactive substances such as ^{51}Cr.

If the factors controlling red-cell production are normal, the bone marrow is capable of increasing erythropoiesis to six to eight times the normal rate. Under some circumstances, the red-cell life-span may be as short as 15 days without development of anemia. Increased production results in an increase in erythroid elements in the bone marrow, and in reticulocytes and nucleated red cells in the blood.

Red-cell production may be quantitated by the use of radioactive iron, permitting determination of the rate and sites of erythropoiesis (Finch *et al.*, 1969). Ferrokinetic studies are helpful in some diagnostic problems, but are not routinely available because of the time they require and the need for specialized equipment.

Red-cell production is partly regulated by a humoral factor, erythropoietin, that is largely, if not exclusively, derived from the kidney (Erslev, 1964). The formation of erythropoietin is increased in the presence of hypoxia (due either to lowered plasma oxygen tension [e.g., at high altitudes] or to anemia). Erythropoietin stimulates the production of bone marrow stem cells which differentiate into red cells. Other actions on erythropoiesis are also possible; an increased level of erythropoietin has been found in many types of anemia, but not in that associated with renal failure (Mann *et al.*, 1965). Erythropoiesis has been reviewed in detail (Finch, 1969).

Factors Necessary for Erythrocyte Production.
Iron. Iron is an integral part of the hemoglobin molecule, essential for the transport of oxygen. The body economy of iron is rather stringent; only about 1 mg of iron is absorbed and lost

daily by the average adult male in spite of a daily turnover of more than 20 mg (Bothwell and Finch, 1962; Crosby, 1966). The body can salvage iron by transporting it from sites of red-cell breakdown in the reticuloendothelial system. In plasma, iron is transported by a beta globulin, transferrin (normally one-third saturated with iron), to the bone marrow for incorporation into hemoglobin. The reticuloendothelial cells in the marrow, liver, and spleen can also act as storage sites for iron. In the storage form it is bound to apoferritin to form the complex known as ferritin, aggregates of which form a yellow-brown pigment, hemosiderin. In this form it is detectable in bone marrow smears or sections.

Gastrointestinal absorption of iron is most efficient in the duodenum and upper jejunum and is favored by an acid intestinal pH. Partial gastrectomy or achlorhydria decreases iron absorption, as do diseases of the intestine associated with malabsorption. The iron content of the small intestinal mucosa is thought to regulate iron absorption. About 5 to 10% of dietary iron is absorbed in the normal adult male. In iron deficiency, up to 20% of dietary iron may be absorbed. Because of this limitation on maximum absorption, and the iron content of most diets, many patients with iron deficiency require supplemental iron therapy.

The iron requirements of the premenopausal female are about twice those of the male because of the monthly menstrual flow, which averages about 35 ml of blood, or 18 mg of iron. An extra 0.5 to 1 mg of iron per day is therefore required. During pregnancy, iron requirements increase greatly because of expanded maternal blood volume and red-cell mass, the iron needs of the fetus and placenta, and blood loss at delivery. Approximately 600 mg of extra iron are needed during the average pregnancy. If the

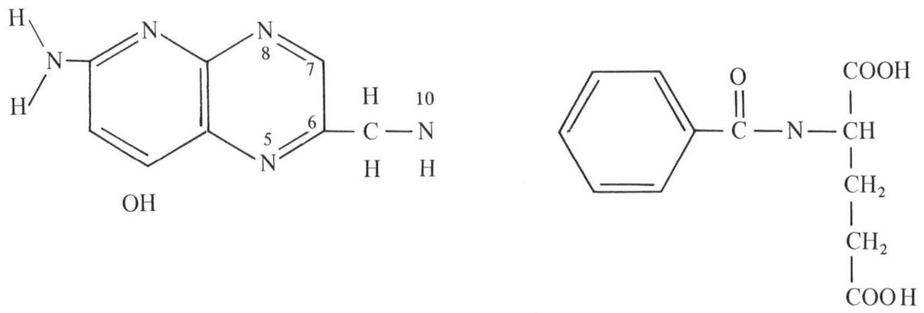

Folic acid
(pteroylglutamic acid)

Figure 8–2. Folates.

infant is nursed, 1 to 2 mg of iron per day are lost via the milk. In spite of increased efficiency of intestinal iron absorption during this time, the demands of pregnancy are usually in excess of the dietary sources, and iron supplementation is advisable.

Folates. Folic acid or, more correctly, the coenzyme forms of folic acid are required for purine and thymidylate synthesis and, therefore, for cell replication (Bertino and Johns, 1968; Huennekens, 1968; Blakley, 1969). Folic acid, a stable, therapeutically useful folate, does not appear to occur naturally and is probably an artifact of isolation (Figure 8–2). Reduced

Table 8–1. BIOSYNTHETIC REACTIONS REQUIRING FOLATE COENZYMES

FOLATE COENZYME	REACTION
N^5-methyl FH_4*	Methionine biosynthesis
N^{10}-formyl FH_4	Purine biosynthesis
N^5,N^{10}-methenyl FH_4	Purine biosynthesis
N^5-formimino FH_4	Histidine degradation
N^5,N^{10}-methylene FH_4	Thymidylate biosynthesis, serine biosynthesis

* 5,6,7,8-tetrahydrofolic acid.

folates, particularly N^{10}-formyltetrahydrofolate, N^5-methyltetrahydrofolate, and their polyglutamates, are probably the major folates found in the diet. Fresh fruits and vegetables, liver, and kidney are major sources of the vitamin. The fate of ingested folates and their polyglutamates is not yet clear; however, studies with the polyglutamate forms of folic acid have demonstrated that conjugase enzymes in the intestinal mucosa convert the polyglutamates to the monoglutamate form before or during absorption (Butterworth *et al.*, 1969). Intestinal conjugase activity may be inhibited in patients receiving either oral contraceptives (Streiff, 1969) or diphenylhydantoin (Hoffbrand and Necheles, 1968; Rosenberg *et al.*, 1968).

Absorption of folates probably occurs throughout the small intestine (Herbert and Shapiro, 1962; Ziemlanski *et al.*, 1968). The average daily folate requirement in adults is estimated to be 25 to 50 μg per day (Herbert, 1963). Increased requirements are present during infancy and pregnancy, and when blood cell production is increased; in these circumstances folate supplementation may be necessary. Folates are stored in liver as polyglutamates, probably of 5-methyltetrahydrofolate (Bird *et al.*, 1965). These stores are sufficient for only one to two months if folate intake ceases, thus explaining the rapidity with which folate deficiency can occur, as contrasted to vitamin B_{12} deficiency.

Folate coenzymes play an important role in cell metabolism by facilitating transfer of one-carbon adducts to acceptor molecules for the synthesis of purines (C_2, C_8), thymidylate, and methionine (Table 8–1). Methionine biosynthesis is of particular importance in that a vitamin B_{12} coenzyme (methylcobalamin) is also required, as well as a catalytic amount of S-adenosyl-methionine (Takeyama *et al.*, 1961; Weissbach *et al.*, 1963).

$$\begin{array}{c} \text{L-Homocysteine} + N^5\text{-methyltetrahydrofolate} \\ \text{(homocysteine methyl-} \\ \text{transferase)} \\[4pt] \text{Methylcobalamin} \,\Big|\Big|\, \text{S-adenosyl-methionine} \qquad (1) \\[4pt] \text{Methionine} + \text{tetrahydrofolate} \end{array}$$

The involvement of coenzymes of both B_{12} and folate in this reaction may explain the hematologic response of B_{12}-deficient patients to large doses of folate and vice versa.

Microbiologic assay with *Lactobacillus casei* may be used to measure serum folate activity and is a useful laboratory aid in assessing the folate status of a patient (Baker *et al.*, 1959). The major form of folate found in plasma is probably N^5-methyltetrahydrofolate (Herbert *et al.*, 1962), whereas most of the folate content of erythrocytes appears to be N^5-methyltetrahydrofolate polyglutamates (Noronha and Aboobaker, 1963). Assay of red-cell folates may provide a better assessment of tissue folate stores.

Vitamin B_{12}. Vitamin B_{12} is necessary for blood-cell formation and for central nervous system function (Herbert, 1963; Beck, 1964).

The daily requirement for vitamin B_{12} is estimated to be between 0.2 and 0.3 μg per day, making it the most potent nutrient known. The cobalamin content of the average daily diet has been estimated at 1 to 85 μg. Liver and kidney contain large amounts of this vitamin, and muscle contains somewhat smaller amounts. Dairy products contain only small quantities of B_{12}; fruits and vegetables are almost devoid of this vitamin. B_{12} probably occurs in a coenzyme form in meats, presumably as methyl or adenosyl cobalamin, but on exposure to light, heat, or acid, it may be converted to hydroxycobalamin, a more stable form utilizable by man (Toohey and Barker, 1961). Cyanocobalamin, the commercially available form of B_{12}, is a stable artifact of isolation.

The mechanism of absorption of vitamin B_{12} is unique (Glass, 1963). Intrinsic factor, a glycoprotein, is secreted by the stomach and strongly binds B_{12}. This complex is carried to the terminal ileum, where absorption takes place in the presence of calcium. After absorption, vitamin B_{12} is transported in the serum, bound primarily to an alpha-1 globulin called transcobalamin. Another binding protein, a beta globulin, has also been described (Hall and Finkler, 1963). Vitamin B_{12} is then avidly taken up by tissues, particularly the liver. Stores of vitamin B_{12} in the liver may be sufficient to sustain body requirements for a year or more if exogenous B_{12} is not available. Conversion of cyanocobalamin (vitamin B_{12}) or hydroxycobalamin to their coenzyme forms probably takes place primarily in the liver, but details of this conversion are lacking.

Bacterial extracts contain at least nine enzymes that require a coenzyme form of vitamin B_{12}, but only two vitamin-B_{12}-requiring enzymes have been identified in mammalian tissue (Jaenicke, 1964; Huennekens, 1968): the enzyme homocysteine methyltransferase (equation 1) and the enzyme methylmalonyl isomerase (Lengyel et al., 1960):

$$\text{Methylmalonyl-CoA} \xrightleftharpoons[]{\text{Adenosyl-cobalamin}} \text{Succinyl-CoA} \quad (2)$$

The physiologic role of this enzymic reaction has not been elucidated, although it has been speculated that this conversion is necessary for neurologic function. However, infants who are unable to carry out this reaction as a result of a hereditary defect do not have the neurologic dysfunction characteristic of adult pernicious anemia (Rosenberg, 1970). The detection of an increased amount of methylmalonic acid in the urine is useful in establishing the diagnosis of vitamin B_{12} deficiency (White and Cox, 1964). The need for vitamin B_{12} in blood-cell production appears to be a consequence of methionine synthesis (equation 1); this reaction may play a key role in control of folate coenzymes. The reaction catalyzed by the enzyme N^5,N^{10}-

methylenetetrahydrofolate reductase, which leads to the formation of N^5-methyltetrahydrofolate, is believed to be essentially irreversible.

$$N^5,N^{10}\text{-methylenetetrahydrofolate} + 2NADPH$$
$$\downarrow \quad\quad (3)$$
$$N^5\text{-methyltetrahydrofolate} + 2NADP$$

Since N^5-methyltetrahydrofolate plays no known role in biosynthetic reactions except for methionine biosynthesis, regeneration of tetrahydrofolate from this inactive storage form may be via methionine biosynthesis. Without an adequate supply of the vitamin B_{12} coenzyme, folate coenzyme deficiency ensues (except for N^5-methyltetrahydrofolate). This concept has been referred to as the "methyl trap" hypothesis (Noronha and Silverman, 1961; Herbert and Zalusky, 1962; Silber and Moldow, 1970). The megaloblastic anemia of B^{12} deficiency, therefore, may be due to an inability to utilize N^5-methyltetrahydrofolate.

Other Factors. It is doubtful that the anemia seen in patients with scurvy is due entirely to lack of *ascorbic acid* (vitamin C), as controlled studies of induced deficiency have not resulted in anemia (Crandon et al., 1940). Vitamin C may play an indirect role in hematopoiesis by helping to maintain folate coenzymes in a reduced form (Nichol and Welch, 1950). *Vitamin C deficiency may therefore intensify folic acid deficiency.* In addition, many scorbutic patients are folate deficient because a vitamin-C-deficient diet is generally deficient in folic acid as well (Herbert and Zalusky, 1962). Vitamin C has also been implicated in iron metabolism, again through its role as a reducing agent (Bothwell et al., 1964). Since scorbutic patients have increased capillary fragility, the consequent blood loss may produce iron deficiency anemia. An anemic patient with scurvy should be investigated for both iron and folic acid deficiency, and appropriate replacement therapy, as well as vitamin C, should be given.

It has not been established that anemia in man can result from dietary deficiency of *riboflavin* alone. Administration of a riboflavin antagonist, galactoflavin, and of a riboflavin-deficient diet produced anemia in patients with neoplastic disease (Lane and Alfrey, 1965; Alfrey and Lane, 1970). This anemia was characterized by vacuolization of early red-cell precursors (similar to that seen with alcohol or chloramphenicol), with no effect on platelets. The cause of the anemia has not been defined. Interference with the formation of the red-cell stroma or with erythropoietin was postulated.

In some patients with pellagra (deficiency of nicotonic acid, or *niacin*), particularly in alcoholics, macrocytic anemia is found. Since

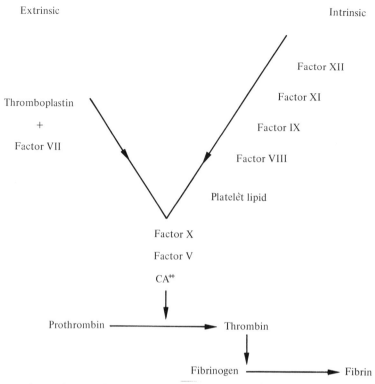

Figure 8-3. The extrinsic and intrinsic coagulation pathways. (From Hillman, R. S.: *Hematology Laboratory Manual.* University of Washington, Seattle, 1969.)

anemia is not characteristically observed in nonalcoholic pellagrins, this disorder may be due to a concomitant folate deficiency.

Pyridoxine (*vitamin B_6*), in the form of the cofactor pyridoxal phosphate, is required for the formation of delta-aminolevulinic acid, the precursor of the porphyrin that is the prosthetic group of hemoglobin. Patients with a dietary deficiency of pyridoxine, or with deficiency resulting from the administration of isoniazid, rarely become anemic. Some patients, however, have a pyridoxine-responsive anemia, responding to 100 to 200 mg of the vitamin per day, a dose approximately 100 times the normal daily requirement (Raab *et al.*, 1961; Horrigan and Harris, 1964). Some of these patients exhibit the characteristics of the anemia produced in swine by vitamin B_6 deficiency: high serum iron, lowered total iron-binding capacity with resultant increased transferrin saturation, increased iron in iron stores (liver and marrow), and "ringed sideroblasts" (i.e., normoblasts with small iron granules surrounding their nuclei). There seems to be a decreased rate of heme synthesis, with resultant accumulation of iron that is not used for hemoglobin formation.

The anemia is often, but not always, hypochromic and microcytic. The bone marrow of some patients is megaloblastic rather than normoblastic. As the pathogenesis is not known, the diagnosis can be made only by therapeutic trial. In some patients, hemoglobin concentration is not restored to normal; if normalization occurs, some morphologic red-cell abnormalities often remain. Most patients relapse when therapy is stopped.

Abnormal Erythropoiesis

Anemia, a decrease in the hemoglobin content of the blood, is due to (1) decreased production of red cells, (2) increased destruction or loss of red cells, or (3) a combination of these two factors. The following discussion outlines the frequently encountered causes of anemia. Polycythemia, an increase in the hemoglobin content of the blood, is also considered.

Anemia Due to Decreased Production of Erythrocytes. *Iron-Deficiency Anemia.* The iron storage compartment is initially depleted, followed by a decreased plasma transferrin saturation (decreased plasma iron and increased total iron-binding capacity). A decrease in the quantity of red cells, then in their size, and then in their content of hemoglobin, ensues. This process results in the characteristic morphologic abnormalities of microcytosis and hypochromia. Tissue changes, such as koilonychia (spoon nails), glossitis, and dysphagia due to a peculiar hypopharyngeal web or membrane formation (Plummer-Vinson syndrome), and menorrhagia (Taymor *et al.*, 1964) develop with severe iron deficiency. Hypochromic red cells are not specific for iron deficiency, but are also found in other disorders of hemoglobin synthesis, such as thalassemia and pyridoxine-responsive anemia.

Because of the increased iron loss in women due to menstruation or pregnancy, iron deficiency (often manifested only by a diminution in storage iron) is extremely common in adult females, and iron supplementation should be a routine part of prenatal treatment. However, iron deficiency in females should not always be considered "physiologic," since a heavy menstrual flow (menorrhagia) and abnormal menstrual timing (metrorrhagia) may be symptoms of important gynecologic disease requiring further evaluation and additional therapy.

Borderline iron supplies in pregnancy may produce iron deficiency in the infant. An all-milk diet, low in iron, aggravates this situation. Prematurity is almost always associated with iron deficiency, since there is less time to acquire iron *in utero* and since rapid growth increases the iron requirement. Such infants need supplemental iron.

In contrast to women, men can easily maintain their stores in the absence of blood loss. *The demonstration of iron deficiency in a man signifies blood loss, which is almost always from the gastrointestinal tract.* A thorough evaluation is mandatory in such a circumstance, since a life-threatening lesion, such as carcinoma of the colon or peptic ulcer, can be successfully treated at an early stage. The stool should be tested for occult blood in *any* patient with iron deficiency, and in males, radiologic evaluation of the gastrointestinal tract is required. Less common causes of chronic blood loss are defective blood-clotting or hereditary lesions such as hemorrhagic telangiectasia.

Anemia Due to Deficiency of Folate and Vitamin B_{12}. Tissue depletion of folate coenzymes or B_{12} coenzymes may lead to inhibition of cell maturation and replication. Although marrow-cell production may be increased, the number of mature cells delivered to the blood may be decreased. This condition has been called "ineffective erythropoiesis" (Giblett *et al.*, 1956). Morphologic abnormalities may occur in the cells of any tissue characterized by rapid "turnover" (e.g., bone marrow or gastrointestinal epithelium). These cells increase in size owing to an increase in intracellular RNA and in other cytoplasmic contents, and the nucleus becomes larger, more reticular, and lacy in appearance, but the DNA content does not increase. These changes characterize the "megaloblast," a term that describes the changes in developing red-cell forms in stained marrow smears. Since B_{12} and folate are also required for platelet and leukocyte production, quantitative changes in these cells (giant platelets, giant metamyelocytes, and an increase in the number of lobes in polymorphonuclear leukocytes) usually accompany the macrocytic anemia. Folate deficiency may also cause megaloblastic changes in small bowel epithelium (Bianchi *et al.*, 1970). In establishing the diagnosis of folate or B_{12} deficiency, the physician should consider (1) inadequate intake, (2) insufficient absorption, (3) relative insufficiency due to increased requirements, (4) metabolic or drug-induced deficiency, and (5) enzymic defects. In the United States, the major cause of folate deficiency is inadequate dietary intake secondary to alcoholism, whereas pernicious anemia is the most common cause of B_{12} deficiency. Colchicine, neomycin, para-aminosalicylic acid, and antiepilepsy drugs may interfere with folate and B_{12} absorption (Webb *et al.*, 1968; Neubauer, 1970).

The diagnosis of a nuclear maturation defect and the determination of its cause require a careful history and physical examination and appropriate laboratory tests. If the patient has a smooth tongue and posterolateral column disease, B_{12} deficiency is suggested. A therapeutic trial may be performed to establish the diagnosis, but with the current laboratory tests available, a trial is usually unnecessary (Herbert, 1963; Wintrobe, 1967; Hillman, 1969).

Subclinical folate deficiency is relatively common, if serum folate measurements are used as an indicator. Clinical deficiency exists when tissue folate stores are also depleted, leading to megaloblastosis and anemia. Determination of folate concentration in erythrocytes may help to indicate depletion in tissues. However, the erythrocyte folate levels reflect conditions present at the time of cell formation, rather than at the time of sampling.

The administration of pharmacologic doses of folic acid (400 μg per day or more) can lead to reticulocytosis and to improvement of anemia in patients with B_{12} deficiency. This relationship appears to be the result of some role of vitamin B_{12} coenzyme in folate metabolism, as discussed previously. Folate administration does not prevent the development or the progression of the neurologic disease sometimes associated with vitamin B_{12} deficiency (Will *et al.*, 1959). Vitamin B_{12} may therefore play a role in the nervous system that is independent of its function in folate metabolism (Vilter *et al.*, 1950; Herbert, 1963). *Principle: If a patient with megaloblastic anemia shows hematologic response to pharmacologic doses of vitamin B_{12} or folate, vitamin deficiency is not established.* Physiologic doses must be administered if a therapeutic trial is conducted to establish the diagnosis.

Aplastic Anemia. The condition characterized by anemia, neutropenia, and thrombocytopenia with a hypocellular marrow, and by absence of lymph gland or organ enlargement, is most commonly referred to as "aplastic anemia." This disorder primarily involves decreased blood-cell production, although some transitions into the relatively rare hemolytic disorder, paroxysmal nocturnal hemoglobinuria (PNH), have been observed (Quagliana *et al.*, 1964). Some patients may eventually develop acute leukemia. Aplastic anemia may occur as a constitutional disorder, associated at times with other congenital anomalies (e.g., retarded growth, abnormal pigmentation, or kidney and eye defects) (Shahidi and Diamond, 1961). More frequently, the disorder is acquired and due either to a variety of agents that are toxic to the bone marrow or to unknown causes. In sufficient quantities, certain agents regularly produce marrow damage. These include ionizing radiation, benzene and related solvents, inorganic arsenic, and drugs used in the treatment of neoplastic diseases (alkylating agents, plant alkaloids, purine, pyrimidine and folic acid analogs, antitumor antibiotics, etc.). In addition, many chemicals and drugs are more insidiously toxic to the marrow, seemingly on the basis of individual sensitivity. Chloramphenicol and phenylbutazone are commonly involved; the anticonvulsants trimethadione (Tridione) and methylphenylethylhydantoin (Mesantoin), less frequently. Organic arsenicals and gold compounds, used in the treatment of arthritis, are also important in this regard. Insecticides, such as DDT, parathion, and chlordane, have been implicated, as have many other drugs often used in clinical medicine (e.g., other antibiotics, sulfa drugs, phenothiazines [which more commonly produce neutropenia alone], other tranquilizers, oral antidiabetic agents, and certain antithyroid agents). *Principle: The physician should consider any chemical compound to which a patient has been exposed as a possible cause of pancytopenia, since removal of the offending drug is a crucial therapeutic step.*

Anemia Due to Underlying Disease. A variety of acquired diseases produce anemia, usually mild, which may be corrected by treating the underlying disease rather than by supplying some deficient nutrient or reducing destruction of red cells. This type of anemia is not usually characterized by marked hypocellularity of the marrow and may be associated with cancer, renal or liver disease, chronic infection, or inflammation such as arthritis.

The anemia of chronic disorders (Cartwright, 1966) is perhaps the most common variety found in medical practice. Usually mild (packed red-cell volume of 25 to 38%), usually normocytic and normochromic, but at times microcytic and/or hypochromic, it is associated with *low* values for serum iron and therefore is often mistaken for iron deficiency. However, the total iron-binding capacity is also low, in contrast to the elevated values found in iron deficiency, and the tissue iron stores are increased rather than decreased. Many types of infection, malignant disease with and without bone metastases, and arthritis are associated with this type of anemia. Iron therapy is useless. Although red-cell life-spans are modestly shortened, this alone cannot account for the anemia, as normal bone marrow can easily compensate for this degree of hemolysis. There is an apparent defect in the transfer of iron from storage depots into the plasma pool and then into hemoglobin. The cause of this defect is unknown. The anemia improves with successful treatment of the underlying disease; transfusions are usually not necessary.

A normocytic, normochromic anemia is often found in renal insufficiency (Adamson *et al.*, 1968; Erslev, 1970). There are no specific changes in serum iron or iron-binding capacity, but incorporation of radioactive iron into red cells is depressed. The severity of the anemia is proportional to the severity of the renal disease. In severe renal disease, platelet numbers and/or function may also be depressed (Rabiner and Molinas, 1970), leading to bleeding and iron deficiency. Apparent anemia may be accentuated or hidden because of changes in plasma volume that frequently occur in kidney disease. The anemia of chronic renal disease is usually a complex disorder combining defective production of erythropoietin by the kidney, increased red-cell destruction (extracorpuscular), and sluggish red-cell production. The latter two factors may improve with dialysis, whereas the former improves only with successful renal transplantation.

Anemia is very common in patients with chronic liver disease (Kimber *et al.*, 1965; Kilbridge and Heller, 1969; Keller *et al.*, 1971). Portal cirrhosis may result in anemia owing to one or more factors. A deficiency of iron may be present owing to blood loss from esophageal varices, hemorrhoids, or peptic ulcer, or to a dietary deficiency of folate. Alcohol may exert a direct depressant effect upon marrow production of all formed elements (McFarland and Libre, 1963; Sullivan and Herbert, 1964; Lindenbaum and Hargrove, 1968; Douglass and Twomey, 1970). Red-cell destruction may be increased owing to splenomegaly caused by portal hypertension. Incorporation of iron into red cells is usually impaired, indicating impaired marrow function, particularly in those patients who should have an elevated rate of erythropoiesis because of hemolysis or blood loss. Treatment consists of supplying deficient factors and correcting poor nutrition and alcoholism.

Anemia may be associated with endocrine disease (Daughaday et al., 1948). Patients with hypothyroidism may demonstrate a mild anemia, usually macrocytic or normochromic, with a normoblastic marrow (Tudhope and Wilson, 1960). The anemia responds slowly over a period of months to the daily administration of thyroid extract or L-thyroxine (130 to 195 mg or 200 to 300 μg, respectively). Patients with myxedema may sometimes have pernicious anemia as well, and the response to B_{12} may be slow unless the hypothyroidism is concurrently treated. Androgen or adrenocortical hormone deficiency may be associated with a mild normocytic anemia that responds to replacement therapy (Baez-Villaseñor et al., 1948).

Anemia Secondary to Blood Loss or to Increased Destruction of Erythrocytes. If anemia is accompanied by normal or increased blood-cell production, hemolysis or blood loss via hemorrhage should be suspected. Thus, the reticulocyte count may be elevated, and the bone marrow shows normoblastic proliferation. *Principle: When there is a sudden massive drop in the hematocrit, the physician should search for blood loss or a hemolytic process in order to identify a potentially reversible situation.*

Anemia Due to Blood Loss. The presence of internal or external hemorrhage can usually be detected by a careful history and physical examination, by examination of the stool for blood, and by appropriate x-rays or endoscopy. The anemia of sudden hemorrhage is normocytic and normochromic, but signs of iron deficiency may appear as iron stores become depleted. Sudden massive hemorrhage is usually associated with a decrease in total blood volume.

Hemolytic Anemia. Acute hemolysis resulting in a sudden drop in the volume of packed red cells is usually an intravascular event due to the presence of an extracellular agent. Intravascular hemolysis can be rapidly docu-

mented by the presence of free hemoglobin in the blood and urine, by the absence of haptoglobin in the serum, and by the presence of methemalbumin in serum. Free haptoglobin in serum can bind an amount of hemoglobin equal to that liberated from the hemolysis of about 20 ml of packed erythrocytes; the complex is cleared by the reticuloendothelial system in about 8 hours. When this binding capacity is exceeded, free hemoglobin may be detected in the serum and urine. Haptoglobin may be lacking for 1 to 3 days, until new synthesis restores normal levels (Reerink-Brongers et al., 1962). If the amount of hemolysis exceeds the haptoglobin concentration, the excess hemoglobin may be oxidized to methemoglobin, then bound to albumin. This methemalbumin complex may be detected for several days following severe hemolysis. Documentation of intravascular hemolysis should be accompanied by a search for possible external agents. A mismatched transfusion, certain bacterial toxins (e.g., *Clostridium welchii*), protozoal infections such as malaria, or severe burns may produce sudden intravascular hemolysis. Intravascular hemolysis may also result from destruction of erythrocytes by prosthetic heart valves (examples of "microangiopathic hemolytic anemia") or during severe hypertension. Occasionally, cells with an intracellular enzyme defect may also be destroyed intravascularly.

Extravascular hemolysis is usually due to antibodies or to intrinsic red-cell defects. This more common type of hemolytic anemia may be accompanied by a positive Coombs test, or by an enzyme, hemoglobin, or membrane abnormality in the erythrocyte. In this type of hemolysis, the serum haptoglobin is normal or low (but not absent), and hemoglobinemia or methemalbuminemia cannot be demonstrated.

The diagnosis of a compensated hemolytic state often requires specialized tests. Initial efforts should be made to document decreased red-cell survival, (e.g., after radioactive chromium [^{51}Cr] tagging). This measurement should be accompanied by the determination of radioactivity over the liver and spleen by external scintillation counting. If there is an increased ratio of counts over the spleen as compared to liver, splenectomy may be advisable (Veeger et al., 1962).

Congenital hemolytic anemia is usually due to an intrinsic red-cell defect; this condition is indicated if compatible normal erythrocytes survive for a normal period of time in the patient, and if the patient's cells have a shortened survival when infused into a normal compatible recipient.

The exact diagnosis of a congenital hemolytic

defect depends upon careful examination of the smear (e.g., for sickle cells, target cells, and spherocytes). This may suggest further procedures such as hemoglobin electrophoresis (which will detect most hemoglobinopathies), tests for membrane defects such as determination of osmotic fragility and autohemolysis, or the acid hemolysin test for paroxysmal nocturnal hemoglobinuria, an *acquired* hemolytic anemia (Crosby, 1951). The most frequent red-cell enzyme defect, glucose-6-phosphate dehydrogenase deficiency, may be detected by procedures available in most laboratories, but elucidation of less common defects, such as pyruvate kinase deficiency, may require the help of a research laboratory (Ranney, 1970; Westerman, 1970).

Acquired hemolytic anemia is almost always due either to the presence of an extracellular agent that produces red-cell destruction (e.g., an antibody or a toxin) or to hyperactivity of the reticuloendothelial system (e.g., hypersplenism).

The term "hypersplenism" has been used most frequently to define a state characterized by enlargement of the spleen, a decrease in the concentration of one or more of the formed elements of the blood, a normally cellular or hypercellular bone marrow, and improvement or cure of the cytopenia with splenectomy (Doan, 1949; Dameshek, 1955). The term implies that the spleen, enlarged by disease such as tumor, increased portal pressure, or infection, performs its normal function of blood-cell sequestration and destruction in an exaggerated way. An inhibitory effect on the bone marrow is less likely but not entirely ruled out.

Warm-reacting antibodies that cause hemolytic anemias usually are IgG-(7S)-incomplete antibodies that may be identified by the Coombs test with IgG-specific antisera. These antibodies usually stimulate extravascular removal of red cells by the reticuloendothelial system. This type of hemolytic anemia may be encountered in lymphomas, in lupus erythematosus, after transfusions, and with certain drugs, such as alpha-methyldopa (Worlledge *et al.*, 1966). Many patients with autoimmune hemolytic anemia do not have recognizable associated diseases.

Hemolytic anemias related to diseases such as *Mycoplasma* pneumonia, infectious mononucleosis, and macroglobulinemia are associated with complete antibodies, which react in the cold either to agglutinate red cells or, in some cases, to bind complement, resulting in hemolysis. These antibodies are macroglobulins (19S, IgM), and identification requires an anti-IgM Coombs serum (MacKenzie and Creevy, 1970).

With careful clinical and laboratory examination, most hemolytic anemias can be characterized and appropriate therapy can be instituted, although sometimes the exact cause cannot be ascertained by the usual tests.

Polycythemia.   Normal values for the volume of packed red cells are 42 to 52% for males and 37 to 47% for females, at sea level (Wintrobe, 1967). These figures encompass 95% of the normal population. In higher altitudes, arterial oxygen saturation is reduced and red-cell mass is increased. An increased packed-cell volume does not necessarily indicate a true increase in the red-cell mass; the latter must be confirmed by actual measurement. A similar change in the packed-cell volume could result from a decreased plasma volume with a normal red-cell mass. This relative polycythemia has been termed "stress polycythemia" and does not require therapy (Lawrence and Berlin, 1952).

A true increase in red-cell mass (erythrocytosis) may occur as a physiologic response to various stimuli, or as part of the hyperproliferative disease of the bone marrow known as polycythemia vera. The latter is usually accompanied by an increase in the other formed elements of the blood, whereas the other disorders producing erythrocytosis are not.

The most common stimulus for erythrocytosis is arterial hypoxia, which may be due to low atmospheric pressure of oxygen at high altitude or to impaired pulmonary ventilation, most commonly found in pulmonary emphysema. Arterial oxygen tension is also lowered in congenital heart disease associated with right-to-left shunting of blood or in pulmonary vascular shunting, which may have the same physiologic result (i.e., some venous blood is never oxygenated). A defect in the oxygen-carrying capacity of the blood may cause polycythemia; these defects include such congenital forms of hemoglobin disease as hemoglobin Chesapeake (Charache *et al.*, 1966). Polycythemia may also be associated with hereditary disorders (hemoglobin M or methemoglobin reductase deficiency) *or with oxidant drugs that produce methemoglobinemia by overcoming the normal mechanisms of methemoglobin reduction.* These drugs include many coal tar derivatives, such as phenacetin, acetanilid, sulfa drugs, chlorates, nitrates, and nitroglycerin (see Chapter 15). Various dyes used in crayons, shoe polish, and laundry marks have also been implicated, especially in children, whose methemoglobin reduction mechanisms may not be as effective as those in adults.

Normal Leukopoiesis

The number of leukocytes in peripheral blood, the percentage of each leukocyte type, and the morphologic characteristics of the individual cells can be easily determined. Clues to disease states may be afforded by an increase or decrease in the total leukocyte concentration or in a specific cell type. Morphologic abnormalities or the presence of cells not usually found in the peripheral blood may also be of great importance (Boggs, 1968).

Granulocyte Physiology (Cartwright *et al.*, 1964). Neutrophilic granulocytes, which make up the majority of the circulating leukocytes, are the most important in terms of susceptibility to infection (see Chapter 10). In contrast to red cells, which fulfill their function intravascularly, neutrophils simply pass through the blood in a brief time (average of 10 hours) on their way to the tissues, where they clear foreign materials by phagocytosis and intracellular catabolism (see Chapter 9). Only about half of the total blood neutrophils are measured in a leukocyte count, the others being marginated along the walls of small vessels. Neutrophils are produced during a 5- to 7-day period in the bone marrow, through an orderly sequence of cell division of immature precursors, maturation, and release from a storage pool of mature cells. Relatively few immature (nonsegmented) neutrophils are released normally, but during infection there may be an increased demand for cells, reflected in the blood as a "shift to the left." Following their passage through the blood, neutrophils apparently serve their function in the tissues and die there or are lost in various body secretions and excretions.

Much of the information on granulocyte function has been derived from studies of labeled cells (e.g., with radioactive diisopropylfluorophosphate, $DF^{32}P$). Estimates of blood transit time ($t_{1/2}$) can be obtained. No true estimate of cell life-span is yet available, since the time spent in the tissues has not been adequately quantitated. A measure of the neutrophil storage pool in the marrow (marrow granulocyte reserve) can be obtained with injections of either bacterial endotoxin or etiocholanolone (Vogel *et al.*, 1967), which cause release of granulocytes from the marrow into the blood. Exercise or epinephrine increases the size of the circulating neutrophil pool by a different mechanism, causing demargination of cells from capillary and venule walls into the circulation (Athens *et al.*, 1961). Adrenal steroids such as prednisone increase the blood granulocyte concentration both by increasing marrow release and by decreasing egress of cells into the tissues (Bishop *et al.*, 1968). Changes in blood neutrophil concentration may therefore result from changes in the rate of marrow input to blood, changes in the rate of outflow from blood to tissues or redistribution of cells between the marginal and circulating blood neutrophil pool.

Useful techniques for evaluating neutrophil kinetics include bone marrow aspiration and biopsy, total leukocyte count and differential, test of marrow reserve with endotoxin or etiocholanolone, test of rapidity and completeness of appearance of cells in an induced inflammation (skin window), and cell labeling, such as with $DF^{32}P$. The use of ^{51}Cr as a granulocyte label has the theoretic advantage of permitting external body counting to evaluate disposition in tissues (especially the spleen), but this technique is still under investigation.

Lymphocyte Physiology (Gowans, 1968). Lymphocytes, which are formed in lymphoid tissue (nodes, spleen, and bone marrow), enter the blood via large lymphatics, such as the thoracic duct, and recirculate. The thymus seems to play an important role in the early development of lymphoid tissue. Lymphocytes probably function both by forming plasma cells capable of producing antibodies and by mounting a cellular response to foreign substances ("cellular immunity"). Interference with this cellular response is useful in preventing graft rejection (e.g., in kidney transplantation). Methods of inhibition include thoracic duct drainage and the use of antilymphocyte serum or of immunosuppressive drugs such as azathioprine or prednisone (see Chapter 12). One of the potential hazards of such treatment is the development of tumors (Deodhar *et al.*, 1969), since lymphocytes may function as part of a surveillance mechanism to prevent proliferation of neoplastic clones (Burnet, 1961).

Though the lymphocyte is a resting cell, it is capable of protein, RNA, and DNA synthesis as well as mitosis when appropriately stimulated. Phytohemagglutinin and specific antigens cause this phenomenon (transformation) *in vitro*; some aspects of lymphocyte function may be measured in this way. Antibody synthesis may be measured *in vivo* following administration of an appropriate antigen. Cellular immunity as an indicator of lymphocyte function may be measured by skin graft rejection time, by certain skin tests (e.g., tuberculin, mumps) if the person has been previously exposed to the antigen, or by sensitization with a chemical such as dinitrochlorobenzene (DNCB). Antibody synthesis and transformation are defective in some cases of chronic lymphatic leukemia; defective cellular immunity has been demonstrated in Hodgkin's disease and sarcoidosis.

Abnormal Leukopoiesis

Leukopenia. *Granulocytopenia* (Kauder and Mauer, 1966). Folic acid and vitamin B_{12} are required for leukocyte formation. Moderate leukopenia, primarily due to a decrease in neutrophilic granulocytes, is commonly noted in association with megaloblastic anemias due to folate or B_{12} deficiency. Examination of the blood smear may be helpful, as an increase in the number of lobes of the neutrophilic granulocytes ("Arneth count") may be the earliest sign of such a vitamin deficiency. Iron deficiency rarely may be associated with hypersegmentation of neutrophils (Beard and Weintraub, 1969), but neutropenia does not always accompany this morphologic change. Alcohol may also inhibit proper production or release of neutrophils (McFarland and Libre, 1963).

Neutropenia may be caused by marrow infiltration by leukemia, lymphoma, or other neoplastic cells, or replacement by fibrosis. In addition to cell crowding of the normal marrow, an inhibitor of normal granulocytopoiesis may be elaborated by tumor cells.

Certain drugs (alkylating agents, plant alkaloids, antimetabolites) usually produce granulocytopenia when given in therapeutic doses, as does radiation therapy when the dose and the extent of bone marrow exposure are sufficient. This risk must be judged in relation to the potential therapeutic benefit. For example, extensive radiation treatment of localized Hodgkin's disease often produces reversible pancytopenia, but since this therapy may produce a cure in a substantial number of patients, the adverse effect of treatment is acceptable. As discussed previously, many drugs used for more benign conditions can cause bone marrow depression, sometimes limited to the granulocyte series.

Occasionally, patients may have persistent or cyclic granulocytopenia without other known disease. During periods of severe neutropenia, they may develop bacterial infection requiring antibiotic treatment. Chronic neutropenia may be familial, and in its most severe form may be associated with overwhelming sepsis and death.

Granulocytopenia associated with normal cellularity or with myeloid hyperplasia may result from increased destruction or utilization of granulocytes. As in the case of red cells, hypersplenism may cause increased destruction or sequestration of circulating leukocytes. Diseases characterized by splenomegaly and neutropenia include cirrhosis with portal hypertension, sarcoidosis, lymphoma, and rheumatoid arthritis ("Felty's syndrome"). Neutropenia is common in viral and rickettsial infections, as well as in certain bacterial infections such as typhoid fever and brucellosis. The mechanism that causes decreased production or increased utilization of neutrophils is not clear. In overwhelming infection, such as severe pneumococcal pneumonia, neutropenia may occur as a result of peripheral utilization of the cells, which eventually overcomes marrow granulocyte reserves (Marsh et al., 1967).

Neutropenia. Immune processes have been implicated in the pathogenesis of neutropenia caused by a transplacentally acquired antibody (Lalezari et al., 1960), neutropenia due to sensitization with aminopyrine (Moeschlin, 1955), and neutropenia associated with antileukocyte antibodies in diseases such as lupus erythematosus (Tullis, 1958).

Lymphopenia. Lymphopenia is less common than neutropenia. A decrease in the absolute lymphocyte count is often found in advanced Hodgkin's disease, systemic lupus erythematosus, and miliary tuberculosis. The leukocytosis usually noted with bacterial infection is commonly associated with a mild absolute lymphopenia. Drugs such as corticosteroids and alkylating agents and irradiation therapy can cause lymphopenia. Certain genetically determined immunologic deficiency states are characterized by lymphopenia and by lack of both humoral antibody and cellular immunity responses (Seligmann et al., 1968). Patients with these disorders commonly die of infection in infancy or childhood (see Chapter 10).

Leukocytosis. An elevated leukocyte count is most often caused by infection. Patients who do not respond to a severe bacterial infection with an elevated neutrophil count usually have some defect in cell formation, which may be due to limited stores of folic acid or may be secondary to inhibition of production by drugs, alcohol, or the infection itself.

Other causes of leukocytosis include malignancies (especially those associated with cell necrosis), necrosis of muscle or myocardium, administration of corticosteroids, severe burns, acidosis, and uremia. Administration of epinephrine or severe muscular exercise may cause neutrophilia by demargination of cells adherent to capillary walls, rather than by direct release of cells from bone marrow.

The lymphocyte count may be elevated in certain infections (e.g., pertussis or infectious lymphocytosis). The diagnosis of infectious mononucleosis is based on a rise in atypical mononuclear cells.

Acute and chronic leukemia are discussed in Chapter 12.

Normal Thrombopoiesis

Platelets (thrombocytes) are the third formed element in the blood. Their concentration in the blood normally ranges from 150,000 to 350,000/cu mm, using the newer direct methods of counting (Hillman, 1969; Harker, 1970). An approximation of their number may also be made by comparing the patient's stained blood smear with a normal blood smear.

If the platelet count is increased or decreased, or if morphologic abnormalities are found in platelets (e.g., diameters larger than 5μ), the bone marrow should be examined to evaluate megakaryocytes. Immature and mature megakaryocytes may be distinguished in the marrow and probably are derived from the same stem cell as are neutrophils and red cells. Although megakaryocytes are found in the lungs and spleen, it is not clear whether they develop *in situ* or migrate from the marrow. Disappearance rates of labeled platelets have shown that platelets remain in the circulation for 8 to 11 days (Kotilainen, 1969). It has not yet been determined whether they disappear from the blood after a finite life-span (as do red cells), or randomly, without regard to age (as do neutrophils), though the former seems probable. The liver and spleen seem to be important in the removal of nonviable platelets. The spleen also appears to serve as a pool for about one-third of the viable platelets (Aster, 1966). Epinephrine can effect release of platelets from the spleen. Splenic enlargement may cause thrombocytopenia by shortening their life-span or by sequestering unusual numbers of viable platelets. Splenectomy may ameliorate various thrombocytopenic states caused by increased platelet destruction or sequestration, but not those associated with decreased production. Labeling of platelets with ^{51}Cr may aid in differentiating thrombocytopenia caused by a production defect from that caused by shortened survival, analogous to the information derived from red-cell chromium labeling.

The production of platelets seems to be determined by the demand for circulating platelets. These demands are met by appropriate changes in megakaryocyte number and size (Harker and Finch, 1969). When platelet production is increased, megakaryocyte changes include an increased number of nuclei within the individual cells, as well as an increased number of immature cells (presumably owing to an increased rate of differentiation of pluripotential stem cells into megakaryocytes). These changes may be regulated by a humoral factor or factors, analogous to erythropoietin, but the actual factors have not been identified.

Adequate platelet function is essential for control of hemorrhage, These functions include adhesion to the site of injury of vessel endothelium, ADP-mediated aggregation at the injury site to form a plug, and acceleration of the formation of fibrin at the injury site by providing a membrane lipoprotein ("platelet factor 3") that acts as a catalytic surface for the interaction of plasma coagulation factors (Marcus, 1969). Dipyridamole blocks ADP-induced platelet aggregation and may be useful in preventing thrombosis or embolism in certain high-risk patients (Sullivan *et al.*, 1968). Aspirin prolongs the bleeding time, probably by blocking the release of ADP from platelets, thus preventing further aggregation (Weiss and Kochwa, 1968). Useful tests for the evaluation of platelet function include the tourniquet test, bleeding time, clot retraction, platelet adhesiveness, platelet factor 3 function, and prothrombin consumption.

Abnormal Thrombopoiesis

Thrombocytopenia. The most common hematologic cause of severe abnormal bleeding is thrombocytopenia. Serious spontaneous hemorrhage does not generally occur until the platelet concentration falls to 20,000/cu mm or less (Gaydos *et al.*, 1962). Proper management depends not only on appropriate replacement therapy but also on recognition of the mechanism and cause of the disorder (Harker, 1969).

Thrombocytopenia may be due to a disorder of production (e.g., marrow replacement by tumor, as in leukemia, carcinoma, lymphoma), radiation damage, drugs, chemicals, or infection (e.g., miliary tuberculosis). Ineffective thrombopoiesis may occur in B_{12} and folate deficiency, analogous to ineffective erythropoiesis associated with these conditions. Thus, total megakaryocyte mass may be increased without significant delivery of platelets to the circulation. Splenomegaly may also result in thrombocytopenia owing to increased splenic trapping of platelets.

Increased destruction of platelets may result from immunologic mechanisms or from consumption in coagulation. "Autoimmune" destruction of platelets may be unaccompanied by other disease ("idiopathic thrombocytopenic purpura") or may result from underlying disorders such as lymphoma, lymphatic leukemia, or systemic lupus erythematosus. Certain drugs (e.g., quinidine, quinine, and sulfonamides) may act as haptenes to induce antiplatelet antibodies, with consequent sudden thrombocytopenia (see Chapter 15).

When disseminated intravascular coagulation occurs owing to abnormal activation of the clotting mechanism (as in promyelocytic leukemia, gram-negative sepsis, meningococcemia, certain obstetric complications, and carcinoma of the prostate), thrombocytopenia usually results along with depletion of other coagulation factors.

Thrombocytosis. An increased concentration of platelets in blood may be found in many disorders, especially malignancies; at times this predisposes to thrombosis or, paradoxically, to hemorrhage. Treatment with an alkylating agent such as busulfan may occasionally be necessary in instances of extreme thrombocytosis.

Functional Platelet Disorders. Several conditions may be associated with abnormal platelet function in the presence of a normal platelet count in blood. Significant bleeding may accompany these functional platelet defects. A defect in "platelet factor 3," as well as interference with ADP-induced platelet

Table 8–2. PROPERTIES OF CLOTTING FACTORS*

FACTOR	NAME	APPROXIMATE PLASMA DISAPPEARANCE ($t_{1/2}$) (HOURS)	CLINICAL SYNDROME DUE TO DEFICIENCY	INHERITANCE OF DEFICIENCY (PER MILLION)
I	Fibrinogen	90	+	<0.5
II	Prothrombin	60	+	<0.5
III	Tissue thromboplastin	—	0	—
IV	Calcium	—	0	—
V	Proaccelerin, labile factor	15	+	<0.5
VII	Proconvertin, stable factor	5	+	<0.5
VIII	Antihemophilic globulin (AHG)	15	+	60–80
IX	Christmas factor, plasma thromboplastin component (PTC)	25	+	15–20
X	Stuart or Stuart-Prower factor	40	+	<0.5
XI	Plasma thromboplastin antecedent (PTA)	—	+	~1.0
XII	Hageman factor, contact factor	40	0	~1.0
XIII	Fibrin stabilizing factor	90	+	<0.5

* From Harker, L. A.: *Hemostasis Manual.* University of Washington, Seattle, 1969.

aggregation, has been described in uremia; this abnormality may be related to dialyzable plasma factors (Marcus, 1969). Platelet aggregation by ADP and thrombin is defective in some patients with portal cirrhosis (Thomas *et al.*, 1967). Thrombocytopenia may also be present in cirrhosis or uremia.

Some abnormalities of platelet function may be congenital. Thrombocytopathy has been defined as a defect in platelet factor 3 (Ulutin, 1965). Thrombasthenia is a disorder associated with prolonged bleeding time, poor clot retraction, lack of aggregation with ADP, but otherwise normal platelet adhesion and concentration (Weiss and Kochwa, 1968). Mild bleeding occurs in skin or mucous membranes, but the disorder tends to become less severe with age. Von Willebrand's disease is genetically determined, characterized variably by a long bleeding time and by an apparent factor VIII deficiency that is correctable by normal or even hemophilic plasma (Weiss, 1968). Thrombopathia is characterized by mild bleeding (spontaneous bruising), a prolonged bleeding time, defective platelet aggregation induced by collagen, and defective release of ADP by platelets.

Normal and Abnormal Coagulation

Once thrombocytopenia is ruled out as a cause of spontaneous bleeding, attention should be directed to deficiency of a clotting factor (or factors). A deficiency of certain factors may also accompany thrombocytopenia (disseminated intravascular clotting), but in this circumstance the clinical situation should alert the physician to this possibility. A careful history is especially important in evaluation of inherited bleeding disorders (Bithell and Wintrobe, 1970).

The clotting process involves a series of reactions that lead to the formation of insoluble fibrin from soluble fibrinogen. Twelve factors have been identified (Table 8-2), many by careful study of patients lacking one of these substances. Two important procedures used to screen for a coagulation defect and to indicate the need for further specific tests are the prothrombin time and the partial thromboplastin time.

The prothrombin time tests the extrinsic coagulation pathway, initiated by tissue thromboplastin activity, and the partial thromboplastin time tests the intrinsic clotting system (Figure 8–3). In the intrinsic clotting system, several reactions must occur before prothrombin is activated, a process requiring several minutes; in contrast, the extrinsic pathway requires only the reaction of thromboplastin with factor VII to activate prothrombin and is complete in 12 to 15 seconds. Since the *in vitro* prothrombin time tests this system by the addition of thromboplastin, a deficiency of factors VII, X, V, II (prothrombin), or I (fibrinogen) increases the prothrombin time. These factors are produced in the liver and some require vitamin K for synthesis. Conditions that may give rise to an abnormal prothrombin time are vitamin K deficiency, defective absorption, or defective synthesis as in liver disease. The partial thromboplastin time tests factors XII, XI, IX, VIII, X, V, II, and I. Kaolin is used to activate factor XII and initiate the test, and cephalin is used instead of platelets.

When both tests are abnormal, the defect may be localized to those factors common to both pathways (i.e., to a stage below factor X). Additional specific tests may then be used to further define the abnormality.

Diagnosis is emphasized, since appropriate therapy depends on the localization of the defect or, more commonly, on detection of multiple defects, as in liver disease or in disseminated intravascular clotting. Therapy must then be directed not only to the clotting problem, which is often an emergency, but also to the underlying disease (e.g., promyelocytic leukemia). Adequate replacement therapy requires knowledge of the half-life of the factor administered, a carefully designed treatment program, and monitoring of the effects of therapy.

SPECIAL CONSIDERATIONS

Therapeutic Use of Blood Components

The administration of blood and blood products may be lifesaving on many occasions, but is always hazardous (Young, 1964). The major hazards of transfusion are excessive expansion of blood volume with precipitation of congestive heart failure, administration of incompatible blood leading to severe allergic reactions and/or hemolysis, and transmission of serum hepatitis or malaria (Brooks and Barry, 1969; Baker and Nyhus, 1970; Ward, 1970; Sturgeon, 1971).

Transfusion of whole blood is required when acute hemorrhage leads both to volume depletion and to a decrease in red cells necessary for oxygen transport. In extreme emergencies, volume expanders such as dextran or albumin may be used until typing and cross-matching are completed and blood is obtained. Severe burns, with loss of blood volume, may also require transfusion (see Chapter 5). If thrombocytopenia or deficiencies of clotting factors accompany red-cell loss, the administration of fresh blood may be desirable. Specific components, such as platelets or factor VIII, may be given in concentrated form, when indicated, without imposing the threat of volume overload. Although blood administration may be required in cases of acute hemolysis, the transfused blood may also be rapidly destroyed. As many such patients reach an equilibrium compatible with survival without blood transfusion, efforts to correct the cause of the hemolysis may be more fruitful. In most instances of chronic anemia, the patient has made physiologic adjustment to the disease, and the use of transfusions should be conservative. *Principle: There is no arbitrary level of hemoglobin or packed-red-cell volume below which a patient must be transfused, and such variables as age, state of the vasculature, and activity of the patient determine the symptoms that suggest a need for transfusion.*

Symptoms including dyspnea, weakness, fatigue, and angina (or asymptomatic ischemic changes recorded on the electrocardiogram) may indicate the need for transfusion. Adults rarely require transfusion of red cells when the hemoglobin is more than 8 g/100 ml (hematocrit of 25%), and children tolerate even lower hemoglobin concentrations. The cause of the anemia influences the necessity for transfusion: If anemia is due to the lack of a specific sub-stance, such as iron or vitamin B_{12}, appropriate treatment often makes transfusion unnecessary. Induction of remission in leukemia or administration of steroids in autoimmune hemolytic anemia may improve the hemoglobin level.

If anemia has developed slowly, it is preferable to transfuse with packed red cells, rather than with whole blood (Chaplin, 1969). There are two advantages to packed-red-cell therapy: (1) as the volume is about half that of whole blood, there is less danger of inducing congestive heart failure; and (2) the danger of hepatitis may be less when plasma is not given. The chances of sensitization to foreign leukocytes, platelets, and immune globulins may also be diminished by the use of washed packed cells. The plasma that is saved can be processed into specific components such as platelets or purified factor VIII and used fresh or frozen. Frozen red cells offer considerable promise for circumventing the storage problems of refrigerated blood, which is generally not useful after about 21 days. One unit (500 ml) of blood or the equivalent amount of packed red cells (200 ml) may be expected to elevate the packed-red-cell volume of the adult recipient by about 4%, if there is no accelerated destruction or continuing loss of red cells.

Use of Adrenocorticosteroids

Many diseases of the blood respond to administration of adrenal steroids. However, the responses are not predictable, and undesirable effects may overshadow the benefits.

Summary Principles: (1) The response to and need for continued administration of steroids are extremely variable; the smallest effective dose should be given for the shortest possible time. (2) A single dose or brief course (1 to 2 weeks) of even high doses of corticosteroids is unlikely to be associated with significant toxicity (see Chapters 6, 7, and 9). *(3) Steroids are usually only palliative and are unlikely to produce a permanent cure* (see Chapters 6 and 9). *(4) Long-term administration of steroids is associated with an increased frequency of side effects* (see Chapter 7). Therefore, other means of treatment must be considered to avoid the prolonged use of steroids. For example, certain types of autoimmune hemolytic anemia or thrombocytopenic purpura may be ameliorated by splenectomy or other drugs, allowing either cessation of steroids or a reduction in dose. *(5) Latent infection, particularly tuberculosis, may be reactivated when a patient is given steroids* (see Chapter 10).

When steroids are given to hematologically normal individuals, certain changes occur in the blood. Although reticulocytosis, erythroid hyperplasia in the bone marrow, and appearance of nucleated red cells in the peripheral blood may follow administration of steroids, it is not certain that they stimulate erythropoiesis directly (Wintrobe *et al.*, 1951). Neutrophilia occurs, owing to increased release of neutrophils by the marrow into the blood and to inhibition of their egress into the tissues (Boggs *et al.*, 1964; Bishop *et al.*, 1968). The inhibition of lymphocyte migration into tissues may in part explain the increased incidence of infection seen in patients treated with steroids. Lymphocytopenia and eosinopenia also occur, the former due at least in part to a direct toxic effect on lymphoid tissue and lymphocytes. Lymphocytopenia is most marked following an acute dose of steroids and may not be sustained during chronic administration (Forsham *et al.*, 1948).

CLINICAL THERAPY

Treatment of Erythrocyte Disorders

Treatment of Anemia. Adequate therapy of anemia requires an exact diagnosis. Once an etiology is determined, treatment of the anemia may not be necessary if the underlying defect is corrected (e.g., a bleeding ulcer or resectable carcinoma). If the patient's blood volume or tissue oxygenation is seriously compromised, administration of iron or appropriate blood transfusion may be helpful. *Principle: An underlying cause for the anemia must always be considered before therapy is initiated.*

  Treatment of Deficiency Anemias. Successful therapy of *iron-deficiency anemia* requires that its cause be found; once this is identified, iron may be administered orally or sometimes parenterally. To verify the accuracy of diagnosis and the adequacy of treatment, the response to iron should be assessed by frequent measurement of reticulocyte counts and of the hemoglobin concentration (Charlton and Bothwell, 1970).

For most patients, oral iron therapy is preferable because it is usually more effective, safer, and cheaper than parenteral therapy. Iron is absorbed from the duodenum in the ferrous form. Therefore, ferrous salts are more easily absorbed than ferric salts, which must be converted to a ferrous form before absorption. Ferrous sulfate is the cheapest and most efficacious preparation available. There is no justification for using combinations of iron with cobalt, molybdenum, folate, B_{12}, or intrinsic factor to treat iron deficiency. These other substances are unnecessary and add to the cost, but, most important, may lead to confusion, since response to the drug may be interpreted as being predominantly related to iron. The diagnostic value of response to iron is lost if combinations with other hematinics are used. Sustained-release preparations of iron are expensive and are often not available to the intestine (i.e., dissolved) until they have passed beyond the region of maximum absorption. Enteric-coated tablets are well tolerated, but may also be poorly absorbed. *Principle: If a preparation is absorbed at a specialized site, the dosage form should be such that the preparation is available for absorption when it reaches the site* (see Chapter 2).

Most of the effective iron preparations may produce disagreeable gastrointestinal side effects, such as nausea, vomiting, constipation, diarrhea, cramps, and epigastric distress. These effects may sometimes be psychologic, since they also accompany placebo administration (see Chapter 14). Initial therapy consists of 300 mg of ferrous sulfate daily with one meal (or 200 mg of the anhydrous salt; each contains 60 mg of elemental iron). The dose should be increased every 1 to 2 days by one tablet to a total of three tablets daily. The medication should then be given between meals and at bedtime, until a maximum of six tablets daily is achieved. There is no reason to exceed this number, and if signs of gastrointestinal irritation appear, fewer doses may be adequate. Other salts (ferrous gluconate or fumarate) have been reported to be less irritating than ferrous sulfate, but the evidence for this is not convincing. The patient should be warned that the iron will cause dark stools. When a response occurs, reticulocytosis may be observed within 4 to 5 days with a peak at 7 to 10 days. The hemoglobin concentration increases at the maximum rate of about 1 g per week. If the hemoglobin concentration does not rise, the diagnosis should be questioned, and the possibility of continued blood loss or of poor iron absorption should be considered. After restoration of normal hemoglobin concentration, treatment should be continued for 3 to 4 months to replete the tissue stores. Further therapy is not required if blood loss has ceased. *Principle: The duration of therapy used to replace stores of a substance (e.g., iron) cannot be based solely on the most sensitive and direct response of an end-organ (e.g., reticulocytosis or hemoglobin concentration), but must also include the total pool size and knowledge of the kinetics of the substance.*

An elixir of ferrous sulfate (containing 30 mg of iron per 5 ml) is useful in children and in patients with dysphagia. Black staining of the teeth and tongue may occur. *Principle: Both the meaningful and the inconsequential results of therapy should be explained to patients before starting a therapeutic regimen.*

Failure to respond to oral iron therapy is usually due to misdiagnosis of the anemia, which may be due to (1) chronic disease (infection, arthritis, cancer), (2) renal disease, (3) hypothyroidism, (4) failure of the patient to take the medication, or (5) failure of iron intake to exceed that which continues to be lost (e.g., from continued bleeding).

Parenteral iron should be used only when clearly required. Valid indications for parenteral iron include continued bleeding that may be aggravated by oral iron therapy (e.g., in a patient with ulcerative colitis), the need for rapid correction of anemia (e.g., in late pregnancy), intestinal malabsorption or the effects of gastrectomy, unreliability of the patient (e.g., in the case of a child or a psychotic), and, rarely, intolerance of oral iron.

Iron dextran (Imferon), which contains 50 mg of iron per milliliter, is the most frequently used parenteral preparation. The iron deficit can be calculated from the hemoglobin deficit (in grams per 100 ml), blood volume (70 ml/kg), and iron content per gram of hemoglobin (3.38 mg). For example, if the hemoglobin concentration is to be increased from 10 g/ 100 ml to 14 g/100 ml in a 70-kg man, the calculation would be:

$$(14-10) \text{ g/100 ml} \times \frac{70 \text{ ml/kg} \times 70 \text{ kg}}{100} \times 3.38$$
$$= 662 \text{ mg of iron}$$

An extra 1000 mg should be given to replenish tissue stores. The initial dose should be small (1 ml) in the event of allergic reaction. Intramuscular administration of 5 ml is the usual daily dose until the calculated total dose has been administered. Anaphylactic reactions may occur (see Chapter 15). More common side effects are pain at the injection site and staining of the skin. Arthralgia, urticaria, nausea, vomiting, and hypotension may also accompany parenteral iron therapy. Although sarcomas have been reported in a few animals chronically injected with this preparation, none have been reported in humans.

An intravenous preparation, iron dextrin, is available, but this route of administration is rarely necessary. Iron dextran may also be given intravenously.

Illustrative Case 1

A 43-year-old woman, with a history of seven pregnancies, six live births, and one abortion, complained to her physician of fatigue and shortness of breath, which had been progressive over a 3-month period. Her menstrual periods had always been rather profuse but had become increasingly so for the last 2 months. There was a history of sporadic iron therapy during her pregnancies but none during lactation. Her youngest child was 2 years old. Her diet seemed adequate and there was no history of weight loss. She denied abdominal pain, change in

bowel habits, or other gastrointestinal symptoms. The rest of the history was noncontributory. On physical examination, the vital signs were normal except for a pulse of 100. There was generalized pallor. Lymphadenopathy, purpura, sternal tenderness, abdominal tenderness, masses, or organomegaly was not present. Pelvic and rectal examination, as well as sigmoidoscopy, were negative. Examination of the blood showed a hematocrit of 18%, hemoglobin of 4.5 g/100 ml, and red-cell count of 2,650,000/cu mm. The mean corpuscular volume (MCV) was 68 μ^3, and the mean corpuscular hemoglobin concentration (MCHC) was 25%. The total leukocyte count was 4,500/cu mm, with a normal differential, and the platelet count was 150,000/cu mm. Examination of the blood smear showed marked anisocytosis, microcytosis, and hypochromia. The reticulocyte count was 1%. The serum iron was 25 μg/100 ml and the total iron-binding capacity was 450 μg/100 ml (5.5% saturation). Examination of the bone marrow showed normoblastic hyperplasia; no iron was seen on examination of the unstained smear or after a Prussian blue stain. The stool guaiac reaction was strongly positive. Liver function tests were normal. Upper gastrointestinal series was normal, but a barium enema showed a constant irregularity, 4 cm in diameter, in the region of the ascending colon. The patient was given 5 units of packed red cells and underwent a laparotomy. An adenocarcinoma of the ascending colon was found and resected. It had not extended into the serosa, regional lymph nodes were not involved, and the liver was normal grossly and by biopsy.

Following surgery the patient was placed on ferrous sulfate, 300 mg three times daily for 6 months. She has been examined every 6 months by her physician for the last 5 years and is in good health, with normal blood and serum iron values. Her menstrual periods are normal and less profuse than they had been.

Comment. The diagnosis of iron-deficiency anemia was easy in this patient, in that she had typical hypochromic microcytic anemia with confirmatory serum iron and marrow findings. It would have been tempting to ascribe her iron deficiency to multiple pregnancies and heavy menstrual flow, and indeed this may have contributed to its severity, but her survival depended on the fact that her bleeding gastrointestinal lesion was found and treated definitively before either massive hemorrhage or metastasis occurred. Simple iron therapy without detailed investigation of the cause would have been palliative but lethal. In retrospect, her recent menorrhagia may have been a result, rather than a cause, of the iron deficiency.

Folate-deficiency anemia may be treated most appropriately if the cause of deficiency and daily folate requirements are understood. A nutritious diet rich in fresh fruits and vegetables may be sufficient to treat patients with dietary folate deficiency. If increased demands for folates are present, as in pregnancy, hemolytic anemia, or infancy, folate supplements may be required to ensure rapid repletion of stores. If the diagnosis is clearly established, large doses of folic acid (1 to 5 mg per day) should correct the deficiency in almost every patient. If impaired absorption is the cause of the deficiency, parenteral folate therapy (Folvite) may be necessary; this may be administered intravenously or intramuscularly. Most multiple-vitamin preparations do not contain folic acid, because such preparations may produce a response in people with B_{12} deficiency and important specific therapy may be ignored. Some vitamin preparations used in pregnant patients do contain folic acid, but the incidence of folate deficiency is relatively high and vitamin B_{12} deficiency very low in pregnancy. Should the diagnosis of folate deficiency not be clearly established by laboratory tests, a therapeutic trial with small physiologic amounts (50 to 400 μg per day) of folic acid may be undertaken. Larger doses of folate may cause a reticulocyte response in B_{12} deficiency, but this small dose will not. The low dose is adequate for true folate deficiency. Treatment should be continued for several weeks after the hematocrit returns to normal in order to replete folate stores. Cessation of therapy depends on the circumstances of the individual patient. For example, if a pregnant patient develops a megaloblastic anemia due to folate deficiency during the third trimester of pregnancy, treatment should be continued for several weeks after delivery. *Principle: The therapist must know the amount of each substance contained in a fixed-dose combination preparation (e.g., multivitamins). Otherwise inadequate replacement of a substance or misinterpretation of a therapeutic result may occur* (see Chapters 2 and 15).

Two preparations are available for treatment of B_{12}-*deficiency anemia*: cyanocobalamin (vitamin B_{12}) and hydroxycobalamin. Although cyanocobalamin has been used to treat B_{12} deficiency for many years, it is not a naturally occurring compound (the cyanide is incorporated into the vitamin as an artifact of isolation). The hydroxycobalamin compound may be preferable, since it is more slowly absorbed and less rapidly excreted.

The purposes of B_{12} therapy are to correct the anemia and neurologic abnormalities due to the deficiency, and to replenish liver stores. Since the daily requirement of B_{12} is about 0.2 to 0.3 μg per day, treatment with 100 μg parenterally per day for 5 to 10 days, followed by 100 μg per month, should accomplish these purposes. If a therapeutic trial is necessary to establish the correct diagnosis, 1 μg per day should be administered intramuscularly for 10 days, and the reticulocyte count and hematocrit should be carefully followed. This small dose is used since

large doses of B_{12} may cause reticulocytosis in patients with folate deficiency. If a therapeutic trial with B_{12} is attempted, the diet during this time should be essentially devoid of folate (Herbert, 1963).

Treatment of Hemolytic Anemias. Acute *hemolysis* constitutes a medical emergency and its evaluation should proceed rapidly. Hemorrhage must be ruled out; the differentiation between an intravascular and an extravascular process must then be made. An intravascular process (e.g., due to incompatible blood transfusion) may result in renal shutdown owing to circulatory collapse and changes in the kidney. Attempts to increase renal blood flow with an osmotic diuretic such as mannitol may be lifesaving (Barry and Malloy, 1962). Extravascular hemolysis due to antibodies is often associated with an underlying disease such as chronic lymphatic leukemia, lymphoma, or systemic lupus erythematosus. The administration of corticosteroids during an acute hemolytic episode may markedly reduce the rate of hemolysis. Many patients may be completely withdrawn from the drug after several weeks, but others may respond poorly or may require chronic administration of small doses. The mechanism of corticosteroid action is not understood, but it may be related to inhibition of proliferation of antibody-forming cells (presumably lymphoid) and to inhibition of phagocytosis of erythrocytes by reticuloendothelial cells.

Splenectomy must be considered if there is no response to steroids, or if a large daily dose is required for control of the hemolytic anemia (20 mg or more of prednisone or its equivalent). The demonstration of splenic sequestration of labeled red cells correlates fairly well with response to splenectomy (Veeger et al., 1962; Allgood and Chaplin, 1967) and may be useful in selecting patients for this procedure. Improvement of the hemolytic anemia may also result from successful treatment of an underlying process, such as lymphoma or lupus erythematosus.

Patients with *sickle-cell anemia* often require treatment for the painful crises secondary to intravascular thrombosis. The pain may be ameliorated by analgesics, but the disease process is more specifically reversed by oxygen. Encouraging results are also obtained with limited exchange transfusions (Brody et al., 1970); 500 to 750 ml of packed red blood cells can be given in association with removal of 500 ml of the patient's blood. In this way, the cells containing the abnormal hemoglobin S are replaced with normal cells, thus breaking the cycle of hypoxia-sickling-hypoxia and vascular occlusion. Phlebotomy also avoids the iron overload that might occur with ordinary transfusion. Occasionally, splenectomy may be of benefit, although these patients usually have small spleens or functional aplasia of the spleen (Pearson et al., 1969). *Principle: Whenever possible, specific therapy should be used. If it is inadequate, efficacious symptomatic therapy is justified.*

Splenectomy is usually indicated for *hereditary spherocytosis*. The condition may be quite mild or may intermittently be associated with severe hemolytic episodes. Anemia may rapidly occur if marrow function diminishes (e.g., as a result of drugs or infections), since the marrow may be working at maximum capacity to maintain the hemoglobin concentration. Because of marrow hyperactivity, these patients may have an increased folate requirement, and folate supplements may be required to maintain erythropoiesis. Removal of the spleen essentially cures the anemia without affecting the intrinsic abnormality of the cell. However, splenectomy before the age of 2 has been associated with an increased risk of serious infection (Smith et al., 1962); if possible, this operation should be postponed until the patient is 2 years old (Eraklis et al., 1967).

Hemolytic anemia may be present in *hereditary elliptocytosis*, another generally benign familial disorder of unknown etiology, characterized by oval or elliptic red cells. This anemia is also usually cured by splenectomy.

The treatment of hemolysis due to *glucose-6-phosphate deficiency* is relatively simple: drugs that induce hemolysis should be avoided (Jaffé, 1970). These include the antimalarials (primaquine and pamaquine) and many other oxidant drugs (Beutler, 1969) (see Chapter 15). Hemolysis is usually self-limiting; it mainly involves older cells, and when these cells are gone, the remaining younger cells are more resistant to oxidation. Transfusion is usually unnecessary.

The hemolytic anemia due to *pyruvate kinase deficiency* may be improved by splenectomy, although the hemoglobin concentration does not return to normal. *Principle: Sometimes the only definite therapy of a disease lies in genetic counseling. The therapist must not ignore the possibility of making life better for the patient by improving the health of his family* (see Chapter 13).

Steroids are usually employed initially to treat the hemolytic anemias associated with underlying diseases, such as *chronic lymphatic leukemia, lymphoma, or lupus erythematosus.* Corticosteroids are also useful for controlling but not curing other manifestations of these diseases (see Chapter 9). Corticosteroids should be used initially to treat *idiopathic autoimmune hemolytic anemias.* Splenectomy is successful in some patients who do not respond to steroids or who require large daily doses. Splenectomy in autoimmune hemolytic anemia is usually more successful in patients with the "warm-antibody" type of anemia and in those with palpable spleens (Wintrobe, 1967).

In patients who fail to respond to splenectomy or to moderate doses of corticosteroids, "immunosuppressive" agents such as azathioprine (Imuran) and cyclophosphamide (Cytoxan) may be effective (Dameshek and Schwartz, 1960; Taylor, 1963). Frequent blood counts (one or two times weekly) should be performed in order to prevent serious bone marrow depression (see Chapter 12).

There has been no consistently satisfactory treatment for *paroxysmal nocturnal hemoglobinuria* (PNH). Washed red cells have been advocated when transfusion is necessary (Dacie, 1948), as increased hemolysis and thrombosis may follow the transfusion of whole blood. The coumarin anticoagulants have also been suggested to prevent the frequent thrombosis seen in this disease, although long-term use has been disappointing. Iron therapy may be necessary if significant urinary loss of this element has occurred. Androgens may also be useful (Hartmann et al., 1966).

Treatment of Aplastic Anemia. Removal and avoidance of the offending agent are crucial. Transfusion of packed red cells to maintain the hematocrit in the region of 30% is generally adequate. Prophylactic antibiotics should not be used, since the possibility of superinfection with resistant organisms is greatly enhanced and since each antibiotic has its own side effects. The use of nonabsorbable oral antibiotics to sterilize the intestinal flora is being evaluated. Appropriate antibiotics should be used when bacterial infections are identified. Specific antibiotic therapy has improved the treatment of infections but, as in acute leukemia, sepsis is still the most important cause of death in patients with aplastic anemia. The frequency of serious infection is increased when the blood neutrophil count is less than 500/cu mm (Vincent and deGruchy, 1967). *Principle: In patients with granulocytopenia who develop fever and chills, bacterial infection should be suspected; after appropriate cultures are taken, antibiotic coverage should be instituted. Delay in antibiotic therapy for report of cultures is unwise because of the danger of rapidly fatal septicemia* (see Chapter 10).

The onset of serious infection may be associated with a further lowering of the neutrophil and platelet count and with increased bleeding, owing perhaps to further depression of marrow function. Granulocyte transfusions are not a practical reality. Platelet transfusions should be reserved for major bleeding episodes or for situations in which major bleeding is likely. The likelihood of serious bleeding is enhanced greatly when the platelet count is less than 20,000/cu mm (Gaydos et al., 1962). Multiple platelet transfusions may lead to nonresponsiveness as well as to febrile reactions because of isoimmunization, but improved methods of platelet typing to select compatible donors may help to solve this problem (Yankee et al., 1969).

Corticosteroids have been used for many years in the therapy of aplastic anemia, employed alone or in association with androgens. The agents usually used are prednisone or triamcinolone, approximately 1 mg/kg daily. The response to steroids alone has been disappointing. Remissions have been rare (Scott et al., 1959; Silink and Firkin, 1968) or have not occurred at all (Shahidi and Diamond, 1961). The major benefit seems to be that bleeding is reduced in some patients, perhaps because capillary fragility is decreased. Corticosteroids do not improve platelet counts. Serious risks accompanying the use of corticosteroids are hypertension and increased susceptibility to infection in patients already compromised by neutropenia. Weight gain, acne, moonface, and truncal obesity are less important. Although adrenal steroids were routinely used until the introduction of androgen therapy and are still extensively used in combination with androgens, their efficacy (if any) is not clear. The response rate in a recent large series was the same in androgen-treated patients with or without adrenal steroids (Sanchez-Medal et al., 1969), and the incidence of undesirable side effects was higher in the corticosteroid-treated group.

The use of cobalt as an erythropoietic stimulus is not efficacious (Berk et al., 1949).

The anemia of hypogonadism in males responds to androgenic therapy (McCullagh and Jones, 1942). Increases in red-cell mass, even to polycythemic levels, were observed in women with breast carcinoma treated with androgens (Kennedy and Gilbertsen, 1957). Androgens have been administered in combination with adrenal corticosteroids to children with aplastic anemia (Shahidi and Diamond, 1961; Desposito et al., 1964). Almost half of those with acquired disease responded, and in many patients therapy could ultimately be stopped; of those with congenital aplastic anemia, about 90% responded but seemingly became dependent on continuous use of androgens. In responsive patients, the anemia and granulocyte count approached normal, but platelet counts tended to remain subnormal. The androgens used have included testosterone enanthate, testosterone propionate, methyltestosterone, and fluoxymesterone, 1 to 2 mg/kg daily. They are usually given orally for convenience, and because parenteral administration is attended by the risk of hematoma formation in the thrombocytopenic patients. Testosterone has been disappointing in adults with aplastic anemia (Seligmann, 1966).

Oxymetholone (Adroyd), a semisynthetic steroid, is claimed to have fewer masculinizing effects than testosterone but to be more effective in stimulating hematopoiesis. Several groups have reported that it is effective in children and adults (Allen et al., 1968). Remission was achieved in all six adult patients treated with this compound in one series (Silink and Firkin, 1968), and in about 50% of 55 adults in another series (Sanchez-Medal et al., 1969). Since this disease may improve spontaneously, these encouraging results must be accepted with reservations (see Chapter 1). As with the use of other androgens, the anemia is most often improved and thrombocytopenia is the least responsive. Although granulocytes and platelets may not completely return to normal levels with therapy, infection and hemorrhage generally are less severe. Oxymetholone is given orally in a dose of 1 to 5 mg/kg per day. Other related steroids such as methalone and methenolone also appear to be active. Side effects of all androgen preparations include hoarseness, hirsutism, acne, amenorrhea, and clitoral enlargement. Eighty percent of patients treated with oxymetholone showed some alteration in liver function (Sanchez-Medal et al., 1969). Patients with aplastic anemia may develop hemosiderosis with liver damage from transfusions, as well as viral hepatitis; thus, liver disease is not necessarily drug induced in this group of patients.

The mechanism of action of androgens in promoting erythropoiesis is not entirely clear. Androgens increase blood and urine levels of erythropoietin, which may in turn stimulate erythropoiesis (Rishpon-Meyerstein et al., 1968; Alexanian, 1969). A direct effect of androgens upon bone marrow is also possible (Reisner, 1966). Androgens have also been used with some success in other types of anemia, particularly in myelofibrosis (Gardner and Nathan, 1966) and multiple myeloma (Cline and Berlin, 1962; Rishpon-Meyerstein et al., 1968).

In most patients with hypocellular bone marrows, splenectomy is not helpful. An occasional patient with aplastic anemia has, however, been improved by the procedure (Scott et al., 1959), especially when there is some evidence of increased red-cell destruction (shortened half-life of ^{51}Cr-labeled red cells) and of splenic sequestration of such cells. Splenectomy should be reserved for those patients who have not responded to androgens. Transfusion of adequate numbers of red cells and platelets is important during surgery.

Illustrative Case 2

A 12-year-old girl was referred because of weakness, pallor, and easy bruising of 3 weeks' duration. The parents were fearful that she had acute leukemia. Six months previously she had been given chloramphenicol for 6 days for an upper respiratory infection. Physical examination revealed pallor, an infected throat, numerous ecchymoses and petechiae, and a temperature of 102° F. Lymphadenopathy, sternal tenderness, and enlargement of the liver or spleen were not present. Packed-red-cell volume was 25%, hemoglobin 8 g/100 ml, and red-cell count 2,900,000/cu mm. Red-cell indices, calculated from the above values, were normal. The reticulocyte count was 0.5%. Total leukocyte count was 2,000/cu mm, with 35% neutrophilic granulocytes, 50% lymphocytes, 10% monocytes, 4% eosinophils, and 1% basophils. The platelet count was 15,000/cu mm. Examination of the blood smear showed moderate anisocytosis but no hypochromia or abnormal cells. Platelets were markedly reduced. Serum iron was 200 μg/100 ml with a total iron-binding capacity of 300 μg/100 ml. Bone marrow aspiration was productive of only a few drops of very sparsely cellular material. Bone marrow biopsy revealed a hypocellular marrow. Stool guaiac test was negative. A throat culture revealed beta-hemolytic *Streptococcus* and a blood culture was negative. The patient was begun on oral penicillin, 250,000 units three times daily for 10 days. She became afebrile within 2 days. On the third hospital day, a severe nosebleed developed that responded briefly to packing but recurred after 3 days. The packed-cell volume fell to 19% and the platelet count was 10,000/cu mm. The patient was given 2 units of fresh whole blood and 6 units of platelets with cessation of the nosebleed. The platelet count was 10,000/cu mm and packed-red-cell volume 30% on the day following transfusion. The patient was begun on 100 mg of oxymetholone daily (2.5 mg/kg) and was able to be discharged from the hospital after 10 days. Three weeks later another nosebleed developed, and red-cell and platelet transfusions were necessary. The patient remained afebrile. After 8 weeks of therapy, her reticulocyte count was 5%, hemoglobin 10 g/100 ml, platelet count 50,000/cu mm, and leukocyte count 4,000/cu mm with 30% neutrophils. After 6 months, her hemoglobin had risen to 12 g/100 ml, leukocytes were normal, but platelets remained somewhat low at 75,000/cu mm. No further bleeding had occurred and purpura was no longer present. Her voice had become somewhat deeper and she had developed acne and an increase in pubic hair. Oxymetholone was discontinued.

Comment. Chloramphenicol is the drug most frequently associated with aplastic anemia, and a history of exposure to this drug is an important clue. However, the diagnosis of leukemia could not be excluded with certainty until the bone marrow biopsy had demonstrated hypoplasia, since pancytopenia without blasts in the blood and a marrow that is difficult to obtain by aspiration may occur with leukemia as well ("aleukemic leukemia"). Supportive care, in terms of appropriate antibiotic treatment of specific infections and red-cell and platelet transfusions, is necessary in many patients during the time required to effect an improvement with androgen therapy (often several weeks or months). The response to androgen may not be complete or may be much less satisfactory than was the case in this patient. Some degree of mild virilization generally occurs. Androgen therapy may be stopped following a good response, but relapse may occur. Restoration of all blood values to normal is not always necessary for the patient to become asymptomatic.

Treatment of Polycythemia. The symptoms of *polycythemia vera* are usually related to the hyperviscosity and slowing of blood flow caused by increased blood volume. These include headache, dizziness, tinnitus, visual disturbances, dyspnea, and thrombosis. The most rapid means of producing relief is withdrawal of 1 or more units of blood every 2 to 3 days until the volume of packed cells is less than 55%. Some patients may be entirely managed with occasional phlebotomy (Dameshek, 1968). Chronic iron deficiency is usually found in this disease, both at the time of diagnosis and as a result of phlebotomy. Supplemental iron should not be given since the iron deficiency contributes to a decreased production of red cells and possibly of white cells and platelets (Dameshek, 1968).

The basic problem in this disease is an overproduction of blood cells; phlebotomy does not deal with this directly. Phlebotomy also does not generally affect the leukocytosis or thrombocytosis, which probably contributes to other major problems such as pruritus, hyperuricemia, as well as to uncomfortable splenic enlargement. For these reasons, other measures may be required.

Ionizing radiation has been used to control this disease. It is administered as small doses (3 to 6 mc) of radioactive phosphorus (^{32}P) (Osgood, 1968), at intervals of 3 to 6 months, depending on the response. Doses should be increased until the packed-red-cell volume is normal. Advocates of this therapy claim that patients so treated survive longer than those who are treated only with phlebotomy, but the comparisons cited were between different series of patients, treated in a noncontrolled fashion. A serious problem is the frequent development of acute leukemia in patients treated with ^{32}P (Modan and Lilienfeld, 1965). Whether the risk of leukemia is outweighed by the increased survival obtained from therapy is uncertain. A controlled study in which patients are randomly selected for radiation or nonradiation therapy is now in progress (Wasserman, 1968).

At least four alkylating agents (chlorambucil, cyclophosphamide, busulfan, and melphalan) may control this disease (Gilbert, 1968; Laszlo, 1968). The duration of follow-up is not yet sufficient to state that development of leukemia will not be a problem, but these drugs are reasonable alternatives to radiation. Of these agents, busulfan is associated with fewer non-hematologic side effects such as gastrointestinal distress, hair loss, or hematuria at any degree of leukopenia or thrombocytopenia. It may therefore be the agent of choice, particularly when leukocytosis and thrombocytosis are present. Initially 4 to 6 mg are given daily until the desired effect is achieved. Patients respond in 1 to 9 months, with the median response occurring at 3 months. At first, most patients also require phlebotomy for symptomatic relief. Cyclophosphamide is useful in patients with thrombocytopenia since it has less tendency to depress platelet production. Treatment with antimetabolites of nucleic acid biosynthesis is being investigated (De Conti and Calabresi, 1970).

Hyperuricemia in polycythemia is mainly treated by a xanthine oxidase inhibitor, allopurinol (see Chapters 7, 9, and 12). In doses of 300 to 800 mg daily, it effectively decreases urate production, hyperuricemia, and urinary urate excretion. Allopurinol is remarkably free from undesirable side effects except for the occasional development of skin rash.

The treatment of secondary polycythemia depends on its cause. A cyst or tumor associated with aberrant erythropoietin production should be removed when possible (Waldmann et al., 1961), but most of the time secondary polycythemia develops as a physiologic response to the need for additional oxygen-carrying capacity. Myelosuppressive agents are generally not indicated, and phlebotomy may be needed if there are symptoms attributable to hyperviscosity. *Principle: Laboratory values must be put into perspective with pathophysiology. Before instituting therapy, the patient's general condition must be carefully considered.*

Treatment of Leukocyte Disorders

Patients with a decreased granulocyte count have an increased risk of bacterial infection, in proportion to the severity of the granulocytopenia (Bodey et al., 1966; Vincent and deGruchy, 1967). If fever develops in patients with severe neutropenia, it must be assumed that infection exists, and antibiotics should be started after cultures of the blood, urine, stool, nose, throat, and sputum are obtained. When the organism is identified, appropriate changes in the antibiotic regimen may be made, but vigilance should not be relaxed since superinfection with other organisms may occur, especially gram-negative bacteria and fungi. Attempts have been made to decrease bacterial exposure by using isolated rooms, "life islands" (plastic isolators), or laminar airflow rooms with air filtered free of bacteria (Perry, 1969), but results have been discouraging. Various regimens of nonabsorbable oral antibiotics intended to reduce the patient's endogenous bacterial flora are being evaluated (Bodey et al., 1968). *Principle: Any drug to which a patient with granulocytopenia has been exposed should be suspected in the pathogenesis of this disorder. All drugs that are not absolutely essential should be discontinued.*

It is impossible to achieve a useful increase in granulocytes by transfusion of fresh normal whole blood, since there are not enough granulocytes present to be of value to the granulocytopenic patient. Moreover, the intravascular survival of mature compatible granulocytes is estimated to be only 10 to 12 hours (Kauder et al., 1965). Large numbers of granulocytes in varying stages of maturity have been obtained from patients with chronic granulocytic leukemia and transfused into granulocytopenic individuals (usually with acute leukemia), with apparent benefit in treating serious bacterial infections (Freireich et al., 1964). Methods to increase the quantity of normal granulocytes from a donor using a continuous-flow cell separator are being explored (Freireich et al., 1965). Granulocyte concentrates obtained in this way were shown to be effective in the therapy of bacterial infection in neutropenic animals and perhaps in man (Epstein et al., 1969; Graw et al., 1971). Optimum granulocyte survival may depend upon the use of immunologically compatible donors (Graw et al., 1969).

Granulocytopenia due to specific deficiencies such as folate or B_{12} is usually not severe or life threatening and responds readily to administration of the correct vitamin.

Certain types of neutropenia associated with splenomegaly, such as rheumatoid arthritis (Felty's syndrome), sarcoidosis, portal hypertension with splenomegaly (Banti's syndrome), and systemic lupus erythematosus, may respond to splenectomy.

Treatment of Bleeding Disorders

Platelet Disorders. *Thrombocytopenia.* Platelet transfusions are generally more useful when there is a defect in production than when there is increased destruction, since the administered platelets will survive longer. Infection and bleeding, as well as immunologic incompatibilities, shorten the survival of transfused platelets. In circumstances where isoimmunization causes rapid destruction of transfused platelets, close relatives, especially siblings, are more effective donors (Yankee *et al.*, 1969). Platelets can be given in whole fresh blood or as concentrates derived from plasma. Platelet transfusions should be used for bleeding associated with thrombocytopenia, and probably as prophylaxis, if the platelet count is below 10,000/cu mm, when a production deficit is present. Under optimal circumstances, a unit of platelets (the amount derived from one unit of blood) produces an increment of 25,000/cu mm/sq m of body surface in the recipient (Yankee *et al.*, 1969).

The cause of the thrombocytopenia must be sought and treated appropriately (e.g., induction of remission in leukemia, or heparin administration in disseminated intravascular coagulation).

Idiopathic thrombocytopenic purpura may be acute and self-limiting, requiring no treatment, or it may respond to a brief course of corticosteroids. If the response to corticosteroids is poor or if large doses are required for more than 6 months to control bleeding or severe bruising, splenectomy is indicated. Patients who do not respond to these measures may benefit by the use of immunosuppressive agents such as azathioprine (Sussman, 1967; Bouroncle and Doan, 1969).

Some patients with chronic thrombocytopenia may not have serious bleeding episodes and it is not possible to maintain "safe" platelet levels for very long, since transfused platelets generally do not survive in the circulation longer than 3 to 4 days. Since transfusion increases the risks of reaction and loss of effectiveness of platelet transfusions, this treatment is best reserved for acute bleeding episodes.

Thrombocytosis. Platelet counts greater than 1,000,000/cu mm may be encountered in various conditions, including infection, trauma, malignancy (especially carcinoma of the lung), and following splenectomy. These situations are generally not accompanied by thrombosis or bleeding and do not require specific therapy. In contrast, polycythemia vera, chronic myelocytic leukemia, or idiopathic thrombocythemia may be associated with bleeding or thrombosis, usually the former. In these instances, it may be beneficial to lower the platelet count with such agents as radioactive phosphorus (Fountain and Losowsky, 1962), busulfan (Silverstein, 1968), or uracil mustard (Robertson, 1970).

Coagulation Factor Disorders (Figure 8–3). *Disseminated Intravascular Coagulation ("Consumption Coagulopathy")* (Bachmann, 1969). Heparin, which can cause bleeding when given

in excess, may be the treatment of choice in certain hemorrhagic disorders associated with depletion of coagulation factors owing to their consumption by continuous intravascular clotting. Intravascular coagulation may occur in many conditions, including certain malignancies (especially promyelocytic leukemia), drug reactions, gram-negative sepsis and shock, transfusion of incompatible blood, septic abortion or *abruptio placentae*, and retained dead fetus (Merskey *et al.*, 1967). These disorders presumably are all capable of causing the release of thromboplastin, thus activating the clotting mechanism. Thrombosis may or may not be observed in association with hypocoagulability. The most significant laboratory findings, which are variably present, include low levels of fibrinogen, platelets, and factors V, VIII, X, and XIII, as well as prolonged thrombin, partial thromboplastin, and prothrombin times.

Heparin is a sulfated mucopolysaccharide occurring naturally in mast cells, especially in the lungs and liver. It is a potent inhibitor of coagulation, having detectable activity against all three stages; generation of thromboplastin, formation of thrombin from prothrombin, and formation of fibrin from fibrinogen, catalyzed by thrombin. Its activity probably resides in its strong negative charges, which react with many proteins (clotting factors) involved in the clotting process. Heparin is metabolized by a liver enzyme, heparinase, and is excreted in the urine when given in large doses. Its plasma half-life increases with the size of the dose (Olsson *et al.*, 1963). It is poorly absorbed orally but is effective when injected intravenously, intramuscularly, or subcutaneously, although the risk of hematoma formation makes the latter two routes less desirable. In the absence of liver or renal disease, heparin may be given as a dose of 10,000 units every 8 hours or 1000 units per hour by continuous intravenous infusion (Merskey *et al.*, 1967). The fibrinogen level, platelet count, and thrombin, prothrombin, and partial thromboplastin times may all become normal following such therapy (Rock *et al.*, 1969). Disseminated intravascular coagulation, particularly when accompanying obstetric complications, may be self-limiting and may not require therapy. However, when coagulation is more severe and prolonged, the use of heparin may allow sufficient time for the underlying process to be treated. Heparin itself may prolong most clotting tests.

Hemorrhage is the expected complication of an overdose of heparin. Because of variations in individual response, patients should be carefully monitored with appropriate coagulation studies. The postoperative state, cancer, and the presence of various drugs (digitalis, tetracyclines, and antihistamines) have been reported to be associated with drug resistance (Levine, 1965). If heparin overdosage occurs, it may be neutralized by the administration of the strongly basic protein, protamine. One to one and one-half milligrams of protamine neutralize approximately 120 units of heparin if administered shortly after the heparin dose; a smaller amount is required if more time has elapsed, since some of the heparin has been metabolized (see Chapter 2). No more than 50 mg should be given over 10 minutes; slow injection of protamine prevents the flushing, bradycardia, and hypotension that may otherwise occur. The clotting time is an adequate measurement of the adequacy of the protamine dose. When given in excess, protamine is an anticoagulant. If the question arises as to whether continued bleeding is due to excess heparin or to excess protamine, the patient's blood may be titrated *in vitro* with heparin or protamine. Sensitivity to heparin, manifested by asthma, urticaria, fever, and rhinitis, may occur in rare instances.

Fibrinolysis. Active bleeding may arise as an uncommon result of primary fibrinolysis. Plasma fibrinogen levels are low in both intravascular coagulation and fibrinolysis, but the latter situation is associated with an increased amount of circulating plasminogen activator and plasmin (Merskey *et al.*, 1967). Tests of the speed of dissolution of a euglobin clot or of fibrin on plates are valuable in making this distinction. Platelets are usually normal in primary fibrinolysis. Conditions associated with fibrinolysis include metastatic prostatic carcinoma (which is rich in plasminogen activator), release of large amounts of activator (which may occur after extensive surgery, shock, or anoxia), poor inactivation of activator in liver disease (such as cirrhosis), and certain leukemias (where increased proteolytic enzymes may also degrade fibrinogen) (Sherry, 1968). The administration of plasmin, thrombokinase, or urokinase produces fibrinolysis; these agents are currently being evaluated in the therapy of thrombosis and embolism. Excess administration of these agents may result in bleeding secondary to generalized fibrinolysis. Both spontaneous and therapeutically induced fibrinolysis may be treated with an inhibitor of this process, epsilon-aminocaproic acid (EACA). A suggested regimen (Sherry, 1968) is a loading dose of 5 g followed by 20 to 30 g daily in four divided doses, either intravenously or orally. Usually 2 or 3 days of treatment are sufficient, although in metastatic carcinoma of the prostate, longer treatment may be required. Nausea, vomiting, and dizziness have been reported as occasional side effects. EACA is excreted largely in the urine (Lewis

and Doyle, 1964). This agent should not be used unless disseminated intravascular coagulation has been ruled out (see Chapter 5).

Vitamin-K-Dependent Coagulation Factor Deficiency. Vitamin K is a fat-soluble naphthoquinone necessary for hepatic synthesis of coagulation factors (II, VII, IX, and X). Its mechanism of action in the liver is not understood. Since there is little storage of the vitamin, it must be continuously absorbed from the gastrointestinal tract, a bile-salt-dependent process. Vitamin K is found in many plant foods and is also synthesized by intestinal bacteria. Dietary deficiency is rare unless accompanied by alteration in the bacterial flora, as after treatment with certain antibiotics (e.g., tetracycline). Vitamin K therapy is indicated (1) when there is a deficiency of bile salts, as in obstructive jaundice due to biliary cirrhosis, stone, or tumor; (2) when absorption of the vitamin is limited by intestinal disease, as in ulcerative colitis or sprue (alterations in flora may also occur when antibiotics are used to treat these disorders); (3) when vitamin K antagonists, such as bishydroxycoumarin or warfarin, given as anticoagulants, have excessively lowered the level of coagulation factors; and (4) in the prophylaxis or treatment of hemorrhagic disease of the newborn, due to a lack of vitamin K at birth.

Vitamin K naturally occurs in two forms, vitamin K_1 and vitamin K_2. The former is used therapeutically, either orally or parenterally, under the name Mephyton. Menadione is a synthetic derivative fully active on a molar basis and is available in two water-soluble forms, the sodium bisulfite (Hykinone) and the sodium diphosphate (Synkavite). These are also available as oral and parenteral preparations.

The prothrombin time is the most rapid index of vitamin K deficiency; a normal value is obtained with adequate replacement therapy and restoration of liver function.

Parenteral therapy is required for treatment and prophylaxis of hemorrhagic disease of the newborn, intestinal disorders, and obstructive liver disease. If oral therapy is used in the presence of biliary obstruction, bile salts must be given concomitantly. In hepatocellular liver disease, the liver cannot utilize vitamin K normally for clotting-factor synthesis. Thus, portal cirrhosis generally does not respond well to vitamin K. To the degree that some obstructive component exists, however, a partial correction of the prothrombin time may occur with treatment. Vitamin K_1 (1 to 3 mg) is given intravenously and the prothrombin time measured again 4 to 8 hours later. If the prothrombin time is corrected, the diagnosis of obstructive jaundice is likely. Large doses of vitamin K may actually worsen the hypoprothrombinemia of hepatocellular disease through an unknown mechanism.

The prophylactic dose of vitamin K_1 recommended for all newborn infants is 0.5 to 1 mg intramuscularly soon after delivery. Menadione is somewhat hazardous since in large doses in premature infants it has been associated with hemolytic anemia and kernicterus.

Twenty to fifty milligrams of intravenous vitamin K_1 may be needed to combat hemorrhage due to overdose of oral anticoagulants. When the vitamin is injected more rapidly than 5 mg per minute, flushing, cyanosis, sweating, and hypotension may occur.

Diseases Due to Lack of Other Coagulation Factors. A variety of purified components of plasma are available for transfusion in situations where they are specifically needed. These factors include fibrinogen, albumin, gamma globulin, factor VIII (antihemophilic globulin, AHG), and factor IX (plasma thromboplastin component, Christmas factor). All except gamma globulin carry the risk of serum hepatitis. The use of plasma components has the advantage of avoiding the volume expansion that might occur with the use of plasma or whole blood.

Hemophilia A has been treated with fresh frozen plasma that contains factor VIII. Unfortunately, the amount required to halt severe bleeding often involves dangerously large volumes. Concentrates of factor VIII prepared by cold precipitation (Pool and Shannon, 1965) and by amino acid precipitation (Webster *et al.*, 1965) have been shown to be effective. The relative hazards of serum hepatitis in the various fractions now available have not been completely evaluated.

A 25% level of factor VIII is generally required for adequate hemostasis to be achieved in spontaneous hemorrhage, and a 50% level for surgery or trauma. This value has been obtained by the administration of 10 to 40 units/kg of factor VIII (1 ml of fresh plasma contains about 1 unit) (Abildgaard *et al.*, 1966). The partial thromboplastin time is a valuable monitor of the efficacy of therapy.

The relative stability of factor IX compared to factor VIII makes it possible to use the plasma derived from bank blood for the therapy of the less common *hemophilia B*. A factor IX concentrate is also available if small volumes are needed.

The congenital *deficiency of factor XI* (plasma thromboplastin antecedent, PTA) responds to the administration of stored plasma.

Hypofibrinogenemia may rarely result from decreased production of fibrinogen in very severe liver disease or as a congenital defect. The transfusion of blood, plasma, or 5 to 10 g of purified fibrinogen may be undertaken for therapy of acute bleeding episodes. Most acquired cases of hypofibrinogenemia are the result of either disseminated intravascular coagulation or fibrinolysis, in which fibrinogen is destroyed at an accelerated rate. Therapy with either heparin or EACA is indicated.

Illustrative Case 3

A 54-year-old nurse was admitted to the hospital because of hematuria, epistaxis, and purpura. She was said to have been in good health until these symptoms began 2 days before admission. There was no history of prior bleeding disorder in herself or in her family. Alcohol ingestion and ingestion of medications were denied. She had recently been separated from her husband. Physical examination revealed only a pulse of 110 and many scattered bruises. The volume of packed red cells was 35%, leukocyte count 12,000/cu mm with a normal differential, and platelet count 300,000/cu mm. The blood smear was not unusual. Liver function tests and blood urea nitrogen were normal. The following clotting studies were done:

	NORMAL VALUE	PATIENT
Clotting time	6–17 min	25 min
Bleeding time	1–9 min	7 min
Clot retraction	55–95%	80%
Prothrombin time	14–16 sec	23 sec
Thrombin time	15–20 sec	18 sec
Partial thromboplastin time	35–53 sec	85 sec
Factor V assay	50–150%	125%
Prothrombin time using 1:1 patient and normal plasma	14–16 sec	15 sec
Prothrombin time using 1:1 patient and normal adsorbed plasma	14–16 sec	24 sec
Prothrombin time 24 hours after vitamin K_1	14–16 sec	16 sec

Comment. The bleeding diathesis in this patient was localized in the coagulation system, because of the normal tests of platelet number and function (bleeding time, clot retraction) and the abnormal tests on plasma. The deficiency was shown not to be an isolated factor VII deficiency, since both PTT and prothrombin time were abnormal. Deficiencies of the intrinsic system of clotting (factors XII, XI, IX, and VIII) alone would not have resulted in an abnormal prothrombin time. The normal thrombin time ruled out a defect in the conversion of fibrinogen to fibrin, either by low fibrinogen levels or by an inhibitor of the process. The presence of a circulating anticoagulant was ruled out by correction of the prothrombin time by normal plasma. Factors II,

VII, IX, and X (the "prothrombin group") are not present in adsorbed plasma, and the use of this reagent did not correct the abnormality. Factor V is present in adsorbed plasma but was not helpful since a defect did not exist, as shown by the assay. The response to vitamin K established the diagnosis of vitamin K deficiency or of antagonism by an intact liver. In liver disease, the response would not have been so complete, and an abnormal level of factor V would have been present.

Later investigation showed a normal xylose absorption test, rendering malabsorption of vitamin K unlikely. A serum specimen obtained on admission later showed an elevated level of dicumarol. The patient later admitted ingestion of large amounts of this drug during her despondence over her marital difficulties. This clinical picture has been described many times in patients, especially women, with access to anticoagulants.

REFERENCES

Abildgaard, C. F.; Simone, J. V.; Corrigan, J. J.; Seeler, R. A.; Edelstein, G.; Vanderheiden, J.; and Schulman, I.: Treatment of hemophilia with glycine-precipitated factor VIII. *New Eng. J. Med.*, 275:471–75, 1966.

Adamson, J. W.; Eschbach, J.; and Finch, C. A.: The kidney and erythropoiesis. *Amer. J. Med.*, 44:725–33, 1968.

Alexanian, R.: Erythropoietin and erythropoiesis in anemic man following androgens. *Blood*, 33:564–72, 1969.

Alfrey, C. P., and Lane, M.: The effect of riboflavin deficiency on erythropoiesis. *Semin. Hematol.*, 7:49–54, 1970.

Allen, D. M.; Fine, M. H.; Necheles, T. F.; and Dameshek, W.: Oxymetholone therapy in aplastic anemia. *Blood*, 32:83–89, 1968.

Allgood, J. W., and Chaplin, H., Jr.: Idiopathic acquired autoimmune hemolytic anemia: review of 47 cases treated from 1955 through 1965. *Amer. J. Med.*, 43:254–73, 1967.

Aster, R. H.: Pooling of platelets in the spleen: role in the pathogenesis of "hypersplenic" thrombocytopenia. *J. Clin. Invest.*, 45:645–57, 1966.

Athens, J. W.; Raab, S. O.; Haab, O. P.; Mauer, A. M.; Ashenbrucker, H.; Cartwright, G. E.; and Wintrobe, M. M.: Leukokinetic studies. III. The distribution of granulocytes in the blood of normal subjects. *J. Clin. Invest.*, 40:159–64, 1961.

Bachmann, F.: Disseminated intravascular coagulation. *D.M.*, Dec., 1969.

Baez-Villaseñor, J.; Rath, C. E.; and Finch, C. A.: The blood picture in Addison's disease. *Blood*, 3:769–73, 1948.

Baker, H.; Herbert, V.; Frank, O.; Pasher, I.; Hutner, S. H.; Wasserman, L. R.; and Sobotka, H.: A microbiologic method for detecting folic acid deficiency in man. *Clin. Chem.*, 5:275–80, 1959.

Baker, R. J., and Nyhus, L. M.: Diagnosis and treatment of immediate transfusion reaction. *Surg. Gynecol. Obstet.*, 130:665–72, 1970.

Barry, K. G., and Malloy, J. P.: Oliguric renal failure. Evaluation and therapy by the intravenous infusion of mannitol. *J.A.M.A.*, 179:510–13, 1962.

Beard, M. E. J., and Weintraub, L. R.: Hypersegmented neutrophilic granulocytes in iron deficiency anaemia. *Brit. J. Haemat.*, 16:161–63, 1969.

Beck, W. S.: The metabolic basis of megaloblastic erythropoiesis. *Medicine*, 43:715–26, 1964.

Benesch, R.: How do small molecules do great things? *New Eng. J. Med.*, 280:1179–80, 1969.

Berk, L.; Burchenal, J. H.; and Castle, W. B.: Erythropoietic effect of cobalt in patients with or without anemia. *New Eng. J. Med.*, 240:754–61, 1949.

Bertino, J. R., and Johns, D. G.: Folate metabolism in man. In *Proceedings, XII Congress, International Society of Hematology, 1968*, pp. 133–43.

Beutler, E.: Drug-induced hemolytic anemia. *Pharmacol. Rev.*, 21:73–103, 1969.

Bianchi, A.; Chipman, D. W.; Dreskin, A.; and Rosensweig, N. S.: Nutritional folic acid deficiency with megaloblastic changes in the small-bowel epithelium. *New Eng. J. Med.*, 282:859–61, 1970.

Bird, O. D.; McGlohon, V. M.; and Vaitkus, J. W.: Naturally occurring folates in the blood and liver of the rat. *Anal. Biochem.*, 12:18–35, 1965.

Bishop, C. R.; Athens, J. W.; Boggs, D. R.; Warner, H. R.; Cartwright, G. E.; and Wintrobe, M. M.: Leukokinetic studies. XIII. A non-steady-state kinetic evaluation of the mechanism of cortisol-induced granulocytosis. *J. Clin. Invest.*, 47:249–60, 1968.

Bithell, T. C., and Wintrobe, M. M.: The bleeding history is the best "screening test" for the presence of a hemorrhagic disorder. *Hosp. Med.*, 96–109, May, 1970.

Blakley, R. L.: *The Biochemistry of Folic Acid and Related Pteridines.* John Wiley & Sons, Inc., New York, 1969.

Bodey, G. P.; Buckley, M.; Sathe, Y. S.; and Freireich, E. J.: Quantitative relationships between circulating leukocytes and infection in patients with acute leukemia. *Ann. Intern. Med.*, 64:328–40, 1966.

Bodey, G. P.; Loftis, J.; and Bowen, E. W.: Protected environment for cancer patients. Effect of a prophylactic antibiotic regimen on the microbial flora of patients undergoing cancer chemotherapy. *Arch. Intern. Med. (Chicago)*, 122:23–30, 1968.

Boggs, D. R.: *White Cell Manual.* Rutgers Medical School, New Brunswick, N.J., 1968.

Boggs, D. R.; Athens, J. W.; Cartwright, G. E.; and Wintrobe, M. M.: The effect of adrenal glucocorticosteroids upon the cellular composition of inflammatory exudates. *Amer. J. Path.*, 44:763–73, 1964.

Bothwell, T. H.; Bradlow, B. A.; Jacobs, P.; Keeley, K.; Kramer, S.; Seftel, H.; and Zail, S.: Iron metabolism in scurvy with special reference to erythropoiesis. *Brit. J. Haemat.*, 10:50–58, 1964.

Bothwell, T. H., and Finch, C. A.: *Iron Metabolism.* F. A. Churchill, Ltd., London, 1962.

Bouroncle, B. A., and Doan, C. A.: Treatment of refractory idiopathic thrombocytopenic purpura. *J.A.M.A.*, 207:2049–52, 1969.

Brody, J. I.; Goldsmith, M. H.; Park, S. K.; and Soltys, H. D.: Symptomatic crises of sickle cell anemia treated by limited exchange transfusion. *Ann. Intern. Med.*, 72:327–30, 1970.

Brooks, M. H., and Barry, K. G.: Fatal transfusion malaria. *Blood*, 34:806–10, 1969.

Burnet, F. M.: Immunologic recognition of self. *Science*, 133:307–11, 1961.

Butterworth, C. E., Jr.; Baugh, C. M.; and Krundieck, C.: A study of folate absorption and metabolism in man utilizing carbon-14-labeled polyglutamates synthesized by the solid phase method. *J. Clin. Invest.*, 48:1131–42, 1969.

Cartwright, G. E.: The anemia of chronic disorders. *Semin. Hematol.*, 3:351–75, 1966.

Cartwright, G. E.; Athens, J. W.; and Wintrobe, M. M.: The kinetics of granulopoiesis in normal man. *Blood*, 24:780–803, 1964.

Chaplin, H., Jr.: Packed red blood cells. *New Eng. J. Med.*, 281:364–67, 1969.

Charache, S.; Weatherall, D. J.; and Clegg, J. B.: Polycythemia associated with a hemoglobinopathy. *J. Clin. Invest.*, 45:813–22, 1966.

Charlton, R. W., and Bothwell, T. H.: Iron deficiency anemia. *Semin. Hematol.*, 7:67–85, 1970.

Cline, M. J., and Berlin, N. I.: Studies of the anemia of multiple myeloma. *Amer. J. Med.*, 33:510–25, 1962.

Crandon, J. H.; Lund, C. C.; and Dill, D. B.: Experimental human scurvy. *New Eng. J. Med.*, 223:353–69, 1940.

Crosby, W. H.: Paroxysmal nocturnal hemoglobinuria: a classic description by Paul Strübing in 1882, and a bibliography of the disease. *Blood*, 6:270–84, 1951.

——: Iron and anemia. *D.M.*, Jan., 1966.

Dacie, J. V.: Transfusion of saline-washed red cells in nocturnal haemoglobinuria. *Clin. Sci.*, 7:65–75, 1948.

Dameshek, W.: Hypersplenism. *Bull. N. Y. Acad. Med.*, 31:113–36, 1955.

——: The case for phlebotomy in polycythemia vera. *Blood*, 32:488–91, 1968.

Dameshek, W., and Schwartz, R.: Treatment of certain "autoimmune" diseases with antimetabolites: a preliminary report. *Trans. Amer. Ass. Phys.*, 73:113–27, 1960.

Daughaday, W. H.; Williams, R. H.; and Daland, G. A.: The effect of endocrinopathies on the blood. *Blood*, 3:1342–66, 1948.

DeConti, R. C., and Calabresi, P.: Treatment of polycythemia vera with azauridine and azaribine. *Ann. Intern. Med.*, 73:575–79, 1970.

Deodhar, S. D.; Kuklinca, A. G.; Vidt, D. G.; Robertson, A. L.; and Hazard, J. B.: Development of reticulum-cell sarcoma at the site of antilymphocyte globulin injection in a patient with renal transplant. *New Eng. J. Med.*, 280:1104–1106, 1969.

Desposito, F.; Akatsuka, J.; Thatcher, L. G.; and Smith, N. J.: Bone marrow failure in pediatric patients. I. Cortisone and testosterone treatment. *J. Pediat.*, 64:683–96, 1964.

Doan, C. A.: Hypersplenism. *Bull. N. Y. Acad. Med.*, 25:625–50, 1949.

Douglass, C. C., and Twomey, J. J.: Transient stomatocytosis with hemolysis: a previously unrecognized complication of alcoholism. *Ann. Intern. Med.*, 72:159–64, 1970.

Epstein, R. B.; Clift, R. A.; and Thomas, E. D.: The effect of leukocyte transfusions on experimental bacteremia in the dog. *Blood*, 34:782–90, 1969.

Eraklis, A. J.; Kevy, S. V.; Diamond, L. K.; and Gross, R. E.: Hazard of overwhelming infection after splenectomy in childhood. *New Eng. J. Med.*, 276:1225–29, 1967.

Erslev, A. J.: The role of erythropoietin in the control of red cell production. *Medicine*, 43:661–65, 1964.

——: Anemia of chronic renal disease. *Arch. Intern. Med. (Chicago)*, 126:774–80, 1970.

Finch, C. A.: *Red Cell Manual.* University of Washington, Seattle, 1969.

Finch, C. A.; Deubelbeiss, K.; Cook, J. D.; Eschbach, J. W.; Harker, L. A.; Funk, D. D.; Marsaglia, G.; Hillman, R. S.; Slichter, S.; Adamson, J. W.; Ganzoni, A.; and Giblett, E. R.: Ferrokinetics in man. *Medicine*, 49:17–53, 1969.

Forsham, P. H.; Thorn, G. W.; Prunty, F. T. C.; and Hills, A. G.: Clinical studies with pituitary adrenocorticotropin. *J. Clin. Endocr.*, 8:15–66, 1948.

Fountain, J. R., and Losowsky, M. S.: Haemorrhagic thrombocythaemia and its treatment with radioactive phosphorus. *Quart. J. Med.*, 31:207–20, 1962.

Freireich, E. J.; Judson, G.; and Levin, R. H.: Separation and collection of leukocytes. *Cancer Res.*, 25:1516–20, 1965.

Freireich, E. J.; Levin, R. H.; Whang, J.; Carbone, P. P.; Bronson, W.; and Morse, E. E.: The function and fate of transfused leukocytes from donors with chronic myelocytic leukemia in leukopenic recipients. *Ann. N. Y. Acad. Sci.*, 113:1081–89, 1964.

Gardner, F. H., and Nathan, D. G.: Androgens and erythropoiesis. III. Further evaluation of testosterone treatment of myelofibrosis. *New Eng. J. Med.*, 274:420–26, 1966.

Gaydos, L. A.; Freireich, E. J.; and Mantel, N.: The quantitative relation between platelet count and hemorrhage in patients with acute leukemia. *New Eng. J. Med.*, 266:905–909, 1962.

Giblett, E. R.; Coleman, D. H.; Pirzio-Biroli, G.; Donohue, D. M.; Motulsky, A. G.; and Finch, C. A.: Erythrokinetics: quantitative measurements of red cell production and destruction in normal subjects and patients with anemia. *Blood*, 11:291–309, 1956.

Gilbert, H. S.: Problems relating to control of polycythemia vera: the use of alkylating agents. *Blood*, 32:500–505, 1968.

Glass, G. B. J.: Gastric intrinsic factor and its function in the metabolism of vitamin B_{12}. *Physiol. Rev.*, 43:529–849, 1963.

Gowans, J. L.: Immunobiology of the small lymphocyte. *Hosp. Pract.*, 3:34–46, 1968.

Graw, R. G., Jr.; Henderson, E. S.; and Perry, S.: Leukocyte procurement and transfusion into leukopenic patients. In *Proceedings of the International Symposium on White Cell Transfusions of the Centre National de la Recherche Scientifique, Paris, June, 1969.*

Graw, R. G., Jr.; Herzig, G. P.; Eyre, H.; Goldstein, I.; Henderson, E. S.; and Perry, S.: Treatment of gram negative septicemia in granulocytopenic patients with normal granulocyte transfusions. *Clin. Res.*, 19:491, 1971.

Hall, C. A., and Finkler, A. E.: A second vitamin B_{12}-binding substance in human plasma. *Biochim. Biophys. Acta*, 78:234–36, 1963.

Harker, L. A.: *Hemostasis Manual.* University of Washington, Seattle, 1969.

——: Platelet production. *New Eng. J. Med.*, 282:492–94, 1970.

Harker, L. A., and Finch, C. A.: Thrombokinetics in man. *J. Clin. Invest.*, 48:963–74, 1969.

Hartmann, R. C.; Jenkins, D. E.; McKee, L. C.; and Heyssel, R. M.: Paroxysmal nocturnal hemoglobinuria: clinical and laboratory studies relating to iron metabolism and therapy with androgen and iron. *Medicine*, 45:331-63, 1966.

Herbert, V.: Current concepts in therapy, megaloblastic anemia. *New Eng. J. Med.*, 268:368–71, 1963.

Herbert, V.; Larrabee, A. R.; and Buchanan, J. M.: Studies on the identification of a folate compound of human serum. *J. Clin. Invest.*, 41:1134–38, 1962.

Herbert, V., and Shapiro, S. S.: The site of absorption of folic acid in the rat *in vitro*. *Fed. Proc.*, 21:260, 1962.

Herbert, V., and Zalusky, R.: Interrelations of vitamin B_{12} and folic acid metabolism: folic acid clearance studies. *J. Clin. Invest.*, 41:1263–76, 1962.

Hillman, R. S.: *Hematology Laboratory Manual.* University of Washington, Seattle, 1969.

Hoffbrand, A. V., and Necheles, T. F.: Mechanism of folate deficiency in patients receiving phenytoin. *Lancet*, 2:528–30, 1968.

Horrigan, D. L., and Harris, J. W.: Pyridoxine-responsive anemia: analysis of 62 cases. *Adv. Intern. Med.*, 12:103–74, 1964.

Huennekens, F. M.: Folate and B_{12} coenzymes. In Singer, T. P. (ed.): *Biological Oxidations*. Interscience, New York, 1968, pp. 439–513.

Jaenicke, L.: Vitamin and coenzyme function: vitamin B_{12} and folic acid. *Ann. Rev. Biochem.*, 33:287–312, 1964.

Jaffé, E. R.: Hereditary hemolytic disorders and enzymatic deficiencies of human erythrocytes. *Blood*, 35:116–34, 1970.

Kauder, E.; Boggs, D. R.; Athens, J. W.; Vodopick, H. A.; Cartwright, G. E.; and Wintrobe, M. M.: Leukokinetic studies. XII. Kinetic studies of normal isologous neutrophilic granulocytes transfused into normal subjects. *Proc. Soc. Exp. Biol. Med.*, **120**:595–99, 1965.

Kauder, E., and Mauer, A.: Neutropenias of childhood. *J. Pediat.*, **69**:147–57, 1966.

Keller, J. W.; Majerus, P. W.; and Finke, E. H.: An unusual type of spiculated erythrocyte in metastatic liver disease and hemolytic anemia. *Ann. Intern. Med.*, **74**:732–37, 1971.

Kennedy, B. J., and Gilbertsen, A. S.: Increased erythropoiesis induced by androgenic hormone therapy. *New Eng. J. Med.*, **256**:719–26, 1957.

Kilbridge, T. M., and Heller, P.: Determinants of erythrocyte size in chronic liver disease. *Blood*, **34**: 739–46, 1969.

Kimber, C.; Deller, D. J.; Ibbotson, R. N.; and Lander, H.: The mechanism of anaemia in chronic liver disease. *Quart. J. Med.*, **34**:33–64, 1965.

Kotilainen, M.: Platelet kinetics in normal subjects and in haematological disorders. *Scand. J. Haemat.*, 5(Suppl.):1–97, 1969.

Lalezari, P.; Nussbaum, M.; Gelman, S.; and Spaet, T. H.: Neonatal neutropenia due to maternal isoimmunization. *Blood*, **15**:236–43, 1960.

Lane, M., and Alfrey, C. P., Jr.: The anaemia of human riboflavin deficiency. *Blood*, **25**:432–42, 1965.

Laszlo, J.: Effective treatment of polycythemia vera with phenylalanine mustard. *Blood*, **32**:506, 1968.

Lawrence, J. H., and Berlin, N. I.: Relative polycythemia — the polycythemia of stress. *Yale J. Biol. Med.*, **24**:498, 1952.

Lengyel, P.; Mazumder, R.; and Ochoa, S.: Mammalian methylmalonyl isomerase and vitamin B_{12} coenzymes. *Proc. Nat. Acad. Sci. U.S.A.*, **46**:1312–18, 1960.

Levine, W. G.: Anticoagulants. In Goodman, L. S., and Gilman, A. (eds.): *The Pharmacological Basis of Therapeutics*, 4th ed. The Macmillan Co., New York, 1970, pp. 1445–63.

Levitt, M.; Schacter, B. A.; Zipursky, A.; and Israels, L. G.: The nonerythropoietic component of early bilirubin. *J. Clin. Invest.*, **47**:1281–94, 1968.

Lewis, J. H., and Doyle, A. P.: Effects of epsilon aminocaproic acid on coagulation and fibrinolytic mechanisms. *J.A.M.A.*, **188**:56–63, 1964.

Lindenbaum, J., and Hargrove, R. L.: Thrombocytopenia in alcoholics. *Ann. Intern. Med.*, **68**:526–32, 1968.

McCullagh, E. P., and Jones, R.: Effect of androgens on blood count of men. *J. Clin. Endocr.*, **2**:243–51, 1942.

McFarland, W., and Libre, E. P.: Abnormal leukocyte response in alcoholism. *Ann. Intern. Med.*, **59**:865–77, 1963.

MacKenzie, M. R., and Creevy, N. C.: Hemolytic anemia with cold detectable IgG antibodies. *Blood*, **36**:549–58, 1970.

Mahoney, M. J., and Rosenberg, L. E.: Inherited defects of B_{12} metabolism. *Amer. J. Med.*, **48**:584–93, 1970.

Mann, D. L.; Donati, R. M.; and Gallagher, N. I.: Erythropoietin assay and ferrokinetic measurements in anemic uremic patients. *J.A.M.A.*, **194**:1321–22, 1965.

Marcus, A. J.: Platelet function. *New Eng. J. Med.*, **280**:1213–20, 1278–84, 1330–35, 1969.

Marsh, J. C.; Boggs, D. R.; Cartwright, G. E.; and Wintrobe, M. M.: Neutrophil kinetics in acute infection. *J. Clin. Invest.*, **46**:1943–53, 1967.

Merskey, C.; Johnson, A. J.; Kleiner, G. J.; and Wohl, H.: The defibrination syndrome: clinical features and laboratory diagnosis. *Brit. J. Haemat.*, **13**:528–49, 1967.

Modan, B., and Lilienfeld, A. M.: Polycythemia vera and leukemia—the role of radiation treatment—study of 1222 patients. *Medicine*, **44**:305–44, 1965.

Moeschlin, S.: Immunologic granulocytopenia and agranulocytosis. *Le Sang.*, **26**:32–51, 1955.

Neubauer, C.: Mental deterioration in epilepsy due to folate deficiency. *Brit. Med. J.*, **2**:759–61, 1970.

Nichol, C. A., and Welch, A. D.: Synthesis of citrovorum factor from folic acid by liver slices: augmentation by ascorbic acid. *Proc. Soc. Exp. Biol. Med.*, **74**:52–55, 1950.

Noronha, J. M., and Aboobaker, V. S.: Studies on the folate compounds of human blood. *Arch. Biochem.*, **101**:445–47, 1963.

Noronha, J. M., and Silverman, M.: On folic acid, vitamin B_{12}, methionine and formiminoglutamic acid metabolism. In *Proceedings, Second European Symposium on Vitamin B_{12} and Intrinsic Factor*. Ferdinand Enke Verlag, Stuttgart, 1961, p. 728.

Olsson, P.; Lagergren, H.; and Ek, S.: The elimination from plasma of intravenous heparin: an experimental study on dogs and humans. *Acta Med. Scand.*, **173**:619–30, 1963.

Osgood, E. E.: The case for ^{32}P in treatment of polycythemia vera. *Blood*, **32**:492–99, 1968.

Pearson, H. A.; Spencer, R. P.; and Cornelius, E. A.: Functional asplenia in sickle-cell anemia. *New Eng. J. Med.*, **281**:923–26, 1969.

Perry, S.: Reduction of toxicity in cancer chemotherapy. *Cancer Res.*, **29**:2319–25, 1969.

Pool, J. G., and Shannon, A. E.: Production of high-potency concentrates of antihemophilic globulin in a closed-bag system: assay *in vitro* and *in vivo*. *New Eng. J. Med.*, **273**:1443–47, 1965.

Quagliana, J. M.; Cartwright, G. E.; and Wintrobe, M. M.: Paroxysmal nocturnal hemoglobinuria following drug-induced aplastic anemia. *Ann. Intern. Med.*, **61**:1045–52, 1964.

Raab, S. O.; Haut, A.; Cartwright, G. E.; and Wintrobe, M. M.: Pyridoxine-responsive anemia. *Blood*, **18**:285–302, 1961.

Rabiner, S. F., and Molinas, F.: The role of phenol and phenolic acids on the thrombocytopathy and defective platelet aggregation of patients with renal failure. *Amer. J. Med.*, **49**:346–51, 1970.

Ranney, H. M.: Clinically important variants of human hemoglobin. *New Eng. J. Med.*, **282**:144–52, 1970.

Reerink-Brongers, E. E.; Prins, H. K.; and Krijnen, H. W.: Haptoglobin and increased haemolysis. *Vox Sang.*, **7**:619–31, 1962.

Reisner, E. H., Jr.: Tissue culture of bone marrow. II. Effect of steroid hormones on hematopoiesis *in vitro*. *Blood*, **27**:460–69, 1966.

Rishpon-Meyerstein, N.; Kilbridge, T.; Simone, J.; and Fried, W.: The effect of testosterone on erythropoietin levels in anemic patients. *Blood*, **31**:453–60, 1968.

Robertson, J. H.: Uracil mustard in the treatment of thrombocythemia. *Blood*, **35**:288–97, 1970.

Robinson, S. H.: The origins of bilirubin. *New Eng. J. Med.*, **279**:143–49, 1968.

Rock, R. C.; Bove, J. R.; and Nemerson, Y.: Heparin treatment of intravascular coagulation accompanying hemolytic transfusion reactions. *Transfusion*, **9**:57–61, 1969.

Rosenberg, I. H.; Godwin, H. A.; Streiff, R. R.; and Castle, W. B.: Impairment of intestinal deconjugation of dietary folate: a possible explanation of megaloblastic anemia associated with phenytoin therapy. *Lancet*, **2**:530–32, 1968.

Sanchez-Medal, L.; Gomez-Leal, A.; Duarte, L.; and Rico, M. G.: Anabolic androgenic steroids in the treatment of acquired aplastic anemia. *Blood*, **34**:283–300, 1969.

Scott, J. L.; Cartwright, G. E.; and Wintrobe, M. M.:

Acquired aplastic anemia: an analysis of 39 cases and review of the pertinent literature. *Medicine*, 38: 119–72, 1959.

Seligmann, M.: Confrontation therapeutiques: insuffisance medullaire chronique. *Nouv. Rev. Franc. Hemat.*, 6:407–16, 1966.

Seligmann, M.; Fudenberg, H. H.; and Good, R. A.: A proposed classification of primary immunologic disorders. *Amer. J. Med.*, 45:817–25, 1968.

Shahidi, N. T., and Diamond, L. K.: Testosterone-induced remission in aplastic anemia of both acquired and congenital types. *New Eng. J. Med.*, 264:953–67, 1961.

Sherry, S.: Fibrinolysis. *Ann. Rev. Med.*, 19:247–68, 1968.

Silber, R., and Moldow, C. F.: The biochemistry of B_{12}-mediated reactions in man. *Amer. J. Med.*, 48: 549–54, 1970.

Silink, S. J., and Firkin, B. G.: An analysis of hypoplastic anaemia with special reference to the use of oxymethalone ("Adroyd") and its therapy. *Aust. Ann. Med.*, 17:224–35, 1968.

Silverstein, M. N.: Primary or hemorrhagic thrombocythemia. *Arch. Intern. Med. (Chicago)*, 122:18–22, 1968.

Smith, C. H.; Erlandson, M. E.; Stern, G.; and Hilgartner, M. W.: Post-splenectomy infection in Cooley's anemia: an appraisal of the problem in this and other blood disorders, with a consideration of prophylaxis. *New Eng. J. Med.*, 266:737–43, 1962.

Streiff, R. R.: Malabsorption of polyglutamic folic acid secondary to oral contraceptives. *Clin. Res.*, 17:345, 1969.

Sturgeon, P.: Recent developments in blood components therapy. *Ann. Intern. Med.*, 74:113–25, 1971.

Sullivan, J. M.; Harken, D. E.; and Gorlin, R.: Pharmacologic control of thromboembolic complications of cardiac-valve replacement. *New Eng. J. Med.*, 279:576–80, 1968.

Sullivan, L. W., and Herbert, V.: Suppression of hematopoiesis by ethanol. *J. Clin. Invest.*, 43:2048–62, 1964.

Sussman, L. N.: Azathioprine in refractory idiopathic thrombocytopenic purpura. *J.A.M.A.*, 202:259–63, 1967.

Takeyama, S.; Hatch, F. T.; and Buchanan, J. M.: Enzymatic synthesis of methyl group of methionine. II. Involvement of vitamin B_{12}. *J. Biol. Chem.*, 236:1102–1208, 1961.

Taylor, L.: Idiopathic autoimmune hemolytic anemia. *Amer. J. Med.*, 35:130–34, 1963.

Taymor, M. L.; Sturgis, S. H.; and Yahia, C.: The etiological role of chronic iron deficiency in production of menorrhagia. *J.A.M.A.*, 187:323–27, 1964.

Thomas, D. P.; Ream, V. J.; and Stuart, R. K.: Platelet aggregation in patients with Laennec's cirrhosis of liver. *New Eng. J. Med.*, 276:1344–48, 1967.

Toohey, J. I., and Barker, H. A.: Isolation of coenzyme B_{12} from liver. *J. Biol. Chem.*, 236:560–63, 1961.

Tudhope, G. R., and Wilson, G. M.: Anaemia in hypothyroidism. *Quart. J. Med.*, 29:513–37, 1960.

Tullis, J. L.: Prevalence, nature, and identification of leukocyte antibodies. *New Eng. J. Med.*, 258:569–78, 1958.

Ulutin, O. N.: Primary thrombocytopathy. *Israel J. Med. Sci.*, 1:857–60, 1965.

Veeger, W.; Woldring, M. G.; vanRood, J. J.; Eernisse, J. G.; Leeksma, C. H. W.; Verloop, M. C.; and Nieweg, H. O.: The value of the determination of the site of red cell sequestration in hemolytic anemia as a prediction test for splenectomy. *Acta Med. Scand.*, 171:507–20, 1962.

Vilter, R. W.; Horrigan, D.; Mueller, J. F.; Jarrold, T.; Vilter, C. F.; Hawkins, V.; and Seaman, A.: Studies on the relationships of vitamin B_{12}, folic acid, thymine, uracil and methyl group donors in persons with pernicious anemia and related megaloblastic anemias. *Blood*, 5:695–717, 1950.

Vincent, P. C., and deGruchy, G. C.: Complications and treatment of acquired aplastic anemia. *Brit. J. Haemat.*, 13:977–99, 1967.

Vogel, J. M.; Kimball, H. R.; Wolff, S. M.; and Perry, S.: Etiocholanolone in the evaluation of marrow reserves in patients receiving cytotoxic agents. *Ann. Intern. Med.*, 67:1226–38, 1967.

Waldmann, T. A.; Levin, E. H.; and Baldwin, M.: The association of polycythemia with a cerebellar hemangioblastoma. *Amer. J. Med.*, 31:318–24, 1961.

Ward, H. N.: Pulmonary infiltrates associated with leukoagglutinin transfusion reactions. *Ann. Intern. Med.*, 73:689–94, 1970.

Wasserman, L. R.: The treatment of polycythemia. Introduction. *Blood*, 32:483–87, 1968.

Webb, D. I.; Chodos, R. B.; Mahar, C. Q.; and Faloon, W. W.: Mechanism of vitamin B_{12} malabsorption in patients receiving colchicine. *New Eng. J. Med.*, 279: 845–50, 1968.

Webster, W. P.; Roberts, H. R.; Thelin, G. M.; Wagner, R. H.; and Brinkhous, K. M.: Clinical use of a new glycine-precipitated antihemophilic fraction. *Amer. J. Med. Sci.*, 250:643–51, 1965.

Weiss, H. J.: Von Willebrand's disease—diagnostic criteria. *Blood*, 32:668–79, 1968.

Weiss, H. J., and Kochwa, S.: Studies of platelet function and proteins in 3 patients with Glanzmann's thrombasthenia. *J. Lab. Clin. Med.*, 71:153–65, 1968.

Weissbach, H.; Peterkofsky, A.; Redfield, B.; and Dickerman, H.: Studies on the terminal reaction in the biosynthesis of methionine. *J. Biol. Chem.*, 238:3318–24, 1963.

Westerman, M. P.: The common hemoglobinopathies. *Amer. Fam. Physician GP*, 2:86–94, 1970.

White, A. M.; and Cox, E. J.: Methylmalonic acid excretion and vitamin B_{12} deficiency in the human. *Ann. N.Y. Acad. Sci.*, 112:915–21, 1964.

Will, J. J.; Mueller, J. F.; Brodine, C.; Kieley, C. E.; Friedman, B.; Hawkins, V. R.; Dutra, J.; and Vilter, R. W.: Folic acid and vitamin B_{12} in pernicious anemia. *J. Lab. Clin. Med.*, 53:22–38, 1959.

Wintrobe, M. M.: *Clinical Hematology*, 6th ed. Lea & Febiger, Philadelphia, 1967.

Wintrobe, M. M.; Cartwright, G. E.; Palmer, J. G.; Kuhns, W. J.; and Samuels, L. T.: Effect of corticotrophin and cortisone on the blood in various disorders in man. *Arch. Intern. Med. (Chicago)*, 88:310–36, 1951.

Worlledge, S. M.; Carstairs, K. C.; and Dacie, J. V.: Autoimmune haemolytic anemia associated with α-methyldopa therapy. *Lancet*, 2:135–39, 1966.

Yankee, R. A.; Grumet, F. C.; and Rogentine, G. N.: Platelet transfusion therapy: the selection of compatible platelet donors for refractory patients by lymphocyte HL-A typing. *New Eng. J. Med.*, 281:1208–12, 1969.

Young, L. E.: Complications of blood transfusion. *Ann. Intern. Med.*, 61:136–46, 1964.

Ziemlanski, S.; Wartanowicz, M.; Dentyniecka, M.; and Szczygiel, A.: Absorption of folic acid in various segments of the alimentary tract. *Acta Physiol. Pol.*, 19:179–86, 1968.

Chapter 9

INFLAMMATORY DISORDERS

Russell L. Miller and *Kenneth L. Melmon*

The history of inflammation and its therapy is as old and as extensive as the history of medicine. Rather than detailing all aspects of inflammatory processes and of the drugs used to alter them, this chapter provides principles that relate to the therapy of any type of inflammatory process. First, the pathogenesis of inflammation and the morphologic changes that occur in the microcirculation of inflamed tissue are discussed. Then the focus turns to some of the most commonly used anti-inflammatory agents, their mechanisms of action, and the assets and liabilities of their use. The third section of this chapter deals with treatment of diseases that illustrate several types of inflammatory processes. The rational choice and use of any anti-inflammatory agent depend on careful consideration of the mechanisms at work in the inflammatory state, as well as on detailed knowledge of how drugs can alter those mechanisms. Even when present knowledge fails to provide ready answers to the difficult questions posed by most of these diseases, therapy must not be based on guesses, intuition, or "trial and error," but rather on determination of reasonable therapeutic goals, weighed against the known efficacy of anti-inflammatory agents.

The inflammatory process is complex and dynamic, consisting of many interdependent cellular and humoral events directed at neutralization of noxious agents and repair of tissue injury. The clinical expression of the process was described by Celsus as *calor, rubor, tumor,* and *dolor*. We now know that each observable manifestation of inflammation represents several homeostatic adjustments and complex biochemical changes. The process is necessary for survival and is an elemental reaction to injury. However, many diseases are characterized by loss of control of homeostatic mechanisms—the severe inflammatory state may be one. If the inflammatory reaction is poorly controlled and becomes excessive in relation to its stimulus, it causes more harm to the host than does the triggering stimulus. Conversely, if the inflammatory response is unable to neutralize the stimulus, the host is unprotected. Therapeutically we usually try to limit the inflammatory response, but some diseases of man (e.g., granulomatous disease of children, agammaglobulinemia, disorders of degranulation of white cells, and severe uremia) characteristically produce a subnormal response to stimuli that elicit inflammation. In addition, drugs used for diseases other than inflammation can limit or prevent an appropriate inflammatory response. These include agents that interfere with leukocyte production or function, deplete the body of endogenous mediators of inflammation, or prevent the release, synthesis, or peripheral effects of the mediators. *Principle: The physician who uses drugs to alter inflammatory states undertakes the same sort of risks as his colleague who treats hypertension by altering homeostatic mechanisms controlling the heart and blood vessels. Both must attempt to understand the physiologic controls and must define therapeutic goals carefully. If they do so their treatment will at least not prove worse than the disease; at best the longevity and quality of life of their patients will be improved.*

The expression of inflammation represents a spectrum depending on the stimulus, the state of the host, and the use of drugs. Tissues need not respond to injury by fully developing all aspects of an inflammatory process. Many different types of stimuli can produce inflammation (Table 9–1). However, despite the diversity of these stimuli only minor variations have been noted in the gross and microscopic pattern of the inflammatory process. These variations usually are attributable to differences between species, the anatomic location of the lesion, or the specific chemical effects of the predominant irritant. The manifestations of the inflammatory processes represent a common pathway of expression of a variety of insults. *Principle: A thorough knowledge of the morphology of an inflammatory process and an understanding of its potential beneficial and detrimental effects is necessary in order to decide when to use drug therapy to alter the process; understanding of the chemical pathogenesis of the process allows proper choice of pharmacologic agents. Thorough knowledge of the pathogenesis also removes some*

Table 9–1. CONDITIONS IN WHICH ELEMENTS OF AN INFLAMMATORY PROCESS MAY BE PRESENT

Infections: viral, bacterial, rickettsial, parasitic
Immune reactions: anaphylaxis, serum sickness, Arthus' reaction, autoimmune diseases, graft rejection, Shwartzman phenomenon, drug reactions related to hypersensitivity
Collagen diseases
Various arthritides
Thermal and radiation injury
Trauma
Neoplasm
Conditions of tissue ischemia
Exposure to drugs, chemicals, or toxins (e.g., endotoxemia, potassium-induced lesions of the small intestine)

---

empiricism from treatment and may allow unconventional anti-inflammatory agents to be introduced.

Knowledge of both the pathogenesis and the pharmacotherapy of inflammation is often fragmentary and intellectually unsatisfying (as compared, for example, with our knowledge of disorders of glucose homeostasis and management of disorders of glucose metabolism). However, there is no excuse for taking action before thought; "empiric" treatment can be just as demanding for the physician and as useful to the patient as therapy grounded in knowledge of biochemistry.

THE INFLAMMATORY PROCESS

The morphologic similarities among all types of inflammation suggest common control mechanisms and mediators that initiate, sustain, and terminate the inflammatory responses in tissues. Early workers traced the major threads of similarity in events and the sequence of the gross pattern of the inflammatory process in various animal species. They found at the anatomic center of an acute inflammatory process the capillaries, terminal arterioles, and venules (Cohnheim, 1889). More recent evidence demonstrates that the regional circulation usually shows a biphasic response to acute inflammation (Burke and Miles, 1958; Sevitt, 1958; Zweifach, 1965). The early phase is usually brief (10 minutes in some cases) and is associated with vasodilation and increased capillary permeability to plasma proteins. The delayed phase is prolonged, lasting hours or days, and is characterized by infiltration of leukocytes into the inflamed tissues, slowed blood flow, hemorrhage, and extensive tissue damage. The phases of an inflammatory process are not always easily distinguishable and may merge. For example, with a relatively strong stimulus the early phase may be transient, overlapping the more prolonged and destructive late phase.

The cardiovascular responses to an inflammatory process are determined by the character and distribution of the "noxious agent." A strong and diffuse stimulus produces widespread changes in the microcirculation as well as stimulation of the autonomic nervous system, resulting in tachycardia, tachypnea, and systemic metabolic changes. With a weaker or localized stimulus, the only observable changes occur in a localized area of the microcirculation.

The microcirculation is the focus of the local changes of inflammation. The earliest event usually is transient arteriolar constriction in the vicinity of the irritant (Spector and Willoughby, 1963). After a few seconds, the blood flow through affected tissues is remarkably increased.

As the precapillary sphincters are opened, some of the blood flow is "shunted" into capillary side channels. At this point the precapillary sphincters are maximally dilated and do not respond to usual vasoconstrictor stimuli. Vascular permeability is increased and plasma proteins are lost into the tissues, causing edema (Zweifach, 1965). Studies of vascular ultrastructure indicate that during experimentally induced inflammatory processes, the endothelial cells become separated from one another, permitting the extravasation of plasma proteins (Majno and Palade, 1961; Majno et al., 1961; Marchesi, 1962). The endothelial cells themselves may be damaged and become swollen, narrowing the vessel lumen. The vessel lumen becomes more narrowed by the adherence of leukocytes, platelets, and erythrocytes to the endothelial surface. Loss of protein-containing fluid and narrowing of the vascular lumen probably account for the progressively slowed blood flow and sludging in the affected capillaries and venules (Landis and Pappenheimer, 1963).

Following the early vascular events, the cellular phase of inflammation begins as more granulocytes in the affected vessels become adherent to the endothelial wall. The mechanisms by which these cells become adherent to the endothelium and subsequently migrate across the vascular wall are not well understood. The initial vascular changes of inflammation involve the venules, but later the capillaries are affected. Petechial hemorrhages develop in the area of severely affected vessels in which stasis and sludging are present. As the blood flow through the capillary bed is reduced, tissue metabolism becomes anaerobic and necrosis eventually ensues. During tissue damage, the microcirculation responds unpredictably to the ordinary exogenous mediators of change in regional blood flow (Zweifach, 1965). The therapist should recognize that the inflammatory state can alter pharmacologic responses. Consequently a desired change must always be measured to determine whether it occurs as a consequence of drug administration.

Although vascular phenomena and the formation of an exudate are important, they represent only part of the pathology of an inflammatory process. Degeneration and/or proliferative changes in tissue also occur. Exposure to an intense irritant results in tissue destruction; a mild irritant causes tissue proliferation. Usually the processes overlap, i.e., tissue degeneration may predominate at the center of an inflamed area, while at the periphery proliferation may occur. The stimulant action of the inflammatory process is necessary for tissue repair or healing.

The morphologic changes described are most characteristic for an acute inflammatory process; similar but less striking changes may be observed when the inflammatory process evolves more slowly. Acute and chronic inflammatory lesions follow similar patterns of tissue repair, but quantitatively more fibrous tissue is usually formed in the course of tissue healing following prolonged inflammatory processes.

Initiation and Termination of the Inflammatory Process

An inflammatory process may be initiated either by obvious and direct mechanical physical damage to the vascular endothelium or by introduction of an inflammatory agent. Most evidence suggests that whatever the initiating agent, a series of intermediate events leads to the activation, release, or production of vasoactive substances that mediate the vascular response. Four key features of the inflammatory reaction imply that chemicals are involved: (1) inflammatory changes occur only in living tissues and are often reversible; (2) the inflammatory process is consistent and orderly; (3) the reaction can be suppressed at least partly by drugs; and (4) there is a latent period between the injury and the reaction (Spector and Willoughby, 1963). A major function of the chemical factors related during an inflammatory process is probably to promote the microcirculatory response and the aggregation of formed elements of the blood, both of which lead first to tissue damage and later to tissue repair. In this perspective, an inflammatory process is the automatic, predictable, and orderly consequence of nonspecific tissue injury and only needs triggering by the etiologic agent. ***Principle: The orderly process of inflammation allows logical interruption of the process.*** Thus a number of agents interfere with different components of inflammation but are additive in their effects only if (1) the process is incompletely antagonized by one agent; (2) the antagonizing processes are interdependent; and (3) the agents can produce their effects after the inflammatory sequence has already been initiated. In considering use of anti-inflammatory agents some attempt should be made to classify drugs that specifically or nonspecifically *prevent* initiation of the process (e.g., allopurinol for gout) or nonspecifically *limit* the reaction once it has been initiated (e.g., salicylates for rheumatoid arthritis or colchicine for gout).

The factors that might limit and modulate the inflammatory process have not been defined. Recent data implicate a relationship between the adenyl cyclase system in granulocytes (Bourne et al., 1970; Bourne and Melmon, 1971; Bourne et al., 1971), lymphocytes (Bourne et al., 1970), and platelets (Wolfe and Shulman, 1969) and anti-inflammatory effects. If this were verified, a molecular explanation of the anti-inflammatory effects of such drugs as theophylline, isoproterenol, and prostaglandin (which potentiate the adenyl cyclase system) might be defined (Miller and Melmon, 1970). Likewise, discovery of endogenous substances and drugs that limit the theoretically continuous cycle of inflammation will be most important (Hinman, 1970; Cuthbert, 1971). Considerable information is available on the common chemical mechanisms responsible for initiation and continuation of the inflammatory process. Surprisingly few studies have attempted to define the processes that terminate an inflammatory reaction. The termination must represent an active process that, if understood, would open new approaches to the therapy of inflammation, in the same way that knowledge of the metabolism of glucose has made the treatment of diabetes more effective. However, the authors do not advocate catecholamines, theophylline, or prostaglandin as useful anti-inflammatory agents.

Possible Mediators of the Inflammatory Process: Amines, Polypeptides, and Proteins

Many of the drugs used to modify an inflammatory process have been directed at altering the metabolism, release, or peripheral effects of endogenous chemical substances potentially capable of mediating aspects of an inflammatory process.

Histamine. The notable actions of histamine are its effects on the vascular system, smooth muscle, and exocrine glands (Goodman and Gilman, 1970). Histamine dilates arterioles and venules in most species. Histamine-induced vasodilation is independent of innervation and is only partly suppressed by antihistamines, but may be completely overcome by sympathomimetic amines (Goodman and Gilman, 1970).

Increases in capillary permeability have been attributed to histamine, but there is no evidence that it affects the smallest blood vessels (those containing a single layer of endothelium with a basement membrane). Histamine increases the permeability of small veins (up to 50 mμ in diameter) by causing separation of the endothelial cells (Majno and Palade, 1961; Majno et al., 1961; Marchesi, 1962).

When histamine is injected into human skin, a characteristic triple response occurs (Lewis, 1927). This series of events involves the local venules, arterioles, capillaries (vessels up to 50 mμ in diameter that may lack thick muscle coats), and sensory nerves. The triad consists of (1) a localized red spot representing the immediate and direct vasodilatory effect of histamine; (2) a bright red flush or "flare" of irregular outline extending for 1 cm or more beyond the original red spot (believed to be produced by the reflex vasodilation of the adjacent small vessels); and (3) a localized collection of edema fluid (a wheal) secondary to the extravasation of plasma fluid through the abnormally permeable wall of the small vessel. Other important effects of histamine include pruritus, but not pain, when the amine is applied to a blister base or injected intradermally; unusually high doses of the amine may produce diapedesis of a small number of leukocytes (Spector and Willoughby, 1964a). In many species, repeated doses of histamine result in tachyphylaxis (Naranjo, 1966). *Principle: The properties of histamine make it a candidate for influencing the acute phase of inflammation. Antihistamines, if useful at all, would have their major effects in this early phase. Whether late phases of inflammation are cause-and-effect related to the early phases is unknown, but this consideration may become fundamental for the proper use of anti-inflammatory agents.*

Histamine is formed by decarboxylation of histidine and is widely distributed in the body. Free histamine is found only in trace amounts in most tissues but may be quite active in terms of the role it can play during an inflammatory process (Ivy and Bachrach, 1966; Erjavec et al., 1967). Mast cells provide the major storage site for histamine (Riley and West, 1966), but the amine is also present in granulocytes. Histamine is stored in the mast-cell granules in a physiologically inactive form. Current evidence indicates that histamine release correlates with degranulation of the mast cell (Uvnas, 1964, 1967). The extrusion of granules is associated with events that alter the mast-cell membrane, such as decreases in pH and changes in the ionic milieu and in temperature. Factors involved in histamine release from the granulocyte include similar changes, plus phagocytosis and damage of its cell membrane produced by antigen-antibody reaction. Histamine release of substances contained in the granular fraction of the cell (lysozyme, myeloperoxidase, alkaline phosphatase, cathepsin, etc.) is capable of contributing to inflammation and are inhibited by drugs that activate the adenyl cyclase system or interfere with degranulation. These observations, and the fact that inhibitors of proteolytic enzymes decrease granule extrusion, indicate an enzymatic basis for release of granules and their contents, presumably including histamine (Lichtenstein and Margolis, 1968; Bourne et al., 1970; Miller and Melmon, 1970; Bourne and Melmon, 1971; Bourne et al., 1971). Anoxia and lack of glucose slow the extrusion of granules; therefore, the process requires energy (Beraldo et al., 1966; Uvnas, 1967). Histamine release may involve activation of an enzyme, located on the mast-cell membrane, that alters the permeability characteristics of the membrane and results in entry of the mast-cell granules into the extracellular fluid. Almost any agent that causes tissue injury also liberates histamine (Spector and Willoughby, 1963, 1964; Beraldo et al., 1966). Proof of the relevance of release of a mediator in the inflammatory process requires serial measurements and correlation of changes in concentration of the substance with morphologic abnormalities (Reichgott and Melmon, 1971).

The role of histamine during an inflammatory process may be defined in part by the effects of pharmacologic antagonists on the peripheral effects of the amine. By heating the skin of a guinea pig, an early and delayed phase of increased small vessel permeability was demonstrated (Sevitt, 1958). Two phases of inflammation may be observed in many other types of injury. The initial phase can be suppressed by pretreatment of the experimental animals with antihistamines (Spector and Willoughby, 1965). In some types of inflammation, such as severe tissue destruction produced by high temperatures or prolonged heating, the early response is less noticeable, and the overall response may appear to be an accelerated late phase that is not altered by antihistamines. X-ray damage to rat intestine causes abnormal vascular permeability within 24 hours. If antihistamines are given at the time of irradiation, the increased vascular permeability is delayed for an additional 24 hours; however, by 72 hours, the severity of the reaction is equal to that of controls (Spector and Willoughby, 1964a). *Principle: The role histamine plays in the development of an inflammatory process is early, transient, incomplete, and not essential for the development of the most characteristic changes that produce lasting tissue alteration.* Therefore, antihistaminics or inhibitors of histidine decarboxylase have limited but specific usefulness as anti-inflammatory agents. Conversely, if an agent that alters mast-cell or granulocyte function also affects the development or maintenance of an inflammatory process, the drug may affect substances in addition to or other than histamine.

Serotonin (5-Hydroxytryptamine). The cardiovascular effects of exogenously administered serotonin are complex and variable because the direct and reflex actions of the amine may occur sequentially or sometimes almost simultaneously. In addition, the response varies depending on the route, speed, and frequency of administration (Page, 1958; Erspamer, 1966). When serotonin is administered, the resultant vasodilation and increased blood flow resemble the changes observed during inflammation. Infusion of serotonin into the brachial artery of normal subjects causes the fingers to redden and then become a dusky blue color. The color changes are thought to be related to dilation and later constriction of the minute vessels of the skin. In rodents, the combination of arteriolar dilation, venular constriction, and separation of endothelial cells occurring after subcutaneous administration of serotonin produces leakage of plasma from venules (Majno and Palade, 1961; Majno et al., 1961). In man serotonin has no prominent effects on vascular permeability (Page, 1958). When applied to the base of a blister, serotonin causes severe pain, which may be delayed in onset but persists for long periods (Spector and Willoughby, 1965). The amine has only a modest and most likely unimportant effect on the emigration of leukocytes from blood vessels (Spector and Willoughby, 1964b). The results of studies on inflammation in different species show variability between species and often little relation to the changes seen in man. Implied is the need for studies of inflammation in man, the need for skepticism about facts extrapolated from animals to man but not tested in man, and the need to recognize the inadequacies of *in vitro* preparations used to screen new anti-inflammatory drugs.

Most serotonin in man (90 to 95%) is synthesized and localized in the enterochromaffin cells of the gastrointestinal mucosa and the serotoninergic cells of the brain; some is present in blood platelets and spleen (Sjoerdsma, 1959). Platelets acquire the free amine by active transport from the blood. Once inside the platelet, serotonin is protected from metabolism until the platelet disintegrates (Melmon and Sjoerdsma, 1963). The mechanism for the release of stored serotonin is not well understood but appears to be related to platelet aggregation (possibly dependent on ATP and ADP), platelet

breakdown (related to death, physical damage, or antigen-antibody alteration of its membrane), or direct damage to enterochromaffin cells.

Serotonin is present in inflammatory exudates for as long as one hour after injury. Whenever serotonin is present in inflammatory exudates, histamine is also present. Inhibitors of serotonin fail to influence the vascular changes of an inflammatory process in man (Spector and Willoughby, 1963).

The limited permeability-enhancing properties of serotonin are species dependent (Sparrow and Wilhelm, 1957). During inflammatory processes in man, this property seems negligible. However, because of the limited information available regarding possible interactions of serotonin with other vasoactive substances, the precise role of the amine in inflammation must be kept open for review. *Principle: The active contribution of a mediator may not be dramatic, but it may be critical for the direct effects of other mediators.*

There is ample evidence that the mediators are physically, chemically, and pharmacologically interrelated (Miller and Melmon, 1970; Kaplan et al., 1971). Under such circumstances it would not be surprising to find that antiserotonin activities may inconsistently be manifested clinically as antihistaminic or antiadrenergic effects.

Catecholamines. The catecholamines are not generally considered as mediators of inflammation. In certain situations, however, they, like serotonin, may alter the manifestations of inflammation. Epinephrine may contribute to the development of hemorrhagic lesions observed in some types of inflammatory processes, such as the Shwartzman phenomenon (Thomas, 1956; Gatling, 1958; McKay et al., 1969). The catecholamines may act locally during inflammatory processes as endogenous anti-inflammatory hormones (see Chapter 5) (Miller and Melmon, 1970). Experimental studies suggest that tissue injury results in augmented synthesis and destruction of catecholamines (Spector and Willoughby, 1965). Presumably, the locally augmented synthesis and release of these substances exert anti-inflammatory effects, and the increased local degradation limits systemic effects. More information is required, however, before the direct and indirect roles of the catecholamines during inflammatory processes can be defined.

Peptides and Proteins. Understanding the roles of peptides and proteins during an inflammatory process is a fascinating but difficult task. These substances serve as a bridge between the humoral theory and the cellular theory of inflammation. They are intimately involved in the pathogenesis of inflammation. The intrinsic coagulation system, components of complement, and components of the kinin-generating system are complex serum proteins. Each system is usually suppressed by inhibitors, and activation requires a number of complex intermediary steps. The systems and processes of activation are interrelated and share key components, so that activation of one leads to activation of components of the other systems. For example, kallikrein and C_1' esterase probably have a common inhibitor. Activation of Hageman factor can lead to the activation of

C_1' esterase and may cause kinin formation in plasma and granulocytes (Donaldson, 1968; Keller-meyer and Graham, 1968; Melmon and Cline, 1968; Webster, 1968).

Kinins. The term "kinin" refers to several polypeptides similar to bradykinin in structure and pharmacologic effect (Melmon and Cline, 1967). The three that occur naturally in man include brady-kinin, lysyl-bradykinin (kallidin), and methionyl-lysyl-bradykinin. Bradykinin may be considered a prototype for the kinins. It is a linear nonapeptide with a molecular weight of 1060 that has been isolated from plasma and synthesized (Boissonnas et al., 1963; Webster and Pierce, 1963). In man, bradykinin is one of the most potent endogenous vasodilators known. The peptide produces arterial and venular dilation by direct action (independent of alpha and beta receptors) on smooth muscle (Gokhale et al., 1966; Kellermeyer and Graham, 1968). Bradykinin increases venular permeability, causing formation of a wheal at intradermal concentrations as low as 10^{-9} M. On a molar basis, the peptide is said to be 15 times more active than histamine in producing this effect (Elliot et al., 1960).

Bradykinin is a very powerful pain-producing agent when applied to a blister base or injected intra-arterially or intradermally in humans (Keller-meyer and Graham, 1968). The peptide may also cause leukocyte adherence and migration during inflammation, but the evidence for these effects is inconclusive and may be dependent on the model chosen for experimental study.

Potentially, 4 to 11 mg of bradykinin can be derived from 1 liter of human plasma. Under normal conditions almost all of the peptide exists in an inactive precursor form and is liberated from a plasma alpha-2-globulin (kininogen) by the peptidase or esterolytic action of enzymes called kallikreins. Presumably, kininogen is produced by the liver, but the factors controlling its production have not been defined. The highest concentrations of kallikreins are in glandular tissue (parotids, pancreas, sweat glands, etc.), plasma, urine, and probably granulocytes in man.

Many of the reactions involved in kinin generation are well characterized (Erdos, 1966b; Webster, 1968; Schachter, 1969). Plasma kallikrein ordinarily exists in an inactive form called prekallikrein and requires activation by other enzymes. Activation of kallikrein is usually associated with the manifestations of acute inflammation, as summarized in Table 9–2. Hageman factor (factor XII) is usually activated first and is responsible for conversion of prekalli-krein to kallikrein. Certain components of the complement system can also be involved in peptide formation. Figure 9–1 depicts the known steps and interrelations with other systems involved in brady-kinin generation. As with histamine release, almost any process causing tissue injury can trigger the series of events resulting in the production of bradykinin. All such stimuli may not effect kinin generation by similar sequences, but activation of surface-active clotting factors, plasmin, or thrombin, or disturbances of granulocyte membranes, can contribute to kinin generation (Kaplan et al., 1971).

Once formed, bradykinin has a very short half-life in the circulation (measured in seconds). Blood plasma, erythrocytes, granulocytes, and most tissues contain enzymes called kininases, which are capable of rapidly inactivating bradykinin (Erdos, 1966a).

A bradykinin-like substance that produces pain has been isolated from human blister fluid and from inflammatory exudates and synovial fluid during acute arthritides of varying etiologies (Nies and Melmon, 1968). Bradykinin may play a role in the

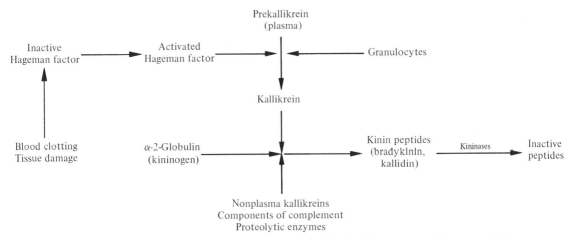

Figure 9–1. Kinin activation and destruction. The kallikrein-kinin system is intimately related and has many parallels to the blood clotting and complement systems. Activated Hageman factor can activate kallikrein and components of the complement system; activated components of complement can also participate in kallikrein activation. The kinins have no known secondary or tertiary structures and are rapidly destroyed by plasma and tissue enzymes collectively termed kininases.

Table 9–2. METHODS OF KALLIKREIN ACTIVATION DURING INFLAMMATION

1. Plasma kallikrein
   a. Initiation of blood clotting
   b. Temperature changes
   c. Immunologic mechanisms
2. Glandular kallikrein
   a. Acute inflammation of organs containing pre-kallikrein
   b. Undefined effects of catecholamines
3. Granulocyte kallikrein or kallikrein activator
   a. Phagocytosis
   b. Alteration of the cell surface
4. Kinin generation by enzymes other than kallikrein
   a. Trypsin
   b. Plasmin
   c. Components of the complement system

development of thermic edema (Rocha e Silva, 1964) and may be important in the pathogenesis of endotoxic shock (Nies et al., 1968a, 1968b; Nies and Melmon, 1971; Nies et al., 1971).

Activated Complement Components. The human complement system consists of at least 11 distinct serum proteins and 2 inhibitors (those of C_1' and C_3' esterase). Complement has long been recognized as important in many inflammatory processes (Müller-Eberhard, 1968; Schur and Austin, 1968). Activation of the complement system need not inevitably progress to its full expression of cell membrane lesions and cytotoxicity, but intermediate reaction products and complexes are formed that have pharmacologic properties important to the inflammatory process.

Anaphylatoxin is a substance of low molecular weight that can release histamine from mast cells and cause smooth-muscle contraction and changes in vascular permeability. It has been implicated in the development of anaphylaxis and other allergic reactions, but its precise biologic significance has not been fully determined. The activated C_1' component of complement promotes activation of other complement components and causes degranulation of mast cells, resulting in the release of histamine and in smooth-muscle contraction. Initially the C_1' esterase was thought to be anaphylatoxin; however, recent studies have demonstrated that C_3' and/or C_5' components of complement may serve as parent molecules for anaphylatoxin (Lepow et al., 1968, 1969). Some investigators have shown that anaphylatoxin may be formed independently of the complement system (Vogt, 1969). There probably are several anaphylatoxins that have distinctive chemical characteristics; yet they may be intimately related in terms of the mechanisms by which they are formed. Activated components of complement can also participate in the inflammatory process by virtue of their chemotactic properties and their ability to enhance phagocytosis. In addition to forming anaphylatoxin, C_3' causes immune adherence, conglutination, chemotaxis, and enhanced phagocytosis by granulocytes. C_5', C_6', and C_7' can form complexes that are chemotactic and can release histamine

independently of anaphylatoxin formation (Müller-Eberhard, 1968). *Principle: The complex interrelationships among proteins, peptides, and amines demonstrate that there is no simple approach to the inflammatory process or its treatment.*

Deficiency of C_1' esterase inhibitor can be demonstrated in a unique clinical syndrome: hereditary angioneurotic edema (Donaldson and Rosen, 1966; Schur and Austin, 1968). Patients with this genetically determined serum protein abnormality may have life-threatening symptoms and signs similar to those of severe allergy and unresponsive to the therapy used for the more common varieties of angioneurotic edema (Thorvaldsson et al., 1969). Although the biochemical hallmark of this disease is deficiency of C_1' esterase, the relationship of the protein deficiency to the pathogenesis of the angioneurotic edema remains unclear. It is not known whether the activated components of the complement system or other vasoactive substances (e.g., activation of kallikrein and production of kinin resulting from the deficiency) account for the manifestations of the disease (Landerman et al., 1962; Klemperer et al., 1968). Thus not only may the active components of a system be involved in an inflammatory response, but malfunction of the modulators of the system must also be considered as key disturbances in an inflammatory reaction.

Components of the Blood-Clotting System. The coagulation system is extremely complex. Activation of the intrinsic clotting system is initiated by activation of Hageman factor (factor XII); this agent then interacts with the complement and kinin-kallikrein systems. In addition to promoting the generation of vasoactive substances, activated Hageman factor by itself is capable of producing increased vascular permeability. Other components of the clotting system may have important functions in the development of an inflammatory process, e.g., fibrin, which can be leukotactic and is an essential component for the development of the classic Shwartzman reaction (Vassalli and McCluskey, 1964; McKay et al., 1969). Plasmin interacts with other plasma proteins such as components of complement, fibrin, and kallikrein. Such interactions might be significant in terms of an inflammatory process, but proof of the relevance of these interactions to the inflammatory process has not yet been obtained (Eisen, 1969; Hamberg, 1969). In diffuse intravascular coagulation (e.g., associated with endotoxemia), the interrelationships of the inflammatory process with abnormalities of coagulation may be critical to the outcome of the disease. The best "anti-inflammatory agent" in such a clinical setting is the drug that can stop the coagulation process—heparin.

There undoubtedly are additional contributors to the inflammatory process but their roles and identification are only now emerging (Miller and Melmon, 1970).

Cellular Contributors to the Inflammatory Process

Mast Cells. Mast cells are mainly found in loose connective tissue, frequently near vascular channels. Their most distinguishing features are their membrane-bound, spheroid, basophilic secretory granules, which may be so numerous that other cytoplasmic structures are obscured. These granules contain large amounts of heparin and other mucopolysaccharides, histamine, and several proteolytic and esterolytic enzyme systems. Serotonin is present in the mast cells of some species, man being a notable exception. The mast cell has been studied for many years (Riley, 1959; Bloom, 1965; Benditt, 1968). Much is known of its structure and composition, but its physiologic function remains unidentified. However, it seems certain that the cell contributes to the development of an inflammatory process.

Changes in mast-cell density and mast-cell granules are thought to be characteristic of many inflammatory lesions. Mast-cell preparations (either *in vitro* or *in vivo* during anaphylaxis) have been used as experimental models of inflammation. The mast cell is readily degranulated (see previous section on histamine), and the granule-bound chemical substances are released into the extracellular fluid. Histamine and probably heparin can have important influences on an inflammatory process, but much less is known about the granule esterases and proteases that are also released from the granules of the mast cell (Benditt, 1968). These enzymes may alter the course of inflammation by interactions with other substances to release or destroy kinins, to activate or destroy complement, to activate blood coagulation factors, to alter membranes of other cells such as granulocytes so that additional intracellular constituents are released, or to alter the structure and characteristics of adjacent connective tissue. Thus not only are the chemical mediators of inflammation interrelated, but so are the cellular components that contain those mediators likely to interact or influence each other's function during the inflammatory process. There is a considerable body of knowledge related to the mechanisms of inflammation. However, we have not yet seen extensive application of this information to therapeutics. Because use of basic pathogenetic information in other areas has been fruitful, we can logically expect major advances in anti-inflammatory therapeutics in the future.

Neutrophilic Polymorphonuclear Leukocytes. Neutrophilic leukocytes protect the body by ingesting and ultimately destroying potentially harmful organisms and foreign material. Phagocytosis occurs after the leukocytes have marginated along the endothelium at the site of the inflammatory process. They then emigrate through the vessel wall, attracted by many substances released or activated by the inflammatory stimulus, and ingest and digest or kill the "noxious" agent. Unfortunately, little is known of the mechanisms responsible for each of these steps, but the process is probably directly influenced by the presence of serum factors such as complement.

The leukocytes can also influence other aspects of the inflammatory response in addition to the destruction of a harmful stimulus. Leukocytes are essential in the Shwartzman phenomenon, Arthus' reaction, the acute inflammatory process of gout, and probably in other conditions (Stetson and Good, 1951; Page and Good, 1958; Cochrane et al., 1959).

Although the extent of the participation of leukocytes is not fully defined, release of their chemical contents appears to be one mechanism of action.

Leukocytes contain granules or lysosomes. These heterogeneous cytoplasmic organelles contain more than a dozen proteins that have diverse activities on tissues. Lysosomes are involved in intracellular digestive function. During an inflammatory process they can injure the cell that contains them or leave the cell so that the surrounding tissues are exposed to their contents. The lysosomal substances can influence inflammatory processes by disrupting mast cells, increasing permeability of vessels, furthering chemotaxis, or injuring normal tissue. Some proteins in the lysosome, including myeloperoxidase, are fungicidal and bactericidal (Weissmann, 1967).

There is evidence that kinin-generating activity or a kallikrein activator is present in the cytoplasm, and a kininase in the granules of neutrophils and eosinophils (Melmon and Cline, 1968). The kinin-generating capability of these cells can account for the delayed appearance of kinin-like substances in experimental inflammatory processes (Kellermeyer and Graham, 1968). Although the optimal pH of kinin generation from the cytoplasm is 7 to 8, cathepsins are active in the potentially acid environment of inflammatory foci, and granulocyte kinin production continues at pH 5.5 (Greenbaum et al., 1966).

Mononuclear Cells. *Mononuclear Phagocytes.* Polymorphonuclear leukocytes are the predominant cells in inflamed tissues during the early phases of an inflammatory process. Later, monocytes and macrophages are more numerous. The factors that attract and stimulate the mononuclear cells seem to differ from those that influence the polymorphonuclear leukocytes. The mononuclear phagocytes (monocytes and macrophages) ingest cellular debris, injured cells, some types of bacteria, fungi, protozoa, and other factors that stimulate inflammation. The mononuclear phagocytes contain many potent hydrolytic enzyme systems that are capable of degrading most of the known macromolecular constituents of tissue cells and bacteria (Cohn, 1965). Mononuclear phagocytes probably contribute to various immune phenomena by processing antigen into immunogenic complexes (Cohn, 1965; Sell and Asofsky, 1968; Weiser et al., 1969). The monocytic phagocytes are important factors in the body's resistance against certain types of infection as well as during tissue repair and healing. Although the role of the monocyte in inflammation has been extensively described, we have little information on ways to influence its function by pharmacologic means.

Lymphocytes. Little is known about the activities of lymphocytes in the inflammatory process. These cells are probably not attracted by the same stimuli that attract polymorphonuclear leukocytes and other mononuclear cells. The lymphocyte is important as a determinant of the course of the immune process because it initiates antibody production, recognizes self-antigens, contains an immunologic memory, and is critical in cellular immunity (Sell and Asofsky, 1968; Parker and Vavra, 1969).

Almost any process causing tissue injury can trigger the series of events included in the inflammatory process. Such stimuli may not produce inflammation by identical mechanisms. The release or activation of histamine, serotonin, bradykinin, complement components, and coagulation factors may contribute to inflammation; many other factors (e.g., slow-reacting substances, prostaglandins, changes in hydrogen ion concentration and oxygen tension), undoubtedly play some part in an inflammatory process. The emigration of granulocytes and mononuclear cells and their interaction have early direct and indirect effects by causing release of cellular contents. In a later phase of inflammation, these cells may be primarily involved in the immune process. *Principle: The complexity of these interlocking systems makes it unlikely that any single drug can (1) act on only one aspect of inflammation or (2) be useful in more than a few of the several varieties of inflammation. Rather, the complexity recalls a lesson learned from evolution: those functions or protective mechanisms that are most important are associated with several fail-safe systems.* In the case of inflammation, the physician must decide whether interference by use of therapeutic agents is desirable or possible. Control systems are not to be tampered with lightly (see Chapter 7), lest one problem be traded for another.

DRUGS USED IN INFLAMMATORY DISORDERS

The drugs used in inflammatory disorders have been studied extensively (Liddle, 1961; Domenjoz, 1966; Eichler and Farah, 1966; Winter, 1966; Janoski *et al.*, 1968; Kuzell, 1968). They are a heterogeneous group with differing chemical and physical properties. Generally speaking, their clinical usefulness as anti-inflammatory agents could not be predicted before they were tested for this purpose. The therapist must be wary about his knowledge of the mechanism of action of anti-inflammatory agents, because (1) they are multipotential substances that have many different properties and effects, and it is difficult to isolate a predominant anti-inflammatory effect; (2) knowledge of the inflammatory process and therefore of potential sites and modes of drug action is incomplete and has been partly based on experimental models that may bear no definite or consistent relationship to the mechanisms of inflammation in human disease; (3) anti-inflammatory agents rarely reverse the entire process of a specific inflammatory disease (e.g., during treatment of rheumatoid arthritis with corticosteroids, the swelling may diminish, the redness and pain

may disappear, and the patient may feel better, but the destruction of his joints continues. In contrast cyclophosphamide [not ordinarily considered an anti-inflammatory drug] may reverse the course of the pathology [Coop. Clinics Comm. of Amer. Rheumatism Ass., 1970]); and (4) diseases that superficially share many pathogenetic and clinical features may not respond to the same anti-inflammatory agent. For example, preparations of gold, when properly used, may ameliorate the manifestations of rheumatoid arthritis, but are without effect in other types of inflammatory disorders.

Yet anti-inflammatory drugs share many properties (e.g., they are acidic, often bind avidly to protein, uncouple oxidative phosphorylation, and competitively antagonize a number of potential mediators of inflammation). *Principle: The pharmacologic properties shared by many anti-inflammatory agents may be unimportant to their in vivo effects since these drugs are so rarely equally useful in a variety of disease states.*

Although we cannot completely categorize these drugs, the process of inflammation has been dissected into many of its components. Continued study of the anti-inflammatory agents, including factors related to their disposition, may define their categories of effectiveness, allowing more rational use of these drugs.

For the present, the drugs used to treat inflammatory disorders can be placed into two groups: agents whose major action is directed against potential mediators (e.g., the antihistamines), and agents with broader but ill-defined anti-inflammatory action (e.g., the salicylates).

Drugs That Antagonize Specific Mediators of Inflammation

Some drugs are useful in certain well-defined types of inflammation. The antihistamines can ameliorate inflammatory processes associated with some types of allergic conditions (e.g., anaphylaxis, blood transfusion reactions, and hypersensitivity phenomena). In some species, such as the guinea pig, histamine release is an important factor in producing anaphylaxis. In humans, probably many other vasoactive substances and alternate mechanisms can contribute to anaphylaxis, and histamine does not seem to account for the total anaphylactic process (Miller and Melmon, 1970). Patients with carcinoid tumors may release large amounts of serotonin into the circulation, but many of the manifestations of the carcinoid syndrome are not entirely related to the large amounts of circulating serotonin but rather to the release or activation of other substances (Melmon, 1968). *Principle: Until a single chemical is proved responsible for a symptom complex, the use of specific antagonists of a single substance can have only limited clinical usefulness.*

There is another important limitation to the use of these drugs. In addition to their ability to prevent the release, activation, or pharmacologic actions of the agonist, this class of drugs may have potentially serious extraneous pharmacologic effects. Several classes of specific antagonists (Table 9–3) have been used to block the effects of a specific chemical mediator. None of the drugs are completely selective or specific, and each can alter the release, metabolism, or effect of several local mediators. Anticomplementary substances have been used experimentally, but as yet these agents are nonspecific and are too toxic for human use (Müller-Eberhard, 1968). However, their use in clinical medicine is predicated on the hypothesis that complement has an important function in the inflammatory process. When more specific and less toxic compounds become available, (1) they may prove effective as anti-inflammatory agents, or (2) if they are ineffective but are capable of preventing complement activity or activation *in vivo*, (a) the critical effects of complement in inflammation will be questioned, or (b) the homeostatic role for complement may outweigh its role in inflammation.

Agents with Anti-inflammatory Properties of Uncertain Mechanism of Action

A number of anti-inflammatory agents were used empirically and successfully before their pharmacologic effects were studied. *Principle: The definition of the mechanism of action of a drug is not a prerequisite for its rational and successful use in clinical medicine; empiric observations may have heuristic value for the therapist.*

Salicylates. Aspirin is hardly new to clinical medicine with regard either to its use as a drug or to knowledge of its pharmacologic activity, which had been described before the Christian era. Initially, preparations of various barks were used for treatment of sepsis, pain, fluid retention, gout, "corns," sciatica, and erysipelas. Even today we know of few additional pharmacologic properties or uses for aspirin.

After Galen, an era of disrepute for therapeutics followed, mainly because of St. Augustine's dictum that all diseases of Christians were due to punishment by demons; physicians were reluctant to interfere with God's will, and most available data on aspirin were suppressed. Aspirin was rediscovered in an English country kitchen by Edward Stone, who was in search of a substitute for imported cinchona bark. His search was based on an old wives' tale about the willow: "As this tree delights in a moist or wet soil where aches chiefly abound, the general maxim that many natural maladies carry their cures along with them, or that their remedies lie not far from their

Table 9–3. INTERACTIONS OF SOME OF THE ANTAGONISTS USED AGAINST SPECIFIC MEDIATORS OF INFLAMMATION*

	REFERENCES †
Antihistamines: mepyramine, phenothiazine	1,2,3,5
Initially release histamine	
Prevent liver necrosis due to hepatotoxins	
Affect ion transport	
Act as stabilizers (lysosomes)	
Possess anticholinergic and antiserotonin properties	
Interact with catecholamines	
Block some of the effects of bradykinin	
Cause central nervous system changes	
Antiadrenergic alpha-blockers: phenoxybenzamine	2
Initially release catecholamines	
Inhibit responses to acetylcholine	
Cause central nervous system stimulation	
Antiserotonin agents: methysergide	2,4
Cause degranulation of basophilic leukocytes	
Possess vasoconstrictor properties	
Cause central nervous system effects	
Anticoagulants: heparin, coumarin	2
Strong acids—combine with any basic substance, e.g., proteins	
Affect several enzyme systems	
Uncouple oxidative phosphorylation	

* The classes of drugs presented are composed of several types of drugs with differing pharmacologic properties. The effects listed apply to the class of drugs and may not be specific for any single agent.

† 1. McLean, A. E. M.; Ahmed, K.; and Judah, J. D.: Cellular permeability and the reaction to injury. *Ann. N.Y. Acad. Sci.*, **116**:986–89, 1964.
  2. Goodman, L. S., and Gilman, A. (eds.): *The Pharmacologic Basis of Therapeutics*, 4th ed. The Macmillan Co., New York, 1970.
  3. Lish, P. M.; Robbins, S. I.; and Peters, E. L.: Specificity of antihistamine drugs and involvement of the adrenergic system in histamine deaths in guinea pig. *J. Pharmacol. Exp. Ther.*, **158**:538–43, 1966.
  4. Graham, J. R.; Suby, H. I.; LeCompte, P. R.; and Sadowsky, N. L.: Fibrotic disorders associated with methysergide therapy for headache. *New Eng. J. Med.*, **274**:359–68, 1966.
  5. Becker, E. L.; Mota, I.; and Wong, D.: Inhibition by antihistamines of the vascular permeability increase induced by bradykinin. *Brit. J. Pharmacol.*, **34**:330–36, 1968.

causes, was so very apposite to this particular case that I could not help applying it. That this might be the intention of Providence had some little weight with me" (Roueché, 1957; Smith, 1966).

Stone was able to gather 50 patients who were victims of agues and intermittent disorders. Although their seizures varied in severity, all were placed on the same regimen, reminiscent of modern studies. Each patient received 20 g of powdered willow bark dissolved in a dram of water administered every 4 hours. The results were "uniformly excellent" (Smith, 1966a, 1966b, 1966c). Studies of other anti-inflammatory agents have not been much more carefully designed.

Thus we returned to the use of salicylates. In the nineteenth century, people became interested in the compounds contained in these natural materials that made them so useful in clinical medicine. In Italy, Fontana and coworkers began to isolate the active principles from willow bark. Later, in France, Larue found that he could isolate and purify the substance responsible for the therapeutic effect. In 1838 this substance was identified in Italy as salicylic acid. Finally in Germany, Kolb managed to synthesize salicylic acid, and today most salicylates have been synthesized.

Kolb found that salicylic acid alone was efficacious but highly toxic, and several of its toxic manifestations were reported by him some time ago. While working in Germany he went to the Bayer Company to join a group of qualified organic chemists interested in the interrelationship between organic and inorganic compounds. They very rapidly synthesized sodium salicylate and phenylsalicylate. However, the prize was left to Felix Hoffmann, a junior in the Bayer Company, whose father had severe rheumatoid arthritis. Hoffmann found that the new synthetics did help his father but that they were much too irritating to the gastric area for consistent ingestion. In his search for a better medication he rediscovered and synthesized yet another derivative, acetylsalicylic acid. He then made the conventional move. Having satisfied himself by laboratory tests and domestic trial of the worth of acetylsalicylic acid, he assembled his notes and carried them dutifully to the Bayer Company's director of pharmacologic research, Heinrich Dreiser. Dreiser had been the architect of diacetylmorphine, or heroin, and was an imposing figure in European science.

Reacting to the data set before him in a manner befitting his rank, Dreiser took one look and took over. It was he who piloted acetylsalicylic acid through its first full clinical evaluation, and it was he who discarded the natural name as being hard to pronounce, hard to remember, and impossible to patent. He replaced it with the commercially seemlier name, aspirin. He cheerfully wrote and signed the pioneering report, confidently entitled "Aspirin," which first brought the compound to the attention of medicine. These events occurred toward the end of 1899; fortunately aspirin's merits took it from there.

Thus aspirin is one of the oldest compounds, senior to quinine, colchicine, and digitalis. It is also one of the least expensive and most widely used drugs in the world. At present the consumption of aspirin in the United States ranges between 26 and 74 million pounds a year. This massive consumption is alarming because aspirin is a dangerous drug. Between 17,000 and 100,000 cases of serious intoxication in children occur each year. Toxicity must not be taken lightly, for from 1 to 10% of these cases of intoxication result in death (see Chapter 17).

Absorption, Fate, and Excretion of Salicylates. Acetylsalicylic acid is usually administered orally. Its rate of absorption is dependent upon the amount of available nonionized and non-protein-bound drug and the surface area of the absorptive membrane (Levy and Leonards, 1966). Once absorbed, the salicylates are converted to salicylic acid within a few minutes. Concentrations of salicylic acid persist long after the acetylsalicylic acid has been metabolized. Thus for practical purposes aspirin is a convenient means of achieving high concentrations of salicylic acid in tissues, without causing the unpleasant side effects associated with ingestion of salicylic acid (Melmon *et al.*, 1969). Salicylic acid and aspirin have comparable anti-inflammatory properties.

In the circulation, salicylic acid is extensively bound to plasma protein. The binding involves an interaction with albumin (Levy and Leonards, 1966), and it is likely that only the free drug mediates therapeutic activity and toxicity. The bound drug acts as a reservoir and is in equilibrium with the free chemical (Stafford, 1963) (see Chapter 2). Clinically, in conditions associated with decreased serum concentrations of albumin, the apparent volume of distribution of salicylate is increased and total concentration of drug in blood is relatively low. Thus the relatively low concentration of albumin in the plasma of infants results in lower concentrations of drug in blood but higher concentrations of the drug in tissues. Evidence of salicylate toxicity may be apparent even when comparatively low doses of the drug are administered. Protein binding may also be influenced by the use of other drugs that can compete with salicylate for protein-binding sites (see Chapters 2 and 16).

Renal excretion of salicylate is influenced by the factors listed in Table 9–4. At physiologic pH, salicylates exist in a completely ionized form and the nonprotein-bound salicylate diffuses slowly across the glomerulus. Salicylic

Table 9–4. FACTORS DETERMINING RATE OF RENAL EXCRETION OF SALICYLATES

Polyuria ↑
Alkaline urine ↑
Renal failure ↓
Oliguria ↓
Acid urine ↓
Presence of other organic acids ↓

↑ Excretion of salicylates is increased.
↓ Excretion of salicylates is decreased.

acid is secreted by the proximal tubule of the kidney, probably by the same mechanisms that govern secretion of other organic acids. If the distal tubular urine is acidic, a significant amount of nonionized salicylate easily diffuses (is reabsorbed) across the distal tubular cell. When flow is rapid, back diffusion is decreased. In an alkaline urine the salicylate molecules exist in an ionized form that diffuses poorly across the renal tubular epithelium (Milne, 1963) (see Chapter 17). *Principle: The multiple factors that operate in the absorption, distribution, metabolism, and excretion of salicylates demonstrate how cookbook recipes for administration of salicylates or even reliance on the meaning of the absolute concentrations of drug in whole blood are inadequate to predict the effective or safe dosage of salicylate. Concentrations of salicylate in blood are not the sole determinants of the adequacy or safety of a dose regimen, but they can be used as therapeutic guides to proper dose.* Other factors that must be considered include the goals of therapy, the simultaneous use of other drugs, the patient's responsiveness, the effect of disease on the kinetics and pharmacology of the drug(s), and the presence of other factors that can modify the drug's action (see Chapters 2 and 15). The rate of decline of the concentration of salicylate in blood is a useful determinant of the optimum frequency of salicylate administration (Levy and Leonards, 1966) (see Chapters 2 and 17).

Mechanism of Anti-inflammatory Action of Salicylates. The efficacy of salicylates in modifying acute inflammation is unquestioned. Definition of the pharmacologic properties by which salicylates produce their effects is necessary so that (1) other agents might be designed or selected as more potent anti-inflammatory drugs; (2) clear objectives can be set in order to base the proper dose of the drug on specific aspects of the inflammatory process; and (3) more can be learned about the mechanisms of inflammation. An enumeration of the pharmacologic effects of the salicylates can be found in any standard textbook of pharmacology; only a brief description of some of the proposed mechanisms of their anti-inflammatory effects is presented here. The pharmacologic effects of salicylate that can alter tissue response to inflammation include (1) the drug's metabolic effects; (2) its interactions with proteins; (3) its action on protein synthesis; (4) its interactions with specific mediators of inflammation; and (5) its ill-defined effects (unrelated to 1 through 4 but definitely present). The last item may be the most important.

The energy derived from the oxidation of food is stored in the form of chemical bonds of pyrophosphates such as adenosine triphosphate (ATP). Hydrolysis of these phosphate bonds releases energy that can be used for cellular functions, e.g., protein synthesis. An agent that disrupts the link between the processes that derive energy by the oxidation of material and by its coupling to storage chemicals in phosphate bonds is called an uncoupling agent. At rather high but therapeutically attainable tissue concentrations, salicylates uncouple oxidative phosphorylation (Whitehouse, 1964; Smith, 1966a, 1966b). The increased vascularity at the site of an inflammatory process allows considerable perfusion of the site and can result in selectively high concentrations of drug in that tissue. By virtue of their uncoupling ability, the salicylates deprive irritated tissues of their normal energy supply. Such deprivation may impair many metabolic and other energy-dependent activities of inflamed tissues.

For example, one hypothesis holds that salicylate interference with energy sources retards the incorporation of inorganic sulfate (^{35}S) into connective tissue (Bostrom *et al.*, 1964). A serious objection to this hypothesis for the primary anti-inflammatory effects of salicylates is that thyroxine, bishydroxycoumarin, and 2,4-dinitrophenol can also uncouple oxidative phosphorylation, but these agents do not possess significant anti-inflammatory effects. However, these drugs may have differing abilities to produce the uncoupling effects in selected tissues at standard concentrations, and salicylates may possess additional and either additive or synergistic anti-inflammatory effects.

Another hypothesis is based on the capacity of salicylates to interact with proteins. Salicylic acid can penetrate the lipoidal membranes of cells, produce intracellular acidosis, disrupt enzyme systems and alter cytoplasmic proteins. By combining with lysyl, amine, thiol, and probably other groups (Skidmore and Whitehouse, 1967), high concentrations of salicylates interfere with enzymatic reactions that may be essential to the development of an inflammatory process (Smith, 1966a, 1966b; Skidmore and Whitehouse, 1967). More important, perhaps, is the binding of salicylates to plasma and tissue proteins. The salicylate-protein complex may have entirely different biochemical and physical properties than the native protein and thus may alter the internal milieu in which the inflammatory process occurs (Mizushima and Kobayashi, 1968).

Salicylates also can nonspecifically inhibit the release or the peripheral effects of the chemical mediators of inflammation. Under some circumstances, salicylates inhibit the generation of kinins by interfering with the activation of kallikrein (Nies and Melmon, 1968). Such an action may be no different from the interaction of the drug with other proteins. Acetylsalicylic acid also antagonizes some of the peripheral actions of kinins, slow-reacting substances, and probably other newly discovered vasoactive substances (Collier, 1963; Piper and Vane, 1969). Finally, salicylates stabilize lysosomal membranes and prevent the release of the lysosomal substances that can contribute to inflammatory processes (Weissmann, 1967; Kuzell, 1968).

Toxicology and Side Effects of Salicylates. Usually the term "side effect" pertains to pharmacologic effects apart from those necessary for therapeutic function. ***Principle: As long as the precise mechanism of action of a drug is unknown, those effects that are truly unrelated to the drug's desirable action will be difficult to determine.*** For example, the two most common side effects experienced with therapeutic doses of aspirin are hypersensitivity reactions and gastrointestinal bleeding, but the mechanisms for these reactions and their relation to the anti-inflammatory action of the drug are unclear.

Aspirin is far more likely to be associated with hypersensitivity reactions than are other forms of salicylate (Smith, 1966c). Hypersensitivity to aspirin is a poorly understood phenomenon but may be related to the drug's protein interactions (see Chapter 15). The symptoms may be manifested as anaphylaxis, skin eruptions, or asthma. The incidence of aspirin sensitivity in asthmatics is relatively low (2.3%), and aspirin is rarely the sole cause of asthmatic attacks (Pearson, 1963). Because the drug is rapidly eliminated, when evidence of hypersensitivity appears, withdrawal of the drug may suffice. More vigorous intervention is not usually necessary unless anaphylaxis occurs.

Gastrointestinal bleeding is a common problem associated with aspirin therapy. The stomach bears the brunt of assault, partly owing to the high concentration of the drug on the relatively small gastric surface area (see Chapters 2 and 4). After passing through the pylorus the drug is diluted, dispersed, and exposed to a much larger absorptive area. In addition, aspirin can cause pylorospasm so that the gastric mucosa is exposed to the drug for prolonged periods. Approximately 70% of patients taking 3 to 6 g of aspirin daily experience minor blood loss (less than 5 ml daily). Larger loss of blood and massive gastrointestinal hemorrhage have been reported, but the incidence of these effects is unknown in relation to total drug use (Salter, 1968). However, because enough aspirin is sold each year literally to provide the average American with pounds of it, massive gastrointestinal bleeding must be relatively rare. The blood loss usually stops after a short period of time; if it continued, most patients on chronic salicylate therapy would be iron deficient, but this has not been the case. Changes in hematocrit during salicylate therapy may not be a manifestation of bleeding. Normochromic, normocytic "anemia" can be associated with salicylate ingestion and may be due to the expansion of the extracellular fluid space by the drug (Bachman *et al.*, 1963). The mechanism for this relatively common expansion of plasma volume has not been well studied.

Salicylate toxicity is also related to the therapeutic or intentional ingestion of excess salicylate. The syndrome is complex and may involve many organ systems. Tinnitus, deafness, nausea, vomiting, and hyperventilation are common but not dangerous symptoms of salicylate intoxication. These symptoms should not be used as a clinical guide to "adequate salicylization" any more than premature ventricular beats should be used routinely to indicate "digitalization," because the appearance of symptoms usually indicates serious salicylate intoxication (Smith, 1966c). Fortunately, the serious complications of salicylate intoxication are relatively rare. The appearance of gastrointestinal hemorrhage, acid-base and electrolyte disturbances, hyperthermia, mental dysfunction, and severe vertigo (Smith, 1966c; Lamont-Havers and Wagner, 1968; Melmon *et al.*, 1969) often requires vigorous countermeasures (see Chapter 17).

Other Nonsteroid Anti-inflammatory Agents. *Phenylbutazone.* Phenylbutazone is an acidic (pK_a 4.5) anti-inflammatory substance that is rapidly absorbed following oral administration. After a single dose, phenylbutazone can be detected for 4 to 5 days. After termination of an extended course of therapy, blood levels of over 2 mg/100 ml may be maintained for 10 days (Rechenberg, 1962). Phenylbutazone is extensively bound to plasma protein. The unbound drug is either rapidly excreted or metabolized (Rechenberg, 1962). One of the major metabolites formed by the hydroxylation of phenylbutazone in man is oxyphenbutazone. Oxyphenbutazone has anti-inflammatory properties and disappears slowly from the body. Much of the ensuing discussion of phenylbutazone applies equally to oxyphenbutazone.

The mechanisms by which phenylbutazone exerts its anti-inflammatory effects are not known, but many of the proposed mechanisms are similar to those of the salicylates.

Phenylbutazone interferes with several enzymes and/or cofactors involved in cellular metabolism. The drug can uncouple oxidative phosphorylation (Whitehouse and Leader, 1967). The uncoupling properties of the drug may at least in part be related to interactions with reactive lysyl, amine, and thiol groups, since enzymes involved in oxidative phosphorylation contain these groups. The biosynthesis of mucopolysaccharide-containing tissues, such as cartilage, is affected because the incorporation of sulfur is inhibited (Domenjoz, 1966).

Complications are estimated to occur in 20 to 40% of all patients treated with phenylbutazone (Rechenberg, 1962) (Table 9–5). This statistic is not surprising because phenylbutazone and other anti-inflammatory drugs that are avidly bound to proteins displace endogenous or other drugs from binding sites and therefore increase the intensity and duration of action of these other agents. The mechanisms of these interactions are definitively explained only in selected cases (Morrelli and Melmon, 1968) (see Chapter 16). Because phenylbutazone has so many pharmacologic effects, pinpointing the reason for a reported side effect may be difficult. For example, a decrease in hematocrit in a patient receiving phenylbutazone could be related to hemodilution, depression of erythropoiesis, or gastrointestinal blood loss. As more

Table 9–5. SIDE EFFECTS OF PHENYLBUTAZONE

Sensitivity reactions

Exanthemata, dermatitis, systemic allergic reactions, toxic or allergic reactions in liver or kidneys

Gastrointestinal effects

Stomatitis, parotitis, epigastric pain, ulcer activation, gastrointestinal bleeding, diarrhea, constipation

Hematopoietic effects

Leukopenia, agranulocytosis, thrombocytopenia, anemia

Renal and cardiovascular reactions

Glucosuric and uricosuric effects, fluid retention, congestive failure

Central nervous system effects

Autonomic disturbances, lethargy, euphoria, vertigo, visual disturbances, fever, convulsant effects

sophistication is gained in recognizing and reporting untoward effects of drugs, we may find that the spectrum of drug-induced lesions is very different from that currently accepted (see Chapter 18).

Gold. Parenteral administration of gold salts can be used to treat certain inflammatory disorders. Several mechanisms to explain the anti-inflammatory effect of gold salts have been suggested, but none have been verified. Uncoupling of oxidative phosphorylation has been invoked (Whitehouse and Leader, 1967), as have inhibition of sulfhydryl systems (Goodman and Gilman, 1970), stabilization of lysosomal membranes, and inhibition of lysosomal enzymes (Weissmann, 1967) (Table 9–6).

The toxicity of gold preparations is manifested by mucocutaneous lesions and hematopoietic, hepatic, renal, and nervous system disorders. The incidence of these toxic reactions again is uncertain. Concentrations of gold in plasma do not correlate well with the development of many of its toxic manifestations (Kuzell, 1968), but toxicity may be related to the total-body content of the metal.

Indomethacin. Indomethacin is a relatively new synthetic anti-inflammatory agent. Very little is known about how it exerts its anti-inflammatory effects. Indomethacin can uncouple oxidative phosphorylation (Whitehouse and Bostrom, 1965), inhibit leukocyte migration (Phelps and McCarty, 1966), and possibly alter serum proteins (Gerber *et al.*, 1967). Indomethacin may have vasoactive properties independent of its other effects (Sicuteri, 1965) and suppresses the vascular permeability-enhancing properties of bradykinin (Willoughby and Spector, 1965). These latter properties may account for its efficacy during inflammatory conditions with exudative features (Ballabio, 1965). Indomethacin is a weak organic acid and can bind and react with serum and probably tissue proteins.

The most severe side effects of indomethacin therapy are headaches, dizziness, giddiness, gastric distress, gastrointestinal bleeding, diarrhea, edema, dermatitis, bronchial asthma, and possibly activation of latent infections (Ballabio, 1965; Kuzell, 1968).

Colchicine. Currently the major clinical use of colchicine is in the treatment and prevention of acute gouty arthritis, even though the drug does not affect uric acid metabolism or excretion. Many theories about its site of action have evolved as more is learned about the pathogenesis of gouty arthritis. Both granulocytes and uric acid crystals are vital for the production of an attack of gouty arthritis. Colchicine does not prevent phagocytosis of the urate crystals but does suppress some cellular activities subsequent to phagocytosis, involved with approximation of the phagosome to the lysosome and release of lysosomal contents into the phagosome. These activities include increased metabolic functions such as cellular respiration, granulocyte mobility, digestive vacuole formation, and lysosomal degranulation (Malawista, 1965, 1968; Malawista and Bodel, 1967). The drug may also alter the inflammation associated with gouty arthritis by interfering with the activation of the granulocyte kallikrein system (Melmon and Cline, 1968) and by preventing the release of histamine (Gillespie *et al.*, 1968).

The toxic effects of colchicine usually result from overdosage. The usual symptoms of

Table 9–6. CHARACTERISTICS OF SOME ANTI-INFLAMMATORY DRUGS*

DRUG	EFFECTS ON POTENTIAL MEDIATORS	METABOLIC EFFECTS	LEUKOCYTES	LYSOSOMES	PROTEIN	IMMUNOLOGIC SYSTEM
Salicylates	1. Interferes with kinin-forming enzymes 2. Antagonizes some of the effects of kinins 3. Nonspecifically interferes with release of histamine and alters its effect on small vessels 4. Inhibits 5-hydroxytryptophan decarboxylase	1. Uncouples oxidative phosphorylation resulting in several metabolic changes, e.g., alteration in membrane permeability to fluids and electrolytes 2. Inhibits muco-polysaccharide biosynthesis 3. Inhibits cellular respiration: mitochondrial oxidation of α-oxoacid		Stabilizes lysosomal membranes *in vitro*	Can react with serum and tissue protein, e.g., sulfhydryl, thiol and lysine groups	1. Suppresses antibody production 2. Interferes with antigen-antibody reaction 3. Inhibits antigen-induced histamine release *in vitro*
Phenylbutazone	1. Interferes with some of the effects of bradykinin 2. Nonspecifically inhibits histamine release 3. Inhibits 5-hydroxytryptophan decarboxylase	1. Uncouples oxidative phosphorylation 2. Inhibits muco-polysaccharide biosynthesis 3. Inhibits cellular respiration when linked to α-oxoacids		1. Stabilizes lysosomal membranes 2. Decreases tissue responses to released lysosomal enzymes	Reacts with several tissue and serum enzymes to alter their properties	

Drug					
Indomethacin	1. Suppresses permeability enhancing activity of kallikrein 2. Inhibits 5-hydroxytryptophan decarboxylase	1. Uncouples oxidative phosphorylation 2. Inhibits mucopolysaccharide biosynthesis	Inhibits ameboid motility of PMNs		Reacts with serum and tissue proteins
Gold		1. Uncouples oxidative phosphorylation 2. Inhibits cellular respiration		1. Is concentrated in lysosomal membrane and stabilizes the membrane 2. Inhibits action of lysosomal enzymes	Reacts with protein, e.g., sulfhydryl groups
Colchicine	1. Interferes with kinin formation 2. Prevents release of histamine *in vitro*		1. Inhibits ameboid motility of PMNs and response to chemotactic stimuli 2. Decreases cellular respiration of PMNs 3. Diminishes digestive vacuole formation	Stabilizes lysosomes	
Chloroquine	1. Antagonizes some of the effects of histamine 2. Inhibits cholinesterase activity of plasma and erythrocytes 3. Inhibits protease-induced release of peptides	1. Inhibits activity of NADH 2. Inhibits mucopolysaccharide biosynthesis	1. Inhibits response to chemotactic stimuli 2. Decreases phagocytosis of leukocytes	Stabilizes lysosomes	1. Binds with nucleic acids 2. Reacts with other tissue and serum proteins

397

* Although many of the anti-inflammatory drugs may share common properties, no single action or combination of effects satisfactorily explains their anti-inflammatory actions. The effects listed here have been observed in experimental models and may occur in man when the drugs are administered in therapeutic amounts.

toxicity are abdominal discomfort, nausea, and diarrhea. Hemorrhagic gastroenteritis is a rare occurrence. Chronic administration may result in agranulocytosis or aplastic anemia.

Colchicine's effectiveness in acute gouty arthritis has been used as a diagnostic test for the presence of gout. Yet aspirin, which has many similar pharmacologic effects, does not produce such dramatic amelioration of symptoms unless the patient has a disease (e.g., rheumatic fever) in which colchicine has little effect. Colchicine may be dramatically effective in gout because granulocyte activity plays such a prominent role in the inflammatory process and because the drug so profoundly affects the granulocyte. In fact, the granulocyte is actually thought to perpetuate gouty inflammation by increasing lactic acid production after ingestion of urate crystals. The lactic acid causes a decrease in local pH, and consequently further crystallization of urates, which leads to further phagocytosis and inflammation. Colchicine interrupts this vicious cycle by preventing the increased metabolic activity and decreased local pH that follow phagocytosis (Seegmiller et al., 1962). However, many additional factors related more to the chemistry of the drugs than to their pharmacologic effects may be important determinants of their clinical efficacy. Such factors as the distribution of the drug to affected tissues, maintenance of effective concentrations of the drug in tissues, pH requirements for pharmacologic activity or inactivation, or other factors in the milieu of the inflamed tissue that change with the state, location, and etiology of the process may also severely modify anti-inflammatory actions.

Chloroquine. Although chloroquine is well known as an antimalarial agent and is also useful in the treatment of certain inflammatory disorders (e.g., rheumatoid arthritis, systemic lupus erythematosus, and photoallergic reactions), we do not know whether common pharmacologic properties of the drug are operative in these diseases. The drug may exert its anti-inflammatory effects at several possible sites of action. Proteins that can interact with DNA are found in these diseases, and such interaction may play a role in their pathogenesis. Chloroquine combines with DNA and thereby changes the protein's physicochemical properties and biologic activity (O'Brien et al., 1966; Sams, 1967). The drug can also inhibit sulfate and mucopolysaccharide metabolism in a manner different from other drugs with similar qualitative but different temporal effects (Whitehouse and Bostrom, 1965). Release of lysosomal substances is inhibited by chloroquine (Ward, 1966; Sams, 1967); chloroquine also possesses antihistaminic properties (Sams, 1967).

Chloroquine is deposited in tissues and slowly disappears from the body after cessation of therapy (McChesney et al., 1967). The high doses and prolonged therapy necessary for an anti-inflammatory effect may result in the appearance of side effects not ordinarily encountered when the drug is used as an antimalarial agent; it may cause dermatitis and gastrointestinal disturbances. One serious side effect is severe damage to the retina, where the drug is preferentially concentrated. The retinopathy may ultimately be reversible, but may initially progress for long periods even though treatment with chloroquine has been stopped (see Chapter 15). The development of retinal changes seems to be partly related to the total amount of drug given during the course of treatment (Arden and Kolb, 1966). A few cases of chloroquine ototoxicity and neuromyopathy have been reported, but the incidence of these changes is unknown. *Principle: A number of drugs sharing common pharmacologic properties have anti-inflammatory potential. The listed effects do not describe all the effects of the drug, and few if any of the tested effects may be important clinically. In fact, when so many drugs are described by the same phrases, but each is used in different clinical states, it is likely that the pharmacologic effects critical to the usefulness of the various drugs have not been discovered.*

Corticosteroids. These drugs, the consequences of their use, and their proper administration are discussed in Chapters 6 and 7. Cortisol and its synthetic analogs have the capacity to suppress many manifestations of an inflammatory process. The quantity of corticosteroid necessary to produce anti-inflammatory effects results in a number of profound metabolic aberrations (Goodman and Gilman, 1970). Most physiologic processes are directly or indirectly influenced by these drugs. The effects of corticosteroids on experimental inflammatory processes include preservation of vascular tone and endothelial integrity and reversal of increased capillary permeability and the exudative process. Possible mechanisms of corticosteroid action include lysosomal stabilization (Weissmann, 1967), inhibition of kinin generation (Cline and Melmon, 1966), inhibition of leukocyte responses (Ketchel et al., 1958; Ward, 1966), alteration of connective-tissue metabolism and biosynthesis (Goodman and Gilman, 1970), and alteration of the immune response (Sell and Asofsky, 1968; Parker and Vavra, 1969).

High doses of corticosteroids are usually necessary to suppress an inflammatory process. The chronicity of many inflammatory diseases may require the use of an anti-inflammatory agent for long periods. When corticosteroids are used, chronicity of administration forces acceptance of a high incidence of inevitable "side effects," e.g., hyperglycemia, peptic ulceration, osteoporosis, infections, fluid retention, Cushing's medicamentosa, growth retardation, and suppression of normal adrenal-pituitary axis function (Goodman and Gilman, 1970) (see Chapter 7). Only moderately successful attempts have been made to modify the incidence of side effects, without compromising the therapeutic effects of the drug, by giving a large single dose of the drug on alternate days (see Chapters 6 and 7). Most of the corticosteroids used systemically as anti-inflammatory agents (cortisone, hydrocortisone, prednisone, prednisolone, methylprednisolone, dexamethasone, and triamcinolone) are rapidly absorbed from the gut or skin, ordinarily have a half-life in the circulation of 1 to 3 hours and maximum biologic effects in 2 to 8 hours after a given dose, and are metabolized and conjugated by the liver before they are eliminated from the body (Liddle, 1961). Theoretically, therapy on alternate days may result in decreased side effects but may also result in decreased effectiveness if relatively consistent concentrations in tissues are required (Liddle, 1961). A reduction in side effects might more logically be achieved by giving smaller repeated doses of the drug so that the total daily dose is reduced, but therapeutic concentrations in tissues could be obtained during most of the day. Because data on the efficacy and toxicity of alternate-day therapy are incomplete, the therapist must watch carefully as evidence accumulates and must make his own decision.

Immunosuppressants

"Immunosuppression" has become one of the therapeutic obsessions of immunologists (see Chapter 12). Although the search for genuine immunosuppressive agents is intense, no drugs have been discovered that selectively suppress aspects of the immune response without excessively damaging other vital functions of the host (e.g., hematopoiesis, epithelial regeneration, and important immune processes). A review of current concepts of normal immunologic function is presented in Figure 9–2. Several of the drugs clinically used to alter immunologic processes before antigen-antibody reactions occur are 6-mercaptopurine, azathioprine, methotrexate, nitrogen mustard, and corticosteroids. By the nature of their pharmacologic effects, these drugs are prophylactic agents in the treatment of inflammation. Theoretically, their effects would be unnoticeable during chronic administration unless the antigen-antibody reaction were continuous and directly responsible for maintaining the inflammatory process.

There are many individual peculiarities among the immunosuppressive drugs, but in general those drugs used to alter the immune response fall into two categories: (1) agents that are especially effective when administered before the antigen, e.g., corticosteroids and alkylating agents such as cyclophosphamide; and (2) those that are effective if administered within 48 hours after antigenic exposure, e.g., 6-mercaptopurine, azathioprine, methotrexate, and alkylating agents such as nitrogen mustard. Generalized cytotoxicity is not the mechanism of immunosuppression by these drugs. The first category of agents is lympholytic and may act by damaging antigen-sensitive cells (Sell and Asofsky, 1968). The second group of drugs can affect nucleic acid synthesis and interfere with multiplication, transformation, or differentiation of cells involved in antibody synthesis (Parker and Vavra, 1969). Neither group interferes with the productive phase of antibody synthesis, antibody-antigen interaction, or subsequent sequelae. *Principle: Although the anti-inflammatory effects of immunosuppressants may be related in part to interference with the immune response, the usefulness of the drugs often may be unrelated to these properties. They may be efficacious during chronic disease when antibody titers continue to rise and complement titers in serum remain low.*

Purine Antagonists: 6-Mercaptopurine and Azathioprine. Azathioprine is converted to 6-mercaptopurine *in vivo* and has a spectrum of activity generally similar to that of 6-mercaptopurine (Parker and Vavra, 1969). 6-Mercaptopurine blocks the interconversions of nucleotides, especially the conversion of inosinic acid to adenylic acid, thus preventing the development of the immunoblast (Figure 9–2). This drug is more effective in suppressing delayed hypersensitivity than in reducing synthesis of humoral antibodies. Azathioprine has the additional effect of binding sulfhydryl groups. The two agents are metabolized in tissues containing xanthine oxidase and must be used carefully in patients receiving xanthine oxidase inhibitors and in xanthinuric patients, because high concentrations of drug persist for a long time after standard doses are administered (see Chapter 16).

Folic Acid Antagonists: Methotrexate. Methotrexate inhibits the enzyme dihydrofolate reductase, blocking the conversion of folic acid to tetrahydrofolic acid, which functions as a coenzyme in one-carbon transfer reactions. Transmethylation reactions are necessary for the biosynthesis of purines, pyrimidines, and certain amino acids. Therapy with folic acid antagonists seems to have its greatest effect on the formation of lymphocytes and plasma cells

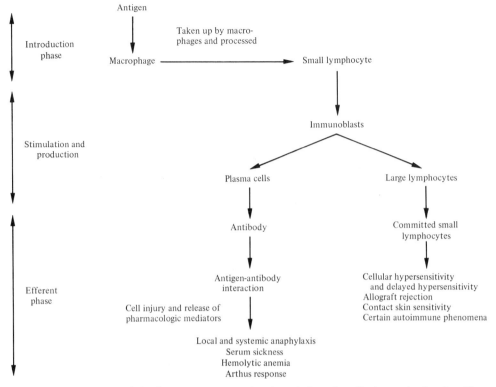

Figure 9–2. Phases of the immune response. Our knowledge of antibody production is still incomplete. Antigen is taken up and processed into highly antigenic complexes by macrophages. Antigen-sensitive cells having the appearance of small lymphocytes can be stimulated by the complexes. Stimulation apparently takes place in lymphoid tissues where macrophages and lymphocytes are in close proximity. After a latent period, large blast cells appear and give rise to antibody-producing cells (probably plasma cells). Small lymphocytes are also formed, but probably arise from different precursor blast cells than do the cells responsible for antibody production. The small lymphocytes have a long life-span and are responsible for cellular immunity and immunologic memory. Antibody titers fall as a consequence of antigen depletion, cellular death, and the failure to stimulate new cells (Sell and Asofsky, 1968; Parker and Vavra, 1969; Weiser *et al.*, 1969).

from the immunoblasts (Parker and Vavra, 1969).

Polyfunctional Alkylating Agents: Nitrogen Mustard and Cyclophosphamide. The alkylating agents can interact directly with cellular proteins, including DNA, and can produce denaturation of each. The polyfunctional alkylating agents inhibit both proliferation and differentiation of cells (see Chapter 12). Note that in Chapter 12 the "side effects" of these agents are described in relation to immunosuppression, and in this chapter in relation to diffuse interference with cell growth (responsible for the antineoplastic actions). *Principle: The "side effect" is only in the eyes of the beholder and usually describes a predictable pharmacologic effect that might be put to therapeutic use. A critical factor determining the predominant effect may be the disease state itself.*

Corticosteroids. Corticosteroids interfere with delayed and immediate hypersensitivity responses. The cellular basis for the action of corticosteroids is not well understood. These drugs produce lymphocytopenia, but antibody production continues when lymphocyte counts are low (Sell and Asofsky, 1968), and antigen-antibody interaction is not known to be affected by corticosteroids. A possible site of action for the effect of corticosteroids in immediate sensitivity reactions is inhibition of the release, activation, or effects of pharmacologic mediators. The drug may thereby reduce or prevent cell damage during antigen-antibody interactions. High doses of corticosteroids are very effective in suppressing delayed sensitivity, but prolonged drug therapy is required for continued suppression.

Side Effects of Immunosuppressants. Side effects of therapy may occur at any time in the course of treatment. The early effects are probably most familiar and include depression of bone marrow function, gastrointestinal disturbances due to interrupted cell regeneration, alopecia, and sepsis (any time during treatment). All these effects have a common pharmacologic basis. Most information on the late sequelae of immunosuppressants has been derived from studies using the drugs as antitumor agents (Watson and Johnson, 1969). The late effects of the drugs seem related to the compensatory response of the body to the constant suppression of cell reproduction and are expressed by induction of tumors, lymphomas, and possibly autoimmune diseases. These effects of drug therapy must be considered when immunosuppressants are to be used therapeutically.

Immunosuppressant Drugs as Anti-inflammatory Agents. Although these drugs can modify certain immune processes, their precise mechanisms of action during all types of inflammation are not well defined. They affect many enzyme systems and alter cellular responses to many stimuli. Many possess anti-inflammatory properties independent of immunosuppressant or antitumor effects. When used in patients with inflammatory lesions, they may exert beneficial effects unrelated to their immunosuppressant activities (Page *et al.*, 1964). For example, salicylates are effective anti-inflammatory agents; they also have mild but definite immunosuppressant qualities (Austen, 1963); yet no one suggests that salicylates are effective treatment against inflammatory lesions as a result of their effects on the immune system. Conversely, because salicylates are effective therapy for a given disorder, it would be erroneous to assume that the disorder necessarily has an immunologic basis. *Principle: Immunosuppressant drugs are multipotential. At the present time there is no direct evidence demonstrating improvement in any inflammatory disorder solely as a direct effect of the immunosuppressive activities of these drugs* (Watson and Johnson, 1969).

The rational use of anti-inflammatory drugs is based primarily on common sense and logic. In most inflammatory conditions the ideal treatment would be to remove or treat the underlying cause of the inflammatory process. Unfortunately, this approach to therapy is limited by the present lack of knowledge of the interrelationships of the multiple etiologic and pathogenetic mechanisms and of factors that determine individual tissue reponsiveness, all of which determine the nature of the inflammatory process. Because we lack complete understanding of these factors, we are frequently required to treat the consequences of tissue injury and to attempt to ameliorate the symptomatic manifestations of an inflammatory process. This approach is justifiable to maintain and preserve as much of the individual's functional capacity and well-being as possible. Symptomatic therapy does not require complete suppression of the inflammatory process.

The use of symptomatic therapy must be individualized. The vigor and aggressiveness of therapy should be governed by the severity and chronicity of the underlying condition as manifested in each patient. Acute inflammatory processes should usually be treated more vigorously but for shorter times than chronic processes. The designation of a process as "acute" implies that the condition changes rapidly and that therapy must be prompt and effective to preserve the involved tissues from extensive damage. In chronic inflammatory processes the acute damage usually is not predominant and the major consequences are related to the reparative processes (as in scleroderma); drugs used to suppress the symptoms of acute inflammation therefore have less dramatic effects. Whether drugs can be used in scleroderma or other chronic inflammatory processes to ultimately reduce the effects of extensive collagen deposits or change the relationship between the reparative process and complement and blood-clotting activation awaits evaluation (LeRoy, 1968; Wilner *et al.*, 1968a, 1968b; Nossel *et al.*, 1969).

Obviously, severe or potentially life-threatening illnesses require more vigorous therapy than do benign conditions. When potent anti-inflammatory drugs are used, the physician must be prepared to accept and manage the hazardous toxic reactions that are likely to occur. The wide spectrum of anti-inflammatory agents available for clinical use makes the use of toxic drugs in benign conditions unnecessary and unacceptable. The casual choice of corticosteroids for all problems is unjustified and dangerous. Drugs must be selected on an individual basis to obtain maximum beneficial effects and minimum toxicity.

As in any therapeutic setting, establishing therapeutic goals and evaluating the response to treatment are mandatory. The symptomatic expressions of many inflammatory processes may be vague; often, therefore, the effects of therapy cannot be evaluated by definite objective parameters. Frequently the enthusiasm and responsiveness of the physician may determine the patient's response to therapy, and the placebo effect must be considered before attributing changes in a patient's condition to drug therapy (see Chapter 14).

EXAMPLES OF
THERAPEUTIC PRINCIPLES

Although we do not understand all the pathogenetic mechanisms of an inflammatory process, or the manner in which anti-inflammatory drugs alter the process, these therapeutic agents can and should be used rationally. In this section selected diseases are used to demonstrate therapeutic principles. Each disease has been selected because it is representative of a specific type of inflammatory process. The details of therapy are not discussed, since they vary in individual cases, but the principles can be applied to most situations, even in other categories of disease.

Infectious Disease: Acute Inflammatory Disease of Known Etiology

In the presence of an acute inflammatory disease of known etiology, the treatment should be specific and directed at the underlying infection. Isolation and characterization of the infectious agent prior to initiation of therapy are helpful in selecting the appropriate chemotherapeutic agent. When anti-inflammatory agents are given during the course of an infectious process, they may mask signs and symptoms that can be useful indicators of the patient's response to antibiotic therapy: (1) if aspirin reverses the patient's fever, the therapist must consider whether the defervescence is related to specific antibiosis or to the antipyretic; (2) anti-inflammatory drugs are nonspecific in their effects and can alter the appearance of other inflammatory disorders not previously recognized; for example, a patient being treated with antibiotics for bacterial arthritis may develop gout when he is given small doses of salicylate as an analgesic; (3) anti-inflammatory agents may cause drug interactions (see Chapter 16) and may result in antagonism of the antibiotic effects; (4) anti-inflammatory agents may alter the course of an infectious process by producing bone marrow suppression. *Principle: During infectious processes, anti-inflammatory drugs can change the manifestations and course of the disease state.*

The use of anti-inflammatory drugs during an infectious process can interfere with natural and vitally important defense mechanisms against infection (see Chapter 10). For example, normal function of the leukocyte and immune processes, which may be critical in containing an infection, is affected by a number of anti-inflammatory drugs. Under most circumstances, antibiotics are only adjunctive to natural defense mechanisms in eradicating the infectious process. Although anti-inflammatory agents may ameliorate pain or pyrexia, if they are unwisely used they may interfere with necessary protective mechanisms and may prolong the duration or increase the severity of infection. Inappropriate use of corticosteroids may produce particularly glaring examples of such adverse effects (see Chapter 4 on the effects of corticosteroids used during infectious hepatitis).

Conversely, consider the rationale for "triple therapy" plus anti-inflammatory agents in patients with tuberculous encephalitis and meningitis (Weiss and Flippin, 1965; Dastur and Udani, 1966; Conner, 1967). This disease illustrates an inappropriate and life-threatening inflammatory response (expressed as either an edematous encephalopathy or allergic encephalitis or meningitis) during an infectious process. Inflammation, fibroblastic proliferation, and organization of necrotic tissue and exudation may progress after bacterial growth has been arrested. When treating this disease, the physician administers both effective antibiotics (isoniazid, para-aminosalicylic acid, and streptomycin) and sometimes anti-inflammatory agents (corticosteroids). In fact the corticosteroids, which can decrease the efficacy of antituberculous agents, may actually be life-saving, particularly when increased intracranial pressure is due to edematous encephalopathy (O'Toole *et al.*, 1969). Apparently when the antibiotics and corticosteroids are carefully managed, effective killing of the acid-fast bacilli may continue. When possible, thoughtful baseline measurements should be made before corticosteroid therapy is initiated. *Principle: Anticipate the most threatening complications of steroid therapy and plan to use measurements that will allow recognition of them. If complications cannot be reversed, set your limits (before initiating therapy) for withdrawal of the drug if the risk begins to exceed benefits.*

Determinations for blood in the stool, hematocrit, eosinophil and electrolyte concentration in blood, concentrations of glucose in blood or glucose tolerance tests, observations of blood pressure and body weight, and estimation of muscle mass and strength and deep tendon reflexes are excellent observations that can serve as guides for therapy. In addition to the amelioration of inflammation, if the drug is given in proper doses, efficacy should be accompanied by eosinopenia. If toxicity is imminent, blood may appear in the stool, the hematocrit may begin to fall, glucose intolerance may become apparent and hypokalemia, decreased reaction of deep tendon reflexes, or weakness may ensue. If blood appears in the stool, antacid therapy may be indicated (see Chapter 4); if therapy is unsuccessful, corticosteroids may have to be withdrawn. Clear-cut toxicity expressed by frank bleeding, psychosis, Cushingoid features, severe hypokalemia, muscle weakness, and loss of muscle mass can be tolerated only if the corticosteroids are likely to be lifesaving. If chronic administration of drug is planned, serious but subtle toxicity must be anticipated. For example, radiologic examination of bones for developing osteoporosis may indicate the need to withdraw the drug, since osteoporotic bones may heal poorly.

During an infectious process, the use of anti-inflammatory agents (1) must not preclude appropriate and specific chemotherapy; (2) may adversely affect the course of the infectious disease by altering normal protective mechanisms or by causing drug reactions; but (3) may be necessary to selectively suppress the "malignant" component of the inflammatory process. *Principle: During infectious processes, change in the character of the disease state caused by anti-inflammatory agents should be anticipated.*

Urticaria: Release of Mediators of Inflammation with Local Effects

Urticaria and angioedema are believed to have a common pathogenesis, and treatment is usually similar for each condition. Acute urticaria may result from immediate hypersensitivity reactions, but in over 70% of chronic cases of urticaria no primary causative factor can be found (Champion *et al.*, 1969; Michaelsson, 1969). Treatment may not be required if the urticaria is relatively mild or self-limited. However, when the lesions are strategically located they can compromise airways and must be treated. The pathogenesis of chronic urticaria has some characteristics in common with the acute disease. Histamine is released from mast cells, components of complement are activated, acetylcholine appears to be released during the production of the lesions, and release of kinins may be important (Thompson, 1968; Michaelsson, 1969).

Many drugs are considered "useful" in the treatment of both acute and chronic urticaria. However, the results of any therapy employed in this disease are extremely difficult to evaluate because so many extratherapeutic factors influence the course of the disease, which in most cases is self-limited. *Principle: The natural history of the disease must always be recalled when deciding upon therapy and before attributing any remission of the disease to drug therapy.*

The development of urticarial lesions may be brought about by many factors, including allergy, sensitivity to drugs, the presence of other systemic disease, and psychologic stress. Frequently a change in just one factor may be sufficient to modify or prevent the development of further lesions and to alleviate the patient's symptoms. When specific causal factors can be identified, ideal therapy is to avoid or eliminate these factors. If this is impossible, e.g., when generalized urticaria or angioedema follows insect stings and the patient is at high risk of further exposure to the insect, hyposensitization is indicated (Sheldon *et al.*, 1967). Most commonly the specific causal factors cannot be identified and nonspecific symptomatic therapy must suffice. When the disease is manifested by edema of the mouth, tongue, pharynx, or larynx, treatment must be immediate and is directed against vasodilation and increases in capillary permeability. Mechanical preservation of an adequate airway, sympathomimetic amines, and occasionally corticosteroids are useful.

Urticaria usually is mild and self-limited, and only antihistamines are required to make the patient comfortable. Antihistamines are efficacious because they competitively inhibit the peripheral effect of histamine. Although they have little effect on established lesions, they may prevent extension and development of new lesions. Even though the trigger mechanism producing the urticaria is unaffected by the drugs, they are efficacious because they directly antagonize a specific mediator (histamine). The side effects of the drugs are well tolerated by most patients who also appreciate their sedative properties. For obvious reasons, corticosteroids are usually not necessary or desirable in the treatment of chronic urticaria, although these drugs are justifiable in acute urticaria of allergic etiology during severe acute reactions.

Anaphylaxis: Release of Mediators of Inflammation with Systemic Effects

In man, the signs and symptoms of anaphylaxis are bronchial muscle contraction, widespread increased capillary permeability, and peripheral vascular collapse, due to the release of multiple chemicals during antigen-antibody interaction. Mediators that most likely participate in human disease include histamine, slow-reacting substance A, and bradykinin (Kaplan *et al.*, 1971). The severity of the reaction should influence treatment. Although anaphylaxis shares many common pathogenetic factors with urticaria, life-threatening respiratory involvement and/or severe hypotension and subsequent cardiac abnormalities may occur at any time during the course of anaphylaxis. Major determinants of the severity of the reaction appear to be the nature, rate, and magnitude of the antigen-antibody reaction.

The most desirable, rewarding, and specific therapy for anaphylaxis is its prevention.

Knowledge of the drugs that are most likely to precipitate an attack and routine identification of those patients who have a predisposition to atopy or past history of reactions to drugs can avert many instances of anaphylaxis (see Chapter 15). Anaphylactic reactions to penicillin account for 100 to 300 deaths annually in the United States (Feinberg, 1961). It is very difficult to avoid exposure to penicillin because so many foods contain the drug (see Chapter 15). Other dangerous drugs, foods, or sensitizing agents may be more easily avoided. Patients with known allergy should carry identification tags or cards, and their records should be prominently labeled with appropriate warnings. Whenever possible, specific tests should be employed for detecting hypersensitivity to a drug to preclude its use (see Chapter 15).

When anaphylaxis has been induced by the parenteral administration of antigen, a tourniquet should be placed on the extremity above the site of injection and vasoconstrictors should be infiltrated locally. These procedures may retard the rate of absorption of antigen at subcutaneous or intramuscular depots and may modify the severity of the reaction (Falleroni, 1968). If the reaction has commenced, its most life-threatening sequelae should be anticipated and treated.

Airway obstruction leading to hypoxia, hypoxemia, cardiac arrhythmias and peripheral vascular collapse may occur, with rapidly fatal consequences. Simple measures should be taken to maintain an open airway and assist ventilation to prevent hypoxia. Use of bronchodilator agents (see Chapter 6) may be lifesaving. *Principle: Sometimes the "ancillary" measures aimed at preservation of vital organ function are of paramount importance and should precede more specific measures.* This principle differs little from those applied to poisoning (see Chapter 17), respiratory disease (see Chapter 6), and cardiovascular shock (see Chapter 5).

Despite the possible contribution of histamine to anaphylaxis, the use of antihistamines is usually futile. Many mediators are responsible for the disorder, and antagonism of only one may have little noticeable effect; the histamine may already be present at receptor sites before antihistamine can be administered. Antihistaminics are effective only when the lesions are not established or when the drugs are administered prior to the complete absorption of the antigen. Even when antihistaminic drugs are given early, they offer only partial protection from the development of new lesions or the delayed complications of anaphylaxis. *Principle: Because anaphylaxis is produced by several mediators of inflammation, specific antagonists of only a single*

substance do not have a critical role in its treatment.

When bronchoconstriction is prominent during anaphylaxis, the principles of therapy for asthma described in Chapter 6 relating to choice of agents and assessment of efficacy should be applied. Rapid administration of rationally chosen drugs is essential. Epinephrine is the standard to which alternative agents must be compared (Sheldon *et al.*, 1967). Epinephrine has stood the test of time, and its beta-stimulating properties can contribute to bronchodilation and to inotropic and chronotropic effects on the heart, but its alpha-stimulating effects may cause systemic vasoconstriction that may be detrimental. Although the latter effect probably is not critical in most patients, there is a clear need for comparison of the standard agent with drugs that produce more prominent and exclusive beta sympathomimetic action (e.g., isoproterenol) (see Chapter 5). If respiratory function is severely impaired, and the response to drug therapy is not immediate or satisfactory, tracheostomy should be performed. *Principle: Limitations of drug therapy must be recognized. Severe airway obstruction may require more vigorous therapy than can be obtained with the use of drugs alone.*

Large doses of corticosteroids may be beneficial in reducing bronchospasm and inflammatory edema associated with anaphylaxis. The maximum biologic effect of corticosteroids does not occur until minutes to hours after administration. They may be useful but are not primary drugs in reducing the immediate danger of respiratory failure or edema.

Hypotension in anaphylaxis may be caused by vasodilation related to hypoxia, by the release of the mediators described above, by vasodilation caused by drugs used to treat bronchospasm, by hypovolemia associated with the formation of edema, or by sudden decreases in cardiac output. Whether this complication requires treatment depends on the adequacy of tissue perfusion. Proper treatment of "shock" depends on accurate assessment of the contributory factors; the principles of therapy are identical to those stated in Chapter 5.

Myocarditis: Inflammation of a Vital Organ

A number of diseases are associated with myocarditis. Infectious processes of viral, bacterial, rickettsial, fungal, and parasitic etiology can involve the heart. Even serum sickness is an example of an allergic disease associated with myocardial inflammatory changes. Diseases that produce myocarditis by unknown mechanisms but are believed to involve immune reactions include rheumatic fever, connective-tissue diseases and postcommissuro-tomy syndrome. Frequently the myocarditis is not recognized and is an unimportant feature in the course of the disease; at other times myocarditis may be the dominant process. If the underlying etiology is unknown, the diagnosis of isolated or primary myocarditis may be made. Many types of myocardial inflammation are benign and self-limited and require no anti-inflammatory therapy.

The heart cannot regenerate its tissues, and when an inflammatory process affects it, irreversible tissue damage and impairment of cardiac function can occur. When therapy is indicated, an attempt should always be made to eliminate or neutralize any known underlying cause for the myocarditis. When no specific etiology can be identified but the myocardial inflammation is severe enough to cause cardiac dysfunction, symptomatic treatment with anti-inflammatory drugs is justifiable and may prevent the acute complications of edema, myocardial failure, and abnormalities in conduction.

The treatment of rheumatic fever illustrates principles in the use of anti-inflammatory agents in myocarditis. Salicylates may strikingly decrease the acute inflammatory components of rheumatic fever and are the preferred treatment in most cases. Their effects are so rapid and impressive that some have mistakenly considered response to the drug to be useful in diagnosing rheumatic fever. However, salicylates can also produce dramatic benefits in myocarditis of other origins and, not surprisingly, fail to improve some patients with definite rheumatic fever. Salicylates and corticosteroids are effective anti-inflammatory drugs, but not specific agents against rheumatic carditis. Despite their palliative effects, these drugs can neither terminate the myocardial inflammation completely nor ultimately prevent cardiac fibrosis or scarring (Kuttner, 1965; Rutstein and Densen, 1965). This fact should emphasize that prevention is much more critical than the nonspecific effects of anti-inflammatory agents. *Principle: From the complex pharmacology of most anti-inflammatory drugs we can predict both their nonspecific effects on most inflammatory states and the limitations of diagnostic implications based on response to them.*

In rheumatic fever, salicylate is the drug of choice although intensive therapy is frequently required before worthwhile effects are seen. Available studies have failed to demonstrate conclusively the superiority of corticosteroids or other anti-inflammatory drugs over the salicylates (Kuttner, 1965; Rutstein and Densen, 1965). In addition, toxic effects of salicylate therapy are generally minor and well known and

often can be prevented without compromising anti-inflammatory effects. When they cannot be prevented (e.g., fluid retention associated with corticosteroids or salicylate therapy that precipitates congestive heart failure), they can be easily recognized and managed.

Salicylates should be administered cautiously to patients with severe carditis in which the inflammatory edema of the myocardium may be life threatening. Corticosteroids may produce a more rapid decrease of inflammatory manifestations than salicylates, but should be reserved for critical clinical settings because the risk involved in chronic use of corticosteroids far outweighs the risks of salicylates.

Gout: A Chronic Disease of Known Etiology with Acute, Intermittent Manifestations of Inflammation

Acute gouty arthritis is precipitated when leukocytes ingest urate crystals (Klinenberg, 1969). Although the exact contribution of leukocytes to the inflammatory process is not known, at least part of the inflammation is associated with release of the mediators of inflammation and release or activation of chemical mediators that may lie dormant in synovial fluid.

The treatment of acute gout should be directed toward the rapid relief of the inflammatory synovitis and arthritis. Colchicine, which has no effect on urate metabolism or excretion or on tophi or urate deposits in tissues, is one of the most valuable drugs for treatment of an acute attack of gout or for prevention of exacerbations of the arthritis. The drug seems to be relatively specific for acute gout (acute sarcoid arthritis responds nearly as well). The relative specificity may be due in part to the intensity of the leukocyte response and to the extremely important role of this cell in mediating and perpetuating the inflammatory response of gout by decreasing extracellular pH and causing further precipitation of urate crystals (Malawista, 1968). Colchicine may alter other inflammatory states, but the effect seems less dramatic when the process is indolent and characteristically less severe than gout (Klinenberg, 1969; Mikkelsen and Robinson, 1969). Another advantage of colchicine in treatment of acute gout is its lack of interference with diagnostic studies related to serum and urine urate concentrations. *Principle: Take advantage of valid therapeutic observations in selecting drugs that appear to be specific for a given disease. Knowledge of the pathogenesis of disease and the pharmacology of the drug may lead to discovery of more specific drugs that may replace the time-honored primary agent.*

There are considerable variations in individual sensitivity to colchicine, and on occasion its gastrointestinal side effects preclude its effective use. Phenylbutazone, oxyphenbutazone, and indomethacin are alternate drugs that have a wider spectrum of anti-inflammatory effects than colchicine (Scott, 1969).

Salicylates are less effective than any of the above drugs in the management of acute gouty arthritis, perhaps because low doses decrease urate excretion and may precipitate or aggravate an acute attack of gout. When daily salicylate administration exceeds 5 g, uricosuria ensues (Yu and Gutman, 1959), but such large amounts of the drug are not usually well tolerated. These effects of salicylate are mentioned not because the drugs should be used to treat gout, but because they are readily available and are frequently used by patients who seek symptomatic relief prior to seeing a doctor. *Principle: An inadequate history or an inadequate appreciation for the pharmacology and use patterns of proprietary agents may be a deterrent to therapy.*

Once the acute inflammatory manifestations of gout are controlled, the underlying mechanisms contributing to accumulation of uric acid in tissues should be evaluated. Several known mechanisms can cause hyperuricemia and gout, but each involves either overproduction or underexcretion of uric acid (Klinenberg, 1969; Mikkelsen and Robinson, 1969) (see Chapter 7). The long-term management of gout is aimed at reducing hyperuricemia and thereby reducing deposits of urate. Control of hyperuricemia with chemical agents may work in one of two ways: (1) drugs may increase the rate of uric acid excretion by the kidney (e.g., probenecid and sulfinpyrazone); or (2) drugs can decrease the synthesis rate of uric acid (e.g., allopurinol). Allopurinol is a powerful inhibitor of xanthine oxidase, an enzyme responsible for the oxidation of xanthine and hypoxanthine to uric acid. The drug is most attractive because it can result in benefit regardless of the mechanism leading to accumulation of uric acid.

Neither class of agent is useful in the treatment of acute gouty arthritis, but prolonged administration may reduce the number of acute attacks. As long as the total body pools of urate are expanded and in equilibrium with plasma, the concentration of uric acid in plasma may remain elevated, even though synthesis rates are diminished. Persistent high concentrations in plasma imply that (1) there may be a persistent need for agents such as colchicine to prevent acute attacks of gouty arthritis (Mikkelsen and Robinson, 1969); and (2) changes of uric acid concentration in plasma are not necessarily good indices of the effectiveness of inhibitors of synthesis. Gout can be produced when cells turn over rapidly, as in some leukemias.

Rheumatoid Arthritis: A Chronic, Systemic, Incurable Disease That Usually Is Not Life Threatening

Rheumatoid arthritis is a systemic disease usually manifested clinically by inflammation of the joints and connective tissues (Goetzl *et al.*, 1971). Our knowledge of the inflammatory process in rheumatoid arthritis is limited but useful in selecting anti-inflammatory drugs. The disease usually develops gradually and is indolent; only in rare instances is the severity of the disease such that it can be mistaken for gout. Drugs to ameliorate acute gout are unlikely to affect the indolent process of rheumatoid arthritis. Factors responsible for the inflammatory process may include phagocytosis by leukocytes of rheumatoid factor complexed to aggregated IgG, or initiation by an immunologic response of local production of mediators of inflammation. The pathogenesis of rheumatoid arthritis is not well understood, and we do not know how the acute inflammation is related to the eventual destruction of joints. The anti-inflammatory and cytotoxic agents used to treat rheumatoid arthritis affect only the inflammation and do not prevent joint destruction. A recent important exception to this statement is cyclophosphamide (Coop. Clinics Comm. of Amer. Rheumatism Ass., 1970). The intensity of the disease fluctuates, as does the relative involvement of different joints at the same time. The evaluation of any type of drug therapy in this unstable disease is extremely difficult. Spontaneous remissions and exacerbations are a part of the natural history of rheumatoid arthritis, and the spontaneous change can easily be mistaken for drug effect. The disease is usually benign, and even with the most conservative treatment a large number (up to 50%) of patients with rheumatoid arthritis improve (Short and Bauer, 1948). The response of the patient to any type of drug therapy is frequently related to the desire of the patient to find some relief from his symptoms and to the enthusiasm of the physician for the effectiveness of the chemical agent (see Chapter 14). Placebo effects are common; in one study 71% of patients with arthritis demonstrated some type of response to placebo adminstration (Morison *et al.*, 1961). Such favorable responses to any type of intervention have led many uncritical investigators " down the garden path" and many physicians to report enthusiastically on harmful drugs such as corticosteroids and dimethylsulfoxide. *Principle: When the course of a disease is variable in severity and long in duration: (1) modest therapeutic goals should be set; (2) study of the individual patient is mandatory before any therapeutic regimen associated with substantial risk is begun; (3) conservatism should be a guiding principle, as any therapeutic plan chosen may be required for long periods and even moderate measures (physiotherapy) may maintain functional capacity as well as do toxic drugs; (4) the full potential of the most conservative therapy should be explored and continued before additional measures are chosen; (5) the need for therapy should be evaluated frequently, particularly if any risk is associated with the regimen; and (6) drug interactions should be anticipated as additional diseases appear that require drug treatment.*

A strong doctor-patient relationship, physical therapy, and vocational rehabilitation may be the most meaningful long-term measures in all patients. If the disease is mild but the inflammation is unresponsive to these measures, drugs must be considered. Their use is primarily aimed at controlling the inflammation, pain, and systemic symptoms and at minimizing immobilization. The most useful drugs for the treatment of rheumatoid arthritis are aspirin, antimalarial agents, intra-articular or parenteral gold, corticosteroids, and "immunosuppressants" or cytotoxic agents. They are used in sequence and in combination as the severity and resistance to remissions increase.

If chemotherapy is needed, salicylates should initially be used; a considerable number of patients require no further treatment. Both the anti-inflammatory and the analgesic effects are beneficial in rheumatoid arthritis (Short and Bauer, 1948; Decker *et al.*, 1964; Duthie *et al.*, 1964; Bayles, 1968; Christian, 1968). As demonstrated by pharmacokinetic data (see Chapters 2 and 17) and the clinical response to aspirin, the drug has its greatest anti-inflammatory and analgesic effects when administered regularly, e.g., every 4 hours (Ansell, 1963). There is no established optimum therapeutic concentration of salicylate in blood, but high concentrations are required for optimum beneficial effects. Some circumstances in rheumatoid arthritis require attention to dosage. Albumin concentrations in blood may be low and protein binding of salicylates diminished; thus increased tissue concentrations and both therapeutic and toxic effects may occur at unusually low blood levels of salicylates. *Principle: The disease state may alter the absorption, distribution, or metabolism of drugs and may result in enhanced beneficial or toxic effects after standard doses.*

Salicylate concentrations in blood should be frequently measured after a given dose to obtain the rate of disappearance of the drug and to guide the dose and frequency of drug administration. Attempts to adjust salicylate dosage by using amounts slightly below the dose that produces toxic symptoms (e.g., tinnitus) are irrational. Symptoms of toxicity vary in different patients, and serious salicylate toxicity can occur before tinnitus appears. If indomethacin is considered, remember that its effects have not been demonstrably superior to those of the salicylates (O'Brien, 1967).

If other anti-inflammatory drug therapy is required in addition to salicylates, the choice is empiric, but gold and the antimalarials are usually preferred when salicylates prove inadequate and when corticosteroids seem unnecessary or undesirable. These agents are used as *supplemental* drug therapy and should not be substituted for salicylates. The major indication for either drug is the continuing presence of active inflammation despite the use of salicylates. Neither gold compounds nor the 4-aminoquinolines affect deformity, ankylosis, or other noninflammatory components of rheumatoid arthritis, and they should not be used for this purpose.

Controlled studies documented gold-induced improvement by all criteria, except radiologic, after 3 months of therapy; but 2 years after the completion of the course of therapy most of the improvement had disappeared (Empire Rheumatism Council, 1960, 1961a). Prolongation of the initial effectiveness of gold therapy has been attempted by administration of "monthly" maintenance therapy. However, there is no convincing evidence that such a schedule of supplemental treatments prevents relapse. These studies also refuted the theory that toxic reactions were associated with greater therapeutic benefit from gold (Empire Rheumatism Council, 1961a, 1961b). The controlled studies of the 4-aminoquinoline antimalarial drugs have demonstrated that prolonged periods of drug administration can gradually reduce symptoms related to the inflammatory components of rheumatoid arthritis (Zvaifler, 1968). The choice between antimalarial agents and gold therapy is equivocal. The clinical usefulness of each agent is limited by its respective toxicity and the prolonged period before beneficial or toxic effects occur. Gold can cause mucocutaneous lesions or hematopoietic, renal, and liver damage at any time during treatment and in some cases after treatment is terminated. It should not be used in patients with dermatitis or pre-existing renal or hepatic impairment. Chloroquine can cause retinal damage and severe visual impairment and should not be used in patients with pre-existing retinal disease or significant visual disturbances, or in patients who cannot be repeatedly examined by an ophthalmologist.

If no response to gold or antimalarials is observed at the recommended low doses of these agents, worthwhile benefits will not be obtained at higher doses, but toxic manifestations are more likely to occur. If the response to either of the drugs is disappointing, measures other than increasing the dose of the drug should be attempted. Such measures might include the use of alternate drugs. *Principle: If a small dose is beneficial a large dose is not necessarily more beneficial but does expose the patient to a greater risk of toxicity.*

In few patients with rheumatoid arthritis can long-term corticosteroid therapy be justified. This class of drugs should not be used until a prolonged trial of conservative management employing less hazardous drugs has proved ineffective. The physician must be sure that the results he hopes to attain will be justified when the patient develops sodium retention and Cushing's medicamentosa, loses muscle mass, bruises easily, bleeds from his ulcer, becomes psychotic, breaks his osteoporotic bones, and is unable to control his diabetes. In most clinical settings corticosteroids should not be used alone or as an initial drug in the treatment of rheumatoid arthritis. *Principle: There is no excuse for substituting an incurable and disabling complication of therapy for a moderately disabling but tolerable disease.*

The choice among corticosteroid preparations is wide but not too difficult to make. Newer, more potent agents appear frequently, but increasing potency per se is no asset. Chemical modification of the corticosteroid molecule has produced compounds that retain anti-inflammatory properties but have only minimal effects on fluid and electrolyte metabolism. Unfortunately all preparations retain the ability to produce metabolic abnormalities. The principles of use of corticosteroids as pharmacologic agents are discussed in Chapters 6 and 7.

Corticosteroid therapy is adjunctive to a carefully planned comprehensive program of individualized care. The corticosteroids do not stop or significantly alter the natural course of the underlying disease (Medical Research Council and Nuffield Foundation, 1955; Empire Rheumatism Council, 1957); both the physician and the patient must understand the goals and the limitations of corticosteroid therapy. The primary goal is to suppress the rheumatic inflammatory process (fever, rash, exudation) when less hazardous drugs have not proved adequate. These drugs do not correct existing deformities, but they can cause further deformity, muscle wasting, and debility.

In order to suppress the inflammatory process without producing less easily controllable diseases, certain guidelines are useful: (1) the smallest amount of drug that attains the therapeutic goal is the optimum dose; (2) complete suppression of the rheumatic process by corticosteroids is neither necessary nor desirable; (3) the use of these drugs is supplemental (patients receiving corticosteroid therapy should also be maintained on a full program of more conservative treatment); (4) increases in activity of disease frequently can be managed successfully by altering other components of the program (e.g., salicylates) without increasing the dose of steroid; (5) patients should be cautioned against self-treatment (changing their dose of medication in order to achieve greater symptomatic relief); (6) the toxicity of these drugs should be minimized by keeping the dose at the lowest possible level; and (7) corticosteroids should be withdrawn as soon as possible after symptomatic manifestations of the inflammatory process have been reduced.

Cytotoxic or immunosuppressive drugs including nitrogen mustard, azathioprine, 6-mercaptopurine, chlorambucil, cyclophosphamide, and methotrexate are frequently used to treat patients with rheumatoid arthritis (Fosdick, 1968; Baum and Vaughn, 1969). The results have been variable and difficult to assess. Part of the variability may be attributed to the hypothesis that forms the basis for use of "immunosuppressive therapy." Although aberrations of components of the immune mechanisms do exist in many patients with rheumatoid arthritis, a cause-and-effect relationship has not been demonstrated between the immune disturbance and the initiation or continuation of the rheumatic process. These abnormalities of the immune system may be a result of the disease process rather than a cause, and they may be protective rather than destructive.

The site and mechanism of action of this class of drugs are not known. Ostensibly these agents might reverse the immune abnormalities that might have some pathogenetic role. Yet when they are used in rheumatoid arthritis there is no demonstrable change in the abnormal immune functions as judged by changes in the latex titer, sensitized sheep-cell agglutination, isoagglutinin titer, and anti-D titers (Brocteur and Moens, 1965; Moens and Brocteur, 1965). On the basis of such evidence the drugs may act by exerting nonspecific anti-inflammatory effects or generalized low-grade toxic effects on cells. Hence they should be designated as "cytotoxic" rather than as "immunosuppressive."

Additional difficulties are encountered in evaluating the efficacy of cytotoxic therapy in rheumatoid arthritis. The definition of the terms "active disease," "improvement," and "remission" is imprecise. In general, most patients in whom the cytotoxic drugs are used represent therapeutic failures to all other drug therapy, including corticosteroids. Thus it is difficult to assess what effect these drugs may have had if they had been used earlier or whether this type of patient is the ideal candidate for cytotoxic therapy. Most patients treated with cytotoxic agents have also been maintained on additional drug therapy, usually low-dose corticosteroids. The beneficial effects of the cytotoxic drugs are based on the reduction in corticosteroid requirements. There are many pitfalls in this type of evaluation. Even if such criteria were acceptable, there are other drugs available (e.g., salicylates) that also could effect a reduction of corticosteroid requirements (Christian, 1968). Another point that must be settled is whether the slight reduction of corticosteroids in patients who are usually already taking low doses justifies exposure to the potential toxicity of cytotoxic drugs. *Principle: The cytotoxic drugs, like all other currently available drug therapy for the treatment of the rheumatic diseases, are nonspecific; their effects usually are suppressive and not curative. These drugs do not alter the natural history of the disease. Their therapeutic value, therefore, must constantly be assessed in terms of their limited suppressive effect and their great toxic potential.*

Well-tolerated, relatively benign drug therapy should be used until more is known about the pathogenetic mechanisms of the disease and the mechanism of the anti-inflammatory effects of the cytotoxic drugs. The use of these drugs in rheumatoid arthritis should be reserved for unusual circumstances, such as well-disciplined investigational use or, in some cases, as a last resort to preserve life or vital organ function when all other measures have been used appropriately without worthwhile benefit.

Rheumatoid arthritis is only one of several chronic debilitating diseases for which there is no definitive cure. These situations are potential traps to the well-meaning but uncritical investigator or therapist; witness the development of dimethylsulfoxide (DMSO) (Editorial, 1965). DMSO is a close relative of acetone and is an excellent solvent. Solutions of 70% concentration and above, when applied to the epidermis, markedly increase the penetration of various substances through the skin. This chemical was also alleged to possess anti-inflammatory and analgesic properties. Clearly this agent deserved serious, careful consideration and investigation. Preliminary reports of its effects were touted by the lay press, and the chemical was lionized before adequate information clearly defined its toxic and therapeutic potential. Patients demanded to have this agent to relieve their pain and improve their activity. Worthwhile and disciplined scientific study was compromised without reason. Later, when some of the serious toxic effects of the chemical were found, the drug was completely withdrawn even from investigational use. This is only one example of what did happen as opposed to what can and should happen in the development of a potentially useful anti-inflammatory agent. There is no good reason to proceed through the wild swings of popularity and debasement usually accorded any new drug on the market (Figure 9–3).

Systemic Lupus Erythematosus: A Chronic Life-Threatening Systemic Disease

Many of the principles relating to the treatment of rheumatoid arthritis can be applied to systemic lupus erythematosus. Both diseases

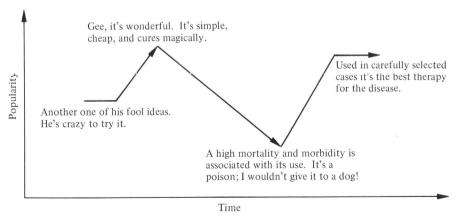

Figure 9–3. What may happen in the course of clinical trials during the development of a drug.

represent active inflammatory lesions; both are chronic but have variable courses with exacerbations and remissions; both are characterized by abnormalities of the immunologic system, but in each instance the pathogenic importance of immunologic anomalies is unclear; and both diseases have inflammatory activity that affects a number of organs. However, in lupus erythematosus the function of vital organs (heart, kidneys, brain, lungs, and hematopoietic system) is likely to be so impaired that the inflammation threatens survival. Specific therapy is not available for either disease and anti-inflammatory therapy does not produce definitive cures. Both diseases respond to the same anti-inflammatory agents, but frequently patients with lupus erythematosus require more vigorous treatment with the most potent and potentially more toxic anti-inflammatory agents. The comparison is superficial, but the available therapy is directed only against the superficial similarities of the two diseases. *Principle: Classification of diseases by the characteristics that may be reversed by treatment may be helpful for developing a logical approach to therapy.* Such classification may be most useful when specific and definitive therapy is not available. This principle should become obsolete as we learn more about the dissimilarities between inflammatory diseases and can design specific and definitive therapy.

Salicylates may be the only drug therapy required for patients with mild disease. The drug often ameliorates mild arthralgia and febrile states in systemic lupus erythematosus as effectively as in acute rheumatic fever or rheumatoid arthritis (Dubois, 1967). Patients with systemic lupus erythematosus or rheumatoid arthritis may develop renal tubular acidosis (RTA) (Morris, 1969) (see Chapter 3). If present, the effects of RTA on excretion of salicylate must be considered; doses may have to be increased and given at frequent intervals to obtain a therapeutic effect. Without knowledge of the disease's effects on the pharmacokinetics of salicylates, the therapy might be judged ineffective when in fact the dose is inadequate.

The antimalarials are valuable in the treatment of skin lesions and mild arthritis in patients with lupus erythematosus. When the antimalarials are used they usually supplement other drug therapy, such as salicylates. They are used for the same purposes as in rheumatoid arthritis and require the same delay period before the drug response develops. If no worthwhile response occurs to standard doses of one antimalarial, it is unlikely that higher doses or a congener will be effective. Periodic examinations by an ophthalmologist who is familiar with the ocular signs of antimalarial toxicity are required, and the drug must be discontinued at the first sign of such toxicity.

When the course of the disease is fulminant, the function of several vital organs may be compromised, and therapy should be vigorous enough to suppress most of the disease's activity. During a crisis in lupus erythematosus, relatively large amounts of corticosteroids should be used initially. Experience, but not controlled experiments, has demonstrated that the corticosteroids can terminate a lupoid crisis. When only a single organ is threatened, e.g., in patients with isolated but severe nephritis, some physicians recommend doses of corticosteroids that are sufficient to suppress not only the general systemic manifestations of the disease but also all the renal abnormalities (Pollak *et al.*, 1964). Other studies have shown no advantage in using doses of steroid higher than those necessary to suppress the general manifestations of the disease. Although the debate is unresolved, the objectives of therapy with steroids are the suppression of inflammation and the preservation of organ function, and the dose should be set according to the severity of the disease and the organ that is affected.

The immunologic abnormalities in patients with lupus erythematosus have made the use of immunosuppressive drugs fashionable, if not efficacious. Objections to this therapy are analogous to those associated with rheumatoid arthritis. At the present time there are no controlled studies evaluating the efficacy of this treatment. Hopes are based on sporadic and incomplete clinical reports that are difficult to interpret. However, the immunologic aberrations and clinical manifestations of the disease can be affected independently by these drugs. Thus even if they are efficacious, they may not significantly affect the immune system but, as in rheumatoid arthritis, may act by nonspecific anti-inflammatory effects or cytotoxic activity.

An additional principle should be stressed: although the disease may not be caused by immunologic abnormalities, laboratory tests measuring some aspect of the quantitation of the abnormality are often used as criteria for judging the benefits or failure of therapeutic interventions. Such criteria may be legitimate, but measurements related to objective changes in the function of the damaged organs are more meaningful. In few instances can therapy be rationalized to treat only the abnormalities found in laboratory tests that do not directly represent change in function of a vital organ.

Psoriasis: A Local Chronic Inflammation

Psoriasis is a chronic, recurrent, generally benign disease that usually is isolated to the skin.

Because the disease is localized and usually neither life threatening nor severely incapacitating, it is susceptible to mild local therapy. Daily applications of crude coal tar to the lesions followed by ultraviolet irradiation of the lesions represents the standard treatment of most cases of psoriasis. The mechanisms whereby these maneuvers suppress the disease are unknown. However, no other therapy offers equivalent success or safety (Scott, 1966; Perry et al., 1968).

When the standard treatment fails or is impractical, corticosteroids applied topically are efficacious. Corticosteroids are absorbed percutaneously (Feldmann and Maibach, 1966). The amount of drug absorbed depends on the type, frequency, and amount of corticosteroid used, the vehicle or base in which it is contained, the thickness of the skin upon which it is applied, the condition of the skin (denuded or inflamed areas allow more absorption than normal skin), and the use of occlusive dressings that enhance tissue maceration and drug absorption. Topical corticosteroids can suppress the hypothalamic-pituitary-adrenocortical axis even before features of Cushing's medicamentosa appear (Carr and Tarnowski, 1968). Such an effect is usually insidious and is potentially dangerous if the patient undergoes stress requiring unusual corticosteroid secretion or if his therapy is suddenly withdrawn and he becomes adrenally insufficient. *Principle: Local administration of a drug does not guarantee local restriction of effects. Always be aware of systemic effects of a drug regardless of its route of administration. The converse is also applicable: if a drug is administered systemically, there is no guarantee that it will reach all tissue sites of concern.*

Examples of the first part of the principle include absorption of neomycin from the gut, absorption of corticosteroids from inflamed joint spaces, and absorption of epinephrine from injections into the gingiva. Examples of the inability of drugs to reach all critical sites are numerous (see Chapter 2), but an instance that is often overlooked is transport of antibiotics to joint spaces or to the lumen of bronchi. The systemic effects frequently may be minimized by using the drug sparingly so that only the desired local effect is predominant.

Corticosteroids may be directly injected into psoriatic lesions when the lesions are resistant to other therapy. Although such treatment may be temporarily beneficial, the injections must be repeated at regular intervals. This mode of therapy may also produce systemic effects and may suppress the pituitary-adrenal axis (Berger and Orentreich, 1968).

Systemic administration of corticosteroids should be reserved for patients who develop acute psoriatic erythroderma or systemic toxemia caused by psoriasis. Ordinarily, the chronic, recurrent, benign nature of psoriatic lesions and the limited and palliative effects of the drug do not warrant the unavoidable side effects associated with long-term use of steroids or the severe exacerbations of the disease when corticosteroid therapy is terminated.

Methotrexate has been used extensively and successfully in patients with psoriasis (Rees et al., 1967). It is used on an empiric basis, and like the other agents discussed, it has nonspecific and palliative effects. Although the pathogenetic mechanisms of psoriasis are not fully understood, methotrexate is probably effective because of its toxic cellular and antimetabolic properties. Although the success of methotrexate has been impressive, so have its toxic effects; if it is indicated at all, its use should probably be restricted to potentially life-threatening forms of psoriasis (Caron, 1969). In addition, some investigators suggest that the drug be used in disease that is socially crippling or emotionally disabling. This suggestion may be a therapeutic "cop-out," and its worthiness awaits critical evaluation of relevant studies.

The optimal dose, route of administration, and long-term effects of methotrexate in this disease have not been established. Recent reports have suggested that methotrexate causes irreversible structural damage to the liver, although a cause-and-effect relationship has not yet been demonstrated. The liver damage seems to be insidious and is not reflected in most of the usual laboratory tests of liver function until advanced changes have occurred (Baker and Dahl, 1969; Epstein and Croft, 1969; Weinstein et al., 1970). Methotrexate can have dangerous effects on all actively growing cells, e.g., bone marrow and gastrointestinal tract, and may cause fetal abnormalities when used in pregnant women.

The drug's toxic effects may at times be intensified by use of other medications. Methotrexate is partly protein bound (Dixon et al., 1965). In patients with hypoalbuminemia or in patients taking other drugs that can displace the methotrexate from plasma proteins (e.g., salicylates or sulfonamides), tissue concentrations of drug are higher than those found after standard doses in normal people. The drug's toxic effects may also be intensified by the presence of other diseases. Relatively large amounts of unchanged methotrexate are excreted in the urine. The presence of renal disease could result in retention of the drug and an increased incidence of toxicity after standard doses. A number of deaths have been related to use of methotrexate for the treatment of psoriasis (Caron, 1969). Unless the disease is exceptionally severe, this toxicity seems unwarranted. Until more is learned of the nature of the drug's effects in psoriasis and its long-term effects, its use should be reserved for investigational purposes or for situations in which supervision can be maintained by a competent investigator. *Principle: The mere availability of a drug does not mean that all who have access to the drug are qualified to use it in innovative ways.* Unless the investigation is well conceived, the plan approved by an ethical, objective panel of experts, and the FDA notified of the project (see Chapter 1), the data will likely be personal at best and damning at worst, and the patient can only suffer from the consequences of "clandestine" use of drugs.

COMPLICATIONS OF THERAPY

Certain principles should be considered in regard to anti-inflammatory drugs: (1) Complications of drug therapy are more likely to occur during chronic administration than during short-term use. For example, the bone marrow depression associated with the use of phenylbutazone is related to the length of treatment with the drug. Try to limit the duration of administration to as short a time as possible. (2) Because many inflammatory conditions are chronic and require drug therapy for extended periods, nonpharmacologic measures should be employed whenever possible. (3) Proper timing of drug administration during the day may be an important determinant of both therapeutic and toxic effects. For example, administration of small amounts of corticosteroids (up to 20 mg of cortisol or its equivalent) in a single dose in the morning does not interfere significantly with nocturnal activation of the adrenocortical system. Used in this way the medication supplements the intrinsic daily production of cortisol. In contrast, if corticosteroids are given in divided doses and the last dose is given close to midnight, activation of the pituitary-adrenal system is prevented (Forsham, 1968). Ultimately this regimen may suppress the adrenal cortex and may abolish the diurnal variation of endogenous steroid secretion. Unless there is compelling reason to give the drug in divided doses, the toxicity is unjustified.

The timing of drug administration in relation to daily activities may also be critical. When administered with meals, salicylates tend to cause less gastric irritation. Other drugs, such as tetracyclines, which can bind with Ca^{++} in the intestine and are poorly absorbed in this combined form, are usually best administered between meals (see Chapter 2). *Principle: The therapeutic and toxic effects of a drug are deter-* *mined not only by its intrinsic properties but also by how the drug is used.*

Although a drug's therapeutic and side effects are not always predictable, toxic reactions are usually minimized when the drug is used in a knowledgeable and cautious manner (see Chapter 15). Usually the most important single factor in limiting undesirable drug effects is the physician. The knowledgeable physician knows which unwanted drug reactions are likely to occur in patients receiving the drug; by use of frequent observations and appropriate laboratory tests he can alter drug therapy at the earliest indication of undesirable effects. In order to do this he must be aware of the common and uncommon side effects of the anti-inflammatory agent he is using. He must realize that the presence of coexistent diseases may change the response to drugs and may intensify undesirable effects. The physician should know his patients, obtain their cooperation, and ensure that they understand the nature of their disease and the therapy that will be employed. If the physician is cognizant of all these variables he will encounter fewer side effects and improved therapeutic benefits when he uses anti-inflammatory drugs.

REFERENCES

Ansell, B. M.: Relationship of dosage and type of salicylate therapy to plasma levels in patients with rheumatoid arthritis. In Dixon, A. St. J.; Martin, B. K.; Smith, M. J. H.; and Wood, P. H. N. (eds.): *Salicylates: An International Symposium.* J. & A. Churchill, Ltd., London, 1963, pp. 35–37.

Arden, G. B., and Kolb, H.: Antimalarial therapy and early retinal changes in patients with rheumatoid arthritis. *Brit. Med. J.*, 1:270–73, 1966.

Austen, K. F.: Immunological aspects of salicylate action. In Dixon, A. St. J.; Martin, B. K.; Smith, M. J. H.; and Wood, P. H. N. (eds.): *Salicylates: An International Symposium.* J. & A. Churchill, Ltd., London, 1963, pp. 161–69.

Bachman, D.; Calkins, E.; and Bauer, W.: Effects of acetylsalicylic acid upon body water distribution in man. In Dixon, A. St. J.; Martin, B. K.; Smith, M. J. H.; and Wood, P. H. N. (eds.): *Salicylates: An International Symposium.* J. & A. Churchill, Ltd., London, 1963, pp. 113–19.

Baker, H., and Dahl, M. G. C.: Drug reactions. VI. Methotrexate and the liver. *Brit. J. Derm.*, 81:465–67, 1969.

Ballabio, C. B.: Clinical properties of indomethacin. In Garattini, S., and Dukes, M. N. G. (eds.): *International Symposium on Non-Steroidal Anti-Inflammatory Drugs.* Excerpta Medica Foundation, Amsterdam, 1965, pp. 342–52.

Baum, J., and Vaughn, J.: Immunosuppressive drugs in rheumatoid arthritis. *Ann. Intern. Med.*, 71:202–204, 1969.

Bayles, T. B.: Salicylate therapy in rheumatoid arthritis. *Med. Clin. N. Amer.*, 52:703–706, 1968.

Benditt, E. P.: Mast cell function: chemical and structural aspects. In Austen, K. F., and Becker, E. L. (eds.): *Biochemistry of the Acute Allergic Reactions.* F. A. Davis Co., Philadelphia, 1968, pp. 119–30.

Beraldo, W. T.; Dias da Silva, W.; Vugman, I.; Rothschild, A. M.; Rocha e Silva, M.; Giertz, Von H.;

Hahn, F.; Mota, I.; Higginbotham, R. D.; and Moussatche, H.: Release of histamine. In Eichler, O., and Farah, A. (eds.): *Handbuch der Experimentellen Pharmakologie*, Vol. 18/1: *Histamine and Antihistaminics*. Springer-Verlag, Berlin, 1966, pp. 334–656.

Berger, R. A., and Orentreich, N.: Local injection of steroids in dermatologic disorders. In Waisman, M. (ed.): *Pharmaceutical Therapeutics in Dermatology*. Charles C Thomas Co., Springfield, Ill., 1968, pp. 36–43.

Bloom, G. D.: Structural and biochemical characteristics of mast cells. In Zweifach, B. W.; Grant, L.; and McCluskey, R. T. (eds.): *The Inflammatory Process*. Academic Press, Inc., New York, 1965, pp. 355–88.

Boissonnas, R. A.; Guttman, S.; Jaquenoud, P. A.; Pless, J.; and Sandrin, E.: The synthesis of bradykinin and of related peptides. *Ann. N.Y. Acad. Sci.*, 104:5–14, 1963.

Bostrom, H.; Berntsen, K.; and Whitehouse, M. W.: Biochemical properties of anti-inflammatory drugs. II. Some effects on sulfate ^{35}S metabolism *in vivo*. *Biochem. Pharmacol.*, 13:413–20, 1964.

Bourne, H. R.; Lehrer, R. I.; Melmon, K. L.; and Cline, M. J.: Cyclic 3′,5′-adenosine monophosphate in the human leukocyte: synthesis, degradation, and effects on neutrophil candidacidal activity. *J. Clin. Invest.*, 50:920–29, 1971.

Bourne, H. R., and Melmon, K. L.: Adenyl cyclase in human leukocytes: evidence for activation by separate beta-adrenergic and prostaglandin receptors. *J. Pharmacol. Exp. Ther.* In press, 1971.

Bourne, H. R.; Melmon, K. L.; and Lichtenstein, L. M.: Histamine stimulates leukocyte adenyl cyclase and blocks antigenic histamine release. *Science.* In press, 1971.

Brocteur, J., and Moens, Chr.: Treatment of rheumatoid arthritis with immunosuppressive drugs. II. Immunological study. *Acta Rheum. Scand.*, 11:221–30, 1965.

Burke, J. F., and Miles, A. A.: The sequence of vascular events in early infective inflammation. *J. Path. Bact.*, 76:1–19, 1958.

Caron, G. A.: Methotrexate: a calculated risk. *Arch. Derm.* (*Chicago*), 99:627–28, 1969.

Carr, R. D., and Tarnowski, W. M.: Percutaneous absorption of corticosteroids. *Acta Dermatovener.*, 48:417–28, 1968.

Champion, R. H.; Roberts, S. O. B.; Carpenter, R. G.; and Roger, J. H.: Urticaria and angio-edema: a review of 554 patients. *Brit. J. Derm.*, 81:588–97, 1969.

Christian, C. L. (ed.): Eighteenth rheumatism review: review of American and English literature for the years 1965 and 1966. *Arth. Rheum.*, 11, Suppl. 3, 1968.

Cline, M. J., and Melmon, K. L.: Plasma kinins and cortisol: a possible explanation of the anti-inflammatory action of cortisol. *Science*, 153:1135–38, 1966.

Cochrane, C. G.; Weigle, W. O.; and Dixon, F. J.: The role of polymorphonuclear leukocytes in the initiation and cessation of the Arthus vasculitis. *J. Exp. Med.*, 110:481–94, 1959.

Cohn, Z. A.: The metabolism and physiology of the mononuclear phagocytes. In Zweifach, B. W.; Grant, L.; and McCluskey, R. T. (eds.): *The Inflammatory Process*. Academic Press, Inc., New York, 1965, pp. 323–53.

Cohnheim, J.: *Lectures on General Pathology*, Sections 1–6 in 3 vols. Translated by A. B. McKee from the 2nd ed. The Syndenham Society, London, 1889–1890.

Collier, H. O. J.: Antagonism by aspirin and like-acting drugs of kinins and SRS-A in guinea-pig lung. In Dixon, A. St. J.; Martin, B. K.; Smith, M. J. H.; and Wood, P. H. N. (eds.): *Salicylates: An International Symposium*. J. & A. Churchill, Ltd., London, 1963, pp. 120–26.

Conner, E. B.: Tuberculous mengingitis in adults. *Southern Med. J.*, 60:1061–67, 1976.

Cooperating Clinics Committee of the American Rheumatism Association, Decker, J. L. (chmn.): A controlled trial of cyclophosphamide in rheumatoid arthritis. *New Eng. J. Med.*, 283:883–89, 1970.

Cuthbert, M. F.: Bronchodilator activity of aerosols of prostaglandins E_1 and E_2 in asthmatic subjects. *Proc. R. Soc. Med.*, 64:15–16, 1971.

Dastur, D. K., and Udani, P. M.: The pathology and pathogenesis of tuberculous encephalopathy. *Acta Neuropath.*, 6:311–26, 1966.

Decker, J. L.; Bollet, A. J.; Duff, I. F.; Shulman, L. E.; and Stollerman, G. H.: Primer on the rheumatic diseases, Parts 1–4. *J.A.M.A.*, 190:127–40, 425–44, 509–30, 741–51, 1964.

Dixon, R. L.; Henderson, E. S.; and Rall, N. I. H.: Plasma protein binding of methotrexate and its displacement by various drugs. *Fed. Proc.*, 24:454, 1965.

Domenjoz, R.: Synthetic anti-inflammatory drugs: concepts of their mode of action. *Advance Pharmacol.*, 4:143–217, 1966.

Donaldson, V. H.: Mechanisms of activation of C_1' esterase in hereditary angioneurotic edema plasma *in vitro*: the role of Hageman factor, a clot-promoting agent. *J. Exp. Med.*, 127:411–29, 1968.

Donaldson, V., and Rosen, F. S.: Hereditary angioneurotic edema: a clinical survey. *Pediatrics*, 37:1017–27, 1966.

Dubois, E. L.: Management and prognosis of systemic lupus erythematosus. *Bull. Rheum. Dis.*, 18:477–82, 1967.

Duthie, J. J. R.; Brown, P. E.; Truelove, L. H.; Baragar, F. D.; and Lawrie, A. J.: Course and prognosis in rheumatoid arthritis, a further report. *Ann. Rheum. Dis.*, 23:193–204, 1964.

Editorial: The story of DMSO. *J.A.M.A.*, 192:320–21, 1965.

Eichler, O., and Farah, A. (eds.): *Handbuch der Experimentellen Pharmakologie*, Vol. 18/1: *Histamine and Anti-Histaminics*. Springer-Verlag, Berlin, 1966.

Eisen, V.: Relation of the fibrinolytic mechanism to other proteolytic systems in plasma. *Proc. Roy. Soc. Biol.*, 173:407–10, 1969.

Elliot, D. F.; Horton, E. W.; and Lewis, G. P.: Actions of pure bradykinin. *J. Physiol.*, 153:473–80, 1960.

Empire Rheumatism Council: Multi-centre controlled trial comparing cortisone acetate and acetyl salicylic acid in the long-term treatment of rheumatoid arthritis. *Ann. Rheum. Dis.*, 16:277–89, 1957.

———: Gold therapy in rheumatoid arthritis: report of a multi-centre controlled trial. *Ibid.*, 19:95–119, 1960.

———: Gold therapy in rheumatoid arthritis: final report of a multi-centre controlled trial. *Ibid.*, 20:315–34, 1961a.

———: Relation of toxic reactions in gold therapy to improvement in rheumatoid arthritis: a report. *Ibid.*, 20:335–40, 1961b.

Epstein, E. H., and Croft, J. D., Jr.: Cirrhosis following methotrexate administration for psoriasis. *Arch. Dermatol.*, 100:531–34, 1969.

Erdos, E. G.: Hypotensive peptides: bradykinin, kallidin and eledoisin. *Advance Pharmacol.*, 4:1–90, 1966a.

———: Release and inactivation of kinins. *Gastroenterology*, 51:893–900, 1966b.

Erjavec, F.; Beaven, M. A.; and Brodie, B. B.: Uptake and release of H^3-histamine in cat submaxillary gland. *Fed. Proc.*, 26:237–42, 1967.

Erspamer, V.: Peripheral physiological and pharmacological actions of indolealkylamines. In Eichler, O., and Farah, A. (eds.): *Handbuch der Experimentellen Pharmakologie*, Vol. 19: *5-Hydroxytryptamine and Related Indolealkylamines.* Springer-Verlag, Heidelberg, 1966, pp. 245–359.

Falleroni, A. E.: Treatment of allergic emergencies. *Mod. Treatment*, 5:782–91, 1968.

Feinberg, S. M.: Allergy from therapeutic products: incidence, importance, recognition and prevention. *J.A.M.A.*, 178:815–18, 1961.

Feldmann, R. J., and Maibach, H. I.: Percutaneous penetration of ^{14}C-hydrocortisone in man. *Arch. Derm. (Chicago)*, 4:649–51, 1966.

Forsham, P. H.: The adrenal cortex. In Williams, R. H. (ed.): *Textbook of Endocrinology*. W. B. Saunders Co., Philadelphia, 1968, pp. 287–379.

Fosdick, W. M.: Cytotoxic therapy in rheumatoid arthritis. *Med. Clin. N. Amer.*, 52:747–57, 1968.

Gatling, R. R.: Altered reactivity to epinephrine in the hypersensitive rabbit. *J. Exp. Med.*, 108:441–52, 1958.

Gerber, D. A.; Cohen, N.; and Guistra, R.: The ability of nonsteroid anti-inflammatory compounds to accelerate a disulfide interchange reaction of serum sulfhydryl groups and 5,5'-dithiobis-(2-nitrobenzoic acid). *Biochem. Pharmacol.*, 16:115–23, 1967.

Gillespie, E.; Levine, L. J.; and Malawista, S. E.: Histamine release from rat peritoneal mast cells: inhibition by colchicine and potentiation by deuterium. *J. Pharmacol. Exp. Ther.*, 164:158–65, 1968.

Goetzl, E. J.; Falchuk, K. H.; Zeiger, L. S.; Sullivan, A. L.; Herbert, C. L.; Adams, J. P.; and Decker, J. L.: A physiological approach to the assessment of disease activity in rheumatoid arthritis. *J. Clin. Invest.*, 50:1167–80, 1971.

Gokhale, S. D.; Gulati, O. D.; Kelkar, L. V.; and Kelkar, V. V.: Effect of some drugs on human umbilical artery *in vitro*. *Brit. J. Pharmacol.*, 27:332–46, 1966.

Goodman, L., and Gilman, A. (eds.): *The Pharmacological Basis of Therapeutics*, 4th ed. The Macmillan Co., New York, 1970.

Greenbaum, L. M.; Freer, R.; and Kim, K. S.: Kinin forming inactivating enzymes in polymorphonuclear leucocytes. *Fed. Proc.*, 25: 287, 1966.

Hamberg, U.: Influences on the kinin system by proteolysis in plasma. *Proc. Roy. Soc. Biol.*, 173:393–406, 1969.

Hinman, J. W.: Prostaglandins: a report on early clinical studies. *Postgrad. Med. J.*, 46: 562–75, 1970.

Ivy, A. C., and Bachrach, W. H.: Physiological significance of the effects of histamine on gastric secretion. In Eichler, O., and Farah, A. (eds.): *Handbuch der Experimentellen Pharmakologie*, Vol. 18/1: *Histamine and Antihistaminics*. Springer-Verlag, Heidelberg, 1966, pp. 810–91.

Janoski, A. H.; Shaver, J. C.; Christy, N. P.; and Rosner, W.: On the pharmacologic actions of 21-carbon hormonal steroids ("glucocorticoids") of the adrenal cortex in mammals. In Deane, H. W., and Rubin, B. L. (eds.): *Handbuch der Experimentellen Pharmakologie*, Vol. 14/3: *The Adrenocortical Hormones*, Part 3. Springer-Verlag, Berlin, 1968, pp. 256–368.

Kaplan, A. P.; Gigli, I.; and Austen, K. F.: Immunologic activation of Hageman factor and its relationship to fibrinolysis, bradykinin generation, and complement. *J. Clin. Invest.*, 50:51a, 1971.

Kellermeyer, R. W., and Graham, R. C., Jr.: Kinins— possible physiologic and pathologic roles in man. *New Eng. J. Med.*, 279:754–59, 802–807, 859–66, 1968.

Ketchel, M. M.; Favour, C. B.; and Sturgis, S. H.: The *in vitro* action of hydrocortisone on leucocyte migration. *J. Exp. Med.*, 107:211–18, 1958.

Klemperer, M. R.; Donaldson, V. H.; and Rosen, F. S.: Effect of C$_1'$ esterase on vascular permeability in man: studies in normal and complement-deficient individuals and in patients with hereditary angioneurotic edema. *J. Clin. Invest.*, 47:604–11, 1968.

Klinenberg, J. R.: Current concepts of hyperuricemia and gout. *Calif. Med.*, 110:231–43, 1969.

Kuttner, A. G.: Current status of steroid therapy in rheumatic fever. *Amer. Heart J.*, 70:147–49, 1965.

Kuzell, W. C.: Non-steroid anti-inflammatory agents. *Ann. Rev. Pharmacol.*, 8:357–76, 1968.

Lamont-Havers, R., and Wagner, B. M.: Proceedings, Conference on Effects of Chronic Salicylate Administration, New York, 1966. U.S. Govt. Printing Office, Washington, D.C., 1968.

Landerman, N. S.; Webster, M. E.; Becker, E. L.; and Ratcliffe, H. E.: Hereditary angioneurotic edema. II. Deficiency of inhibitor for serum globulin permeability factor and/or plasma kallikrein. *J. Allergy*, 33:330–41, 1962.

Landis, E. M., and Pappenheimer, J. R.: Exchange of substances through the capillary walls. In Hamilton, W. F., and Dow, P. (eds.): *Handbook of Physiology*, Sec. 2: *Circulation*. American Physiological Society, Washington, D. C., 1963, pp. 961–1034.

Lepow, I. H.; Dias da Silva, W.; and Eisele, J. W.: Nature and biological properties of human anaphylatoxin. In Austen, K. F., and Becker, E. L. (eds.): *Biochemistry of Acute Allergic Reactions*. F. A. Davis Co., Philadelphia, 1968, pp. 265–82.

Lepow, I. H.; Dias da Silva, W.; and Patrick, R. A.: Biologically active cleavage products of components of complement. In Movat, H. Z. (ed.): *Third International Symposium on Cellular and Humoral Mechanisms of Anaphylaxis and Allergy*, October 3–5, 1968. S. Karger, Basel, 1969, pp. 237–52.

LeRoy, E. C.: Precipitating and complement-fixing antibodies to collagen with species and collagen subunit specificity. *Proc. Soc. Exp. Biol. Med.*, 128:341–47, 1968.

Levy, G., and Leonards, J. R.: Absorption, metabolism and excretion of salicylates. In Smith, M. J. H., and Smith, P. K. (eds.): *The Salicylates: A Critical Bibliographic Review*. Interscience Publications, a division of John Wiley & Sons, New York, 1966, pp. 5–48.

Lewis, T.: *The Blood Vessels of the Human Skin and Their Responses*. Shaw & Sons, Ltd., London, 1927.

Lichtenstein, L. M., and Margolis, S.: Histamine release *in vitro*: inhibition by catecholamines and methylxanthines. *Science*, 161:902–903, 1968.

Liddle, G. W.: Clinical pharmacology of the anti-inflammatory steroids. *Clin. Pharmacol. Ther.*, 2:615–35, 1961.

McChesney, E. W.; Fasco, M. J.; and Banks, W. F., Jr.: The metabolism of chloroquine in man during and after repeated oral dosage. *J. Pharmacol. Exp. Ther.*, 158:323–31, 1967.

McKay, D. G.; Muller-Berghaus, G.; and Cruse, V.: Activation of Hageman factor for ellagic acid and the generalized Shwartzman reaction. *Amer. J. Path.*, 54:393–420, 1969.

Majno, G., and Palade, G. E.: Studies on inflammation. I. The effect of histamine and serotonin on vascular permeability: an electron microscopic study. *J. Biophys. Biochem. Cytol.*, 11:571–605, 1961.

Majno, G.; Palade, G. E.; and Schoefl, G. I.: Studies on inflammation. II. The site of action of histamine and serotonin along the vascular tree: a topographic study. *J. Biophys. Biochem. Cytol.*, 11:607–26, 1961.

Malawista, S. E.: The action of colchicine in acute gout. *Arth. Rheum.*, 8:752–56, 1965.

———: Colchicine: a common mechanism for its anti-inflammatory and anti-mitotic effect. *Arth. Rheum.*, 11:191–97, 1968.

Malawista, S. E., and Bodel, P. J.: The dissociation by

colchicine of phagocytosis from increased oxygen consumption in human leukocytes. *J. Clin. Invest.*, **46**:786–96, 1967.

Marchesi, V. T.: The passage of colloidal carbon through inflamed endothelium. *Proc. Roy. Soc. Biol.*, **156**:550–52, 1962.

Medical Research Council and Nuffield Foundation: A comparison of cortisone and aspirin in the treatment of early cases of rheumatoid arthritis. *Brit. Med. J.*, **2**:695–700, 1955.

Melmon, K. L.: Kinins—one of many mediators of the carcinoid syndrome. *Gastroenterology*, **55**:545–48, 1968.

Melmon, K. L., and Cline, M. J.: Kinins. *Amer. J. Med.*, **43**:153–60, 1967.

———: The interaction of leukocytes and the kinin system. *Biochem. Pharmacol.*, *Suppl.*, 271–81, 1968.

Melmon, K. L.; Morrelli, H.; and Rowland, M.: The clinical pharmacology of salicylates. *Calif. Med.*, **110**:410–22, 1969.

Melmon, K. L., and Sjoerdsma, A.: Serotonin in platelets, its uptake and disappearance after administration of the amine by mouth. *Lancet*, **2**:316–18, 1963.

Michaelsson, G.: Chronic urticaria: a clinical study with special reference to vascular reactions mediated by the kallikrein-kinin system. *Acta Dermatovener.*, **49**:404–16, 1969.

Mikkelsen, W. M., and Robinson, W. D.: Physiologic and biochemical basis for the treatment of gout and hyperuricemia. *Med. Clin. N. Amer.*, **53**:1331–47, 1969.

Miller, R. L., and Melmon, K. L.: The related roles of histamine, serotonin, and bradykinin in the pathogenesis of inflammation. *Series Haematol.*, **3**:5–38, 1970.

Milne, M. D.: The excretion of salicylate and its metabolism. In Dixon, A. St. J.; Martin, B. K.; Smith, M. J. H.; and Wood, P. H. N. (eds.): *Salicylates: An International Symposium.* J. & A. Churchill, Ltd., London, 1963, pp. 18–27.

Mizushima, Y., and Kobayashi, M.: Interaction of anti-inflammatory drugs with serum proteins, especially with some biologically active proteins. *J. Pharm. Pharmacol.*, **20**:169–73, 1968.

Moens, Chr., and Brocteur, J.: Treatment of rheumatoid arthritis with immunosuppressive drugs. I. Clinical study. *Acta Rheum. Scand.*, **11**:212–20, 1965.

Morison, R. A. H.; Woodmansey, A.; and Young, A. J.: Placebo responses in an arthritis trial. *Ann. Rheum. Dis.*, **20**:179–85, 1961.

Morrelli, H. F., and Melmon, K. L.: The clinician's approach to drug interactions. *Calif. Med.*, **109**:380–89, 1968.

Morris, C. R.: Renal tubular acidosis: mechanisms, classification and implications. *New Eng. J. Med.*, **281**:1405–13, 1969.

Müller Eberhard, H. J.: Chemistry and reaction mechanisms of complement. *Advance Immunol.*, **8**:1–80, 1968.

Naranjo, P.: Toxicity of histamine: lethal doses. In Eichler, O., and Farah, A. (eds.): *Handbuch der Experimentellen Pharmakologie*, Vol. 18/1: *Histamine and Anti-Histaminics.* Springer-Verlag, Berlin, 1966, pp. 179–201.

Nies, A. S.; Cline, M. J.; and Melmon, K. L.: Mechanism of activation of human plasma kallikrein by endotoxin. *Clin. Res.*, **16**:157, 1968a.

Nies, A.; Forsyth, R.; Williams, H.; and Melmon, K.: Contributions of kinins to endotoxic shock in unanesthetized rhesus monkeys. *Circ. Res.*, **22**:155–64, 1968b.

Nies, A. S.; Greineder, D. K.; Cline, M. J.; and Melmon, K. L.: The divergent effects of endotoxin fractions on human plasma and leukocytes. *Biochem. Pharmacol.*, **20**:39–46, 1971.

Nies, A., and Melmon, K.: Kinins and arthritis. *Bull. Rheum. Dis.*, **19**:512–17, 1968.

Nies, A. S., and Melmon, K. L.: Mechanism of endotoxin-induced kinin production in human plasma. *Biochem. Pharmacol.*, **20**:29–37, 1971.

Nossel, H. L.; Wilner, G. D.; and LeRoy, E. C.: Importance of polar groups for initiating blood coagulation and aggregating platelets. *Nature*, **221**:75–76, 1969.

O'Brien, M. W.: A three month trial of indomethacin in rheumatoid arthritis with special reference to analysis and inference. *Clin. Pharmacol. Ther.*, **8**:11–37, 1967.

O'Brien, R. L.; Olenick, J. G.; and Hahn, F. E.: Reactions of quinine, chloroquine, and quinacrine with DNA and their effect on the DNA and RNA polymerase reactions. *Proc. Nat. Acad. Sci.*, **55**:1511–17, 1966.

O'Toole, R. D.; Thornton, G. F.; Muckherjee, M. K.; and Nath, R. L.: Dexamethasone in tuberculous meningitis: relationship of cerebrospinal fluid effects to therapeutic efficacy. *Ann. Intern. Med.*, **70**:39–48, 1969.

Page, A. R.; Condie, R. M.; and Good, R. A.: Suppression of plasma cell hepatitis with 6-mercaptopurine. *Amer. J. Med.*, **36**:200–13, 1964.

Page, A. R., and Good, R. A.: A clinical and experimental study of the function of neutrophils in the inflammatory response. *Amer. J. Path.*, **34**:645–69, 1958.

Page, I. H.: Serotonin (5-hydroxytryptamine): the last four years. *Physiol. Rev.*, **38**:277–335, 1958.

Parker, C. W., and Vavra, J. D.: Immunosuppression. *Prog. Hemat.*, **6**:1–81, 1969.

Pearson, R. S. B.: Hypersensitivity to aspirin. In Dixon, A. St. J.; Martin, B. K.; Smith, M. J. H.; and Wood, P. H. N.: *Salicylates: An International Symposium.* J. & A. Churchill, Ltd., London, 1963, pp. 170–73.

Perry, H. O.; Soderstrom, C. W.; and Schulze, R. W.: The Goeckerman treatment of psoriasis. *Arch. Derm. (Chicago)*, **98**:178–82, 1968.

Phelps, P., and McCarty, D. J.: Suppression of crystal-induced synovitis in canine joints by indomethacin. Demonstration of inhibition of leucocyte mobility. *Arthritis Rheum.*, **9**:532, 1966.

Piper, P. J., and Vane, J. R.: Release of additional factors in anaphylaxis and its antagonism by anti-inflammatory drugs. *Nature*, **223**:29–35, 1969.

Pollak, V. E.; Pirani, C. L.; and Schwartz, F. D.: The natural history of the renal manifestations of systemic lupus erythematosus. *J. Lab. Clin. Med.*, **63**:537–50, 1964.

Rechenberg, H. K. (ed.): *Phenylbutazone and Butazolidin.* Edward Arnold, Ltd., London, 1962.

Rees, R. B.; Bennett, J. H.; Maibach, H. I.; and Arnold, H. L.: Methotrexate for psoriasis. *Arch. Derm. (Chicago)*, **95**:2–11, 1967.

Reichgott, M. J., and Melmon, K. L.: Bradykinin: physiology, hormonal effects; bradykinin: regulation of peptide generation; bradykinin: clinical evaluation of hormonal excess and deficiency. In Berson, S. A., and Yalow, R. S. (eds.): *Methods in Investigative and Diagnostic Endocrinology.* North-Holland Publishing Co. In press, 1971.

Riley, J.: *The Mast Cells.* Livingstone, Ltd., Edinburgh, 1959.

Riley, J. F., and West, G. B.: The occurrence of histamine in mast cells. In Eichler, O., and Farah, A. (eds.): *Handbuch der Experimentellen Pharmakologie*, Vol. 18/1: *Histamine and Anti-Histaminics.* Springer-Verlag, Berlin, 1966, pp. 116–35.

Rocha e Silva, M.: Chemical mediators of the acute inflammatory reaction. *Ann. N. Y. Acad. Sci.*, 116:899–911, 1964.

Roueché, B.: *The Incurable Wound and Further Narratives of Medical Detection.* Little, Brown & Co., Boston, 1957.

Rutstein, D. D., and Densen, E.: The natural history of rheumatic fever and rheumatic heart disease: ten-year report of a cooperative clinical trial of ACTH, cortisone, and aspirin. *Circulation*, 32:457–76, 1965.

Salter, R. H.: Aspirin and gastrointestinal bleeding. *Amer. J. Dig. Dis.*, 13:38–58, 1968.

Sams, W. M., Jr.: Chloroquine: mechanisms of action. *Mayo Clin. Proc.*, 42:300–309, 1967.

Schachter, M.: Kallikreins and kinins. *Physiol. Rev.*, 49:509–47, 1969.

Schur, P. H., and Austin, J. K.: Complement in human disease. *Ann. Rev. Med.*, 19:1–24, 1968.

Scott, A. I.: Psoriasis. In MacKenna, R. M. B. (ed.): *Modern Trends in Dermatology.* Butterworths, Washington, D.C., 1966, pp. 294–304.

Scott, J. T.: Management of gout. *Brit. Med. J.*, 3:456–57, 1969.

Seegmiller, J. E.; Howell, R. R.; and Malawista, S. E.: Mechanism of action of colchicine in acute gouty arthritis. *J Clin. Invest.*, 41:1399, 1962.

Sell, S., and Asofsky, R.: Lymphocytes and immunoglobulins. *Prog. Allergy*, 12:86–160, 1968.

Sevitt, S.: Early and delayed oedema and increase in capillary permeability after burns of the skin. *J. Path. Bact.*, 75:27–37, 1958.

Sheldon, J. M.; Lovell, R. G.; and Mathews, K. P.: *A Manual of Clinical Allergy.* W. B. Saunders Co., Philadelphia, 1967.

Short, C. L., and Bauer, W.: The course of rheumatoid arthritis in patients receiving simple medical and orthopedic measures. *New Eng. J. Med.*, 238:142–48, 1948.

Sicuteri, F.: Indomethacin as a new vasoconstrictor and therapeutic agent in migraine. In Garattini, S., and Dukes, M. M. G. (eds.): *International Symposium on Non-Steroidal Anti-Inflammatory Drugs.* Excerpta Medica Foundation, Amsterdam, 1965, pp. 335–39.

Sjoerdsma, A.: Serotonin. *New Eng. J. Med.*, 261:181–88, 231–39, 1959.

Skidmore, I. F., and Whitehouse, M. W.: Biochemical properties of anti-inflammatory drugs. X. The inhibition of serotonin formation in vitro and inhibition of the esterase activity of α-chymotrypsin. *Biochem. Pharmacol.*, 16:737–51, 1967.

Smith, M. J. H.: Anti-inflammatory activity of salicylates. In Smith, M. J. H., and Smith, P. K. (eds.): *The Salicylates: A Critical Bibliographic Review.* Interscience Publishers, a division of John Wiley & Sons, New York, 1966a, pp. 203–32.

———: Metabolic effects of salicylates. *Ibid.*, 1966b, pp. 49–105.

———: Toxicology. *Ibid.*, 1966c, pp. 233–306.

Sparrow, E. M., and Wilhelm, D. L.: Species differences in susceptibility to capillary permeability factors: histamine, 5-hydroxytryptamine, and compound 48/80. *J. Physiol.*, 137:51–65, 1957.

Spector, W. G., and Willoughby, D. A.: The inflammatory response. *Bact. Rev.*, 27:117–54, 1963.

———: Vasoactive amines in acute inflammation. *Ann. N. Y. Acad. Sci.*, 116:839–46, 1964a.

———: The effect of vascular permeability factors on the emigration of leucocytes. *J. Path. Bact.*, 87:341–46, 1964b.

———: Chemical mediators. In Zweifach, B. W.; Grant, L.; and McCluskey, R. T. (eds.): *The Inflammatory Process.* Academic Press, Inc., New York, 1965, pp. 427–48.

Stafford, W. L.: Protein binding of salicylates. In Dixon, A. St. J.; Martin, B. K.; Smith, M. J. H.; and Wood, P. H. N. (eds.): *Salicylates: An International Symposium.* J. & A. Churchill, Ltd., London, 1963, pp. 74–78.

Stetson, C. A., and Good, R. A.: Studies on the mechanism of the Shwartzman phenomenon. Evidence for the participation of polymorphonuclear leukocytes in the phenomenon. *J. Exp. Med.*, 93:49–64, 1951.

Thomas, L.: The role of epinephrine in the reactions produced by the endotoxins of gram negative bacteria. I. Hemorrhagic necrosis produced by epinephrine in the skin of endotoxin treated animals. *J. Exp. Med.*, 104:865–80, 1956.

Thompson, J. S.: Urticaria and angioedema. *Ann. Intern. Med.*, 69:361–80, 1968.

Thorvaldsson, S. E.; Sedlack, R. E.; Gleich, G. J.; and Ruddy, S. J.: Angioneurotic edema and deficiency of C_1' esterase inhibitor in a 61-year-old woman. *Ann. Intern. Med.*, 71:353–58, 1969.

Uvnas, B.: Release processes in mast cells and their activation by injury. *Ann. N. Y. Acad. Sci.*, 116:880–90, 1964.

———: Mode of binding and release of histamine in mast cell granules from the rat. *Fed. Proc.*, 26:219–21, 1967.

Vassalli, P., and McCluskey, R. T.: The pathogenic role of fibrin deposition in immunologically induced glomerulonephritis. *Ann. N. Y. Acad. Sci.*, 116:1052–62, 1964.

Vogt, W.: Anaphylatoxin formation, problems of its relation to complement and identity in various species. In Movat, H. Z. (ed.): *Third International Symposium on Cellular and Humoral Mechanisms of Anaphylaxis and Allergy*, Toronto, October 3–5, 1968. S. Karger, Basel, 1969, pp. 260–64.

Ward, P. A.: The chemosuppression of chemotaxis. *J. Exp. Med.*, 124:209–30, 1966.

Watson, D. W., and Johnson, A. G.: The clinical use of immunosuppression. *Med. Clin. N. Amer.*, 53:1225–41, 1969.

Webster, M. E.: Human plasma kallikrein, its activation and pathological role. *Fed. Proc.*, 27:84–89, 1968.

Webster, M. E., and Pierce, J. V.: The nature of the kallidins released from human plasma by kallikreins and other enzymes. *Ann. N. Y. Acad. Sci.*, 104:91–107, 1963.

Weinstein, G. D.; Cox, J. W.; Suringa, D. W. R.; Millard, M. M.; Kalser, M.; and Frost, P.: Evaluation of possible chronic hepatotoxicity from methotrexate for psoriasis. *Arch. Dermatol.*, 102:613–18, 1970.

Weiser, R. S.; Myrvik, Q. N.; and Pearsall, N. N.: *Fundamentals of Immunology for Students of Medicine and Related Sciences.* Lea & Febiger, Philadelphia, 1969, pp. 37–71.

Weiss, W., and Flippin, H. F.: The changing incidence and prognosis of tuberculous meningitis. *Amer. J. Med. Sci.*, 250:46–59, 1965.

Weissmann, G.: Role of lysosomes in inflammation and disease. *Ann. Rev. Med.*, 18:97–112, 1967.

Whitehouse, M. W.: Biochemical properties of anti-inflammatory drugs. III. Uncoupling of oxidative phosphorylation in a connective tissue (cartilage) and liver mitochondria by salicylate analogues: relationship of structure to activity. *Biochem. Pharmacol.*, 13:319–36, 1964.

Whitehouse, M. W., and Bostrom, H.: Biochemical properties of anti-inflammatory drugs. VI. The effects of chloroquine (resochin), mepacrine (quinacrine) and some of their potential metabolites on cartilage metabolism and oxidative phosphorylation. *Biochem. Pharmacol.*, 14:1173–84, 1965.

Whitehouse, M. W., and Leader, J. E.: Biochemical

properties of anti-inflammatory drugs. IX. Uncoupling of oxidative phosphorylation and inhibition of a thiol enzyme (papain) by some cyclic β-diones and ninhydrin. *Biochem. Pharmacol.*, **16**:537–51, 1967.

Willoughby, D. A., and Spector, W. G.: The lymph node permeability factor in delayed hypersensitivity reactions. In Garattini, S., and Dukes, M. N. G. (eds.): *International Symposium on Non-Steroidal Anti-Inflammatory Drugs*. Excerpta Medica Foundation, Amsterdam, 1965, pp. 107–13.

Wilner, G. D.; Nassel, H. L.; and LeRoy, E. C.: Aggregation of platelets by collagen. *J. Clin. Invest.*, **47**:2616–21, 1968a.

————: Activation of Hageman factor by collagen. *J. Clin. Invest.*, **47**:2608–15, 1968b.

Winter, C. A.: Nonsteroid anti-inflammatory agents. *Ann. Rev. Pharmacol.*, **6**:157–74, 1966.

Wolfe, S. M., and Shulman, N. R.: Adenyl cyclase activity in human platelets. *Biochem. Biophys. Res. Commun.*, **35**:265–72, 1969.

Yu, T. F., and Gutman, A. B.: Study of the paradoxical effects of salicylates in low, intermediate, and high dosage on the renal mechanism for excretion of urate in man. *J. Clin. Invest.*, **38**:1298–1315, 1959.

Zvaifler, N. J.: Antimalarial treatment of rheumatoid arthritis. *Med. Clin. N. Amer.*, **52**:759–64, 1968.

Zweifach, B. W.: Microvascular aspects of tissue injury. In Zweifach, B. W.; Grant, L.; and McCluskey, R. T. (eds.): *The Inflammatory Process*. Academic Press, Inc., New York, 1965, pp. 161–96.

Chapter 10

INFECTIOUS DISEASE

Howard F. Morrelli

When deciding on therapy for a patient with a suspected infectious disease, the physician must assess the host, the infection, and the interaction between the two. Host assessment requires evaluation of the adequacy of normal defense mechanisms to detect processes that might predispose to infection. Assessment of the infectious process involves considerations of anatomic site and of the specific agent known or thought to be responsible. The interaction between host and infectious agent may be evaluated by observing the local and systemic patterns of response, at times including the immunologic reaction to the infectious process.

The most important decision in the use of antibiotics is whether they should be used at all. Antibiotics may be toxic, even when properly used. Before instituting therapy, the physician must consider (1) whether infection definitely is present; (2) whether the infection is amenable to available antibotic therapy; and (3) whether the indications for antibiotic use are compelling enough to warrant risking the replacement of the patient's normal flora by organisms resistant to relatively nontoxic antibiotics.

Specific antibiotic selection is determined by the organism responsible for the infection. Clinical judgment and bacteriologic methods for isolation and identification must be employed before institution of therapy. Abundant literature on mechanisms of action of antibiotics and listings of "agents of choice" recommended for specific organisms may be employed to select appropriate treatment (Feingold, 1963; Medical Letter, 1968c; Parker, 1969; Goodman and Gilman, 1970). However, rational selection of antibiotics involves more than a consideration of "the bug and a drug." Other factors influencing therapeutic decisions include (1) the pharmacology of the drug, including its undesirable effects; (2) features of the patient that influence the drug's pharmacokinetics or his unique responses to drugs; and (3) how the infectious process should respond. Strictly pharmacologic data are significant, particularly in selected infections or in use of combinations of agents, but features of the patient that interact with the organism and with the antibiotic are equally important in managing patients with infectious disease.

NORMAL DEFENSE MECHANISMS AGAINST INFECTION AND THEIR KNOWN DEFECTS

Skin and Mucous Membranes

Intact skin and mucous membranes physically protect against infection by pathogenic organisms. The importance of intact skin is demonstrated by the high incidence of local and systemic bacterial infection following burns or the use of indwelling venous catheters for more than two days (Druskin and Siegel, 1963; Stein and Pruitt, 1970). The most common portals of entry for staphylococcal sepsis are the skin and respiratory tract (Cluff et al., 1968), and "secondary" bacterial pneumonia often follows viral damage to the respiratory mucosa. Other local tissue factors in the skin and the respiratory and gastrointestinal mucosa may be important in preventing invasion of organisms; e.g., infections are rare in richly vascular and cellular granulation tissue, but relatively common in less vascular lesions such as decubitus ulcers.

Humoral and Secretory Antibodies

In addition to the bactericidal or inhibitory effects of gamma G and gamma M antibodies, the actions of gamma A globulins appear to be important in defending against infections. Deficiencies of either circulating IgA or of the secretory form of IgA (two molecules of circulating IgA plus a "secretory piece") have been associated with high rates of bacterial infection, particularly of the respiratory tract (Tomasi, 1967, 1968).

A variety of syndromes of congenital and acquired antibody deficiency have been described. Quantitative assay of gamma globulins is necessary to identify these patients, who are subject to repeated bouts of pyogenic infections or to chronic infections of the respiratory tract. These infections may be ameliorated or prevented by gamma globulin therapy, but commercially available gamma globulin contains more IgG than IgM or IgA globulin; deficiency of immunoglobulins other than IgG can be corrected transiently and with difficulty by administration

of plasma (Prasad et al., 1964; Alper et al., 1966; Craddock et al.,1966; Merler and Rosen, 1966; Robbins et al., 1966; Rosen and Janeway, 1966; Durant et al., 1968; Janeway, 1968; Kretschmer et al., 1969).

A congenital form of severe agammaglobulinemia, associated with thymic aplasia, is not ameliorated by gamma globulin therapy. This suggests a lymphocytic defect in immunologic competence (Rosen et al., 1966; Rosen, 1968). A few such patients have apparently responded to bone marrow transplantation, a means of producing syngenic or allogenic lymphocyte stem cells (Good, 1969; Meuwissen et al., 1969).

Patients with certain diseases associated with immunologic defects, e.g., lymphoma, multiple myeloma, Hodgkin's disease, lupus erythematosus, or sarcoidosis, or patients taking corticosteroids or "immunosuppressive" drugs (see Chapter 9) are susceptible to infection with a variety of conventional and exotic organisms, such as DNA viruses (e.g., cytomegalic virus), fungi (e.g., Cryptococcus neoformans), or protozoa (e.g., Toxoplasma gondii and Pneumocystis carinii) (Torack, 1957; Louria et al., 1960; Fahey et al., 1963; Aisenberg, 1964; Sokal and Firat, 1965; Duvall and Carbone, 1966; Murray et al., 1966; Rifkind et al., 1966; Brown et al., 1967; Hall et al., 1967; Vogel et al., 1968; Barlotta et al., 1969; Hart et al., 1969). Immunoprophylaxis for these disorders with gamma globulin may seem theoretically attractive, but a trial in hypogammaglobulinemic patients with multiple myeloma failed to show a significant decrease in incidence of pneumonias between the treated and control groups (Salmon et al., 1967). Patients with acute leukemia commonly have infections, but prophylactic administration of gamma globulin to these patients is apparently not successful (Bodey et al., 1964). Interpretation of these studies requires caution. Commercially available gamma globulin may not provide the specific antibodies that are deficient in the patient (e.g., antibodies to many types of pneumococci in myeloma patients, IgM or IgA antibodies in others). *Principle: The efficacy of gamma globulin therapy in some cases of hypogammaglobulinemia does not justify its use in superficially analogous circumstances. Nor does the failure of gamma globulin or plasma therapy to prevent infection under certain circumstances (e.g., pneumococcal pneumonia in myeloma) invalidate its use to prevent infection in other hypogammaglobulinemic patients. The efficacy of gamma globulin therapy must be demonstrated in a given patient prior to its repeated use.* Conventional and hyperimmune gamma globulins have been utilized prophylactically in patients exposed to the viruses of viral hepatitis or measles to prevent or attenuate the disease. Their prophylactic use in other viral infections such as mumps has not been rewarding. Clinical studies on the efficacy of gamma globulins in disorders other than globulin deficiency states frequently are disappointing (Janeway and Rosen, 1966; Conrad, 1969). Multiple exposure to commercially available gamma globulin may be associated with allergic reactions, including anaphylaxis; its casual use cannot be recommended (Ellis and Henney, 1969; Miller, 1969).

Polymorphonuclear Leukocytes

Quantitative and qualitative defects in polymorphonuclear leukocytes (PMNs) allow dissemination of bacterial infection. The incidence of bacterial infection is inversely correlated with the number of circulating polymorphonuclear leukocytes per milliliter of blood. Infections are most common in patients with PMN counts of 100 to 500/ml; a gradual decrease in rate of infection is associated with PMN counts of 500 to 1500/ml or more (Bodey et al., 1966; Fernbach et al., 1969). Attempts to prevent infections in such patients with prophylactic use of "broad-spectrum" or multiple antibiotics virtually always fail; resistant bacterial strains or fungi fill the bacteriologic vacuum created by eradication of sensitive strains. Attempts to cure severe infections with antibiotics in such patients are frequently unsuccessful. Severe infections in patients with neutropenia may be treated by transfusion of PMNs; further trials comparing antibiotics and PMN transfusions are necessary, as PMN transfusions must be frequent, are expensive, and are not devoid of adverse effects (Freireich et al., 1964; Graw et al., 1971).

Polymorphonuclear leukocytes may be defective in their ability to kill bacteria or fungi. Some defects are restricted to a single bacterial or fungal type; others are more generalized. Abnormal PMNs may also be associated with severe viral infections (Lux et al., 1970). Defective PMNs have most commonly been found in children with unusual or recurrent infections (Moeschlin, 1956; Lawrence, 1957; Stefanini et al., 1958; Page et al., 1962; Cutting and Lang, 1964; Krill et al., 1964; Zuelzer, 1964; Blume et al., 1968; Davis et al., 1968; Kyle and Linman, 1968; Douglas, 1970; Salmon et al., 1970). Neutrophil dysfunction may be associated with burn injuries (Alexander and Wixson, 1970). The mechanisms involved in these rare defects have not been fully clarified (Quie, 1969).

Other Defense Mechanisms

Patients deficient in the third or fifth component of complement are subject to recurrent episodes of bacterial infection (Alper et al., 1970; Miller and Nilsson, 1970). Other means of preventing infection are afforded by tissue and circulating histiocytes, monocytes, the reticuloendothelial system, and the lymphatic system. Opsonins and specific antitoxins (e.g., diphtheria antitoxin, antistreptolysin) formed in response to injection of toxoids, vaccines, or infection may prevent or attenuate future infections.

Interferon is a generic term descriptive of soluble proteins of molecular weight 20,000 to 160,000 produced by cells infected by viruses. Interferon can also be induced by a variety of organic and synthetic substances (Weinstein and Chang, 1968). Interferon has a broad spectrum of antiviral activity, possibly by interfering with the capability of viruses to cause a cell to replicate viral protein structure. Because antibiotics have a very limited role in most viral infections, therapy with interferon or induction of interferon production is being vigorously investigated (Finter, 1966; Finkelstein and Merigan, 1968; Rita, 1968; Wolstenholme and O'Connor, 1968; Merigan, 1969).

Principle: The patient's defense mechanisms must be considered in addition to the infecting organism and the antibiotic agent appropriate for the organism. A patient with normal defense mechanisms may manage some infections without antibiotic therapy. In patients with severely compromised defense mechanisms, even antibiotics that are potently bactericidal in vitro may fail to eradicate the infection in vivo. One cannot render a patient bacteriologically sterile by antibiotic therapy. A physician's expectations of antibiotic therapy must be realistic: antibiotics alone may not be curative.

HOST RESPONSES OFFERING CLUES TO THE ETIOLOGY OF THE INFECTION

The suspicion of bacterial infection should be confirmed by bacteriologic methods. Methods range from a simple gram stain for gonococcal urethritis to determination of the antibacterial activity of dilutions of the treated patient's serum against the causative organism. Pending bacteriologic confirmation and, if necessary, sensitivity testing of antibiotic activity, the pattern of the patient's local or systemic response to infection may provide clues as to whether the infection is bacterial or viral, and even as to what type of organism is responsible. Inflammatory responses are discussed in Chapter 9. Specific patterns of response to infection may assist the physician in determining whether bacterial infection is likely and in selecting antibiotics prior to bacteriologic confirmation (when the patient is too ill to permit delay).

For example, the pattern of physical findings versus radiologic demonstration of pulmonary involvement by bacterial, viral, rickettsial, and *Chlamydia* (*Mycoplasma* or Eaton agent) infections may be impressive. Physical findings of pneumonia are ordinarily present in bacterial pneumonias but may be absent or elusive in viral and rickettsial pneumonias. In patients with pneumonia of uncertain etiology, presence or absence of physical findings and other clues to be mentioned later should influence decisions about antibiotic therapy. Absence of physical findings may justify delay in antibiotic therapy until further observation of the patient and results of cultures provide additional evidence.

Immunologic Responses to Infection and Prophylactic Therapy

Streptococcal infections elicit responses in tissues that may depend in part on the age of the patient and may be variably prevented by penicillin prophylaxis; e.g., rheumatic fever occurs mostly in children and can be prevented (Taranta *et al.*, 1964), whereas glomerulonephritis cannot be prevented. Pharyngeal infections with streptococci elicit different immunologic responses than does skin infection (Wannamaker, 1970). Immunologic evidence supports the epidemiologic link between streptococcal infections and acute rheumatic fever and its recurrences (Cantanzaro *et al.*, 1954; Seelers, 1966). Almost all recurrences of acute rheumatic fever in children and adults can be prevented by the prophylactic use of oral or parenteral penicillin. Monthly parenteral injections of penicillin are somewhat more effective than oral therapy, possibly because of more reliable drug administration (Doyle *et al.*, 1967; Feinstein *et al.*, 1968; Pansegrau *et al.*, 1968; Feinstein and Levitt, 1970). The recurrence rate of acute rheumatic fever diminishes with age. The efficacy of prophylactic therapy with penicillin in older patients is unresolved (Taranta and Griffith, 1966). A high risk of exposure to streptococci and the difficulties in diagnosing rheumatic fever in adults or in establishing the hemodynamic significance of a valve lesion during active rheumatic carditis may justify continuing prophylaxis. On the other hand, many patients would be treated to prevent recurrences in a few, as recurrences are uncommon in the elderly. If bacterial endocarditis occurs during penicillin prophylaxis, resistant organisms may be responsible. Only one-half the organisms responsible for endocarditis during penicillin prophylaxis for rheumatic fever are

susceptible to penicillin (Doyle *et al.*, 1967). Pending evidence from a long-term and sizable, controlled clinical trial, the decision for or against prophylactic therapy is arbitrarily made on an individual basis, taking into account the likelihood of exposure of the patient to streptococci, the age of the patient, and the severity of cardiac involvement.

In some patients the initial attack of acute glomerulonephritis is related to extrarenal streptococcal infections. Clinically, it is difficult to distinguish an initial attack of acute glomerulonephritis from exacerbations of a pre-existing latent or chronic glomerulonephritis. By consensus, initial episodes of acute glomerulonephritis are treated by antibiotic therapy for known or suspected streptococcal infection; there is no evidence to support the use of chronic prophylactic therapy to prevent recurrences. Recurrences of glomerulonephritis appear to be related to a variety of stresses other than nephritogenic streptococcal infection (Dixon, 1968; Dodge *et al.*, 1968; Pollak *et al.*, 1968). Acute glomerulonephritis in the elderly occurs infrequently and is difficult to recognize (Schwartz and Kassirer, 1963; Boswell and Eknoyan, 1968). Particularly in older patients, the possible association of bacterial endocarditis with glomerulonephritis should be considered, as the renal lesion may respond to therapy of the endocarditis (Heptinstall and Joekes, 1963; Stickler *et al.*, 1968).

Other patterns of reaction to infection, such as erythema nodosum, the Arthus and Shwartzman phenomena, and various "allergic" manifestations, are discussed in Chapter 9.

Patterns of Systemic Response

The patient's systemic response to infection may provide clues to its etiology. These patterns should be carefully considered in the decision to begin or to withhold antibiotic therapy. Fever and hematologic abnormalities are discussed here to exemplify the use of systemic signs to diagnose and follow the course of infections; general patterns of response are discussed to present differences commonly found among the actions of infectious agents.

Fever. Although fever is a nonspecific sign in many disorders, it offers the physician a means of following the course of some infections. Fever is a systemic reaction to a pyrogen, which *may* be due to bacterial infection. Excessive anxiety about the possibility of sepsis can mislead inexperienced clinicians to the conclusion that high fever *means* bacterial infection. The presence of fever may lead to the premature and inappropriate administration of antibiotics to a patient with a disorder unresponsive to, or even complicated by, antibiotic therapy. Considerably more evidence of bacterial infection than the presence of fever is required before antibiotic therapy is initiated.

In the past, patterns of fever were used as clues to the etiology of disease (Osler, 1918); today this exercise is relatively unrewarding. High spiking fevers with impressive zeniths and nadirs suggest intermittent release of pyrogenic substances and classically occur in circumstances of "pus under pressure" or ascending cholangitis. Regrettably, many bacterial or nonbacterial infections may also produce this pattern. The so-called "hectic febrile course" can also be caused by sarcoidosis (Nolan and Klatskin, 1964), drugs (Cluff and Johnson, 1964), and a large array of other disorders (Keefer and Leard, 1955; Petersdorf and Beeson, 1961). Tachypnea and dyspnea out of proportion to fever may suggest pulmonary embolism as opposed to bacterial pneumonia (Israel and Goldstein, 1957; Fred, 1969). Rarely, periodic or recurrent fevers are seen that suggest a specific disorder (e.g., malaria, Colorado tick fever, familial Mediterranean fever).

The majority of fevers due to bacterial infection respond to appropriate antibiotic therapy within a few days. Even the fevers of disseminated tuberculosis and bacterial endocarditis frequently improve during the first week of therapy. Use of the fever index (degrees of fever multiplied by the hours per day of fever) has been suggested as a more precise means of following a febrile course (Fekety and McDaniel, 1968). Failure of the daily fever spike or fever index to diminish should lead the physician to reconsider his original diagnosis and his therapy. He should also look for complications of infection or types of infection (e.g., abscess, osteomyelitis) that respond poorly to antibiotic therapy alone and should consider the possibility of drug fever. *Principle: Although febrile patterns are of limited value in the diagnosis of a specific bacterial infection, the fever's course during antibiotic therapy may provide valuable information as to the appropriateness of diagosis and therapy.*

Hematologic Abnormalities. Bacterial infection is usually accompanied by polymorphonuclear leukocytosis, but in overwhelming infections or during early gram-negative sepsis, leukopenia may occur (see Chapter 5). Classically, the polymorphonuclear leukocyte count is low in viral infections, but there are many exceptions to this observation. Some viral infections, notably acute pericarditis, are associated with a brisk polymorphonuclear leukocytosis (McGuire *et al.*, 1954). Tuberculosis may mimic virtually any hematologic abnormality, including acute leukemia (Cooper, 1959; Hughes *et al.*, 1959; Lowther, 1959; Dawborn and Cowling, 1961; Milder *et al.*, 1961; Finch and Castleman, 1963). Thrombocytopenia and hemolytic anemia should suggest the possibility of disseminated intravascular coagulation, particularly in patients with gram-negative bacterial infections (McKay, 1969). The physician must know whether the antibiotic he uses has effects on the hematopoietic system, lest he attribute changes in the patient's blood to a manifestation of the disease instead of to his therapy.

Adequate antibiotic therapy frequently controls the leukocytosis of acute simple bacterial infections within a week. Failure of the leukocytosis to diminish should alert the physician to the possibility of incorrect diagnosis, inadequate therapy, or a complication of the infection.

Anatomic Location of Infection

The anatomic location of an infection may influence its bacteriologic type and its response to antibiotic therapy. Devascularized tissues may harbor anaerobic or microaerophilic organisms; delivery of antibiotics to such areas may be impossible. Obstruction of a normal drainage route may cause retention of infected fluids. These infections respond poorly, if at all, to antibiotic therapy alone. The failure of antibiotics to kill bacteria in purulent collections may be due to (1) slow growth of bacteria (antibiotics being most effective against rapidly multiplying organisms), or (2) inactivation of the antibiotic by purulent fluid. Surgical drainage may be required to allow recovery, even in tissues as vascular as the liver (where a priori one might wrongly anticipate excellent delivery of defense mechanisms and antibiotics to the site of infection).

Other infections that may resist antibiotic therapy alone are endocarditis and osteomyelitis. The valvular lesions of endocarditis are relatively avascular, possibly accounting for the need for relatively high concentrations of antibiotics to effect a cure. If response to therapy in endocarditis is not adequate despite appropriate antibiotic therapy, a complication such as cardiac abscess or peripheral mycotic aneurysm may be present. Involucrum formation in osteomyelitis may reduce access of blood and antibiotics to the infection site. In diabetics with vascular disease, osteomyelitis of the lower extremity regularly fails to respond to antibiotic therapy; amputation is required to effect a "cure" (Waldvogel *et al.*, 1970). *Principle: Débridement of devascularized tissue and surgical drainage of infected spaces or abscesses may be requisite to adequate therapeutic response, despite the* in *vitro sensitivity of the bacteria to the antibiotic being administered. Failure of a patient to respond to appropriate antibiotics demonstrates a need for other definitive therapy.*

HOST FACTORS PREDISPOSING TO SPECIFIC INFECTIONS OR TO ALTERED RESPONSE TO INFECTIONS

Age of the Patient

The incidence and/or mortality of a variety of infections is greatest in the first or declining decades of life. This has been demonstrated in staphylococcal sepsis (Cluff *et al.*, 1968), gram-negative bacteremia (Udhoji and Weil, 1965; Altemeier *et al.*, 1967), and pneumococcal meningitis (Wilson and Lerner, 1964; Swartz and Dodge, 1965). Although infants have high rates of infection, their mortality from infection is less than that of elderly patients. Reasons for these differences in morbidity and mortality are not known. The relative immaturity of the infant's immunologic mechanisms may predispose him to infection, but his lack of associated diseases may allow recovery. Cardiovascular disease is correlated with fatal infections in the elderly (Cluff *et al.*, 1968), but these patients are more likely to have other disorders, such as diabetes, malignancy, uremia, cirrhosis, or hematologic disease, that adversely affect the outcome of infections (McHenry *et al.*, 1962; Altemeier *et al.*, 1967; McHenry, 1969).

The elderly patient may have comparatively little fever with bacterial infections. Trivial signs of infection in the elderly should be pursued vigorously to permit early diagnosis, in the hope that earlier therapy will improve survival.

Nosocomial Infections

Hospital-acquired infections are often due to antibiotic-resistant strains of staphylococci or gram-negative organisms. These infections commonly involve postoperative wounds, the urinary tract, the lungs, or the skin (Rosenblatt *et al.*, 1969). The organisms prevalent in a hospital and/or their antibiotic sensitivities change with time, possibly as a result of changing local practices of antibiotic use (McNamara *et al.*, 1967; Barrett *et al.*, 1968a; Bulger and Sherris, 1968; Bulger *et al.*, 1970; Dans *et al.*, 1970; Feingold, 1970; Scheckler and Bennett, 1970; Selden *et al.*, 1971). Knowledge of the hospital's flora may allow earlier recognition of infections likely to be resistant to antibiotics. Unusual organisms such as *Serratia marcescens* may be involved in nosocomial infections (Magnuson

and Elston, 1966). Minor epidemics may be caused by a resistant organism, e.g., a methicillin-resistant strain of *Staphylococcus aureus* (Barrett *et al.*, 1968b; O'Toole *et al.*, 1970). These infections are particularly odious because they sometimes require use of toxic antibiotics and subject the patient to risk of superinfection with fungi.

Hospital use of antibiotics alters the bacterial ecology of the patient and physician. The hospital is a dangerous place for a patient initially free of infection (see Chapter 14). The number of serious and fatal staphylococcal infections in many hospitals has greatly increased, and other microorganisms that are ordinarily considered saprophytic or of low virulence may cause infections. Since the introduction of chemotherapy, there has been a progressive and alarming increase in bacteremic deaths caused by *E. coli*, *Aerobacter*, etc. Strains of these organisms may produce superinfections in surface wounds, or in the alimentary, urinary, or respiratory tract of patients under treatment with multiple antibiotics. These organisms are usually resistant to all the antibiotics previously administered to the patient and often to all the antibiotics commonly used in hospitals.

There has been a substantial absolute as well as relative increase in deaths from nosocomial infections. These deaths are not noted to suggest that the overall influence of antibiotics has been deleterious. It is clear, however, that the gains in therapy from antibiotics do not constitute a "free ride"; their cost to the community at large is infection and death of certain patients who would otherwise have survived. The physician's responsibility is to know the proper indications for antibiotics and to use them effectively. *Principle: Antibiotics are necessary for the treatment of bacterial infections, but excessive use of antibiotics needlessly exposes the patient to drug toxicity and alters the hospital flora to favor appearance of resistant pathogenic organisms.*

Diabetes Mellitus

A variety of metabolic disorders or complications may predispose to infection in diabetics. Definite proof of the role of the metabolic disorders of mild diabetes in increased infections is not available. Chronic monilial intertrigo is common in early diabetes mellitus and subsides with control of hyperglycemia. Bacterial infection seems to be more common and slower to respond to therapy in patients with mild diabetes. Diabetes mellitus is associated with gram-negative bacteremia much more often than with meningitis or staphylococcal sepsis (Dodge and Swartz, 1965;

Altemeier *et al.*, 1967; Cluff *et al.*, 1968). This relationship may be due to the high rate of renal infection in diabetes mellitus; the kidney (particularly after bladder catheterization) commonly is the portal of entry of gram-negative bacteria.

Infection worsens glucose tolerance and may precipitate diabetic ketoacidosis. Acidosis impairs the function of polymorphonuclear leukocytes in animals (Sheldon and Bauer, 1958, 1959; Perillie *et al.*, 1962). Diabetic patients in ketoacidosis may develop necrotizing fungal infections of the head (rhinocerebral mucormycosis) (Ackerman and Vickery, 1968). Pyelonephritis in diabetics may be complicated by acute renal papillary necrosis. Diabetics are susceptible to both acute and chronic severe bacterial and fungal infections. The frequency and severity of these infections may be reduced by control of hyperglycemia and prevention of diabetic ketoacidosis.

Adrenocorticosteroids and Congeners

Interrelations exist between adrenal function and the effects of corticosteroids on bacterial infection (Beisel and Rapoport, 1969). The anti-inflammatory effects of corticosteroids on lymphocytes, the lymphatics, the reticuloendothelial system, localized inflammation, the complement system, and fibroblast function sometimes permit reactivation of tuberculosis and favor dissemination of bacterial infection (see Chapter 9).

Corticosteroids may be utilized to suppress the inflammatory response to an infection, as in tuberculous meningitis, provided appropriate antibiotics against the infecting organism are given (O'Toole *et al.*, 1969). The use of corticosteroids in tuberculous meningitis has resulted in equivocal long-term results (Toole and McCall, 1969; Klastersky *et al.*, 1971). The decision to use or to withhold corticosteroids in tuberculous meningitis should be considered open, pending further studies, unless acute reduction in cerebrospinal fluid pressure is necessary.

Patients taking corticosteroids for noninfectious disease require particularly close scrutiny to permit early diagnosis of infection. Corticosteroids may modify a patient's conventional responses to bacterial infection, reducing the fever and local tenderness, and may even alter the radiographic findings in bacterial pneumonias. Conditions ordinarily easy to recognize, such as septic peritonitis, may be manifested very subtly in patients taking corticosteroids. Steps to diagnose infections should be liberally undertaken in such patients. The use of corticosteroids to manage patients with adrenal insufficiency during the stress of infection is discussed in Chapter 7.

Nephrotic Syndrome

Nephrotic patients tend to develop bacterial infections such as primary pneumococcal peritonitis. Subsequent to the introduction of antibiotics, "abdominal crises" in nephrotics have more often been attributed to staphylococcal or antibiotic-induced enterocolitis (Schreiner, 1963). Nephrotic patients may remit during corticosteroid therapy, but they are at high risk of fatal infection (Pollak *et al.*, 1968).

Prednisone regularly increases the polymorphonuclear white-blood-cell count in nephrotics. The degree of the leukocytosis is dose dependent (Floyd *et al.*, 1969); even 30 mg prednisone daily increases PMN counts to 13,700 (range 7400 to 24,000), and patients with the nephrotic syndrome are often given much larger doses. This therapy not only obscures some signs of infection, but introduces one itself. Careful observation of the patient may provide clues, but the physician may be required to make an intuitive decision about the presence or absence of infection. Such a decision is actually a guess, and careful observations should be continued to re-evaluate the need for antibiotic therapy.

Hepatic Cirrhosis

Hepatic cirrhosis is occasionally associated with gram-negative bacterial sepsis, but is associated less frequently with staphylococcal bacteremia or purulent meningitis (Swartz and Dodge, 1965; Altemeier *et al.*, 1967; Cluff *et al.*, 1968). Gastrointestinal mucosal edema and portal shunting of blood may be responsible for gram-negative sepsis or peritonitis in cirrhosis (Conn, 1964). Peritonitis due to pneumococci has also been reported (Epstein *et al.*, 1968). The hypersplenism of cirrhosis does not commonly induce neutropenia to a degree associated with very high rates of bacterial infection (i.e., less than 1000/ml). The severe and transient leukopenia observed in some cirrhotic patients is possibly due to bone marrow depression by ethanol (McFarland and Libre, 1963) or folate deficiency.

Hematologic Disorders

A number of hematologic disorders appear to predispose patients to bacterial infection. Patients with Hodgkin's disease have impaired delayed hypersensitivity responses and are liable to viral and fungal infections (Aisenberg, 1964; Sokal and Firat, 1965; Casazza *et al.*, 1966; Brown *et al.*, 1967; Perry *et al.*, 1967); they are also subject to infection with organisms that elicit a granulomatous reaction, such as *M.*

tuberculosis, Listeria, Brucella, or *Salmonella.* The frequency of tuberculosis in Hodgkin's disease led early workers to the incorrect assumption that tuberculosis was the cause of Hodgkin's disease. In contrast, patients with hypogammaglobulinemia are subject to infection with pyogenic organisms. Hodgkin's disease appears to differ immunologically from leukemias, lymphomas, and leprosy in that the correction of the defect in delayed hypersensitivity is more resistant to cell transfer (Paradisi *et al.*, 1969). Pneumococcal pneumonia is commonly recurrent in patients with multiple myeloma (Zimmerman and Hall, 1954; Lawson *et al.*, 1955; Lippincott *et al.*, 1960; Fahey *et al.*, 1963; Linton *et al.*, 1963; Solomon *et al.*, 1963; Caggiano *et al.*, 1967; Salmon *et al.*, 1967).

Patients with thymoma may have quantitative or qualitative defects in gamma globulins and/or pancytopenia, resulting in recurrent bacterial infections or uncommon infections (Jacox *et al.*, 1964; Mongan *et al.*, 1966; Korn *et al.*, 1967).

Salmonella osteomyelitis and fulminant pneumococcal meningitis occur in patients with sickle-cell anemia (Hook *et al.*, 1957; Robinson and Watson, 1966). Perhaps the enhanced susceptibility to infection may be analogous to that reported to occur after splenectomy (Smith *et al.*, 1962). Functional asplenia, as determined by splenic uptake of radioactive technitium (Pearson *et al.*, 1969), and deficiency in serum opsonizing pneumococcal activity have been demonstrated in patients with sickle-cell disease (Winkelstein and Drachman, 1968).

Thyroid Disease

Either thyroid storm or myxedema coma may be precipitated by bacterial infection. Signs of infection may be obscured by myxedema or thyrotoxicosis, but the signs should be carefully evaluated, as the catabolic effects of infection are devastating in either setting.

Thoracic Disease

Recurrent pneumonia should alert the clinician to the possibility of both intrathoracic and extrathoracic disorders. Intrathoracic diseases (chronic obstructive airway disease, cardiovascular disease, bronchiectasis, asthma, prior lung diseases, etc.) are as common in recurrent pneumonias as are extrathoracic diseases (alcoholism, diabetes, sinusitis, malignancies, neurologic and hematologic abnormalities, etc.) (Winterbauer *et al.*, 1969). In chronic pulmonary disease, pulmonary infection is occasionally induced by anoxia, cardiac failure, or respiratory acidosis (Stone *et al.*, 1953). Intoxication with ethanol, hypoxia, or acute starvation in animals depresses the ability of the lungs to clear

bacteria (Green and Kass, 1964; Brunstetter *et al.*, 1971; Cross *et al.*, 1971; Gee *et al.*, 1971; Menzel, 1971). Atelectasis, bronchial obstruction, or aspiration predisposes to severe, resistant, or recurrent pneumonias. Obstructive lesions may require surgical therapy in addition to use of antibiotics to prevent recurrences. The use of intermittent and prophylactic antibiotics and of other forms of therapy in these chronic conditions is discussed in Chapter 6.

Renal Disease

Uremic patients have impaired inflammatory responses (see Chapter 9) and may have little fever during a bacterial infection. Sepsis is a common problem during acute renal failure, probably owing in part to the common use of intravenous and indwelling bladder catheters. A bladder catheter in acute renal failure is usually unnecessary (Swann and Merrill, 1953; Bluemle *et al.*, 1959; Franklin and Merrill, 1960; Kiley *et al.*, 1960; Wells *et al.*, 1960; Maher and Schreiner, 1962; Levinsky, 1966). Indwelling intravenous catheters should be rotated every two to three days to reduce the rate of infections introduced by this route.

Both hemodialysis and peritoneal dialysis are complicated by infections, including septic pulmonary embolism from an infected shunt that must be removed despite antibiotic therapy (Maher and Schreiner, 1965; Goodwin *et al.*, 1969; Miller and Tassistro, 1969).

Patients who have undergone renal transplantation usually require "immunosuppressive" therapy and are subject to infection with conventional and opportunistic organisms (Hill *et al.*, 1964; Rifkind *et al.*, 1967; Ginn, 1969).

Drugs of Abuse

Alcohol may predispose to infection by causing neutropenia or defective leukocyte mobilization into traumatized skin (Brayton *et al.*, 1970). Infections may be related to the general debility of the alcoholic patient or to the tendency of infection to follow any episode of central nervous system depression (pulmonary atelectasis with infection, aspiration pneumonia).

Other drugs of abuse are associated with a variety of skin, cardiovascular, and pulmonary infections, sometimes with unusual organisms. These infections are due to contamination of drug and to unsterile injection equipment (Louria, 1969).

This section does not include all factors that may predispose to bacterial infection. It has omitted, for example, a discussion of prophylaxis for endocarditis in cardiovascular disease, the role of otitis media or of the age of the patient in determining the type of organism to be expected in purulent meningitis (Swartz and Dodge, 1965), and topics such as eradication of the carrier state in meningococcal disease (Deal and Sanders, 1969; Artenstein *et al.*, 1970). These subjects are well covered in texts on infectious disease.

Although medicine has long recognized that a host deficiency in nutritional state enhances the risk of an acquired infection (Gordon and Scrimshaw, 1970), the merits of "hyperalimentation" with massive doses of vitamin C are not established, and may be toxic (Pauling, 1970; Thornton, 1970; Lambden, 1971).

ANTIBIOTICS

A brief discussion of the chemistry, antibacterial spectrum, advantages, and liabilities of commonly used antibiotics follows. The dosage and use of uncommonly utilized antibiotics are discussed in textbooks of pharmacology and medicine. Many of the recommendations of "first-choice" antibiotics listed here for specific organisms have been abstracted from a review (Medical Letter, 1968c). For less common bacterial infections, in which the opportunity to compare various drugs is infrequently available, some dispute continues about the relative efficacy of one or more antibiotics. Areas of contention are cited. The physician is assisted by reviews such as those provided by the *Medical Letter*, but if a patient does not respond well to a "first-choice" drug, a detailed review of the medical literature may be required to determine whether new studies indicate preference for another antibiotic. Sensitivity testing is also helpful in decisions of antibiotic choice.

The Penicillins

The penicillins are derivatives of 6-aminopenicillanic acid. Benzyl penicillin (penicillin G) is available as the potassium salt (about 1.6 mEq potassium per 1,000,000 units) or as the sodium salt (about 2.0 mEq sodium per 1,000,000 units). The salt form selected is important during renal disease or congestive heart failure.

Penicillin G is painful on intramuscular injection and has a short duration of action; procaine penicillin G is relatively painless intramuscularly and has a 24-hour duration of action (with low concentrations in blood). Benzathine penicillin G is a "slow-release" preparation of penicillin that provides low concentrations in blood for 14 to 30 days.

Alphaphenoxymethylpenicillin (penicillin V) and alphaphenoxyethylpenicillin (phenethicillin) were developed to provide acid stability and allow oral administration. Although the relatively inexpensive penicillin G is degraded by gastric acid, increasing the dose may result in satisfactory blood concentrations. Gastrointestinal absorption of the penicillins is usually greatest when the drug is taken on an empty stomach.

The route of penicillin administration depends upon the nature of the infection being treated. Low concentrations of penicillin in the blood are adequate for prophylaxis against recurrences of rheumatic fever, allowing oral administration of penicillin or use of benzathine penicillin G intramuscularly. Uncomplicated pneumococcal pneumonia responds to the relatively low blood concentrations achieved by intramuscular procaine penicillin, 1,000,000 units given every 12 hours. In bacterial endocarditis, a sustained high concentration of penicillin in blood may be necessary; constant intravenous infusions of penicillin G are ordinarily recommended. The rapid renal clearance of penicillins accounts for their short half-life in blood and results in urinary concentrations of antibiotic that are quite high (higher than the concentrations usually employed for bacteria sensitivity testing), allowing their use in pyelonephritis due to *E. coli*.

Antibacterial Spectrum. The penicillins are either bactericidal or bacteriostatic, depending upon dose and organism. Their principal antibiotic action appears to be interference with bacterial cell-wall synthesis. The following organisms are thought to be most appropriately treated by one of the penicillins just described (Medical Letter, 1968c):

Gram-positive cocci
> *Streptococcus pyogenes*
> *Streptococcus viridans* (streptomycin may be required for resistant strains)
> *Streptococcus anaerobius*
> *Enterococcus* (with streptomycin)
> *Staphylococcus aureus* (nonpenicillinase-producing)
> *Diplococcus pneumoniae*

Gram-negative cocci
> *Neisseria meningitidis*
> *Neisseria gonorrheae* (relatively resistant strains occur, requiring higher doses of penicillin)

Gram-positive bacilli
> *Bacillus anthracis*
> *Bacillus perfringens*
> *Clostridium tetani* (local therapy of infection, antitoxin, and immunization are required)

Gram-negative bacilli
> *Fusobacterium fusiforme*

Spirochetes
> *Spirillum minus*
> *Treponema pallidum*

Treponema pertenue

Actinomycetes

Actinomyces israelii

2,6-Dimethoxyphenyl penicillin (methicillin) and the remaining penicillin derivatives to be discussed are resistant to the penicillinase produced by some strains of *Staphylococcus aureus*. Current preparations of methicillin are quite soluble and stable in water or saline (earlier preparations were unstable, requiring infusion shortly after solution). Methicillin's antimicrobial spectrum is similar to penicillin G's, but on a weight basis, 20 to 30 times more methicillin than penicillin G is required to kill pneumococci, group A streptococci, and penicillin-sensitive staphylococci. Methicillin is resistant to the action of penicillinase, inhibiting the growth of penicillinase-producing staphylococci in a minimum inhibitory concentration between 1.5 and 6.2 μg/ml. It is bactericidal in almost the same concentration at which it is bacteriostatic. Resistance of staphylococci to the drug can be demonstrated *in vitro*, and methicillin-resistant staphylococci have been reported clinically (Barrett *et al.*, 1968b).

Methicillin must be given parenterally. It is rapidly excreted by the kidneys and some appears in the bile. Its rapid clearance requires that it be administered every four hours intramuscularly (unless probenecid is given). Methicillin is bound to serum proteins in approximately the same percentage as penicillin G, but this binding does not interfere with its antibacterial activity. As methicillin crosses the blood-brain barrier poorly, it is relatively ineffective in staphylococcal meningitis.

Patients allergic to penicillin G may show cross-hypersensitivity to methicillin, but independent of this phenomenon, about 5% of patients receiving the drug develop rashes, fever, and angioneurotic edema. Because it is expensive, methicillin should be reserved for use in severe penicillin-resistant staphylococcal infections.

Other synthetic penicillins in this category include 3-phenyl-5-methyl-4-isoxazolyl penicillin (oxacillin); 3-chlorophenyl-5-methyl-4-isoxazolyl penicillin (cloxacillin); 6-(2-ethoxy-1) naphthamido penicillin (nafcillin); and 2,6-dichlorophenyl-5-methyl-4-isoxazolecarboxamido penicillin (dicloxacillin). Oxacillin is as effective as methicillin against staphylococci and has the advantage of oral absorption. The minimal inhibitory concentration (MIC) for resistant staphylococci is 0.8 μg/ml. Although this MIC is considerably less than methicillin's, some of this advantage is presumably lost because 75 to 80% of the drug is bound to serum proteins. In practice, oxacillin is virtually obsolete, having been replaced by its congeners, cloxacillin and dicloxacillin, which chemically differ from oxacillin only in their content of chloride. *In vitro*, cloxacillin has about the same degree of activity as does oxacillin, but because the drug is more rapidly absorbed and more slowly excreted, higher antibacterial levels are achieved. The dosage of cloxacillin is about 2.0 g per day. Dicloxacillin is nearly twice as active as cloxacillin, but otherwise there is little difference between these two drugs. Nafcillin has been alleged by some to be superior to methicillin, but when they are used in equivalent dosages, there is little difference between them. Furthermore, the oral dosage form of nafcillin may be absorbed more erratically than cloxacillin or dicloxacillin.

The only organism for which this category of penicillin is recommended as a "first choice" antibiotic is a penicillinase-producing *Staph. aureus* (Medical Letter, 1968c). No particular advantages in antibiotic efficacy are known for any of these penicillins. Some are available for oral or parenteral use only. Cloxacillin and dicloxacillin are much better absorbed after oral administration than oxacillin or nafcillin. Pending bacteriologic diagnosis of the type of gram-positive coccal infection present, one of these penicillins may temporarily be used to cover the possibility of a resistant staphylococcal infection, particularly in ill patients (Petersdorf and Turck, 1966). ***Principle: The treatment of ill patients with proven or suspected staphylococcal infections must begin with a penicillinase-resistant penicillin, and one should change to penicillin G only if the organism is sensitive to that drug.***

Alpha-amino penicillin (ampicillin) has relatively less antibiotic activity against organisms sensitive to penicillin G and is *not active against penicillinase-producing staphylococci*. It has activity against certain gram-negative bacteria and has been recommended as the antibiotic of initial choice for the following organisms (Medical Letter, 1968c):

Gram-negative bacilli

Shigella (resistance may occur)

Escherichia coli (resistance may occur)

Proteus mirabilis

Hemophilus influenzae

Bordetella pertussis

Actinomycetes

Actinomyces muris ratti

Ampicillin is active against *E. coli* and *Proteus mirabilis*, possesses intermediate activity against the paracolon group, but is relatively ineffective against *Klebsiella*, *Pseudomonas*, and indole-positive strains of *Proteus*. Ampicillin is active *in vitro* against *E. coli* and *Proteus mirabilis* and is useful in urinary tract infections

(Lee and Hill, 1968), but it is relatively ineffective against *Klebsiella-Aerobacter* and is totally inactive against indole-positive strains of *Proteus* and *Pseudomonas*. The *in vitro* sensitivity of enterococci to ampicillin is greater than to penicillin G. When ampicillin is used orally, the dosage in adults should probably not exceed 2 to 3 g per day because a higher dose often produces diarrhea. Parenteral doses as high as 12 g per day are usually well tolerated and may be necessary in severe infections.

Ampicillin may be used for initial therapy of bacteriologically undiagnosed meningitis in children and for chronic typhoid carriers (Simon and Miller, 1966). Ampicillin is considerably more stable in acid than is penicillin G (Hou and Poole, 1969). Hetacillin is an investigational antibiotic similar to ampicillin (Tuano *et al.*, 1966; Kirby and Kind, 1967; Sabath and Finland, 1967; Steigbigel *et al.*, 1967). Carbenicillin is an investigational drug active in high doses against some strains of *Pseudomonas* (Brumfitt *et al.*, 1967; Marks and Eickhoff, 1970; Hoffman and Bullock, 1970; Hoffman *et al.*, 1970).

Adverse Reactions. The important problem of penicillin allergy (Idsoe *et al.*, 1968) is discussed in Chapter 15. In addition to hypersensitivity or "meta reactions," a number of rare toxic reactions have been described for the penicillins, including psychosis and convulsions from high doses (Seamans *et al.*, 1968); transverse myelitis (Shaw, 1966); bone marrow depression from methicillin (McElfresh and Huang, 1962); cholestatic jaundice from oxacillin (Freedman, 1965); hyperkalemia from potassium salts of penicillin G in renal failure (Stewart, 1964); pulmonary emboli from inadvertent use of procaine penicillin G intravenously (Hoigne and Krebs, 1964; Popper, 1964); meningeal irritation from intrathecal administration; Herxheimer reactions in the therapy of syphilis (Knudsen and Aastrup, 1965); nephritis during therapy with penicillin G or methicillin (Feigin and Fiascone, 1965; Baldwin *et al.*, 1968); induction of lupus erythematosus-like syndrome (Alarcon-Segovia *et al.*, 1965); development of a positive Coombs test and hemolytic anemia (Petz and Fudenberg, 1966; Swanson *et al.*, 1966); and appearance of agranulocytosis with monohistiocytosis (Graf and Tarlov, 1968). Penicillin G may alter laboratory tests, including urinary glucose, protein, and phenolsulfonphthalein; methicillin may cause an elevation in blood ammonia and a reduction in serum calcium (Elking and Kabat, 1968). Increases in serum glutamic oxaloacetic transaminase have been reported with ampicillin, nafcillin, and oxacillin (Wirth and Thompson, 1965). Skin rashes are more common with ampicillin than with the other penicillins. Bacterial or fungal superinfections are not uncommon, whereas severe gastrointestinal irritation or thrombophlebitis from intravenous administration is rare.

The Cephalosporins

Cephalothin is a derivative of 7-aminocephalosporanic acid, which resembles the 6-aminopenicillanic acid structure of penicillin. Cephaloridine is a congener of cephalothin; both drugs must be given by the parenteral route. Cephaloridine is less painful on intramuscular injection than cephalothin.

The cephalosporins inhibit bacterial cell-wall synthesis and are generally useful in patients allergic to penicillin who harbor a penicillin-sensitive organism. Allergic reactions to cephalosporins occur in some patients allergic to penicillin. Cephalosporins, with notable exceptions, are generally less active than penicillin G, the semisynthetic penicillins, or the ampicillin group against organisms sensitive to these antibiotics. The cephalosporins have a somewhat broader spectrum of antibiotic activity than ampicillin; they are active against a variety of organisms, including penicillinase-producing staphylococci (Perkins and Saslaw, 1966). Staphylococci are exceedingly sensitive, but as the *in vitro* inoculum size is increased, sensitivity diminishes. This effect is generally true for the cephalosporins and in a sense puts them at a relative disadvantage to the penicillins. Cephalosporins are also active against gram-negative organisms, particularly *Proteus mirabilis*, *E. coli*, and *Klebsiella-Aerobacter*. Cephalothin is ineffective against most strains of *Aerobacter* but is very active against *Klebsiella*. As cephalothin is totally inactive against *Pseudomonas*, superinfection with this organism is a special problem when the drug is used. Cephalosporins are not the *most* active of available antibiotics against gram-negative bacteria, but they have some activity against most of these organisms. Cephalothin is particularly useful in bacteremia and other severe infections of unknown etiology, provided *Pseudomonas* is not the causative agent. The drug usually can be given to patients with uremia (see comments on toxicity) (Perkins *et al.*, 1969). Although not cross-allergenic with the penicillins *in vitro*, cephalothin itself induces hypersensitivity reactions, more commonly in patients allergic to penicillin. The *in vitro* activity of cephaloridine is identical to that of cephalothin, with two exceptions: (1) Cephaloridine is more active than cephalothin against *E. coli*; approximately 90% of strains are inhibited by concentrations of 10 μg/ml or less.

Conversely, cephalothin is predictably more active against penicillinase-producing staphylococci. This difference, however, only becomes manifest with a high inoculum of organism, and its clinical significance is as yet unknown. (2) Cephaloridine has some clear-cut advantages over cephalothin, as it is much better tolerated intramuscularly or intravenously and gives higher and more sustained blood levels. On the other hand, cephaloridine is potentially nephrotoxic when doses exceed 4 g per day. Various types of renal toxicity, including both tubular and glomerular damage, have been reported; the use of cephaloridine may be more hazardous in patients with pre-existing renal disease. In practice, cephaloridine does not appear to offer a significant advantage over cephalothin (Medical Letter, 1968a).

A cephalosporin is recommended as an antibiotic of first choice only for infections due to *Klebsiella pneumoniae* (resistant strains occur), and as an alternative drug for other organisms (Medical Letter, 1968c). Both cephalothin and cephaloridine have been used successfully in a variety of severe infections (Merrill *et al.*, 1966; Benner and Morthland, 1967; Martin *et al.*, 1967; Parker *et al.*, 1967; Tempest and Austrian, 1967). Cephalothin crosses the blood-brain barrier in patients with meningitis only if cerebrospinal fluid protein concentrations are in excess of 50 mg/100 ml (Lerner, 1969), and it is therefore not ordinarily recommended for meningitis; but it enters the uninflamed eye of man (Riley *et al.*, 1968).

Hypersensitivity reactions similar to those seen with penicillin have been reported, especially in patients allergic to penicillin. A positive Coombs test and hemolytic anemia may be found in patients taking cephalothin (Molthan *et al.*, 1967). Thrombophlebitis at the intravenous infection site is described for both cephalothin and cephaloridine and may prevent their further administration. An oral cephalosporin (cephalexin) is available for use (Kabins *et al.*, 1970).

The Macrolide Antibiotics

The Erythromycins. The erythromycins contain a large lactone ring (hence the term "macrolide"). Five erythromycin preparations are available, including erythromycin (free base), erythromycin ethylsuccinate, erythromycin ethylcarbonate, erythromycin stearate, and erythromycin estolate.

The antibacterial spectra of these formulations are identical. They are active against many gram-positive cocci, including penicillinase-producing organisms, and against some gram-negative cocci and rods, probably by interfering with protein synthesis. The erythromycins are recommended as the antibiotics of first choice for infection with *Listeria monocytogenes* (resistance may occur), but clinical experience with this rare infection is limited and some investigators prefer to use tetracycline or ampicillin. *Corynebacterium diphtheriae* (antitoxic therapy is mandatory) may respond to an erythromycin or to penicillin G. *Chlamydia* (*Mycoplasma*) *pneumoniae* appears sensitive to the erythromycins or to tetracycline. Erythromycins are useful as drugs of "second choice" for many bacterial infections (Medical Letter, 1968c), particularly if there is penicillin allergy or known resistance of the infecting organism to the "first-choice" antibiotic.

Adverse reactions to the erythromycins include rare allergic responses and occasional instances of stomatitis or gastrointestinal disturbances (Medical Letter, 1968b). Cholestatic jaundice and/or elevation of the serum glutamic oxaloacetic transaminase may occur with the estolate formulation of erythromycin (Gronroos *et al.*, 1967; Medical Letter, 1968b; Sabath *et al.*, 1968).

Lincomycin and Oleandomycin. Other macrolide antibiotics, including lincomycin and oleandomycin, share with erythromycin the ability to inhibit protein synthesis of bacteria, but have a narrower spectrum of antibiotic action. Lincomycin-resistant strains of *Neisseria gonorrhoeae* may be sensitive to an erythromycin, implying some difference in action between the drugs (Kutscher *et al.*, 1968). The toxicities of lincomycin and oleandomycin are similar to those of the erythromycins. There appears to be no obvious reason to prescribe these drugs in preference to an erythromycin (Sanders, 1969).

The Tetracyclines

The tetracyclines have a polycyclic structure with a variety of simple ring substituents. They include tetracycline, chlortetracycline, oxytetracycline, demethylchlortetracycline, methacycline, and doxycycline.

These antibiotics have a common spectrum of activity (inhibiting protein synthesis of bacteria) and resistance. All are relatively well absorbed from the gastrointestinal tract and are largely excreted unchanged in the urine. Substantial differences exist among the tetracyclines in their gastrointestinal absorption, protein binding, and rates and degree of renal versus hepatic clearance. These variations account for differences in dose size and frequency of administration. Gastrointestinal absorption of the tetracyclines is incomplete, and major reductions in absorption occur if they are given with foods or medications containing divalent cations (as they are chelating agents). The pharmacokinetics of the tetracycline preparation selected for a patient should be known by the physician to ensure appropriate dosage (Goodman and Gilman, 1970). Major differences in cost to the patient also exist.

Tetracyclines have been recommended as drugs of first choice for *Pseudomonas pseudomallei* (with or without a sulfonamide), *Brucella*, *Mima*, *Herrellea*, and *Bacteroides* species, but resistance to tetracyclines may be seen with these infections and sensitivity testing is required. Tetracyclines also are recommended for infection with *Hemophilus influenzae* (meningitis) (many experts strongly advocate the use of chloramphenicol or ampicillin), *Pasteurella pestis*, *Hemophilus ducreyi* (chancroid), *Calymmatobacterium granulomatis* (granuloma inguinale), *Vibrio cholerae* (adjunctive to fluid-electrolyte therapy), *Borrelia recurrentis*, *Leptospira*, *Rickettsia*, the virus of psittacosis, *Lymphogranuloma venereum* (lymphopathia venereum), *Chlamydia trachomatis* (trachoma) (topically with oral sulfonamide), and the virus of inclusion conjunctivitis (Medical Letter, 1968c).

The physician should note the variety of *rare* organisms for which tetracyclines are recommended as agents of first choice. The tetracyclines may also be used as alternate drugs for a variety of gram-positive and gram-negative infections, including many group A streptococci and pneumococci, *if sensitivity tests confirm their activity*. Regrettably, resistance of organisms to the tetracyclines is not uncommon.

The use of the descriptive term "broad spectrum" is very unfortunate, as it can lead to the uncritical use of these drugs as an "umbrella" in bacteriologically undiagnosed infections. Patients are better treated by more specific and potent antibiotics on the basis of clinical and bacteriologic evidence than by the "broad-spectrum" approach. *Principle: There is no "panaceamycin" available to relieve the physician of his task in making as specific an etiologic diagnosis as possible and in prescribing the most specific and potent antibiotic available.*

The term "broad spectrum" may be used equally well to describe the toxic effects of the tetracycline antibiotics. These drugs commonly induce nausea, vomiting, diarrhea, pruritus ani, overgrowth of *Candida albicans*, appearance of resistant organisms, deposition in bone, and staining of the teeth if given to children (or to a fetus via a pregnant patient). Less frequently they induce malabsorption or photosensitivity reactions (particularly with demethylchlortetracycline), and when administered parenterally they may cause fatal liver disease (particularly in renal disease during pregnancy) (Schultz *et al.*, 1963; Medical Letter, 1968b).

Other reactions to the tetracyclines include allergic reactions (anaphylactic shock has been produced by demethylchlortetracycline), blood dyscrasias, interference with protein metabolism (increasing the blood urea nitrogen in renal failure), increased intracranial pressure in infants, and a Fanconi-like syndrome resulting from use of outdated tetracycline (Medical Letter, 1968b; Furey and Tan, 1969). The defect in renal acidification may be associated with severe sodium or potassium wasting (Fulop and Drapkin, 1965). *Principle: The use of the phrase "broad spectrum" for antibacterial agents should be abandoned, as its connotations may falsely lead a physician to substitute drug use for critical analysis of a patient's infection. If the phrase is retained in clinical parlance, it may equally well be applied to the toxicity of antibiotics.*

The Aminoglycoside Antibiotics

Kanamycin, neomycin, streptomycin, and gentamicin have similar chemical composition and probably have similar mechanisms of antibacterial action. They interfere with bacterial transcription of messenger RNA in protein synthesis (Suzuki *et al.*, 1970). These drugs are highly polar, necessitating their parenteral administration if systemic effects are desired. They are excreted almost exclusively by the kidney, and severe toxicity occurs in renal dysfunction unless the dose is reduced. Their limited lipid solubility probably accounts for their slow entry into cells and cerebrospinal fluid unless the meninges are inflamed. Streptomycin, kanamycin, and neomycin in high concentrations in blood may cause apnea due to a curariform action on neuromuscular end plates. Gentamicin should be considered a candidate for similar reactions, based on its chemical similarity.

Streptomycin. Streptomycin alone is recommended as the agent of first choice only in *Francisella* (*Pasteurella*) *tularensis* infections, in which the superiority of streptomycin to penicillin or to tetracycline seems verified (Young *et al.*, 1969). Streptomycin is also very useful in combination with penicillin for infections due to enterococci, and with a tetracycline for the rare infection glanders (Medical Letter, 1968c). Streptomycin is a potent antibiotic, but resistant strains of bacteria may appear within a few days if it is used alone. Other than in enterococcal infections, streptomycin's chief use is in infections due to sensitive mycobacteria.

Streptomycin causes dose-dependent eighth-nerve damage. In uremia toxicities may occur at normal doses owing to retention of the drug. The toxicity of dihydrostreptomycin precludes its use.

Neomycin, Kanamycin, and Gentamicin. Neomycin, with its wide bactericidal spectrum against both gram-positive and gram-negative bacteria, is highly effective but more toxic than kanamycin. It may be of value when used locally in wounds or abscess cavities.

Closely related biochemically to neomycin, kanamycin has a wide antibacterial spectrum and is active against certain species of gram-positive and gram-negative bacteria, as well as tubercle bacilli. It is inactive against streptococci and pneumococci. Although initially advertised as a potent antistaphylococcal drug, kanamycin should not be used in staphylococcal infections because so many effective and less toxic agents are available. Its biggest asset appears to be its effectiveness in certain gram-negative infections, especially those due to *E. coli*, *Klebsiella-Aerobacter*, the paracolon group, and *Proteus*. It is a poor antituberculous drug and should not be used in preference to streptomycin, PAS, and INH. Kanamycin must be used parenterally to achieve therapeutic blood levels. It is rapidly excreted and should be administered no less often than every 6 to 9 hours in dosage of 0.5 g (some therapists give 7.5 mg/kg body weight every two hours). Like neomycin, it is poorly absorbed from the gastrointestinal tract but is a potent intestinal antiseptic and may be used to reduce intestinal flora in hepatic coma.

When given intramuscularly, kanamycin has two major toxic side effects: (1) Severe, sometimes irreversible deafness may occur if a total dose of more than 20 g is administered. The onset of toxicity may be insidious because auditory function in the high-frequency range is lost first. The high-frequency end of the hearing scale is uncommonly used in ordinary conversation; clinical deafness may occur rather suddenly and is not always reversible. Some therapists make it a practice to limit the total dose of kanamycin to 20 g and then to withhold the drug for at least 6 months following a course, to reduce the incidence of severe deafness. (2) A second toxic effect of kanamycin is deterioration in renal function, with diminution in creatinine and PAH clearance and in PSP excretion, and appearance of casts in the urinary sediment. In patients with uremia the dosage should be reduced drastically or the drug avoided (Falco *et al.*, 1969; Gingell *et al.*, 1969).

Gentamicin is bactericidal, primarily against gram-negative pathogens (Hahn and Sarre, 1969). It is also very active against staphylococci, but its activity against pneumococci and group A streptococci is relatively slight, and it is ineffective against enterococci. Gentamicin is very potent *in vitro* and inhibits most strains of *E. coli*, *Klebsiella-Aerobacter*, and *Pseudomonas*. Activity against *Proteus mirabilis* is probably less than that of ampicillin, but indole-positive strains of *Proteus* are inhibited in lower concentrations than with any other drug. On the basis of these *in vitro* data, gentamicin should be useful against *Aerobacter*, *Klebsiella*, indole-positive strains of *Proteus*, and *Pseudomonas* (Kirby and Standiford, 1969; Waitz and Weinstein, 1969).

When this agent was initially tested, a number of patients with pyelonephritis and uremia developed severe vestibular toxicity. As a result, the doses subsequently recommended were too low to achieve the minimum inhibitory concentrations necessary for the antibacterial effect of the drug in tissues. When gentamicin is used in patients with normal renal function, dosage can be increased to 3 to 5 mg/kg per day, given every 6 to 8 hours. With this dose, the concentration of drug in blood and tissue is approximately 10 μg/ml, which is sufficient to kill most gram-negative bacteria. Furthermore, the preliminary clinical evidence suggests that this drug has been highly effective in some patients with severe *Pseudomonas* and other gram-negative infections. There is also some evidence that the combination of gentamicin and cephalothin produces the best clinical results in patients with undiagnosed gram-negative bacteremia (Martin *et al.*, 1969).

Gentamicin must be given intramuscularly but is relatively painless. It is toxic, primarily to the vestibular portion of the eighth nerve, and the toxicity is often not reversible. The drug must be given with care in patients with diminished renal function. Because this agent is excreted via the kidneys, urine levels are very high and the drug is effective in urinary tract infections.

Because of their toxicity, these drugs are best reserved for use in life-threatening infections due to gram-negative organisms (sepsis, severe pneumonia, meningitis, acute bacterial endocarditis), pending culture and sensitivity testing of the organism responsible for the infection (Maiztegui *et al.*, 1965; Weinstein and Klainer, 1966; Darrell and Waterworth, 1967; Newman and Holt, 1967; Curtis *et al.*, 1967; Leedom *et al.*, 1969; Louria *et al.*, 1969; McHenry, 1969).

Polymyxin and the Colistins

These basic polypeptides include polymyxin B and polymyxin E (which is very similar to colistin) (Nord and Hoeprich, 1964). They are water soluble and may be considered toxicologically and therapeutically equivalent except for differences in dose. Their sole clinical indication is for serious systemic infection that is thought or known to be due to *Pseudomonas* or to rare organisms resistant to other antibiotics. Available forms of the drugs include polymyxin B sulfate, colistin sulfate, and colistimethate sodium (a repository form). Polymyxin E (or colistimethate sodium for intramuscular injection) contains dibucaine, precluding its intravenous or intrathecal use. These drugs require parenteral administration for systemic effects and intrathecal administration for meningitis and are dependent on renal clearance. Excretion is almost entirely by way of the urinary tract and urinary levels are extremely high, but only relatively low tissue levels are achieved with the polymyxins, perhaps because of their extensive binding to plasma proteins. The polymyxins are highly effective in urinary tract infections, but are much less so in deep-seated tissue infections, such as endocarditis or meningitis. When indicated, the drug should be instilled directly into abscess cavities; when used for meningitis, polymyxin B should be given intrathecally. In addition to the toxicities shared with the aminoglycosides, skin rashes, paresthesias, and visual and speech disorders may be seen (Goodman and Gilman, 1970). Apnea may occur if these drugs are used in patients with renal failure (Koch-Weser *et al.*, 1970).

Principle: Unless major advantages are demonstrated for a single agent among a similar group of antibiotics (such as antibacterial activity against organisms resistant to other antibiotics), it is reasonable to group similar drugs to facilitate recall of their utility and toxicities. Early clinical reports sometimes tend to exaggerate therapeutic claims and to minimize adverse effects. Be cautious in interpreting early claims for new antibiotics.

Drugs for Chemotherapy of Tuberculosis

In addition to streptomycin, isoniazid (INH) and p-aminosalicylic acid (PAS) are the most commonly used drugs for tuberculosis.

Isoniazid has a relatively simple chemical structure, is well absorbed and enters cells. It is acetylated in the liver at varying rates, depending on the genetic constitution of the individual (see Chapter 13).

Side effects include dizziness, ataxia, optic neuritis, convulsions, paresthesias, and peripheral neuropathy. The symptoms are dose related, thought to be due to competition of INH with vitamin B_6, and the peripheral manifestations may be prevented by simultaneous use of the vitamin. Glossitis, gastrointestinal irritation, and hepatic damage occasionally occur (Martin and Arthaud, 1970). Folate deficiency, a positive Coombs test, and other blood dyscrasias may appear. Isoniazid toxicity may account for a syndrome reminiscent of rheumatoid arthritis or of lupus erythematosus (Good *et al.*, 1965). INH may slow the metabolism of diphenylhydantoin, causing the latter's toxicity (Kutt *et al.*, 1966).

p-Aminosalicylic acid (PAS) also has a simple chemical structure. The drug is readily absorbed and partly acetylated by the liver in competition with INH, but most appears unaltered in the urine.

PAS is relatively ineffective when given alone, but prolongs the half-life of INH by competition for hepatic acetylation and slows the appearance of acid-fast bacilli resistant to INH or to streptomycin.

Gastrointestinal disturbances (mostly nausea) are frequently seen with PAS. Allergic reactions, a lupus-like syndrome, liver damage, renal damage (possibly due to crystallization of the relatively insoluble acetylated metabolite of PAS), blood dyscrasias, goiter, and a malabsorption syndrome may be seen with chronic PAS therapy. Administration of PAS with meals or with antacids may reduce the incidence of gastrointestinal symptoms (Moser, 1969).

Chemotherapy of tuberculosis ordinarily utilizes at least two of the above drugs and in serious infections all three are initially given. An apparently highly effective and relatively nontoxic analogue of INH, rifampin, is under investigation and may be useful in the chemotherapy of tuberculosis (Leading Article, 1968; Hobby *et al.*, 1969).

Some strains of *M. tuberculosis* and some species of *Mycobacterium* are resistant to these agents, necessitating sensitivity testing and therapy with one of the effective but more toxic alternate drugs: cycloserine (confusion, coma, peripheral neuropathy, folate deficiency, liver damage, malabsorption, seizures, or psychosis); ethambutol (optic neuritis, renal damage, peripheral neuritis, or allergic reactions); ethionamide (gastrointestinal disturbances, liver damage, peripheral neuropathy, allergic reactions, gynecomastia, glucose intolerance, or psychic disturbances); pyrazinamide (liver damage, sideroblastic anemia, photosensitivity reactions, hyperuricemia, or gout); or viomycin (eighth-cranial-nerve damage, rashes, renal damage, or electrolyte disturbances). For example, *M. balnei* is best treated with cycloserine; *M. leprae*, with a sulfone (McCurdy *et al.*, 1966; Medical Letter, 1968b,c).

Combined drug therapy of tuberculosis may be necessary (Johnston and Hopewell, 1969). Problems in drug resistance are the subject of many articles (Hobby *et al.*, 1964; USPHS Cooperative Investigation, 1964; Radenbach, 1968; Neff and Coan, 1969).

Chemoprophylaxis for tuberculosis may be required in patients exposed to tuberculosis, those patients with a positive skin test to tuberculosis who are placed on corticosteroid therapy, or young tuberculin reactors (Curry, 1965; American Thoracic Society Ad Hoc Committee, 1967).

The diagnostic and prognostic importance of skin testing in tuberculosis and in atypical acid-fast infections may be obtained from the following reviews: Wier and Schless, 1959; Edwards, 1963; Kent and Schwartz, 1967; Smith, 1967.

The general features of tuberculosis as presently detected in medical practice are well covered by the following articles: Myers, 1959; Arrington *et al.*, 1966; Stead *et al.*, 1968. The diagnostic problems of tuberculosis peritonitis and pericarditis have been reviewed (Singh *et al.*, 1969; Rooney *et al.*, 1970); disseminated intravascular coagulation has been reported in miliary tuberculosis (Goldfine *et al.*, 1969).

The public health aspects of tuberculosis continue to be of interest (Horwitz, 1969). Difficulties in the diagnosis and treatment of atypical acid-fast infection are covered in the following reviews and articles: Runyon, 1959; Lewis *et al.*, 1960; Chapman *et al.*, 1962; Phillips and Larkin, 1964; Curry, 1965; Klinenberg *et al.*, 1965; Bates, 1967; Hobby *et al.*, 1967; Chapman, 1969; Johanson and Nicholson, 1969.

Other Antibiotics

Chloramphenicol. A discussion of this antibiotic has purposefully been deferred to emphasize its relative role in clinical practice. It is a simple chemical with limited water solubility, allowing rapid absorption from the intestine and distribution to tissues. It is normally hydrolyzed and glucuronidated by the liver. Its antibacterial action creates an imbalance between ribonucleic acid (RNA) and protein synthesis that leads to bacterial accumulation of RNA (resembling messenger RNA). Some of the toxic effects of the drug are thought to be due to altered protein synthesis.

Although activity of chloramphenicol can be demonstrated against a variety of infecting organisms, its important toxicities should nearly always preclude its use save for infections with *Salmonella* (*Salmonella* gastroenteritis does not necessarily require therapy). It is an alternative to other antibiotics for certain uncommon bacterial, rickettsial, or filterable agent infections (Medical Letter, 1968c). Ampicillin is an alternative drug for therapy of known salmonellosis.

Adverse reactions to chloramphenicol include severe blood dyscrasias, such as a lethal "gray syndrome" in infants who are unable to metabolize the drug (Burns *et al.*, 1959; Kent and

Wideman, 1959; Weiss *et al.*, 1960; Lischner *et al.*, 1961), as well as gastrointestinal disturbances, sideroblastic anemia, allergic and febrile reactions, peripheral neuropathy, and optic neuritis. The hematologic reactions to chloramphenicol may be severe; complete blood counts should be performed at least every other day during therapy.

Four types of blood dyscrasia may appear in patients given chloramphenicol: (1) Slight transient leukopenia may occur; this is of little consequence. (2) Megaloblastic cells may appear in the bone marrow. Whether this stage of chloramphenicol toxicity is a forerunner of aplastic anemia is unknown. (3) Deleterious effects of chloramphenicol are seen in anemic patients. For example, patients with iron-deficiency anemia fail to respond to iron as long as they receive chloramphenicol, but when the drug is withdrawn, blood values return to normal. Similar observations have been made with respect to the response to vitamin B_{12} in pernicious anemia. (4) Complete necrosis of the bone marrow may appear with consequent aplastic anemia, agranulocytosis, and, more rarely, thrombocytopenia. This relatively rare but most dreaded side effect may represent a "hypersensitivity" rather than a toxic effect of chloramphenicol.

A number of clues should lead the clinician to suspect that chloramphenicol is interfering with erythropoiesis. A high serum iron is the early hallmark of chloramphenicol toxicity, but absence of reticulocytes is a helpful indicator and is a less cumbersome test than the measurement of serum iron. Ingestion of phenylalanine may ameliorate the sideroblastic anemia induced by chloramphenicol (Ingall *et al.*, 1965; Scott *et al.*, 1965; Brauer and Dameshek, 1967; Medical Letter, 1968b; Wallerstein *et al.*, 1969).

Chloramphenicol was introduced into clinical practice prior to the availability of equally effective and far less toxic antibiotics. Chloramphenicol is undoubtedly prescribed more frequently than necessary. Over 500,000 prescriptions for chloramphenicol and chloramphenicol palmitate were purchased, by persons 65 years of age or older, in 1966 alone (Task Force on Prescription Drugs, 1968). At least some practitioners of medicine prescribe chloramphenicol inappropriately; steps must be taken to correct these errors. ***Principle: Times change. The availability of antibiotics and the relative preference of one or another for a specific infection will hopefully continue to develop toward enhanced efficacy and reduced toxicity. Diligent continuing education enables a physician to prescribe drugs appropriately.***

Other Drugs. Vancomycin is an effective

drug against all gram-positive organisms, particularly staphylococci resistant to other antibiotics. The agent is bactericidal at almost the same concentration at which it is bacteriostatic, and no cross-resistance between it and other agents has been encountered. The intramuscular preparation is extremely painful and oral absorption of the agent is negligible. Its chief disadvantage lies in the fact that it must be given intravenously to achieve effective blood levels. Intravenous administration consists of 0.5 g every 6 hours (dissolved in 100 to 200 ml of glucose). Toxic effects have been limited to chills, fever, thrombophlebitis, flushing sensations, and circumoral paresthesias. These can be prevented to some degree by adding small amounts of hydrocortisone to the infusion and by premedicating the patient with antihistamines and aspirin. Although vancomycin has been used relatively infrequently in recent years, it may again be in ascendancy as methicillin-resistant staphylococcal infections appear.

Vancomycin is also useful in the treatment of staphylococcal enterocolitis. The parenteral form of the drug is dissolved in water and given by stomach tube or mixed in orange juice. Two grams are given in a single dose. If diarrhea does not stop, this dose may be readministered within 12 hours. Only one or two doses are generally necessary to eliminate staphylococci from the bowel.

A number of other antibiotics (bacitracin, paramomycin, novobiocin, *etc.*) are of some historical interest and are discussed in Goodman and Gilman, 1970. These drugs may be used topically and, in very rare circumstances, for unusual bacteria resistant to less toxic antibiotics. When used topically or for wound irrigation, they may be absorbed and cause systemic toxicity (Davia *et al.*, 1970). The antifungal antibiotics and drugs for parasitic infestations are well covered elsewhere (Medical Letter, 1968c, 1969; Goodman and Gilman, 1970).

SULFONAMIDES

The development and early use of sulfonamides are reviewed in Goodman and Gilman, 1970.

Sulfonamides are presently used chiefly in therapy of acute bladder infections and as nonspecific, but probably efficacious, treatment in ulcerative or granulomatous colitis. A few uncommon infections, such as *Nocardia*, are somewhat amenable to sulfonamide therapy.

Sulfonamides, nitrofurantoin, methenamine mandelate, and nalidixic acid are frequently used to prevent recurrences of acute urinary tract infection in chronic pyelonephritis. They appear to reduce the incidence of acute infections, but it has not been demonstrated that they influence the course of the renal disease (Freeman *et al.*, 1968).

There are differences among these agents, in terms of both their efficacy and their toxicity. Methenamine mandelate may be more effective (if urine pH is consistently acid) than nitrofurantoin or sulfamethizole in preventing recurrences, but no suppressive therapy succeeds unless control of bacteriuria is initially achieved with a "broad-spectrum" antibiotic (Freeman *et al.*, 1968). Nalidixic acid readily permits the appearance of resistant organisms (Ronald *et al.*, 1966); oxalinic acid is less subject to this phenomenon (Atlas *et al.*, 1969). Nitrofurantoin has a narrow spectrum of antibacterial activity but resistance does not develop; the drug does not appear in the urine in patients with renal failure (McCabe *et al.*, 1959; Sachs *et al.*, 1968).

Some investigators consider sulfisoxazole (Gantrisin) to be the drug of choice for suppression of urinary tract infections, as it is rapidly absorbed, results in high blood levels, and is rapidly excreted in the urine, where it is quite soluble. The entire question of success rates of various programs for suppression of recurrent urinary tract infection remains controversial; men may respond to treatment more favorably than women (Lindemeyer *et al.*, 1963; Turck *et al.*, 1966). Sulfamethoxypyridazine is excreted and metabolized slowly and can be administered infrequently. Side reactions with this drug have occurred in 6 to 10% of patients and have included nausea, rash, photosensitivity, fever, headache, abdominal pain, eosinophilia, albuminuria, and crystalluria. A number of deaths have been attributed to this drug, due to hypersensitivity myocarditis, aplastic anemia, thrombocytopenic purpura, or the Stevens-Johnson syndrome. Because of these side effects, long-acting sulfonamides should probably not be used (Mitchell, 1970). Sulfonamides are now thought to be contraindicated in meningococcal meningitis and meningococcemia, as most of these infections are now due to type B and D meningococci, which are resistant to sulfonamides.

Prior to initiation of therapy with one of these drugs, a physician should review their merits and liabilities, pharmacology, and pharmacokinetics to be certain he has selected the best available drug. He must also, in view of the chronicity of therapy, periodically review the medical literature to discover the "new" side effects that may occur in his patients. For example, acute and chronic pleuropneumonic reactions have been described in patients taking nitrofurantoin

(Rosenow et al., 1968; Hailey et al., 1969); bilateral ureteral obstruction has been encountered during therapy with sulfamethoxazole (Schainuck and Hano, 1967); severe jaundice with sulfamethizole (Plotkin and Jones, 1965); temporal arteritis with sulfisoxazole (Lee and Andrews, 1967); salivary gland enlargement with sulfisoxazole (Nidus et al., 1965); a serum-sickness-like illness with sulfapyridine (Han et al., 1969); and erythema multiforme gravis with long-acting sulfonamides (Baker, 1968). *Principle: A physician who intends to place a patient on chronic therapy must make his initial therapeutic selection optimal. He must keep current with the medical literature to enable recognition of unusual drug effects (even those tenuously related to the drugs he has prescribed).*

PATIENT'S MODIFICATION OF ANTIBIOTIC PHARMACOKINETICS

The physician must consider how his patient may differ from others in antibiotic pharmacokinetics and in responses not related to the intended antibiotic effect. These topics have been completely and elegantly reviewed and are presented here in simple table form (Weinstein and Dalton, 1968). Table 10–1 summarizes the known patient features that alter pharmacokinetics of antibiotics. Table 10–2 lists modified patient responses to certain drugs. The condensed format of this presentation should not lead one to underestimate the critical importance of these features in the outcome of therapy or the appearance of drug toxicity.

A concise discussion of renal dysfunction and antibiotic dose is available (Kunin, 1967, 1968). Discussions of the relation of uremia to doses of newer antibiotics should be reviewed before these drugs are used in a patient with renal disease (Ruedy, 1966; Lindholm, 1967; McCloskey and Hayes, 1967; Goodwin and Friedman, 1968; Gingell et al., 1969). Table 10–3 briefly summarizes some of these data.

ANTIBIOTIC RESISTANCE AND SENSITIVITY TESTING

Bacteria may be intrinsically resistant to the bactericidal or bacteriostatic action of antibiotics. Many gram-negative organisms and resistant staphylococci possess an enzyme, beta lactamase (penicillinase), that inactivates penicillin G. Chloramphenicol and the aminoglycosides are inactivated by bacteria by phosphorylation, acetylation, or adenylation (McDermott, 1958; Sabath, 1969; McDermott, 1970).

Bacteria uncommonly acquire resistance to antibiotic action by genetic mutation. Resistance factors (R factors) are nonchromosomal bacterial cytoplasmic substances that can be transferred from one organism to another, conferring upon the recipient strain resistance to one or many antibiotics. Epidemiologic studies indicate that this process may occur in patients on antibiotic therapy. The spread of the resistant strain of organisms in a hospital population appears to be a function of conventional bacteriologic contamination, rather than by the simultaneous appearance of resistance via bacterial transfer of R factors (Gardner and Smith, 1969).

Bacteria may be present in patients in resting form and be resistant to antibiotics that are most active against multiplying organisms. Bacteria may also exist in modified form as spheroplasts, protoplasts, or L-forms (special cultural techniques are required to demonstrate their presence). Since these forms of bacteria have no conventional cell wall, they are highly resistant to the antibacterial effects of drugs that inhibit cell-wall synthesis (e.g., penicillins and cephalosporins), but remain sensitive to the bacteriostatic effects of tetracyclines, macrolides, and aminoglycosides (Guze, 1968). The clinical importance of L-forms in relapsing bacterial infections has not been established (Feingold, 1969).

Sensitivity testing of antibiotics against bacteria may be done by serial dilutions of antibiotics in fluid culture media to determine the minimum concentration of antibiotic that inhibits bacterial proliferation (MIC) or kills bacteria (MBC). Another method utilizes discs containing antibiotic that are placed on culture plates of the organism. The diameter of the zone of inhibition of bacterial growth around the antibiotic disc reflects the effect of the antibiotic on bacterial growth. Careful bacteriologic techniques have been described that overcome some of the liabilities of the disc method (diffusibility of the antibiotic into the culture medium, variable antibiotic content of discs, effect of the bacterial inoculum size, etc.) (Bauer et al., 1966). Although the tube dilution method probably gives more accurate information, the disc method is generally more available, and despite its relative liabilities offers useful information in terms of the probability that an antibiotic concentration similar to that efficacious *in vitro* can be attained *in vivo* (Ryan et al., 1970). Sensitive organisms are those whose growth is inhibited by low concentrations of the antibiotic in tube dilution testing, or those demonstrating a large zone of inhibition in disc sensitivity testing. Neither method determines whether the antibiotic effect is bactericidal. Inoculation of bacteria from tube dilution

Table 10–1. FEATURES OF THE PATIENT THAT MODIFY ANTIBIOTIC PHARMACOKINETICS

PATIENT FEATURE	DRUG AFFECTED	PHARMACOKINETIC CHANGE
Age		
Premature infants and neonates	Penicillins	Impaired renal clearance
Premature infants and neonates	Chloramphenicol	Impaired hepatic clearance
Premature infants and neonates	Sulfonamides	Decreased protein binding, kernicterus
		Decreased acetylation
Premature infants	Cephalothin	Impaired clearance
Premature infants	Streptomycin	Impaired clearance
Premature infants	Neomycin	Decreased renal clearance
Premature infants and neonates	Kanamycin	Decreased renal clearance
Premature infants and neonates	Colistin, bacitracin	Decreased serum levels
Premature, fetus, neonates and infants	Tetracyclines	Dental staining
Elderly	Dihydrostreptomycin	Impaired clearance
Elderly	Tetracyclines	Impaired clearance
Gastric acidity		
Decreased acid (infants, senile patients)	Penicillin	Increased G.I. absorption
Genetic constitution	Isoniazid	Rate of acetylation
Pregnancy	Penicillins, streptomycin, chloramphenicol, cephalothin, sulfonamide, tetracyclines, isoniazid	Drugs cross placental barrier
	Sulfobromophthalein	Impaired hepatic clearance
Diabetes mellitus	Penicillins, sulfas	Slow absorption from intramuscular injections
Mucoviscidosis	Neomycin, polymyxin	*In vitro* inactivation by sputum
Hepatic function		
Cirrhosis	Chloramphenicol	Impaired hepatic clearance
	Neomycin	Increased G.I. absorption
	Lincomycin	
Liver disease	Methicillin, nafcillin, ampicillin, penicillin G, streptomycin	Impaired clearance
		Decreased bile concentration
Renal function		
Renal failure	Penicillins Cephalothin Kanamycin Vancomycin Polymyxin B Tetracyclines p-Aminosalicylic acid Isoniazid Colistin Lincomycin Gentamicin Nitrofurantoin Amphotericin B	Impaired renal clearance

Table 10–2. FEATURES OF THE PATIENT THAT MODIFY HIS RESPONSE TO ANTIBIOTICS

PATIENT FEATURES	DRUG	ALTERED EFFECT
Age		
Prematurity and infancy	Chloramphenicol Sulfonamides	Kernicterus, gray syndrome
Fetal to young children	Tetracyclines	Teeth staining
Glucose-6-phosphate dehydrogenase deficiency	Sulfas Nitrofurantoin Furazolidone Furaltadone Nitrofurazone Sulfoxone Thiazolsulfone Diaminodiphenylsulfone Chloramphenicol	Hemolysis
Hemoglobinopathy		
Hemoglobin Zurich	Sulfas	Hemolysis
Hemoglobin H	Sulfas	Hemolysis
Pregnancy	Sulfonamides	Neonatal kernicterus
	Isoniazid	Fetal brain damage
		Fetal damage (bone and teeth)
	Tetracyclines	Jaundice, renal failure in patients with pyelonephritis
		Increasing blood urea nitrogen in uremia
	Chlortetracycline	Jaundice
Pernicious, folic-acid, and iron-deficiency anemia	Chloramphenicol	Poor response to hematinic therapy
Atopic allergy	Many drugs	Allergic reactions
Central nervous system disease	Penicillin	Seizures
Myasthenia gravis	Streptomycin	Muscle weakness
Hepatitis or cirrhosis	Chlortetracycline	Increased hepatic fat
Prior hepatitis	Tetracyclines	Increased serum concentration of glutamic oxaloacetic and glutamic pyruvic transaminase
Cirrhosis	Lincomycin	Half-life of drug doubled
	Nafcillin Ampicillin Tetracyclines Lincomycin Erythromycin	Use with care in hepatic disease
Starvation	Sulfisoxazole	Impaired drug metabolism
Uremia	Sulfisoxazole	Impaired drug metabolism
Tissue autolysis	Sulfonamides	Intracellular constituents impair antibiotic action

Table 10-3.   EXCRETION OF ANTIBIOTICS IN RENAL FAILURE

DRUG	APPROXIMATE PERCENT RENAL EXCRETION	NORMAL HALF-LIFE IN BLOOD	HALF-LIFE IN BLOOD IN ANURIA	DANGER OF USING WITH RENAL DISEASE	SUGGESTED DOSE IN NORMALS	SUGGESTED INTERVAL BETWEEN DOSES IN ANURIA
Penicillins except ampicillin	Normally subject to renal clearance. Hepatic excretion in anuria	IV half-life 0.5 ± 0.17 hr	3.5 to 21.2 hr	Hyperkalemia from potassium penicillin G	Depends on type of infection and level necessary	Same as in normal (may need sodium salt). Excreted in bile
Ampicillin			11 to 15 hr			12 hr
Tetracycline	18–70	5.8 hr IV 7.2 hr orally	T max. 110 hr Chlortetracycline longest	Increased BUN Liver damage	0.5–1.0 g IV and 0.5 q 6–9 hr	0.5 gm q 3–4 days; avoid chlortetra-cycline
Streptomycin	30–80	2.4 to 2.7 hr	50 to 110 hr	Labyrinthine damage and deafness	1 g q 12 hr	1–2 g initially and 1/2 initial dose q 3–4 days
Kanamycin and neomycin	52–90	3 hr	3 to 4 days	Renal, curariform	Parenteral 1 g qd; oral 1 g q 4 hr	Loading dose and 1/2 loading dose q 3–4 days
Gentamicin	86–100	2.5 to 5.7 hr	45 hr	Labyrinthine damage	80 mg qd	80 mg every 48 hr
Polymyxin B	Large amounts in urine	6 hr	2 to 3 days	Kidney damage Apnea	1.5–2.5 mg/kg qd 3 doses δ > 0.2 g qd	Loading dose, then 1/2 loading dose q 3 to 4 days

438

Colistin	40–80	1.6 to 2.7 hr	2 to 3 days	Apnea Nephrotoxicity	3 to 4 days
Cephalothin	60–90	0.5 to 0.85 hr	2.9 to >18 hr		Daily
Cephaloridine	70	1.5	20 to 23 hr		Daily
Erythromycin	15	1.2 to 1.6 hr	4.0 to 5.8 hr	No danger	200–300 mg PO q 4–6 hr — Same as in normal
Lincomycin	10–15	4.4 to 4.7 hr	20 to 13 hr		12 hr
Nitrofurantoin	36	20 min			Do not use
Chloramphenicol		1.6 to 3.3 hr	3.2 to 4.3 hr	No danger except in infancy	2–4 g qd in divided doses — Same dose with caution if liver or hematologic abnormality present
Novobiocin	Inactivated by non-renal means	2.3	?		No modification
Bacitracin	9–31	1.5 hr	?	Nephrotoxicity	Max. dose 100,000 U/day not greater than 25,000 U/dose — Unknown
Vancomycin	30–100	6 hr	9 days	Deafness	9 days

studies into antibiotic-free media determines whether growth was inhibited by a bactericidal or a bacteriostatic effect.

Methods of sensitivity testing have clear limitations: (1) laboratory assays of sensitivity and resistance do not necessarily correlate with clinical results, as access of antibiotic to the form of the organisms responsible for infection in the patient is not tested; (2) the *in vitro* methods of testing for antibiotic sensitivity do not necessarily simulate the conditions of infected tissue; (3) the antibiotic effect seen *in vitro* may be not attainable in infected tissue; and (4) the antibiotic concentration *in vivo* may be much greater than the MIC reported by the laboratory (urinary concentration of antibiotic may greatly exceed the antibiotic concentration utilized in testing). The nature of the infectious process should influence antibiotic choice, in addition to the sensitivity tests. Life-threatening infections may justify the use of a toxic antibiotic if it is rapidly bactericidal *in vitro*, whereas minor infections may warrant a trial with a less potent but less toxic drug. *Principle: Antibiotic sensitivity testing is of great importance in selection of an antibiotic, but it must be placed in appropriate clinical context. The ultimate antibiotic sensitivity test in infectious disease is the patient's clinical response to therapy.*

COMBINATIONS OF ANTIBIOTICS IN INFECTIOUS DISEASE

Based on clinical grounds, an experienced clinician can often ascertain the organism likely responsible for a patient's infection, and he can select a single antibiotic for therapy, pending verification by culture. At times, the type of infection cannot be easily determined, and elements of games theory enter into the therapeutic decision. The games theory of therapeutics consists of the inquiry, "What will happen to the patient if I fail to cover the possibility of an infection with bacteria resistant to the antibiotic I have selected?" Infections such as sepsis, acute endocarditis, and massive pneumonia may require initial use of several antibiotics to cover the possibility of infection with penicillinase-producing organisms or gram-negative bacteria, including *Pseudomonas* species. The latter organism should be suspected if a patient has a nosocomially acquired infection in a hospital with a recent high recovery rate of *Pseudomonas* from clinical specimens, or if a patient develops the infection while on "broad-spectrum" antibiotic therapy. Following blood cultures, in a less critically ill patient with pneumonia in whom it has been impossible to acquire an adequate sputum specimen for gram stain examination, the physician might be justified in initiating therapy with a penicillinase-resistant penicillin to cover the possibility of a penicillinase-producing organism (but only pending cultural verification and sensitivity testing). Neither multiple antibiotics nor the so-called "broad-spectrum" antibiotics should be continued when the issue is clarified, as more specific and less toxic therapy is usually available. The appearance of resistant strains of organisms is fostered by use of multiple antibiotics. *Principle: The decision to utilize a toxic antibiotic with activity against several organisms or to embark upon therapy with multiple antibiotics must consider the potential for inducing drug toxicity in the individual patient and for increasing the hospital's flora of highly resistant bacteria. The use of multiple antibiotics is never justifiable as an alternative to careful clinical analysis and adequate bacteriologic studies.*

Combinations of antibiotics may have indifferent, antagonistic, additive, or synergistic effects in antibacterial action (Dowling, 1965; Jawetz, 1967). Tetracyclines interfere with the bactericidal action of penicillin against streptococci *in vitro* (Jawetz, 1967a; 1967b). In a small series of patients with pneumococcal meningitis, the mortality was greater in patients receiving penicillin and a tetracycline than in those receiving penicillin alone (Lepper and Dowling, 1951; Olsson *et al.*, 1961); similar antagonism in human meningitis has been shown for ampicillin versus the combination of ampicillin, chloramphenicol, and streptomycin (Mathies *et al.*, 1967). Chloramphenicol reduces the efficacy of penicillin in experimental pneumococcal meningitis (Wallace *et al.*, 1967). The antagonistic effect may be due to failure of the cell-wall-free organism (induced by penicillin) to rupture during the inhibited synthesis of protein (elicited by the tetracycline). As a general rule, a bactericidal antibiotic should not be used with a bacteriostatic agent (Jawetz, 1967).

A synergistic effect of penicillin with streptomycin against some streptococci has been demonstrated *in vitro* and verified in cases of endocarditis due to enterococci. Penicillin alone is bacteriostatic in enterococcal infections, but the combination of penicillin with streptomycin is bactericidal (Jawetz, 1967). Ampicillin is potentiated by streptomycin in enterococcal infections.

Combinations of penicillinase-sensitive and resistant penicillin derivatives have been studied *in vitro* and employed to a limited extent clinically, in infections with organisms that produce penicillinase (gram-negative organisms and resistant strains of *Staph. aureus*). Penicillinase-resistant penicillins may form relatively stable complexes with the organism's penicillinase, inactivating it for sufficient periods of time to permit the antibiotic action of the penicillinase-sensitive penicillin (Farrar *et al.*, 1967; Sabath *et al.*, 1967; Maniar, 1969). Other combinations under investigation include carbenicillin plus either gentamicin, polymyxin, or colistin for *Pseudomonas* infections (Smith *et al.*, 1969), fucidin plus either erythromycin, novobiocin, or rifampin for methicillin-resistant staphylococci (Jensen and Lassen, 1969), dicloxacillin and hetacillin for gram-negative organisms (McKee and Turck, 1967), and ampicillin with cloxacillin for *E. coli* and *Staph. aureus* (Nishida and Mine, 1969). These findings are of interest and may prove to be of therapeutic importance, but such combinations should be reserved for infections known to be due to a resistant organism that is synergistically antagonized by a specific combination of antibiotics. *Principle: The synergistic effects of antibiotics against a few bacteria should not imply that this effect is common. Only when an infection is known to be due to an organism responsive to a combination of antibiotics, and not to a single antibiotic, should combination therapy be initiated.*

The limitations and hazards of multiple-antibiotic therapy have been stressed. Fixed-dose combinations of antibiotics are commercially available but there are no apparent grounds for their prescription (National Academy of Sciences, 1969). The availability of fixed-dose combinations tends to imply that combined therapy is somehow "better" than therapy with a single drug, but this is infrequently the case. The fixed-dosage form may contain an amount of antibiotic unsuitable for the infection being treated. The hazards of a drug reaction are increased when multiple drugs are used, potentially making it necessary to discontinue all antibiotic therapy in a patient who is infected (as one may not be certain which drug caused the reaction). Furthermore, the improper connotation that the combination provides "broad-spectrum" antibacterial activity may lull the physician into a false sense of security that blunts his diagnostic acumen.

Some surgeons have the bad habit of prescribing combinations of penicillin and streptomycin in fixed-dosage form for prophylaxis against postoperative wound infections. The habit stems from early days of antibiotic therapy, when relatively few specific agents were available for therapy of infections of enteric origin, and before controlled clinical trials disproved the emotionally attractive notion that postoperative wound infections in surgically uncontaminated cases could be prevented by antibiotic therapy.

This habit is so firmly entrenched in some physicians and reinforced by their uncontrolled observational experience that they are unable to accept adequate data that should dissuade them from the routine use of antibiotics following surgery in uninfected tissues (McKittrick and Wheelock, 1954; Sanchez-Ubeda *et al.*, 1958; Barnes *et al.*, 1959, 1961, 1962; Cole and Barnard, 1961; Rocha, 1962; Karl *et al.*, 1966). To summarize the studies briefly, McKittrick's study comparing 80 controls with prophylactically treated patients showed hospital stays averaging 2 days longer for the treated group, and complications in 14 of the control group compared with 26 complications in the treated group. In reviewing the incidence of infections following hernia repair or hysterectomy, a slightly higher infection rate was found since antibiotics have become available (Barnes *et al.*, 1959). Antibiotic therapy for patients with nonperforated appendicitis resulted in infections in 5.3% of the patients, whereas only 2% of patients without antibiotic therapy developed infection postoperatively. Sanchez-Ubeda's study showed a higher infection rate in prophylactically treated patients after surgically clean operations. Following abdominal hysterectomy, Barnes reported a 3.8% infection rate in patients on prophylactic therapy, and a 3.5% rate in those without antibiotics. In a study comparing approximately 300 patients in each group, Rocha found the infection rate to be 4.36% in treated patients, and only 3% in controls. Barnes described a variety of surgical procedures in which 449 patients received antibiotics prophylactically and 558 did not; infections occurred in 70 of the treated patients and in 44 of the controls. Karl's study showed wound infections in 12 of 65 patients on antibiotics and in 9 of 70 patients on a placebo.

PNEUMONIA, A DISEASE STATE DEMONSTRATING PRINCIPLES IN INFECTIOUS DISEASE

The differential features in presentation, management, complications, and prognosis in pneumonia of several etiologies are presented here to demonstrate how the therapist should utilize clinical signs diagnostically, estimate severity of infection, establish therapeutic goals, and evaluate the patient's progress.

Pneumonia due to *Chlamydia pneumoniae*, adenovirus, or other viruses tends to occur sporadically in student or military populations. The patient with adenovirus infection is twice as likely as the patient with *Chlamydia* pneumonia to complain or show evidence of upper respiratory tract involvement. Both groups of patients have fever, cough, chilliness, muscle fatigue, malaise, and headache. Few have chest pain or purulent sputum; very few show bloody streaking of the sputum. Fever over 102° F is present in about one-half of the cases; some signs of pulmonary consolidation, particularly râles, are found in about two-thirds at some point in the course. Laboratory studies show white-blood-cell counts greater than 10,000/ml in 10 to 20% of patients. Chest x-ray shows a highly variable pattern, usually of migratory or lower lobar involvement. *Chlamydia* pneumonia responds to tetracycline or erythromycin (George *et al.*, 1966). A rapid, quantitative, cold agglutination titer test has been developed. This procedure may help identify the patient with *Chlamydia* pneumonia to allow administration of antibiotics solely to patients with this infection (Griffin, 1969).

Pneumococcal pneumonia is the most common bacterial pneumonia. Frequently it follows an upper respiratory tract infection. The onset of symptoms typically is abrupt, with rigors, fever, cough, chest pain, "rusty" sputum, and development of physical findings and radiographic evidence of lobar involvement, but a more diffuse bronchopneumonia may occur. The white-blood-cell count usually is more than 15,000/ml. Fever less than 102° F or frankly bloody sputum should alert the physician to the possibility of pulmonary embolus (Israel and Goldstein, 1957; Fred, 1969). The physician who takes the responsibility for ordering drugs should personally examine the patient's sputum. It is useful for the physician to witness the patient's production of sputum to determine whether the specimen is sputum (thoracic in origin) or spittle (oral or nasopharyngeal in origin). Obtaining a specimen of sputum by transtracheal aspiration may be necessary in some cases (Kalinske *et al.*, 1967; Hahn and Beaty, 1970). Rusty or "prune juice" sputum is characteristic, but some types of pneumococci produce a mucoid sputum similar to that usually seen with *Klebsiella pneumoniae* infections. Less commonly, gray-green, yellow, or blood-streaked sputum may be found, particularly in smokers or in patients with chronic bronchitis. Gram stain examination should be done to assure that purulent material is examined and that the predominant flora is associated with polymorphonuclear leukocytes. Blood cultures should always be obtained to confirm the diagnosis.

Unless the pneumonia is complicated by meningitis (lumbar puncture should be performed on all delirious patients, even if delirium tremens is strongly suspected), endocarditis,

arthritis, emphysema, or lung abscess, small doses of penicillin G (less than 1,000,000 units per day in divided doses) should result in clinical improvement in 2 to 3 days. Higher doses of penicillin G or prolonged administration (more than 2 to 3 days after the patient is completely afebrile) probably is unnecessary and may increase the chance of superinfection with resistant organisms (Louria and Brayton, 1963). The patient taking penicillin often has gram-negative organisms on follow-up gram stain or culture of the sputum, but changes in therapy are not required unless there are definite signs of infection due to these organisms. Alternative drugs for pneumococcal pneumonia are erythromycin and cephalothin. Some pneumococci are resistant to tetracycline (Schaffner *et al.*, 1966).

Causes of prolonged fever in pneumococcal pneumonia include empyema, sterile pleural effusions, pulmonary atelectasis, and scarring in patients with chronic lung disease, slow resolution due to bronchial obstruction, drug fever, or underlying chronic infection, such as tuberculosis. Recurrent pneumonias should suggest the possibility of associated intrathoracic or extrathoracic disease.

Inadequate pulmonary drainage may slow the resolution rate in pneumococcal pneumonia. Analgesics to allow coughing and sputum evacuation and avoidance of cough-depressing drugs are recommended. Endotracheal suction or even tracheotomy may be required to permit adequate drainage.

The mortality in pneumococcal pneumonia has been reduced from about 30% in the preantibiotic era to 5 to 10% in treated patients. The principal reduction in mortality has been in young adults, particularly in men (Reimann, 1967). The continuing high death rate in the very young and elderly eloquently demonstrates the following. ***Principle: Bactericidal antibiotic therapy alone is not a sole determinant of the outcome of bacterial infections; defects in the individual patient's ability to deal with infection must be found and corrected, whenever possible, for optimal therapy.***

Staphylococcal pneumonia may also follow upper respiratory tract infections and is generally more severe and rapid in evolution of clinical signs than pneumococcal pneumonia. Radiographic evidence of pneumothorax, pneumatoceles, abscess formation, emphysema about the pulmonary infiltrate, or early loculation of pleural exudate is a clue to this etiology. In staphylococcal sepsis multiple pulmonary nodules with cavitation may be seen. Pregnant patients, those with valvular heart disease or influenza infection, those taking "broad-spectrum" antibiotic therapy, elderly patients, those with other staphylococcal infections, and post-operative patients are candidates for staphylococcal pneumonia (Shulman *et al.*, 1965). Therapy with a penicillinase-resistant antibiotic is required, pending sensitivity testing, and assiduous attention must be paid to ancillary measures to enable the patient to cope with the infection.

Pneumonia due to *Pseudomonas* occurs principally in patients with chronic lung or cardiovascular disease; in a few, prior antibiotic therapy may have predisposed to the infection (Tillotson and Lerner, 1968a). Apprehension, confusion, cyanosis, relative bradycardia, reversal of the diurnal fever curve, and abnormal liver and kidney function may be found. Chest x-rays may show a diffuse, nodular, lower-lobe bronchopneumonia with microabscesses. The mortality rate is 50% in patients with this pneumonia; bacteremic patients show necrotizing bacillary vasculitis and thrombosis of pulmonary vessels (Tillotson and Lerner, 1968a). Disseminated intravascular coagulation may occur during gram-negative sepsis and may respond to heparin therapy (Clarkson *et al.*, 1969).

Pneumonia due to the anaerobe *Bacteroides* occurs in young women with pelvic infections with this organism and in older men with significant chronic pulmonary disease. Severe illness with lower-lobe bronchopneumonia, subacute, protracted but progressive complaints, and massive, putrid, and rapidly reaccumulating pleural effusions dominate the clinical picture (Tillotson and Lerner, 1968b). Surgical drainage as well as appropriate antibiotic therapy is necessary for recovery.

Pneumonia due to *E. coli* occurs in patients with bacteremia of gastrointestinal or renal origin, diabetes mellitus, and pyelonephritis. Many patients have cardiac disease, but chronic lung disease is not usual. Lower-lobe bronchopneumonia with metapneumonic emphysema is characteristic; abscesses are rare. Multiple-antibiotic resistance is common, and patient recovery (40% in one study) is ascribed to clinical recognition and appropriate antibiotic therapy (Tillotson and Lerner, 1967). The underlying disease is another important determinant of the outcome of therapy.

Predisposing features to pneumonia with *Proteus* species are chronic lung disease and alcoholism. The onset is heralded by a period of altered consciousness, often stupor or delirium tremens, with aspiration pneumonia producing dense lobar consolidation with multiple abscesses. The involved lung is contracted in volume, and when an upper lobe is infected the trachea is ipsilaterally deviated. The duration of pneumonia, despite adequate antibiotic therapy, is long (15 to 43 days). Clinical recognition and appropriate antibiotic therapy result in a relatively low mortality rate (Tillotson and Lerner, 1968c). *Proteus* may also cause pneumonia by apparent hematogenous spread of infection and may be associated with emphysema (Seriff, 1969).

Hemophilus influenzae uncommonly causes pneumonia in adults, except in patients with chronic lung disease. A review of six cases found a high correlation with chronic bronchitis, but no distinctive clinical features facilitating clinical recognition (Goldstein *et al.*, 1967).

Friedländer's pneumonia, due to *Klebsiella pneumoniae*, is usually found in alcoholics or in other patients whose defense mechanisms against bacterial infection are compromised. The acute form of this pneumonia is a fulminating infection with dense lobar infiltration and extreme toxicity. Leukopenia, high fever, and shock may be present. Gram stain of the mucoid sputum reveals short, stubby gram-negative rods. Chest x-rays may show bulging of the interlobar fissure. The pneumonia may pursue a more chronic course with cavitation, abscess formation, and scarring (Hamburger, 1967; Reimann, 1968). Early recognition and therapy of the acute pneumonic process are essential to survival (Shulman *et al.*, 1965).

Occasionally, outbreaks of pulmonary infection due to highly resistant and/or rare bacteria have been related to contamination of respiratory equipment with organisms. A high incidence of such infections in a hospital population should lead to investigation of this potential source of infection (Ringrose *et al.*, 1968; Grieble *et al.*, 1970). *Principle: Some bacterial pneumonias may occur in certain types of patients and may elicit fairly characteristic findings. When clinical signs are present, they may allow early prediction of the type of bacterial infection, its likely complications and its course, and specific antibiotic therapy. These clues may indicate what interventions other than antibiotic therapy may be necessary to enhance survival. Poor results in treating pneumonias in infants and in the elderly demonstrate the need to explore and improve means of therapy in addition to antibiotic use. The physician can take only limited comfort from the knowledge that the patient is infected with an organism sensitive to his antibiotic therapy.*

The errors most commonly cited as being of crucial importance in the management of bacterial pneumonia are (Shulman *et al.*, 1965):

1. The frequency with which the etiologic agent is missed on gram smears of sputum.

2. Failure to suspect the appropriate organism in certain clinical situations.

3. Delay in recognition of superinfections.

4. Tardy appreciation of the systemic complications of bacterial pneumonia, particularly meningitis.

5. Inappropriate use of antibiotics, particularly because mechanical factors interfering with bronchial drainage remain undetected.

6. Failure to appreciate the alterations in flora of the sputum in patients receiving antibiotics.

7. The propensity of nonbacterial complications of pneumonia, such as sterile pleural effusions or atelectasis, to produce fever.

Each of the above errors should be rephrased in a positive sentence to provide a list of principles for management of bacterial pneumonias.

This chapter has indicated the variety of considerations important to therapeutic decisions in infectious disease. A review of patient features that predispose to infection with certain organisms in pneumonia and their clinical picture has been provided to demonstrate the applicability of the general principles described in the earlier sections. Similar information should be sought for any infection, and application of the general principles or approach to infections as illustrated here should be rewarding.

REFERENCES

Ackerman, I. P., and Vickery, A. L., Jr.: Case records of the Massachusetts General Hospital: weekly clinicopathological exercises. Case 48-1968: facial pain, ophthalmoplegia and obtundation with hyperglycemia and uremia. New Eng. J. Med., 279:1220–29, 1968.

Aisenberg, A. C.: Hodgkin's disease: prognosis, treatment and etiologic and immunologic considerations. New Eng. J. Med., 270:508–14, 565–70, 617–22, 1964.

Alarcon-Segovia, D.; Worthington, J. W.; Ward, E. L.; and Wakim, K. G.: Lupus diathesis and the hydralazine syndrome. New Eng. J. Med., 272:462–66, 1965.

Alexander, J. W., and Wixson, D.: Neutrophil dysfunction and sepsis in burn injury. Surg. Gynecol. Obstet., 130:431–38, 1970.

Alper, C. A.; Abramson, N.; Johnston, R. B., Jr.; Jandl, J. H.; and Rosen, F. S.: Increased susceptibility to infection associated with abnormalities of complement-mediated functions and of the third component of complement (C3). New Eng. J. Med., 282:349–54, 1970.

Alper, C. A.; Rosen, F. S.; and Janeway, C. A.: The gamma globulins. II. Hypergammaglobulinemia. New Eng. J. Med., 275:591–96, 652–58, 1966.

Altemeier, W. A.; Todd, J. C.; and Inge, W. W.: Gram-negative septicemia: a growing threat. Ann. Surg., 166:228–40, 1967.

American Thoracic Society Ad Hoc Committee: Chemoprophylaxis for the prevention of tuberculosis. Amer. Rev. Resp. Dis., 96:558–60, 1967.

Arrington, C. W.; Hawkins, J. A.; Richert, J. H.; and

Hopeman, A. R.: Management of undiagnosed pleural effusions in positive tuberculin reactors. Amer. Rev. Resp. Dis., 93:587–93, 1966.

Artenstein, M. S.; Gold, R.; Zimmerly, J. G.; Wyle, F. A.; Schneider, H.; and Harkins, C.: Prevention of meningococcal disease by group C polysaccharide vaccine. New Eng. J. Med., 282:417–20, 1970.

Atlas, E.; Clark, H.; Silverblatt, F.; and Turck, M.: Nalidixic acid and oxolinic acid in the treatment of chronic bacteriuria. Ann. Intern. Med., 70:713–21, 1969.

Baker, H.: Drug reactions IV. Erythema multiforme gravis and long-acting sulphonamides. Brit. J. Dermatol., 80:844–46, 1968.

Baldwin, D. S.; Levine, B. B.; McCluskey, R. T.; and Gallo, G. R.: Renal failure and interstitial nephritis due to penicillin and methicillin. New Eng. J. Med., 279:1245–52, 1968.

Barlotta, F. M.; Ochoa, M., Jr.; Neu, H. C.; and Ultmann, J. E.: Toxoplasmosis, lymphoma, or both? Ann. Intern. Med., 70:517–28, 1969.

Barnes, B. A.; Behringer, G. E.; Wheelock, F. C., Jr.; and Wilkins, E. W.: An analysis of factors associated with sepsis in two operative procedures, 1937–1957. New Eng. J. Med., 261:1351–57, 1959.

————: Postoperative sepsis: trends and factors influencing sepsis over a 20-year period reviewed in 20,000 cases. Ann. Surg., 154:585–98, 1961.

————: Surgical sepsis: analysis of factors associated with sepsis following appendectomy (1937–1959). Ann. Surg., 156:703–12, 1962.

Barrett, F. F.; Casey, J. I.; and Finland, M.: Infections and antibiotic use among patients at Boston City Hospital, February, 1967. New Eng. J. Med., 278:5–9, 1968a.

Barrett, F. F.; McGehee, R. F., Jr.; and Finland, M.: Methicillin-resistant Staphylococcus aureus at Boston City Hospital: bacteriologic and epidemiologic observations. New Eng. J. Med., 279:441–48, 1968b.

Bates, J. H.: A study of pulmonary disease associated with mycobacteria other than Mycobacterium tuberculosis: clinical characteristics. XX. A report of the Veterans Administration–Armed Forces Cooperative Study on the Chemotherapy of Tuberculosis. Amer. Rev. Resp. Dis., 96:1151–57, 1967.

Bauer, A. W.; Kirby, W. M. M.; Sherris, J. C.; and Turck, M.: Antibiotic susceptibility testing by a standardized single disk method. Amer. J. Clin. Path., 45:493–96, 1966.

Beisel, W. R., and Rapoport, M. I.: Inter-relations between adrenocortical functions and infectious illness. New Eng. J. Med., 280:541–46, 596–604, 1969.

Benner, E. J., and Morthland, V.: Cephaloridine therapy of infections caused by penicillin-resistant Staphylococcus aureus. Antimicrob. Agents Chemother., 1967, pp. 159–63.

Bluemle, L. W., Jr.; Webster, G. D., Jr.; and Elkinton, J. R.: Acute tubular necrosis. Analysis of one hundred cases with respect to mortality, complications, and treatment with and without dialysis. Arch. Intern. Med. (Chicago), 104:180–97, 1959.

Blume, R. S.; Bennett, J. M.; Yankee, R. A.; and Wolff, S. M.: Defective granulocyte regulation in the Chediak-Higashi syndrome. New Eng. J. Med., 279:1010–15, 1968.

Bodey, G. P.; Buckley, M.; Sathe, Y. S.; and Freireich, E. J.: Quantitative relationships between circulating leukocytes and infection in patients with acute leukemia. Ann. Intern. Med., 64:328–40, 1966.

Bodey, G. P.; Nies, B. A.; Mohberg, N. R.; and Freireich, E. J.: Use of gamma globulin in infection in acute-leukemia patients. J.A.M.A., 190:1099–1102, 1964.

Boswell, D. C., and Eknoyan, G.: Acute glomerulonephritis in the aged. *Geriatrics*, 23:73–80, 1968.

Brauer, M. J., and Dameshek, W.: Hypoplastic anemia and myeloblastic leukemia following chloramphenicol therapy. Report of three cases. *New Eng. J. Med.*, 277:1003–1005, 1967.

Brayton, R. G.; Stokes, P. E.; Schwartz, M. S.; and Louria, D. B.: Effect of alcohol and various diseases on leukocyte mobilization, phagocytosis and intracellular bacterial killing. *New Eng. J. Med.*, 282:123–28, 1970.

Brown, R. S.; Haynes, H. A.; Foley, H. T.; Godwin, H. A.; Berard, C. W.; and Carbone, P. P.: Hodgkin's disease: immunologic, clinical and histologic features of 50 untreated patients. *Ann. Intern. Med.*, 67:291–302, 1967.

Brumfitt, W.; Percival, A.; and Leigh, D. A.: Clinical and laboratory studies with carbenicillin: a new penicillin active against *Pseudomonas pyocyanea*. *Lancet*, 1:1289–93, 1967.

Brunstetter, M.; Hardie, J. A.; Schiff, R.; Lewis, J. P.; and Cross, C. E.: The origin of pulmonary alveolar macrophages. *Arch. Intern. Med. (Chicago)*, 127:1064–68, 1971.

Bulger, R. J.; Larson, E.; and Sherris, J. C.: Decreased incidences of resistance to antimicrobial agents among *Escherichia coli* and *Klebsiella-Enterobacter*. Observations in a university hospital over a 10-year period. *Ann. Intern. Med.*, 72:65–71, 1970.

Bulger, R. J., and Sherris, J. C.: Decreased incidence of antibiotic resistance among *Staphylococcus aureus*. A study in a university hospital over a 9-year period. *Ann. Intern. Med.*, 69:1099–1108, 1968.

Burns, L. E.; Hodgman, J. E.; and Cass, A. B.: Fatal circulatory collapse in premature infants receiving chloramphenicol. *New Eng. J. Med.*, 261:1318–21, 1959.

Caggiano, V.; Cuttner, J.; and Solomon, A.: Myeloma proteins, Bence Jones proteins and normal immunoglobulins in multiple myeloma. *Blood*, 30:265–87, 1967.

Cantanzaro, F. J.; Stetson, C. A.; Morris, A. J.; Chamovitz, R.; Rammelkamp, C. H.; Stolzer, B. L.; and Perry, W. D.: The role of the streptococcus in the pathogenesis of rheumatic fever. *Amer. J. Med.*, 17:749–56, 1954.

Casazza, A. R.; Duvall, C. P.; and Carbone, P. P.: Infection in lymphoma. *J.A.M.A.*, 197:710–16, 1966.

Chapman, J. S.: Atypical mycobacteria: alteration of the host, either at a local site or immunologically, may be a prerequisite to the development of significant disease. *Hosp. Med.*, 5:30–38, May, 1969.

Chapman, J. S.; Dewlett, H. J.; and Potts, W. E.: Cutaneous reactions to unclassified mycobacterial antigens: a study of children in household contact with patients who excrete unclassified mycobacteria. *Amer. Rev. Resp. Dis.*, 86:547–52, 1962.

Clarkson, A. R.; Sage, R. E.; and Lawrence, J. R.: Consumption coagulopathy and acute renal failure due to gram-negative septicemia after abortion. *Ann. Intern. Med.*, 70:1191–99, 1969.

Cluff, L. E., and Johnson, J. E., III: Drug fever. *Progr. Allergy*, 8:149–94, 1964.

Cluff, L. E.; Reynolds, R. C.; Page, D. L.; and Breckenridge, J. L.: Staphylococcal bacteremia and altered host resistance. *Ann. Intern. Med.*, 69:859–73, 1968.

Cole, W. R., and Barnard, H. R.: A reappraisal of the effects of antimicrobial therapy on the course of appendicitis in children. *Amer. Surg.*, 27:29–32, 1961.

Conn, H. O.: Spontaneous peritonitis and bacteremia in Laennec's cirrhosis caused by enteric organisms: a relatively common but rarely recognized syndrome. *Ann. Intern. Med.*, 60:568–79, 1964.

Conrad, M. E.: Infectious hepatitis in military populations: problems encountered with gamma globulin prophylaxis. *Bull. N.Y. Acad. Med.*, 45:167–80, 1969.

Cooper, W.: Pancytopenia associated with disseminated tuberculosis. *Ann. Intern. Med.*, 50:1497–1501, 1959.

Craddock, C. G.; Arquilla, E. R.; Hildemann, W. H.; Skoog, W. A.; Sparkes, R. S.; and Winkelstein, A.: The immune system, immunoglobulins, and some disorders of the lymphatic system. *Ann. Intern. Med.*, 64:687–708, 1966.

Cross, C. E.; Mustafa, M. G.; Peterson, P.; and Hardie, J. A.: Pulmonary alveolar macrophage. *Arch. Intern. Med. (Chicago)*, 127:1069–77, 1971.

Curry, F. J.: Atypical acid-fast mycobacteria. *New Eng. J. Med.*, 272:415–17, 1965.

Curtis, J. R.; McDonald, S. J.; and Weston, J. H.: Parenteral administration of gentamicin in renal failure: patients undergoing intermittent haemodialysis. *Brit. Med. J.*, 1:537–39, 1967.

Cutting, H. O., and Lang, J. E.: Familial benign chronic neutropenia. *Ann. Intern. Med.*, 31:876–87, 1964.

Dans, P. E.; Barrett, F. F.; Casey, J. I.; and Finland, M.: *Klebsiella-Enterobacter* at Boston City Hospital, 1967. *Arch. Intern. Med. (Chicago)*, 125:94–101, 1970.

Darrell, J. H., and Waterworth, P. M.: Dosage of gentamicin for *Pseudomonas* infections. *Brit. Med. J.*, 1:535–37, 1967.

Davia, J. E.; Siemsen, A. W.; and Anderson, R. W.: Uremia, deafness, and paralysis due to irrigating antibiotic solutions. *Arch. Intern. Med. (Chicago)*, 125:135–39, 1970.

Davis, W. C.; Douglas, S. D.; and Fudenberg, H. H.: A selective neutrophil dysfunction syndrome: impaired killing of staphylocci. *Ann. Intern. Med.*, 69:1237–43, 1968.

Dawborn, J. K., and Cowling, D. C.: Disseminated tuberculosis and bone marrow dyscrasias. *Aust. Ann. Med.*, 10:230–36, 1961.

Deal, W. B., and Sanders, E.: Efficacy of rifampin in treatment of meningococcal carriers. *New Eng. J. Med.*, 281:641–45, 1969.

Dixon, F. J.: The pathogenesis of glomerulonephritis. *Amer. J. Med.*, 44:493–98, 1968.

Dodge, P. R., and Swartz, M. N.: Bacterial meningitis —a review of selected aspects. II. Special neurologic problems, postmeningitic complications and clinicopathological correlations. *New Eng. J. Med.*, 272:954–60, 1965.

Dodge, W. F.; Spargo, B. H.; Bass, J. A.; and Tarvis, L. B.: The relationship between the clinical and pathologic features of poststreptococcal glomerulonephritis. A study of the early natural history. *Medicine*, 47:227–67, 1968.

Douglas, S. D.: Analytic review: disorders of phagocyte function. *Blood*, 35:851–66, 1970.

Dowling, H. F.: Present status of therapy with combinations of antibiotics. *Amer. J. Med.*, 39:796–811, 1965.

Doyle, E. F.; Spagnuolo, M.; Taranta, A.; Kuttner, A. G.; and Markowitz, M.: The risk of bacterial endocarditis during antirheumatic prophylaxis. *J.A.M.A.*, 201:807–12, 1967.

Druskin, M. S., and Siegel, P. D.: Bacterial contamination of indwelling intravenous polyethylene catheters. *J.A.M.A.*, 185:966–68, 1963.

Durant, J. R.; Eisner, J. W.; Tassoni, E. M.; and Smalley, R. V.: "Asymptomatic" type I dysgammaglobulinemia in siblings. *Ann. Intern. Med.*, 68:867–71, 1968.

Duvall, C. P., and Carbone, P. P.: *Cryptococcus neoformans* pericarditis associated with Hodgkin's disease. *Ann. Intern. Med.*, 64:850–56, 1966.

Edwards, L. B.: Current status of the tuberculin test. *Ann. N.Y. Acad. Sci.*, **106**:32–42, 1963.

Elking, Sister M. P., and Kabat, H. F.: Drug-induced modifications of laboratory test values: a summary in tabular form of commonly ordered laboratory tests, their normal values and as altered by various drugs. *Amer. J. Hosp. Pharm.*, **25**:485–519, 1968.

Ellis, E. F., and Henney, C. S.: Adverse reactions following administration of human gamma globulin. *J. Allergy*, **43**:45–54, 1969.

Epstein, M.; Calia, F. M.; and Gabudza, G. J.: Pneumococcal peritonitis in patients with postnecrotic cirrhosis. *New Eng. J. Med.*, **278**:69–73, 1968.

Fahey, J. L.; Scoggins, R.; Utz, J. P.; and Szwed, C. F.: Infection, antibody response and gamma globulin components in multiple myeloma and macroglobulinemia. *Amer. J. Med.*, **35**:698–707, 1963.

Falco, F. G.; Smith, H. M.; and Arcieri, G. M.: Nephrotoxicity of aminoglycosides and gentamicin. *J. Infect. Dis.*, **119**:406–409, 1969.

Farrar, W. E.; O'Dell, N. M.; and Krause, J. M.: Use of penicillinase-resistant penicillins to increase the susceptibility of gram-negative bacteria to antibiotics. *Ann. Intern. Med.*, **67**:733–43, 1967.

Feigin, R. D., and Fiascone, A.: Hematuria and proteinuria associated with methicillin administration. *New Eng. J. Med.*, **272**:903–904, 1965.

Feingold, D. S.: Antimicrobial chemotherapeutic agents: the nature of their action and selective toxicity. *New Eng. J. Med.*, **269**:900–906, 957–64, 1963.

————: Biology and pathogenicity of microbial spheroplasts and L-forms. *New Eng. J. Med.*, **281**:1159–68, 1969.

————: Hospital-acquired infections. *New Eng. J. Med.*, **283**:1384–91, 1970.

Feinstein, A. R., and Levitt, M.: Tonsils, streptococcal infections and recurrences of rheumatic fever. *New Eng. J. Med.*, **282**:285–91, 1970.

Feinstein, A. R.; Spagnuolo, M.; Jonas, S.; Kloth, H.; Tursky, E.; and Levitt, M.: Prophylaxis of recurrent rheumatic fever: therapeutic-continuous oral penicillin vs. monthly injections. *J.A.M.A.*, **206**:565–68, 1968.

Fekety, F. R., and McDaniel, E.: The fever index in evaluation of the course of infectious diseases, with special reference to pneumococcal pneumonia. *Yale J. Biol. Med.*, **41**:282–88, 1968.

Fernbach, D. J.; Nora, A. H.; and Simonsen, L. G.: Recognizing and treating neutropenic infection. *Postgrad. Med.*, **45**:167–73, 1969.

Finch, S. C., and Castleman, B.: Case records of the Massachusetts General Hospital: weekly clinicopathological exercises. Case 12–1963: pancytopenia and purpura. *New Eng. J. Med.*, **268**:378–85, 1963.

Finkelstein, M. S., and Merigan, T. C.: Interferon—1968: how much do we understand? *Calif. Med.*, **109**:24–34, 1968.

Finter, N. B. (ed.): *Interferons*. W. B. Saunders Co., Philadelphia, 1966.

Floyd, M.; Muckle, T. J.; and Kerr, D. N. S.: Prednisone-induced leucocytosis in nephrotic syndrome. *Lancet*, **1**:1192–93, 1969.

Franklin, S. S., and Merrill, J. P.: Acute renal failure. *New Eng. J. Med.*, **262**:711–18, 761–67, 1960.

Fred, H. L.: Bacterial pneumonia or pulmonary infarction? *Dis. Chest*, **55**:422–25, 1969.

Freedman, M. A.: Oxacillin—apparent hematologic and hepatic toxicity. *Rocky Mountain Med. J.*, **62**:34–36, 1965.

Freeman, R. B.; Bromer, L.; Brancato, F.; Cohen, S. I.; Garfield, C. F.; Griep, R. J.; Hinman, E. J.; Richardson, J. A.; Thurm, R. H.; Urner, D.; and Smith, W. M.: Prevention of recurrent bacteriuria with continu-

ous chemotherapy. U.S. Public Health Service Cooperative Study. *Ann. Intern. Med.*, **69**:655–72, 1968.

Freireich, E. J.; Levin, R. H.; Whang, J.; Carbone, P. P.; Bronson, W.; and Morse, E. E.: The function and fate of transfused leukocytes from donors with chronic myelocytic leukemia in leukopenic recipients. *Ann. N.Y. Acad. Sci.*, **113**:1081–89, 1964.

Fulop, M., and Drapkin, A.: Potassium-depletion syndrome secondary to nephropathy apparently caused by "outdated tetracycline." *New Eng. J. Med.*, **272**:986–89, 1965.

Furey, W. W., and Tan, C.: Anaphylactic shock due to oral demethylchlortetracycline. *Ann. Intern. Med.*, **70**:357–58, 1969.

Gardner, P., and Smith, D. H.: Studies on the epidemiology of resistance (R) factors. I. Analysis of *Klebsiella* isolates in a general hospital. II. A prospective study of R factor transfer in the host. *Ann. Intern. Med.*, **71**:1–9, 1969.

Gee, J. B. L.; Vassallo, C. L.; Vogt, M. T.; Thomas, C.; and Basford, R. E.: Peroxidative metabolism in alveolar macrophages. *Arch. Intern. Med. (Chicago)*, **73**:1046–49, 1971.

George, R. B.; Ziskind, M. M.; Rasch, J. R.; and Mogabgab, W. J.: *Mycoplasma* and adenovirus pneumonias. Comparison with other atypical pneumonias in a military population. *Ann. Intern. Med.*, **65**:931–42, 1966.

Gingell, J. C.; Chisholm, G. D.; Calnan, J. S.; and Waterworth, P. M.: The dose, distribution, and excretion of gentamicin with special reference to renal failure. *J. Infect. Dis.*, **119**:396–401, 1969.

Ginn, H. E.: Late medical complications of renal transplantation. *Arch. Intern. Med. (Chicago)*, **123**:537–42, 1969.

Goldfine, I. D.; Schachter, H.; Barclay, W. R.; and Kingdon, H. S.: Consumption coagulopathy in miliary tuberculosis. *Ann. Intern. Med.*, **71**:775–77, 1969.

Goldstein, E.; Daly, A. K.; and Seamans, C.: *Haemophilus influenzae* as a cause of adult pneumonia. *Ann. Intern. Med.*, **66**:35–40, 1967.

Good, A. E.; Green, R. A.; and Zarafonetis, C. J. D.: Rheumatic symptoms during tuberculosis therapy: a manifestation of isoniazid toxicity? *Ann. Intern. Med.*, **63**:800–807, 1965.

Good, R. A.: Immunologic reconstitution: the achievement and its meaning. *Hosp. Practice*, **4**:41–47, April, 1969.

Goodman, L. S., and Gilman, A. (eds.): *The Pharmacologic Basis of Therapeutics*, 4th ed. The Macmillan Co., New York, 1970.

Goodwin, N. J.; Castronuovo, J. J.; and Friedman, E. A.: Recurrent septic pulmonary embolization complicating maintenance hemodialysis. *Ann. Intern. Med.*, **71**:29–38, 1969.

Goodwin, N. J., and Friedman, E. A.: The effects of renal impairment, peritoneal dialysis, and hemodialysis on serum sodium colistimethate levels. *Ann. Intern. Med.*, **68**:984–94, 1968.

Gordon, J. E., and Scrimshaw, N. S.: Infectious disease in the malnourished. *Med. Clin. N. Amer.*, **54**:1495–1508, 1970.

Graf, M., and Tarlov, A.: Agranulocytosis with monohistiocytosis associated with ampicillin therapy. *Ann. Intern. Med.*, **69**:91–95, 1968.

Graw, R. G.; Herzig, G. P.; Eyre, H.; Goldstein, I.; Henderson, E. S.; and Perry. S.: Treatment of gram negative septicemia in granulocytopenic patients with normal granulocyte infusions. *Clin. Res.*, **19**:491, 1971.

Green, G. M., and Kass, E. H.: Factors influencing the clearance of bacteria by the lung. *J. Clin. Invest.*, **43**:769–76, 1964.

Grieble, H. G.; Colton, F. R.; Bird, T. J.; Toigo, A.; and Griffity, L. G.: Fine-particle humidifiers and *Pseudomonas aeruginosa* infections. *New Eng. J. Med.*, **282**:531–35, 1970.

Griffin, J. P.: Rapid screening for cold agglutinins in pneumonia. *Ann. Intern. Med.*, **70**:701–705, 1969.

Gronroos, J. A.; Saarimaa, H. A.; and Kalliomaki, J. L.: A study of liver function during erythromycin estolate treatment. *Curr. Ther. Res.*, **9**:589–94, 1967.

Guze, L. B.: *Microbial Protoplasts, Spheroplasts and L-Forms.* Williams and Wilkins Co., Baltimore, 1968.

Hahn, F. E., and Sarre, S. G.: Mechanism of action of gentamicin. *J. Infect. Dis.*, **119**:364–69, 1969.

Hahn, H. H., and Beaty, H. N.: Transtracheal aspiration in the evaluation of patients with pneumonia. *Ann. Intern. Med.*, **72**:183–87, 1970.

Hailey, F. J.; Glascock, H. W.; and Hewitt, W. F.: Pleuropneumonic reactions to nitrofurantoin. *New Eng. J. Med.*, **281**:1087–90, 1969.

Hall, T C.; Choi, O. S.; Abadi, A.; and Krant, M. J.: High-dose corticoid therapy in Hodgkin's disease and other lymphomas. *Ann. Intern Med.*, **66**:1144–53, 1967.

Hamburger, M.: Pitfalls in management of pneumococcal pneumonia. All strains of pneumococcus are sensitive to penicillin, but recovery may be slower than expected. *Hosp. Med.*, **3**:24–32, Nov., 1967.

Han, T.; Chawla, P. L.; and Sokal, J. E.: Sulfapyridine-induced serum-sickness-like syndrome associated with plasmacytosis, lymphocytosis and multiclonal gamma-globulinopathy. *New Eng. J. Med.*, **280**:547–48, 1969.

Hart, P. D.; Russell, E., Jr.; and Remington, J. S.: The compromised host and infection. II. Deep fungal infection. *J. Infect. Dis.*, **120**:169–91, 1969.

Henney, C. S., and Ellis, E. F.: Antibody production to aggregated human γG-globulin in acquired hypogammaglobulinemia. *New Eng. J. Med.*, **278**:1144–46, 1968.

Heptinstall, R. H., and Joekes, A. M.: Focal glomerulonephritis. In Strauss, M. B., and Welt, L. G. (eds): *Diseases of the Kidney.* Little, Brown and Co., Boston, 1963, pp. 306–19.

Hill, R. B.; Rowlands, D. T.; and Rifkind, D.: Infectious pulmonary disease in patients receiving immunosuppressive therapy for organ transplantation. *New Eng. J. Med.*, **271**:1021–27, 1964.

Hobby, G. L.; Johnson, P. M.; Boytar-Papirnyik, V.; and Wilber, J.: Primary drug resistance: a continuing study of tubercle bacilli in a veterans population within the United States. *Amer. Rev. Resp. Dis.*, **99**:777–79, 1969.

Hobby, G.; Johnson, P. M.; Lenert, T. F.; Crawford-Gagliardi, L.; Greetham, L.; Ivaska, T.; Lapin, A.; Maier, J.; O'Malley, P.; and Trembley, C.: A continuing study of primary drug resistance in tuberculosis in a veteran population within the United States. *Amer. Rev. Resp. Dis.*, **89**:337–49, 1964.

Hobby, G. L.; Redmond, W. B.; Runyon, E. H.; Schaefer, W. B.; Wayne, L. G.; and Wichelhausen, R. H.: A study on pulmonary disease associated with mycobacteria other than *Mycobacterium tuberculosis*: identification and characterization of the mycobacteria. XVIII. A report of the Veterans Administration–Armed Forces Cooperative Study. *Amer. Rev. Resp. Dis.*, **95**:954–71, 1967.

Hoffman, T. A., and Bullock, W. E.: Carbenicillin therapy of Pseudomonas and other gram-negative bacillary infections. *Ann. Intern. Med.*, **73**:165–71, 1970.

Hoffman, T. A.; Cestero, R.; and Bullock, W. E.: Pharmacodynamics of carbenicillin in hepatic and renal failure. *Ann. Intern. Med.*, **73**:173–78, 1970.

Hoigne, R., and Krebs, A.: Simultaneous allergic (anaphylactic) and embolictoxic reactions by accidental intravascular injection of procaine-penicillin. *Int. Arch. Allergy*, **24**:48–49, 1964.

Hook, E. W.; Campbell, G. G.; Weens, H. S.; and Cooper, G. R.: *Salmonella* osteomyelitis in patients with sickel-cell anemia. *New Eng. J. Med.*, **257**:403–407, 1957.

Horwitz, O.: Public health aspects of relapsing tuberculosis. *Amer. Rev. Resp. Dis.*, **99**:183–93, 1969.

Hou, J. P., and Poole, J. W.: Kinetics and mechanism of degradation of ampicillin in solution. *J. Pharmaceut. Sci.*, **58**:447–54, 1969.

Hughes, J. T.; Johnstone, R. M.; Scott, A. C.; and Stewart, P. D.: Leukaemoid reactions in disseminated tuberculosis. *J. Clin. Path.*, **12**:307–11, 1959.

Idsoe, O.; Guthe, T.; Wilcox, R. R.; and DeWeck, A. L.: Nature and extent of penicillin side-reactions, with reference to fatalities from anaphylaxis. *Bull. W.H.O.*, **38**:159–88, 1968.

Ingall, D.; Sherman, J. D.; Cockburn, F.; and Klein, R.: Amelioration by ingestion of phenylalanine of toxic effects of chloramphenicol on bone marrow. *New Eng. J. Med.*, **272**:180–85, 1965.

Israel, H. L., and Goldstein, F.: The varied clinical manifestations of pulmonary embolism. *Ann. Intern. Med.*, **47**:202–26, 1957.

Jacox, R. F.; Mongan, E. S.; Hanshaw, J. B.; and Leddy, J. P.: Hypogammaglobulinemia with thymoma and probable pulmonary infection with cytomegalovirus. *New Eng. J. Med.*, **271**:1091–96, 1964.

Janeway, C. A.: Progress in immunology: syndromes of diminished resistance to infection. *J. Pediat.*, **72**:885–903, 1968.

Janeway, C. A., and Rosen, F. S.: The gamma globulins. IV. Therapeutic uses of gamma globulin. *New Eng. J. Med.*, **275**:826–31, 1966.

Jawetz, E.: Combined antibiotic action: some definitions and correlations between laboratory and clinical results. *Antimicrob. Agents Chemother.*, 1967a, pp. 203–209.

———: The use of combinations of antimicrobial drugs. *Hosp. Med.*, **3**:48–51, Dec., 1967b.

Jensen, K., and Lassen, H. C. A.: Combined treatment with antibacterial chemotherapeutical agents in staphylococcal infections. *Quart. J. Med.*, **38**:91–106, 1969.

Johanson, W. G., and Nicholson, D. P.: Pulmonary disease due to *Mycobacterium kansasii*: an analysis of some factors affecting prognosis. *Amer. Rev. Resp. Dis.*, **99**:73–85, 1969.

Johnston, R. F., and Hopewell, P. C.: Chemotherapy of pulmonary tuberculosis. *Ann. Intern. Med.*, **70**:359–67, 1969.

Kabins, S. A.; Kelner, B,; Walton, E.; and Goldstein, E.: Cephalexin therapy as related to renal function. *Amer. J. Med. Sci.*, **259**:133–42, 1970.

Kalinske, R. W.; Parker, R. H.; Brandt, D.; and Hoeprich, P. D.: Diagnostic usefulness and safety of transtracheal aspiration. *New Eng. J. Med.*, **276**:604–608, 1967.

Karl, R. C.; Mertz, J. J.; Veith, F. J.; and Dineen, P.: Prophylactic antimicrobial drugs in surgery. *New Eng. J. Med.*, **275**:305–308, 1966.

Keefer, C. S., and Leard, S. E.: *Prolonged and Perplexing Fevers.* Little, Brown and Co., Boston, 1955.

Kent, D. C., and Schwartz, R.: Active pulmonary tuberculosis with negative tuberculin skin reactions. *Amer. Rev. Resp. Dis.*, **95**:411–18, 1967.

Kent, S. P., and Wideman, G. L.: Prophylactic antibiotic therapy in infants born after premature rupture of membranes. *J.A.M.A.*, **171**:1199–1203, 1959.

Kiley, J. E.; Powers, S. R., Jr.; and Beebe, R. T.: Acute renal failure; eighty cases of renal tubular necrosis. *New Eng. J. Med.*, **262**:481–86, 1960.

Kirby, W. M. M., and Kind, A. C.: Clinical pharmacology of ampicillin and hetacillin. *Ann. N.Y. Acad. Sci.*, **145**:291–97, 1967.

Kirby, W. M. M., and Standiford, H. C.: Gentamicin: *in vitro* studies. *J. Infect. Dis.*, **119**:361–63, 1969.

Klastusky, J.; Coppel, R.; and Debusscher, L.: Betamethasone in the management of severe infections. *New Eng. J. Med.*, **284**:1248–50, 1971.

Klinenberg, J. R.; Grimley, P. M.; and Seegmiller, J. E.: Destructive polyarthritis due to a photochromogenic mycobacterium. *New Eng. J. Med.*, **272**:190–93, 1965.

Knudsen, E. A., and Aastrup, B.: Jarisch-Herxheimer reactions in the treatment of early syphilis with penicillin and bismuth-arsphenamine. *Brit. J. Vener. Dis.*, **41**:177–80, 1965.

Koch-Weser, J.; Sidel, V. W.; Federman, E. B.; Kanarek, P.; Finer, D. C.; and Eaton, A. E.: Adverse effects of sodium colistimethate. Manifestations and specific reaction rates during 317 courses of therapy. *Ann. Intern. Med.*, **72**:857–68, 1970.

Korn, D.; Gelderman, A.; Cage, G,; Nathanson, D.; and Strauss, A. J. L.: Immune deficiencies, aplastic anemia and abnormalities of lymphoid tissue in thymoma. *New Eng. J. Med.*, **276**:1333–39, 1967.

Kretschmer, R.; August, C. S.; Rosen, F. S.; and Janeway, C. A.: Recurrent infections, episodic lymphopenia and impaired cellular immunity. *New Eng. J. Med.*, **281**:285–90, 1969.

Krill, C. E., Jr.; Smith, H. D.; and Mauer, A. M.: Chronic idiopathic granulocytopenia. *New Eng. J. Med.*, **270**:973–79, 1964.

Kunin, C. M.: A guide to use of antibiotics in patients with renal disease. A table of recommended doses and factors governing serum levels. *Ann. Intern. Med.*, **67**:151–58, 1967.

————: More on antimicrobials in renal failure. *Ann. Intern. Med.*, **69**:397–98, 1968.

Kutscher, E.; Southern, P. M., Jr.; and Sanford, J. P.: Clinical significance of lincomycin-resistant *Neisseria gonorrhoeae*. *Antimicrob. Agents Chemother.*, 1968, pp. 331–34.

Kutt, H.; Winters, W.; and McDowell, F. H.: Depression of parahydroxylation of diphenylhydantoin by antituberculosis chemotherapy. *Neurology*, **16**:594–602, 1966.

Kyle, R. A., and Linman, J. W.: Chronic idiopathic neutropenia: a newly recognized entity? *New Eng. J. Med.*, **279**:1015–19, 1968.

Lambden, M. P.: Dangers of massive vitamin C intake. *New Eng. J. Med.*, **284**:336–37, 1971.

Lawrence, J. S.: Leukopenia: its mechanism and therapy. *J. Chron. Dis.*, **6**:351–64, 1957.

Lawson, H. A.; Stuart, C. A.; Paull, A. M.; Phillips, A. M.; and Phillips, R. W.: Observations on the antibody content of the blood in patients with multiple myeloma. *New Eng. J. Med.*, **252**:13–18, 1955.

Leading Article: The macrolides and lincomycin. *Brit. Med. J.*, **2**:233–34, 1968.

Lee, D. K., and Andrews, J. M.: Temporal arteritis developing in the course of sulfonamide therapy. *J.A.M.A.*, **200**:720–21, 1967.

Lee, H. A., and Hill, L. F.: The use of ampicillin in renal disease. *Brit. J. Clin. Pract.*, **22**:354–57, 1968.

Leedom, J. M.; Wehrle, P. F.; Mathies, A. W., Jr.; Ivler, D.; and Warren, W. S.: Gentamicin in the treatment of meningitis in neonates. *J. Infect. Dis.*, **119**:476–80, 1969.

Lepper, M. H., and Dowling, H. F.: Treatment of pneumococcic meningitis with penicillin compared with penicillin plus aureomycin: studies including observations on an apparent antagonism between penicillin and aureomycin. *Arch. Intern. Med. (Chicago)* **88**:489–94, 1951.

Lerner, P. I.: Penetration of cephalothin and lincomycin into the cerebrospinal fluid. *Amer. J. Med. Sci.*, **257**:125–31, 1969.

Levinsky, N. G.: Management of emergencies. V. Acute renal failure. *New Eng. J. Med.*, **274**:1016–18, 1966.

Lewis, A. G.; Lasche, E. M.; Armstrong, A. L.; and Dunbar, F. P.: A clinical study of the chronic lung disease due to non-photochromogenic acid-fast bacilli. *Ann. Intern. Med.*, **53**:273–85, 1960.

Lindemeyer, R. I.; Turck, M.; and Petersdorf, R. G.: Factors determining the outcome of chemotherapy in infections of the urinary tract. *Ann. Intern. Med.*, **58**:201–16, 1963.

Lindholm, D. D.: Antibiotic persistence during renal failure and dialysis. *Amer. Heart J.*, **73**:841–42, 1967.

Linton, A. L.; Dunnigan, M. G.; and Thomson, J. A.: Immune responses in myeloma. *Brit. Med. J.*, **2**:86–89, 1963.

Lippincott, S. W.; Korman, S.; Fong, C.; Stickley, E.; Wolins, W.; and Hughes, W. L.: Turnover of labeled normal gamma globulin in multiple myeloma. *J. Clin. Invest.*, **39**:565–72, 1960.

Lischner, H.; Seligman, S. J.; Krammer, A.; and Parmlee, A. H., Jr.: Outbreak of neonatal deaths among term infants associated with administration of chloramphenicol. *J. Pediat.*, **59**:21–34, 1961.

Louria, D. B.: Medical complications of pleasuregiving drugs. *Arch. Intern. Med. (Chicago)*, **123**:82–87, 1969.

Louria, D. B., and Brayton, R. G.: The efficacy of penicillin regimens, with observations on the frequency of superinfection. *J.A.M.A.*, **186**:987–90, 1963.

Louria, D. B.; Fallon, N.; and Browne, H. G.: The influence of cortisone on experimental fungus infections in mice. *J. Clin. Invest.*, **39**:1435–49, 1960.

Louria, D. B.; Young, L.; Armstrong, D.; and Smith, J. K.: Gentamicin in the treatment of pulmonary infections. *J. Infect. Dis.*, **119**:483–85, 1969.

Lowther, C. P.: Leukemia and tuberculosis. *Ann. Intern. Med.*, **51**:52–56, 1959.

Lux, S. E.; Johnston, R. B.; August, C. S.; Say, B.; Penchaszadeh, V. B.; Rosen, F. S.; and McKusick, V. A.: Chronic neutropenia and abnormal cellular immunity in cartilage-hair hypoplasia. *New Eng. J. Med.*, **282**:231–36, 1970.

McCabe, W. R.; Jackson, G. G.; and Grieble, H. G.: Treatment of chronic pyelonephritis. II. Short-term intravenous administration of single and multiple antibacterial agents; acidosis and toxic nephropathy from preparation of intravenous nitrofurantoin. *Arch. Intern. Med. (Chicago)*, **104**:710–19, 1959.

McCloskey, R. V., and Hayes, C. P.: Plasma levels of dicloxacillin in oliguric patients and the effect of hemodialysis. *Antimicrob. Agents Chemother.*, 1967, pp. 770–72.

McCurdy, P. R.; Donohoe, R. F.; and Magovern, M.: Reversible sideroblastic anemia caused by pyrazinoic acid (Pyrazinamide). *Ann. Intern. Med.*, **64**:1280–84, 1966.

McDermott, W.: Microbial persistence. *Yale J. Biol. Med.*, **30**:257–91, 1958.

————: The John Barnwell lecture: microbial drug resistance. *Amer. Rev. Resp. Dis.*, **102**:857–76, 1970.

McElfresh, A. E., and Huang, N. H.: Bone-marrow depression resulting from the administration of methicillin. *New Eng. J. Med.*, **266**:246–47, 1962.

McFarland, W., and Libre, E. P.: Abnormal leukocyte response in alcoholism. *Ann. Intern. Med.*, **59**:865–77, 1963.

McGuire, J.; Kotte, J. H.; and Helm, R. A.: Acute pericarditis. *Circulation*, **9**:425–42, 1954.

McHenry, M. C.: Bacteremic shock due to gram-negative bacilli. Some concepts of pathogenesis and management based on recent developments. *Geriatrics*, **24**:101–11, 1969.

McHenry, M. C.; Martin, W. J.; and Wellman, W. E.: Bacteremia due to gram-negative bacilli: review of 113 cases encountered in the five-year period of 1955 through 1959. *Ann. Intern. Med.*, **56**:207–19, 1962.

McKay, D. G.: Progress in disseminated intravascular coagulation. *Calif. Med.*, **111**:186–99, 1969.

McKee, W. M., and Turck, M.: Susceptibility of gram-negative pathogens to the combination of dicloxacillin and hetacillin. *Antimicrob. Agents Chemother.*, 1967, pp. 705–10.

McKittrick, L. S., and Wheelock, F. C., Jr.: The routine use of antibiotics in elective abdominal surgery. *Surg. Gynec. Obstet.*, **99**:376–77, 1954.

McNamara, M. J.; Balows, A.; and Tucker, E. B.: A study of the bacteriologic patterns of hospital infections. *Ann. Intern. Med.*, **66**:480–88, 1967.

Magnuson, C. W., and Elston, H. R.: Infections caused by nonpigmented *Serratia:* report of seven cases. *Ann. Intern. Med.*, **65**:409–18, 1966.

Maher, J. F., and Schreiner, G. E.: Cause of death in acute renal failure. *Arch. Intern. Med. (Chicago)*, **110**:493–504, 1962.

————: Hazards and complications of dialysis. *New Eng. J. Med.*, **273**:370–77, 1965.

Maiztegui, J. I.; Biegeleisen, J. Z., Jr.; Cherry, W. B.; and Kass, E. H.: Bacteremia due to gram-negative rods. A clinical, bacteriologic, serologic and immunofluorescent study. *New Eng. J. Med.*, **272**:222–29, 1965.

Maniar, A. C.: Combined effects of ampicillin and methicillin on cell wall morphology of a methicillin-resistant staphylococcus. *J. Antibiot.*, **22**:248–52, 1969.

Marks, M. I., and Eickhoff, T. C.: Carbenicillin: a clinical and laboratory evaluation. *Ann. Intern. Med.*, **73**:179–87, 1970.

Martin, C. E., and Arthaud, J. B.: Hepatitis after isoniazid administration. *New Eng. J. Med.*, **282**:433–34, 1970.

Martin, C. M.; Cuomo, A. J.; Geraghty, M. J.; Zager, J. R.; and Mandes, T. C.: Gram-negative rod bacteremia. *J. Infect. Dis.*, **119**:506-17, 1969.

Martin, C. M.; Donohoe, R. F.; and Saia, J. S.: Controlled trial of cephaloridine, lincomycin, and nafcillin in severe gram-positive coccal infections. *Antimicrob. Agents Chemother.*, 1967, pp. 118–26.

Mathies, A. W.; Leedom, J. M.; Ivler, D.; Wehrle, P. F.: and Portnoy, B.: Antibiotic antagonism in bacterial meningitis. *Antimicrob. Agents Chemother.*, 1967, pp. 218–24.

Medical Letter: Cephaloridine (Loridine). **10**:45–48, 1968a.

————: Principal toxic, allergic, and other adverse effects of antimicrobial drugs. *Ibid.*, **10**:73–76, 1968b.

————: The choice of systemic antimicrobial drugs. *Ibid.*, **10**:77–84, 1968c.

————: Drugs for parasitic infections. *Ibid.*, **11**:21–28, 1969.

Menzel, D. B.: Alveolar macrophage. *Arch. Intern. Med.*, **74**:1044–45, 1971.

Merigan, T. C., Jr.: Interferon and interferon inducers: the clinical outlook. *Hosp. Practice*, **4**:42–49, March, 1969.

Merler, E., and Rosen, F. S.: The gamma globulins. I. The structure and synthesis of the immunoglobulins. *New Eng. J. Med.*, **275**:480–86, 536–42, 1966.

Merrill, J. P.: Kidney disease: acute renal failure. *Ann. Rev. Med.*, **11**:127–50, 1960.

Merrill, S. L.; Davis, A.; Smolens, B.; and Finegold, S. M.: Cephalothin in serious bacterial infection. *Ann. Intern. Med.*, **64**:1–24, 1966.

Meuwissen, H. J.; Gatti, R. A.; Terasaki, P. I.; Hong, R.; and Good, R. A.: Treatment of lymphopenic hypogammaglobulinemia and bone-marrow aplasia by transplantation of allogeneic marrow. *New Eng. J. Med.*, **281**:691–97, 1969.

Milder, E.; Oxenhorn, S.; Schlecker, A.; Naji, A.; and Nieporent, H. J.: A case of miliary tuberculosis simulating acute blastic leukemia. *J.A.M.A.*, **177**:116–20, 1961.

Miller, M. E.: Uses and abuses of gamma globulin. *Hosp. Practice*, **4**:38–43, Jan., 1969.

Miller, M. E., and Nilsson, U. R.: A familial deficiency of the phagocytosis-enhancing activity of serum related to a dysfunction of the fifth component of complement (C5). *New Eng. J. Med.*, **282**:354–58, 1970.

Miller, R. B., and Tassistro, C. R.: Peritoneal dialysis. *New Eng. J. Med.*, **281**:945–49, 1969.

Mitchell, R. G.: The sulphonamides in children. *Practitioner*, **204**:20–26, 1970.

Moeschlin, S.: Immunological granulocytopenia and agranulocytosis: clinical aspects. *Acta Med. Scand.*, **154** (Suppl. 312): 518–40, 1956.

Molthan, L.; Reidenberg, M. M.; and Eichman, M. F.: Positive direct Coombs test due to cephalothin. *New Eng. J. Med.*, **277**:123–25, 1967.

Mongan, E. S.; Kern, W. A.; and Terry, R.: Hypogammaglobulinemia with thymoma, hemolytic anemia, and disseminated infection with cytomegalovirus. *Ann. Intern. Med.*, **65**:548–59, 1966.

Moser, R. H.: *Diseases of Medical Progress, A Study of Iatrogenic Disease*, 3rd ed. Charles C Thomas, Springfield, Ill., 1969.

Murray, J. F.; Haegelin, H. F.; Hewitt, W. L.; Latta, H.; McVickar, D.; Rasmussen, A. F., Jr., and Rigler, L. G.: Opportunistic pulmonary infections. *Ann. Intern. Med.*, **65**:566–94, 1966.

Myers, J. A.: The natural history of tuberculosis in the human body. I. The demonstrable primary pulmonary infiltrate. *Amer. Rev. Tuberc.*, **79**:19–30, 1959.

National Academy of Sciences–National Research Council Division of Medical Sciences Drug Efficacy Study: Fixed combinations of antimicrobial agents. *New Eng. J. Med.*, **280**:1149–54, 1969.

Neff, T. A., and Coan, B. J.: Incidence of drug intolerance to antituberculosis chemotherapy. *Dis. Chest*, **56**: 10–12, 1969.

Newman, R. L., and Holt, R. J.: Intrathecal gentamicin in treatment of ventriculitis in children. *Brit. Med. J.*, **1**:539–42, 1967.

Nidus, B. D.; Field, M.; and Rammelkamp, C. H.: Salivary gland enlargement caused by sulfisoxazole. *Ann. Intern. Med.*, **63**:663–65, 1965.

Nishida, M., and Mine, Y: Protective effect of cloxacillin on enzymatic degradation of ampicillin by penicillinase, and therapeutic activity of mixtures of ampicillin and cloxacillin. *J. Antibiotic*, **22**:144–50, 1969.

Nolan, J. P., and Klatskin, G.: The fever of sarcoidosis. *Ann. Intern. Med.*, **61**:455–61, 1964.

Nord, N. M., and Hoeprich, P. D.: Polymyxin B and colistin: a critical comparison. *New Eng. J. Med.*, **270**:1030–35, 1964.

Olsson, R. A.; Kirby, J. C.; and Romansky, M. J.: Pneumococcal meningitis in the adult: clinical, therapeutic and prognostic aspects in forty-three patients. *Ann. Intern. Med.*, **55**:545–49, 1961.

Osler, W.: *The Principles and Practice of Medicine*. D. Appleton and Co., New York, 1918.

O'Toole, R. D.; Drew, L.; Dahlgren, B. J.; and Beaty, H. N.: An outbreak of methicillin-resistant *Staphylococcus aureus* infection. Observations in hospital and nursing home. *J.A.M.A.*, **213**:257–63, 1970.

O'Toole, R. D.; Thornton, G. F.; Mukherjee, M. K.; and Nath, R. L.: Dexamethasone in tuberculous meningitis. Relationship of cerebrospinal fluid effects to therapeutic efficacy. *Ann. Intern. Med.*, **70**:39–48, 1969.

Page, A. R.; Berendes, H.; Warner, J.; and Good, R. A.: The Chediak-Higashi syndrome. *Blood*, **20**:330–43, 1962.

Pansegrau, D. G.; Rosenfeld, W. C.; Calvelo, M. G.; Kioschos, J. M.; and Kroetz, F. W.: The management of patients with prosthetic heart valves. *Med. Clin. N. Amer.*, **52**:1133–43, 1968.

Paradisi, E. R.; deBonaparte, Y. P.; and Morgenfeld, M. C.: Response in two groups of anergic patients to the transfer of leukocytes from sensitive donors. *New Eng. J. Med.*, **280**:859–61, 1969.

Parker, R. H.: Antimicrobial agents: selection and use. *J. Chron. Dis.*, **21**:719–36, 1969.

Parker, R. H.; Kalinske, R. W.; and Hoeprich, P. D.: Cephaloridine therapy of endocarditis and other life-threatening infections. *Antimicrob. Agents Chemother.*, 1967, pp. 150–58.

Pauling, L. C.: *Vitamin C and the Common Cold.* W. H. Freeman Co., San Francisco, 1970.

Pearson, H. A.; Spencer, R. P.; and Cornelius, E. A.: Functional asplenia in sickle-cell anemia. *New Eng. J. Med.*, **281**:923–26, 1969.

Perillie, P. E.; Nolan, J. P.; and Finch, S. C.: Studies on the resistance to infection in diabetes mellitus: local exudative cellular response. *J. Lab. Clin. Med.*, **59**: 1008–15, 1962.

Perkins, R. L., and Saslaw, S.: Experiences with cephalothin. *Ann. Intern. Med.*, **64**:13–24, 1966.

Perkins, R. L.; Smith, E. J.; and Saslaw, S.: Cephalothin and cephaloridine: comparative pharmacodynamics in chronic uremia. *Amer. J. Med. Sci.*, **257**:116–24, 1969.

Perry, S.; Thomas, L. B.; Johnson, R. E.; Carbone, P. P.; and Haynes, H. A.: Hodgkin's disease: combined clinical staff conference at the National Institutes of Health. *Ann. Intern. Med.*, **67**:424–42, 1967.

Petersdorf, R. G., and Beeson, P. B.: Fever of unexplained origin: report on 100 cases. *Medicine*, **40**:1–30, 1961.

Petersdorf, R. G., and Turck, M.: *Ann. Intern. Med.*, **64**:207–12, 1966.

Petz, L. D., and Fudenberg, H. H.: Coombs-positive hemolytic anemia caused by penicillin administration. *New Eng. J. Med.*, **274**:171–78, 1966.

Phillips, S., and Larkin, J. C.: Atypical pulmonary tuberculosis caused by unclassified mycobacteria. *Ann. Intern. Med.*, **60**:401–408, 1964.

Plotkin, G. R., and Jones, W. A.: Case records of the Massachusetts General Hospital: weekly clinicopathological exercises. Case 37–1965: progressive jaundice and death in a previously well man. *New Eng. J. Med.*, **273**:440–46, 1965.

Pollak, V. E.; Rosen, S.; Pirani, C. L.; Muehrcke, R. C.; and Kark, R. M.: Natural history of lipoid nephrosis and of membranous glomerulonephritis. *Ann. Intern. Med.*, **69**:1171–96, 1968.

Popper, M.: Unintentional intravascular injection of penicillin. *Public Health Rep.*, **79**:610–12, 1964.

Prasad, A. S.; Aboud, M. A.; Salawi, A.; and Schulert, A. R.: Hypogammaglobulinemia: iodinated gamma globulin studies. *Ann. Intern. Med.*, **61**:319–25, 1964.

Quie, P. G.: Intracellular killing of bacteria. *New Eng. J. Med..*, **280**:502–503, 1969.

Radenbach, K. L.: Chemotherapy of chronic pulmonary tuberculosis with polyresistant bacteria with reference to ethambutol and capreomycin. *Scand. J. Resp. Dis.*, **65**:195–206, 1968.

Reimann, H. A.: Acute respiratory tract infections in the aged. *Geriatrics*, **22**:160–67, March, 1967.

——: Viral versus bacterial and other pneumonias: diagnostic and therapeutic problems. *Hosp. Med.*, **4**:36–54, Sept., 1968.

Rifkind, D.; Faris, T. D.; and Hill, R. B., Jr.: *Pneumocystis carinii* pneumonia: studies on the diagnosis and treatment. *Ann. Intern. Med.*, **65**:943–56, 1966.

Rifkind, D.; Goodman, N.; and Hill, R. B., Jr.: The clinical significance of cytomegalovirus infection in renal transplant recipients. *Ann. Intern. Med.*, **66**:1116–28, 1967.

Riley, F. C.; Boyle, G. L.; and Leopold, I. H.: Intraocular penetration of cephaloridine in humans. *Amer. J. Ophthal.*, **66**:1042–49, 1968.

Ringrose, R. E.; McKown, B.; Felton, F. G.; Barclay, B. O.; Muchmore, H. G.; and Rhoades, E. R.: A hospital outbreak of *Serratia marcescens* associated with ultrasonic nebulizers. *Ann. Intern. Med.*, **69**:719–29, 1968.

Rita, G. (ed.): *The Interferons, An International Symposium.* Academic Press, Inc., New York, 1968.

Robbins, J. B.; Eitzman, D. V.; and Ellis, E. F.: Immunochemical evidence for the development of an "acquired" hypogammaglobulinemic state. *New Eng. J. Med.*, **274**:607–10, 1966.

Robinson, M. G., and Watson, R. J.: Pneumococcal meningitis in sickle-cell anemia. *New Eng. J. Med.*, **274**:1006–1008, 1966.

Rocha, H.: Postoperative wound infections. *Arch. Surg. (Chicago)*, **85**:457–59, 1962.

Ronald, A. R.; Turck, M.; and Petersdorf, R. G.: A critical evaluation of nalidixic acid in urinary-tract infections. *New Eng. J. Med.*, **275**:1081–89, 1966.

Rooney, J. J.; Crocco, J. A.; and Lyons, H. A.: Tuberculous pericarditis. *Ann. Intern. Med.*, **72**:73–78, 1970.

Rosen, F. S.: The lymphocyte and the thymus gland—congenital and hereditary abnormalities. *New Eng. J. Med.*, **279**:643–48, 1968.

Rosen, F. S.; Gotoff, S. P.; Craig, J. M.; Ritchie, J.; and Janeway, C. A.: Further observation on the Swiss type of agammaglobulinemia (alymphocytosis): the effect of syngeneic bone-marrow cells. *New Eng. J. Med.*, **274**:18–21, 1966.

Rosen, F. S., and Janeway, C. A.: The gamma globulins. III. The antibody deficiency syndromes. *New Eng. J. Med.*, **275**:709–15, 769–76, 1966.

Rosenblatt, M. B.; Zizza, F.; and Beck, I.: Nosocomial infections. *Bull. N.Y. Acad. Med.*, **45**:10–21, 1969.

Rosenow, E. C.; DeRemee, R. A.; and Dines, D. E.: Chronic nitrofurantoin pulmonary reaction: report of five cases. *New Eng. J. Med.*, **279**:1258–62, 1968.

Ruedy, J.: The effects of peritoneal dialysis on the physiological disposition of oxacillin, ampicillin and tetracycline in patients with renal disease. *Canad. Med. Ass. J.*, **94**:257–61, 1966.

Runyon, E. H.: Anonymous mycobacteria in pulmonary disease. *Med. Clin. N. Amer.*, **43**:273–90, 1959.

Ryan, K. J.; Schoenknecht, F. D.; and Kriby, W. M. M.: Disc sensitivity testing. *Hosp. Practice*, **5**:91–100, Feb., 1970.

Sabath, L. D.: Drug resistance of bacteria. *New Eng. J. Med.*, **280**:91–94, 1969.

Sabath, L. D.; Elder, H. A.; McCall, C. E.; and Finland, M.: Synergistic combinations of penicillins in the treatment of bacteriuria. *New Eng. J. Med.*, **277**:232–38, 1967.

Sabath, L. D., and Finland, M.: Resistance of penicillins and cephalosporins to beta-lactamases from gram-negative bacilli: some correlations with anti-bacterial activity. *Ann. N.Y. Acad. Sci.*, **145**:237–47, 1967.

Sabath, L. D.; Gerstein, D. A.; and Finland, M.: Serum glutamic oxalacetic transaminase. False elevations during administration of erythromycin. *New Eng. J. Med.*, **279**:1137–39, 1968.

Sachs, J.; Geer, T.; Noell, P.; and Kunin, C. M.: Effect of renal function on urinary recovery of orally administered nitrofurantoin. *New Eng. J. Med.*, **278**:1032–35, 1968.

Salmon, S. E.; Cline, M. J.; Schultz, J.; and Lehrer, R. I.: Myeloperoxidase deficiency: immunologic study of a genetic leukocyte defect. *New Eng. J. Med.*, **282**:250–53, 1970.

Salmon, S. E.; Samal, B. A.; Hayes, D. M.; Hosley, H.; Miller, S. P.; and Schilling, A.: Role of gamma globulin for immunoprophylaxis in multiple myeloma. *New Eng. J. Med.*, **227**:1336–40, 1967.

Sanchez-Ubeda, R.; Fernand, E.; and Rousselot, L. M.: Complication rate in general surgical cases. *New Eng. J. Med.*, **259**:1045–50, 1958.

Sanders, E.: Lincomycin versus erythromycin: a choice or an echo. *Ann. Intern. Med.*, **70**:585–90, 1969.

Schaffner, W.; Schreiber, W. M.; and Koenig, M. G.: Fatal pneumonia due to a tetracycline-resistant pneumococcus. *New Eng. J. Med.*, **274**:451–52, 1966.

Schainuck, L. I., and Hano, J. E.: Bilateral ureteral obstruction following sulfamethoxazole. *J. Urol.* **98**:466–69, 1967.

Scheckler, W. E., and Bennett, J. V.: Antibiotic usage in seven community hospitals. *J.A.M.A.*, **213**:264–67, 1970.

Schreiner, G. E.: The nephrotic syndrome. In Strauss, M. B., and Welt, L. G. (eds.): *Diseases of the Kidney.* Little, Brown and Co., Boston, 1963, pp. 335–444.

Schultz, J. C.; Adamson, J. S.; Workman, W. W.; and Norman, T. D.: Fatal liver disease after intravenous administration of tetracycline in high dosage. *New Eng. J. Med.*, **269**:999–1004, 1963.

Schwartz, W. B., and Kassirer, J. P.: Clinical manifestations of acute glomerulonephritis. In Strauss, M. B., and Welt, L. G. (eds.): *Diseases of the Kidney.* Little, Brown and Co., Boston, 1963, pp. 268–305.

Scott, J. L.; Finegold, S. M.; Belkin, G. A.; and Lawrence, J. S.: A controlled double-blind study of the hematologic toxicity of chloramphenicol. *New Eng. J. Med.*, **272**:1137–42, 1965.

Seamans, K. B.; Gloor, P.; Dobell, A. R. C.; and Wyant, J. D.: Penicillin-induced seizures during cardiopulmonary bypass: a clinical and electroencephalographic study. *New Eng. J. Med.*, **278**:861–68, 1968.

Seelers, T. F., Jr.: Etiology of rheumatic heart disease. In Hurst, J. W., and Logue, R. B. (eds.): *The Heart.* McGraw-Hill Book Co., New York, 1966, pp. 491–94.

Selden, R.; Lee, S.; Wang, W. L. L.; Bennett, J. V.; and Eickhoff, T. C.: Nosocomial *Klebsiella* infections: intestinal colonization as a reservoir. *Ann. Intern. Med.*, **74**:657–64, 1971.

Seriff, N. S.: Lobar pneumonia due to *Proteus* infection in a previously healthy adult. *Amer. J. Med.*, **46**:480–88, 1969.

Shaw, E. B.: Transverse myelitis from injection of penicillin. *Amer. J. Dis. Child.*, **111**:548–51, 1966.

Sheldon, W. H., and Bauer, H.: Activation of quiescent mucormycotic granulomata in rabbits by induction of acute alloxan diabetes. *J. Exp. Med.*, **108**:171–77, 1958.

———: The development of the acute inflammatory response to experimental and cutaneous mucormycosis in normal and diabetic rabbits. *J. Exp. Med.*, **110**:845–52, 1959.

Shulman, J. A.; Phillips, L. A.; and Petersdorf, R. G.: Errors and hazards in the diagnosis and treatment of bacterial pneumonias. *Ann. Intern. Med.*, **62**:41–58, 1965.

Simon, H. J., and Miller, R. C.: Ampicillin in the treatment of chronic typhoid carriers: report on fifteen treated cases and a review of the literature. *New Eng. J. Med.*, **274**:807–15, 1966.

Singh, M. M.; Bhargava, A. N.; and Jain, K. P.: Tuberculous peritonitis: an evaluation of pathogenetic mechanisms, diagnostic procedures and therapeutic measures. *New Eng. J. Med.*, **281**:1091–94, 1969.

Smith, C. B.; Dans, P. E.; Wilfert, J. N.; and Finland, M.: Use of gentamicin in combinations with other antibiotics. *J. Infect. Dis.*, **119**:370–77, 1969.

Smith, C. H.; Erlandson, M. E.; Stern, G.; and Hilgartner, M. W.: Postsplenectomy infection in Cooley's anemia: appraisal of problems in this and other blood disorders, with consideration of prophylaxis. *New Eng. J. Med.*, **266**:737–43, 1962.

Smith, D. T.: Diagnostic and prognostic significance of the quantitative tuberculin tests. The influence of subclinical infections with atypical mycobacteria. *Ann. Intern. Med.*, **67**:919–46, 1967.

Sokal, J. E., and Firat, D.: Varicella-Zoster infection in Hodgkin's disease: clinical and epidemiological aspects. *Amer. J. Med.*, **39**:452–63, 1965.

Solomon, A.; Waldmann, T. A.; and Fahey. J. L.: Metabolism of normal 6.6S gamma globulin in normal subjects and patients with macroglobulinemia and multiple myeloma. *J. Lab. Clin. Med.*, **62**:1–17, 1963.

Stead, W. W.; Kerby, G. R.; Schlueter, D. P.; and Jordahl, C. W.: The clinical spectrum of primary tuberculosis in adults. Confusion with reinfection in the pathogenesis of chronic tuberculosis. *Ann. Intern. Med.*, **68**:731–45, 1968.

Stefanini, M.; Mele, R. H.; and Skinner, D.: Transitory congenital neutropenia: a new syndrome. *Amer. J. Med.*, **25**:749–58, 1958.

Steigbigel, N. H.; McCall, C. E.; Reed, C. W.; and Finland, M.: Antibacterial action of "broad-spectrum" penicillins, cephalosporins and other antibiotics against gram-negative bacilli isolated from bacteremic patients. *Ann. N.Y. Acad. Sci.*, **145**:224–36, 1967.

Stein, J. M., and Pruitt, B. A., Jr.: Suppurative thrombophlebitis. A lethal iatrogenic disease. *New Eng. J. Med.*, **282**:1452–55, 1970.

Stewart, G. T.: Toxicity of the penicillins. *Postgrad. Med.*, **40** (Suppl.):160–65, 1964.

Stickler, G. B.; Shin, M. H.; Burke, E. C.; Holley, K. E.; Miller, R. H.; and Segar, W. E.: Diffuse glomerulonephritis associated with infected ventriculoatrial shunt. *New Eng. J. Med.*, **279**:1077–82, 1968.

Stone, D. J.; Schwartz, A.; Newman, W.; Feltman, J. A.; and Lovelock, F. J.: Precipitation by pulmonary infection of acute anoxia, cardiac failure and respiratory acidosis in chronic pulmonary disease: pathogenesis and treatment. *Amer. J. Med.*, **14**:14–22, 1953.

Suzuki, J.; Kunimoto, T.; and Hori, M.: Effects of kanamycin on protein synthesis: inhibition of elongation of peptide chains. *J. Antibiot.*, **23**:99–101, 1970.

Swann, R. C., and Merrill, J. P.: The clinical course of acute renal failure. *Medicine*, **32**:215–92, 1953.

Swanson, M. A.; Chanmougan, D.; and Schwartz, R. S.: Immunohemolytic anemia to antipenicillin antibodies. *New Eng. J. Med.*, **274**:178–81, 1966.

Swartz, M. N., and Dodge, P. R.: Bacterial meningitis —a review of selected aspects. I. General clinical features, special problems and unusual meningeal reactions mimicking bacterial meningitis. *New Eng. J. Med.*, **272**:725–31, 779–87, 842–48, 898–902, 1965.

Taranta, A., and Griffith, G. C.: Should adults with rheumatic heart disease be kept on continuous penicillin prophylaxis? *Amer. J. Cardiol.*, **18**:627–29, 1966.

Taranta, A.; Kleinberg, E.; Feinstein, A. R.; Wood, H. F.; Tursky, E.; and Simpson, R.: A long-term epidemiologic study of subsequent prophylaxis, streptococcal infections, and clinical sequelae. V. Relation of the rheumatic fever recurrence rate per streptococcal infection to pre-existing clinical features of the patients. *Ann. Intern. Med.*, **60** (Suppl. 5):58–67, 1964.

Task Force on Prescription Drugs: Background Papers:

The Drug Users. U.S. Department of Health, Education and Welfare, U.S. Government Printing Office, Washington, D.C., 1968.

Tempest, B., and Austrian, R.: Cephaloridine and penicillin G in the treatment of pneumococcal pneumonia. *Ann. Intern. Med.*, 66:1109–15, 1967.

Thornton, P. A.: Influence of exogenous ascorbic acid on calcium and phosphorus metabolism in the chick. *J. Nutr.*, 100:1479–86, 1970.

Tillotson, J. R., and Lerner, A. M.: Characteristics of pneumonias caused by *Escherichia coli*. *New Eng. J. Med.*, 277:115–22, 1967.

———: Characteristics of nonbacteremic Pseudomonas pneumonia. *Ann. Intern. Med.*, 68:295–307, 1968a.

———: Bacteroides pneumonias: characteristics of cases with empyema. *Ann. Intern. Med.*, 68:308–17, 1968b.

———: Characteristics of pneumonias caused by *Bacillus proteus*. *Ann. Intern. Med.*, 68:287–94, 1968c.

Tomasi, T. B.: The gamma A globulins: first line of defense. *Hosp. Practice*, 2:26–35, July, 1967.

———: Human immunoglobulin A. *New Eng. J. Med.*, 279:1327–30, 1968.

Toole, J. F., and McCall, C. E.: Brain inflammation and steroids: two double-edged swords. *Ann. Intern. Med.*, 70:221–22, 1969.

Torack, R. M.: Fungus infections associated with antibiotic and steroid therapy. *Amer. J. Med.*, 22:872–82, 1957.

Tuano, S. B.; Johnson, L. D.; Brodie, J. L.; and Kirby, W. M. M.: Comparative blood levels of hetacillin, ampicillin and penicillin G. *New Eng. J. Med.*, 275:635–37, 1966.

Turck, M.; Anderson, K. N.; and Petersdorf, R. G.: Relapse and reinfection in chronic bacteriuria. *New Eng. J. Med.*, 275:70–73, 1966.

Udhoji, V. N., and Weil, M. H.: Hemodynamic and metabolic studies on shock associated with bacteremia. *Ann. Intern. Med.*, 62:966–78, 1965.

United States Public Health Service Cooperative Investigation: Prevalence of drug resistance in previously untreated patients. *Amer. Rev. Resp. Dis.*, 89:327–36, 1964.

Vogel, C. L.; Cohen, M. H.; Powell, R. D., Jr.; and DeVita, V. T.: *Pneumocystis carinii* pneumonia. *Ann. Intern. Med.*, 68:97–108, 1968.

Waitz, J. A., and Weinstein, M. J.: Recent microbiological studies with gentamicin. *J. Infect. Dis.*, 119:355–60, 1969.

Waldvogel, F. A.; Medoff, G.; and Swartz, M. N.: Osteomyelitis: a review of clinical features, therapeutic considerations and unusual aspects. *New Eng. J. Med.*, 282:198–206, 260–66, 316–22, 1970.

Wallace, J. F.; Smith, R. H.; Garcia, M.; and Petersdorf, R. G.: Studies on the pathogenesis of meningitis. VI. Antagonism between penicillin and chloramphenicol in experimental pneumococcal meningitis. *J. Lab. Clin. Med.*, 70:408–18, 1967.

Wallerstein, R. O.; Condit, P. K.; Kasper, C. K.; Brown, J. W.; and Morrison, F. R.: Statewide study of chloramphenicol therapy and fatal aplastic anemia. *J.A.M.A.*, 208:2045–50, 1969.

Wannamaker, L. W.: Differences between streptococcal infections of the throat and of the skin. *New Eng. J. Med.*, 282:23–31, 78–85, 1970.

Weinstein, L., and Chang, T. W.: Interferon: nonviral infections and nonviral inducers. *Ann. Intern. Med.*, 69:1315–19, 1968.

Weinstein, L., and Dalton, A. C.: Host determinants of response to antimicrobial agents. *New Eng. J. Med.*, 279:467–73, 524–31, 580–88, 1968.

Weinstein, L., and Klainer, A. S.: Management of emergencies. IV. Septic shock—pathogenesis and treatment. *New Eng. J. Med.*, 274:950–53, 1966.

Weiss, C. F.; Glazko, A. J.; and Weston, J. K.: Chloramphenicol in newborn infants: physiologic explanation of its toxicity when given in excessive doses. *New Eng. J. Med.*, 262:787–94, 1960.

Wells, J. D.; Margolin, E. G.; and Gall, E. A.: Renal cortical necrosis: clinical and pathologic features in twenty-one cases. *Amer. J. Med.*, 29:257–67, 1960.

Wier, J. A., and Schless, J. M.: The tuberculin reactions of 530 patients admitted to the tuberculin service, Fitzsimons Army Hospital. *Amer. Rev. Resp. Dis.*, 80:569–74, 1959.

Wilson, F. M., and Lerner, A. M.: Etiology and mortality of purulent meningitis at the Detroit Receiving Hospital. *New Eng. J. Med.*, 271:1235–38, 1964.

Winkelstein. J. A., and Drachman, R. H.: Deficiency of pneumococcal serum opsonizing activity in sickle-cell disease. *New Eng. J. Med.*, 279:459–66, 1968.

Winterbauer, R. H.; Bedon, G. A.; and Ball, W. C., Jr.: Recurrent pneumonia: predisposing illness and clinical patterns in 158 patients. *Ann. Intern. Med.*, 70:689–700, 1969.

Wirth, W. A., and Thompson, R. L.: The effect of various conditions and substances on the results of laboratory procedures. *Amer. J. Clin. Path.*, 43:579–90, 1965.

Wolstenholme, G. E. W., and O'Connor, M. (eds.): *Interferon, Ciba Foundation Symposium*. Little, Brown and Co., Boston, 1968.

Young, L. S.; Bicknell, D. S.; Archer, B. G.; Clinton, J. M.; Leavens, L. J.; Feeley, J. C.; and Brachman, P. S.: Tularemia epidemic: Vermont, 1968. Forty-seven cases linked to contact with muskrats. *New Eng. J. Med.*, 280:1253–60, 1969.

Zimmerman, H. H., and Hall, W. H.: Recurrent pneumonia in multiple myeloma and some observations on immunologic response. *Ann. Intern. Med.*, 41:1152–63, 1954.

Zuelzer, W. W.: "Myelokathexis"—a new form of chronic granulocytopenia: report of a case. *New Eng. J. Med.*, 270:699–704, 1964.

Chapter 11

PSYCHIATRIC AND NEUROLOGIC DISORDERS

Leo E. Hollister

DRUGS FOR TREATING PSYCHIATRIC DISORDERS

General Considerations

Psychiatric diagnosis is almost completely based on inference. With the exception of those acute and chronic brain syndromes associated with neuropathologic abnormalities, most psychiatric disorders leave none of the visible marks that provide confirmatory feedback from the necropsy room. The data upon which we make our inferences are "soft," being based on what patients tell us, what we infer from what they tell or how they act, or what other people tell us about them. Even the most precise psychologic testing makes only the grossest sort of distinctions, such as a "functional" rather than an "organic" disorder.

Despite these difficulties, clinical data of the type mentioned can at least be handled in a standardized fashion. Psychometric codification of these data and criteria for their evaluation can be developed to permit a semiquantitative appraisal of the degree of departure from normal as well as a qualitative profile of the type of psychopathology present. Numerous psychiatric rating scales have been developed to assess most psychiatric disorders in an "objective" way, especially since the advent of psychotherapeutic drugs. Experience with these methods indicates that psychometric assessments approach the validity and the level of consensual agreement between raters that one might expect from interpretations of abnormal electrocardiograms or chest x-rays (Hamilton, 1968). Even "soft data" can be objective if relevant.

Not only do we lack the ability to verify our diagnoses by the ultimate demonstration of some pathological change, but we have little concept of the pathogenesis of the illness we are treating. Theories of pathogenesis for the functional psychiatric disorders abound, but evidence for any of these is relatively scanty. At times, frustration with psychiatric nomenclature has led to the suggestion that all psychiatric diagnosis be abandoned and that patients be described in terms of disturbances in psychodynamics. To many, this suggestion is analogous to substituting the intangible for the nebulous. Recently, the tendency has been to classify empiric groupings of psychiatric disorders based on the presenting clinical symptoms and signs and the demographic variables in patients (Overall and Hollister, 1964; Lorr and Klett,

1969). Such groupings have verified the major traditional diagnostic categories of psychiatric patients, but have decreased the subdivisions. They appear to have some value in differentiating between responses to drugs. Still, such empiric classifications probably will not add to our basic understanding of functional psychiatric disorders. *Fortunately, one does not need to understand the pathophysiology of a psychiatric disorder to treat it effectively.*

Therapeutic Considerations in Diagnostic Categories

Anxiety Reactions. Anxiety is believed to be a reaction to psychologic stimuli, either external or internal. When external stimuli are clearly identifiable and consciously appreciated, the subjective response is called fear. If the stimuli are largely internal, such as unresolved conflicts, and are triggered by external events whose associations are not recognized, the stimuli are not consciously identified and the responses tend to be more diffuse, less intense, and usually chronic. In such instances, anxiety is often called "free floating" and its causes may lie buried in the unconscious. Further distinctions may be made between "current" anxiety (induced, acute, phasic, or state anxiety) and "character" anxiety (trait, basic, or chronic anxiety). The latter aspect includes the "normal" level of anxiety for a particular person, as well as his susceptibility to increased anxiety, but only when it is severe enough to cause dysfunction or discomfort. Few physicians would take the position that such anxiety should be treated solely by drugs or solely by psychotherapy. The case for nondrug treatment seems well established by the abundant evidence that anxiety may result from unresolved intrapsychic conflicts or environmental stresses. To the extent that conflicts may be resolved or the environment improved, anxiety may be relieved. On the other hand, many clinical studies indicate that drug therapy may be effective in providing symptomatic relief, at least compared with no drug therapy or with placebo. One study indicates that drugs may provide as much relief as psychotherapy (Brill *et al.*, 1964). The choice should not be "either/or" but "both," providing two points of therapeutic attack. *Principle: When two different approaches to treatment are effective and do not interfere with each other, it is unwise to rely solely on one.*

Depressive Reactions. Feelings of depression and sadness are such common human experiences that most of us can easily identify with patients suffering from the manifold symptoms of depressive reactions. However, the symptom of depression should not be confused with the

various syndromes that, depending upon their severity, constitute depressive disorders. The latter seem to have clear roots in both the patient's personality and life experiences, but not all persons subjected to similar stresses develop depression.

Following the clinical observation that reserpine can evoke depression and the subsequent demonstration that reserpine depletes the brain stores of serotonin, norepinephrine, and dopamine, biogenic amines in the brain have been linked to depressive disorders (see Chapter 18). The "norepinephrine hypothesis" has proposed not only a biochemical substrate for depression, but also an explanation of the modes of action of some antidepressant drugs (Schildkraut *et al.*, 1967).

The norepinephrine hypothesis is attractive but compelling exceptions to it exist. In fact, almost an equally convincing case can be made for the participation of indoleamines in affective disorders (Glassman, 1969). Still, it is one of the very few promising leads for establishing a biochemical explanation for an emotional illness.

Depressive illness may represent an interaction between environmental stress and some biochemical alteration in an individual. The person with a defect in the mechanism that supplies norepinephrine might be "depression prone." Given the proper environmental stresses, his coping mechanisms mediated by the central adrenergic pathways are inadequate and a depressive disorder ensues. A normal person subjected to the same stresses might merely experience a transient feeling of the "blues" but is able to cope adequately. As with anxiety reactions, depressive disorders may be treated both with drugs and with measures designed to alleviate emotional stresses, usually psychotherapy. *Principle: A hypothesis for the pathogenesis of a disease may be useful in describing the disease and in predicting responses to a group of drugs. However, hypothesis is not fact until responses to drugs can be predicted a priori without post-facto explanations or exceptions.*

Schizophrenic Reactions. Whatever else schizophrenia may be, it is an unmitigated disaster. Few illnesses take a comparable toll of the most useful years of life. Few illnesses have been so frustrating to explain or to treat, and cures are rare indeed. A great tragedy is that so little effort is expended on this most serious psychiatric problem; it is as though a dermatologist were more concerned with treating patients with dandruff than those with skin cancer.

One of the most frustrating aspects of schizophrenia is that its manifestations may be very subtle, and if the affected individual has good native intelligence and/or a high socioeconomic status, he may never come to medical attention, but simply may be described as an eccentric. Still, there are many individuals whose illness is clearly apparent. They are socially withdrawn, their thinking is disturbed, and their ability to function is severely impaired. Unfortunately, probably less than 15% of individuals who are seriously affected and who require any kind of prolonged hospitalization ever function "normally." Drug therapy has made a great impact on the management of schizophrenics, and indeed may be the only effective treatment, but better drugs are desperately needed. *Principle: The efficacy of drug therapy must be judged not only on immediate results but also on its effect on the quality of the patients's life.*

Schizophrenic reactions have been ascribed either to social-family relationships or to biochemical-genetic influences. One hypothesis considers that schizophrenia represents a disordered learning process, initiated and sustained by conflicting messages coming from the mother. Such messages constantly put the child on the horns of a dilemma (the "double-bind" hypothesis). Another theory attributes schizophrenia to a genetically determined biochemical abnormality, in which a normal biogenic amine may be transmuted into an endogenous psychotogen. Despite extensive investigation, evidence for such biochemical substrates of schizophrenia is still tenuous (Hollister, 1968a). Nonetheless, the fact that chemical methods of treatment clearly ameliorate the disease has supported the belief that schizophrenia is primarily a biologic rather than a psychologic disorder.

Other Psychiatric Disorders. Increased interest in mental deficiency has led to several promising developments. Mongolism is no longer a mystery, but is identified clearly as a genetic disorder; although this new understanding has not yet been of therapeutic value, it may be of help in prophylaxis. An increasing number of metabolic defects, mainly disorders of amino acid metabolism, have been identified as causes of mental deficiency; some are amenable to management (e.g., phenylalanine-poor diets may be used to manage phenylketonuria). Still, most cases of mental deficiency are not explainable on the basis of quantitative or qualitative abnormalities of chemistry or physics. The more severe cases are usually untreatable. Drug therapy, at least with those agents currently available, has offered very little to these patients.

Alcoholism and drug addiction are probably second only to schizophrenia as the most important problems in psychiatry. Few psychiatrists are involved either in research or in treatment of these disorders; very little is known about the determinants of drug-seeking behavior or about the characteristics of drugs that provoke such behavior (Chapter 15).

The widespread abuse of drugs is not simply a drug problem, but has many social ramifications. The rapid increase in social use of drugs in the past decade constitutes one of the most volatile social phenomena in contemporary society (Melmon, 1971). Further, the epidemiology of narcotic abuse is clearly related to the poverty and desolation of the ghetto. Fortunately, some promising approaches to therapy of narcotic abuse have been recently developed, one employing pharmacologic means, the other employing sociopsychologic principles ("encounter groups" as exemplified by Synanon).

Acute and chronic brain syndromes associated with neuropathological abnormalities may range from disorders whose pathogenesis is understood and can be treated, to disorders whose pathogenesis is not understood, making any drug therapy entirely empiric. The discovery that general paresis is a late complication of syphilis and the availability of adequate diagnostic measures and specific treatment have virtually eradicated this formerly common mental disease. If the manifestations of nutritional deficiency can be recognized early enough, some instances of the Wernicke syndrome or Korsakoff psychosis can be ameliorated with appropriated vitamin therapy. On the other hand, the great number of patients with presenile, senile, and arteriosclerotic brain disease, or mixtures thereof, defies our attempts at specific therapy. Drug therapy is largely symptomatic, although atherosclerosis may foreseeably yield to drug therapy.

Categories of Drugs and Therapeutic Principles

Classification of Psychotherapeutic Drugs. The least complex and most realistic classification of these agents is based on their putative clinical uses. In general, drugs used for treating anxiety, in all its clinical guises, are referred to as antianxiety agents; those used for treating depressive syndromes are called antidepressants; and those used for treating schizophrenic reactions or other psychoses are termed antipsychotics. Even this classification has defects; each of the drug types may, under certain circumstances, be used for the other two purposes. Besides these three important classes of psychotherapeutic drugs, a mixed group is available for specific purposes.

Antianxiety Drugs. *Chemical Classes.* Older drugs in this series include the barbiturates; newer drugs are shown in Figure 11–1. Meprobamate and its congeners are substituted glycerol derivatives. Some members of this group

ANTIANXIETY DRUGS

Glycerol Derivatives

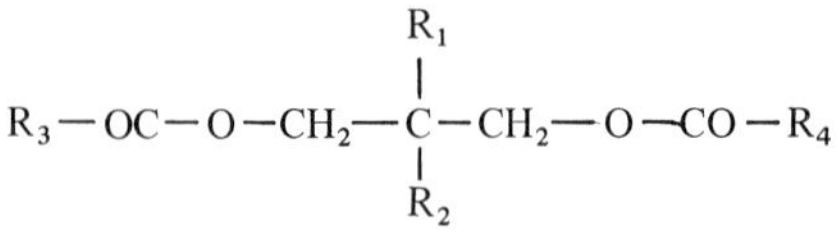
R1
R3—OC—O—CH2—C—CH2—O—CO—R4
R2

Meprobamate (Miltown, Equanil); tybamate (Solacen, Tybatran)

Benzodiazepine Derivatives

Chlordiazepoxide (Librium)

Diazepam (Valium)

Oxazepam (Serax)

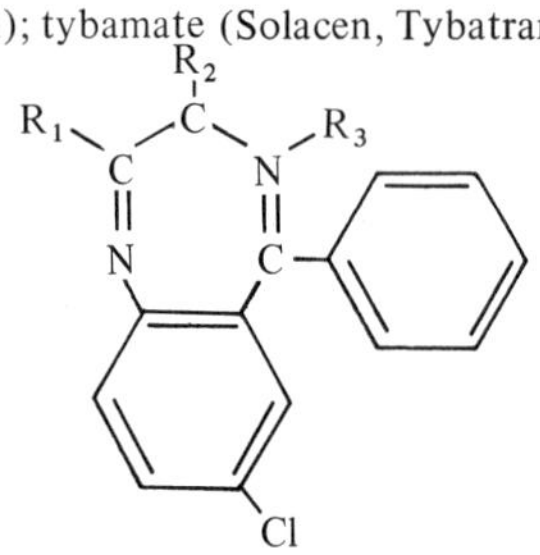
R2
R1
C
R3
C
N
N
C
Cl

Diphenylmethane Derivatives

Diphenhydramine (Benadryl)

Hydroxyzine (Atarax, Vistaril)

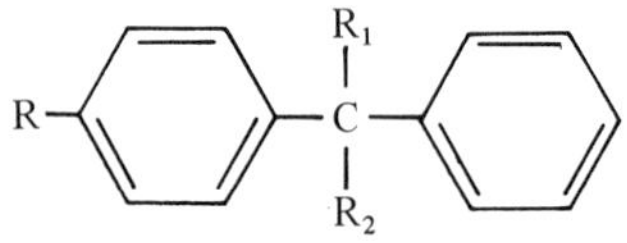
R1
R
C
R2

ANTIDEPRESSANTS

Tricyclic Type

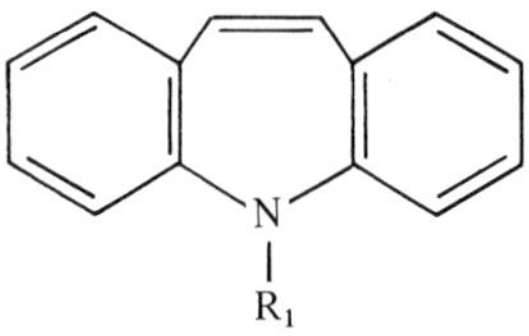
N
R1

Imipramine (Tofranil)
Desipramine
(Pertofrane)

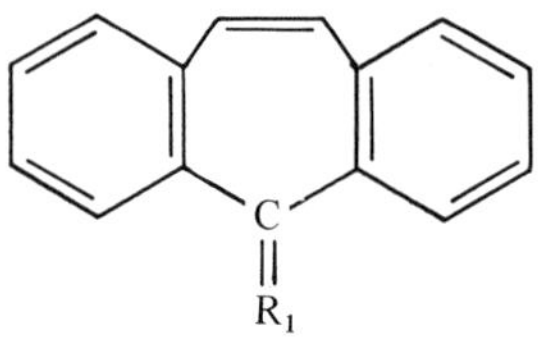
C
R1

Amitriptyline (Elavil)
Nortriptyline (Aventyl)
Protriptyline (Vivactil)

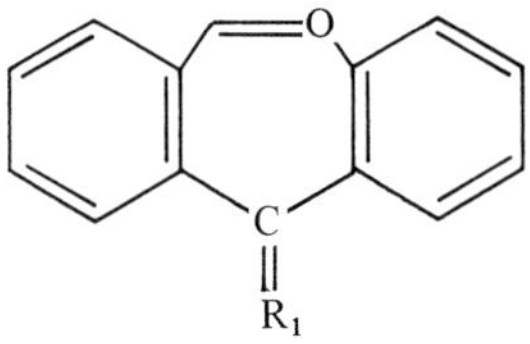
O
C
R1

Doxepine (Sinequan)

Monoamine Oxidase Inhibitors

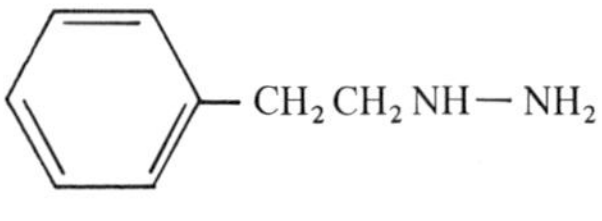
CH2 CH2 NH— NH2

Phenelzine (Nardil)
Isocarboxazide (Marplan)
Nialmide (Niamid)

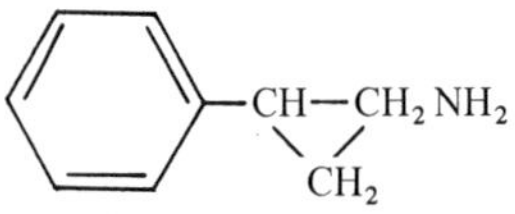
CH—CH2 NH2
CH2

Tranylcypromine (Parnate)

Sympathomimetic Stimulants

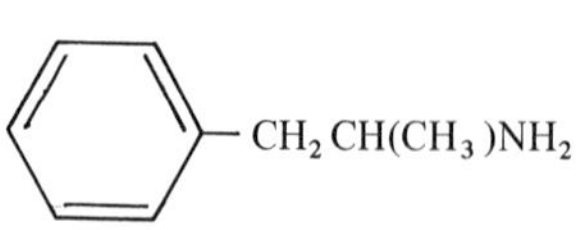
CH2 CH(CH3)NH2

Dextroamphetamine (Dexedrine)
Methamphetamine (Desoxyn, Methedrine)

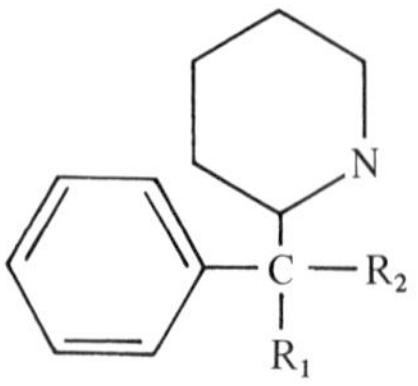
N
C
R2
R1

Pipradrol (Meratran)

Methylphenidate
(Ritalin)

Figure 11–1. Classes of antianxiety and antidepressant drugs based on chemical structures. Generic names of drugs are given in parentheses.

have been promoted primarily for nonsedative purposes, such as carisoprodol (Soma) as a centrally acting muscle relaxant or mebutamate (Capla) as an antihypertensive, but it seems likely that they are far more alike than different. Difference in half-life of the drugs may be of some clinical importance (see Chapter 2); the mean plasma half-life of tybamate is approximately one-third that of meprobamate. Chlordiazepoxide and its congeners belong to a new chemical group, the benzodiazepines. A vague structural relationship to the diphenylmethane derivatives can also be discerned. Diazepam is a more potent variant of the chlordiazepoxide structure; oxazepam is an active metabolite of diazepam. The pharmacologic profiles of these three drugs are virtually identical. Diphenylmethane antihistaminics have enjoyed a revival as antianxiety agents, diphenhydramine being well known as an antihistaminic, whereas hydroxyzine has been introduced primarily as an antianxiety drug. As antihistaminics can be sold over the counter, a number of widely used proprietary "tranquilizers" or "nonbarbiturate" hypnotics are members of this class. Some of these preparations are compound formulations that include scopolamine; overuse has led to acute toxic deliria.

Pharmacologic Properties. Antianxiety agents have pharmacologic effects resembling those of the older sedatives (Irwin, 1968). Their depressive effects on the central nervous system are dependent upon dosage, milder depression often resulting in the desired therapeutic effect (relief of anxiety), along with some impairment of psychologic functions. Larger doses may induce sleep, and toxic doses produce deep coma. Many of these drugs are anticonvulsant by virtue of depression of the motor cortex. Block of spinal cord internuncial neurons, as well as the sedative effects, contributes to a weak muscle relaxant action; overdoses are manifested by weakness, incoordination, and flaccidity. The development of tolerance after repeated use, as well as the tendency of some persons to abuse these drugs, may lead to physical dependence manifested by withdrawal reactions on abrupt discontinuation. In these respects, most of the newer antianxiety agents share some of the pharmacologic properties of the barbiturates.

These resemblances may be an artifact of the animal pharmacologic screening tests used for detecting potential antianxiety drugs. Diminution of spontaneous activity, prolongation of hexobarbital sleeping time, increased seizure threshold, hind limb ataxia, and many other animal tests employ the barbiturate model. It is not surprising that most other drugs resemble them. In fact, a truly different type of anti-

anxiety drug probably would not have passed the usual preclinical screening tests. If propranolol (Inderal) proves to be an effective antianxiety agent, as preliminary evidence suggests, it will be necessary to re-evaluate many of the traditional screening tests for antianxiety drugs (Granville-Grossman and Turner, 1966; Wheatley, 1969). *Principle: Once a pharmacologic model has been established for a class of drugs, it is relatively easy to discover new agents that resemble the old, but discovery of completely novel approaches to treatment is unlikely.* Clinicians often have the chance to observe potentially useful pharmacologic properties overlooked in the pharmacologic screening of a drug.

Clinical Use. Drug therapy is most logically considered as adjunctive rather than primary in the management of anxiety reactions, psychophysiologic disorders, or simply the nervousness of everyday life. Reliance on drugs to ameliorate symptoms may deprive patients of other types of treatment, resulting in more harm than benefit.

Administration of a symptomatic treatment should be limited to the prevalence of symptoms causing some degree of discomfort or disability. Consequently, some traditional concepts of treatment may be abandoned in the case of antianxiety drugs. One of these concepts is that a fixed dosage schedule, of the classical t.i.d. or q.i.d. type, should be followed. Insomnia is a frequent symptom of anxiety, and the therapeutic value of "sleep which knits up the ravelled sleeve of care" has long been recognized. As most antianxiety agents are also hypnotic in large doses and have rather long plasma half-lives, the major dose might be given at bedtime to exploit the hypnotic effects. Rather than viewing the extended effects into the next day as "drug hangover," one could take the position that this type of mild central nervous system depression is precisely what is aimed for as daytime sedation. Additional small doses of drug may be taken during the day as needed, depending upon the presence of symptoms.

Another tradition that might be questioned is continuous treatment. Anxiety is often episodic in intensity. Instead of prolonged administration of drugs, brief courses should be utilized to relieve each particular episode. Interrupted therapy decreases the tendency to develop tolerance with return of symptoms despite continued drug treatment, or the need for steadily increasing doses to maintain control of symptoms. The fact that the patient knows he can obtain relief may often sustain him quite adequately over periods without drug. Futhermore, *placebo responses are frequent and definite in anxious patients.* Placebo responses may confound the clinical pharmacologist attempting to evaluate drugs, but offer a potential advantage in the practical management of anxious patients (see Chapter 14).

Patients vary considerably in their dose requirements. Variations of two- to threefold have been observed in concentrations of meprobamate in plasma 4 hours after a single dose, or in the plasma half-time of disappearance following chronic administration (Hollister and Levy, 1964). Fixed doses or dosage schedules are not appropriate for these drugs. *Principle: The therapeutic goal should determine the dose.*

Efficacy of Antianxiety Drugs. Although some studies have failed to show any differences between some of the newer drugs and placebos, most controlled evaluations have demonstrated beneficial effects (Rickels *et al.*, 1959; McNair *et al.*, 1965). In view of the many sources of negative bias that may be introduced in controlled studies of antianxiety drugs, more weight must be given to those studies that have shown differences. Very few studies have demonstrated the superiority of newer drugs over phenobarbital. Although antianxiety drugs are effective, the self-limiting nature of the illness, as well as the influence of nondrug factors, makes demonstration of efficacy difficult.

Several problems have become evident as clinical experience with these drugs has accumulated: (1) anxious patients respond favorably to any attention, including placebo; (2) differences between drugs and placebo are often subtle and transient; and (3) drugs, but not placebos, may interact with nonspecific factors in the treatment situation (Uhlenhuth *et al.*, 1959). Among the metapharmacologic influences that interact in this way are characteristics of patients (initial level of anxiety, social class, degree of compliance), of physicians (degree of confidence in drug therapy, rapport with patient), and of the locale in which the drug is given (private practice office, pay or charity clinic) (Rickels, 1968). The best possible combination of circumstances to produce a good result from an antianxiety drug would involve a patient with a high level of anxiety and a compliant personality from a low social class being treated by a physician who is warm and friendly and believes in drug therapy. *Principle: Drug effects may be augmented by considering those aspects of the treatment situation that interact with drugs to produce the most favorable results.*

Choice of Antianxiety Agent. In order of efficacy, the benzodiazepines and meprobamate may have a slight edge over barbiturates, all probably being superior to placebo. The fact that placebo alone is so often effective must affect the choice of drug. If there is a high prob-

ability of some degree of remission from any proffered treatment, the most familiar and cheapest antianxiety drug might be used first. Consequently, phenobarbital might first be tried in relatively small doses, as it is cheaper than placebo and almost as innocuous. Should the patient respond satisfactorily, fine; if he does not, the dose may be increased to tolerance. Failing still, one of the newer drugs should be tried. *Principle: Familiarity with a drug need not breed contempt, but may be an asset, in that the physician may be more alert to unwanted effects and more able to assess therapeutic effects.*

Among the glycerol derivatives, meprobamate is probably the most useful. Its congener, tybamate, has a very short duration of action, which limits its usefulness for chronic treatment (Shelton and Hollister, 1967). The short half-life of tybamate could become an advantage for as-needed daytime doses, although another drug should be used for the major nighttime dose. Other drugs of this series have similar, if not identical, actions to meprobamate.

The three available benzodiazepines, chlordiazepoxide, diazepam, and oxazepam, are also essentially identical except for dose and duration of action, chlordiazepoxide being the longest-acting and oxazepam the shortest-acting drug (Randall and Schallek, 1968). All rank with the moderate or long-acting barbiturates in duration of action. Although oxazepam is an active metabolite of diazepam, larger doses must be used, possibly owing to poorer absorption of oxazepam. *Principle: Congeners may be similar in their pharmacologic effects, but chemical differences may alter their kinetics and may provide useful choices among them for specific needs.*

Antihistaminics with sedative activity, such as hydroxyzine, have generally been disappointing. A number of nonbarbiturate hypnotics, such as glutethimide (Doriden), are commonly used in small doses for daytime sedation. Such drugs have no superiority over those mentioned above, and, in the case of glutethimide, the increased risks from physical dependence or increased hazards when the drug is used with suicidal intent are scarcely justified by any possible benefits.

Another drug primarily promoted as a hypnotic, methaqualone (Quaalude), is used for daytime sedation. This drug has been widely abused in other countries and its repetitive use should be discouraged. The promotion of phenothiazine antipsychotics in smaller-than-usual doses as antianxiety agents seems unwarranted in view of the generally disappointing results from controlled studies. This use of such powerful agents seems analogous to using a sledge hammer to drive a tack; such a method demands an exceedingly careful touch lest a hole be put in the wall.

Summary Principles: (1) The decision to treat anxiety should be based on the degree of disability or discomfort produced. (2) Treatment with drugs should be symptomatic and adjunctive; drugs should not deprive patients of psychotherapy when it is appropriate. (3) Treatment with drugs should be limited in time and maximal dose, preferably with interrupted courses. (4) Doses should be individualized for each patient. (5) Dosage schedules should be flexible. (6) Favorable nondrug influences should be exploited as much as possible. (7) Choice of drug is largely empiric, but ordinarily treatment should begin with the most effective and least toxic drug.

Antidepressants. *Chemical Structures.* Two new classes of chemical compounds, the tricyclics and the monoamine oxidase (MAO) inhibitors, as well as the older sympathomimetic stimulants, may be considered as antidepressants. Other drug classes may also vie for this description, but these are described elsewhere.

The dibenzazepine nucleus resembles the phenothiazine nucleus, although the spatial configuration may differ more than is apparent in a two-dimensional representation (Figure 11–1). A group of dibenzocycloheptadiene derivatives, made by substituting a carbon atom for the nitrogen atom in the nucleus, has also appeared. Because of the confusing chemical names for such similar compounds, the simpler term, tricyclic, is preferred when referring to these drugs. The discovery that the monodemethylated derivative of imipramine is a metabolic product of imipramine with apparent antidepressant activity led to great interest in these derivatives, which now outnumber the dimethylated compounds (Brodie *et al.*, 1961). This situation seems to differ from that of phenothiazines, where monodemethylation markedly weakens all pharmacologic actions.

The MAO inhibitors are of two chemical types, hydrazides and nonhydrazides. The first hydrazide drug was iproniazid (Marsilid), a drug formerly employed for its tuberculostatic activity. A later member of the series was pheniprazine (Catron). Both have subsequently been removed from the market because of intolerable toxicity. As part of the toxicity was believed to result from the formation of free hydrazine, later variants of this group included structures that protected the hydrazine moiety, as in the case of isocarboxazide and nialamide. The nonhydrazide MAO inhibitor, tranylcypromine, chemically resembles dextroamphetamine, having a cyclopropyl rather than an isopropyl side chain. This chemical difference markedly enhances its ability to inhibit monoamine oxidase as compared with dextroamphetamine, which possesses only weak monoamine oxidase inhibitory properties. However, tranylcypromine retains some of the sympathomimetic actions of dextroamphetamine.

The older sympathomimetic stimulants, exemplified by dextroamphetamine, were phenalkylamines. Newer members of this group, such as methylphenidate or pipradrol, contain a piperidine ring in a structure resembling the diphenylmethanes; on close inspection one can discern a portion of the molecule with a phenethylamine structure.

Pharmacologic Actions. The modes of action of some of the antidepressants in terms of the norepinephrine hypothesis of depression are described in Chapter 18. This hypothesis, however attractive, is based primarily on indirect evidence. Consequently, judgment should be withheld on whether the mechanisms of action of antidepressant drugs can be fully explained within the framework of their ability to interfere with catecholamine metabolism. *Principle: Most drugs have complex pharmacologic effects. To attribute a priori all their clinical effects to one of their actions may be misleading.* Thus the monoamine-oxidase-inhibiting effects of iproniazid are not equated with its antituberculous effects.

Although dextroamphetamine is a sympathetic stimulant, it is necessary to differentiate between stimulation and antidepressant effects. There is very little reason clinically to believe that the two actions are necessarily related. Amphetamines cause sympathetic stimulation by releasing norepinephrine (Carr and Moore, 1969). In terms of the norepinephrine hypothesis, such an action might be antidepressant. Curiously, severe depression may follow withdrawal from amphetamines after high doses taken over brief periods. To make matters even more complex, a psychosis quite similar to paranoid schizophrenia may be evoked during a chronic period of amphetamine abuse (Hawks *et al.*, 1969). Both these complications of amphetamine abuse support the theory that biogenic amines play an important role in these two naturally occurring emotional disorders.

Tolerance to dextroamphetamine is attributed in part to development of a false neurotransmitter *p*-hydroxynorephedrine (Groppetti and Costa, 1969). Thus if doses are not graduated upward, the effects of the drug may be lost. This consideration may explain why dextroamphetamine is not highly regarded as an antidepressant in practice. The drug is usually given at a low fixed dose. For brief periods some relief of depression may be obtained, but in severe, chronic depressions, the effects are neither adequate nor sustained. To date, no clinical trials have been undertaken with larger-than-customary doses. Theoretically, cocaine should be an antidepressant, but its effects have not been tested.

Inhibition of MAO is slow in onset and long in duration. In man, the extent of MAO inhibition in brain is always uncertain, as most techniques measure only peripheral MAO activity. Now techniques to measure inhibition of MAO in the brain are available (Tozer *et al.*, 1966), but relatively few clinical studies have correlated MAO inhibition with efficacy in relieving depressive symptoms. The argument has been made that many of the failures of MAO inhibitors occur because the customary doses of these drugs are inadequate. *Principle: For most drugs a dose-response curve can be drawn that has a sigmoid configuration. Whenever a desired response is not observed, the dose must be increased until the desired therapeutic effect is attained, until an unwanted side effect limits treatment, or until chemical determinations (e.g., quinidine levels in plasma) indicate that the maximum safe level of drug has been reached.*

Although the drugs are efficacious, they so readily inhibit MAO in peripheral tissues that their use has declined. MAO inhibition has caused a number of unexpected, though wholly predictable, interactions with other drugs and foods (Sjoqvist, 1965) (see Chapter 16). Sympathomimetic drugs, such as epinephrine, norepinephrine, ephedrine, metaraminol (Aramine), phenylephrine (Neosynephrine), amphetamines, and methylphenidate, interact with MAO inhibitors to evoke acute hypertension with central nervous system and circulatory complications (subarachnoid hemorrhage or acute pulmonary edema). Foods such as cheeses, yeast extracts, pickled herring, chicken livers, or broad beans, which contain pressor amines (usually tyramine), have caused similar interactions. The same is true of alcoholic beverages. As might be expected, MAO inhibition adds to the central sympathetic stimulation from tricyclic antidepressants, and concurrent use in high doses has produced agitation, hyperpyrexia, convulsions, coma, and death. The action of many sedatives, such as barbiturates, meperidine (Demerol), chlordiazepoxide, and chloral hydrate, has also been enhanced, leading to unexpectedly severe central nervous system depression. Because of these interactions and their serious consequences, many clinicians are loath to use MAO inhibitors. Those few who are still favorably disposed emphasize the need to employ adequate doses; some even recommend concurrent use with the tricyclics to obtain an additive effect.

Imipramine, which so resembles chlorpromazine chemically, and to a lesser extent pharmacologically, was first thought to be a possible antipsychotic drug. Actually, the chemical resemblance to phenothiazines may be less than it seems, for the ethylene bridge in the central ring removes the coplanar structure of the phenothiazines (Figure 11–1). The chief pharmacologic difference between phenothiazines and imipramine is that imipramine and the other tricyclics sensitize central adrenergic synapses, whereas phenothiazines block central adrenergic transmission. Curiously, both types of drugs are thought to achieve these apparently diametric effects by the same process, that of stabilizing the membrane of the nerve ending. In the case of chlorpromazine, permeability to the release of norepinephrine is reduced, whereas in the case of imipramine, the permeability to reuptake is impaired (Glowinski and Axelrod, 1965). As all intra- and extracellular membrane surfaces may not be symmetric, and because of the different spatial geometry of the drug molecules, one type of drug may affect the internal side of the cell membrane and another the external side.

Another important difference is that the tricyclics are more potent anticholinergics than the phenothiazines. Indeed, the anticholinergic action usually limits dosage, the usual doses of tricyclics being far lower than doses of phenothiazines. The possible relevance of central anticholinergic action to antidepressant effects is still uncertain, but this rather distinct pharmacologic difference should not be overlooked. The tricyclics are similar to phenothiazines, however, in their sedative effect. When the drugs are given to normal subjects in equivalent doses, it is difficult to distinguish the sedation produced by either type of drug. The role of sedation in antidepressant action is also questionable, but the most sedative tricyclic, amitriptyline, is often regarded as the best antidepressant, and phenothiazines may have a definite antidepressant action. Individual drugs have more than a single pharmacologic effect. Antidepressant action may be contingent upon a combination of effects rather than upon any single one.

Efficacy of Antidepressants. Several difficulties arise in evaluating drug therapy of depression. Besides the distinction that must be made between the ubiquitous symptom of depression and depressive illnesses, the physican is faced with assessing the severity of the illness. Some depressions may require no treatment, whereas others demand urgent intervention to avoid a fatal outcome. To confuse matters, the terminology for describing depressive syndromes is so poorly defined that even expert psychiatrists often interpret terms differently. The term "antidepressant" is a bit misleading in suggesting that a drug so labeled is effective in all types of depressions. Increasing clinical evidence indicates that the wide range of drugs may have specific and limited uses for depressed patients.

Although drugs have a role in the treatment of depressions, two other approaches to management have also been valuable: convulsive therapy and psychotherapy. Preoccupation with drug therapy may deprive patients of the benefits of other treatments. It is of particular importance in choosing the proper treatment to keep in mind the severity of the illness:

1. Some patients, even those admitted to a hospital, improve rapidly within a week or two of admission if given only supportive treatment by psychotherapy. In general, these patients have depressions that are not severe, external precipitating causes for depression are evident, and few, if any, psychotic symptoms are present.

2. The severely depressed patient, especially if suicidal, should be considered for convulsive therapy with little delay. Convulsions may be induced electrically (ECT) or by the convulsant chemical flurothyl (Indoklon). Antidepressant drugs may be used concurrently or following remission from convulsive therapy to prevent relapse.

3. Patients with depressions of moderate severity may benefit from a combination of drug therapy and psychotherapy. The choice of drug is based primarily on the clinical manifestations of the depression.

Although the total number of large-scale controlled studies of antidepressants is small, a consistent pattern seems to be emerging (Overall et al., 1962; Wittenborn et al., 1962; Greenblatt et al., 1964; Clinical Psychiatry Committee, 1965). Electroconvulsive therapy (ECT), even when studied "unblind" and with negative bias, appears to be a reliable effective treatment. Imipramine is usually found superior to placebo or MAO inhibitors, but the latter rarely exceed the effects of placebo. Smaller-scale controlled studies suggest that amitriptyline is either equal or slightly superior to imipramine, and that the demethylated analogs are either equal or somewhat inferior to the parent compounds (Burt et al., 1962; Hollister et al., 1963). Treatments may be listed in the following order of effectiveness: ECT, amitriptyline, imipramine, demethylated tricyclics, MAO inhibitors, and placebo. Placebo should be listed in the rank ordering, because patients given placebo often respond favorably (see Chapter 14). Although the therapeutic results of placebo are statistically less significant than those of the tricyclics, the practical difference between the drugs and placebo in clinical use is less impressive (Raskin et al., 1970).

There is a plausible explanation for the difficulty in demonstrating more-than-slight differences in efficacy between the tricyclics and placebo. The tricyclics are highly effective, but in only a small proportion of patients with depression. The true difference in response in these patients is diluted by uncritical or unqualified patient selection, thus nullifying the sensitivity of the test situation. A false conclusion here involves a type II error (see Chapter 1). Three separate controlled studies, in which depressed patients were classified empirically into three diagnostic subtypes, have consistently revealed the superiority of tricyclics, both imipramine and amitriptyline, in depressions categorized as "retarded." Usually such patients compose less than 20% of a heterogeneous group of hospitalized patients with depression. However, in four studies, antipsychotics have been consistently more effective in "anxious" depression, a major depressive subtype. Anxious depressions account for more than 50% of admissions to hospitals (Overall et al., 1969). Curiously, a third class of depressions categorized as "hostile" seems to respond equally well to both tricyclics and phenothiazines. *Principle: Controlled clinical trials are fraught with many hazards. If the population under test is not homogeneous, falsely negative results may be obtained. Rigorous diagnostic criteria are required to reduce the incidence of type II errors.*

Choice of Antidepressants. The clearest indication for the tricyclics is in retarded, endogenous, or possibly psychotic depressions characterized by blunted affect, lack of motor movements, and emotional withdrawal. As imipramine and amitriptyline are the oldest tricyclics and as the newer members have no demonstrated superiority over them, either drug might be used. The choice should be based on the therapist's degree of experience with each; doses are the same, however, so that interchanging these drugs should create few problems. The demethylated congeners of tricyclics do not appear to have any more therapeutic efficacy than the parent compounds, nor do compounds with active metabolites seem to exhibit increased efficacy.

Increasingly, physicians are combining phenothiazines with tricyclics, so that commercially available combinations of perphenazine and amitriptyline (Triavil, Etrafon) in a variety of dose ratios have been introduced. The major indication for such combinations has been in depressions with accompanying agitation or psychotic symptoms (Hollister *et al.*, 1967a). Initially, such combinations should be made extemporaneously, but once a suitable ratio has been found, substitution of the fixed combination might be considered on the basis of convenience and reduced cost. Although depressed patients with predominant symptoms of anxiety, tension, somatic complaints, and some self-recrimination have been best managed by phenothiazine derivatives, these drugs should not be prescribed initially to outpatients (Overall *et al.*, 1962). As antianxiety drugs are widely used for treating such depressions in clinical practice, it might be worthwhile to try one of these agents prior to using the potent phenothiazines. Controlled trials indicate that antianxiety drugs may be useful in these types of depressions (Hollister *et al.*, 1971).

Because of the danger of inhibition of monoamine oxidase, MAO inhibitors should be considered last-choice agents to be used only when other drugs have failed. The most widely used of these drugs, tranylcypromine, should be specifically limited to severely depressed hospitalized patients. If MAO inhibitors are used, the patient must be scrupulously instructed regarding their hazards in combination with a variety of foods and drugs, especially some agents that may be used as self-medicaments, such as "cold capsules" containing phenylpropanolamine (Propadrine) or other vasoconstrictors.

A few patients, especially those with reactive depressions following a loss or secondary to a physical illness, may respond to the euphoriant effects of stimulants such as dextroamphetamine, methylphenidate, or pipradrol. These drugs should be limited in amount and duration of treatment, lest habituation and dependence occur.

Patterns of dosage may vary considerably depending upon the antidepressant. Tricyclics usually are prescribed initially in relatively small divided doses. Later, doses are rapidly increased, until toxicity or therapeutic effect is seen. The sedative and anticholinergic pharmacologic properties often limit dosage. Studies of plasma concentrations of one of the demethylated analogs, desipramine, revealed wide variations obtained from the same doses of drug (Hammer and Sjoqvist, 1967). The variation was as much as 30-fold, with an average variation of eightfold. Such variation in plasma levels is genetically determined, for later studies have revealed very similar plasma concentrations in steady-state conditions in identical, as contrasted with fraternal, twins (Alexanderson *et al.*, 1969). There should be no uniform dose of these drugs. Evidence suggests that plasma levels of these drugs may parallel clinical efficacy or toxic

effects. Pharmacokinetic studies may be helpful in preventing toxicity, reassuring the physician that extraordinary amounts may be necessary in certain cases, and revealing possible genetic predisposition to variation in metabolism. In some patients who do not experience a pharmacologic effect despite sizeable oral doses, administration of the drug parenterally or in a different oral form, such as liquid concentrates, may be rational (see Chapter 2). *Principle: Variation in physiologic availability of a drug, as well as unusual metabolism or elimination, should be sought as a reason for poor clinical response before discarding a potentially useful drug.*

MAO inhibitors presumably produce their clinical effects to the degree that monoamine oxidase inhibition is attained. Some commonly used dosage schedules may fail to inhibit MAO sufficiently. A clinical criterion that might be used to assay the degree of MAO inhibition is evidence of sympathetic inhibition, such as orthostatic hypotension, slowed heart rate, increased bowel sounds, or abnormal responses to Valsalva's maneuver or the cold pressor test (see Chapter 5). Chemical evidence of MAO inhibition is manifested by increased urinary excretion of tyramine or tryptamine, neither of which is normally metabolized when MAO is inhibited. *Principle: When the mechanism of a drug action is known and can be documented objectively, therapeutic dosage schedules should be related to demonstrable pharmacologic effects.*

Sedatives or antianxiety drugs are used in treatment of depressions in much the same way that they are used for treating anxiety. While most experimental studies of phenothiazines in depression have used rather large doses, usually in the antipsychotic range, it is possible that much smaller doses would suffice and would be less toxic. Sympathomimetic stimulants may be given in a single dose in the morning, as their span of action is far longer than ordinarily believed. Persistence of the effects of a single dose may interfere with sleep and may be harmful rather than helpful.

It is customary to treat with antidepressants for several weeks following clinical remission. The actual duration of treatment is best judged by the natural history of the disorder. If depression has recurred at closely spaced intervals, the drugs may be given for a protracted period.

Summary Principles: (1) The decision to use antidepressant drugs hinges mainly upon the severity of the depressive reaction; the least severe may require no drug treatment and the most severe should be considered for electroconvulsive therapy, possibly with concurrent drug therapy. (2) The choice of antidepressant should not be re-

stricted only to drugs usually considered as "anti-depressants," such as tricyclics or MAO inhibitors, but should include antianxiety agents and some antipsychotic drugs. (3) The drug to be used in a particular patient chiefly depends on the type of depressive reaction. Tricyclics are clearly indicated for depressions that might be classified as "retarded," "endogeneous," or "psychotic"; antianxiety drugs or phenothiazine derivatives may be preferred agents for depressions associated with anxiety or agitation. (4) MAO inhibitors and stimulants are of limited value, the former in rare instances of hospitalized patients refractory to all other treatment, and the latter in patients whose illness is expected to be self-limited. (5) Doses may be used over a very wide range depending upon the response of patients. (6) Dosage regimens should be determined by the type of drug being employed. (7) Duration of treatment is best gauged by the previous course of the disorder in the individual patient.

Antipsychotics. *Chemical Structures.* At present, seven chemical classes of compounds are known that ameliorate psychoses and evoke extrapyramidal reactions, the two unique properties of antipsychotic drugs (Figure 11-2). Although some close resemblances between the chemical structures of the phenothiazines and thioxanthenes are apparent, resemblances between reserpine and the benzoquinolizine derivatives or the butyrophenones and phenylpiperazines are less obvious. No representative of the benzoquinolizine, phenylpiperazine, or indolic derivatives is available on the American market, and the rauwolfia alkaloids have become virtually obsolete. Thus for practical purposes, we are concerned only with three chemical classes.

The structures of most antipsychotic drugs can be viewed as tertiary or, rarely, secondary amines derived from methylethylamine (–C–C–N–C). Phenothiazine antipsychotics have a common S-shaped configuration, regardless of which subfamily they belong to (R–N–C–C–C–N–C). The thioxanthenes show a similar nucleus (R–C–C–C–C–N–C), as do the butyrophenones (R–C–C–C–C–N–C). This conformation of the molecule may be critical to its effect (Stach and Poldinger, 1966; Janssen, 1970).

The phenothiazine derivatives are the oldest and the most popular antipsychotics. Partly because of chemical differences but also because of variations in pharmacologic actions and potency, distinction between the phenothiazines should be made. Compounds with an aliphatic dimethylaminopropyl side chain, such as chlorpromazine, are relatively low in potency and high in sedative effects. Substitution at the 2-position of the phenothiazine nucleus creates a more potent compound; for example, chlorpromazine is more potent than promazine (Sparine). Some substituents such as the trifluoromethyl group confer more potency than a simple chlorine atom (triflupromazine < chlorpromazine). The nuclear substituents may increase potency by increasing fat solubility of the molecule. The piperidine side chain is represented by thioridazine and piperacetazine. Piperacetazine is more potent than thioridazine and has pharmacologic properties that are more like those of the piperazine group, to which it has a closer spatial configuration. Thioridazine and its side chain sulfoxide metabolite, mesoridazine (Serentil), are most different from other phenothiazines in pharmacologic actions. Three variants of the piperazine side chain, along with variations of the ring substituent, create a large class of piperazinyl phenothiazines. These compounds are much more potent than their ring-substituted analogs in the aliphatic series. They possess less sedative effects than the other two classes, but are more likely to produce extrapyramidal reactions at equivalent therapeutic doses. *Principle: Chemical classification of drugs within a large group allows some prediction of pharmacologic differences between the subgroups.*

Pharmacologic Actions. Neither the exact mechanism of antipsychotic action nor the pathogenetic basis for schizophrenia is known. Schizophrenia is peculiarly human and is not found in most animal models. However, most antipsychotic drugs have common pharmacologic properties when given to animals: (1) they induce a cataleptic state; (2) they induce palpebral ptosis; (3) they specifically inhibit operant and exploratory behavior; (4) they specifically inhibit intracranial self-stimulation, amphetamine- or apomorphine-induced stereotyped behavior, and apomorphine-induced vomiting; and (5) they protect against epinephrine- or norepinephrine-induced mortality (Janssen, 1967). *Principle: Pharmacologic events in animals may correlate with entirely unrelated actions in man. Nonetheless, such correlations may be useful in predicting therapeutic effects.*

Phenothiazines are believed to act by blocking access of norepinephrine and dopamine to receptors in the brain. This action is ascribed to stabilization of the membranes of the synaptic clefts so that release is impeded. Using fluorescent techniques, a number of anatomically discrete monoaminergic systems (dopamine, norepinephrine, and serotonin) have been demonstrated in the brain (Andén et al., 1969). Blockade by antipsychotics could decrease neural transmission in these systems and may correlate with the antipsychotic effects.

Phenothiazines

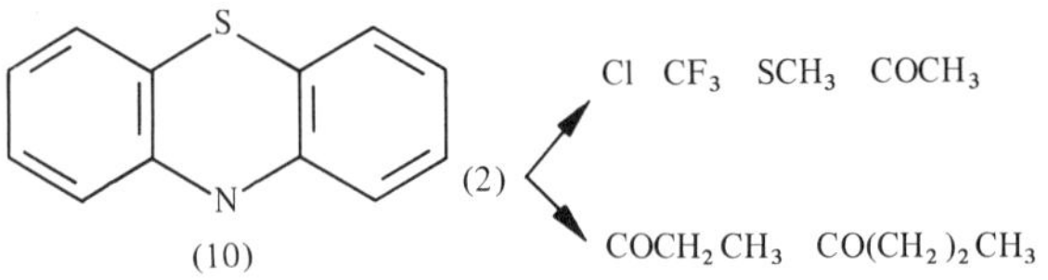

(2)

Cl   CF$_3$ SCH$_3$ COCH$_3$

COCH$_2$CH$_3$ CO(CH$_2$)$_2$CH$_3$

(10)

Aliphatic Group   (10)   CH$_2$—CH$_2$—CH$_2$—N—(CH$_3$)$_2$

Chlorpromazine (Thorazine); triflupromazine (Vesprin)

Piperidine Group   (10)   CH$_2$—CH$_2$—   or   CH$_2$—CH$_2$—CH$_2$—N

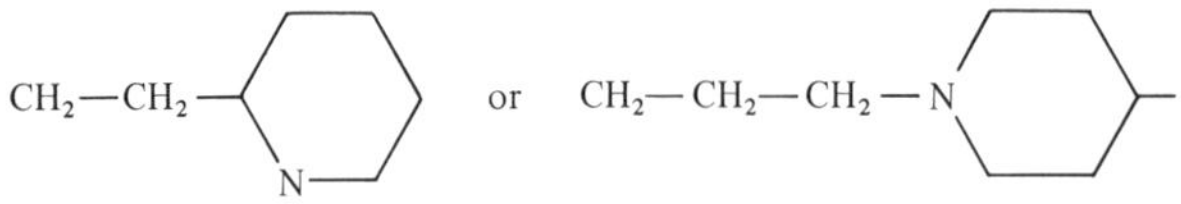

Thioridazine (Mellaril); piperacetazine (Quide)

Piperazine Group   (10)   CH$_2$—CH$_2$—CH$_2$—N   N—

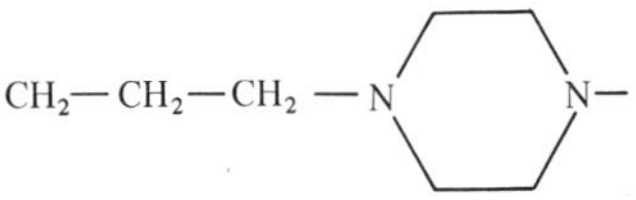

Acetophenazine (Tindal): carphenazine (Proketazine); prochlorperazine (Compazine); perphenazine (Trilafon); butaperazine (Repoise); thiopropazate (Dartal); trifluoperazine (Stelazine); fluphenazine (Prolixin, Permitil)

Thioxanthenes

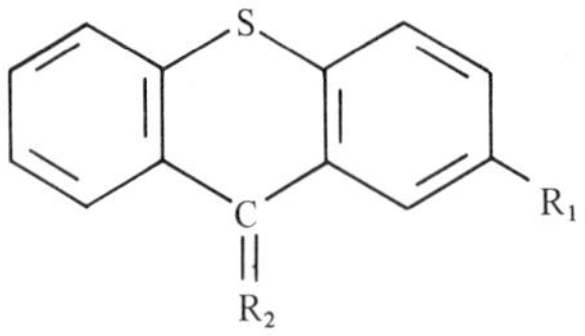

R$_1$

C

R$_2$

Aliphatic   Chlorprothixene (Taractan)
Piperazine   Thiothixene (Navane)

Butyrophenone

Haloperidol (Haldol)

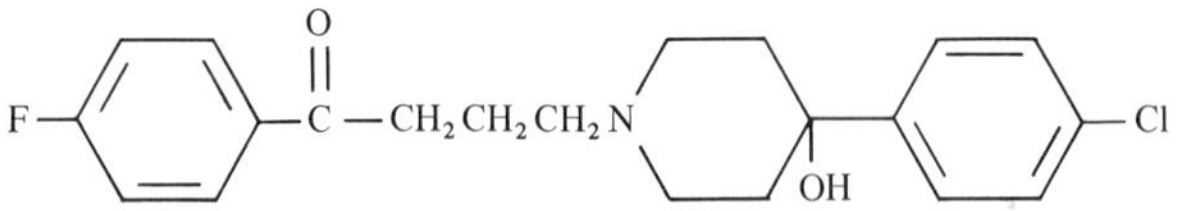

F—   —C—CH$_2$CH$_2$CH$_2$N   —Cl
OH

Figure 11–2. Three chemical classes of antipsychotic drugs. Six of the possible substituents at the 2-position of the phenothiazine are shown, but separation into different subgroups is usually on the basis of the side chains at the 10-position. The same possibilities for chemical changes apply to the thioxanthenes. Many variants of the butyrophenone structure are under investigation, as this class of drugs is very different chemically from the other two.

Blockade is manifested by increased amounts of amines in cell bodies, or by an increased turnover of these amines as indicated by increased urinary excretion of their metabolic end products, homovanillic acid, normetanephrine, and 3-methoxytyramine. The development of extra-pyramidal reactions, a frequent and unique concomitant effect of antipsychotics, may be mediated by the dopaminergic blockade.

From an anatomic point of view, antipsychotic drugs appear to affect three of the major integrating systems of the brain to diminish the emotional response to external or internal stimuli. The drugs may reduce sensory input by altering the function of the brain stem reticular activating system, a monitoring system for sensory input (Himwich, 1958). The limbic system may provide the emotional set to incoming messages, and its functions are believed to be disrupted by the production of seizure patterns in the amygdaloid nucleus. Chemical blockade of norepinephrine-mediated transmission may decrease the activity of central sympathetic systems, especially in the hypothalamus, thereby diminishing peripheral somatic responses to emotional signals. Chlorpromazine concentrates in the limbic and hypothalamic areas as well as in the cortex. In addition to the subcortical actions, some degree of cortical depression may occur when chlorpromazine is given. The subcortical depressive action, however, produces sedation that differs from the effect of conventional sedatives.

Efficacy of Antipsychotic Drugs. Unique prejudices against drug therapy of schizophrenia existed when antipsychotic drugs were first introduced. Subsequently, experimental verification of their efficacy has been unrivaled. In virtually all studies, the results were clear: antipsychotic drugs were far more effective than placebo or other drugs such as barbiturates, and these favorable results could be obtained regardless of the stage of the illness, the type of hospital in which the patients were being treated, or the other ancillary types of treatment offered (Casey *et al.*, 1960; Adelson and Epstein, 1962; Lasky *et al.*, 1962; Michaux *et al.*, 1964; NIMH-PSC Collaborative Study Group, 1964).

Although phenothiazines have been the most thoroughly studied and the most frequently used, other classes of antipsychotics are also effective (e.g., reserpine), but compare unfavorably in efficacy or are more toxic than phenothiazines. Placebo controls have been discontinued in clinical studies with these drugs. New antipsychotics are appropriately evaluated using some standard agent as the comparison drug. Even the demonstration of equal efficacy must be critically evaluated. The possibility that a difference between treatments may not be detected is great if comparative studies do not use homogeneous groups and large populations (see Chapter 1). *Principle: A new drug should not be accepted simply on the basis of its superiority to a placebo; it should at least be the equal of standard drugs in regard to efficacy and toxicity.*

Benefits from antipsychotics are not simply due to sedation. Many prominent symptoms of schizophrenia that have previously resisted sedatives are ameliorated. Disturbed thinking, paranoid symptoms, delusions, emotional and social withdrawal, and personal neglect may improve. Regardless of how it is accomplished, the alleviation of such characteristic psychotic symptoms by these drugs justifies the epithet antipsychotic.

Antipsychotic drugs have been used effectively and safely in conjunction with most other psychiatric therapies. Although lack of improvement of patients treated with placebos has cast doubt upon the efficacy of group or individual psychotherapy and occupational and industrial therapy, these therapies have not been completely evaluated in the treatment of schizophrenics. In any case, drugs do not prevent any benefits from therapies, and vice versa. Electroconvulsive therapy, which may be indicated for agitated schizophrenics who do not respond to drugs alone, can be used simultaneously with phenothiazines, so long as the lowered convulsive threshold produced by the drugs is appreciated. *Principle: Proper testing of a drug includes its evaluation within the total therapeutic program; a drug that might be effective alone might possibly interfere with other therapeutic measures.*

Choice of Antipsychotics. When tested in large groups of patients, most antipsychotic drugs have been equally efficacious, although individual patients respond differently to different drugs. Such an observation is consistent with experience with other types of drugs, such as antihypertensives, anti-inflammatory agents, and diuretics. One of the early clinical postulates was that the more sedative phenothiazines, such as chlorpromazine and thioridazine, would be preferable for patients with agitation, whereas less sedative drugs, such as trifluoperazine and perphenazine, would be best for patients with symptoms of withdrawal and retardation. More recently, formal attempts have been made to discover a rationale for selecting the right drug for the right patient, but thus far these have met with little success (Klett and Moseley, 1965; Hollister *et al.*, 1967b; NIMH-PRB Collaborative Study Group, 1967). No matter how appealing an untested rationale may initially be, objective tests must be conducted to prove it.

An array of drugs is available for empiric trial in a given patient. The usual dictum has been to learn to use a few drugs well rather than all drugs poorly. Such a dictum is based on the assumption that differences between the proper and improper use of a drug probably exceed any pharmacologic differences between drugs. A rational way to narrow the choice of antipsychotics is to master the pharmacology and use of one of each of the three types of phenothiazines, one of the two thioxanthenes, and a butyrophenone. For example, the choice of drugs could include triflupromazine, thioridazine, acetophenazine, thiothixine, and haloperidol. Many other combinations are possible, although haloperidol is the only available member of its class. With five such drugs, the full range of pharmacologic differences between the various antipsychotics can be exploited.

Many patients may improve with administration of a single drug, but remission may be incomplete. Thus it is tempting to try various combinations of drugs. Some combinations stagger the imagination. At one time, a single patient may receive two phenothiazines, a tricyclic antidepressant, an antiparkinsonian drug (usually gratuitously), a nighttime hypnotic, and a daytime stimulant. No evidence supports the superiority of any combination of drugs over the proper use of a single antipsychotic drug, but much evidence suggests that irrational polypharmacy may increase the problems of toxicity and unwanted interactions (Merlis *et al.*, 1970) (see Chapter 16). The possibility that combination of two or more phenothiazines in proportionately lower doses may result in fewer side effects (analogous to the reasoning behind the use of triple-sulfonamide combinations) has not been adequately tested to justify widespread clinical adoption.

Few drugs have such great therapeutic margins and so wide a range of doses as the antipsychotics. Differences in daily therapeutic doses of 20- to 30-fold have been recorded. Although requirements of most patients fall within a fairly narrow range, occasional patients may require rather high doses. Chronic schizophrenics under the age of 40 who have been hospitalized less than 10 years seem most likely to benefit from high-dose regimens (Prien and Cole, 1968; Curry *et al.*, 1970a, 1970b). No patient should be considered a drug failure without an intensive course of therapy. Routine use of massive doses may represent overtreatment for many patients. Phenothiazine concentrations in blood are difficult to measure. It is still uncertain whether unchanged drug is the sole active component or whether metabolites also contribute to therapeutic efficacy. Consequently, the significance of such measurements is uncertain, although it may be possible to define an optimal range of chlorpromazine levels in plasma (Curry and Marshall, 1968; Curry *et al.*, 1970a). Fuller understanding of the pharmacokinetics of these drugs may provide better guides to regulation of dose than purely clinical criteria. In the meantime, *the proper dose is a quantity sufficient to maximize therapeutic goals and to minimize unwanted effects.*

When can a therapeutic effect be expected? Responses of patients newly treated with drugs are variable. Onset ranges from days to weeks. Most clinicians consider that failure of acute or newly recognized schizophrenics to improve after 6 to 8 weeks of adequate treatment is an indication to try another compound. Newly treated chronic schizophrenics may require 12 to 24 weeks of treatment before a change of medication is warranted. *Principle: Expectations from an efficacious drug should be set in relation not only to the disease but also to its duration, rate of spontaneous change or progress, previous therapeutic attempts, and possible interactions with other drugs currently or recently used.*

Assuming that complete or partial remission is attained, how long should treatment be continued? The substitutive model of treatment is illustrated by the use of insulin in an insulin-dependent diabetic. Treatment is constructed as being indefinite and uninterrupted, although the requirements for insulin might shift considerably, depending on many extrinsic variables. The palliative model of therapy is illustrated by the treatment of duodenal ulcers (see Chapter 4). Therapy may be continued well past symptomatic remission, when drugs can be gradually minimized. Although a high percentage of patients with duodenal ulcer relapse within five years of an initial remission, rigid treatment over the five years may be unnecessary, may not prevent recurrence, and may cost more than retreating when needed. Arguments are made for both approaches in managing schizophrenics with drugs. Most evidence supports the substitutive model. A sizeable number of readmissions to hospitals can be traced to some breach in drug treatment initiated by either the patient or the doctor. Supervised continued treatment delays rehospitalization (Engelhardt *et al.*, 1967). *Principle: Therapeutic failure during treatment of a chronic disease does not necessarily mean the drug is of little value. Besides tachyphylaxis to the drug, actual withdrawal on a voluntary basis could explain exacerbation of disease.*

Summary Principles: (1) Antipsychotics are the most strongly established of all psychotherapeutic drugs. (2) Increasing evidence suggests that they may contribute most, if not all, the measurable improvement in hospitalized schizophrenics. (3) These agents should not be used for trivial purposes; their use for minor emotional disorders should be discouraged. (4) The great number of drugs available creates some practical problems in choosing drugs. By using single members of various chemical classes, each of which has the basic pharmacologic properties of the whole class, one can exploit the full range of actions with only five drugs. (5) Doses are highly variable and they must be individualized. (6) Maintenance therapy probably should be indefinite and uninterrupted, although doses may generally be smaller than the doses initially used. (7) No known combination of these drugs has been clearly shown to be superior to adequate amounts of the proper single drug; polypharmacy is not required.

Clinical Therapy

Manic or Cyclic Affective Disorders: Lithium Therapy. The bizarre increase in psychomotor activity, grandiosity, and emotional lability that characterizes the acute manic state is a dramatic symptom that has been effectively controlled by antipsychotic drugs, such as phenothiazines, reserpine, and haloperidol, or by electroconvulsive therapy. Since the introduction in 1949 of lithium carbonate as a treatment, interest in this novel approach has steadily grown. As these disorders are frequently repetitive, either with recurrent attacks of mania or with alternating attacks of mania and depression, lithium therapy has been extended beyond the management of the acute manic episode to prophylactic treatment (Baastrup and Schou, 1967; Noyes, 1969; Gershon, 1970). The concept of an effective prophylaxis against a major psychiatric disorder is intriguing, but is not fully supported by the evidence presently at hand.

The peculiarly episodic nature of cyclic affective disorders has prompted inquiry into possible changes in electrolytes, neuroendocrines, or catecholamines to explain the rapid development of symptoms. As yet no pathogenetic mechanism of manic disorders is known. Extracellular water tends to be low during both mania and depression, and plasma cortisol levels in manics tend to rise as episodes subside, contrary to what has been reported in depression. All these changes are slight and fall within the normal range of variation (Coppen et al., 1966). The norepinephrine hypothesis has been postulated in reverse for mania; i.e., an excess of norepinephrine occurs at central adrenergic synapses during manic attacks. Withdrawal from treatment with alpha-methylparatyrosine, a specific inhibitor of tyrosine hydroxylase, has been associated with transient hypomanic states, suggesting a rebound phenomenon following suppression of synthesis of norepinephrine (Schildkraut and Kety, 1967).

Evidence of Efficacy. Lithium therapy appears effective in managing acute manic episodes (Maggs, 1963; Schou, 1968). Success has varied, but in most instances ranges to 70% remission. The onset of action may be slow as adequate plasma lithium concentrations are being attained. In severe attacks when relief is urgent, anti-psychotic drugs or ECT may be preferred. A controlled comparison of chlorpromazine and lithium revealed essentially no difference in therapeutic effects in acute manic patients (Spring et al., 1970). Unlike the antipsychotic drugs whose efficacy seems dependent upon their sedative effects, remissions obtained with lithium appear to be independent of mental dulling; lithium might be a preferred treatment, all else being equal.

Uncontrolled studies assert that lithium may prevent recurrent episodes of mania, cyclic manic and depressive attacks, or even recurrent depression (Baastrup and Schou, 1967; Angst et al., 1969). The methodologic problems in proving such use are enormous (Blackwell and Shepherd, 1968). Results from a large, cooperative controlled study of this question may not be available for years. *Principle: Early enthusiasm for a new drug may lead to uncritical acceptance of its therapeutic value. Controlled studies are mandatory when doubts remain about efficacy based on historic controls.*

Kinetics and Elimination. A considerable amount of data is available regarding the absorption, distribution, and elimination of lithium. To prevent toxicity, concentrations in plasma must be maintained within a critical and narrow range. Lithium carbonate (the preferred salt) is largely absorbed within minutes following an oral dose and absorption is virtually complete within 6 to 8 hours. Peak concentrations in serum occur within 2 to 4 hours after the oral dose. The half-life in serum is about 24 hours in the adult (somewhat longer in the elderly). The long half-life indicates that a steady state should be attained within a few days (3 to 5) following single daily doses and that therapy may be maintained by a single daily dose. Still, divided doses may be safer for preventing any unusual variations in concentrations of drug in plasma (see Chapter 2).

The ion is initially distributed in total body water, but later shifts intracellularly against a concentration gradient. Various tissues concentrate the drug to different degrees. There is no evidence of protein binding. Passage into the brain is slow, but when a steady state has been reached, the cerebrospinal fluid contains about 40% of the serum lithium level (Platman and Fieve, 1968).

Lithium appears in the urine within 15 minutes of a dose, peak excretion occurring in 1 to 2 hours followed by a slow decline over the next 6 to 7 hours. About 50 to 75% of the dose may be excreted within a 24-hour period, and eventually about 95% of administered lithium can be accounted for by urinary excretion. Clearance of lithium is about 20% that of creatinine, with clearance rates ranging from 15 to 30 ml per minute. About 80% of filtered lithium is reabsorbed, somewhat similar to potassium ion. Ordinarily, the rate of excretion is independent of urine flow and dietary sodium, but with marked deficiency of sodium much greater amounts of lithium may be retained (accounting for the disastrous poisonings that occurred when lithium chloride was employed as a salt substitute in sodium-depleted patients being treated for congestive heart failure). Once lithium therapy is established, the clearance rate for an individual is quite constant (Platman *et al.*, 1968). Determination of lithium clearance is a recommended procedure for establishing the proper maintenance dose during prolonged therapy. *Principle: Pharmacokinetic studies may provide data for judging routes of administration of drugs, intervals between doses, and doses that attain therapeutic levels of drug in the blood.*

Clinical Use. The goal in treatment is to attain a serum lithium level of between 0.8 and 1.6 mEq per liter; the lower level may be inadequate for therapeutic results and the higher level is likely to be accompanied by side effects. Once remission has occurred, lower serum levels (0.4 to 0.8 mEq per liter) may be adequate to maintain benefits.

Side effects commonly occur when concentrations in serum range from 1.6 to 2.0 mEq per liter. Then nausea, vomiting, diarrhea, abdominal pain, thirst, sluggish, dazed feelings, muscle weakness, and hand tremors may occur. When concentrations exceed 2.0 mEq per liter, more serious toxicity is manifested by drowsiness, coarse tremors or muscle twitching, slurred speech, vomiting, and diarrhea (Allgén, 1969). These may be prodromal symptoms of lethal toxicity and the drug should be stopped immediately on their appearance. In a few instances in which the usual doses were given in the face of probable impaired renal function, serious toxicity has occurred; progressive impairment of consciousness, increased muscle tone, hyperreflexia, muscle fasciculation, and somatically triggered or spontaneous tetanic seizures have resulted. Deaths have occurred from complications of these toxic manifestations.

As the ion is more stable in the body than is sodium or potassium it is not as easily removed by water diuresis, diuretics, or potassium chloride (see Chapter 17). Increased sodium chloride hastens elimination, but the response is slow (Platman *et al.*, 1969; Schou, 1969; Ho *et al.*, 1970). Osmotic diuresis with urea, sodium bicarbonate, acetazolamide (Diamox), and aminophylline increases lithium excretion under experimental conditions (Thomsen and Schou, 1968) and is probably worth trying when toxicity

occurs in patients with normal renal function. When renal function is impaired, peritoneal dialysis may be worth a trial, with careful replacement of other electrolytes. *Principle: The physician not only should be constantly alert to toxic manifestations of a drug, but also should have a plan for their management, even when such experience is limited.*

Thyroid enlargement with diminished function has occurred in some patients on long-term lithium treatment, such as prophylaxis of recurrent manic attacks. A careful initial evaluation of thyroid size and function should be made when treatment is contemplated, and repeated observations should be made during treatment.

Summary Principles: (1) The use of lithium for managing acute manic attacks is acceptable, provided one does not forget other treatments that may be more immediately effective. (2) Lithium as a prophylactic treatment for cyclic manias or for alternating mania and depression is experimental and so far unproved. (3) Concentration of lithium in serum and lithium clearance can be used as rather specific guides to doses and are especially important for any program of prolonged treatment. (4) Concentrations in serum should be kept within the recommended range for best therapeutic effects; nothing is gained and much may be lost by exceeding these concentrations.

Childhood and Adolescent Behavior Disorders. These disorders cannot be classified into the same diagnostic categories applied to adults. Childhood and adolescent behavior disorders fit into four major categories: (1) behavior disorders such as hyperactivity, delinquency, or sociopathic-aggressive behavior; (2) organic brain syndromes, such as epilepsies, brain damage from birth, trauma or disease, or so-called minimal brain damage with only borderline neurologic signs and EEG abnormalities; (3) schizophrenias of the usual types, in addition to childhood autism; and (4) affective disorders, chiefly depression, in postpubertal children. Many young patients do not fall into these categories, so that a purely empiric approach is necessary in some, using graded ratings of symptoms and signs. Such standardization of descriptive aspects of these disorders might be helpful in allaying the present confusion engendered by multiple, ill-defined diagnostic terms and subsequent therapeutic manipulations (Fish, 1968a, 1968b).

Childhood schizophrenia and depression are probably best treated with the same drugs used to treat these disorders in adults. Just as in adults, the severity of these disorders covers a broad range. Severely autistic children, such as those unable to talk or make social contact, or those with destructive behavior, may show limited responses to antipsychotic drugs. Less severely schizophrenic children may respond better to drugs, along with a program of social rehabilitation. In general, one starts with low doses of drugs, gradually increasing them until such time as side effects limit further increases or until therapeutic effects are attained. Dystonic reactions are especially common in children being treated with antipsychotic drugs, but are often quite amenable to treatment or prevention by use of elixir of diphenhydramine, which has enough anticholinergic action to be effective. The latter type drug is also a preferred sedative for children who often do not tolerate barbiturates well (Van Praag, 1969).

The "hyperkinetic" or "minimal brain dysfunction" child is characterized by poor attention span, distractability, emotional lability, aggressiveness, and hyperactivity. This syndrome is estimated to affect 3 to 4% of school-age children, most often becoming evident during the early school years. Boys are much more frequently diagnosed as having this disorder than girls. Minor neurologic abnormalities or EEG abnormalities may be found, as well as some history of difficult birth or early injury or infection which might be viewed as a possible cause for brain damage. Although some children seem to undergo a spontaneous remission at about age 12, especially if they have been adequately treated, those children who are untreated have a much higher risk of later becoming delinquent, schizophrenic, or having some other psychiatric disorder (Weiss et al., 1971). Thus, proper recognition of the disorder and its early treatment are highly desirable. Because the diagnosis of borderline cases is difficult, some children are probably undiagnosed, while others may be diagnosed inappropriately. Sometimes the diagnosis is established on the basis of a therapeutic trial with stimulant drugs.

Dextroamphetamine was first used to treat this syndrome in 1937. Since then sympathomimetic stimulants have remained the drugs of choice over sedatives or antipsychotics (Conners et al., 1969). Recently the preferred drug has become methylphenidate, largely because of unjustified fears that use of dextroamphetamine may predispose to its later abuse; no such sequence has been documented. The customary doses of dextroamphetamine range between 10 and 30 mg daily, with those of methylphenidate being approximately double. Doses are usually divided. Some patients seem to require more frequent dosage than others to avoid brief periods of emotional lability as the effect of the drug wears off. In such cases, it might make

sense to attempt to prolong the span of action of dextroamphetamine by administering a dose of sodium bicarbonate to alkalinize the urine and decrease its rate of excretion. Fortunately, any beneficial effects from stimulant drugs are usually evident fairly soon, usually within the first three weeks of treatment. Courses of treatment are often geared to the school year, with vacation periods being used for testing possible withdrawal of drug. The drug program may be resumed only if relapse occurs. Pharmacologic treatment may be expected to help from one half to two thirds of those treated. In general, it seems to be more likely to succeed in those instances in which there is more clear-cut evidence of some organic brain impairment (Lasagna and Epstein, 1970). Other treatments which must be included in any reasonable therapeutic program include family counseling and special teaching for any specific learning disabilities.

Drugs should not be used in acute stress or adjustment reactions where the cause is clearly apparent, such as a change in home or school, an illness, or separation from a friend. These episodes are usually self-limiting and it might be best for the child's future development to work through them psychologically rather than to seek help from a bottle. *Principle: Too many people in our society seek solace through drugs. Be careful about encouraging it unnecessarily, particularly in the young.*

Although the usefulness of drugs is clear in some young patients, drug selection is complicated by the vast array of possible combinations of symptoms and by the great number of drugs for which efficacy has been claimed. In general, drugs seem to be most effective for reducing psychomotor excitement. Such reduction may produce secondary benefits of more organized behavior and improved attention span (Fish, 1968a, 1968b; Kornetsky, 1970).

Summary Principles: (1) Drugs should be chosen on the basis of the target symptoms being attacked; potent drugs are reserved for severe disorders. (2) As with the elderly, paradoxic reactions, such as sedation from stimulants or excitation from sedatives, may be more common in children. (3) Doses of drugs should be individualized; although conservative doses are first employed, children may be more tolerant of many of these drugs than anticipated. Side effects must be actively searched for in children and may be a limiting factor. (4) Duration of treatment depends on the past history of the disorder, or the chance that it may undergo spontaneous remission. (5) Drug therapy in behavior disorders of this age group should be accompanied by intensive psychotherapeutic training and rehabilitative programs.

Mental Deficiency. The great hope for a drug that increases mental capacity has not yet been realized. Drugs currently available can influence the mentally retarded only by indirect actions, such as controlling motor behavior and distractability, which in turn may lead to increased attention span and better intellectual performance. Treatment is entirely symptomatic and any gains are likely to be small.

The earliest reports of the effects of reserpine and chlorpromazine in treating mentally retarded children and adults were quite glowing: behavior was controlled, self-care markedly increased, and intelligence quotients raised. The more sober view of recent years is that while most of these changes may occur, their degree is far less than originally thought and a sizeable number of patients obtain none of these benefits. In any case, treatment with drugs is symptomatic. Large doses of drugs may be required and treatment may be prolonged. *Principle: Symptomatic relief that does not alter the course of the illness must always be weighed against the risks and costs of therapy.*

Psychoses Associated with Old Age. These disorders include presenile, senile, arteriosclerotic, and mixed types of brain syndromes. Treatment has been aimed at postulated specific causes: general malnutrition (vitamins, amino acid supplements, digestive enzymes, anabolic steroids), deficiency of specific nutrients (glutamic acid, yeast ribonucleic acid, adenosine-5-monophosphate), circulatory disorders (niacin, nicotinic acid alcohol [Roniacol], cyclandelate [Vasodilan]), or arteriosclerosis (heparin and other anticoagulants, thyroxine analogs, vegetable oils, and other lipid-lowering agents). No specific proof of the efficacy of any of these measures is available, nor is there any reason to believe that these postulated mechanisms are valid, with the exception of impaired circulation in the case of cerebral arteriosclerosis.

An organic basis for senile psychoses is suggested by the spotty neurofibrillary degeneration and senile plaque formation, but the cause and site of the defect are unknown. The multiple areas of small cerebral infarcts, which may cause brain sections to resemble a Swiss cheese, are associated with local vascular occlusion or thrombosis. In either case, the damage to the nervous system is irreversible. Treatment, no matter how specific it might be, is more likely to prevent future injury than to repair past damage.

The fact that some "senile" patients show improvement following improved social care has weakened the correlation between brain damage and the level of impairment. Poverty, isolation, and physical illness may impair the mental capacity of the aged, mimicking the senile state. When these causes are excluded, however, the degree of impairment correlates positively with the degree of pathology.

Analeptic-stimulant therapy with pentylenetetrazole (Metrazole) still has its proponents, but almost all adequately controlled studies have been negative (Haydu *et al.*, 1961). Sympathomimetic stimulants may be dangerous or may even aggravate irritability or psychotic symptoms. Tricyclic antidepressants may be used, but with great caution, in patients with a concurrent retarded depression. The peripheral and central anticholinergic actions of these drugs may cause severe side effects, including aggravation of the confused mental state. In addition hypotension has resulted in physical injuries due to falls, or possibly has precipitated myocardial infarctions.

Most symptomatic control of the psychoses of the aged has come from the judicious use of phenothiazines, such as acetophenazine or thioridazine. Irritability, disturbed sleep, and careless personal hygiene may be alleviated. As with tricyclic antidepressants, doses must be very low initially and adjusted with great care. The well-known propensity for paradoxic reactions to conventional sedatives in the elderly, with agitation often being precipitated by drugs such as phenobarbital, should be considered in the use of such drugs. Until the basic mechanisms of these disorders are better understood, treatment will be limited to a purely empiric approach.

Alcohol and Drug Abuse. Despite the renewed concern about drugs of abuse, alcohol is most abused of all. In contrast to the estimated 200,000 heroin addicts in this country, there are approximately six million alcoholics. The number of persons using stimulants and sedatives is probably somewhere between these two extremes. The distinguishing aspects of the different types of drug abuse have been well described elsewhere (WHO Expert Committee, 1964). We know relatively little about the pharmacologic effects requisite for a drug of abuse, except that the drug usually is a euphoriant to which tolerance can readily develop. Recent evidence suggests that alkaloids may be formed from endogenous catecholamines in the presence of alcohol and that some of these, such as tetrahydropapaveroline, might provide the basis for the addictive effects of this drug (Cohen and Collins, 1970; Davis and Walsh, 1970). Biogenic amines that act as neurotransmitters are also involved in addiction to opiate drugs (Dole, 1970). In addition, little is known about the psychologic and social factors that enter into the choice of the drug of abuse. Although some of the principles of treatment are similar among the various types of drug abuse, each presents some special problems.

Abuse of Alcohol and Sedative Drugs. Previously this classification was called alcohol-barbiturate-type abuse but the introduction of many new sedatives in the past 20 years has extended the range beyond barbiturates. Glutethimide, methaqualone, meprobamate, and others among the new sedatives have been "abused." Still, barbiturates are the most widely misused among the sedatives, quite possibly because of their lower price (AMA Committee on Alcoholism and Addiction, 1965). Problems associated with the newer agents, which resemble barbiturates pharmacologically, are quite similar.

Drugs play a role in the management of alcohol withdrawal syndromes, as well as in attempts to mitigate drinking by aversive or prophylactic treatments. Acute alcoholic intoxication may require drugs for the control of disturbed behavior, but careful use of sedatives in the presence of high levels of blood alcohol is required lest fatalities occur. Supportive treatment often suffices, and, when toxic levels of alcohol have been taken, dialysis by any technique may be lifesaving by rapidly removing alcohol from the body.

Alcohol withdrawal syndromes vary from the "shakes" to hyperthermic, and possibly fatal, delirium tremens. As the term implies, these syndromes appear in the presence of a declining or absent level of plasma alcohol. Consequently, many anonymous alcoholics become manifest only when some intercurrent injury puts them into a hospital and removes the source of their drug. *There are two major principles of treatment: (1) replacement of alcohol with a pharmacologically or physiologically equivalent drug, and (2) gradual withdrawal of the equivalent drug.*

For many years, drugs such as pentobarbital sodium, paraldehyde, and chloral hydrate have been standard agents for substitution, but sedatives that may be somewhat safer in regard to respiratory depressant effects, such as chlordiazepoxide or chlormethiazole (Heminevrin), have recently been introduced (Kaim *et al.*, 1969). Other new drugs, such as promazine (Sparine), chlorpromazine, and hydroxyzine, are not the physiologic equivalents required and are considerably less efficacious than equivalent agents. Further, by lowering the seizure threshold, they may aggravate the normal tendency toward withdrawal seizures.

The goal of treatment is to keep the patient in a state of light sleep until symptoms are controlled and gradual withdrawal of drug can be undertaken. Doses of substitutive drugs must be flexible to meet the varying needs of the patient. Exceedingly large doses, at least by

usual standards, may be required; for example, doses of chlordiazepoxide of 600 to 800 mg daily are frequently necessary. Weaning from drug should be gradual and guided by the patient's clinical state. Most patients can be managed by conventional sedative doses within a week.

Treatment of withdrawal reactions from conventional sedatives employs the same principles already mentioned. Shorter-acting sedatives, such as secobarbital sodium or meprobamate, are more likely to be abused than are longer-acting sedatives, such as phenobarbital or chlordiazepoxide. The process is easier and the chances of secondary dependence are reduced. The course of withdrawal reactions depends to a great extent on the half-time of disappearance of the drug in question. Those with the longest half-time, such as the benzodiazepines, may not produce symptoms for as long as 48 hours following withdrawal, and the reaction may be attenuated over time, with seizures not appearing until a week or more following discontinuation of the drug. Meprobamate and short-lived barbiturates produce acute reactions quite similar to those from alcohol.

The principles and practice of aversive therapy depend on the clinical pathogenesis of the symptoms produced by the abusive drug. Treatment has been well described (Lader, 1967). The unpleasant interaction between disulfiram (Antabuse) or calcium cyanamide and alcohol may be used both as a deconditioning device and as a deterrent. The interval, or prophylactic, treatment of alcoholics leaves much to be desired. Based on the hypothesis that the compulsion to drink is due to a mounting level of anxiety, a number of sedative drugs have been substituted for alcohol with varying degrees of success. The early enthusiasm for antianxiety agents has been tempered because it is relatively easy to convert an addict from one drug to another. Although there may be some advantage in doing this, if the new drug is safer than the old, the possibility of dangerous additive effects from combining alcohol with many of these drugs is a limiting factor (Melville *et al.*, 1966; Trenholm *et al.*, 1970).

Abuse of Heroin and Opiates. Drugs are useful both in treating opiate withdrawal reactions and in prophylaxis. The principles in treating withdrawal reactions to opiates are essentially similar to those used for alcohol withdrawal: the substitution of a physiologically equivalent drug and gradual weaning. Methadone (Dolophine) is the preferred agent for such substitution, the dose being based on the estimated daily intake of the addicting drug.

The prophylactic use of methadone for

rehabilitating narcotic addicts is one of the more exciting developments in drug therapy of the past decade (Dole *et al.*, 1966). One addicting drug is deliberately substituted by another that has less euphoriant effect and that blocks those effects of heroin. Presumably, drug-seeking behavior will be diminished, or, at least, continued use of heroin will become unrewarding.

Results from methadone maintenance programs have been variable but mostly favorable. As heroin addiction has a fairly high mortality and an enormous social morbidity, any approach as promising as methadone maintenance should be fully exploited. Some of the drawbacks to widespread application have been the extensive medical and paramedical resources needed to carry out present treatment programs. More simplified techniques of treatment, including the use of longer-acting methadone homologs, such as *dl*-acetylmethadol or *l*-methadyl acetate, may facilitate the extension of this form of treatment (Jaffe and Senay, 1971). In the long run, one would prefer to use true narcotic antagonists, such as cyclazocine or naloxone. The former drug shares with other antagonists the propensity to produce some psychotomimetic symptoms, thus not being widely acceptable to patients. The latter drug would be ideal, in that it has no clinical action other than narcotic antagonism, except for the fact that it is brief in action and requires monumental oral doses to be effective. A search for some long-acting preparation of naloxone or similar drugs is underway. The possibilities for sharply reducing the numbers of heroin addicts are great, but the problem will not be solved until the powerful influences of ghetto misery on the one hand and large profits for organized crime on the other have been eliminated.

Abuse of Stimulants. Stimulant abuse has rapidly grown in the United States during the past decade. Stimulant abuse may be the most serious drug problem of our youth. The most widely abused stimulant is methamphetamine, probably because it is the simplest for illicit chemists to make. Any other amphetamine-like drug, such as methylphenidate, may be similarly abused, including some that are promoted solely as anorexic agents, such as phenmetrazine (Preludin) (AMA Committee on Alcoholism and Addiction, 1966).

Modest levels of abuse of stimulants do not produce any withdrawal reactions of consequence, but withdrawal from some of the monumental doses used (as much as 4 g of methamphetamine daily, taken intravenously) is usually accompanied by severe restlessness, depression, and malaise. The use of sedatives to encourage sleep or of tricyclic antidepressants to combat withdrawal depression is still controversial. In any case, tricyclics should not be considered for use until all amphetamines have been excreted, to avoid potentiation of the effects of the latter drug.

Many of the dangers of stimulant abuse are physical. Nutritional deficiency may follow prolonged appetite suppression with remarkable losses of weight. Possibly abetted by the nutritional disturbance, but more likely owing to the practice of using contaminated injection equipment, viral hepatitis is a frequent complication. The most serious complication is mental. Psychotic reactions that mimic paranoid schizophrenia may appear insidiously (Kramer *et al.*, 1967). Although it was formerly thought that many of these reactions were exaggerations of pre-existing psychopathology, recent experimental evidence suggests that amphetamine psychosis can be quickly induced in previously unaffected volunteer subjects (Griffith *et al.*, 1970). The amphetamine psychosis may be the best available model for research into the mechanisms of schizophrenia. Persistent or severe psychotic reactions require management with antipsychotic drugs.

Unwanted Effects

Pharmacokinetics of Clinical Importance. *Antianxiety Drugs.* The major metabolite of phenobarbital is a hydroxylated form, but 30% is excreted unchanged in the urine. Of all barbiturates, phenobarbital has the largest renal excretion. Consequently, it might be the preferred barbiturate in cases of liver impairment, but not in cases of renal insufficiency (see Chapter 3).

The benzodiazepines (chlordiazepoxide, diazepam, oxazepam) are also excreted to a large extent by the kidney. The half-life in blood varies with the drug and the duration of administration. Following acute doses, chlordiazepoxide has a $t_{1/2}$ of 24 hours, but after large doses have been administered chronically, the $t_{1/2}$ may be increased to 48 hours. On acute administration, diazepam shows an initial $t_{1/2}$ in the blood of 7 to 10 hours, followed by a slow phase of 3 days. Oxazepam is probably similar. Probably both have longer half-times when chronically administered (Randall and Schallek, 1968). As with phenobarbital, drugs of this class are preferable in patients with impaired liver function, but are to be avoided in patients with renal failure.

Meprobamate is hydroxylated in the liver. The ratio of hydroxylated to free drug in urine is low after a single dose, but increases rapidly with chronic administration, doubling within a week. Such a change is construed as evidence that the drug stimulates its own metabolism, and there is evidence that phenobarbital may also act as an enzyme inducer and increase the rate of metabolism of meprobamate (see Chapter 16). Clinically, this rapid change in rate of metabolism may be manifested by a fairly rapid development of tolerance to the drug's effects. Because most antianxiety drugs may induce similar increases in their metabolism, try to use the drug for brief interrupted periods to avoid losing therapeutic effects. If the drug must be continued without interruption, increasing doses may compensate for increased rate of metabolism, but such large doses have obvious disadvantages.

Antipsychotics. Most knowledge about the metabolism of phenothiazine derivatives in man is derived from studies on chlorpromazine. The drug is quickly metabolized in the liver and metabolites are excreted in bile. Both metabolites and unchanged drug are rapidly excreted by the kidney (Beckett *et al.*, 1963). The apparent plasma $t_{1/2}$ for chlorpromazine is less than 6 hours following a single dose, but may be much longer following chronic administration, as equilibration between concentrations in plasma and tissue stores takes place (Curry and Marshall, 1968). When patients have concurrent liver disease, smaller-than-usual doses may be adequate. Because only 10% of unchanged drug is excreted in the urine, and most pharmacologic activity is in the parent compound, the problem of renal impairment is lessened. The high partition coefficient of chlorpromazine (and, accordingly, its high concentration in fat) and its strong binding to plasma and tissue proteins make rapid elimination of the drug almost impossible, a consideration of importance in overdoses (see Chapter 17). By the same token, tissue stores of the drug are increased during chronic dosage. Drug effects may persist long after the drug has been discontinued. As redistribution from storage sites commences, drug or metabolites can be detected in the urine for days following single doses and for weeks or months following chronic dosage. *Principle: The pharmacokinetic properties of a drug may explain protracted therapeutic or toxic effects long after the drug has been discontinued.*

Antidepressants. The therapeutic considerations for chlorpromazine apply to the tricyclic antidepressants (Christiansen *et al.*, 1967). Unlike chlorpromazine, monodemethylation of the dimethylaminopropyl side chain of imipramine does not produce a markedly weaker compound. Such analogs of imipramine and amitriptyline have been proposed for therapeutic uses on the basis of their being active metabolites of the parent drugs; presumably they should work

more quickly. Another postulated advantage of the active analogs is that some patients may fail to metabolize the parent drug to produce active metabolites. Thus far, the clinical differences between the parent compounds and the demethylated analogs are negligible. *Principle: Although drugs may act through active metabolites, these may not account for all the possible therapeutic effects, and their clinical introduction may not be advantageous.*

The hydrazide MAO inhibitors are largely acetylated in the liver. Patients have been found with genetically determined fast and slow acetylating activity, whose metabolism of phenelzine simulates the varied acetylation rate observed with isoniazid (Price-Evans *et al.*, 1965) (see Chapter 13). A patient who slowly acetylates a drug may become toxic after being given usual doses of the drug.

Organ System Factors Influencing Clinical Effects. *Nervous System.* Although the pharmacologic effects of antipsychotic drugs, such as those blocking dopamine receptors, are consistent with the production of extrapyramidal reactions, such symptoms affect only a few patients. The prevalence of clinically important extrapyramidal syndromes following antipsychotic drugs is determined in part by the presence of advanced age, pre-existing brain damage, and genetically determined susceptibility (Hollister, 1968b) (see Chapter 13). Some patients may develop these reactions to any antipsychotic drug given in small doses, whereas others seem to be completely refractory to this pharmacologic effect. Seizures and late-appearing dyskinesias are also related in part to pre-existing brain lesions and advanced age. The symptoms are related to dose of the drug: seizures to the current daily dose level and dyskinesias to the cumulative dose (Simpson and Angus, 1970). Dyskinesias have been quite difficult to reverse and may constitute a serious obstacle to long-term treatment with these drugs (Crane, 1968). The neuromuscular block produced by chlorpromazine is usually of little significance, except for symptoms of weakness in normal patients and the aggravation of myasthenia gravis in patients with subclinical disease. *Principle: Unusual sensitivity to pharmacologically predictable side effects of a drug may disclose the presence of unsuspected disease.*

The initial "set" of the nervous system may determine the extent of a response to a psychotherapeutic drug. A markedly agitated patient may become calmer when given an antipsychotic drug, whereas a withdrawn patient may show signs of increased activity. Psychoactive drugs interact with the personality of the patient (Di Mascio, 1968). Everyone knows the multiple effects that the single psychoactive drug ethanol has on various personality types. Systematic study of the interactions between personality type and drugs has been vigorously pursued in the case of sedative and stimulant drugs. Patients with personalities characterized by extroversion and physical activity ("doers") may react to a sedative drug with increased anxiety and depression. Presumably the drug impairs their customary way of functioning, which disturbs them. Conversely, patients with personalities characterized by introversion, passivity, and introspection ("thinkers") tolerate these drugs well in the presence of anxiety. The situation is reversed with stimulants; the active personality may feel tranquilized and the passive personality overstimulated.

The response to antipsychotic drugs in a schizophrenic is vastly different from responses in a "normal." Most normal volunteers who take these drugs generally find them disagreeable, particularly when they produce psychotomimetic effects. For this reason, the antipsychotic drugs have generally been poorly received as antianxiety drugs. In contrast, the psychotic patient's behavior often improves and he tolerates enormous doses of the same drug with little complaint. Perhaps one must be crazy, either literally or figuratively, to take antipsychotic drugs. Some schizophrenic patients, especially those who retain insight and who have preponderant somatic complaints, may respond poorly to the drugs and may require special care in establishing a proper dose (UCLA Interdepartmental Conference, 1969).

Liver and Kidney. Disease of the liver and kidneys may influence drug kinetics and pharmacologic effect. Cholestatic jaundice from phenothiazines or tricyclics most often has an allergic basis (Sherlock, 1967). Although the dose of drug may have to be altered, simple hepatocellular disease does not constitute an absolute contraindication to the use of these drugs. Hepatocellular liver disease is not affected by cholestatic jaundice, even should it supervene. On the other hand, hydrazide MAO inhibitors may produce hepatocellular damage and should be avoided under such circumstances. *Principle: Contraindications to a drug should be limited to side effects that definitely aggravate rather than superficially resemble existing pathology.*

No direct toxic or allergic effects of psychotherapeutic drugs are known to affect the kidney.

Hematopoietic System. Agranulocytosis is a direct result of bone marrow toxicity from chlorpromazine and is more likely to occur in patients with initially diminished marrow reserves (Pisciotta, 1968). Preliminary tests of marrow reserve capacity, such as determination of rate of nucleic acid synthesis (incorporation of ^{3}H-thymidine), are possible but too cumbersome for routine clinical use. Before therapy is instituted, particularly in elderly women, leukocyte counts, past history of leukopenia, or evidence of associated chronic illness should be weighed to properly estimate the risk of reaction versus the benefit of therapy. Agranulocytosis has been observed with drugs related to phenothiazines, such as chlorprothixene and the tricyclic antidepressants. The agranulocytosis produced by each of the drugs occurs early in the course of treatment and seems to be relatively independent of dose. Although leukocyte production may resume after cessation of therapy, agranulocytosis often reappears when the drug is reintroduced. Few problems with erythrocytes or platelets have been encountered and none with coagulation mechanisms.

Cardiovascular System. Orthostatic hypotension and rapid resting pulse rates are frequent effects of the phenothiazines. The "high-dose" types may produce alpha-adrenergic blockade (see Chapter 5). Mean arterial pressure, peripheral resistance, and stroke volume have been decreased in patients treated chronically with such drugs (Carlsson et al., 1966). Such effects may be additive when other disorders of the cardiovascular system are present or when other drugs (not used as antipsychotic agents) are used, such as antihypertensives or diuretics (see Chapter 16). Orthostatic hypotension from phenothiazines and tricyclics has precipitated myocardial infarctions. Isolated T-wave abnormalities are therefore of debatable clinical importance. Possibly by prolonging repolarization and decreasing conductivity, phenothiazines may set the stage for the rare instances of sudden, unexpected death from ventricular fibrillation. By depleting endogenous stores of catecholamines, reserpine may unmask occult heart failure. Chlorpromazine has some antidiuretic action and is an alpha-adrenergic blocker. Such drugs might also precipitate heart failure in patients with borderline myocardial function. *Principle: Consideration of the pharmacology of a drug may lead to anticipation of its adverse effects.*

There are no known problems arising from altered regional blood flow during cardiac disorders that affect the tissue distribution of the antipsychotics. Very likely distribution is unaffected because the drugs are strongly protein bound (see Chapter 2). Decreased hepatic or renal blood flow might diminish metabolism and excretion of some of these drugs, but clinical effects due to such changes have been subtle, at best.

Respiratory System. Experimental evidence suggests that many of the new psychotherapeutic drugs, such as the phenothiazines and benzodiazepines, are less depressant to respiration than are other sedatives. Although these observations may be true in normal people or in those with mild respiratory diseases, respiratory depression can be clinically important when the patient has severe respiratory disease, when there is a combination of obesity and hypoventilation, or when consciousness is obtunded from any cause, including alcohol and other drugs. In general, doses of sedatives, hypnotics, tranquilizers, or opiates great enough to produce sleep are very likely to aggravate pre-existing respiratory failure (Hunter, 1967).

Doses, Dosage Schedules, Dosage Forms. The doses of drugs required to produce either similar concentrations in plasma, or, more important, the same clinical effects, vary widely. Dosage schedules should be flexible in each case; nightly administration of the total or major portion of the daily dose of many of these drugs often may be preferable to divided doses during the day, and timing of the dose in relation to administration of other drugs (nonabsorbable antacids markedly adsorb the phenothiazines and interfere with their absorption) or food may be important in determining their availability.

Ordinarily, the dosage form of a drug is not of greater importance than the possible pharmacologic differences between drugs. However, such could be the case with some antipsychotic drugs such as chlorpromazine. Administration of drug by intramuscular injection assures rapid availability, with a potency ratio of approximately 4:1 as contrasted with oral doses. Such treatment cannot be long continued owing to the pain and inflammation produced by injections, but the parenteral route may be an effective way to initiate therapy. Of the oral dosage forms, the liquid concentrate is the most reliable for its physiologic availability. Tablets are most commonly used, and deserve to be in terms of convenience and expense, but one cannot always rely on their availability. A patient who responds less well than expected to a regimen of tablet medication should be tried on another drug form before the drug is termed ineffective. Prolonged-action medications are highly unreliable in terms of their physiologic availability and their use is irrational for such intrinsically long-acting drugs. They are doubly condemned because they are the most expensive oral-dosage form (Hollister *et al.*, 1970).

A very long-acting injectable form of fluphenazine, the enanthate ester, has found increasing use as maintenance therapy for outpatients. A single injection can be repeated every 2 to 3 weeks to assure adequate intake of drug. Fears that this preparation might release large amounts of drug unevenly have not been justified, although acute extrapyramidal reactions of the dystonic type are more common than with oral doses. If this preparation is limited to outpatient treatment of patients previously well stabilized on oral doses of the drug, doses can be determined to prevent untoward reactions. A drug molecule containing a free alcoholic group is esterified with a medium-chain fatty acid; the ester must be hydrolyzed by tissue lipases to release the drug, accounting for the truly prolonged action of the compound. This principle has been applied previously to free-alcohol forms of many hormones, such as corticosteroids and sex hormones, but among the antipsychotics thus far only to fluphenazine.

Drug Interactions. The number of known interactions between drugs is multiplying geometrically (see Chapter 16). Evidence from animal experiments suggests the possibility of many more interactions than have yet been demonstrated in man. The discussion that follows is necessarily incomplete. Only interactions of greatest clinical importance will be mentioned.

Antianxiety Drugs. Phenobarbital or other barbiturates may produce unexpected degrees of sedation or respiratory depression when used in combination with other central nervous system depressants, such as alcohol, other antianxiety drugs, or antihistaminics. The combination with alcohol is especially lethal, leading to unwitting suicides. Pretreatment or concurrent treatment with phenobarbital stimulates drug-metabolizing enzymes not only for the drug itself, but also for meprobamate, coumarin anticoagulants, hydantoin anticonvulsants, griseofulvin (Fulvicin), and steroids (Kuntzman, 1969).

Thus far, the benzodiazepines seem to have only additive sedative effects when given with other depressant drugs and are relatively safe. Meprobamate also has an additive effect combined with other sedatives but it may stimulate its own metabolism or that of its congeners when given chronically.

Paraldehyde, pentobarbital, chloral hydrate, and meprobamate may be used for treating acutely alcoholic patients. Either an additive or a synergistic effect may occur in the presence of high levels of blood alcohol, and fatalities may rapidly ensue with little advance warning (Rubin *et al.*, 1970).

Antidepressants. MAO inhibitors interact with many other drugs and foods. The great variety of such interactions has led many clinicians to the conclusion that this class of drugs is too dangerous for use except under the most meticulous supervision. The tricyclics interact with guanethidine (Ismelin) to negate its antihypertensive action (Pettinger *et al.*, 1968).

Antipsychotics. Phenothiazine derivatives are additive when combined with analgesics (meperidine, morphine), anesthetics, and sedatives (alcohol, barbiturates, antihistaminics). Some members of this class without antipsychotic action, such as promethazine (Phenergan), are used deliberately to exploit this interaction. The antihypertensive effects of reserpine and thiazides may be enhanced by concurrent use of phenothiazines. Haloperidol stimulates the metabolism of phenindione (Hedulin), decreasing its anticoagulant effect.

Interactions Between Psychotherapeutic Drugs. Among the psychoactive agents, the greatest danger of drug interactions occurs with various combinations of psychotherapeutic drugs. Polypharmacy is prevalent and the number of possible combinations of these drugs is enormous. A single hospitalized psychotic patient often is given two phenothiazines (based on the unproved contention that a combination provides full therapeutic effects but only fractional side effects), a tricyclic antidepressant (presumably because the patient may seem withdrawn or depressed), an anticholinergic antiparkinsonian drug (most often gratuitously, either in the absence of any overt Parkinson's syndrome or without awareness that the anticholinergic action of the tricyclic protects against extrapyramidal effects), a hypnotic, such as chloral hydrate (for sleep), and a stimulant, such as dextroamphetamine (to start the next day). Aside from the possibility that opposing effects may attenuate the desired therapeutic action, the greatest danger is that the accumulation of anticholinergic effects from the phenothiazines, the tricyclic, and the antiparkinsonian agent may produce bladder or bowel paralysis or may precipitate an attack of glaucoma. The fact that many patients improve mentally when all such drugs are withdrawn may indicate that they were suffering from mental confusion associated with overdoses of centrally acting anticholinergic drugs. *Principle: Some patients feel that if a little drug is good, more must be better. Too often, physicians believe that if one drug is good, two will be better, or if these are not effective, three will be. Combining drugs constructively, to exploit desired pharmacologic effects, must be predicated upon a thorough knowledge of drug action.*

DRUGS FOR TREATING PARKINSON'S SYNDROME

Types of Disorders

The mechanism of a disorder need not always be understood for its successful treatment.

However, the more we understand the pathologic physiology or biochemistry of a disorder, the more likely we are to treat it effectively. For three-quarters of a century, empiric treatment with anticholinergic drugs has been the mainstay of reasonably effective therapy for Parkinson's disease (Hofmann and Hollister, 1970). Within the past 15 years, as our understanding of the pathogenesis of the disease has increased, a new and very promising treatment has been developed, based on the concept of replacing a deficient biogenic amine, dopamine, in the extrapyramidal areas of the brain. If the initial promise of such treatment is sustained (and it seems likely), it will be the first instance of the *principle of replacement therapy with a neurohumor in the treatment of a neurologic disorder.*

At present, three types of Parkinson's syndrome are recognized (Wilkins and Brody, 1969). A diminishing number of patients are seen with a Parkinson's syndrome presumed to be the sequel of an attack of encephalitis lethargica during the epidemic of this disorder that occurred between 1919 and 1926 (Duvoisin and Yahr, 1965). A larger number of patients are now diagnosed as having a Parkinson's syndrome of unknown cause, the "idiopathic" type. Both syndromes include muscle rigidity, rhythmic tremor, akinesia, loss of associated movements, gait disturbances, and signs of parasympathetic stimulation common to Parkinson's syndrome. Postencephalitic Parkinson's syndrome may be distinguished by a history of encephalitis or by the presence of other typical neurologic residuals, such as hemiplegia, bulbar and ocular palsies, dystonic disorders, tics, or behavioral disorders. Oculogyric crises are especially characteristic of the postencephalitic variety. A third variety, appearing within the past 15 years, is associated with the use of antipsychotic drugs. In many respects, these drug-induced syndromes strongly resemble the naturally occurring Parkinson's syndromes, but in two aspects they are somewhat different: akathisia, or uncontrollable restlessness, and acute dystonic reactions, including oculogyric crises, are seen frequently in the absence of any other clear-cut symptoms of Parkinson's syndrome (Duvoisin, 1968).

Partly as a result of the drug-induced model of Parkinson's syndrome, investigation has led to the current concept of a disorder of biogenic amines as a pathogenetic basis for the illness (Klawans, 1968). Dopamine seems to be of primary importance (see Chapter 18), but acetylcholine must also be considered, possibly in its balance with dopamine in the neuronal pathways (Hornykiewicz, 1966; Barbeau, 1969). The widespread degeneration of neurons in the basal ganglia, especially in the substantia nigra and corpus striatum, is associated with a decreased dopamine content in the same areas. A similar biochemical lesion is produced by treatment of animals with reserpine or similarly acting antipsychotic drugs, each of which may elicit the drug-induced syndrome. Other drug-induced Parkinson's syndromes may be evoked by phenothiazines and butyrophenones, but in these cases, the biochemical defect seems to be a block of access of dopamine to receptor sites rather than its depletion. Fortunately, either type of drug-induced reaction seems to be fully reversible.

Pathogenetic Mechanisms

Neurophysiologic Abnormalities. Two of the most disabling symptoms of Parkinson's syndrome are muscle rigidity and tremors (Lipp, 1967). The continual driving of skeletal muscles impedes both active and passive movements in the waking state. The rigidity is assumed to result from the unbalanced activity of the remaining nerve cells. As certain neurons are destroyed in the circuits regulating muscle tone and posture, other cells in that system not only may be deprived of coordinating signals, but may be "released" so as to cause a stream of spontaneous impulses from the brain to the muscles.

Abnormally rapid firing of neurons might have two explanations, one based on denervation supersensitivity, another on loss of inhibitory stimuli. The disease could remove some incoming excitatory signals to which all nerve cells normally are accustomed. Denervated brain cells may develop supersensitivity to humoral agents and a tendency to become spontaneously active. The net effect might be continuous random firing of deafferented cells. Pharmacologic approaches to remedy this situation would include (1) stabilizing the neuron's intrinsic electrical activity, or (2) blocking the spontaneous impulses at the next motor neuron in the pathway.

Atropine and its analogs stabilize cell membranes by hyperpolarization, making it possible that "conventional" drugs dampen the generation of spontaneous discharges in partly denervated nerve cells. On the other hand, if one of the neural transmitters in the extrapyramidal circuits were acetylcholine, atropine-like drugs could act as they do in peripheral parasympathetic synapses, blocking impulse transmission to the next neuron. These pharmacologic actions might decrease excessive resting muscle tonus but could not fully restore normal neuronal connections and would have little effect on the akinesia or loss of associated movements typical

of Parkinson's disease. Although conventional drugs for the syndrome may act by these mechanisms, the response is incomplete.

Another possible explanation for rigidity depends upon analogy to the inhibitory feedback loop involving Renshaw cells in the spinal cord (Figure 11–3). The excitatory (E) cell receives incoming signals from the intact sources (A and B), as well as those that have been damaged as a result of the disease, represented by the dashed lines (D). The spontaneous overactivity of the latter would produce the denervation of the areas of cell membrane represented by the heavy black strips. The membrane-stabilizing pharmacologic approach described for atropine might apply at the point indicated by the number 1.

The E cell depolarizes along its axon (α) and triggers depolarization at a lower E cell, which is a spinal motor neuron (E^1). Simultaneously, an impulse also passes along a collateral axon (β) to an inhibitory (I) cell, whose axon completes a feedback loop with the upper E cell. If the synapse marked by the number 2 is cholinergic (cross-hatching), it could be blocked by atropine. At the synapse shown between the axon of the I cell and the body of the E cell, an inhibitory transmitter (dots), quite possibly dopamine, might be liberated. At the point indicated by number 3, the rate of synthesis of the inhibitory transmitter might be changed, or at point 4, the rate of release might be altered. If one assumes deficiency of an inhibitory transmitter, dopamine, in Parkinson's disease, its replenishment by levodopa could restore the feedback control and offer still another pharmacologic approach. Such a schema is highly speculative, but it could account for some of the clinical features of rigidity and for its pharmacologic correction.

Tremor is the second major cause of disability. It is usually present at rest, but is appreciably diminished during voluntary activity. Tremor in Parkinson's disease is not the result of a simple undamped oscillation in a segmental stretch reflex loop, as is seen in clonus, but originates in the brain. Like rigidity, tremor is observed only in the waking state. The decrease with voluntary activity is particularly characteristic. Passive joint movements may transiently abolish the tremor as well. Thus alternating bursts of motor activity are evident only when the involved cells are not pre-empted by signals coming from other brain areas or from the periphery.

Brain lesions may cause surrounding neurons to fire rhythmically while undisturbed and yet permit the same units to behave normally when "driven." Neurosurgical and neurophysiologic investigation has demonstrated cells in the

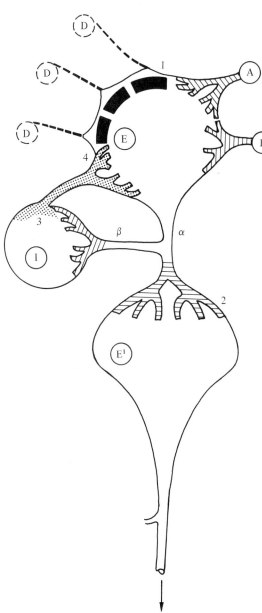

Figure 11–3. Model of postulated pathophysiologic mechanism in Parkinson's disease. *E*, upper motor neuron; E^1, lower motor neuron; *I*, inhibitory cell; *A, B*, normal modulating cells; *D*, diseased cells; *α*, excitatory axon; *β*, inhibitory axon; *1*, possible site of action of atropine as a membrane stabilizer; *2*, cholinergic synapse; *3*, site of dopamine synthesis; *4*, site of dopamine release (see text for complete explanation of model). (From Hofmann, W. W., and Hollister, L. E.: Pharmacotherapy for Parkinson's disease: a new era. *Pharmacol. Physicians*, **4**: No. 7, 1970.)

region of the ventral basal thalamic nuclei that fire rhythmically at tremor frequencies. Destructive lesions in this area abolish tremor while sparing voluntary control. This evidence suggests that the tremor "generator" is within the basal ganglia and may drive neurons primarily responsible for voluntary activity. The disappearance of tremor during purposeful movement suggests either (1) direct overriding of the oscillatory output by phasic impulses or (2) replacement of periodic activity with steady firing as basal ganglia become involved in postural adaptation to the intended movement. If one visualizes the sequence depicted in Figure 11–3 as operative in the substantia nigra, which is most often heavily involved in the rigid patient, and also as operative in the ventral thalamus in the patient with tremor, one can imagine a somewhat similar mechanism for both disorders. During the waking state, the cells would have some minimal activity manifested by the resting tremor. An essential difference from the explanation for rigidity would be one or more additional feedback loops providing an excitatory output to the first *E* cell following a circuit delay of about 150 milliseconds. Under normal circumstances, the *I* cell would depolarize first and the returning excitatory inputs would find the *E* cell inhibited. The loss of such inhibition would provide a mechanism by which *E* cells would receive an excitatory stimulus after a short delay each time they fired, the time required for travel of the returning impulse setting the frequency. Spontaneous oscillations in such a system could be reduced whenever a steady series of impulses from a voluntary motor center occurred, accounting for the reduction in tremor by voluntary movements.

Biochemical Abnormalities. Both cholinergic and dopaminergic mechanisms may be involved in Parkinson's syndrome. Evidence for the importance of cholinergic mechanisms is most direct, based on the therapeutic effectiveness of anticholinergic drugs. A cholinergic model of Parkinson's syndrome has been provided by a cholinomimetic agent, tremorine. Although limited to mice, and therefore not as convincing a model as that provided by antipsychotic drugs in humans, tremorine's effect was shown to be due to a central action, reversible by anticholinergics (Everett, 1956). A more direct test of central cholinergic mechanisms in patients with Parkinson's disease was provided by comparing the effects of anticholinesterases that do and do not pass the blood-brain barrier (Duvoisin, 1967). Symptoms were aggravated by physostigmine, which enters the brain, but not by the quaternary anticholinesterases, which do not. Aggravation of symptoms was reversed by benz-

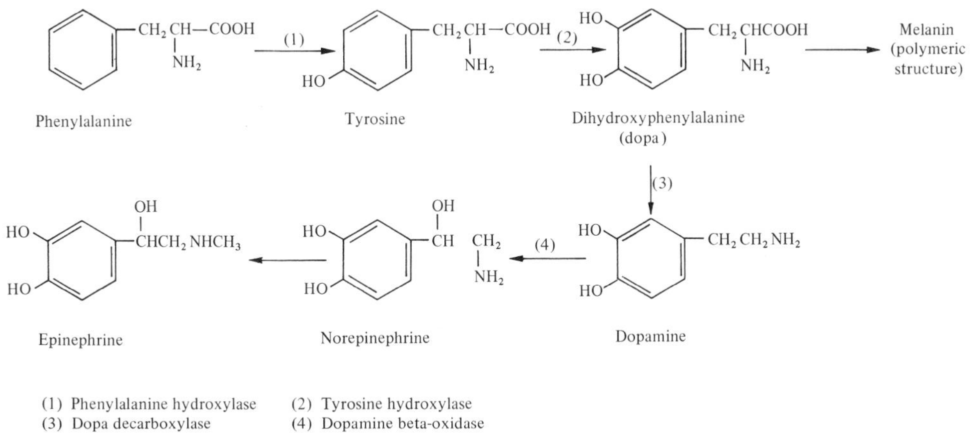

(1) Phenylalanine hydroxylase (2) Tyrosine hydroxylase
(3) Dopa decarboxylase (4) Dopamine beta-oxidase

Figure 11–4. Biosynthetic pathways of catecholamines. Tyrosine hydroxylase step is rate limiting. (From Hofmann, W. W., and Hollister, L. E.: Pharmacotherapy for Parkinson's disease: a new era. *Pharmacol. Physicians*, **4**: No. 7, 1970.)

tropine or scopolamine. Finally, the highest concentrations of acetylcholine, choline acetylase, and acetylcholinesterase in the brain are found in the corpus striatum, and it is tempting to believe that nature did not establish this metabolic "machinery" without purpose.

Most biochemical theories of Parkinson's syndrome now consider dopamine to be of prime importance. The disease process may impair the biosynthesis of dopamine in the central nervous system. The tyrosine hydroxylase reaction may be implicated, as it is usually the rate-limiting step (Figure 11–4). Whether enzyme activity is decreased directly in cells by the disease or by the loss of damaged neurons is still not clear. In any case, administration of phenylalanine has not been effective in treatment. Conversely, administration of melanocyte-stimulating hormone (MSH), by diverting levodopa from dopamine production to melanin synthesis, aggravates the symptoms of Parkinson's disease.

Assuming that the primary defect is a deficiency of dopamine, an imbalance between the cholinergic and dopaminergic systems could be redressed either by decreasing cholinergic activity or by increasing dopaminergic activity by replenishing dopamine. The fact that both treatments provide some degree of relief of symptoms suggests that this imbalance may occur. Other mechanisms by which atropine-like drugs may be effective, such as their effect on membrane potentials, might be independent of the postulated imbalance. If this is the case, it might be appropriate to use both pharmacologic approaches simultaneously, if response to one is less than optimal. Clinical evidence in some patients suggests that combined treatment is better than levodopa alone. ***Principle: In some disorders, the balance between opposing systems (e.g., cholinergic and dopaminergic) may be more relevant than the degree of function; correction of a disturbed balance may be the appropriate treatment goal.***

Clinical Therapy

Conventional Drugs in Parkinson's Syndrome. Until recently, pharmacologic approaches to treating this disease have been limited to variations on an old theme. Hyoscine was used in Charcot's clinic, primarily to treat the symptoms of parasympathetic hyperactivity (excessive salivation, sweating, and sebum production), and proved to be of even greater benefit. Since then, the major emphasis in therapy has been on the development of additional drugs with central anticholinergic actions. Even antihistamines may be effective, as they are also anticholinergics. The conventional antiparkinsonian drugs, grouped according to their chemical structures, are shown in Figure 11–5.

Benztropine is closely related to the belladonna alkaloids, the major chemical modification being the addition of the diphenhydramine group. Trihexyphenidyl retains the diphenylmethane structure; minor variations result in some of its congeners. Phenothiazines in which the nitrogen atom in the aliphatic chain is separated from that in the ring by only two carbons, rather than three (as in the case of chlorpromazine), are more sedating and are potent antihistaminics and anticholinergics, but lack antipsychotic activity. Diphenhydramine has antihistaminic, sedative, and anticholinergic effects; the latter probably account for its utility in Parkinson's disease.

Tropines

Tropine nucleus

Atropine

Benztropine
(Cogentin, 1-6 mg)

Trihexyphenidyl and Congeners

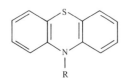

Trihexyphenidyl
(Artane, 5-15 mg)

Cycrimine
(Pagitane, 15-20 mg)

Biperiden
(Akineton, 2-8 mg)

Phenothiazines

$R = CH_2 CH_2 N(C_2 H_5)_2$

Diethazine
(Diparcol, 400-800 mg)

$R = CH_2 CH \; N(C_2 H_5)_2$
$\quad\quad\quad |$
$\quad\quad\quad CH_3$

Ethopropazine
(Parsidol, 100-600 mg)

Phenothiazine nucleus

Diphenylmethanes

$R = CH3$

Orphenadrine
(Disipal, 100-250 mg)

Diphenhydramine
(Benadryl, 75-150 mg)

Figure 11–5. Conventional anticholinergic-type drugs for treating Parkinson's disease. (From Hofmann, W. W., and Hollister, L. E.: Pharmacotherapy for Parkinson's disease: a new era. *Pharmacol. Physicians*, **4**: No. 7, 1970.)

Treatment of common diseases, especially if they are chronic and difficult to manage, may lead to a profuse number of minor modifications of a chemical class of drugs. The intent may be to alter pharmacologic action, as in the case of the phenothiazines described above. Sometimes the intent is simply to make a commercial product. Regrettably, chemical changes have not greatly improved the anticholinergic type of anti-parkinsonian drug. Major differences in response are not likely within a chemical class of drugs. Comparative clinical studies indicate no great differential among chemical congeners or even among members of different chemical classes. *Principle: Whenever a profusion of drugs is available, it is often wise to choose one from each major chemical class and learn to use it well, rather than to use all drugs poorly.*

Tachyphylaxis is a common problem in the use of antiparkinsonian drugs. Substitution with other drugs is usually tried, but the basic similarity of pharmacologic action of these drugs limits the success of the changes. Some reports have suggested specific effects of certain drugs on various symptoms, such as rigidity or akinesia, whereas other drugs have been reported to have broader therapeutic effects, ameliorating all symptoms, including tremors, excessive salivation, etc. Practical experience indicates that symptomatic response is more directly related to the severity, type, and extent of the disease than to unique attributes of a drug.

Current anticholinergic drug therapy provides acceptable symptomatic relief in only about 25% of patients, objective signs being observed in an even smaller fraction. For severely affected patients, however, even a relatively small degree of improvement may result in considerable functional gains, so that these goals of therapy are welcome, even if complete remission is seldom attained. *Principle: The dose of any drug is variable, depending upon the individual patient and his tolerance of side effects. Often the patient is the best judge of his appropriate dose, so that neither doses nor dosage schedules should be fixed.* The proper total management of patients includes nondrug treatments such as exercise, physiotherapy, and a program of physical and social activities.

Surgical treatment, which initially appeared quite promising, is usually limited to younger patients who also may respond well to drug therapy. These qualifications are not intended to demean conventional treatments. Dramatic and sometimes sustained improvement has been obtained in many patients. The prompt relapse of patients whose drug treatment is discontinued is further evidence of efficacy. Still, symptoms progress in many patients despite use of maximally tolerated doses. A more specific pharmacologic approach to treatment is highly desirable.

Treatment with Levodopa. Based on the concept of Parkinson's syndrome as a disorder of the basal ganglia due to dopamine deficiency, a novel approach to treatment has emerged. The biosynthesis of catecholamines is summarized in Figure 11–4. Phenylalanine therapy failed to improve Parkinson's syndrome, presumably because the rate-limiting step in this sequence was between tyrosine and dihydroxyphenylalanine (levodopa). This failure would not, of course, preclude the possibility of increasing levodopa concentrations in brain as a substrate for dopamine synthesis (Cotzias *et al.*, 1967). Dopamine itself cannot be given, as it does not cross the blood-brain barrier. Thus far, the results have been so encouraging that the treatment has been hailed as the most significant advance in the therapy of a neurologic disorder in the past half century.

As with any new treatment, modifications have been made as clinical experience increases (Cotzias *et al.*, 1969; Morgan and Bianchine, 1971):

1. Initially, the racemic mixture of dopa was used, primarily because of the greater expense of the active L-isomer. Now levodopa is employed alone; this may have reduced some of the side reactions initially encountered, including leukopenia. Leukopenia was more likely due to organic solvents contaminating the preparation than to the presence of the D-isomer.

2. The initial dosage schedule has been lengthened to avoid too rapid increments of dose. Doses are administered seven times daily to reduce the size of single doses. Increments are made every other day, from an initial dose of 300 mg daily to a maximum tolerated dose or to an arbitrary maximum dose of 8 g daily. The average optimal dose has been 5.8 g daily. Little improvement has been observed at daily doses less than 3 g.

3. Improvement may not be evident for as long as 6 weeks. Even an effective dose must be maintained for weeks prior to change in symptoms. Once an effective dose is attained, further improvement may occur with the passage of time. Discontinuation of drug seldom results in relapse before several days and often not before several weeks. Symptoms reappear in the reverse order of their disappearance. Retreatment with the same dosage schedule as initially used reverses relapses.

4. Levodopa therapy has also been effective for the extrapyramidal syndrome associated with chronic manganese poisoning, as well as in Parkinson's disease (Cotzias, 1970).

5. Alpha-methyldopa hydrazine is a compound that blocks dopa decarboxylase peripherally but does not enter the brain. It has been used with levodopa therapy in the hope that it would allow a reduction in dose. If levodopa were not converted so rapidly in the rest of the body, a greater fraction of the dose might reach the central nervous system. As the present fraction of administered levodopa that enters the nervous system is no doubt minute, even a slight reduction in decarboxylase activity might permit increased access of levodopa to brain. Fewer limiting gastrointestinal side effects would occur and treatment would become less expensive. This particular dopa decarboxylase inhibitor is currently being tested clinically. If it or other decarboxylase inhibitors prove to be safe, it might be possible to reduce the dose of levodopa to about 10% of that currently used. Another approach has been to try to reduce the urinary excretion of levodopa by giving probenecid. Still another approach has been to give disulfiram to inhibit dopamine beta-oxidase (Figure 11–4). *Principle: A clear definition of the therapeutic goal and an understanding of the biochemical basis of a drug's action and of its*

pharmacokinetic behavior are exceedingly helpful in planning rational therapy.

Unwanted Effects

Anticholinergic drugs must often be used in mildly toxic doses to attain maximum therapeutic benefits. Patients and their families should be alerted to the more dangerous toxic effects. Probably the most dangerous complication of central anticholinergic drugs is heat stroke caused by inhibition of thermoregulatory sweating. The elderly patient may fall into deep stupor with high fever; prompt and vigorous treatment is required. Elderly patients are often quite susceptible to the deliriant actions of anticholinergics; any evidence of confusion or of alternating levels of awareness constitutes an urgent indication for reducing the dose. Acute urinary retention and paralytic ileus are dangerous complications of peripheral anticholinergic blockade. Adjunctive drugs often are used to counter side effects, such as amphetamine to treat drug-induced drowsiness or mental depression. Such drugs are of little value, and their cardiovascular effects may be harmful, especially when added to those of the anticholinergic drugs. *Principle: Whenever possible, avoid treating an unwanted effect of a drug with another drug.*

Moderate and labile hypertension, and clinically insignificant orthostatic hypotension, have been observed as side effects from levodopa therapy, but neither requires treatment. Nausea and vomiting, frequent dose-limiting side effects, may be prevented by gradual increments in dose or by giving the drug with protein-containing foods. Mental symptoms such as sleeplessness, irritability, and paranoid delusions have been encountered, but other patients are stimulated and euphoric. Perhaps euphoria is due to their clinical improvement. About half the patients experience involuntary movements such as choreiform motions of the extremities, grimacing or gnawing movements of the face, or fleeting myoclonus. Mild elevation of blood urea nitrogen and of protein-bound iodine have been encountered without other signs of renal toxicity or of thyroid dysfunction.

As with any new chronic treatment, the possibility of long-term toxicity is uncertain. The occasional incidence of bizarre mental symptoms and choreiform movements that are not amenable to therapy may ultimately have greater importance than at present. Still, some patients are in their third year of continued treatment with levodopa without any major or life-threatening complications (Barbeau, 1969). One would hope that this long-overdue therapeutic advance will continue to be effective and safe for this disorder.

DRUGS AND SLEEP

Diagnostic Considerations

Insomnia. Insomnia may be defined as (1) an inability to induce sleep as readily as desired; (2) an inability to stay asleep, with frequent awakenings; (3) an abbreviated period of sleep with premature awakening; (4) a night of sleep interrupted by nightmares and voluntary arousals; or (5) sleep that is not refreshing. Attempts to categorize sleep disturbances to provide diagnostic criteria for emotional disorders have not been rewarding, although some type of sleep disorder seems to occur in all (Detre, 1966). The patterns of disturbances of sleep are of clinical importance in the treatment of this ubiquitous symptom (Hobson, 1969).

As in constipation, another disturbance of normal function, defining "normal" is difficult. The sleeping time needed per day varies widely from one person to another. In animals, the range extends from the long, deep sleep of the bear or lion to the true insomnia of the antelope or dolphin. Most humans require between 7 and 8 hours nightly. Many require less, although 5 hours is the usual lower limit. Whether one really requires more sleep than this is questionable, although some adults sleep as much as 12 hours daily. One's feeling of well-being and ability to function may be curtailed by a night of poor sleep, but under normal conditions insomnia alone does not lead to physical or mental injury. Insomnia may be associated with many physical or emotional disorders, but is more likely a consequence than a cause. *Principle: "Normal" is never absolute; sometimes the boundaries between normal and disordered functions are poorly defined.*

Many therapeutic approaches other than drug therapy can be taken to manage sleeplessness, but drugs appear to constitute one of the most prevalent methods of treatment, as hypnotic-sedative drugs rank high among drugs prescribed or manufactured. The vast use of such drugs is inappropriate and may lead to harmful consequences. Further, the rapid increase in knowledge about mechanisms of sleep and the effects of drugs upon them have made it imperative that we consider how drugs used for other purposes may affect sleep patterns.

Mechanisms of Sleep. Activity of the ascending reticular activating system of the brain provides a mechanism for the waking state. Various sensory inputs sustain its activity (Moruzzi, 1962; Magoun, 1963). Although decreasing such inputs might provide a passive mechanism for inducing sleep, sleep induction may be an active phenomenon. Transections of the lower brain stem in animals produce a state of insomnia. The median raphe system of nuclei in the brain stem is important for sleep; when it is destroyed or its content of serotonin is diminished by pharmacologic means, insomnia occurs. Further, electrical stimulation of many parts of the brain produces sleep. Thus sleep may be more an active than a passive phenomenon and may be related both to definite anatomic structures and to specific biogenic amines.

The first indication that sleep has variable stages was the observation of a state of sleep characterized by rapid eye movements (REM), usually associated with dreaming. Many laboratories have delineated the various types of sleep seen in both animals and man. Two major types of sleep are now recognized: rapid eye movement (REM) and nonrapid eye movement (NREM), the latter being further subdivided into four stages (Rechtschaffen and Kales, 1968).

The distinguishing features of sleep stages are obvious in electrographic recordings of muscle tone (electromyograph, EMG) and eye movements (electro-oculogram, EOG), and in the electroencephalogram (EEG). The awake state is characterized by sporadic eye movements, high muscle tone, and low-voltage fast EEG activity. Slow eye movements herald the onset of stage 1 sleep, which is often associated with hypnogogic hallucinations. Stage 2 sleep is characterized by "sleep spindles" in the EEG and a considerable decrease in muscle tone. In sleep stages 3 and 4, the EEG becomes progressively slower in frequency and higher in amplitude. Stage 4 sleep is characterized by very-slow-frequency, high-amplitude waves in the EEG. REM sleep somewhat resembles the awake state electrographically; the EEG tracing shows a similar low-voltage fast activity, but eye movements are more frequent and more regular than in the awake state. The major difference in the REM state is a completely flat EMG tracing, indicating marked muscle inhibition. By continual recording throughout the night, it is possible to distinguish these various types of sleep, to record the pattern of their occurrence, and to calculate the total amount of time spent in each state (Kales et al., 1968, 1969).

The pattern of sleep in a normal young adult during an 8-hour night begins with an initial awake period (sleep latency period), followed by a rapid progression through the stages of NREM sleep until a period of sustained stage 4 sleep is reached. This sequence is then followed by a reverse progression into the first period of REM sleep, some 60 to 90 minutes after sleep's onset. The first REM period may last for only a few minutes and is followed by another cycle. During the night, about four such cycles occur, though in the second and succeeding cycles, less time is spent in stage 4 sleep and more in the other stages, including progressively longer periods of REM sleep. Brief awakenings may occur from REM or stage 2 sleep. In the elderly, sleep latency is increased, and stage 4 sleep may be entirely absent; the onset of the first REM period (REM latency) is delayed, REM periods tend to have the same length, and awakenings are more frequent.

The normal duration of REM sleep is about 100 minutes per night, accounting for 20 to 25% of total sleep time. The amount of REM sleep is relatively constant. Stage 4 sleep accounts for less than 1 hour of the total sleep time, the remaining time being spent mainly in stage 2. Disturbances of normal sleep, either by prolonged enforced sleeplessness or by drugs, seem to affect mainly the proportions of stage 4 NREM sleep and REM sleep, which accordingly are of greatest investigational interest. In the pattern of sleep described, the progression is from wakefulness to NREM sleep to REM sleep to wakefulness. The first step is reversible; i.e., one can awaken from slow wave sleep. The latter step is irreversible; i.e., one rarely progresses directly from waking to the REM state.

Combined anatomic and biochemical studies have revealed two systems serving these major divisions of sleep. Destruction of the median raphe system and its serotonin-containing neurons markedly diminishes all stages of sleep (Jouvet, 1969). Depleting this system of serotonin by treatment with parachlorphenylalanine does the same in animals; in man and monkeys, this treatment seems only to decrease REM sleep (Wyatt et al., 1969). Parachlorphenylalanine specifically blocks tryptophan hydroxylase and impairs the synthesis of serotonin. Destruction of the locus caeruleus, with its norepinephrine-containing neurons, greatly reduces the amount of tonic inhibition associated with REM sleep. A number of biochemical mechanisms for depleting this nucleus of norepinephrine achieve the same result. Alpha-methylparatyrosine, a specific inhibitor of tyrosine hydroxylase, and disulfiram, an inhibitor of dopamine beta-oxidase, interfere with the biosynthesis of norepinephrine (Figure 11–4). Alpha-methyldopa, possibly by producing a false transmitter, alpha-methylnorepinephrine, also interferes with this norepinephrine-mediated system that serves REM sleep. *Principle: Pharmacologic "tools," i.e., substances that selectively impair biochemical or neurophysio-*

logic functions, are of great importance in the study of the physiology of the nervous system.

The cause of the shift from NREM to REM sleep is unclear. Treatment with monoamine oxidase inhibitors impairs REM sleep, leading to the hypothesis that a deaminated metabolite of serotonin may be essential for the transition. Atropine also blocks the transition, suggesting that a cholinergic mechanism may trigger the noradrenergic system of the locus caeruleus. *Principle: Various aminergic systems seem to work in concert to produce effects in the central nervous system; one cannot study a single system in isolation.*

The importance of stage 4 and REM sleep has been documented by numerous studies in which subjects have been entirely deprived of all sleep (Gulevich *et al.*, 1966). Under such circumstances, both stage 4 and REM sleep must be "made up" by increasing their proportions in the sleep that follows. Compensation for stage 4 sleep occurs first, suggesting that it has greater restitutive functions. Similar com-

pensatory phenomena occur when either type of sleep is selectively deprived (by awakening subjects as it becomes apparent from their electrographic records that they are entering a specific stage of sleep). The compensatory periods are also of considerable importance in studying the "rebound" effects of drugs that alter sleep patterns, especially those that decrease the total amount of REM sleep.

Hypnotic Drugs

Chemical Structures. Both barbiturates and glutarimides have six-membered ring structures with two possible substituents at the 5-position (Figure 11–6). Modifications of the structures of barbiturates have had little influence on their pharmacologic actions. Despite the traditional classification of short-, intermediate-, and long-acting types of barbiturates, there seems to be relatively little difference between the more prominent groups (Mark, 1969). Secobarbital, pentobarbital, and amobarbital are usually prepared for oral administration as sodium salts,

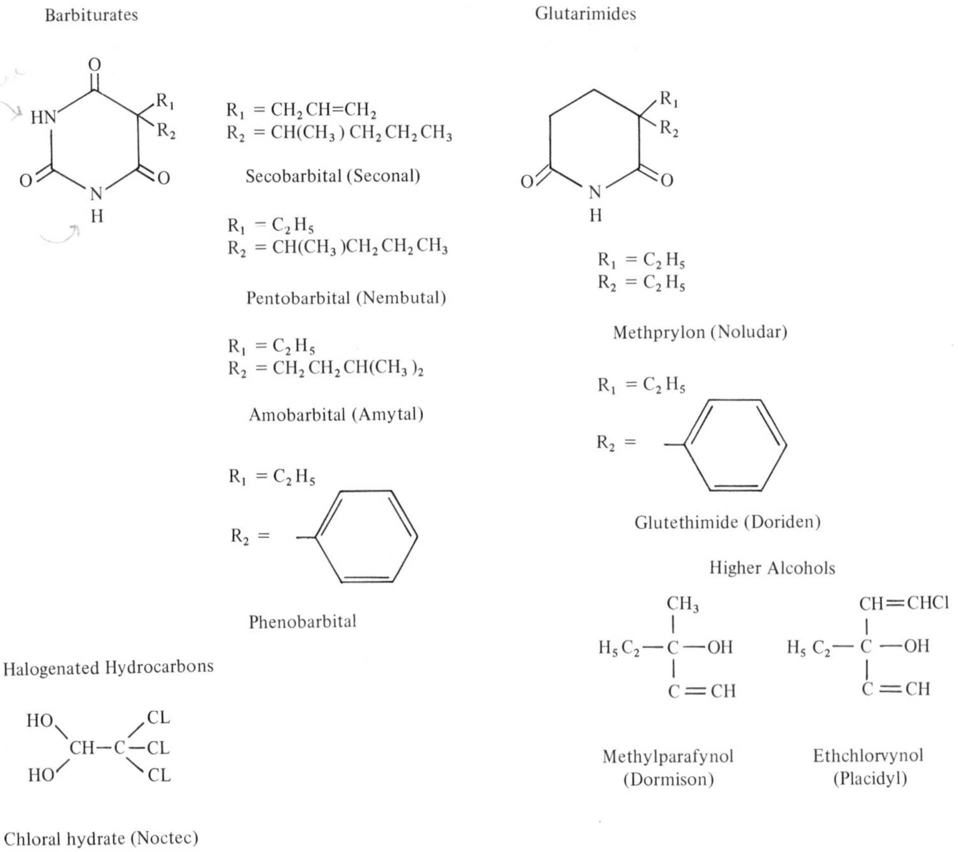

Figure 11–6. Chemical structural relationships between various classes of hypnotic drugs.

which increases their rate of absorption as compared to phenobarbital, which is only available for oral dosage in the acid form. Quite possibly the slower absorption of phenobarbital accounts for its relative unpopularity as a drug of abuse, as it does not intoxicate as quickly as the others.

The structures of the glutarimides are similar to those of barbiturates, despite the fact that these drugs were widely touted as nonbarbiturate sedatives when first introduced. This group differs only slightly from the barbiturates in general pharmacologic properties. They are usually less potent, requiring more milligrams of drug for a given therapeutic effect. One great disadvantage of glutethimide as compared with its barbiturate analog, phenobarbital, is that it must be totally metabolized, which creates serious problems in cases of overdose. *Principle: Molecular modification may at times improve a compound, but it may also create disadvantages. Often such modifications are made primarily for commercial rather than scientific purposes; be skeptical unless a clear advantage can be proved.*

The halogenated hydrocarbon chloral hydrate is enjoying resurgent popularity. It is a weak hypnotic, requiring rather large doses to be effective. The drug is active by way of its metabolite trichlorethanol. Longer-chain alcohols, such as methylparafynol and ethchlorvynol, are also rather weak and offer no price or safety advantages over chloral hydrate.

Pharmacologic Properties. The major effect of these drugs, depression of the central nervous system (CNS) at all segmental levels, accounts for most of their clinical uses, which range from sedation to anesthesia (Shideman, 1961). The dose of drug depends upon the level of CNS depression and the clinical effects desired. Sedative, antianxiety, and hypnotic drugs cannot be clearly separated pharmacologically, as drugs usually classified in one category may act in the others, given an appropriate adjustment of dose. In this regard, it would be proper to consider drugs listed in Figure 11-6 as antianxiety agents and to consider those listed in Figure 11-1 as hypnotics. *Principle: The pharmacologic classification of a drug is often arbitrary and based on some selected clinical use or dose. One must always consider all of a drug's pharmacologic actions, which allow it to be used for different goals, e.g., phenobarbital as an antianxiety agent, an anticonvulsant, and a hypnotic.*

Even small doses of sedative-hypnotic drugs produce varying degrees and duration of impairment of psychologic or motor functions in normal subjects. The impairment may be less obvious in anxious subjects, when relief of anxiety may countervail any drug-induced impairment. Higher doses of these drugs enforce

sleep, whether or not the patient so desires, or may produce release phenomena with signs of drunkenness, emotional disinhibition, or excitement in susceptible individuals. Gross motor impairment may be manifested by ataxia. Hypnotic doses of these drugs may also have analgesic effects, but only with other significant alterations in sensory modalities. Anesthetic doses of these drugs are often close to lethal doses. Even anesthetic barbiturates, such as thiopental (Pentothal Sodium), are seldom used as the sole anesthetic agent, but rather as adjuncts to others. Depression of the motor cortex and anticonvulsant action can be obtained with high doses of most of these drugs, usually well into their hypnotic range; phenobarbital is relatively selective in depressing the motor cortex, especially when given chronically, allowing its use in epilepsy without undue sedation.

Tolerance to CNS effects may rapidly develop, requiring special consideration in the clinical use of these drugs. Cross-tolerance among the various members sharing similar pharmacologic actions is also important, especially in regard to substitution of drugs when treating or preventing withdrawal reactions. Abuse must be substantial (four to six times the usual therapeutic dose daily) and long (days or weeks) to produce withdrawal reactions with most drugs in this class. Additive effects are to be expected when these drugs are taken concurrently with other central nervous system depressants, commonly alcohol.

Effects of Hypnotics on Normal Sleep Patterns. Although laboratory techniques for studying sleep patterns have been applied only to a limited extent in studying the effects of various hypnotic drugs, they have already challenged some previously held premises about these agents.

To study even a single dose of a single drug in a single subject usually requires at least 5 nights in the sleep laboratory: at least two nights for control, the first showing a characteristically abnormal "first-night" effect; 1 night on the drug; and two nights' follow-up for residual effects. These periods can be lengthened in various ways to evaluate extended treatment, sometimes with an intervening period of dosage outside the laboratory. By widely spacing periods of control recordings between drug trials, the effects of different doses of a drug may be studied in the same person. Each night of testing requires continual recordings and supervision, plus an enormous amount of data analysis, not to mention the considerable inconvenience to subjects. It is not surprising that sample sizes of greater than ten subjects are seldom reported for any dose or dosage schedule of a drug. Evaluation of hypnotics in the sleep laboratory uses several criteria: total sleep time, total time awake, number of awakenings, sleep latency, total REM sleep time, number of REM sleep periods, REM latency, and total time in stage 3 or 4 NREM sleep. The sleep laboratory is not the most efficient means for the clinical screening of hypnotic drugs; a simple procedure is to use clinical measurements based on subjective responses of patients and on observations of their sleep patterns (Bloomfield *et al.*, 1967; Jick, 1969). The great value of the sleep laboratory has been in delineating the types of sleep induced by available hypnotic drugs. *Principle: Old techniques for clinical screening of drugs should not be discarded simply because a new technique becomes available; both may offer useful information.*

In single therapeutic doses, most hypnotic drugs have similar actions in decreasing sleep latency, increasing total sleep time, decreasing awake time and number of awakenings, increasing the time spent in stage 3 or 4 NREM sleep, increasing the latency of the first REM period, and decreasing the number of REM periods and the total time in REM sleep. The more rapid onset of sleep, its increased depth, and its better maintenance are generally considered favorable effects for insomniac patients, but the effects on REM sleep might be unfavorable. However, when REM sleep is decreased, there is a strong tendency to "make it up." Compensatory REM sleep seems to occur even when hypnotic drugs are used for periods as short as 3 to 4 days. Although the initial decrease in REM sleep time becomes less on succeeding nights, following discontinuation of the drug REM time immediately increases, then is followed by a slow return toward normal duration. Following more chronic administration of hypnotics, REM rebound may be severe and may be accompanied by vivid nightmares and restlessness. Normal sleep patterns may not be restored for weeks (Oswald, 1968). The clinical implications of such long-lasting alterations are not entirely clear, but although sporadic use of hypnotics may ameliorate a disturbed sleep pattern, chronic use of such drugs may actually create an additional disturbance. The patient may continue to use the drug to avoid the unpleasant consequences of withdrawal. The potential of a drug to reduce REM sleep and to produce sharp rebound upon discontinuation has been proposed as a criterion of its propensity to cause dependence (Hartmann, 1969). Although this hypothesis has much supporting evidence, it is not fully established. *Principle: Sometimes a small amount of drug taken intermittently may provide symptomatic*

relief, whereas a larger dose may undo the beneficial effects and create a new problem equal to or worse than the original one.

Therapeutic Considerations

The Insomniac Patient. Insomnia is a real complaint, although it may merely be one of many psychosomatic complaints or possibly the symptom of a more severe underlying emotional disorder. A comparison of "good" and "poor" sleepers revealed that the latter took longer to fall asleep, slept less, awakened more, had less REM sleep, tended to expend their stage 4 sleep earlier, and had higher physiologic arousal (heart rate, body temperature) than did "good" sleepers (Monroe, 1967). Their responses to the Cornell Medical Index suggested that sleeplessness was one of a cluster of physical and emotional complaints. Many of the deviations in sleep pattern shown by the insomniac are ameliorated by hypnotic drugs, which no doubt explains their vast popularity.

The many other complaints of insomniacs should alert the physician to look for physical or emotional disorders. Pain may disturb sleep, whether it be from mild arthritis, pruritus, the night pain of duodenal ulcer, or the early morning cramps of an irritable bowel. Sudden fearful arousals with palpitation and sweating may be due to thyrotoxicosis, angina, hypoglycemia, pheochromocytoma, or anxiety attacks. If such arousals are accompanied by dyspnea, early heart failure may be present.

Similarly, insomnia may be caused by emotional disorders. Worry over one's job, financial dealings, or love affairs, as well as the excitement of a stimulating evening, may interfere with sleep. Such causes are usually easily uncovered. Chronic anxiety reactions are almost always accompanied by some degree of sleep disturbance, as are depressive reactions. Attempts have been made to classify depressive reactions on the basis of type of sleep disorder (difficulty in starting sleep presumably due to reactive depression; early morning awakening presumably due to endogenous depression), but the only valid statement that can be made is that some degree of sleep disturbance is constantly seen in any clinical depression (Gresham *et al.*, 1965). Sleep disturbances are also seen in schizophrenia, but it is doubtful that they are pathogenic. Rather, schizophrenia with florid symptoms may be accompanied by a basic disturbance in sleep mechanisms, as evidenced by a decreased need to make up REM sleep following deprivation (Zarcone *et al.*, 1968).

The use of drugs, either self-administered by the patient or prescribed by the physician, may interfere with sleep patterns. A careful drug history is imperative in evaluating insomnia. Two commonly taken social drugs may interfere with sleep. Caffeine is generally recognized as having this effect, but for curious reasons, it may not do so until the middle years of life. Therefore, persons who have been able to drink their evening cup of coffee with impunity may begin to find sleep more difficult and may fail to associate the insomnia with ingestion of this drug. Although alcohol is a depressant, and often enhances the onset of sleep, heavy drinkers often find that they awaken in the early morning in a stimulated state. It is speculative whether this is a mild symptom of withdrawal or the result of secondary release of catecholamines from previous alcoholic intake, but alcohol may interfere with sleep in some persons (Johnson et al., 1970). Appetite suppressants, nasal vasoconstrictors, asthma remedies containing sympathomimetics, or antidepressants of the sympathomimetic or monoamine-oxidase-inhibiting type may also interfere with sleep.

Some types of insomnia may be "normal." Persons who travel through several time zones a day may find that their normal biologic rhythms, including that of sleep-awakening, are interrupted. Sleeping in a strange bed or in unusual surroundings may interfere with normal sleep. Any change in the accustomed ambient noise level during the night may temporarily alter one's sleep pattern. Finally, some people simply seem to require less sleep or to require it in a more infantile pattern (by frequent cat naps rather than by sustained sleep). Such individuals may have to learn to live with their peculiarities and try to make the most of them.

Desiderata of Hypnotic Drugs. Ideally, a hypnotic would alter sleep in the following manner: (1) rapid onset with a decrease in sleep latency time; (2) no change in the normal pattern of sleep; (3) duration sufficient to ensure a complete night's sleep with no early morning awakening; (4) little residual daytime sedation; (5) little or no tendency to become habituating or for tolerance to develop; and (6) little danger of successful suicide if an overdose is taken. None of the drugs currently available meet these requirements; some drugs may meet them better than others.

The rapidity of onset may be increased by administering the drug in liquid form, but most hypnotics are available only in a tablet or capsule form. Taking an adequate amount of fluid with the dose, so as to assure prompt disintegration and suspension of the material, may hasten the onset of sleep. Remaining active or upright for a short time after taking the medication may hasten the onset of action; to some degree this can be accomplished by taking the dose approximately 30 minutes prior to retiring.

Although evidence regarding the effect of hypnotics on normal sleep patterns is still fragmentary, chloral hydrate and the benzodiazepines (chlordiazepoxide, flurazepam, and diazepam) may cause less disruption than the barbiturates, glutarimides, or antihistaminics. One must be cautious in interpreting the available data. A drug may have little effect on normal sleep at one dose, but have an adverse effect at a higher dose. Studies of the effects of these drugs in normal subjects may not be entirely relevant to patients with disturbed sleep patterns and a partial deprivation of REM or NREM sleep. Further, most studies have been concerned with relatively brief periods of drug administration.

Both the duration of action and "hangover" effects are more dependent upon the dose of drug and the individual vagaries in patients' responses than upon intrinsic differences between drugs. Any dose that maintains sleep throughout an 8-hour period is also likely to have some degree of daytime carry-over. As mentioned in connection with antianxiety drugs, "hangover" may not be entirely a disadvantage. A hypothetic drug with a rapid onset and a very brief duration of action would be ideal for those patients who are unpredictably troubled with early awakening and inability to return to sleep. Such patients are loath to take conventional hypnotics later in the night lest they be too sleepy during the day. Without drugs, they may be unable to return to sleep and may suffer the impairment of a poor night's rest. No suitable drug of this type is currently available, although some patients empirically use alcoholic beverages to meet this particular need.

Habituation and tolerance may develop to any of these drugs, providing compelling reasons for avoiding their uninterrupted use. Glutethimide and the barbiturates may present serious problems in regard to overdoses, so that prescriptions for relatively few doses of these drugs may provide a lethal single dose. On the other hand, the benzodiazepines are relatively suicide proof.

Choice of Hypnotic Drug. Although an active hypnotic drug can easily be distinguished from placebo at any reasonable dose, differences between active hypnotic drugs are difficult to detect either by preference of patients or by objective criteria, assuming equivalent doses have been given. Consequently, the choice of drug may be empiric, based on the preference of the patient or on his past responses. When the choice between drugs is not clear, as may often be the case, one might first try the oldest and cheapest. Chloral hydrate and the barbiturates qualify on both counts. If hypnotics are used with appropriate infrequency, however, the total cost of such agents over a year should not be excessive.

The beginning dose shall be small and should be increased only if necessary. Once a good night's sleep has been attained, the drug should not be used for 2 or 3 nights. The patient should be told that the goal is to restore his normal sleep rhythm and not to make him dependent on the drug. It should be stressed that sleep during many nights without drug will be good and that occasional imperfect sleeps will do little harm. Sometimes the knowledge that relief is ultimately attainable will tide a patient over a few bad nights. *Principle: Treatment with hypnotics should be on an interrupted basis, to decrease the likelihood of tolerance and habituation and to allow prescription of sublethal amounts of drug.*

Many patients report that aspirin relieves their insomnia. Aside from the possibility that aspirin may facilitate sleep by alleviating discomfort, whether due to concurrent arthritis or simply to the muscle aching that many people develop after a tense day, aspirin may have central effects similar to those of antianxiety drugs. If aspirin is used as a hypnotic, it should be taken with abundant water, preferably well before retiring.

Tricyclic antidepressants may have sedative qualities. Even in normal presurgical patients, 25-mg doses of amitriptyline have hypnotic effects equal to those of 100 mg of secobarbital sodium. As depression may be a cause of insomnia, a trial of a tricyclic antidepressant may be worthwhile if depression is suspected as an etiologic factor. Antianxiety agents can, for the most part, be used interchangeably with hypnotic drugs; the hypnotic effect may be attained by a larger-than-usual bedtime dose of the antianxiety drug. Antipsychotic phenothiazine derivatives are poor hypnotics. Their induction of disagreeable reactions in normal patients is well known. Even in psychotic patients, they often fail to relieve sleep disturbances. Use of conventional hypnotics, such as chloral hydrate, is appropriate for insomnia in patients taking antipsychotic drugs.

Nondrug Management of Insomnia. The relaxation that follows a warm bath, a massage, or the relief of sexual tension can be used to promote sleep. Many insomniacs have developed elaborate rituals for courting sleep, and some seem to work. Boring tasks that do not require close attention, such as watching the innumerable commercials during the late movie on television, often induce sleep. As much of the process of going to sleep has a certain ritual to it anyway (undressing, attending to various items of toilet, etc.), some conditioning of responses may normally occur. It may be worthwhile to plan some sort of ritual for patients who seek relief from insomnia and to link this with drug therapy, to exploit the conditioned reflex aspect of the process of going to sleep. *Principle: To the extent that drug responses can be "conditioned" by their association with habitual activities, habit alone may substitute for the drug or enhance its effect. No drug that affects the mental state works in a vacuum; all interact to some extent with the personality of the patient and the setting in which they are given.*

A regular daily pattern of activities and exercise may facilitate normal sleep. Whereas sleep patterns may be entirely normal in patients who are inactive, simply increasing the activity level to the point of moderate fatigue may afford relief for some insomniacs. Sleeping during the day disrupts the usual nocturnal sleep pattern and should be avoided, even when the urge to sleep is strong. The last full meal of the day should precede retiring by several hours, for some persons experience indigestion if they retire too soon after a heavy meal. At times, a patient may prefer to get out of bed should he awaken and not be able to return to sleep than to fret in the dark about his insomnia. An hour or two of reading in the middle of the night may lead to a shortened but more refreshing sleep during the remainder of the night.

Summary Principles: (1) Insomnia is a symptom. Although it may often be a symptom without a disease, one should be alert to underlying causes that may require more specific treatment. (2) Treatment should be considered only on an intermittent basis. (3) The choice of drug is empiric and may depend upon the preference of the patient. (4) The smallest dose suitable for obtaining the desired effects should be used. (5) Small amounts of these drugs should be prescribed at any single time, to reduce the likelihood of lethal consequences from deliberate or accidental overdoses. (6) All possible factors that may interact with drugs should be considered in exploiting the hypnotic effect.

Unwanted Effects

Extension of Pharmacologic Effects of Hypnotics. Oversedation may not be due solely to excessive dose. Many patients also take daytime sedatives, tranquilizers, antihistaminics, or other drugs that may add to residual effects of the hypnotic. Alcohol is a commonly self-administered drug whose lethal interactions with hypnotics are often not known by patients or even by physicians. Barbiturates in particular synergize with the respiratory depression from alcohol and may lead to unexpected and unintended deaths when taken in the presence of high concentrations of alcohol in plasma.

Excessive daytime sedation may be controlled by reducing the size of the nighttime dose. Despite the fact that the clinical effects of "long-acting" and "medium long-acting" barbiturates are similar, their persistence in plasma differs following single doses. The rate of disappearance of phenobarbital from plasma over a 24-hour period varies between 11% and 23% in man (Butler et al., 1954). On the other hand, approximately 50% of the peak level of sodium pentobarbital is cleared from plasma over 24 hours (Hollister et al., 1963). As with most other drugs used as hypnotics, an appreciable amount of barbiturate remains in plasma for a prolonged period. Whether troublesome clinical symptoms are produced may depend on many other factors.

Habituation is a danger with any drug that produces a pleasant state, as hypnotics often do. As tolerance quickly occurs with most of these drugs, the tendency to increase dose to maintain therapeutic effects is strong. Continued use of therapeutic doses of some of these drugs apparently leads to a secondary disorder of sleep that may promote their chronic use. Withdrawal reactions follow relatively minor levels of prolonged abuse. Consequently, patients suspected of overuse of these drugs should not be withdrawn from them abruptly, lest a withdrawal reaction be precipitated.

Withdrawal reactions to a drug may be an extreme instance of the effects of sleep deprivation. Measurable abnormalities in REM sleep follow the withdrawal of even small single doses of hypnotics used for only 3 nights (Kales et al., 1969). The rebound in REM sleep may exceed the actual loss experienced during the drug state and may persist for some time. The situation differs from experimental REM deprivation, where "makeup" REM is less than the amount deprived.

Hypnotic-sedative drugs are the most common chemical agents used for committing suicide, and as many patients with insomnia may have masked emotional disorders, the physician should try to minimize this danger by prescribing small amounts. The management of the consequences of toxic doses of these drugs is reviewed in Chapter 17. The suppression of REM sleep by many hypnotics may be considered an unwanted effect, as it may be related to the propensity to develop dependence. Still, in some clinical situations, as following various types of ocular surgery, immobilization of the eyes is desirable. Although such immobilization is assiduously carried out during waking hours, until recently little attention has been given to the events that occur during sleep. Currently, experiments are being carried out to determine if the suppression of eye movements during normal sleep by certain hypnotic drugs may be used advantageously in such situations (Kales et al., 1970). *Principle: An unwanted effect of a drug may be desirable in special situations* (see Chapter 18).

Pharmacologic Effects of Nonhypnotic Drugs. As many drugs affect sleep, their effects on normal sleep must be considered along with the patient's response to hypnotics. Caffeine and nicotine produce very little change in REM sleep. In some individuals, modest doses of caffeine (250 mg) may produce disturbances in sleep that increase as the dose is increased. Alcohol has an effect on REM sleep somewhat similar to that of the usual sedative-hypnotic drugs, in that it decreases REM sleep, followed by a rebound of REM makeup time. The latter is especially evident during the stages of severe alcohol withdrawal, when REM time may occupy nearly 100% of sleep time. Its incursion into the waking hours may be the mechanism of some of the hallucinatory phenomena of the alcohol withdrawal state (Yules et al., 1966).

Amphetamines, such as dextroamphetamine in doses of 10 and 15 mg, increase REM latency and decrease REM time; body movements are increased, total sleep time is reduced, and stage 4 sleep is lessened (Rechtschaffen and Maron, 1964). Opposite effects are observed following withdrawal of amphetamine in addicts: REM latency is decreased, REM sleep is increased especially in the early portion of the night, and total sleep time is increased (Oswald and Thacore, 1963). Diethylpropion (Tenuate), phenmetrazine (Preludin), tranylcypromine, and methylphenidate probably have effects similar to those of the amphetamines. Fenfluramine, an anorexiant phenylalkylamine derivative, differs from its analogs in having sedative rather than stimulant effects. It produces little change in sleep patterns except to increase total NREM time (Oswald et al., 1968). *Principle: Chemical modification of drugs to separate desired from undesired pharmacologic effects is rarely successful, but such efforts are valid reasons for creating analogs of existing drugs.*

Heroin impairs sleep in doses of 5 and 10 mg. Awakening is more frequent, as well as shifts to lighter (stage 1) NREM sleep, and REM time is decreased. Morphine in doses of 7.5, 15, and 30 mg has similar effects in previously addicted volunteers. Waking is increased, stage 1 and 2 NREM sleep is increased at the expense of stages 3 and 4, REM latency is increased, and total REM time is decreased, although the pattern of REM periods is not disturbed (Kay et al., 1969). The commonly held notion that morphine puts one into the arms of Morpheus may not be entirely correct.

Psychotherapeutic drugs have variable effects. Vivid dreams and frightening nightmares are reported as side effects of reserpine, which increases REM time, perhaps more consistently over a range of doses than any other drug (Hartmann, 1966). The effects of chlorpromazine have been contradictory, probably because results are dose dependent. REM sleep is depressed by single doses of 100 mg, but increased by doses of 25 mg. Following REM depression, there is no immediate REM make-up, presumably owing to the slow clearance of the drug from the body (Lewis and Evans, 1969). Imipramine and the other tricyclic antidepressants resemble hypnotics in decreasing sleep latency, increasing REM latency, decreasing REM time, increasing stage 3 and 4 NREM sleep, and allowing fewer awakenings. A striking difference is the greatly reduced makeup of REM sleep; the decrease in REM compensation may be related to the antidepressant effects (Hartmann, 1969). *Principle: Automatic conclusions about drugs (e.g., "antidepressant equals stimulant"), though superficially logical, may prove to be contrary to fact.*

DRUGS FOR RELIEF OF PAIN

Aspects of Pain

All of us endure pain to a varying extent, and many times it is considered "normal" or inconsequential. Severe or unusual pain is bothersome, causes concern, and demands explanation or relief. The boundaries between normal discomforts and pathologic pain are often obscure. Prominent cardiologists have often been astounded at their slowness in recognizing the true significance of the pain signaling their first myocardial infarct. Pain is only a symptom, and its importance is determined by the underlying disease state causing it. *Principle: Prior to any attempt to treat pain, or at least concomitant with it, an attempt should be made to determine its biologic significance.*

The sensation of pain is difficult to describe. The same difficulty has been likened to describing colors to a person blind from birth. Fortunately, most of us have experienced a spectrum of pain and can partly describe pain by use of analogy. Patients vary considerably in their tolerance of discomfort; those whose tolerance is low are more likely to visit physicians than are stoics. Pain is usually perceived both as unpleasant and as evidence of ill health. It therefore evokes fear or anxiety. Some have

defined pain as an unpleasant experience that we associate with tissue damage or describe in terms of tissue damage or both (Merskey and Spear, 1967). If "ill health" is substituted for the phrase "tissue damage," such a definition is applicable to the complaints of most patients. In summary, pain is an unpleasant subjective experience symptomatic or symbolic of some underlying disorder that arouses anxiety.

Pathophysiologic Mechanisms

Nerve endings sensitive to pain are widely distributed in tissues (Ruch, 1960). Pathways for pain transmission have been delineated, but central processing of pain is more diffuse; it is difficult to delineate specific areas in the thalamus, for instance, that subserve only sensations of pain. The distribution of central pain pathways may be diffuse and a number of modalities of sensation may be transmitted together. *Principle: There is no specific area in the brain upon which analgesic drugs act.*

Physical stimuli compress or stretch sensitive tissue, whereas chemicals act directly on sensitive nerve endings to cause pain (see Chapter 4). Usually physical stimuli are of brief duration, but may underlie chronic pain, as in a herniated intervertebral disc. Chemical stimuli are most likely to mediate chronic pain. For instance, when one touches a hot object and reflexly withdraws the hand, pain results from the direct action of the heat. If no tissue injury has occurred, the pain rapidly subsides. If a first- or second-degree burn has occurred, chemical stimuli then maintain the pain until the reaction to acute damage subsides.

The source of pain can usually be identified: (1) pain from skin or subcutaneous tissue; (2) pain from skeletal muscle; or (3) visceral pain. Each type of pain may be relieved by nonpharmacologic measures. For example, applications of cold to burned skin or of heat to sore muscles are effective remedies. Angina pectoris may be relieved by rest and the pain of duodenal ulcer by food. However, nitroglycerin or oxygen may be effective for some types of angina pectoris, and pain from duodenal ulcer may quickly respond to antacids. *Principle: Specific therapy for pain depends on correction of the underlying pathophysiologic event.*

If reversal of the pathogenetic factor responsible for pain is not possible, two distinct therapeutic choices exist: drugs that work peripherally and those that act centrally. For example, local anesthetics interrupt transmission of the pain stimulus in the peripheral nerve, whereas general anesthetics reduce brain function to the point where pain is not perceived. Some drugs that work peripherally block impulse generation at chemoreceptors. Some centrally active drugs block central excitatory synaptic transmission or activate inhibiting neurons and synapses. *Principle: The two nonspecific pharmacologic approaches to amelioration of pain are distinct and may be used in combination to treat many types of pain.*

Other analgesics are classified by their modes of action. The nonnarcotic analgesics work primarily in the periphery; the narcotic analgesics (e.g., morphine) act centrally. Drugs that act peripherally are frequently and effectively used for pain originating in integument or musculoskeletal systems; drugs that act centrally are best for pain originating in viscera. Thus morphine is not used for a trivial pain arising from the musculoskeletal system, but may be needed for crushing injuries or burns.

Clinical Evaluation of Analgesics

A standard in the field of evaluation of subjective responses, including pain, was reported by Beecher (1959). The book contained a summary of shortcomings of the laboratory investigations used to evaluate analgesics and stressed the necessity for clinical evaluation of these drugs. It distinguished between the primary sensation of pain and the secondary mental processing or reaction to it and reviewed the valid techniques that may be used to study drugs that alter subjective responses to pain.

Analgesics of the morphine type are usually studied in patients with postoperative pain, who require an analgesic and are closely observed. The main disadvantages of this method are that such patients have been previously exposed to multiple drugs that act on the central nervous system, and their need for a reliably effective drug is so great that placebos are generally not feasible. Elegant techniques have been developed by which patients can be used to compare a new drug against the standard dose of 10 mg of morphine (Bellville *et al.*, 1968; Loan *et al.*, 1968). Drugs used for chronic pain are generally tested in cancer patients (Houde *et al.*, 1960). In these tests, it is usually possible and desirable to compare the effects of several doses of several drugs in the same patient (see Chapter 12).

The study of aspirin-type analgesics is often limited to patients with musculoskeletal disorders, headache, or mild postoperative pain. The general principles of testing are the same and depend on a quantifiable grading of relief of pain. For example, some of the weaker narcotic analgesics may be compared with aspirin in patients with episiotomy pain.

Narcotic Analgesics

Chemical Structures. Although the planar structure of morphine has been known since 1925, our awareness of its three-dimensional structure is more recent and has led to the development of pharmacologically active semisynthetic opiate derivatives as well as synthetic opioids. Some analogs are 10,000 times as potent as morphine, but their clinical utility is not any greater than that of morphine. *Principle: Potency of drugs often has no relationship to therapeutic efficacy or clinical usefulness.*

Two types of alkaloids are found naturally in opium: benzoisoquinolines and phenanthrenes. The former, exemplified by papaverine, are not important as analgesics; the latter include morphine and codeine. The phenyl-N-methyl-piperidine moiety represents the active site for attachment to receptors and is common to most drugs of this type (Gero, 1954). The most notorious semisynthetic derivative of morphine is heroin, the diacetyl derivative. A series of analogs called morphones or codones (based on their respective prototypes) has been created by substituting a ketone for the hydroxyl group at R_2 (Figure 11–7) and eliminating the $\Delta 7$-8 bond. Oxymorphone (Numorphan) and hydromorphone (Dilaudid) are examples of morphones; hydrocodone (Hycodan) and oxycodone (Percodan) are examples of codones. However, morphine and codeine remain the most important members of this group in clinical practice.

Meperidine (Demerol) is a phenylpiperidine with good analgesic action (Figure 11–7). A number of analogs, anileridine (Leritine), piminodine (Alvodine), and diphenoxylate (Lomotil), are made by replacing the N-methyl substituent with other groups attached to the nitrogen, but none are as effective as the parent compound. Diphenoxylate is used orally for its constipating effect. Meperidine's analgesic action makes it the most important member of the group.

The morphinans are derivatives of the natural alkaloids in which the oxygen bridge has been eliminated, making a tetracyclic rather than a pentacyclic configuration. Levorphanol (Levo-Dromoran) and methorphan are the analogs of morphine and codeine, respectively, in this series.

The benzomorphans are further reduced to tricyclic forms while maintaining the crucial phenylpiperidine moiety. The most interesting derivative is a mixed antagonist-agonist derivative, pentazocine (Talwin), which has excited considerable clinical interest (Figure 11–7). The major activity of pentazocine is due to the L-isomer (Forrest *et al.*, 1969).

Methadone (Dolophine) is a diphenylmethane derivative that resembles many anticholinergic

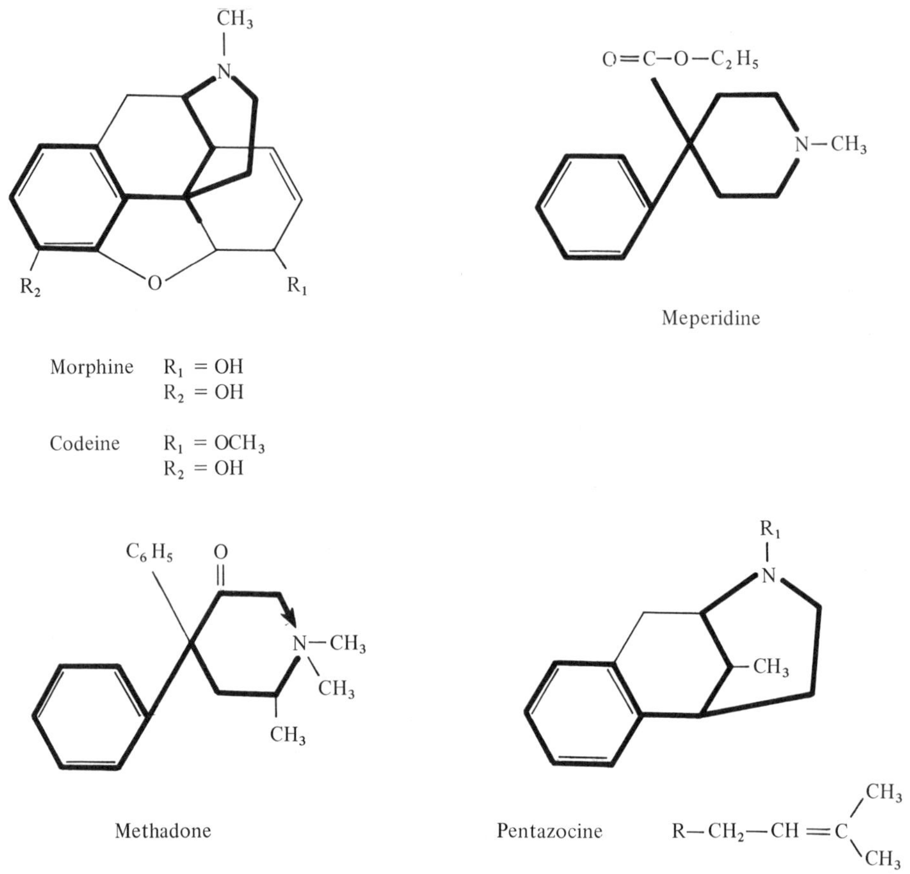

Morphine R_1 = OH
                R_2 = OH

Codeine R_1 = OCH_3
                R_2 = OH

Meperidine

Methadone   Pentazocine $R-CH_2-CH=C\begin{smallmatrix}CH_3\\CH_3\end{smallmatrix}$

Figure 11–7. Representative narcotic analgesics showing common phenylpiperidine moiety.

drugs. As shown in Figure 11–7, it is possible to draw its configuration so that it mimics the phenylpiperidine moiety. An analog, D-propoxyphene hydrochloride (Darvon), retains only minimal pharmacologic properties of narcotic drugs. Nonetheless, it is one of the most widely prescribed drugs in clinical practice. *Principle: The popularity of a drug is not necessarily a reflection of efficacy, especially in situations where the latter is difficult to assess.*

Substitution of the methyl group of the nitrogen atom by an allyl group ($-CH_2-CH-CH_2$) converts morphine to nalorphine (Nalline), a strong narcotic antagonist. The substitution allows maintenance of receptor affinity, but the drug loses intrinsic activity. Other allyl-substituted antagonists include levallorphan (Lorfan), the analog of levorphanol, naloxone, cyclazocine, and pentazocine. The latter drugs have both agonist (morphine-like) and antagonist characteristics and may separate the addictive from the analgesic actions of morphine-like drugs. Such separation has not been proved, as some cases of dependence to pentazocine have occurred. *Principle: Chemical classification of drugs may be used to organize a seemingly diverse group, indicating possible common mechanisms of action, and may lead to the development of new types of drugs.*

Pharmacologic Actions. Narcotic analgesics seem to act centrally, although specific sites of action are not known. They may not abolish pain, but they do reduce the patient's perception of and his affective responses to it. Patients treated with morphine commonly report that they can still feel their pain, but that it is no longer a source of concern. Perhaps pain stimulates a variety of excitatory synapses or transmitters, and the narcotics block excitation. In addition, there seem to be inhibitory synapses or transmitters that provide for central inhibition of pain. Central inhibition may be the mechanism for obtunding pain by hypnosis, Yoga techniques, or placebo responses (Beecher, 1955). Central inhibitory pathways are suggested by experiments in which the aversive and aggressive reactions of monkeys to painful stimulation are blocked by electrical stimulation of the caudate nucleus (Delgado, 1963).

Tolerance to narcotic analgesics is developed fairly rapidly. The number of people who become addicted to the narcotics as a consequence of even prolonged legitimate clinical use is small when compared to the increasing numbers of abusers. When drugs are properly used in hospitals, few of the conditions predisposing to addiction exist. A critical factor predisposing to addiction is self-administration for an immediate and continuing reward (Schuster, 1970). Such situations apply to the "street user" of drugs, who commonly gives himself his own dose and whose reward may be either escape from an unbearable reality or forestalling of abstinence phenomena. *Principle: Narcotics should seldom be withheld simply because of fear of initiating drug dependence. The social use of drugs, unlike the medical use, cannot be viewed solely in the light of pharmacologic and medical considerations.*

It is common practice to screen every new narcotic analgesic for its propensity to induce dependence in animals and in selected humans (Fraser and Harris, 1967). The predictive value of this screening has been good. However, the value of an analgesic is not determined solely by its lack of addictive effects. The search continues for drugs that show a separation of analgesic from addictive properties.

Effects on Specific Systems. *Central Nervous System.* Analgesia, drowsiness, and euphoria are the predominant effects of narcotics in patients with pain. Most subjects who are not in pain, or in emotional distress, experience dysphoria but no analgesia. Whether euphoria or dysphoria is predominant may depend upon the personality of the subject. *Principle: Drugs that alter subjective responses interact with the personality of patients, their expectations, and the existing environmental situation.* Therefore, the predominant effect may be variable. The ideal analgesic drug would specifically and selectively ameliorate pain without having general effects on the central nervous system, such as hypnosis or depression of respiration.

Narcotics also depress respiration by decreasing the responsivity of the respiratory center to carbon dioxide (but not to oxygen). The cough reflex is also depressed, allowing milder narcotics to be used as cough suppressants. The nausea and vomiting produced by narcotics are related to direct stimulation of the chemoreceptor trigger zone and to sensitization to transmission from the vestibular apparatus. These effects are prominent only early in the use of the drug and may be minimized by asking the patient to remain as still as possible in bed. Miosis is a well-known clinical sign of opiate intake; its mechanism is not known. Finally, narcotics lower body temperature and have mild antidiuretic effects.

Gastrointestinal System. Gastrointestinal motility, especially of the large bowel, is decreased. This property has been used clinically, and paregoric (camphorated tincture of opium), is the most widely used preparation for treating diarrhea. Deodorized tincture of opium also is useful to control diarrhea. Although morphine is used for treating the severe pain of biliary colic, it actually increases intrabiliary pressure. The pain is relieved but the underlying disease is exacerbated. The benefit of the former action in this instance outweighs the adverse effect. This action of narcotic analgesics may induce changes in the liver excretory pattern that lead to abnormal tests of hepatic function.

Cardiovascular System. Orthostatic hypotension may be an important clinical effect of morphine. Morphine directly decreases peripheral vascular resistance and redistributes blood flow to the heart and cerebral vessels (Miller *et al.*, 1970). Some of the effect may be related to histamine release, although antihistaminics do not usually prevent morphine-induced hypotension. A positive inotropic action has been ascribed to increased sympathoadrenal discharge (Vasko *et al.*, 1966). As large intravenous doses of morphine, unlike other anesthetics, do not produce cardiac depression, the drug may be used safely as an anesthetic agent in patients with minimal circulatory reserve (Lowenstein *et al.*, 1969).

Clinical Use. *Indications.* The primary indication for narcotic analgesics is the relief of severe, acute pain. Renal or biliary colic, acute myocardial infarction, extensive surgical procedures, burns, or other traumas are clinical situations in which the value of these drugs is unrivaled. Narcotics are also indicated for treating severe chronic pain associated with malignancies. Unfortunately, physicians sometimes think that any patient with malignancy and pain should be treated with narcotics, when nonnarcotic analgesics may be effectively employed. Conversely, the hazards of tolerance, increasing doses, and dependence are not of concern in patients who truly require these drugs.

Acute pulmonary edema is a clinical state in which narcotics are indicated, not for relief of pain but for their cardiovascular-respiratory effects (see Chapters 5 and 6) and to allay anxiety.

The use of narcotic drugs as routine preoperative medication along with anticholinergic drugs is being questioned. Narcotic drugs may not be justified in the absence of pain when apprehension is the only problem. Conventional sedatives or antianxiety drugs given in suitable doses should be equally effective. *Principle: One should always question traditional therapeutic regimens, for tradition often is their only basis for use. When adequate methods are available for assessing the efficacy of a traditional regimen, they should be applied.*

Choice of Narcotic Analgesic. Morphine still ranks as the standard narcotic in most clinical settings (Lasagna, 1964). Meperidine and pentazocine are the chief current competitors. Dependence on these drugs was initially thought to be less than with morphine, but this putative advantage has long since been dispelled for meperidine, and recently, cases of dependence on pentazocine have been documented. *Principle: Dependence is such a minor risk in clinical situations that it should not be a strong factor in making a choice between narcotics.* Rather, such factors as the differential response of patients to side effects or the personal preference of patients are more valid determinants for the choice of drug. Meperidine is somewhat shorter acting than morphine, but pentazocine shows no appreciable difference in duration of action, given in doses that produce equivalent analgesia. Morphone or morphinan derivatives offer no appreciable advantages over these drugs.

Codeine and D-propoxyphene are frequently used analgesics. Although these drugs technically are narcotics, they are ranked with the nonnarcotic analgesics for clinical indications. *Principle: Classification of drugs by their chemical structures has liabilities as well as assets. Drugs of the same chemical class may have different clinical indications* (see Chapter 15).

Doses, Routes of Administration, and Dosage Schedule. The initial analgesic dose of morphine usually is 10 mg given parenterally. Occasionally this dose may be incorrect, depending upon the weight of the patient or the severity of his pain. Often the response to the first dose can be used as a guide for selection of subsequent doses. *Principle: The least dose required to produce satisfactory relief of pain is desirable; no more, and certainly no less.* Meperidine is about one-eighth as potent as morphine when both are given parenterally, and pentazocine one-third to one-fourth as potent (Paddock *et al.*, 1969). The subcutaneous route is usually preferred, but in situations requiring rapid relief of pain, such as severe burns or injuries, slow intravenous administration of drug is necessary. Oral doses of these drugs are three to four times larger than parenteral doses and are seldom used for treating acute severe pain.

Rather than to prescribe routinely "10 mg of morphine sulfate subcutaneously every 4 hours as needed," it is better to consider the clinical condition, possible contraindications, and the actual need of the patient. Then the dose can be better established, and the dosage interval can be based on the patient's need. The patient should initiate the request for medication, and either the physician or nurse should decide when it is necessary. If the patient does not ask for the drug, he should be consulted before a dose is given; he may have perfectly good reasons for not wanting it. A collection of abdominal gas precipitated by an opiate may be more uncomfortable than postoperative pain. A more reasonable order might be "upon request or assent of the patient, but no oftener than every 2 hours." Ludicrous as it sounds, patients have been awakened from sound sleep to be given an analgesic or hypnotic ordered at fixed intervals. Routine fixed orders are seldom satisfactory even when the patient has chronic pain. *Principle: Dosage schedules should meet the needs of the patient.*

Unwanted Effects and Contraindications. Most unwanted effects are extensions of primary pharmacologic actions rather than allergic or idiosyncratic reactions (see Chapter 15). Some contraindications are established by concurrent diseases or by other drugs being given concurrently (see Chapter 16).

Central Nervous System. Patients with myxedema do not tolerate sedatives and narcotics well. Frank coma may be precipitated by even conventional doses of either class of drugs. Untreated myxedema is a definite contraindication to the use of morphine or kindred drugs.

The central depressant effects of morphine are additive with other drugs, such as phenothiazines, tricyclic antidepressants, monoamine oxidase inhibitors, or conventional sedative-hypnotic drugs. Morphine, meperidine, and pentazocine are mainly metabolized in the liver (Berkowitz and Way, 1969). Consequently, in patients with hepatic failure, the prolonged effects of narcotics must be anticipated. As with sedative-hypnotics, some patients react paradoxically to narcotics, becoming excited rather than sedated. Pentazocine, an analog of nalorphine, often elicits psychotomimetic effects that limit the utility of the drug. Oral doses of 240 mg elicit psychotomimetic effects (Beaver *et al.*, 1968).

Respiratory System. The dangers of giving drugs that depress respiration or obtund consciousness in patients with impaired pulmonary function apply with special emphasis to narcotics (see Chapter 6). Pulmonary failure, bronchial asthma, and cor pulmonale are generally considered to be relative contraindications to narcotics, which may be lethal unless blood gases can be measured and artificial ventilation provided.

Nonnarcotic Analgesics

Chemical Structures. The important drugs in this group are derivatives of salicylic acid and aniline. The major salicylic acid derivatives include sodium salicylate, aspirin, and salicylamide and are closely related (top, Figure 11–8). Acetanilid is the simplest modification of the aniline structure; acetophenetidin (phenacetin) has an ethoxy substituent at the para position. Both drugs are metabolized to an active metabolite, acetaminophen (Tylenol) or p-aminophenol (middle, Figure 11–8). The chemical relationship between aminopyrine and phenylbutazone (Butazolidin) and the aniline series is less evident. These drugs are often referred to as pyrazolone derivatives based on the five-membered ring structure (bottom, Figure 11–8). Phenylbutazone also has an active metabolite, oxyphenbutazone (Tandearil), created by para-hydroxylation of the phenyl group. Mefenamic

acid (Ponstel) is related structurally to these compounds.

Pharmacologic Effects. *Analgesia.* Virtually all drugs in this group have analgesic, antipyretic, and anti-inflammatory effects (see Chapter 9), but differ considerably in the relative proportion of each of these actions. Aspirin is the standard drug for comparing analgesic effects and has not been surpassed. Although aspirin has many central actions and may in part modify pain by a central effect, current evidence indicates that its primary site for analgesia is peripheral (Guzman and Lim, 1968; Collier, 1969). Aspirin, sodium salicylate, acetaminophen, and phenylbutazone block the pain response elicited by injection of bradykinin by peripheral effects. The narcotic analgesics are ineffective when they can only reach peripheral sites (Beaver, 1966; Coffman, 1966; Keele, 1969). Such findings suggest that salicylates, anilines, and other nonnarcotic drugs may act directly on receptor sites for pain, antagonize formed chemical mediators, or prevent the formation of pain mediators, of which bradykinin is an example. *Principle: When two classes*

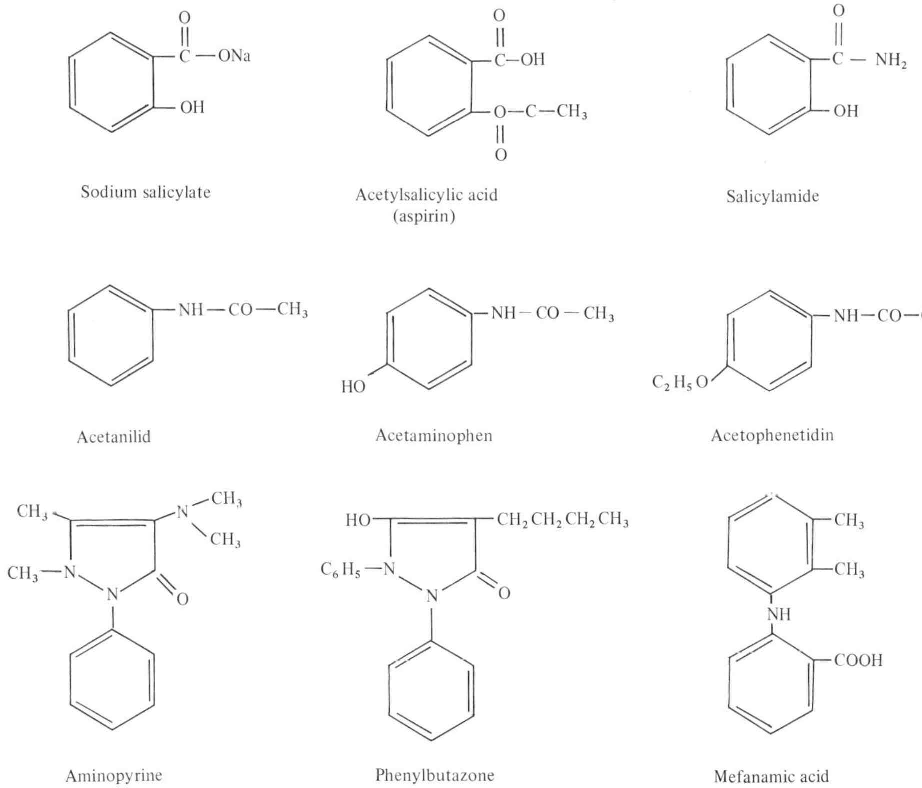

Figure 11–8. Chemical structural relationships between various types of nonnarcotic analgesics.

of drugs act by different mechanisms, their simultaneous use may be both rational and efficacious.

Antipyretic Effect. Before specific remedies were available for diseases that produce fever, antipyretic drugs were used effectively to reduce the detrimental effects of high fever. Some might argue that most fevers should not be lowered except by removal of their cause, as fever is a normal body defense against a number of inciting agents. Still, it is hard to convince a patient suffering the miseries of aching muscles and chills from a viral infection that he should be thankful that the elevated body temperature may impede replication of the virus and that he should abstain from aspirin. Furthermore, very high fever may produce more damage than benefit. The antipyretic effect seems to be entirely due to a central action. Loss of heat is primarily through the skin, mediated by increased cutaneous blood flow and possibly, but not necessarily, by increased sweating.

Anti-inflammatory Effects. This action is often difficult to separate from the analgesic effect. In fact, the anti-inflammatory effects of aspirin were long overlooked until objective comparisons were made between aspirin and corticosteroids in diseases such as rheumatoid arthritis or rheumatic fever. Subsequently, aspirin has been shown to antagonize a great many substances that may play a role in the inflammatory process (see Chapter 9). It is rather remarkable that a single drug has such profound effects against the body's defense mechanisms of pain, fever, and inflammation.

Central Nervous System Effects. Although aspirin has effects on the central nervous system when taken in toxic doses (see Chapter 17), notable central nervous system effects seldom follow normal doses. Some have alleged, but not proved, that aspirin may have some characteristics analogous to those of sedatives (Krumholz *et al.*, 1964). Nausea and vomiting are more likely due to local gastric irritation than to a central action.

Other Effects. Aspirin in large doses stimulates release of adrenocorticotropic hormone, but clinically this action is of no significance. A number of effects on prothrombin time, platelets, bleeding time, and other coagulation processes, as well as its effect on uric acid clearance, are discussed in Chapters 4, 6, 7, 9, 16, and 17.

Clinical Use. The nonnarcotic analgesics are most effective in treating pain arising from the integument or from the musculoskeletal system. They are particularly effective for headache or arthritis. Because pain frequently recurs or is chronic, preference for aspirin over the narcotic analgesics is justified (Beaver, 1970). In addition, the anti-inflammatory effects contribute added benefits. Aspirin may have been overlooked as an analgesic in some types of pain ordinarily treated by narcotics, such as pain from wounds or burns. Aspirin ameliorates most types of pain, with the exception of pain arising from periodic contractions of smooth muscle. When aspirin is used, smaller-than-customary doses of narcotic analgesics may be needed and fewer side effects of both drugs might result. An analogy is the routine use of thiazide diuretics to diminish doses and side effects of antihypertensive agents (see Chapter 5). Because nonnarcotic drugs must be given orally, their routine use is not always feasible, e.g., in postoperative pain following gastric surgery.

As with other drugs, a plateau in response may be reached as doses are increased. Graded responses are observed over a range of 300 to 1200 mg of aspirin, but higher doses simply increase toxicity, including local gastric irritation. When aspirin is given, gastric irritation is almost inevitable. Despite these limitations, aspirin is a widely applicable analgesic.

The constant discussion of aspirin rather than other nonnarcotic drugs as analgesics seems justified on the basis of most clinical comparisons (Beaver, 1966). Aspirin is superior to sodium salicylate and acetophenetidin and equal to acetaminophen as an analgesic or antipyretic. Acetaminophen may not be as toxic as aspirin in certain situations and may be the drug of choice when aspirin is poorly tolerated. Acetanilid and acetophenetidin must be metabolized, and their use in preference to acetaminophen seems irrational.

Aminopyrine lapsed into well-deserved obscurity for many years. However, it has been included in a number of proprietary analgesics and has caused a resurgence of cases of agranulocytosis. Phenylbutazone should not be regarded as an analgesic. Its active metabolite, oxyphenbutazone, is preferred for treatment of rheumatic disorders or gout. Mefenamic acid is a weaker analgesic than aspirin and its toxicity is serious.

Some may argue that to use one aspirin tablet (usually 325 mg) is analogous to using 1 pt of blood for transfusion; each will either do little good or is not indicated. Although a larger dose (650 mg) may not result in markedly higher concentrations of salicylate in plasma, it persists longer (see Chapter 2). The preferred single dose is usually two tablets. Three (975 mg) or four tablets (1300 mg) may be required when pain is severe or when one wishes to sustain relief (as during sleep). There is practically no experience with higher single doses. Within the above range of doses, increasing therapeutic effects may be expected.

Frequency of doses depends on many variables: the half-life of the drug in the particular patient, the amount of fluid intake, the urine pH, and other factors that may affect the concentration of drug in plasma and its rate of urinary excretion. The salicylate half-life varies over a threefold range among different individuals following single doses (Levy and Hollister, 1964). Consequently, it makes little sense to specify an arbitrary interval of time between doses, such as "every 4 hours," without good reason. The patient may offer the best clues, and the interval between doses may be based on his demands. Assuming that single doses are small and the patient's demands genuine, toxicity is not likely to occur. After several doses have been given, the interval between doses may increase as a plateau of salicylate and possibly of unhydrolyzed aspirin concentration in plasma is attained (see Chapter 2). *Principle: The best single dose of aspirin is that adequate to relieve pain; the proper dosage interval is that which sustains relief without causing toxicity.*

Considering that aspirin is an acid, it is taken in a cavalier fashion. Patients who self-administer the drug seem content to wash it down with the fewest possible swallows of water. Nurses dispense it with small amounts of water. Many patients complain of gastric intolerance or show evidence of gastrointestinal blood loss when careful measurements are made. The simple expedient of taking aspirin with 6 or 8 oz of water would probably reduce these difficulties by providing more rapid dissolution of the tablet. Indeed, if warm water is used, the levels of aspirin in plasma are even more rapidly attained.

The dosage form of aspirin must be considered, as discussed in Chapter 2. Because tablets of aspirin are inexpensive, they are most commonly used. The ideal tablet would dissolve quickly enough to prevent retention of irritant at a single point in the stomach. Some brands that disintegrate within seconds may irritate the patient's throat or esophagus. Enteric-coated aspirin has been posed as an alternative to uncoated tablets, but these preparations are often unreliably absorbed. Buffered tablets have no appreciable advantage over "regular" aspirin tablets, although some are more elegant pharmaceutical formulations (in line with their far greater expense) and provide slightly more rapid delivery of drug. Aspirin in solution, buffered with stoichiometric amounts of sodium bicarbonate, might be expected to be the best dosage form, but is a cumbersome formulation with very high sodium content. Other buffered

forms may be better (Leonards and Levy, 1969). Delayed- or prolonged-action formulations of aspirin are of limited value; at the very best, they might provide a more acceptable way of delivering a large single dose of aspirin when one wishes to sustain an effect overnight.

Although classified as narcotic analgesics, codeine, D-propoxyphene, and orally administered pentazocine are often used in clinical situations where nonnarcotic analgesics are indicated. Precisely equivalent therapeutic doses between these drugs and aspirin are estimates at best, but appear to be approximately 60 mg codeine, 65 mg D-propoxyphene, and 50 mg of pentazocine as equal to 650 mg of aspirin (Kantor *et al.*, 1966). Codeine may have some advantage over aspirin in having a higher ceiling of analgesic effect (demonstrable up to 360-mg oral doses), but this advantage has not been proved for the others (Beaver, 1966). Doses of less than 65 mg of D-propoxyphene have been difficult to distinguish from placebo. As preparations of this drug are available that contain only one-half that amount, it seems possible that one is giving little more than placebo (see Chapter 14). In general, nonnarcotic analgesics are preferred to these drugs, but combining the two different types of drugs may be useful in obtaining a greater degree of analgesia than can be obtained from either alone.

Adverse effects of aspirin, including gastrointestinal bleeding, allergic reactions, and the management of accidental or suicidal overdoses, are discussed in Chapters 10 and 17.

Because acetaminophen is less likely to cause gastric irritation or massive gastrointestinal bleeding, it may be the preferred drug for patients for whom aspirin is contraindicated because of ulcer disease. Cross-sensitivity between aspirin and acetaminophen in patients allergic to aspirin has not been demonstrated, but allergy to acetaminophen may occur. Overdoses of acetaminophen are not associated with profound hyperventilation or the severe acid-base imbalance characteristic of aspirin overdose and may be easier to treat.

Chronic interstitial nephritis, renal papillary necrosis, and chronic pyelonephritis have been encountered in patients chronically using analgesic mixtures containing acetophenetidin (Gilman, 1964; Harrow, 1967; Shelley, 1967). As this drug (but also aspirin) was a common denominator in most such mixtures (the most frequently used being aspirin compound or APC), it seemed logical to incriminate it as a pathogenetic factor. Not surprisingly, matters are not that simple. Acetophenetidin produces less renal irritation than aspirin, as judged by renal cell counts in urine. As acetophenetidin is seldom used alone, it is difficult to determine if this drug produces renal complications. The best conclusion at present is that the renal complications may be related to some combined, or possibly synergistic, effect of the components of analgesic mixtures rather than solely to acetophenetidin. There are other compelling reasons why such mixtures should not be used (see below), but unfortunately, a vast number of these analgesic mixtures is available for over-the-counter sale and self-administration.

Acetophenetidin and acetanilid have metabolites that may induce methemoglobinemia. Acetophenetidin is metabolized in small part to aniline, then to ethoxyaniline, both of which produce methemoglobin. Rarely is this complication clinically important. Autoimmune hemolytic anemia, as well as hemolytic anemia in the presence of glucose-6-phosphate dehydrogenase deficiency, may be elicited by acetophenetidin or other aniline derivatives (see Chapter 15).

Aminopyrine and some of its analogs, such as dipyrone, produce agranulocytosis by an immunologic mechanism. These drugs have recently been reintroduced into analgesic mixtures, so that patients and often their physicians are not aware of the risk. A recent upsurge of reports of agranulocytosis attributable to these drugs has disclosed this nefarious practice (Huguley, 1964). Under the circumstances, the risk from aminopyrine and its congeners is not justified by the benefits. *Principle: Patients take many more drugs than physicians prescribe. Always be concerned about what your patient buys over the counter and what such preparations contain* (see Chapters 14, 15, and 16).

Other Drugs That Alleviate Pain

Phenylbutazone was included among the nonnarcotic analgesics because it has some clinical relationship to aminopyrine. It is never used simply for pain. Similarly, indomethacin is used only for its anti-inflammatory effects (see Chapter 9).

Sedatives, antianxiety agents, and phenothiazine derivatives, either alone or in combination with other analgesics, have been used for pain. Use of sedatives alone for pain may lead to delirium, by obtunding consciousness without specifically blocking the transmission of pain. Conversely, relief from pain does not always guarantee relief from anxiety or permit sleep. The addition of phenobarbital, pentobarbital, or chlordiazepoxide to analgesics to manage pain may improve rest. Because most sedative drugs alleviate muscle spasm, they may be especially useful when pain is attributable to spasm of skeletal muscle.

Although chlorpromazine was initially used in a mixture to potentiate narcotic anesthesia, the drug was found to have a more important use as an antipsychotic. As normal persons often poorly tolerate the unusual sedative effects of antipsychotic drugs, another phenothiazine, promethazine (Phenergan), is more commonly used in combination with narcotic analgesics. This combination is particularly useful for preoperative or postoperative pain in surgical or obstetric patients. Another antihistaminic phenothiazine, methotrimeprazine (Levoprome), is a more specific analgesic (Beaver *et al.*, 1966). As this drug is merely a chemical modification of trimeprazine (Temaril), it is difficult to explain its stronger and more specific analgesic action. Methotrimeprazine when given parenterally is comparable in efficacy to morphine and meperidine, and as addiction is not at all likely, methotrimeprazine may have great usefulness in chronic pain states requiring potent analgesics for prolonged periods. Unfortunately, its tendency to produce orthostatic hypotension limits its usefulness (AMA Council on Drugs, 1968).

Recently, the analgesic properties of dextroamphetamine have been recognized, adding even another dimension to this remarkable drug. On the basis of animal tests, the drug might best be used in combination with other analgesics (Evans, 1962). Preliminary studies of a combination of 10 mg of dextroamphetamine with 10 mg of morphine are in progress; it is hypothesized that analgesia will be enhanced and sleepiness and mental confusion reduced as compared with morphine alone.

Combinations of Analgesic Drugs

Combinations of analgesics have a long tradition. If such combinations are extemporaneous rather than fixed, more can be said in their favor than against them. Fixed combinations do not afford the flexibility of dose and timing required for maximum benefits from combination therapy.

Morphine or meperidine has often been used simultaneously with scopolamine, exploiting not only the anticholinergic properties of the latter drug but also its tendency to produce amnesia. Such use has been particularly appropriate in situations when surgical procedures may be relatively brief and extensive general anesthesia is not desirable, such as obstetric delivery. The combination of promethazine and narcotic analgesics is clinically satisfactory, not only because analgesia is increased, but because of the mild anticholinergic and antiemetic properties of the phenothiazine. Although various attempts have been made to combine two or more narcotic analgesics, little evidence supports the superiority of combinations over equivalent doses of single drugs.

Two combinations of oral analgesics have a long tradition. One, the combination of aspirin, acetophenetidin (phenacetin), and caffeine (aspirin compound, APC), makes little sense and may have positive disadvantages. The strongest case against aspirin compound is that it may be erroneously thought to be the equal of aspirin. By combining two similar drugs, aspirin and acetophenetidin, nothing is gained, but as acetophenetidin is less effective than aspirin, something is lost. The minute amount of caffeine in such mixtures is unlikely to have any appreciable effect, especially in the majority of adults who have already developed some degree of tolerance for caffeine. Although combinations of similar drugs are often rationalized on the basis of reduced doses causing fewer side effects from either drug, such a happy consequence is unlikely with this combination. Rather, the patient might be more likely to develop side effects peculiar to each drug.

The combination of aspirin with codeine is of considerable value. The combination is not only clinically effective but also rational. The drugs alleviate pain by different mechanisms; there is every reason to believe that the effects are truly additive. Codeine is easily and readily absorbed when taken orally and has the highest ratio of oral/parenteral potency (0.68) of any narcotic analgesic. Extemporaneous combination of these two drugs is easily managed and provides a broad range of analgesic effect. As codeine has relatively little potential for causing dependence, use of this combination is suitable for chronic as well as acute pain. Unfortunately, fixed combinations of oxycodone or dextropropoxyphene with what is essentially aspirin compound (Percodan and Darvon Compound, respectively) have become quite popular. As neither narcotic is as effective as codeine, and as aspirin compound is less effective than aspirin, it would seem far wiser to rely on extemporaneous combinations of aspirin and codeine. *Principle: Combinations of analgesic drugs are rational when drugs with different mechanisms of action are combined and irrational when drugs with similar mechanisms of action are combined. Extemporaneous combinations provide far more flexibility and range of analgesic effects than do fixed combinations.*

DRUGS FOR TREATING OR PREVENTING SEIZURES

Diagnostic Considerations and Pathogenetic Mechanisms

General Statement of Problem. Epilepsy afflicts between 1 and 2% of the population and the incidence seems to be increasing owing to the prolongation of lives of brain-injured patients. Part of the rise is ascribable to diagnostic refinements, especially in electroencephalographic techniques. Most epileptics, perhaps 90%, develop their initial symptoms during childhood, adolescence, or youth. Many instances of epilepsy developing past age 20 represent an acquired brain disorder such as the residuals of head injury, diseases, or infections affecting the central nervous system, metabolic disorders, or intracranial neoplasms. Even in patients 40 years of age the diagnosis of a newly appearing seizure may ultimately be idiopathic epilepsy. The latter term remains applicable to the majority of epileptic patients, generally exceeding 70%.

Epilepsy constitutes a lifelong disability for many patients, although some, especially those with childhood and posttraumatic seizure disorders, eventually become seizure free.

The patient must contend not only with the possibility of unpredictable and unexpected disability, but also with the embarrassment caused by a seizure in public. The epileptic may be discriminated against in employment opportunities and is usually forbidden to drive a motor vehicle. In addition to the physical dangers of an unpredictable seizure, which may include death by asphyxia, the possibility of closely spaced successive bursts of seizures, as in status epilepticus, constitutes a life-threatening medical emergency. Many epileptic patients must be treated without interruption for the remainder of their lives if they are to be spared these dangers and be fully productive.

Classification and Description of Seizure Disorders. Many isolated seizures, such as those associated with alcoholism, hypoglycemia, or fever in children, are symptomatic and should not be diagnosed as epilepsy. The clinician should regard any transient, recurrent neurologic or psychologic dysfunction as a seizure until proved otherwise. Numerous classifications of seizure patterns have been proposed, usually differing only slightly in point of view. Many are based on characteristic electroencephalographic changes. One might be tempted to adopt a classification based on response to drugs, but this would not be entirely reliable. Consequently, the following modified classification is utilized (Gastaut et al., 1964).

Generalized Seizures. This category includes seizures characterized by motor disturbances or by impaired consciousness.

The most common type of epilepsy is grand mal, manifested by major motor seizures. Grand mal variants include tonic-clonic, tonic or clonic, and atonic motor manifestations. The usual pattern is of a cry, followed by a generalized motor seizure, initially tonic but later with rapidly rhythmic and symmetric jerking movements, with loss of consciousness, lasting for a minute or two. The seizure is followed by complete restoration of function and consciousness within a matter of minutes or hours. Auras, loss of sphincter control, and postictal lethargy or transient paralysis are also features of this type of epilepsy. The electroencephalogram (EEG) may be normal between seizures, but paroxysms of symmetrical slow waves may be evoked by various provocative procedures, such as hyperventilation or sleep. A similar pattern may develop in symptomatic epilepsy, as from a brain tumor, if the focal generator has access to midline structures or to both hemispheres. In such a case, the focal aspect of the seizure may be submerged by the spread to a major convulsive expression and must be carefully sought.

Myoclonic spasms, another epileptic motor symptom, may occur in infancy as sudden, brief, and violent "jackknifing" movements. This disorder is often associated with mental deficiency and is accompanied by a characteristic generalized paroxysmal spike and slow-wave activity (hypsarrhythmia) on the electroencephalogram. Another form occurring in childhood between the ages of 3 and 6 years is less violent and consists of symmetric jerking of muscles of limbs, face, and trunk without loss of consciousness. Gross electroencephalographic abnormalities are also observed. Although many of these children are thought to be mentally defective, the defect may be more apparent than real. Intellectual performance and even psychologic testing may be disturbed by the 200 to 400 electrical "storms" daily, which are not of enough magnitude to evoke a full-blown seizure. Intellectual deficit may show a marked improvement after treatment, owing to diminution of this disruptive electrical activity.

Petit mal is another type of generalized seizure characterized by periods of altered consciousness (absences) lasting for seconds. The seizure is manifested by a blank, staring expression and possibly by minor motor disturbances such as clonic movements of the head or upper extremities. Petit mal attacks, which may recur dozens of times daily, are not recognized by the patient, who is partly amnesic for them. The disorder typically begins in childhood and at puberty may be accompanied or supplanted by grand mal attacks. Lapses or absences that begin past the age of 18 years rarely are petit mal attacks, even though clinically similar. They are most often the result of a focal generator firing in one or both temporal lobes and require different treatment (see below). The EEG pattern evoked by hyperventilation is quite characteristic and shows bilateral synchronous spike and wave patterns at a frequency of about 3 per second. Patients with petit mal attacks account for about 3% of all epileptics, although the frequency is much higher in children than in adults.

Focal Seizures. Simple motor seizures consist of local tonic and clonic movements, often unilateral and sometimes resulting in the patient's assuming strange postural forms. They may spread locally in the "jacksonian march." Focal spikes and sharp or slow waves may be superimposed on a background of generalized abnormal activity in the EEG. Complex seizures, which may be psychomotor or psychosensory, include those arising in the temporal lobes. Psychomotor seizures may consist of sudden bizarre, but often seemingly purposeful, movements of an automatic and repetitive nature. Some typical movements include masticatory, swallowing, or adversive movements. Milder manifestations include lapses, as described above. Such patients often exhibit bizarre behavior between attacks, and many are diagnosed as being schizophrenic. The personality disturbance in these patients may be due either to disturbance of memory and learning or to disordered perception produced by recurrent subclinical bursts of seizures in limbic structures. Early diagnosis and treatment, especially in children, may be important in preventing the mental disorder. Sensory seizures may include visual, auditory, olfactory, or gustatory experiences. At times, the change in mental function during such attacks resembles that produced by psychotomimetic drugs and includes loss of contact with reality, mental confusion, hallucinatory and dream states, illusions, and blocking of normal thought processes.

Psychomotor seizures are generally much more difficult to diagnose than other types of epilepsy and therefore are often missed. The number of afflicted patients is very likely greater than ordinarily supposed. A diagnostic clue is the appearance in the EEG of focal spikes or sharp and slow waves in the anterior temporal and adjacent regions on one or both sides, usually on a background of generalized abnormal activity. Therapeutic response to drugs may also be helpful in establishing the diagnosis. However, the diagnosis may be masked by the anticonvulsants often given to these patients for attendant grand mal attacks.

Epileptic Equivalents. Recurrent attacks of headaches, dizziness, abdominal pains, vomiting, inappropriate laughing spells, and fainting are considered as nonconvulsive manifestations of epilepsy when they are associated with abnormalities in the EEG. The physiologic basis for such equivalents is believed to be either a focal discharge producing a subjective response or a more generalized electrical disturbance that alters perception but does not involve the motor cortex. A therapeutic trial with anticonvulsants often helps to establish the diagnosis. *Accurate diagnosis of the type of epileptic disorder is crucial, because the diagnosis strongly determines the choice of drugs.*

Pathogenetic Mechanisms. The mechanism of seizure production appears to be similar, regardless of whether a specific cause is discovered or whether the condition is diagnosed as "idiopathic" epilepsy. The necessity for discovering specific causes is clear. Some of the causes are remediable or at least require prompt treatment and, if not, add an element of urgency to undertaking treatment with drugs. Urgency in initiating treatment is less in seizure disorders of unknown cause.

The normal brain is unstable, with millions of neurons firing at different times. The brain is relatively resistant to spontaneous seizures because inhibitory feedback loops regulate the frequency of firing of individual neurons. This prevents synchronization of neuronal firing to the degree necessary to cause self-regenerative neuronal firing. During a seizure, many more neurons than normal fire in a synchronous fashion in a particular part of the brain. This explosion, or paroxysm, may spread to contiguous areas and may lead to a generalized discharge of brain neurons. In contrast to the usual EEG pattern (with relatively low-voltage and fairly high-frequency waves), that seen during a major epileptic attack may show peaked high-voltage waves (spikes) with rapid and repetitive firing or, large, wide, high-voltage slow waves. The physiologic fault seems to be the lack of the normal mechanisms by which neurons inhibit each other and desynchronize their activity.

The trigger for seizures may be either focal or diffuse. It acts either by increasing the rate of actively firing neurons, thereby achieving a statistical synchronization with summation, or by interfering with inhibiting connections that regulate the rate of firing. Rarely can the whole brain be considered epileptic; usually the seizure is triggered from a local area. In idiopathic epilepsy, the area producing the abnormal firing shows no manifest histopathology, but is presumed to be abnormal in its fine structural organization, physiology, or biochemistry. Once an epileptogenic lesion is established, many extrinsic factors can trigger it. Among these stimuli are hyperventilation, overeating, hypoglycemia, premenstrual fluid retention, various stages of sleep, rapid blinking or other rhythmic photic stimulation, strong emotional states such as fright or embarrassment, fever, alcohol intake, or a reduction in medication. *Principle: In the total management of the patient with epilepsy, the physician must try to control the extrinsic triggers to which a patient may be responsive.*

To some extent, seizure disorders may be considered self-perpetuating, even though the individual seizure is clearly self-limited. Whether repeated seizures can cause increased disorganization of neural behavior greater than that initially present is still uncertain. Some clinical evidence suggests that treatment may limit disorganization. Many motor seizures are associated with significant cerebral anoxia that may add to neuronal damage. Mental deterioration and gliosis in the region of Ammon's horn, although rare, are clinical and pathologic indicators that repeated uncontrolled major seizures may produce progressive damage.

There are two possible means of pharmacologic attack on the seizure disorders. The capacity of the local trigger area for repetitive, synchronous firing may be diminished by raising the threshold for firing. Drugs such as phenobarbital generally operate at this level. In another approach, the propagation of excessive firing to contiguous areas of the brain is prevented. Drugs such as diphenylhydantoin act in this fashion by diminishing nerve membrane excitability.

Anticonvulsant Drugs

Chemical Structures. The four major groups of anticonvulsant drugs are variations on a similar chemical theme (Figure 11–9). The six-membered barbiturate nucleus comprises one group, but has been truncated to a five-membered ring in the case of the other groups. The hydantoins have a nitrogen atom at the 1-position of the five-membered ring, the oxazolidones have an oxygen atom at this position, and the succinimides have a carbon atom at the 1-position. The substituents at the 5-position in any of these classes may be a combination of aromatic and aliphatic groups (e.g., phenyl and ethyl groups in the case of phenobarbital), two aromatic groups (e.g., diphenylhydantoin [Dilantin]), or a mixture of two aliphatic groups (e.g., mephenytoin [Mesantoin], the oxazolidones, and phensuximide [Milontin]). The non-N-methylated compounds are usually preferred, as N-demethylation very likely occurs quickly in the body. *Principle: When the fate of chemicals in the body is known, rational choice between congeners often can be made.*

Pharmacologic Actions. Despite some of the

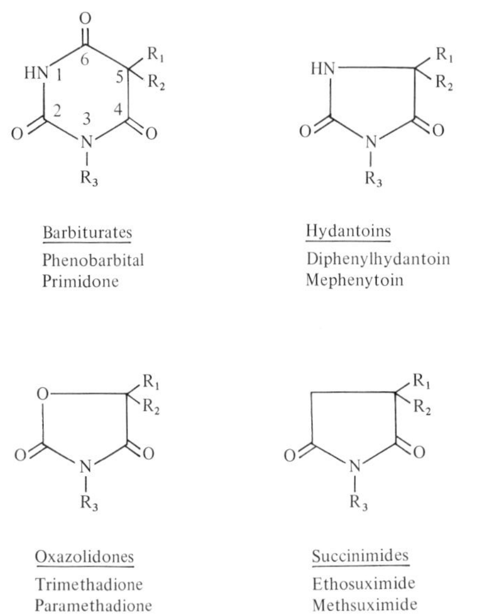

Figure 11–9. Chemical structural relationships of various types of anticonvulsants.

chemical similarities between the four classes of drugs, they differ considerably in their pharmacologic behavior. The usual assay of a drug with potential anticonvulsant activity measures its effect in modifying experimental seizures induced in animals by electroshock or pentylenetetrazole. Both produce both tonic and clonic phases of seizures, and in the case of electroshock, the seizures can be graded in intensity (Millichap, 1969).

All drugs effective against grand mal tonic convulsions protect mice against the tonic component of electroshock seizures. Primidone is the most potent. Seizures induced in mice by pentylenetetrazole are best prevented by phenobarbital and primidone, whereas diphenylhydantoin seems to have little effect. Drugs used in the treatment of petit mal are less potent against experimental seizures than are those employed in the treatment of grand mal. Contrary to previous beliefs, activity against pentylenetetrazole seizures is not a good predictor of clinical efficacy in petit mal; trimethadione is very weak in this regard, whereas phenobarbital is potent, yet trimethadione is much more effective clinically. The majority of drugs advocated for psychomotor seizures have approximately equal activity against both maximal electroshock and pentylenetetrazole seizures. *Principle: The model of induced seizures in animals to screen anticonvulsants leaves much to be desired. Inactivity in such tests does not necessarily mean that the drug has no clinically useful anticonvulsant activity.*

Differences in structure-activity relationships provide only limited clues to the differing clinical effects of anticonvulsant drugs. The substituents at position 5 are important. A phenyl group at this position protects against the tonic phase of electroshock seizures. Diphenylhydantoin, with two phenyl radicals, prevents the cortical spread of focal seizures and clinically protects against generalized tonic-clonic seizures. Alkyl radicals at position 5 confer protection against pentylenetetrazole-induced seizures in animals, but this action is not necessarily predictive of efficacy against petit mal. Drugs having both phenyl and alkyl groups at position 5, such as phenobarbital, mephenytoin, methsuximide (Celontin), and primidone (Mysoline), protect against both types of experimental seizures, but have inconstant clinical effects between grand mal and petit mal attacks.

With one conspicuous exception, the biochemical effects of anticonvulsants do not explain their mode of action. Most do not change respiration of the brain or influence the concentration of biogenic amines in brain. The exception is that diphenylhydantoin enhances the extrusion of sodium from cells. This effect may be of considerable importance in maintaining a state of hyperpolarization of the cell membrane that thereby prevents the spread of firing from seizure foci to other areas of the brain. Acetazolamide also influences ion distribution by diminishing the entry of sodium into cells, such as would occur during depolarization. Considerable work needs to be done to establish the mechanism of action of these drugs. These described effects may be simply measurable but indirect concomitants of another effect. By analogy to the speculations on the antiarrhythmic effects of diphenylhydantoin in cardiac tissue, enhanced repolarization could enhance conduction in depressed inhibitory fibers or prevent the development of abnormal, repetitively firing cyclic pathways. *Principle: Do not accept a known action of a drug as the basis for its therapeutic effect, as this may inhibit exploration of alternative pathophysiologic mechanisms and pharmacologic interventions.*

Special Anticonvulsants and Adjunctive Drugs. A number of drugs are useful for managing epilepsy, either in special situations or as adjuncts to a program including multiple drugs. The carbonic anhydrase inhibitor acetazolamide (Diamox) has been effective in the management of patients with resistant attacks of both grand mal and petit mal. A few investigators regard acetazolamide as the most effective drug for petit mal. Unfortunately, tolerance develops quickly to the inhibition of this enzyme, so that only brief courses of the drug are efficacious.

Further, the drug penetrates brain poorly. Thus some basic program of anticonvulsants must always be given as well. The therapeutic effects are believed to result from the action of the drug on permeability of the cell membrane, but other feasible beneficial effects include the production of a mild metabolic acidosis and possibly an increase in carbon dioxide tension in brain cells.

Use of phenacemide (Phenurone), a 5-phenylacetylurea with an open ring structure between the 1- and 5-positions, is limited to patients with psychomotor attacks completely resistant to other anticonvulsants. Its serious side effects, including mental symptoms, blood dyscrasias, and hepatitis, do not justify its use under other circumstances.

Myoclonic seizures in infants are especially responsive to a benzodiazepine derivative, nitrazepam. This drug, which is chemically and pharmacologically related to the antianxiety drugs chlordiazepoxide and diazepam, probably owes its efficacy to additive sedative, muscle relaxant, and anticonvulsant properties. The drug is not available in the United States, but it is likely that diazepam might be successfully used for the same indication (Snyder, 1968). Diazepam has also been used successfully in the treatment of status epilepticus. It can be administered intravenously and has considerably fewer respiratory depressant effects than other sedatives.

Amphetamines and other sympathomimetic stimulants may be used for alleviating oversedation caused by large doses of phenobarbital or other sedative anticonvulsants. Rather than aggravating seizures, as one might suppose, amphetamine seems to increase the effects of the anticonvulsants, perhaps by decreasing the triggering effect of drowsiness on seizures. Amphetamine is also useful in treating emotional lability, hyperactivity, and behavior disturbances in epileptic children.

Choice of Anticonvulsant Drugs. Satisfactory treatment of patients with generalized or focal motor seizures is generally achieved by the use of one or more of three drugs: phenobarbital, diphenylhydantoin, and primidone (Karnes, 1968). Although treatment should be started with only one drug, and estimates of its effect should be made before addition of a second drug, often a combination of phenobarbital and diphenylhydantoin is finally used. Because phenobarbital is easy to administer, often efficacious, inexpensive, and relatively less toxic than other anticonvulsants, it should be used first. Initial doses must be gauged so as to avoid excessive sedation, but with time, doses of 65 mg two or three times daily may be tolerated. If seizures are controlled by phenobarbital, this drug should be continued alone. For those patients unable to tolerate fully therapeutic doses of phenobarbital, diphenylhydantoin may be added, initially in doses of 100 mg twice daily, but possibly increasing to 200 mg twice daily. Alternatively, a large single loading dose may be given to hasten development of therapeutic levels of drug. Primidone, related to the barbiturates, is a weak second choice to combine with diphenylhydantoin, as it is less potent and more prone to cause side effects. Each of these three drugs is essentially equal in efficacy when used alone. The efficacy of various combinations must be assessed by the response of the patient.

The array of drugs used for treating petit mal seizures is quite different. Acetazolamide is considered by some to be the most effective drug, but it is rarely effective alone for long periods. Usually, treatment is started with ethsuximide, using doses of 250 mg two or three times daily. If the succinimide drugs do not adequately control attacks, one of the oxazolidones, such as trimethadione or paramethadione (Paradione), should be tried, using doses of 300 mg two or three times daily. Phenobarbital may be used prophylactically against latent grand mal seizures in patients with an early age of onset and a clear family history of severe disorders. Acetazolamide or thiazide diuretics may be especially useful in relieving the premenstrual aggravation of attacks in women.

Complex temporal lobe seizures respond better to primidone than to phenobarbital. The usual initial dose should be small, perhaps 250 mg two or three times daily. Often, adequate control requires treatment with a combination of drugs, and methsuximide is the logical second drug to be added, in doses of 300 mg three or four times daily. Diphenylhydantoin and mephenytoin are also effective against psychomotor seizures and are especially indicated when these are mixed with motor seizures. Phenacemide is used solely in patients with this disorder or in those with mixed seizures who are refractory to other drug therapy. Doses of 250 mg three times daily should be tried initially, but this dose may be doubled if necessary.

Myoclonic seizures are best treated initially with a benzodiazepine, as this type of drug is relatively easy and safe to use. Doses of 2.5 to 5 mg of diazepam might be tried twice daily, the major limiting factor being oversedation. If this drug used alone is inadequate, a course of adrenocorticotropin, 20 U.S.P. units intramuscularly, might be given daily for 20 days, strictly empirically. *Principle: Unless there is some compelling need for haste, treatment of patients with seizures should begin with a single drug that is increased to full doses over time. Additional drugs may be added in a similar fashion if adequate control is not achieved by a single drug.*

The treatment of status epilepticus is a true medical emergency, especially when generalized motor seizures occur in close succession. Parenteral medication is required, the intravenous route being preferred. This route is mandatory for diphenylhydantoin, which is poorly absorbed when given intramuscularly. Until recently, sodium phenobarbital and diphenylhydantoin sodium were the mainstays of treatment, but diazepam has added an additional method of control that has proved to be of great value. The intravenous administration of 10 mg of diazepam is frequently sufficient to interrupt the succession of seizures within minutes, with relatively mild and brief impairment of consciousness (Howard *et al.*, 1968). As controlled studies have not yet compared diazepam with intravenous sodium phenobarbital, one cannot be sure that similar control could not be attained with the latter drug in appropriate doses (130 to 260 mg). Although some patients have responded to diazepam after failing to respond to sodium phenobarbital, the favorable result may have been due to an additive effect. A single drug should be used first, with diazepam preferred owing to less sedation. If seizures are not controlled within 15 minutes, a large dose of diphenylhydantoin sodium should be given intravenously, except in infants or patients with cardiac conductive defects. The dose should be between 500 and 1000 mg at a rate not greater than 25 to 50 mg per minute, if adequate concentrations of drug in plasma are to be achieved. Previous failures of this preparation in status epilepticus have probably been due to inadequate doses or to intramuscular administration. Because of the limited solubility of the drug, it must be prepared in solution at pH 11.0. Not only is this solution highly irritating, but when the pH is lowered, the drug may be precipitated in muscle without being absorbed. Additional doses of one of these drugs may be given at hourly intervals if seizures persist, but one must be cautious to avoid drug-induced coma from overtreatment.

Summary Principles: (1) The type of epilepsy must be diagnosed before treatment commences, as many failures to achieve satisfactory control of seizures stem from misdiagnosis. (2) Although the choice of drugs used in the various types of epilepsies may be empiric, proper choice is essential. Thus, managing psychomotor seizures with drugs useful for petit mal may lead to complete failure. Failing to recognize mixed epilepsies also may lead to failure. Mixed epilepsies occur frequently and may require a drug program different from that appropriate for a single disorder. *(3) As a general rule, the safest, most effective, and least expensive drug should be tried first.* Hence considerable emphasis has been placed on phenobarbital. *(4) Although a single drug within a chemical class provides most of the pharmacologic effects of others within that class, occasionally one drug is better tolerated or more effective for individual patients. Rarely should two drugs from the same class be combined unless such a combination might reduce side effects of either while maintaining maximum therapeutic benefits. (5) Except in situations in which rapid control of seizures is deemed of great importance, drugs should be started one at a time and in conservative doses.* The patient should be warned that initial doses may not be fully effective to prevent his becoming discouraged. *(6) The decision to undertake anticonvulsant therapy should not be made lightly, as treatment may last for at least several years, if not a lifetime.* If the patient has had only a single seizure and no obvious cause is determined, the physician might wait to determine the seizure pattern. It might be simpler and safer to forego anticonvulsant therapy than to use it to prevent one seizure a year. *Once the decision to use drugs has been made, the goal should be the suppression of all seizures.* An acceptable level of control is possible in about one half the cases. *In exceptional circumstances, the amount and number of drugs required may cause toxicity to the extent that slightly incomplete control with fewer drugs or lower doses may be an acceptable alternative. The more complete the drug-maintained remission, the more likely remission will be sustained following discontinuation of drugs.* The latter may be attempted after a patient has been seizure free for 2 or 3 years. *(7) Any attempt to discontinue or change treatment should be made slowly and carefully.* Too abrupt a decrease in dose or too rapid a change in medication may provoke seizures. *(8) Combinations of drugs are often required and are very often justified.* The differing points of pharmacologic attack on the pathogenetic mechanisms of seizures, exemplified by phenobarbital and diphenylhydantoin, make such a combination rational. *Aside from supplementing modes of action, combinations may avoid side effects by allowing reduced doses of each single drug used. One must be sure, especially if the side effect is dangerous, that two drugs that produce the same side effect are not used together.* Mesantoin and trimethadione both produce bone marrow depression and are contraindicated in combination. Combinations of drugs are necessary in most cases of mixed epilepsy.

When drugs must be taken continuously for

long periods, lapses in drug-taking may be expected (see Chapter 15). Lapses cannot be great without the possibility of recurrent seizures. To avoid this source of drug failure, reasonable efforts should be made to assure faithful adherence to the drug program. Parents should be actively involved in supervising treatment of children, or responsible adults in supervising patients being treated with anticonvulsants for seizures secondary to a neurologic disorder that might impair judgment or sense of responsibility. In cases of doubt about adherence to drug regimens, determining the concentration of drug in blood or brief hospitalization for observation and control of dosage may be helpful.

Pharmacokinetic Considerations. The two most commonly used anticonvulsant drugs, phenobarbital and diphenylhydantoin, are both rather long acting. Phenobarbital is eliminated at the rate of only 15% in 24 hours, whereas after a steady-state condition has been reached with diphenylhydantoin treatment, the concentration in plasma drops by only 10% in the first 12 hours after discontinuation of treatment. Accordingly, dosage schedules for both drugs need not be frequent; twice-daily schedules should suffice. It may be desirable to give the major part of the daily dose of phenobarbital at night so as to avoid excessive daytime sedation, while equally dividing the daily requirements of diphenylhydantoin.

Concentrations of diphenylhydantoin in plasma can be measured without extreme difficulty and provide a valuable technique for assessing the adequacy of or compliance to therapy. The desired therapeutic concentrations are often 10 μg/ml or more. Mild toxic symptoms occur at concentrations in excess of 15 μg/ml. Consequently a relatively small margin exists for obtaining optimal effects, and the ability to monitor concentration in plasma can be of great practical importance (Gibberd *et al.*, 1970). A wide range of concentrations in plasma is found following similar standard doses of drug in different patients. The mean concentration in plasma was 9.5 μg/ml in 37 patients receiving 4 to 5 mg/kg body weight, but the individual values ranged from 3 to 22 μg/ml. Further, 8 patients had concentrations of 5 μg/ml or less, which might be well below the range of full therapeutic efficacy, and 3 had concentrations well over 15 μg/ml, where toxic effects would be expected. The maximum daily dose usually is 0.5 g or less, as 77% of patients receiving 0.6 g daily develop clinical signs of toxicity.

One of the major metabolic pathways for disposition of diphenylhydantoin is the parahydroxylation of one of the phenyl groups, with subsequent glucuronic acid conjugation and elimination. The urinary output of this compound may account for 50 to 70% of the total amount of drug given, with unmetabolized drug accounting for less than 5%. Some patients have developed toxicity on ordinary doses of the drug owing to a defect in parahydroxylation (Kutt *et al.*, 1964) or due to drug interactions (Kutt *et al.*, 1970). It remains to be seen whether too rapid parahydroxylation in other patients is responsible for unduly low levels of drug. *Principle: The therapeutic and toxic effects of diphenylhydantoin seem to be strongly related to its concentration in plasma, so that close chemical monitoring may lead to more effective use.*

Phenobarbital is an excellent inducer of hepatic-drug-metabolizing enzymes, and levels of diphenylhydantoin are lower following pretreatment with phenobarbital. These findings led to some apprehension that their concurrent use, which is so customary, might materially lessen the efficacy of diphenylhydantoin (Cucinell *et al.*, 1965). Comparison of concentrations of drug in plasma during steady-state conditions in patients taking diphenylhydantoin with or without concurrent phenobarbital (doses of 0.5 to 1.2 mg/kg) revealed only a minor decrease in patients on combined therapy. Further, the addition of phenobarbital to the therapeutic program of patients using diphenylhydantoin led to almost equal numbers of increased, decreased, or unchanged concentrations in plasma. In no instance was the magnitude of change sufficient to be clinically important. Thus it appears that the customary combination is acceptable and advantageous (Kutt *et al.*, 1969).

Unwanted Effects. Few classes of drugs produce a wider array of side effects than do the anticonvulsants. Seldom, however, are side effects of such consequence that effective therapy cannot be continued. The main goal of treatment is to make the patient function optimally. Side effects that lessen normal function cannot be long tolerated. Oversedation is the major problem, especially when phenobarbital is used. Other anticonvulsants cause lesser degrees of sedation, but in the usual combinations, some additive sedative effects may be expected. Doses must be carefully titrated.

A disturbance in folic acid metabolism can be detected in most patients taking anticonvulsant drugs and is seldom recognized clinically (Reynolds *et al.*, 1966). Each of the three major drugs used (phenobarbital, diphenylhydantoin, and primidone) can produce this disorder when used alone, and the disturbance is especially marked when drugs are used in combination. The hematologic consequences of folate deficiency are not too difficult to detect clinically, but the abnormal mental states that accompany folate deficiency are less obvious, ranging from mild confusional states to psychoses resembling schizophrenia (Reynolds, 1967). These disorders may be ameliorated by folic acid treatment.

Principle: With any chronic treatment, the desired effects must be balanced against undesired effects. By keeping the number of drugs used to the minimum, by using combinations of drugs that exploit different pharmacologic actions, and by keeping doses to the lowest adequate to keep the patient seizure free, the therapist can use anticonvulsants with optimum efficacy and minimal toxicity.

REFERENCES

Adelson, D., and Epstein, L. J.: A study of phenothiazines with male and female chronically ill schizophrenic patients. *J. Nerv. Ment. Dis.*, **134**:543–54, 1962.

Alexanderson, B.; Evans, D. A. P.; and Sjoqvist, F.: Steady-state plasma levels of nortriptyline in twins: influence of genetic factors and drug therapy. *Brit. Med. J.*, **4**:764–68, 1969.

Allgén, L-G.: Laboratory experience of lithium toxicity in man. *Acta Psychiat. Scand.*, **207**:98–104, 1969.

AMA Committee on Alcoholism and Addiction: Dependence on barbiturates and other sedative drugs. *J.A.M.A.*, **193**:673–77, 1965.

———: Dependence on amphetamines and other stimulant drugs. *J.A.M.A.*, **197**:1023–27, 1966.

AMA Council on Drugs: A non-narcotic analgesic agent. Methotrimeprazine (Levoprome). *J.A.M.A.*, **204**:161–62, 1968.

Andén, N. E.; Carlsson, A.; and Häggendal, J.: Adrenergic mechanisms. *Ann. Rev. Pharmacol.*, **9**:119–34, 1969.

Angst, J.; Dittrich, A.; and Grof, P.: Course of endogenous affective psychoses and its modification by prophylactic administration of imipramine and lithium. *Int. Pharmacopsychiat.*, **2**:1–11, 1969.

Baastrup, P. C., and Schou, M.: Lithium as a prophylactic agent. Its effect against recurrent depressions and manic-depressive psychosis. *Arch. Gen. Psychiat. (Chicago)*, **16**:162–72, 1967.

Barbeau, A.: L-Dopa therapy in Parkinson's disease: a critical review of nine years' experience. *Canad. Med. Ass. J.*, **101**:791–800, 1969.

Beaver, W. T.: The pharmacologic basis for the choice of an analgesic. II. Mild analgesics. *Pharmacol. Physicians*, **4**: No. 12, 1970.

Beaver, W. T.: Mild analgesics. A review of their clinical pharmacology. *Amer. J. Med. Sci.*, **250**:577–604, 1965; **251**:576–99, 1966.

Beaver, W. T.; Wallenstein, S. L.; Houde, R. W.; and Rogers, A.: A comparison of the analgesic effects of methotrimeprazine and morphine in patients with cancer. *Clin. Pharmacol. Ther.*, **7**:436–46, 1966.

———: A clinical comparison of the effects of oral and intramuscular administration of analgesics: pentazocine and phenazocine. *Clin. Pharmacol. Ther.*, **9**:582–97, 1968.

Beckett, A. H.; Beaven, M. A.; and Robinson, A. E.: Metabolism of chlorpromazine in humans. *Biochem. Pharmacol.*, **12**:779–94, 1963.

Beecher, H. K.: The powerful placebo. *J.A.M.A.*, **159**:1602–1606, 1966.

———: *Measurement of Subjective Responses. Quantitative Effects of Drugs.* Oxford University Press, New York, 1959.

Bellville, J. W.; Forrest, W. H., Jr.; and Brown, B. W., Jr.: Clinical and statistical methodology for cooperative clinical assays of analgesics. *Clin. Pharmacol. Ther.*, **9**:290–302, 1968.

Berkowitz, B., and Way, E. L.: Metabolism and excretion of pentazocine in man. *Clin. Pharmacol. Ther.*, **10**:681–89, 1969.

Blackwell, B., and Shepherd, M.: Prophylactic lithium: Another therapeutic myth? An examination of the evidence to date. *Lancet*, **1**:968–71, 1968.

Bloomfield, S. S.; Tetreault, L.; La Freniere, B.; and Bordeleau, J. M.: A method for the evaluation of hypnotic agents in man. The comparative hypnotic effects of secobarbital, methaqualone and a placebo in normal subjects and in psychiatric patients. *J. Pharmacol. Exp. Ther.*, **156**:375–82, 1967.

Brill, N. Q.; Koegler, R. R.; Epstein, L. J.; and Forgy, E. W.: Controlled study of psychiatric outpatient treatment. *Arch. Gen. Psychiat. (Chicago)*, **10**:581–95, 1964.

Brodie, B.; Dick, P.; Kielholz, P.; Poldinger, W.; and Theobald, W.: Preliminary pharmacological and clinical results with desmethylimipramine (DMI) G-35020, a metabolite of imipramine. *Psychopharmacologia*, **2**:467–74, 1961.

Burt, C. G.; Gordon, W. F.; Holt, N. F.; and Hordern, A.: Amitriptyline in depressive states: a controlled trial. *J. Ment. Sci.*, **108**:711–30, 1962.

Butler, T. C.; Mahaffee, C.; and Waddell, W. J.: Phenobarbital: studies of elimination, accumulation, tolerance, and dosage schedules. *J. Pharmacol. Exp. Ther.*, **111**:425–35, 1954.

Carlsson, C.; Dencker, S. J.; Grimby, G.; and Haggendal, J.: Noradrenaline in blood-plasma and urine during chlorpromazine treatment. *Lancet*, **1**:1208, 1966.

Carr, L. A., and Moore, K. E.: Norepinephrine: Release from brain by *d*-amphetamine *in vivo*. *Science*, **164**:322–23, 1969.

Casey, J. F.; Bennett, I. F.; Lindley, C. J.; Hollister, L. E.; Gordon, M. H.; and Springer, N. N.: Drug therapy in schizophrenia. A controlled study of the relative effectiveness of chlorpromazine, promazine, phenobarbital, and placebo. *Arch. Gen. Psychiat. (Chicago)*, **2**:210–20, 1960.

Christiansen, J.; Gram, L. F.; Kofod, B.; and Rafaelsen, O. J.: Imipramine metabolism in man. A study of urinary metabolites after administration of radioactive imipramine. *Psychopharmacologia*, **11**:255–64, 1967.

Clinical Psychiatry Committee of the Medical Research Council: Clinical trial of the treatment of depressive illness. *Brit. Med. J.*, **1**:881–86, 1965.

Coffman, J. D.: The effect of aspirin on pain and hand blood flow responses to intra-arterial injection of bradykinin in man. *Clin. Pharmacol. Ther.*, **7**:26–37, 1966.

Cohen, G., and Collins, M.: Alkaloids from catecholamines in adrenal tissue: possible role in alcoholism. *Science*, **167**:1749–51, 1970.

Collier, H. O. J.: New light on how aspirin works. *Nature*, **233**:35–37, 1969.

Conners, C. K.; Rothschild, G.; Eisenberg, L.; Schwartz, L. S.; and Robinson, E.: Dextroamphetamine sulfate in children with learning disorders. *Arch. Gen. Psychiat. (Chicago)*, **21**:182, 1969.

Coppen, A.; Shaw, D. M.; Malleson, A.; and Costain, R.: Mineral metabolism in mania. *Brit. Med. J.*, **1**:71–75, 1966.

Cotzias, G. C.: Metabolic modification of some neurologic disorders. *J.A.M.A.*, **210**:1255–62, 1970.

Cotzias, G. C.; Papavasiliou, P. S.; and Gellene, R.: Modification of parkinsonism—chronic treatment with l-dopa. *New Eng. J. Med.*, **280**:337–45, 1969.

Cotzias, G. C.; Van Woert, M. H.; and Schiffer, L. M.: Aromatic amino acids and modification of parkinsonism. *New Eng. J. Med.*, **276**:374–79, 1967.

Crane, G. E.: Dyskinesia and neuroleptics. *Arch. Gen. Psychiat. (Chicago)*, **19**:700–703, 1968.

Cucinell, S. A.; Conney, A. H., Sansur, M.; and Burns, J. J.: Drug interactions in man. I. Lowering effect of phenobarbital on plasma levels of bishydroxycoumarin (Dicumarol) and diphenylhydantoin (Dilantin). *Clin. Pharmacol. Ther.*, **6**:420–29, 1965.

Curry, S. H.; Davis, J. M.; Janowsky, D. S.; and Marshall, J. H. L.: Factors affecting chlorpromazine plasma levels in psychiatric patients. *Arch. Gen. Psychiat. (Chicago)*, **22**:209–15, 1970b.

Curry, S. H., and Marshall, J. H. L.: Plasma levels of chlorpromazine and some of its relatively non-polar metabolites in psychiatric patients. *Life Sci.*, **7**:9–17, 1968.

Curry, S. H.; Marshall, J. H. L.; Davis, J. M.; and Janowsky, D. S.: Chlorpromazine plasma levels and effects. *Arch. Gen. Psychiat. (Chicago)*, **22**:289–96, 1970a.

Davis, V. E., and Walsh, M. J.: Alcohol, amines, and alkaloids: a possible biochemical basis for alcohol addiction. *Science*, **167**:1005–1007, 1970.

de Alarcon, R., and Carney, M. W. P.: Severe depressive mood changes following slow-release intramuscular fluphenazine injection. *Brit. Med. J.*, **3**:564–67, 1969.

Delgado, J. M. R.: Cerebral heterostimulation in a monkey colony. *Science*, **141**:161–63, 1963.

Detre, T.: Sleep disorders and psychosis. *Canad. Psychiat. Ass. J.*, **11** (Suppl):S169–77, 1966.

Di Mascio, A.: Personality and variability of response to psychotropic drugs: relationship to "paradoxical effects". In Rickels, K. (ed.): *Non-Specific Factors in Drug Therapy*. Charles C Thomas, Springfield, Ill., 1968, pp. 40–49.

Dole, V. P.: Biochemistry of addiction. *Ann. Rev. Biochem.*, **39**:821–40, 1970.

Dole, V. P.; Nyswander, M. E.; and Kreek, M. J.: Narcotic blockade. *Arch. Intern. Med. (Chicago)*, **118**:304–309, 1966.

Duvoisin, R. C.: Cholinergic-anticholinergic antagonism in parkinsonism. *Arch. Neurol. (Chicago)*, **17**:124–36, 1967.

———: Neurological reactions to psychotropic drugs. In Efron, D. H. (ed.): *Psychopharmacology. A Review of Progress, 1957–1967*. Public Health Service Publication No. 1836, U.S. Govt. Printing Office, Washington, D.C., 1968, pp. 561–74.

Duvoisin, R. C., and Yahr, M. D.: Encephalitis and parkinsonism. *Arch. Neurol. (Chicago)*, **12**:227–39, 1965.

Engelhardt, D. M.; Rosen, B.; Freedman, N.; and Margolis, R.: Phenothiazines in prevention of psychiatric hospitalization. IV. Delay or prevention of hospitalization—a re-evaluation. *Arch. Gen. Psychiat. (Chicago)*, **16**:98–101, 1967.

Evans, W. O.: Synergism of autonomic drugs in opiate or opioid-induced analgesia: a discussion of its potential utility. *Milit. Med.*, **127**:1000–1003, 1962.

Everett, G. M.: Tremor produced by drugs. *Nature*, **177**:1238, 1956.

FDA Statement (April 1970): Current drug information. Lithium carbonate. *Ann. Intern. Med.*, **73**:291–93, 1970.

Fish, B.: Drug use in psychiatric disorders of children. *Amer. J. Psychiat.*, **124** (Suppl.):31–36, 1968a.

———: Methodology in child psychopharmacology. In Efron, D. H. (ed.): *Psychopharmacology. A Review of Progress, 1957–1967*. Public Health Service Publication No. 1836, U.S. Govt. Printing Office, Washington, D.C., 1968b.

Forrest, W. H. Jr.; Beer, E. G.; Bellville, J. W.; Ciliberti, B. J.; Miller, E. V.; and Paddock, R.: Analgesic and other effects of the *d*- and *l*-isomers of pentazocine. *Clin. Pharmacol. Ther.*, **10**:468–76, 1969.

Fraser, H. F., and Harris, L. S.: Narcotic and narcotic antagonist analgesics. *Ann. Rev. Pharmacol.*, **7**:277–300, 1967.

Gastaut, H.; Caveness, W. F.; Landolt, H.; Lorentz de Haas, A. M.; McNaughton, F. L.; Magus, O.; Merlis, J. K.; Pond, D. A.; Radermecker, J.; and Storm van Leeuwen, W.: A proposed international classification of epileptic seizures. *Epilepsia*, **5**:297–306, 1964.

Gero, A.: Steric considerations on the chemical structure and physiological activity of methadone and related compounds. *Science*, **119**:112–14, 1954.

Gershon, S.: Lithium in mania. *Clin. Pharmacol. Ther.*, **11**:168–87, 1970.

Gibberd, F. B.; Dunne, J. F.; Handley, A. J.; and Hazleman, B. L.: Supervision of epileptic patients taking phenytoin. *Brit. Med. J.*, **1**:147–49, 1970.

Gilman, A.: Analgesic nephrotoxicity: a pharmacological analysis. *Amer. J. Med.*, **36**:167–73, 1964.

Glassman, A.: Indoleamines and affective disorders. *Psychosom. Med.*, **31**:107–14, 1969.

Glowinski, J., and Axelrod, J.: Effects of drugs on the uptake, release, and metabolism of H^3-norepinephrine in the rat brain. *J. Pharmacol.*, **149**:43–49, 1965.

Granville-Grossman, K. L., and Turner, P.: The effect of propranolol on anxiety. *Lancet*, **1**:788–90, 1966.

Greenblatt, M.; Grosser, G. H.; and Wechsler, H.: Differential response of hospitalized depressed patients to somatic therapy. *Amer. J. Psychiat.*, **120**:935–43, 1964.

Gresham, S. C.; Agnew, H. W., Jr.; and Williams, R. L.: The sleep of depressed patients. An EEG and movement study. *Arch. Gen. Psychiat. (Chicago)*, **13**:503–507, 1965.

Griffith, J. D.; Cavanaugh, J. H.; Held, J.; and Oates, J. A.: Experimental psychosis induced by the administration of *d*-amphetamine. In Costa, E., and Garattini, S. (eds.): *International Symposium on Amphetamines and Related Compounds*. Raven Press, New York, 1970, pp. 897–904.

Groppetti, A., and Costa, E.: Tissue concentrations of *p*-hydroxynorephedrine in rats injected with *d*-amphetamine: Effect of pretreatment with desipramine. *Life Sci.*, **8**:653–65, 1969.

Gulevich, G.; Dement, W.; and Johnson, L.: Psychiatric and EEG observations on a case of prolonged (264 hours) wakefulness. *Arch. Gen. Psychiat. (Chicago)*, **15**:29–35, 1966.

Guzman, F., and Lim, R. K. S.: The mechanism of action of the non-narcotic analgesics. *Med. Clin. N. Amer.*, **52**:3–14, 1968.

Hamilton, M.: Observer error in psychiatry. *Proc. Roy. Soc. Med.*, **61**:453–54, 1968.

Hammer, W., and Sjoqvist, F.: Plasma levels of monomethylated tricyclic antidepressants during treatment with imipramine-like compounds. *Life Sci.*, **6**:1895–1903, 1967.

Harrow, B. R.: Renal papillary necrosis: A critique of pathogenesis. *J. Urol.*, **97**:203–208, 1967.

Hartmann, E.: Reserpine: its effect on the sleep-dream cycle in man. *Psychopharmacologia*, **9**:242–47, 1966.

———: Pharmacological studies of sleep and dreaming: chemical and clinical relationships. *Biol. Psychiat.*, **1**:243–58, 1969.

Hawks, D.; Mitcheson, M.; Ogborne, A.; and Edwards, G.: Abuse of methylamphetamine. *Brit. Med. J.*, **2**:715–21, 1969.

Haydu, G. G.; Lange, H. S.; and Whittier, J. R.: Effects of Metrazol-vitamin administration in chronic psychoses. *Curr. Ther. Res.*, **3**:255–61, 1961.

Himwich, H. E.: Psychopharmacologic drugs. *Science,* **127**:59–72, 1958.

Ho, A. K. S.; Gershon, S.; and Pinckney, L.: The effects of acute and prolonged lithium treatment on the distribution of electrolytes, potassium and sodium. *Arch. Int. Pharmacodyn. Ther.,* **186**:54–65, 1970.

Hobson, J. A.: Sleep: physiologic aspects. *New Eng. J. Med.,* **281**:1343–46, 1969.

Hofmann, W. W., and Hollister, L. E.: Pharmacotherapy for Parkinson's disease: a new era. *Pharmacol. Physicians,* **4**:No. 7, 1970.

Hollister, L. E.: Predictable and unpredictable drug responses in man: the nervous system. In Wolstenholme, G., and Porter, R. (eds.): *Drug Responses in Man.* J. and A. Churchill, London, 1967, pp. 155–68.

———: *Chemical Psychoses. LSD and Related Drugs.* Charles C Thomas, Springfield, Ill., 1968a.

———: Human pharmacology of antipsychotic and antidepressant drugs. *Ann. Rev. Pharmacol.,* **8**:491–516, 1968b.

Hollister, L. E.; Curry, S. H.; Derr, J. E.; and Kanter, S. L.: Studies of delayed-action medication. V. Plasma levels and urinary excretion of four different dosage forms of chlorpromazine. *Clin. Pharmacol. Ther.,* **11**:49–59, 1970.

Hollister, L. E.; Kanter, S. L.; and Clyde, D. J.: Studies of prolonged-action medication. III. Pentobarbital sodium in prolonged-action form compared with conventional capsules. Serum levels of drug and clinical effects following acute doses. *Clin. Pharmacol. Ther.,* **4**:612–18, 1963.

Hollister, L. E., and Levy, G.: Kinetics of meprobamate elimination in humans. *Chemotherapia,* **9**:20–24, 1964.

Hollister, L. E.; Overall, J. E.; Bennett, J. L.; Kimbell, I., Jr.; and Shelton, J.: Specific therapeutic actions of acetophenazine, perphenazine and benzquinamide in newly admitted schizophrenic patients. *Clin. Pharmacol. Ther.,* **8**:249–55, 1967b.

Hollister, L. E.; Overall, J. E.; Johnson, M.; Katz, G.; Kimbell, I., Jr.; and Honigfeld, G.: Evaluation of desipramine in depressive states. *J. New Drugs,* **3**:161–66, 1963.

Hollister, L. E.; Overall, J. E.; Pokorny, A.; and Shelton, J.: Acetophenazine and diazepam in anxious depressions. *Arch. Gen. Psychiat. (Chicago),* **24**:273–78, 1971.

Hollister, L. E.; Overall, J. E.; Shelton, J.; Pennington, V.; Kimbell, I., Jr.; and Johnson, M.: Drug therapy of depression. Amitriptyline, perphenazine, and their combination in different syndromes. *Arch. Gen. Psychiat. (Chicago),* **17**:486–93, 1967a.

Hornykiewicz, O.: Dopamine (3-hydroxytryptamine) and brain functions. *Pharmacol. Rev.,* **18**:925–64, 1966.

Houde, R. W.; Wallenstein, M. S.; and Rogers, A.: Clinical pharmacology of analgesics. A method of assaying analgesic effect. *Clin. Pharmacol. Ther.,* **1**:163–74, 1960.

Howard, F. M., Jr.; Seybold, M.; and Reiher, J.: The treatment of recurrent convulsions with intravenous injection of diazepam. *Med. Clin. N. Amer.,* **52**:977–87, 1968.

Huguley, C. M., Jr.: Agranulocytosis induced by Dipyrone, a hazardous anti-pyretic and analgesic. *J.A.M.A.,* **189**:938–41, 1964.

Hunter, C. C., Jr.: Errors in management of patients dying of chronic obstructive lung disease. *J.A.M.A.,* **199**:188–91, 1967.

Irwin, S.: Anti-neurotics: practical pharmacology of the sedative-hypnotics and minor tranquilizers. In Efron, D. H. (ed.): *Psychopharmacology. A Review of Progress, 1957-67.* Public Health Serv. Publication No. 1836, U.S. Govt. Printing Office, Washington, D.C., 1968, pp. 185–204.

Jaffe, J. H., and Senay, E. C.: Methadone and *l*-methadyl acetate. Use in management of narcotics addicts. *J.A.M.A.,* **216**:1303–1305, 1971.

Janssen, P. A. J.: Chemical and pharmacological classification of neuroleptics. In Bobon, D. P.; Janssen, P. A. J.; and Bobon, J. (eds.): *Modern Problems of Pharmacopsychiatry. 5. The Neuroleptics.* S. Karger, Basel, 1970, pp. 33–43.

———: The pharmacology of haloperidol. *Int. J. Neuropsychiat.,* **3** (suppl.): S10–18, 1967.

Jick, H.: Clinical evaluation of hypnotics. In Kales, A. (ed.): *Sleep: Physiology and Pathology. A Symposium.* J. B. Lippincott Co., Philadelphia, 1969, pp. 289–97.

Johnson, L. C.; Burdick, M. A.; and Smith, J.: Sleep during alcohol intake and withdrawal in the chronic alcoholic. *Arch. Gen. Psychiat. (Chicago),* **22**:406–18, 1970.

Jouvet, M.: Biogenic amines and the states of sleep. *Science,* **163**:32–41, 1969.

Kaim, S. C.; Klett, C. J.; and Rothfeld, B.: Treatment of the acute alcohol withdrawal state: a comparison of four drugs. *Amer. J. Psychiat.,* **125**:1640–46, 1969.

Kales, A.; Adams, G. L.; and Pearlman, J. T.: Implications of REM sleep. *Amer. J. Ophthal.,* **69**:615–22, 1970.

Kales, A.; Beall, G.; Berger, R.; Heuser, G.; Jacobsen, A.; Kales, J.; Pharmelee, A., Jr.; and Walter, R.: Sleep and dreams. Recent research on clinical aspects. UCLA Interdepartmental Conference. *Ann. Intern. Med.,* **68**:1078–1104, 1968.

Kales, A.; Malmstrom, E. J.; Scharf, M. B.; and Rubin, R. T.: Psychological and biochemical changes following use and withdrawal of hypnotics. In Kales, A. (ed.): *Sleep: Physiology and Pathology. A Symposium.* J. B. Lippincott Co., Philadelphia, 1969, pp. 331–43.

Kantor, T. G.; Sunshine, A.; Laska, E.; Meisner, M.; and Hopper, M.: Oral analgesic studies: pentazocine hydrochloride, codeine, aspirin and placebo and their influence on response to placebo. *Clin. Pharmacol. Ther.,* **7**:447–54, 1966.

Karnes, W. E.: Medical treatment for convulsive disorders. *Med. Clin. N. Amer.,* **52**:959–75, 1968.

Kay, D. C.; Eisenstein, R. B.; and Jasinski, D. R.: Morphine effects on human REM state, waking state and NREM sleep. *Psychopharmacologia,* **14**:404–16, 1969.

Keele, C. A.: Sites and modes of actions of antipyretic-analgesic drugs. *Proc. Roy. Soc. Med.,* **62**:535–39, 1969.

Klawans, H. L.: The pharmacology of Parkinsonism. A review. *Dis. Nerv. Syst.,* **29**:805–16, 1968.

Klett, C. J., and Moseley, E. C.: The right drug for the right patient. *J. Consult. Psychol.,* **29**:546–51, 1965.

Kornetsky, C.: Psychoactive drugs in the immature organism. *Psychopharmacologia,* **17**:105–36, 1970.

Kramer, J. C.; Fischman, V. S.; and Littlefield, D. C.: Amphetamine abuse. Pattern and effects of high doses taken intravenously. *J.A.M.A.,* **201**:305–309, 1967.

Krumholz, W. V.; Sheppard, C.; and Merlis, S.: Studies with aspirin: psychopharmacologic and methodologic considerations. *Clin. Pharmacol. Ther.,* **5**:691–94, 1964.

Kuntzman, R.: Drugs and enzyme induction. *Ann. Rev. Pharmacol.,* **9**:21–36, 1969.

Kutt, H.; Brennan, R.; Dehejia, H.; and Verebely, K.: Diphenylhydantoin intoxication. A complication of isoniazid therapy. *Amer. Rev. Resp. Dis.,* **101**:377–84, 1970.

Kutt, H.; Haynes, J.; Verebeley, K.; and McDowell, F.: The effect of phenobarbital on plasma diphenylhydantoin level and metabolism in man and in rat liver microsomes. *Neurology,* **19**:611–16, 1969.

Kutt, H.; Wolk, M.; Scherman, R.; and McDowell, F.:

Insufficient parahydroxylation as a cause of diphenyl-hydantoin toxicity. *Neurology*, **14**:524–48, 1964.

Lader, M. H.: Alcohol reactions after single and multiple doses of calcium cyanamide. *Quart. J. Stud. Alcohol*, **28**:468–75, 1967.

Lasagna, L.: The clinical evaluation of morphine and its substitutes as analgesics. *Pharmacol. Rev.*, **16**:47–83, 1964.

Lasagna, L., and Epstein, L. C.: The use of amphet-amines in the treatment of hyperkinetic children. In Costa, E., and Garattini, S. (eds.): *International Symposium on Amphetamines and Related Compounds*. Raven Press, New York, 1970, pp. 849–64.

Lasky, J. J.; Klett, C. J.; Caffey, E. M., Jr.; Bennett, J. L.; Rosenblum, M. P.; and Hollister, L. E.: Drug treatment of schizophrenic patients: a comparative evaluation of chlorpromazine, chlorprothixene, flu-phenazine, reserpine, thioridazine, and triflupromazine. *Dis. Nerv. Syst.*, **23**:698–706, 1962.

Leonards, J. R., and Levy, G.: Reduction or prevention of aspirin-induced occult gastrointestinal blood loss in man. *Clin. Pharmacol. Ther.*, **10**:571–75, 1969.

Levy, G., and Hollister, L. E.: Variation in rate of salicylate elimination by humans. *Brit. Med. J.*, **2**:286–88, 1964.

Lewis, S. A., and Evans, J. I.: Dose effects of chlor-promazine on human sleep. *Psychopharmacologia*, **14**:342–48, 1969.

Lipp, J. A.: Symposium on extrapyramidal disease. Basic neurophysiology. Neuropharmacological aspects of drug therapy. *Appl. Ther. Res.*, **9**:439–47, 1967.

Loan, W. B.; Morrison, J. D.; and Dundee, J. W.: Evaluation of a method for assessing potent analgesics. *Clin. Pharmacol. Ther.*, **9**:765–76, 1968.

Lorr, M., and Klett, C. J.: Psychotic behavioral types. A cross-cultural comparison. *Arch. Gen. Psychiat. (Chicago)*, **20**:592–97, 1969.

Lowenstein, E.; Hothowell, P.; Levine, F. H.; Daggett, W. M.; Austen, W. G.; and Laver, M. B.: Cardio-vascular response to large doses of intravenous mor-phine in man. *New Eng. J. Med.*, **281**:1389–93, 1969.

McNair, D. M.; Goldstein, A. P.; Lorr, M.; Cibelli, L. A.; and Roth, I.: Some effects of chlordiazepoxide and meprobamate with psychiatric outpatients. *Psychopharmacologia*, **7**:256–65, 1965.

Maggs, R.: Treatment of manic illnesses with lithium carbonate. *Brit. J. Psychiat.*, **109**:56–65, 1963.

Magoun, H. W.: *The Waking Brain*, 2nd ed. Charles C Thomas, Springfield, Ill., 1963.

Mark, L. C.: Commentary. Archaic classification of barbiturates. *Clin. Pharmacol. Ther.*, **10**:287–91, 1969.

Melmon, K. L.: Preventable drug reactions—causes and cures. *New Eng. J. Med.*, **284**:1361–68, 1971.

Melville, K. I.; Joron, G. E.; and Douglas, D.: Toxic and depressant effects of alcohol given orally in com-bination with glutethimide or secobarbital. *Toxicol. Appl. Pharmacol.*, **9**:363–75, 1966.

Merlis, S.; Sheppard, C.; Collins, L.; and Fiorentino, D.: Polypharmacy in psychiatry: patterns of differential treatment. *Amer. J. Psychiat.*, **126**:1647–51, 1970.

Merskey, H., and Spear, F. G.: The concept of pain. *J. Psychosom. Res.*, **11**:59–67, 1967.

Michaux, M. H.; Hanlon, T. E.; Ota, K. Y.; and Kur-land, A. A.: Phenothiazines in the treatment of newly admitted state hospital patients: global com-parison of eight compounds in terms of an outcome index. *Curr. Ther. Res.*, **6**:331–39, 1964.

Miller, R. L.; Forsyth, R.; McCord, C.; and Melmon, K. L.: The selective changes in regional blood flow produced by morphine. *Clin. Res.*, **18**:341, 1970.

Millichap, J. G.: Relation of laboratory evaluation to clinical effectiveness of antiepileptic drugs. *Epilepsia*, **10**:315–28, 1969.

Monroe, L. J.: Psychological and physiological dif-ferences between good and poor sleepers. *J. Abnorm. Psychol.*, **72**:255–64, 1967.

Morgan, J. P., and Bianchine, J. R.: The clinical pharmacology of levodopa. *Rational Drug Ther.*, **5**:No. 1, 1971.

Moruzzi, G.: Active processes in the brain stem during sleep. *The Harvey Lectures*, 58. Academic Press, Inc., New York, 1962.

NIMH-PRB Collaborative Study Group: Differences in clinical effects of three phenothiazines in "acute" schizophrenia. *Dis. Nerv. Syst.*, **28**:369–83, 1967.

NIMH-PSC Collaborative Study Group: Phenothiazine treatment in acute schizophrenia. *Arch. Gen. Psychiat. (Chicago)*, **10**:246–61, 1964.

Noyes, R., Jr.: Lithium carbonate: a review. *Dis. Nerv. Syst.*, **30**:318–21, 1969.

Oswald, I.: Drugs and sleep. *Pharmacol. Rev.*, **20**:273–303, 1968.

Oswald, I.; Jones, H. S.; and Mannerheim, J. E.: Effects of two slimming drugs on sleep. *Brit. Med. J.*, **1**:796–99, 1968.

Oswald, I., and Thacore, V. R.: Amphetamine and phenmetrazine addiction. *Brit. Med. J.*, **2**:427–31, 1963.

Overall, J. E., and Hollister, L. E.: Computer pro-cedures for psychiatric classification. *J.A.M.A.*, **187**:583–88, 1964.

Overall, J. E.; Hollister, L. E.; Pokorny, A. D.; Casey, J. F.; and Katz, G.: Drug therapy in depressions. *Clin. Pharmacol. Ther.*, **3**:16–22, 1962.

Overall, J. E.; Hollister, L. E.; Shelton, J.; Kimbell, I., Jr.; and Pennington, V.: Broad-spectrum screening of psychotherapeutic drugs: thiothixene as an anti-psychotic and antidepressant. *Clin. Pharmacol. Ther.*, **10**:36–43, 1969.

Paddock, R.; Beer, E. G.; Bellville, J. W.; Ciliberti, B. J.; Forrest, W. H., Jr.; and Miller, E. V.: Analgesic and side effects of pentazocine and morphine in a large population of postoperative patients. *Clin. Pharmacol. Ther.*, **10**:355–65, 1969.

Pettinger, W. A.; Mitchell, J. R.; and Oates, J. A.: Cardiovascular effects and toxicity of psychotropic agents in man. In Efron, D. H. (ed.): *Psychopharma-cology. A Review of Progress, 1957–67*. Public Health Service Publication No. 1836, U.S. Govt. Printing Office, Washington, D.C., 1968.

Pisciotta, A. V.: Mechanisms of phenothiazine induced agranulocytosis. In Efron, D. H. (ed.): *Psychopharma-cology. A Review of Progress, 1957–67*. Public Health Service Publication No. 1836, U.S. Govt. Printing Office, Washington, D.C., 1968.

Platman, S. R., and Fieve, R. R.: Biochemical aspects of lithium in affective disorders. *Arch. Gen. Psychiat. (Chicago)*, **19**:659–63, 1968.

———: Lithium retention and excretion. The effect of sodium and fluid intake. *Arch. Gen. Psychiat. (Chicago)*, **20**:285–89, 1969.

Platman, S.; Rohrlich, J.; and Fieve, R.: Absorption and excretion of lithium in manic-depressive disease. *Dis. Nerv. Syst.*, **29**:733–38, 1968.

Price-Evans, D. A.; Davison, K.; and Pratt, R. T. C.: The influence of acetylator phenotype on the effects of treating depression with phenelzine. *Clin. Pharmacol. Ther.*, **6**:430–35, 1965.

Prien, R. F., and Cole, J. O.: High dose chlorpromazine therapy in chronic schizophrenia. Report of NIMH-PRB Collaborative Study Group. *Arch. Gen. Psychiat. (Chicago)*, **18**:482–95, 1968.

Randall, L. O., and Schallek, W.: Pharmacological activity of certain benzodiazepines. In Efron, D. H. (ed.): *Psychopharmacology. A Review of Progress, 1957–67*. Public Health Service Publication No. 1836,

U.S. Govt. Printing Office, Washington, D.C., 1968.

Raskin, A.; Schottenbrandt, J. C.; Reatig, N.; and McKeon, J. J.: Differential response to chlorpromazine, imipramine and placebo. A study of subgroups of hospitalized depressed patients. *Arch. Gen. Psychiat. (Chicago)*, 23:164–73, 1970.

Rechtschaffen, A., and Kales, A. (eds.): *A Manual of Standardized Terminology, Techniques and Scoring System for Sleep Stages of Human Subjects.* NIH Publication 204, U.S. Govt. Printing Office, Washington, D.C., 1968.

Rechtschaffen, A., and Maron, L.: The effect of amphetamine on the sleep cycle. *Electroenceph. Clin. Neurophysiol.*, 16:438–45, 1964.

Reynolds, E. H.: Schizophrenia-like psychoses of epilepsy and disturbances of folate and vitamin B_{12} metabolism induced by anticonvulsant drugs. *Brit. J. Psychiat.*, 113:911–19, 1967.

Reynolds, E. H.; Chanarin, I.; Milner, G.; and Matthews, D. M.: Anti-convulsant therapy, folic acid and vitamin B-12 metabolism and mental symptoms. *Epilepsia*, 7:261–70 1966.

Rickels, K. (ed.): *Non-specific Factors in Drug Therapy.* Charles C Thomas, Springfield, Ill., 1968.

Rickels, K.; Clark, T. W.; Ewing, J. H.; Klingensmith, W. C.; Morris, H. M.; and Smock, C. D.: Evaluation of tranquilizing drugs in medical outpatients. Meprobamate, prochlorperazine, amobarbital sodium and placebo. *J.A.M.A.*, 171:1649–56, 1959.

Rubin, E.; Gang, H.; Misra, P. S.; and Lieber, C. S.: Inhibition of drug metabolism by acute ethanol intoxication. *Amer. J. Med.*, 49:801–806, 1970.

Ruch, T. C.: Pathophysiology of pain. In Ruch, T. C., and Fulton, J. F. (eds.): *Medical Physiology and Biophysics.* W. B. Saunders Co., Philadelphia, 1960, pp. 350–68.

Schildkraut, J. J., and Kety, S. S.: Biogenic amines and emotion. *Science*, 156:21–30, 1967.

Schildkraut, J. J.; Schanberg, S. M.; Breese, G. R.; and Kopin, I. J.: Norepinephrine metabolism and drugs used in the affective disorders: a possible mechanism of action. *Amer. J. Psychiat.*, 124:600–608, 1967.

Schou, M.: Lithium: elimination rate, dosage, control, poisoning, goiter, mode of action. *Acta Psychiat. Scand.*, 207:49–54, 1969.

———: Lithium in psychiatric therapy and prophylaxis. *J. Psychiat. Res.*, 6:67–95, 1968.

Schuster, C. R., Jr.: Psychological approaches to opiate dependence and self-administration by laboratory animals. *Fed. Proc.* 29:2–5, 1970.

Shelley, J. H.: Phenacetin, through the looking glass. *Clin. Pharmacol. Ther.*, 8:427–71, 1967.

Shelton, J., and Hollister, L. E.: Simulated abuse of tybamate in man: failure to demonstrate withdrawal reactions. *J.A.M.A.*, 199:338–40, 1967.

Sherlock, S.: The prediction of hepatotoxicity due to therapeutic agents in man. In Wolstenholme, G., and Porter, R. (eds.): *Drug Responses in Man.* J. and A. Churchill, Ltd., London, 1967, pp. 138–54.

Shideman, F. E.: Clinical pharmacology of hypnotics and sedatives. *Clin. Pharmacol. Ther.*, 2:313–44, 1961.

Simpson, G. M., and Angus, J. W. S.: Drug induced extrapyramidal disorders. Controlled studies of the relationship between the behavioural change and the extrapyramidal symptoms produced by psychotropic drugs. *Acta Psychiat. Scand.*, 212:7–58, 1970.

Sjoqvist, F.: Psychotropic drugs. Interaction between monoamine oxidase (MAO) inhibitors and other substances. *Proc. Roy. Soc.*, 58:967–78, 1965.

Snyder, C. H.: Myoclonic epilepsy in children: short-term comparative study of two benzodiazepine derivatives in treatment. *Southern Med. J.*, 61:17–20, 1968.

Spring, G.; Schweid, D.; Gray, C.; Steinberg, J.; and Horwitz, M.: A double-blind comparison of lithium and chlorpromazine in the treatment of manic states. *Amer. J. Psychiat.*, 126:1306–10, 1970.

Stach, K., and Poldinger, W.: Strukturelle Betrachtungen der Psychopharmaka: Versuch einer Korrelation von chemischer Konstitution und clinischer Wirkung. In Jucker, E. (ed.): *Progress in Drug Research.* Birkhauser Verlag, Basel, 1966, pp. 129–90.

Thomsen, K., and Schou, M.: Renal lithium excretion in man. *Amer. J. Physiol.*, 215:823–27, 1968.

Tozer, T. N.; Neff, N. H.; and Brodie, B. B.: Application of steady state kinetics to the synthesis rate and turnover time of serotonin in the brain of normal and reserpine-treated rats. *J. Pharmacol. Exp. Ther.*, 153:177–82, 1966.

Trenholm, H. L.; Maxwell, W. B.; Paul, C. J.; Wiberg, G. S.; and Coldwell, B. B.: Biochemical aspects of the interaction of ethanol with barbiturates. *Canad. J. Biochem.*, 48:706–11, 1970.

UCLA Interdepartmental Conference: Schizophrenia. *Ann. Intern. Med.*, 70:107–25, 1969.

Uhlenhuth, E. H.; Canter, A.; Neustadt, J. O.; and Payson, H. E.: The symptomatic relief of anxiety with meprobamate, phenobarbital and placebo. *Amer. J. Psychiat.*, 115:905–10, 1959.

van Praag, H. M.: Psychotropic drugs in child psychiatry. *Int. Pharmacopsychiat.*, 3:137–54, 1969.

Vasko, J. S.; Henney, R. P.; Brawley, R. K.; Oldham, H. N., and Morrow, A. G.: Effects of morphine on ventricular function and myocardial contractile force. *Amer. J. Physiol.*, 210:329–34, 1966.

Weiss, G.; Minde, K.; Werry, J.; Douglas, V.; and Nemeth, E.: Studies on the hyperactive child. *Arch. Gen. Psychiat. (Chicago)*, 24:409–14, 1971.

Wheatley, D.: Comparative effects of propranolol and chlordiazepoxide in anxiety states. *Int. J. Psychiat.*, 115:1411–12, 1969.

WHO Expert Committee on Addiction-Producing Drugs: Thirteenth Report. World Health Organization Technical Report, Series #273, Geneva, 1964.

Wilkins, R. H., and Brody, I. A.: Parkinson's syndrome. *Arch. Neurol. (Chicago)*, 20:440–41, 1969.

Wittenborn, J. R.; Plante, M.; Burgess, F.; and Maurer, H.: A comparison of imipramine, electro-convulsive therapy, and placebo in the treatment of depressions. *J. Nerv. Ment. Dis.*, 135:131–37, 1962.

Wyatt, R. J.; Engleman, K.; Kupfer, D.; Scott, J.; Sjoerdsma, A.; and Snyder, F.: Effects of parachlorophenylalanine on sleep in man. *Electroenceph. Clin. Neurophysiol.*, 27:529–32, 1969.

Yules, R. B.; Freedman, D. X.; and Chandler, K. A.: The effect of ethyl alcohol on man's electroencephalographic sleep cycle. *Electroenceph. Clin. Neurophysiol.*, 20:109–11, 1966.

Zarcone, V.; Gulevich, G.; Pivik, T.; and Dement, W.: Partial REM phase deprivation and schizophrenia. *Arch. Gen. Psychiat. (Chicago)*, 18:194–202, 1968.

Chapter 12

DISORDERS OF CELL GROWTH

Joseph R. Bertino and *William M. Hryniuk*

GENERAL CONSIDERATIONS

The modern era of cancer chemotherapy began in 1941 when Huggins and Hodges demonstrated that diethylstilbestrol ameliorated carcinoma of the prostate. Subsequently a host of drugs was introduced for chemotherapy. As the history of this field is short, a rational basis for drug therapy of malignancies has developed only recently. Since qualitative, exploitable differences in malignant-cell biochemistry are rare, in contrast to bacterial diseases, most of the drugs available to the cancer chemotherapist affect normal cells, in particular replicating cells. This chapter stresses the principles of chemotherapy of malignant diseases, with emphasis on the kinetics of normal-cell and tumor-cell growth. Detailed information on drugs is not provided; generalizations regarding classes of drugs and principles of use are stressed. Specific examples of how a therapeutic program might be formulated for an individual patient are given. Since these drugs may be used with other treatment modalities, attention is given to combination therapy.

The cancer chemotherapist must answer three questions when he approaches the patient: Should the patient be treated at all? If so, with what drug or drugs? What dosage schedule is optimum?

Should the Patient Be Treated?

The decision to treat the patient should be made like any other therapeutic decision; i.e., the physician must consider whether or not benefit will likely result at a tolerable toxicity. Benefit can be in the form of an increase in lifespan or palliation of physical symptoms, or it can be psychologic (the importance of psychologic benefits of therapy should not be ignored). *Principle: A correct assessment of the benefit likely to accrue from therapy can be made only if the physician has available to him all the facts regarding (1) the type, extent, and grade of the malignancy, (2) its natural history, (3) the most current results of treatment, and (4) the psychologic makeup of the patient.* The toxicity of the proposed treatment must be considered above all, but it must be evaluated in the light of the therapeutic goal. *Principle: Greater risks of drug toxicity are accepted for induction of remission or permanent tumor eradication than the risks accepted for palliation of symptoms alone.*

The chemotherapist must also consider that toxicity that can be managed in one hospital may not be manageable in another. In certain circumstances the availability of supportive facilities may spell the difference between success or failure of chemotherapy. For example, to induce remission in acute leukemia in adults, induction of complete marrow aplasia may be required. Availability of special supportive measures to ensure the patient's survival may allow marrow aplasia to be produced intentionally.

What Drug?

The decision to treat a patient with malignant disease hinges on the availability of a drug that is active against the malignancy. Unfortunately, there are no useful *in vitro* methods that allow the selection of drugs against a specific tumor. Therefore, the therapist must resort to an agent or combination of agents that has been beneficial in similar tumors. This is an unsatisfactory situation; not all drugs have been tried in all combinations against all tumors in large, well-controlled studies. *Principle: The chemotherapist has no assurance that the currently accepted drug for a particular malignancy is the best available, but knows only that it has been reported to have some activity. In view of the toxicity of these agents, controlled trials must be carefully conducted to be meaningful, and to avoid causing suffering in the majority of patients in whom the drug has no antitumor activity* (Holland, 1966b).

Most tumors are resistant to most chemotherapeutic agents in use. In only a few instances is the biochemical basis of this resistance even partly understood. In virtually every instance of initial response to a particular drug the tumor eventually becomes resistant to that drug. The mechanisms of "acquired" resistance have been defined in a variety of experimental systems (Hutchison, 1965), but not to any significant degree in the clinical setting.

What Dosage Schedule?

Even if the chemotherapist is able to choose a drug, he has no precise way of deciding which dose schedule is most appropriate for his patient. Again, he must rely on past experience. This becomes very frustrating when it is realized that dosage and timing may be crucial determinants of response and that adequate data are available for very few drugs. For example, cyclophosphamide has virtually no antitumor activity but does produce toxicity if given in small, divided doses to patients with Burkitt's lymphoma; if it is given in large infrequent doses, complete and long-lasting regression of the tumor may occur with acceptable toxicity (Burkitt and Burchenal, 1969). *Principle: The dose schedule of a cancer chemotherapeutic drug may be a critical determinant of its efficacy and toxicity.*

In view of the major problems in selection of drugs and dosage schedules, it is not surprising

that chemotherapy has been relegated to a relatively minor position in the treatment of malignant disease. Recently, new knowledge has been applied to cancer chemotherapy, resulting in substantial improvement in response to treatment. These advances include (1) the development of several new drugs and re-evaluation of older ones; (2) improvement in supportive techniques, especially the availability of platelet transfusions and newer antibiotics; (3) major advances in tumor immunology; and (4) increased understanding of tumor growth kinetics and the relationship between tumor growth rate and antimetabolite drugs.

THEORETIC CONSIDERATIONS

Tumor and Normal Stem-Cell Kinetics

"Cell-Kill" Hypothesis. The therapeutic benefit of increased life-span resulting from the treatment of malignant disease may be related to the number of tumor cells killed by treatment (Skipper *et al.*, 1964). Cure is possible if every tumor cell is killed; in experimental situations even one tumor cell can eventually result in the death of the animal (Furth and Kahn, 1937). The tumor "cell-kill" hypothesis was derived from a detailed study of a transplantable leukemia (L1210) in mice. When a critical size of tumor (approximately 1×10^9 cells) was reached in each mouse, death occurred. Since the tumor-doubling time was known, and the duration of life was related to the initial tumor inoculum, it was shown that treatment prolonged life in proportion to the number of cells killed. Second, a particular treatment was found to kill a certain percentage of cells, independent of the number of cells present, provided their growth rate was constant (Skipper *et al.*, 1965). This principle was well known to bacteriologists studying the action of germicidal agents (Chick, 1908) and is referred to as "logarithmic order of death," or kill by "first-order kinetics" (Wilcox, 1966) (see Chapter 2).

The problem now involves the selectivity of "cell kill." Certain drugs and combinations are capable of curing experimental mouse leukemias, and even certain tumors in man. It is important to understand how this selectivity can be produced, to permit new approaches to the treatment of human tumors not presently cured. In the cure of the L1210 tumor in mice, up to 10^9 cells must be killed (Skipper *et al.*, 1964). It has been estimated that a 20-kg child, dying of acute lymphoblastic leukemia, has 10^{12} malignant cells (Frei and Freireich, 1965). Assuming that a tumor weighing 1 g is the smallest size detectable, and that it contains 10^9 cells, chemotherapy must eradicate the entire malignant population of 10^9 cells. This must be accomplished without producing an intolerable deficit of normal cells, such as in the bone marrow and gut epithelium. An estimate of the "logs of kill" that these normal cell compartments can withstand has been obtained (Bruce and Bergsagel, 1967). In man, 450 rads of whole body irradiation are probably lethal and 600 rads are lethal for mice. As 600 rads produce 2 logs of reduction of hematopoietic stem cells in mice, the lethality of 450 rads in man may be related to the same factor of reduction (Alexander, 1965). With intensive supportive therapy, perhaps another log of normal-stem-cell kill may be tolerable and reversible.

How can such a marked differential kill (10^9 to 10^{12} tumor cells versus less than 10^3 normal cells) be obtained in man? A few drugs do have some differential effects (i.e., do not appreciably affect normal stem cells in therapeutic doses), but the spectrum of tumors affected by these drugs is small, and the logs of tumor-cell kill possible with these agents appear to be limited. *Principle: In the treatment of cancer, the physician must consider quantitative differences between the responses of normal and tumor cells.*

Cycle-Specific and Noncycle-Specific Drugs. To approach the problem of selectivity, a model system in an experimental animal was devised to quantitate the effects of chemotherapeutic agents on both normal and malignant cells (Bruce et al., 1966). The study revealed a linear relationship between the number of hematopoietic stem cells injected into irradiated mice and the macroscopic colonies produced (Till and Mc-Culloch, 1961). Similarly, transplantable AKR lymphoma cells produced macroscopic colonies in the spleens of syngenic mice in direct relationship to the number of cells inoculated (Bush and Bruce, 1964). This assay has allowed measurements of the effects of dose and duration of treatment on both tumor-cell and hematopoietic stem-cell proliferation. On the basis of effects on these two stem-cell compartments, drugs were classified into three groups (Bruce et al., 1966). The first group of drugs (nitrogen mustard, 1,3-bis-[2-chloroethyl]-1-nitrosourea [BCNU], and x-ray [Figure 12–1]) decimated both the hematopoietic stem cells and the tumor cells to the same

degree. However, the second and third classes of drugs, also given over a 24-hour period, decimated the tumor population to a much greater degree than the normal stem cells. Some drugs in the third class at higher doses produced as much as a 10,000-fold greater kill of lymphoma cells than of normal stem cells. This class included drugs such as cyclophosphamide (Figure 12–1), dactinomycin, and 5-fluorouracil. The remaining drugs tested (methotrexate, vinblastine, azaserine, 6-mercaptopurine, and high-specific-activity tritiated thymidine [^{3}H-TdR]) still achieved a marked differential cell kill (500-fold), but the differences diminished with increased doses. The selectivity of the agents in the last two classes was attributed to a differential effect of the agents on proliferating versus nonproliferating cells. Hematopoietic stem cells were in a state of low proliferative activity compared to the lymphoma cells. However, the susceptibility of the normal stem cells to agents of the second and third class did increase when their proliferative activity increased (e.g., following sublethal irradiation or drug treatment) and reverted to normal only when this increased proliferation subsided (Bruce and Meeker, 1967; Valeriote and Bruce, 1967). It was suggested that class II and III agents were capable of killing cells only if the drug was present when these cells were engaged in active proliferation (DNA synthesis and mitosis). The cells not killed by therapy were considered quiescent during the time of drug exposure. On implantation into animals, however, cells resumed active proliferation and produced splenic colonies. The proliferating cells killed by the class II and III agents were said to be in "cycle." Agents that killed both normal and tumor cells irrespective of their proliferative state (class I) have been referred to as "noncycle-specific" agents, and agents of the second and third class have been called "cycle-specific" agents.* *Principle: Differential cell kill might be expected from a cycle-specific agent if the tumor were growing rapidly, with a short generation*

---

* Actually, Bruce called class II drugs "phase specific" and class III drugs "cycle specific," but since the basis for this difference has not been elucidated, both classes will be referred to as cycle specific.

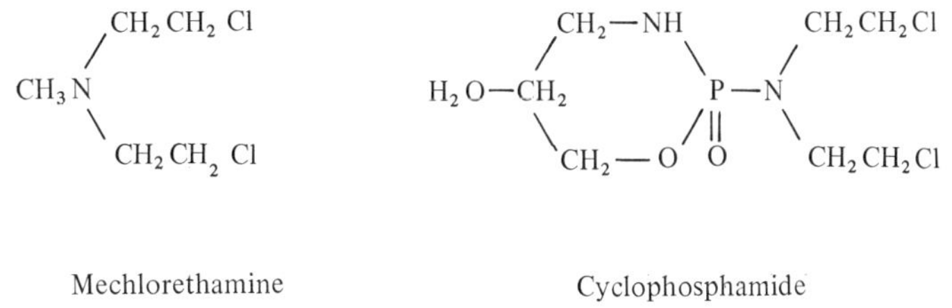

$$CH_3N \diagup^{CH_2CH_2Cl}_{\diagdown CH_2CH_2Cl}$$

$$H_2O-CH_2 \diagup^{CH_2-NH}_{\diagdown CH_2-O} \diagdown P-N \diagup^{CH_2CH_2Cl}_{\diagdown CH_2CH_2Cl} \; \overset{\|}{O}$$

Figure 12–1. Structural formulas of mechlorethamine (Mustargen) and cyclophosphamide (Cytoxan).

Mechlorethamine   Cyclophosphamide

time, and if the marrow and gastrointestinal mucosa were in "resting" condition (i.e., most of the cells not in cycle).

Repeated treatments at intervals long enough to allow the normal stem cells to recover from any increased proliferative activity caused by the agent would produce a net differential kill each time, with eventual cure. In certain experimental conditions, this goal has been achieved (Goldin *et al.*, 1956a, 1956b; Skipper *et al.*, 1967), and in some clinical situations use of this concept has led to improved antitumor effects.

Growth Rate of Tumors. The concepts developed thus far have assumed that tumor growth rate is constant. However, in most circumstances, when tumor size increases, its cell growth slows (Laird, 1964, 1965; McCredie *et al.*, 1965; Mendelsohn, 1965; Laster *et al.*, 1969). This may be due to an increase in the generation time of the tumor, a decrease in the growth fraction of the tumor, and/or an increase in the tumor cell death rate (Steel, 1967). These changes may result from overcrowding and decreased nutrition of the tumor, but the process is poorly understood. In this phase of growth, the tumor population is not in so active a proliferative state; both tumor and normal cells may be in a resting state and the differential "cell kill" of cycle-specific agents is lost. Indeed, if marrow involvement with tumor or infection is present, the marrow may be in a more active proliferative phase than are the tumor cells; even greater toxicity than usual may be produced with drug therapy, with less-than-usual tumor response. Recent studies have shown that DNA synthesis in cells in a plateau phase of growth is less sensitive to the action of at least one cycle-specific drug (methotrexate) than are cells in log phase of growth (Hryniuk *et al.*, 1969). Therefore, when tumors are large and growth has plateaued, attempts to decrease tumor size by the use of noncycle-active agents, surgery, or x-ray therapy should be considered (Rall and Homan, 1967; Hryniuk and Bertino, 1969a, 1969b; Schabel, 1969). The use of a noncycle-active agent is of value if recovery of normal tissue is more rapid than recovery of the tumor tissue. Since the dose-response curve of these agents is steep, a maximum dose should be administered to kill as many cells as possible, keeping in mind the narrow therapeutic index of these compounds. If sufficient tumor cell kill is obtained, the logarithmic phase of tumor growth may be re-established and the cycle-specific agents may regain their value.

Compartmentalization of Cells. Not all tumor-bearing compartments are affected to the same degree by a course of therapy (Skipper *et al.*, 1965). In animal model systems, as well as in man, cells in the central nervous system are least affected by chemotherapy, owing to failure of certain drugs to pass the blood-brain barrier.

The failure of cell kill in the central nervous system may account for relapses in leukemia. Intrathecal administration of chemotherapeutic agents is necessary in patients with manifest central nervous system involvement. In contrast, similar cells in the blood are most sensitive to antimetabolite effects (at least with methotrexate) (Hryniuk and Bertino, 1969b). Furthermore, sensitivity of tumor cells in different organs (e.g., leukemia cells in the spleen, kidney, or liver) may vary depending on the drug employed. Organ-specific differences in sensitivity of cells may be related to binding or metabolism of the drug in the different tissues or to biochemical influences of the organ on cell growth or metabolism.

Drug Resistance. Although a great deal of information is available in bacteria and animal tumor systems concerning the frequency and mechanisms of drug resistance (Welch, 1959; Brockman, 1963; Hutchison, 1965), relatively little is known about resistance in human tumors. On the basis of appearance of drug-resistant mutations in animal tumors, it seems likely that similar mutants occur in human tumors. Attempts to reduce this occurrence by using drugs in high dose and in combinations have not yet been demonstrated to be of clinical value. Further study of this aspect of human malignancy is warranted, since drug resistance almost inevitably limits the success of treatment of those tumors that initially respond dramatically.

Host Immunity to Tumors. The Skipper model does not assign any role to host immunity in controlling the proliferation of cells; however, some evidence supports a role for host immunity in the retardation of growth or the regression of some tumors (Southam, 1967; Hellström and Hellström, 1970). In man, immunity may add to the beneficial effects of chemotherapy in the successful treatment of choriocarcinoma and Burkitt's lymphoma (Klein *et al.*, 1967; Hulka and Mohr, 1968; Klein, 1968). Attempts to augment naturally occurring host immunity by nonspecific therapy (e.g., BCG administration), or to induce immunity by injecting formalin-fixed or irradiated tumor cells from the patient or other patients with leukemia, have been of value (Mathe *et al.*, 1969; Skurkovich *et al.*, 1969). In both the experimental systems (Martin *et al.*, 1964) and in man, the tumor inoculum or tumor size must be reduced markedly, by either surgery, x-ray, or chemotherapy, for immunotherapy to be effective.

Drugs Used in Cancer Chemotherapy

This section emphasizes general principles for use of drugs in cancer chemotherapy. Several excellent reviews deal with the biochemistry and pharmacology of these drugs in greater depth (Calabresi and Welch, 1965; Oliverio and Zubrod, 1965; Sartorelli and Creasey, 1969; Cline, 1971). A list of drugs used in cancer chemotherapy and a current assessment of their value are given in Table 12–1. These results have been obtained empirically for the most part; they should not be interpreted as indicating "standard" therapy, but rather as indicating the sensitivity of certain tumors to available drugs (Hiatt, 1967; Luce *et al.*, 1967).

For purposes of discussion of drug toxicity and combinations of drugs, these agents may be divided into two broad categories, selective and nonselective agents. These drugs are also classified, when possible, as cycle active or noncycle active.

Selective Drugs. A truly selective drug for the treatment of neoplastic disease would eradicate the tumor without harming the host. All known chemotherapeutic agents in therapeutic doses have some untoward host effects. Several compounds have emerged, however, whose side effects are not primarily upon normal replicating tissues; these agents are referred to as selective drugs.

Perhaps the most important selective agents are hormones. Several generalizations apply to the use of these agents: (1) pharmacologic doses are usually required for antitumor effects; thus side effects are primarily those of hormone excess; (2) resistance to these agents occurs; therefore, hormones almost without exception are palliative, not curative; (3) the spectrum of activity of antitumor hormones is limited; and (4) hormones are probably noncycle-active agents.

Estrogens have been useful in the treatment of postmenopausal women with breast cancer (Kennedy, 1965), as well as in the treatment of prostatic cancer. Progestins cause tumor regression in about one-third of patients with endometrial carcinoma (Anderson, 1965; Kelly and Baker, 1965) and have somewhat less but definite activity against breast cancer and hypernephroma. Testosterone and closely related derivatives have been effective against breast cancer (Cooperative Breast Cancer Group, 1964; Kennedy, 1965) and against hypernephroma (Bloom and Wallace, 1964). Androgens are also used in the therapy of bone marrow failure, especially in certain neoplastic diseases such as chronic lymphatic leukemia and multiple myeloma. In these circumstances, the beneficial effects are most likely related to erythropoietin-stimulating properties of the hormones (Kennedy, 1964). Thyroid hormone has produced impressive results in the treatment of metastases from some papillary carcinomas of the thyroid (Crile, 1966).

Adrenocortical hormones also have specific antineoplastic activity against malignancies of the lymphatic system, in particular acute lymphatic leukemia, chronic lymphatic leukemia, and lymphomas (Burningham *et al.*, 1964; Frei and Freireich, 1965). They have limited but well-documented antitumor activity in patients with breast cancer (Lemon, 1959; Kennedy, 1965). Corticosteroids are also extremely useful in the treatment of hemolytic anemia that may develop in patients with malignancy, especially in chronic lymphatic leukemia and lymphomas. Adrenocortical hormones, or synthetic congeners (usually prednisone, because of its lower sodium-retaining effect than hydrocortisone, convenience in available dosage size, and cost), are sometimes used in the treatment of cancer patients for their nonspecific mood-elevating and appetite-stimulating properties, but the serious side effects of steroids may make this hazardous.

Other therapies that result in hormonal changes are ovariectomy, adrenalectomy, and pituitary ablation to treat cancer of the breast (Moore *et al.*, 1967), and orchiectomy for prostatic carcinoma. Radioactive iodine is given to selected patients with metastatic thyroid carcinoma if the isotope is taken up by the metastases.

Aside from the hormones, few other agents have a selective and specific action against neoplasms. A prototype of this class of agent, o,p'-DDD (1,1-dichloro-2-[ortho-chlorophenyl]-2-[para-chlorophenyl]ethane), has been developed. This drug selectively destroys adrenocortical tissue, and its use has resulted in transient tumor regression in approximately one-third of patients with adrenocortical carcinoma (Hutter and Kayhoe, 1966).

To this list may be added the use of surgery and irradiation therapy. In a sense both of these therapies also are selective. Local tumor control or eradication is possible in many instances without significant host toxicity. These therapies always should be kept in mind when specific local problems arise, even in patients with disseminated malignancy.

Two other recently introduced compounds are important selective agents: the vinca alkaloid vincristine and the enzyme L-asparaginase (Figure 12–2). Unfortunately, these agents appear to have a narrow spectrum of activity, but they are extremely important compounds in a heuristic sense. Like any of the aforementioned "selective" therapies, these drugs usually can be employed in situations when bone marrow

Table 12-1. DRUGS USED IN CANCER CHEMOTHERAPY

DRUG	"CYCLE ACTIVE"	TOXICITY			ANTITUMOR RESULTS		
		BONE MARROW	G.I.	OTHER	EXCELLENT	GOOD	FAIR
Alkylating agents							
Mechlorethamine (nitrogen mustard, mustargen, HN₂)	No	+ +	+ +		Hodgkin's disease	Reticulum-cell sarcoma, lymphosarcoma	Melanoma, cervix, head and neck
Cyclophosphamide (Endoxan, Cytoxan)	Yes	+ +	+	Alopecia, chemical cystitis	Burkitt's lymphoma, Hodgkin's disease, reticulum-cell sarcoma, lymphosarcoma	Acute lymphatic leukemia, myeloma, neuroblastoma, retinoblastoma	Lung, melanoma, cervix, head and neck
Chlorambucil (Leukeran)	No	+ +	±		Hodgkin's disease, lymphoma, chronic lymphocytic leukemia		
Busulfan (Myleran)	No	+ +	±	Pulmonary fibrosis, skin pigmentation	Chronic myelocytic leukemia		
Melphalan (L-sarcolysin, Alkeran)	No	+ +	±			Myeloma	
Antimetabolites							
Methotrexate (amethopterin)	Yes	+ +	+ +		Choriocarcinoma, Burkitt's lymphoma, acute lymphatic leukemia	Head and neck cancer	Lung (epidermoid)
Mercaptopurine (Purinethol, 6-mercaptopurine)	Yes	+ +	+		Acute lymphatic leukemia	Acute and chronic myelocytic leukemia	
Fluorouracil (5-fluorouracil)	Yes	+ +	+ +			Gastrointestinal carcinoma	
Cytosine arabinoside (Cytosar)	Yes	+ +	+		Acute leukemia		

Hormones

Drug	Carcinogenic			Toxicity	Indications		
Adrenal steroids	?	++	−	Hormone excess	Acute and chronic lymphatic leukemia	Reticulum-cell sarcoma lymphosarcoma, Hodgkin's disease	Breast carcinoma
Estrogens	?	−	±	Hormone excess		Breast carcinoma Carcinoma of prostate	
Androgens	?	−	−	Hormone excess		Breast carcinoma	Hypernephroma
Progesterone	?	−	−	Hormone excess		Carcinoma of uterine body	
Vinca alkaloids							
Vinblastine (Velban)	Yes	++	++	Neuropathy	Hodgkin's disease	Choriocarcinoma	Breast carcinoma
Vincristine (Oncovin)	Yes	±	±		Acute lymphatic leukemia, Wilms's tumor, reticulum cell sarcoma	Neuroblastoma, retinoblastoma	
Antibiotics							
Actinomycin D (dactinomycin, Cosmegen)	Yes	++	++		Choriocarcinoma, Wilms's tumor, testicular tumors	Rhabdomyosarcoma	Sarcomas
Mithramycin	?	++	++	Liver disease, hypocalcemia, bleeding	Embryonal testicular tumors		Glioblastomas
Bleomycin*	?	−	±	Skin changes, pulmonary fibrosis		Squamous cell carcinoma, lymphoma, embryonal testicular tumors	
Daunorubicin*	?	++	+	Cardiac toxicity		Acute leukemia	
Miscellaneous							
O, p′ − DDD	?	±	++			Adrenal cortical carcinoma	
L-Asparaginase*	?	−	+	Liver toxicity, pancreatitis	Acute lymphatic leukemia		
Procarbazine (Natulan)	?	++	+		Hodgkin's disease		

* Investigational drugs.

517

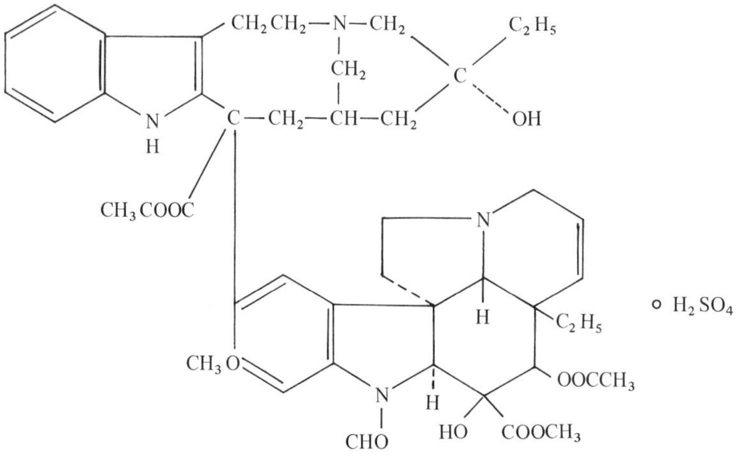

Figure 12–2. Vincristine sulfate (Oncovin). Vinblastine sulfate differs from vincristine sulfate by the replacement of the formyl by a methyl group.

function is poor, or in combination with one or more "nonselective" agents, since as a rule toxicities are not additive. Vincristine must be given intravenously and, like nitrogen mustard or vinblastine, can cause severe local tissue damage if it extravasates. Nevertheless it is an extremely useful drug for producing remissions in acute lymphatic leukemia and it has some definite antitumor effects in patients with lymphoma. Striking antitumor effects have also been noted in patients with Wilms's tumor (Southwest Cancer Chemotherapy Group, 1963) and neuroblastoma (James et al., 1965); less striking but documented antitumor effects have been found in patients with breast carcinoma (Mittleman et al., 1963). Both vincristine and vinblastine are considered to be "cycle-active" agents.

The most recently introduced "selective" agent with a novel mechanism of action is L-asparaginase. This enzyme, first discovered to be the active antitumor principle in guinea pig serum (Kidd, 1953), is now produced commercially from E. coli. This drug produces rapid and profound depletion of asparagine concentrations in serum and marked inhibition of protein synthesis, as evidenced by a decrease in serum concentrations of clotting factors and albumin (Capizzi et al., 1970). These effects on protein synthesis are usually transient and improve despite continued therapy. Little or no toxicity to the replicating cells of the gastrointestinal mucosa or bone marrow is produced by asparagine depletion, but blast cells in patients with acute lymphatic leukemia are rapidly lysed; hence this drug is an effective agent in the treatment of acute lymphatic leukemia (Oettgen et al., 1967). Asparaginase does not appear to be "cycle active." Although the enzyme is a curative agent in the treatment of certain lymphomas in mice (Boyse et al., 1967), even

extremely high doses do not produce long-term remissions in patients with leukemia or lymphoma. Only 10% of patients with acute myelocytic leukemia respond to this drug, as compared to approximately 50% of patients with lymphatic leukemia. Except for a few patients with melanoma who respond to this drug, trials in patients with other solid tumors have been unrewarding (Hill et al., 1967; Haskell et al., 1969; Oettgen and Schulten, 1969). The major side effects encountered with this drug have been allergic; several cases of anaphylactic shock have been reported, but these reactions usually are successfully treated (see Chapter 9). The use of extremely large doses (1000 IU/kg of body weight per day for 10 to 20 days) has resulted in increased toxicity; nausea and vomiting, weight loss, and serum protein depletion have been more severe. Several cases of fatal acute pancreatitis and nonketotic hyperosmotic diabetic acidosis have been reported (Haskell et al., 1969; Capizzi et al., 1970).

Despite these toxicities, the use of this drug in acute lymphatic leukemia in low doses (10 to 200 IU/kg body weight per day) has been a relatively safe, effective method of inducing remission.

"Nonselective Drugs." Most drugs currently used to treat malignancies usually have clinical effects on normal replicating tissues and may be referred to as "nonselective" agents. The alkylating agents (except for cyclophosphamide), BCNU, and perhaps procarbazine are noncyclespecific drugs, whereas the antimetabolites (methotrexate [Figure 12–3], 6-mercaptopurine, thioguanine, 5-fluorouracil, cytosine arabinoside, and azauridine [Figure 12–4]) and other natural products (vincristine, vinblastine, and dactinomycin) are considered to be cyclespecific agents. The noncycle-active drugs have a narrow therapeutic index, and a certain amount

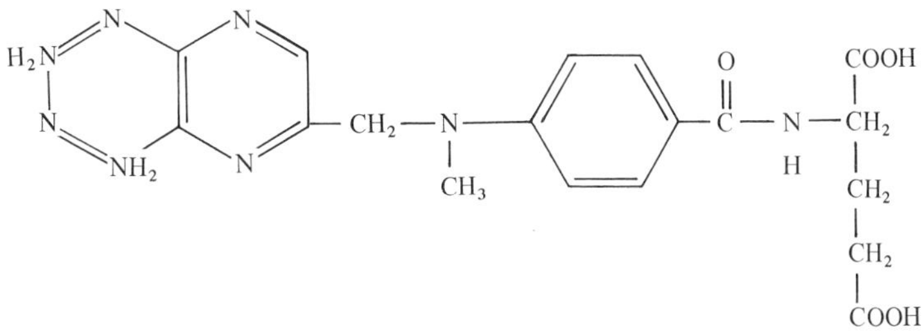

Figure 12–3. Structural formula of the folate antagonist methotrexate.

of toxicity (usually bone marrow depression) is almost invariably produced. However, the degree of toxicity produced by an average therapeutic dose often depends upon the condition of the patient. For example, a patient with leukemia, pancytopenia, and an infiltrated, poorly functioning marrow does not tolerate these agents very well; severe marrow aplasia may result. Yet the same dose of this drug may be administered with minimum risk to a patient with slight bone marrow infiltration, or to a patient in bone marrow remission. Drug dosage may have to be reduced in "poor-risk" patients, regrettably in those patients with a large number of tumor cells who "need" more, rather than less, antineoplastic drug. The condition of the patient is especially important when large doses of cycle-active drugs are desirable over a short interval. Large amounts of drug may be administered in this circumstance if marrow is normal and gastrointestinal mucosa function is intact, resulting in an excellent therapeutic index for certain tumors. *Principle: The features of the individual patient may be crucial in determining the success of therapy. "Average therapeutic dose" is a term appropriate to a population. Knowledge of the pathophysiology of the disease state and the pharmacologic actions of the drug is imperative for optimal chemotherapy.*

Combination Chemotherapy. As chemotherapeutic agents have different toxicities, efforts have been made to combine drugs to improve the antitumor effects without increasing toxicity. In addition to improvement of the drugs' therapeutic indices, combination chemotherapy may prevent or delay the onset of drug resistance (Venditti and Goldin, 1964; Sartorelli, 1965).

From a theoretic point of view, and by analogy to antibiotic therapy of bacterial infections, agents that fall within the same class (cycle active or noncycle active) would not be expected to be synergistic or even additive, contrasted with agents from different classes (Valeriote *et al.*, 1968a, 1968b). For example, the use of an alkylating agent (chlorambucil) and vinblastine has produced additive or synergistic antitumor effects in patients with Hodgkin's disease. A greater percentage of complete remissions was produced with the combination than with either drug alone (Lacher and Durant, 1965). Despite this useful generalization, biochemical events in the cell may allow two cycle-active agents to synergize with each other, or two drugs of different classes to antagonize each other (Sartorelli, 1965). For example, two synergistic combinations of antimetabolites used in the treatment of experimental murine leukemia are methotrexate with 6-mercaptopurine and thioguanine with cytosine arabinoside (Venditti *et al.*, 1956; Burchenal and Dollinger, 1967; Gee *et al.*, 1969). In contrast, the use of asparaginase with methotrexate negates the action of the folate antagonist in experimental tumors (Capizzi *et al.*, 1970). Large doses of prednisone have

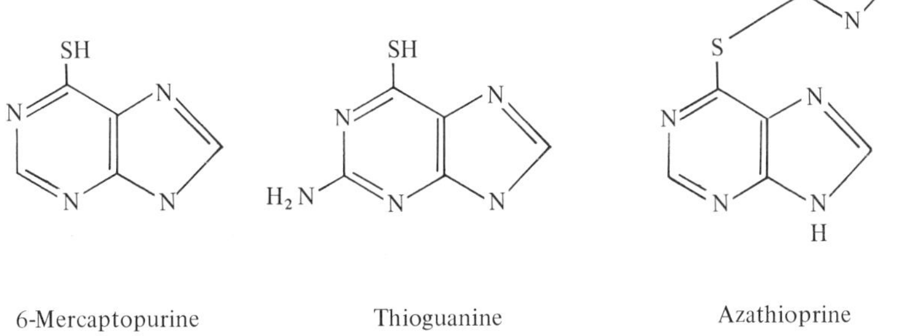

Figure 12–4. Structural formulas of the purine antagonists.

6-Mercaptopurine   Thioguanine   Azathioprine

been used in combination with one or more other drugs (vincristine, cyclophosphamide, methotrexate, or 6-mercaptopurine) in the treatment of acute leukemia and in children with lymphoblastic leukemia. A significant increase has been reported in the percentage of patients achieving remission with one of these combinations as compared to any single drug (Henderson 1969). Thus a "selective" drug may be used with one or more cycle-active "nonselective" drugs to achieve an improved therapeutic result. Since prednisone is not effective in Bruce's assay system, its classification is unclear. Although prednisone in combination with other drugs produces additive or synergistic effects in obtaining remissions, it is not well documented that the combinations produce greater cell kill (i.e., that prednisone plus the antimetabolite produces a longer *duration* of remission than does the antimetabolite alone, assuming that remission duration is a rough measure of cell kill). *Principle: Some therapy remains largely empiric, but this should not inhibit attempts to analyze the type of response obtained. The lympholytic action of corticosteroids could quickly reduce elevated blood-cell counts of relatively mature cells, resulting in a gratifying clinical remission, with no implications as to efficacy related to lymphoblast-cell "log kill," perhaps a more critical determinant of duration of remission.*

Unequivocal demonstration that a combination of drugs is more effective than one drug is always difficult. A large number of patients must be treated so that each drug alone may be compared with the combination. The tumor type should be as homogeneous as possible, in regard to histology, location, and extent of disease. Several dose schedules of each drug used alone and in combination should also be employed, since the optimum dose and schedule for a single drug when used alone may not be the same for that drug in combination. However, the numbers of patients required limit the doses that can be tested. For example, based on encouraging studies of effective combination therapy of the L1210 lymphoma with methotrexate and 6-mercaptopurine (Venditti *et al.*, 1956), a cooperative group carried out a well-designed study of this combination in patients with acute leukemia (Acute Leukemia Group B, 1961). The use of methotrexate in combination with 6-mercaptopurine did not improve the duration of remission as compared to sequential use of methotrexate followed by 6-mercaptopurine, or 6-mercaptopurine followed by methotrexate. However, since only one combination schedule could be used (because of the large number of patients necessary for the study),

improved results yet may be obtained with a different dosage schedule of this combination. Detailed studies of this combination against the L1210 lymphoma emphasize the importance of the dose and schedule of these drugs necessary to obtain additive or synergistic effects (Venditti *et al.*, 1956). The same standards should be applied to evaluation of efficacy and safety of fixed-dose drug combinations used for any purpose. It is also important to realize that if the combinations are given in a single preparation, one is in essence using a "different" or "new" drug. *Principle: Clinical trials of drug combinations can show that one regimen is better than another, but the best possible combination treatment for a given tumor is almost impossible to define. This goal can be best approached by utilizing all available biochemical evidence, knowledge of tumor growth kinetics, and knowledge of the drugs themselves in planning the clinical trial.*

Special Methods to Deliver High Concentrations of Drugs to Isolated Areas. *Regional Perfusion and Infusion.* The rationale for administering drugs to a tumor via its arterial blood supply is that high concentrations of drug may be delivered to the neoplasm. Since there may be a dose effect in tumor-cell kill, the same amount of drug administered intra-arterially rather than intravenously may produce better results by increasing the concentration of drug in the tumor. Intra-arterial therapy has been used to treat tumors in areas of the body difficult to treat by surgical procedures or by x-ray therapy, or tumors that perhaps may be *cured* by these modalities so rarely as not to warrant amputation or disfigurement. Such lesions have been located in the head and neck, the brain, the extremities, the liver, and the organs of the lower abdomen (the rectum, cervix, and bladder) (Lawrence, 1963).

Infusion refers to the administration of a drug via the artery supplying a tumor without attempting to isolate the venous return and thus recirculate the drug. This technique is more commonly used than is perfusion and is associated with fewer exacting technical problems (see Chapter 2).

Perfusion therapy (i.e., administering a drug into the arterial blood supply of a tumor via a closed circuit in which the tumor's venous return is recirculated via a pump) has a great potential advantage: systemic toxicity should be minimal. Even in perfusion of extremities, this ideal is difficult to achieve in practice, since some leakage of drug into the systemic circulation usually occurs (Creech *et al.*, 1958).

These procedures have received a great deal of attention in the past decade. Most of the technical problems of intra-arterial administration have been solved. However, much more research needs to be done on drug selection and scheduling, the use of this procedure as an adjuvant to surgical or x-ray therapy, and the effect of this treatment on the subsequent biologic behavior of the tumor.

The use of alkylating agents or antimetabolites that are rapidly destroyed by blood or liver enzymes allows creation of a very high tumor concentration without a high systemic concentration. Therefore the intra-arterial route may reduce systemic toxicity. Local toxicity limits the dose that may be employed; alkylating agents that react readily (HN_2, etc.) produce toxicity in replicating as well as in nonreplicating tissue, and there is probably little advantage in prolonged administration of drug, except to ensure complete perfusion of the tumor. In this regard, antimetabolites have an advantage over alkylating agents in that local toxicity may be more selective, i.e., limited to replicating tissue. For example, the intra-arterial administration of low continuous doses of fluorouracil into the external carotid artery produces regional mucositis as its major toxicity. Long-term administration of antimetabolites, by encompassing the generation time of most of the tumor cells, might produce the greatest therapeutic benefit. Several approaches have been used to minimize systemic toxicity: (1) infusion of a small concentration of drug, enough to produce an appreciable concentration of the agent in the blood supply of the tumor, but not in the systemic circulation; (2) infusion of a drug that is rapidly metabolized by blood or liver, such as 5-fluorouracil (Sullivan et al., 1960; Burrows et al., 1967) or dichloromethotrexate (Cleveland et al., 1969); or (3) systemic administration of an antidote at the same time the drug is administered intra-arterially (Sullivan et al., 1959).

The role of intra-arterial chemotherapy as an adjunct to subsequent radiation therapy and/or surgery is being evaluated in several centers. Although the tumor response to intra-arterial therapy often is impressive, the ultimate value of this combined approach has not been demonstrated (Lawrence, 1963). *Principle: Even the most logically sound therapeutic intervention must be confirmed by testing in diseased man. A critical study allows rejection of unnecessary methods and establishes the efficacy of others.*

Intrathecal and Intraventricular Drug Administration. The delivery of drugs into the cerebrospinal fluid (CSF) via intrathecal or intraventricular administration has limited usefulness. The principal indication for administration of an antineoplastic drug into the CSF is for the treatment of tumors that grow in suspension in the CSF and/or involve the meninges,

deriving their nutrients from the CSF (Moore et al., 1960). The advantage of intrathecal or intraventricular drug administration in these circumstances is considerable, since high levels of drug are achieved. Furthermore, when given systemically, many drugs do not cross the "blood-brain barrier." Systemic use of the folate antagonist methotrexate is ineffective in meningeal disease. In contrast, intrathecal methotrexate is effective in the treatment of meningeal leukemia (Rieselbach et al., 1963). However, the "blood-brain barrier" is unidirectional for methotrexate as well as for most other drugs. Methotrexate administered intrathecally diffuses out into the systemic circulation, and systemic toxicity can be produced if a high dose is administered.

Inasmuch as most solid tumors of the brain derive their nourishment from the arterial circulation rather than from the CSF, intraventricular administration of drugs is usually not effective in the treatment of brain tumors. Delivery of drugs via the arterial circulation to brain tumors has been attempted but has met with only limited success (Luyendijk and van Beusekom, 1966).

Intracavitary Drug Administration. Chemotherapeutic agents often are administered into the pleural space, peritoneum, or pericardial sac to control malignant effusions. Several irritating agents cause pleural adhesions that obliterate the pleural space, including radioisotopes, nitrogen mustard, quinacrine, tetracycline, and even talc (Ultman, 1962). This inflammatory effect does not depend on any specific antitumor property of the drug, but more upon its irritant properties (see Chapter 9). Absorption of the drug can occur, however, and systemic toxicity has been produced after intrapleural administration of nitrogen mustard. Large-tube pleural drainage carried out for 2 to 3 days also can obliterate the pleural space, obviating the need for sclerosing agents (Lambert et al., 1967). *Principle: When apparently equivalent alternative means to the same therapeutic goal are available, they should carefully be weighed for relative toxicities and advantages in the individual patient.* For a young patient with poor bone marrow reserve, drainage might be preferred. In a "fragile" patient or a patient with blood-clotting defects, intracavitary therapy might be safer.

Thio-TEPA, a slowly reacting alkylating agent, is often used for control of pericardial or abdominal effusions due to malignant disease (Bateman et al., 1955). This drug usually is most effective if the tumor cells derive their nourishment from the effusion fluid. When large masses are present, this approach to control of the effusion is less successful. The intracavitary use of antimetabolites such as 5-fluorouracil also suffers this limitation.

Evaluation of Drug Therapy in Man

Measurement of Normal Stem Cells in Man. Techniques for accurate measurement of tumor and hematopoietic stem-cell kill in the mouse have provided valuable information about differential cell kill, dose response, and rates of recovery of these tissues. Unfortunately, there are no satisfactory methods to measure normal or tumor stem cells in man. The recent development of methods for growing human marrow cells *in vitro* may allow the eventual development of an assay for measurement of normal hematopoietic stem cells before and during therapy. However, the cloning efficiency of bone marrow cells in culture has been low, and only granulocyte colonies have been obtained (Bradley and Metcalf, 1966; Senn *et al.*, 1967). Some estimate of the effect of chemotherapy on the bone marrow and the gut epithelium can be obtained by measuring the consequences of cell kill in these tissues: reduced granulocyte, reticulocyte, and platelet levels for bone marrow stem cells (Valeriote *et al.*, 1968a, 1968b), and mucositis or ulceration for the gastrointestinal mucosa stem cells. Carefully performed blood-cell counts can accurately determine granulocyte concentrations as low as 100/cu mm. Plotting serial granulocyte counts on a logarithmic scale quantitates changes in granulocyte counts of two logs (e.g., 3000 to 30), aiding evaluation of the intensity of therapy (Bergsagel *et al.*, 1968; Hryniuk and Bertino, 1969a, 1969b). Mucositis produced by therapy should be graded on a 1-to-4+ scale, although the degree of tissue damage can only crudely be related to logs of mucosal cell kill by this simple method of evaluation. *Principle: Unavailability of precise means of following a drug's effects should not discourage attempts to utilize the available information. Using the available information in a quantitative manner permits usable estimates of response and provides a solid basis for comparison with other patients or treatments.*

Evaluation of Tumor-Cell Kill. As in the case of normal stem cells, reliable techniques to measure tumor-cell kill in man have not been developed. Whenever possible, quantitation of the tumor mass, expressed as a volume, should be performed, since it is usually the best available guide for following the response to therapy. By using volume measurements, the therapist can estimate the change in cell number, assuming that 1 ml of cells represents approximately 10^9 cells. However, a change in the size of a tumor mass may not accurately reflect the

amount of tumor-cell kill obtained after a course of therapy. For example, in an experimental mouse tumor it was shown that 3 logs of cell kill were obtained by cyclophosphamide therapy, yet no measurable change in tumor size occurred because of the slow removal rate of dead tumor cells and their rapid replacement by new cells (Wilcox *et al.*, 1965).

By analogy with the quantitation of normal granulocytes as a measure of hematopoietic stem-kill, accurate measurement of the peripheral blast-cell count on a logarithmic scale is helpful in assessing the results of treatment in patients with leukemia. A decrease of as much as 3 logs may be measurable (e.g., 100,000 to 100). However, quantitation in the bone marrow, the more important compartment, is not satisfactory.

When tumors produce characteristic enzymes or hormones, concentration of these products in blood may afford valuable guides to tumor-cell kill. If the amount of substance produced is a function of cell number, and if therapy produces a decrease in this substance only by cell kill, the concentration of the product may be related directly to cell kill. The measurement of urinary chorionic gonadotropin titers in patients with choriocarcinoma has been extremely useful in this regard, and accurate quantitation of very low concentrations is possible with a radio-immunoassay (Figure 12-5). Urinary para-protein quantitation in patients with myeloma (Alexanian *et al.*, 1968; Salmon and Smith, 1970) and serum and urinary lysozyme concentrations in patients with monocytic leukemia (Osserman and Lawlor, 1966; Perillie *et al.*, 1968) may be useful measurements of cell kill. Quantitation by sensitive assays of hormones produced by other endocrine and nonendocrine tumors may provide similar useful information during treatment (Midgley, 1966).

The success of therapy and degree of tumor-cell kill should be related directly to an increase in life-span over that expected for an untreated group, as in the L1210 animal model system. However, most human tumors occur in a heterogeneous group of patients (age, sex, heredity, general condition, etc.) and differ as to tumor location and size at the time of discovery. These variations result in a wide range of survival times and obscure the data on the effect of therapy on life-span. However, certain malignancies in humans have a short natural history, affect a relatively uniform patient population, and have similar biologic behavior (e.g., acute lymphatic leukemia in children and choriocarcinoma in women). When patients with these diseases are carefully studied, the increase in survival may be related to tumor-cell

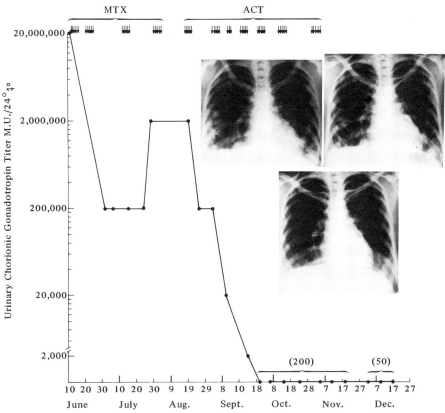

Figure 12–5. Chemotherapy of a patient with metastatic choriocarcinoma. The vertical arrows indicate 5-day courses of methotrexate and actinomycin D. This patient presented with a urinary chorionic gonadotropin (UCG) titer of 20,000,000; with the sensitive assays available, this titer was followed down through 7 logs, allowing therapy to be closely monitored. Methotrexate produced 2 logs of decrease in the UCG titer, but despite continued therapy with this drug, the titer began to rise, indicating that resistance was occurring. Guided by this rise in UCG titer rather than by the chest x-ray (which did not change), therapy was rapidly changed to actinomycin D. This drug decreased the UCG titer markedly, each course resulting in 1 to 2 logs of decrease of UCG titer and presumably of tumor cells. The patient was then treated until the titer was within the normal range. The patient has remained free of disease since 1962. Although the effects on normal tissue are not shown here, the therapy was intensive, and each course of methotrexate or actinomycin D was given to the limit of tolerable toxicity (usually 2 logs of granulocyte or platelet decrease, or mucositis), and therapy was resumed immediately on recovery from toxicity (granulocyte count greater than 1,500/cu mm, platelet count greater than 100,000/cu mm, no liver function abnormalities). Supportive care for this type of regimen must be optimal to avoid drug-related deaths; in this series of 50 patients 37 presumable "cures" were obtained with the use of sequential methotrexate and actinomycin D therapy (or vice versa), with only one toxic death due to methotrexate. (From Ross, G. T.; Goldstein, D. P.; Hertz, R.; Lipsett, M. B.; and Odell, W. D.: Sequential use of methotrexate and actinomycin D in the treatment of metastatic choriocarcinoma and related trophoblastic diseases in women. *Amer. J. Obstet. Gynec.,* **93**:223–29, 1965.)

kill (Ross et al., 1965; Holland, 1966a). *Principle: Careful following of both toxic and therapeutic effects of drug therapy is essential in the treatment of patients with malignancy. As drugs and combinations become more effective, and possibly more toxic, the physician must carefully measure drug effects on the neoplasm and the host and assess the risks with reference to the therapeutic goal, i.e., palliation or cure.*

DISEASES ALLOWING THE DEMONSTRATION OF PRINCIPLES

Human Tumor-Cell Kinetics

On the basis of the principles described, a rational approach to the chemotherapy of human cancer is possible. However, for almost every human malignancy, the information necessary to apply these principles is lacking. The chemotherapist who decides that therapy is likely to benefit a patient with a malignancy does not have information available to him concerning the generation time, the growth fraction, the death rate, or the growth rate of the tumor. Patients with leukemia have been studied with tritium-labeled thymidine (Mauer and Fisher, 1966; Clarkson et al., 1967), but relatively few investigations of solid-tumor-cell kinetics have been performed in man. A double-label *in vitro* technique, utilizing tritium-labeled and ^{14}C-labeled thymidine, may yield information on the cell kinetics of solid tumors (Young et al., 1969; Young and De Vita, 1970).

The observation that a tumor is "slow growing" does not provide sufficient information for therapeutic decision. Some slow-growing tumors may be characterized by a very low growth fraction with a short generation time, or by a very high death rate. These tumors might even be more sensitive to cycle-active drugs than are tumors that enlarge rapidly. In general, tumors that may rapidly enlarge (e.g., choriocarcinoma, Burkitt's lymphoma, reticulum-cell leukemia, and blast crisis of chronic granulocyte leukemia) probably have a short generation time (24 hours or less) and a large growth fraction. On the other hand, certain tumors that grow moderately rapidly may have long generation times but large growth fractions and an insignificant cellular death rate. These respond poorly to cycle-active drugs, as do some slowly growing tumors. *Principle: Because of poorly understood factors, perhaps host immunity, nutrition, or endocrine status, tumor growth may vary considerably in the same patient. Thus some tumor cells may at times exist in a resting phase (G_1 or G_0) and may be insensitive to therapy with cycle-specific agents.*

Specific Drug Therapy

After the patient's general condition is evaluated, the histology of the tumor is identified, and some estimate is made of the progression and amount of tumor present, the chemotherapist is ready to consider specific drug therapy. Since *in vitro* tests have not been developed to a practical point, some judgment must be made on the basis of previous trials as to the sensitivity of the tumor to the various antitumor agents. Aside from the kinetic considerations previously discussed, and a few exceptions (Wolberg, 1969; Hryniuk and Bertino, 1969a, 1969b), the reasons for the differences in tumor sensitivity to certain drugs are only poorly understood.

Assuming a drug or drugs are identified as active, the dose, duration, and route of administration of the compound must then be considered. The therapist must understand the metabolism of the drug, as well as any possible alterations in its metabolism caused by the patient's condition (liver or kidney involvement) or by concurrent use of other drugs. It is extremely important to decide on goals of therapy before treatment, in order to plan a program for the individual patient. The type of tumor, the histologic staging, and the clinical staging are important considerations in this decision. *Principle: The patient and doctor should be aware of the toxic potential of the drug, and the acceptable limits of the intensity of therapy should be set before therapy commences. Thus when cure is a possibility, as in choriocarcinoma, only near-lethal toxicity may be prohibitive (i.e., greater than the LD_{10}). However, if the expected gain is minimal, as in the routine treatment of carcinoma of the colon with 5-fluorouracil, even moderate morbidity may not be acceptable.*

Supportive Therapy

The chemotherapist must anticipate and be prepared to treat the complications of malignant disease. The complications can arise from the tumor per se (Amatruda, 1969; Gellhorn, 1969), by its direct invasion of organs or occasionally by its metabolic activity, or from those problems induced by chemotherapy. Patients with malignancies, in particular those that involve the marrow, are especially susceptible to infection. These infections may result from lowered resistance of the patient, due to depressed host immunity caused by the cancer, due to steroid therapy, or due to depressed leukocyte concentration in blood resulting from either marrow invasion by tumor or chemotherapeutic agents (Bodey, 1966). These infections often may be unusual, i.e., caused by gram-negative bacteria, fungi, protozoa, or viruses (Hutter and Collins, 1962; Bodey, 1966; Bodey et al., 1966; Louria, 1966). *Principle: The physician must be aware of complicating infections during treatment of neoplasms. Recognition of infection is often difficult because host resistance and response to the infection are altered by the disease or its treatment. However, the search should be diligent, since prompt treatment with appropriate antibiotics may be lifesaving.*

Availability of platelet transfusions has considerably improved the therapy of thrombocytopenic bleeding due to marrow invasion by tumor or to drug therapy. Most chemotherapists consider platelet transfusions useful if the platelet count is less than 20,000/cu mm, when active bleeding is likely (Gaydos et al., 1962; Freireich, 1967).

Renal failure is commonly observed in patients with malignant disease and may be due to dehydration, invasion of the kidney or ureteral obstruction by tumor, or uric acid nephropathy secondary to tumor-cell breakdown. Adequate hydration and allopurinol therapy can prevent the potentially catastrophic renal damage due to dehydration or to uric acid accumulation (Krakoff and Murphy, 1968). Chemotherapy or x-ray therapy may be necessary to relieve renal failure caused by kidney or ureteral involvement by tumor.

Hypothetic Examples Illustrating Principles of Chemotherapy of Malignant Tumors

Type 1. The patient has a disseminated malignancy, sensitive to a wide variety of agents. The tumor has a short generation time and a rapid doubling time and is not massive (10 to 100 g).

Some hematologic malignancies fulfill these criteria, e.g., acute lymphatic leukemia, lymphoblastic lymphoma, reticulum-cell sarcoma, and Burkitt's lymphoma. Rapid growth rates are characteristic of these diseases, and doubling times of 24 hours or less are frequently noted. Response to therapy may be rapid, and the potential of hyperuricemia and uric acid nephropathy should be obviated by hydration of the patient and initiation of allopurinol therapy (see Chapters 7 and 9). Other tumors may also be characterized by rapid growth, particularly certain childhood tumors (e.g., Wilms's tumor, neuroblastoma, retinoblastoma, and medulloblastoma). Some solid tumors may grow rapidly in adults (e.g., choriocarcinoma, melanoma, and certain anaplastic tumors). When these tumors are small, therapy should be intensive and prolonged, since a long-term remission or even cure may be possible. If the patient has a tumor in the bone marrow, initial therapy with one or more selective drugs should be considered. When the bone marrow is restored to normal, cycle-active drugs should be given intensively (Bergsagel, 1971). Combination therapy should be considered if an additive or synergistic combination of drugs is available. The current programs for the treatment of acute lymphatic leukemia illustrate this approach: vincristine and prednisone are used as initial agents, followed by intensive therapy with methotrexate in large infrequent doses, and by intermittent retreatment with vincristine and prednisone (Acute Leukemia Group B, 1965; Holland, 1966a; Hryniuk and Bertino, 1969a, 1969b). *Principle: Until known curative regimens are developed for each malignancy, the programs described above should not be considered "standard" or "final" therapy. Patients should be studied carefully at centers equipped to provide maximum patient care and to obtain maximum information. Therapy should be continued for several months, even if complete remission is evident. Estimates of the duration of therapy required to produce cure in patients with acute lymphatic leukemia, if all malignant cells are destroyed, are in the range of 6 to 12 months. After this period, attempts to produce host immunity may be worth considering* (Mathe et al., 1969).

Type 2. A patient has a tumor similar to type 1, but the disease is advanced, with hepatic involvement and widespread lymphadenopathy, i.e., 100 to 1000 g of tumor.

Again, initial therapy may depend on the degree of marrow invasion by the tumor. If the marrow is involved, selective agents may be employed. If one or more large, bulky masses are present, and the tumor is radiosensitive, local x-ray therapy should be considered. If there is no invasion of the bone marrow, initial therapy might include use of a noncycle-active agent, either alone or in combination with a selective agent, to obtain maximum response, since the tumor size may indicate a "plateau" growth phase. Once some regression has been obtained and tumor mass reduced, cycle-specific agents can be instituted provided bone marrow function has returned to normal. The National Cancer Institute programs for the treatment of Hodgkin's disease and reticulum-cell sarcoma illustrate this approach (Serpick et al., 1969; DeVita et al., 1970).

Type 3. The patient has a massive primary tumor with metastatic lesions in lymph nodes. The tumor is growing moderately slowly and is no longer curable by radiation therapy or surgery.

Examples of this type of tumor are epidermoid tumors of the head and neck, lung, and gastrointestinal tract. This problem is common and difficult to treat adequately. Generalizations about these tumors are tenuous, because of the marked differences in their biologic behavior, depending on the cell type and origin of the lesion. All therapeutic modalities should be considered, and a plan developed in conjunction with radiotherapists and surgeons. Surgery or radiation therapy may be palliative, and adjunctive chemotherapy in either of these circumstances should be considered. These tumors are only moderately sensitive to drugs, and as a rule are not sensitive to any of the selective agents. Depending on the bulk of tumor remaining after surgery or radiation, a program employing a noncycle-specific agent followed by or together with a cycle-specific agent might be considered (Schabel, 1969). Unless residual tumor is small, palliation would most likely be the immediate goal with the currently available drugs. In the future, these patients may be treated in a more aggressive manner as effective new drugs or drug combinations are developed. Some progress has been made in the therapy of epidermoid carcinomas of the head and neck, using high-dose methotrexate therapy with leucovorin "rescue" (Mitchell *et al.*, 1968) and in the treatment of lung carcinoma with cyclophosphamide (Bergsagel *et al.*, 1968). Although moderately slowly growing, some epidermoid carcinomas of the head and neck may have small growth fractions, short generation times, and appreciable death rates, rendering them susceptible to cycle-active agents.

Type 4. The patient has a slowly growing tumor that is widely disseminated and very large (10^{12} cells) and is characterized by a long generation time and low growth fraction.

Diseases such as chronic lymphocytic lymphoma, lymphocytic lymphosarcoma, and multiple myeloma (Alexanian *et al.*, 1969) are examples of this type of tumor. Several other tumors may also fall into this category; however, the kinetics of growth in tumors such as carcinoids, certain papillary adenocarcinomas, astrocytomas, basal-cell carcinomas and some sarcomas are not known. The type 4 case poses a difficult problem for chemotherapy. Cycle-active agents, especially antimetabolites, are not effective. Noncycle-active agents are acceptable if given in short, repeated courses, allowing the marrow and gastrointestinal tract to recover fully between courses. A slow, steady response might be possible if the normal stem cells recover faster then the tumor cells (Skipper, 1968). A steady response is often seen when alkylating agents

are used for the treatment of chronic hematologic malignancies. Since these patients may live several years even without treatment, it is important not to overtreat, especially when the patients are asymptomatic. If the marrow has been invaded in a patient with a neoplasm of lymphatic tissues, the selective agent prednisone often is useful.

Principle: In therapy of cancer, the physician must decide whether or not the patient should be treated, by what drug or drug combinations, and by what dose schedule. Therapeutic goals must be defined in advance and balanced against potential drug toxicity. Cancer chemotherapy differs in no important way from similar considerations for any other therapy.

DRUGS USED IN IMMUNOSUPPRESSION

General Considerations

Many of the drugs used for the treatment of malignancy are also effective suppressors of the immune response in man (Berenbaum, 1967a, 1967b; Schwartz, 1967). This property has been of concern to chemotherapists, since augmentation of host defenses against malignant cells is theoretically more desirable than depression of these defenses. However, when suppression of the immune response is desirable, as in host rejection of transplanted organs, suppression of a graft versus host reaction, or suppression of the "autoimmune" response (as may occur in the so-called diseases of autoimmunity), these properties may be useful. Information accrued from the use of these drugs in the treatment of malignant disease has been extremely valuable in the treatment of nonmalignant conditions. Good clinical judgment as to when to treat patients with these drugs is important, for in some circumstances the natural history of the autoimmune diseases is long and life expectancy may not be compromised by the disease. The physician must be aware not only of the acute short-term toxicities of the drugs used but also of the possible long-term effects of these compounds.

This section covers the limited principles that have evolved from animal studies and the use of immunosuppressive drugs in man. This type of therapy, except perhaps in preventing host rejection of transplanted organs, should be considered experimental, and every patient should be carefully evaluated and followed so that the beneficial and hazardous effects of these compounds can be clearly documented, a process that will take many years to complete. Only then can the benefits and risks of drug use in these diseases be appreciated.

Mechanism of Action and Classes of Drugs with Immunosuppressive Properties

Although the rationale for the use of these drugs is ascribed to their immunosuppressive properties, the clinical usefulness of these agents may depend not solely upon these specific immunologic effects, but also upon anti-inflammatory or other unknown properties. Definitive proof of an immunosuppressive mechanism in a given disease depends upon measurements of changes induced by the drug in the specific immunologic abnormality associated with the disease. This circumstance has only rarely been possible.

Mechanism of Action as Related to the Immune Response. An antigenic stimulus, such as an organ graft, may initiate a complex series of events leading to an expression of cellular immunity (delayed hypersensitivity) or humoral immunity (Figure 12–6). Damage to the target cell may result, accompanied by an inflammatory response; the cycle may be continued by formation of new products of cell damage, which may then act to restimulate the system. Drugs may inhibit one or more of these steps; the drug employed, and the timing and dose of the drug in relation to the antigenic stimulus, are important determinants of the degree and type of immunosuppression obtained. By studying antibody production and delayed hypersensitivity in experimental animals and in man, it has been found that antimetabolites (6-mercaptopurine, azathioprine, methotrexate, and 5-fluorouracil) are most effective as immunosuppressive agents when given a day or two after the immune stimulus (Santos, 1967, 1968).

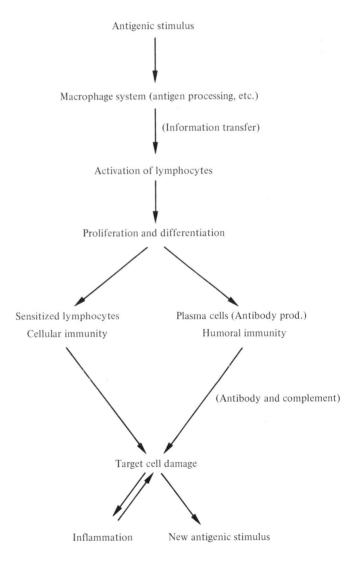

Figure 12–6. Schematic view of mechanisms operating in the immune process. (From Santos, G. W.: The pharmacology of immunosuppressive drugs. *Pharmacol. Physicians*, **2**:1–6, 1968.)

As might be expected from the ability of these drugs to inhibit cell proliferation, they probably act during the stage of proliferation following antigenic activation of lymphocytes (Figure 12-6). X-ray and the alkylating agent busulfan are effective only if given before the immune stimulus. Cyclophosphamide, a potent cytotoxic agent, has been an effective immunosuppressive agent in rodents if given either before or after the antigenic stimulus, although maximum effects are seen when this drug is given one or two days after the antigen.

In man, these drugs have the ability to inhibit (1) delayed hypersensitivity reactions (such as the induction of skin sensitivity to dinitrochlorobenzene); (2) the primary immune response to a specific antigen (e.g., *E. coli* V antigen), primarily IgG and IgM antibodies; and (3) the anamnestic response to an antigen (e.g., tetanus toxoid), primarily IgG serum antibody. Established delayed hypersensitivity and pre-existent antibody titers are usually unaffected (Swanson and Schwartz, 1967).

Corticosteroids probably block the inflammation stage of the immune response. They have proved valuable in the treatment of several autoimmune diseases, but the long-term toxic effects of corticosteroids should not be underestimated (Karnofsky, 1967) (see Chapter 9). Indeed, one of the important uses of an antimetabolite or cyclophosphamide in the treatment of autoimmune disease is to wean the patient from steroid therapy that may be the cause of undesirable side effects.

Enhancement. If an immunosuppressive drug (particularly an antimetabolite) is administered before the antigenic stimulus, enhanced antibody response may result. This paradoxical effect has been noted in experimental animals and occasionally in patients with autoimmune disease, following challenge with a foreign antigen (Chanmougan and Schwartz, 1966; Swanson and Schwartz, 1967). The explanation for this effect is not yet clear, but the result does suggest that pretreatment of patients with immunosuppressive drugs may not be indicated.

Drug-Induced Immunologic Tolerance. Tolerance (nonreactivity to a specific antigen) has been produced in animals and in man by administering large doses of antigen with appropriate timing of the immunosuppressive agent (Aisenberg, 1967; Santos, 1968; Gordon *et al.*, 1969). Tolerance may be desirable to enhance acceptance of grafts, as in bone marrow transplantation, or even to reverse an autoallergic state by producing tolerance of the host to his own antigenic tissue.

Cell Kinetics and the Use of Immunosuppressive Drugs. Certain drugs and dose schedules can inhibit one or more components of the immune response and may even produce immunologic tolerance, leading to the expectation that improvement of dosage schedules in immunosuppressive therapy may provide a better therapeutic index. Antimetabolites used in high intermittent doses at the correct interval after antigenic stimulus may effectively eliminate the antigen-stimulated lymphocytes, which appear to have generation times of 7 to 14 hours (Berenbaum, 1967a, 1967b). These high intermittent doses are less toxic (assuming the marrow is normal) than prolonged schedules; a significant increase in the therapeutic index may result. Some data suggest the effectiveness of such regimens in man (Mitchell *et al.*, 1968), but these regimens have not yet been tested following organ transplantation. As with different types of tumors, dose schedules that might be most effective for one condition, e.g., in organ transplantation, may not be the best schedule for treating an autoimmune disease, e.g., systemic lupus erythematosus. *Principle: Knowledge of the immune response, mechanism of action of drugs, and timing of drug administration and dosage schedules may allow more selective manipulation of the immune response.*

Diseases Treated by Drugs That Inhibit the Immune Response

Organ Transplantation. Renal transplantation is now commonplace, owing to the use of immunosuppressive drugs (particularly the purine antagonists). Although short-term success is likely, immediate and long-term rejections continue. Rejections are due to the limited effectiveness of these agents as immunosuppressive agents and to cumulative toxicity. Fewer rejections occur with better selection of donors by tissue typing, but the use of closely related donors for transplantation remains a problem. In addition to azathioprine (Imuran), the drug usually employed, steroids and x-ray therapy have been used as immunosuppressants for transplant recipients (Michael *et al.*, 1967). Methotrexate, a potent immunosuppressive agent, has not been used in patients receiving transplants, since most of the drug is renally excreted and increased toxicity might therefore result if it were not cleared by the kidney.

Unlike other organ transplants, when the object of therapy following the transplant is to prevent the rejection of the graft by the host, bone marrow transplants involve an additional problem. When bone marrow transplants "take," the immunologically competent cells from the donor may also survive and react against the host, giving a graft-versus-host reaction. This event, characterized by skin rash, diarrhea, liver derangement, and often death, has been approached by the use of posttransplant cytotoxic therapy. Successful treatment requires destruction of the donor lymphocytes (which are reacting against the host) without harming the donor cells producing normal blood cells. Some success has attended the use of methotrexate or cyclophosphamide with intermittent dose schedules. In this circumstance, scheduling appears to be extremely important in order to obtain a differential effect.

Bone marrow transplants have not been successful for treating human leukemia, but have been successful in the treatment of certain hereditary deficiencies (DeKoning et al., 1969). Bone marrow grafts have been obtained, but either a graft-versus-host reaction or the return of the leukemia has led to failure. Nevertheless, this is an area of active experimentation that offers some promise (Mathe et al., 1967; Santos, 1968; Thomas, 1970).

Therapy of Autoimmune Disease. Despite the theoretic objections to the use of immunosuppressive agents in autoimmune disease, moderate success has been obtained in the treatment of diseases such as systemic lupus erythematosus (Miescher and Riethmuller, 1965; Swanson and Schwartz, 1967), rheumatoid arthritis (Kahn et al., 1967; Fosdick, 1968), Wegener's granulomatosis, ulcerative colitis, glomerulonephritis, and other vascular-collagen diseases (Corley et al., 1966). Since the pathophysiology of these diseases is not clear, the exact targets for therapy are difficult to identify. Attempts to correlate the measurement of a defined immune response with therapeutic results have not been successful (Swanson and Schwartz, 1967). *Principle: The clinical effectiveness of immunosuppressive drugs in immunologic disease is not well understood and may depend upon (1) inhibition of one or more steps in the immune response, (2) anti-inflammatory action, and (3) the state of the lesion, i.e., reversible or irreversible.*

Special Problems Associated with Immunosuppressive Therapy

The risks of long-term therapy with cancer chemotherapeutic agents have received more attention in recent years, not only because certain patients with malignant disease live longer and are being treated for longer periods with these agents, but also because these drugs are being increasingly used in nonmalignant disease (Karnofsky, 1967). Hepatic fibrosis caused by methotrexate or 6-mercaptopurine has been reported (Clark et al., 1960; Hutter et al., 1960), but the time incidence is difficult to ascertain, as is the contribution of the underlying disease

(acute leukemia) and/or other drugs to the process. The reported cases of pulmonary fibrosis associated with busulfan therapy are few, but the true incidence is unknown (Karnofsky, 1967). Long-lived aplasia of the bone marrow has occurred after the use of alkylating agents, especially busulfan and thio-TEPA, but is probably uncommon after antimetabolite therapy.

Increased susceptibility to infection, in particular to opportunistic organisms such as cytomegalic virus, *Pneumocystis carinii*, or various fungi, has been observed in patients receiving steroids who are also granulocytopenic (Hill et al., 1964). In patients not receiving steroids or immunosuppressive agents to reduce the granulocyte count below 1000/cu mm, these infections have been less common (Fosdick, 1968).

Another potential hazard is teratogenicity. Although several normal pregnancies have been reported in women receiving azathioprine after a renal transplant (Kaufman et al., 1967), the use of these agents in patients with childbearing potential should be avoided if possible. Several of the antimetabolites, in particular methotrexate and 6-mercaptopurine, are well-known abortifacients, especially if taken during the first trimester of pregnancy.

Probably the most disturbing possibility of long-term administration of these drugs is the production of diminished resistance to or actual induction of cancer by cytotoxic agents. Procarbazine, a methylhydrazine compound useful in the treatment of Hodgkin's disease, and chlornaphazine, an alkylating agent that is no longer used, are potent carcinogenic agents (Videbaek, 1964; Stutman, 1969). Antilymphocyte serum and x-rays have made viral leukemias easier to induce in mice. Several cases of lymphoma have been reported in patients who received renal transplants and immunosuppressive therapy (Penn et al., 1969). Large series of patients with psoriasis treated with methotrexate for long periods have not demonstrated increased incidence of malignancy, but this potential hazard requires further careful study. *Principle: Immunosuppressive agents currently in use are potent chemicals with the capacity to injure or destroy a variety of host cells; the long-term effects of these compounds have not been fully elucidated. Their potential for producing beneficial effects in autoimmune disease should be weighed against the known and theoretic hazards.*

REFERENCES

Acute Leukemia Group B: Studies of sequential and combination antimetabolite therapy in acute leukemia:

6-mercaptopurine and methotrexate. *Blood*, 18:431–54, 1961.

————: New treatment schedule with improved survival in childhood leukemia. Intermittent parenteral versus daily oral administration of methotrexate for maintenance of induced remission. *J.A.M.A.*, 194:75–81, 1965.

Aisenberg, A. C.: Studies on cyclophosphamide-induced tolerance to sheep erythrocytes. *J. Exp. Med.*, 125:833–45, 1967.

Alexander, P.: *Atomic Radiation and Life*, 2nd ed. Penguin Books, Middlesex, England, 1965.

Alexanian, R.; Bergsagel, D. E.; Migliore, P. J.; Vaughn, W. K.; and Howe, C. D.: Melphalan therapy for plasma cell myeloma. *Blood*, 31:1–10, 1968.

Alexanian, R.; Haut, A.; Khan, A. U.; Lane, M.; McKelvey, E. M.; Migliore, P. J.; Stuckey, W. J., Jr.; and Wilson, H. E.: Treatment for multiple myeloma. Combination chemotherapy with different melphalan dose regimens. *J.A.M.A.*, 208:1680–85, 1969.

Amatruda, T. T., Jr.: Non-endocrine secreting tumors. In Duncan, G. G. (ed.): *Diseases of Metabolism*, 6th ed. W. B. Saunders Co., Philadelphia, 1969, pp. 1227–44.

Anderson, D. G.: Management of advanced endometrial adenocarcinoma with medroxyprogesterone acetate. *Amer. J. Obstet. Gynec.*, 92:87–99, 1965.

Bateman, J. C.; Moulton, B.; and Larsen, N. J.: Control of neoplastic effusions by phosphoramide chemotherapy. *Arch. Intern. Med. (Chicago)*, 95:713–19, 1955.

Berenbaum, M. C.: Immunosuppressive agents and the cellular kinetics of the immune response. In Mihich, E. (ed.): *Immunity, Cancer and Chemotherapy*. Academic Press, Inc., New York, 1967a.

————: Immunosuppressive agents and allogenic transplantation. Symposium on Tissue and Organ Transplantation. *J. Clin. Path. (Suppl.)*, 20:471–98, 1967b.

Bergsagel, D. E.: An assessment of massive-dose chemotherapy of malignant disease. *Canad. Med. Ass. J.*, 104:31–36, 1971.

Bergsagel, D. E.; Robertson, G. L.; and Hasselback, R.: Effect of cyclophosphamide on advanced lung cancer and the hematological toxicity of large intermittent intravenous doses. *Canad. Med. Ass. J.*, 98:532–38, 1968.

Bloom, H. J., and Wallace, D. M.: Hormones and the kidney; possible therapeutic role of testosterone in a patient with regression of metastases from renal adenocarcinoma. *Brit. Med. J.*, 2:476–80, 1964.

Bodey, G. P.: Infectious complications of acute leukemia. *Med. Times*, 94:1076–85, 1966.

Bodey, G. P.; Buckley, M.; Sathe, Y. S.; and Freireich, E. J.: Quantitative relationships between circulating leukocytes and infection in patients with acute leukemia. *Ann. Intern. Med.*, 64:328–40, 1966.

Boyse, E. A.; Old, L. J.; Campbell, H. A.; and Mashburn, L. T.: Suppression of murine leukemia by L-asparaginase. Incidence of sensitivity among leukemias of various types: comparative inhibitory activities of guinea pig serum L-asparaginase and *Escherichia coli* L-asparaginase. *J. Exp. Med.*, 125:17–31, 1967.

Bradley, T. R., and Metcalf, D.: The growth of mouse bone marrow cells *in vitro*. *Aust. J. Exp. Biol. Med. Sci.*, 44:287–300, 1966.

Brockman, R W.: Mechanisms of resistance to anticancer agents. *Advance Cancer Res.*, 7:129–234, 1963.

Bruce, W. R., and Bergsagel, D. E.: On the application of results from a model system to the treatment of leukemia in man. *Cancer Res.*, 27:2646–49, 1967.

Bruce, W. R., and Meeker, B. E.: Comparison of the sensitivity of hematopoietic colony-forming cells in different proliferative states to 5-fluorouracil. *J. Nat. Cancer Inst.*, 38:401–405, 1967.

Bruce, W. R.; Meeker, B. E.; and Valeriote, F. A.: Comparison of the sensitivity of normal hematopoietic and transplanted lymphoma colony-forming cells to chemotherapeutic agents administered *in vivo*. *J. Nat. Cancer Inst.*, 37:233–45, 1966.

Burchenal, J. H., and Dollinger, M. R.: Cytosine arabinoside (NSC-63878) in combination with 6-mercaptopurine (NSC-755), methotrexate (NSC-740), or 5-fluorouracil (NSC-19893) in L1210 mouse leukemia. *Cancer Chemother. Rep.*, 51:435–38, 1967.

Burkitt, D. P., and Burchenal, J. H. (eds.): *Treatment of Burkitt's Tumour*. Springer Verlag, New York, 1969.

Burningham, R. A.; Restrepo, A.; Pugh, R. P.; Brown, E. P.; Schlossman, S. F.; Khuri, P. D.; Lessner, H. E.; and Harrington, W. J.: Weekly high dose glucocorticosteroid treatment of lymphocytic leukemias and lymphomas. *New Eng. J. Med.*, 270:1160–66, 1964.

Burrows, J. H.; Talley, R. W.; Drake, E. H.; Dan Diego, E. L.; and Tucker, W. G.: Infusion of fluorinated pyrimidines into hepatic artery for treatment of metastatic carcinoma of liver. *Cancer*, 20:1886–92, 1967.

Bush, R. S., and Bruce, W. R.: The radiation sensitivity of transplanted lymphoma cells as determined by the spleen colony method. *Radiat. Res.*, 21:612–21, 1964.

Calabresi, P., and Welch, A. D.: Cytotoxic drugs, hormones and radioactive isotopes. In Goodman, L. S., and Gilman, A.: *The Pharmacological Basis of Therapeutics*, 3rd ed. The Macmillan Co., New York, 1965, pp. 1345–92.

Capizzi, R. L.; Bertino, J. R.; and Handschumacher, R. E.: L-asparaginase. *Amer. Rev. Med.*, 1970, in press.

Chanmougan, D., and Schwartz, R. S.: Enhancement of antibody synthesis by 6-mercaptopurine. *J. Exp. Med.*, 124:363–78, 1966.

Chick, H.: An investigation of the laws of disinfection. *J. Hyg.*, 8:92–158, 1908.

Clark, P. A.; Hsia, Y. E.; and Huntsman, R. G.: Toxic complications of treatment with 6-mercaptopurine: two cases with hepatic necrosis and intestinal ulceration. *Brit. Med. J.*, 1:393–95, 1960.

Clarkson, B.; Ohkita, T.; Ota, K.; and Fried, J.: Studies of cellular proliferation in human leukemia. I. Estimation of growth rates of leukemic and normal hematopoietic cells in two adults with acute leukemia given single injections of tritiated thymidine. *J. Clin. Invest.*, 46:506–29, 1967.

Cleveland, J. C.; Johns, D.; Farnham, G.; and Bertino, J. R.: Arterial infusion of dichloromethotrexate in cancer of the head and neck: a clinicopharmacologic study. In Zuidema, G. D., and Kinner, D. B. (eds.): *Current Topics in Surgical Research*, Academic Press, Inc., New York, 1969.

Cline, M. J.: *Cancer Chemotherapy*. W. B. Saunders Co., Philadelphia, 1971.

Cooperative Breast Cancer Group: Testosterone propionate therapy in breast cancer. *J.A.M.A.*, 188:1069–72, 1964.

Corley, C. C., Jr.; Lessner, H. E.; and Larsen, W. E.: Azathioprine therapy of "autoimmune" diseases. *Amer. J. Med.*, 41:404–12, 1966.

Creech, O., Jr.; Krementa, E. T.; Ryan, R. F.; and Winblad, J. N.: Chemotherapy of cancer: regional perfusion utilizing an extracorporeal circuit. *Ann. Surg.*, 148:616–32, 1958.

Crile, G., Jr.: Endocrine dependency of papillary carcinomas of the thyroid. *J.A.M.A.*, 195:721–24, 1966.

DeKoning, J.; Dooren, L. J.; Van Bekkum, D. W.; Van Rood, J. J.; Dicke, K. A.; and Raol, J.: Transplantation of bone marrow cells and fetal thymus in an infant with lymphopenic immunological deficiency. *Lancet*, 1:1223–27, 1969.

DeVita, V. T., Jr.; Serpick, A. A.; and Carbone, P. P.: Combination chemotherapy in the treatment of advanced Hodgkin's disease. *Ann. Intern. Med.*, 73:881–96, 1970.

Fosdick, W. M.: Cytotoxic therapy in rheumatoid arthritis. *Med. Clin. N. Amer.*, 52:747–57, 1968.

Frei, E., and Freireich, E. J.: Progress and perspectives in the chemotherapy of acute leukemia. *Advance Chemother.*, 2:269–98, 1965.

Freireich, E. J.: The management of acute leukemia. *Canad. Med. Ass. J.*, 96:1605–10, 1967.

Furth, J., and Kahn, M. C.: The transmission of leukemia of mice with a single cell. *Amer. J. Cancer*, 31:276–82, 1937.

Gaydos, L. A.; Freireich, E. J.; and Mantel, N.: The quantitative relation between platelet count and hemorrhage in patients with acute leukemia. *New Eng. J. Med.*, 266:905–909, 1962.

Gee, T. S.; Yu, K. P.; and Clarkson, B. D.: Treatment of adult acute leukemia with arabinosylcytosine and thioguanine. *Cancer*, 23:1019–32, 1969.

Gellhorn, A.: Ectopic hormone production in cancer and its implication for basic research in abnormal growth. *Advance Intern. Med.*, 15:299–316, 1969.

Goldin, A.; Venditti, J. M.; Humphreys, S. R.; and Mantel, N.: Influence of concentration of leukemic inoculum on the effectiveness of treatment. *Science*, 123:840, 1956a.

———: Modification of treatment schedules in the management of advanced mouse leukemia with amethopterin. *J. Nat. Cancer Inst.*, 17:203–12, 1956b.

Gordon, R. O.; Wade, M. E.; and Mitchell, M. S.: The production of tolerance to human erythrocytes in the rat with cytosine arabinoside or cyclophosphamide. *J. Immunol.*, 103:233–43, 1969.

Haskell, C. M.; Canellos, G. P.; Leventhal, B. G.; Carbone, P. P.; Block, J. B.; Serpick, A. A.; and Selawry, O. S.: L-Asparaginase: therapeutic and toxic effects in patients with neoplastic disease. *New Eng. J. Med.*, 281:1028–34, 1969.

Hellström, K. I., and Hellström, I.: Immunologic defences against cancer. *Hosp. Pract.*, p. 45, Jan., 1970.

Henderson, E. S.: Treatment of acute leukemia. *Seminar Hemat.*, 6:271–319, 1969.

Hiatt, H. H.: Cancer chemotherapy—present status and prospects. *New Eng. J. Med.*, 276:157–66, 1967.

Hill, J. M.; Roberts, J.; Loeb, E.; Khan, A.; MacLellan, A.; and Hill, R. W.: L-Asparaginase therapy for leukemia and other malignant neoplasma. *J.A.M.A.*, 202:882–88, 1967.

Hill, R. B.; Rowlands, D. T.; and Refkind, D.: Infectious pulmonary disease in patients receiving immunosuppressive therapy for organ transplantation. *New Eng. J. Med.*, 271:1021–27, 1964.

Holland, J. F.: Progress in treatment of acute leukemia. In Dameshek, W., and Dutcher, R. M. (eds.): *Perspectives in Leukemia*. Grune & Stratton, New York, 1966a, pp. 217–40.

———: In Lasagna, L. S. (ed.): *International Encyclopedia of Pharmacology and Therapeutics*, Section 6, Vol. II, *Clinical Pharmacology*. Pergamon Press, New York, 1966b, pp. 597–616.

Hryniuk, W. M., and Bertino, J. R.: Rationale for the selection of chemotherapeutic agents. *Advance Intern. Med.*, 15:267–98, 1969a.

———: The treatment of leukemia with large doses of methotrexate and folinic acid: clinical-biochemical correlates. *J. Clin. Invest.*, 48:2140–55, 1969b.

Hryniuk, W. M.; Fischer, G. A.; and Bertino, J. R.: S-phase cells of rapidly growing and resting populations. Differences in response to methotrexate. *Molec. Pharmacol.*, 5:557–64, 1969.

Huggins, C., and Hodges, C. V.: Studies on prostatic cancer. I. The effect of castration, of estrogen and of androgen injection on serum phosphatases in metastatic carcinoma of the prostate. *Cancer Res.*, 1:293–97, 1941.

Hulka, J. F., and Mohr, K.: Trophoblast antigenicity demonstrated by altered challenge graft survival. *Science*, 161:696–98, 1968.

Hutchinson, D. J.: Studies on cross-resistance and collateral sensitivity (1962–1964). *Cancer Res.*, 25:1581–95, 1965.

Hutter, A. M., Jr., and Kayhoe, D. E.: Adrenal cortical carcinoma. Results of treatment with o,p-DDD in 138 patients. *Amer. J. Med.*, 41:581–92, 1966.

Hutter, R. V., and Collins, H. S.: The occurrence of opportunistic fungus injections in a cancer hospital. *Lab. Invest.*, 11:1035–45, 1962.

Hutter, R. V.; Shipkey, F. H.; Tan, C. T. C.; Murphy, M. L.; and Chowahury, M.: Hepatic fibrosis in children with acute leukemia. *Cancer*, 13:288–307, 1960.

James, D. H., Jr.; Hustu, O.; Wrenn, E. L., Jr.; and Pinkel, D.: Combination chemotherapy of childhood neuroblastoma. *J.A.M.A.*, 194:123–26, 1965.

Kahn, M. F.; Bedoiseau, M.; and deSege, S.: Immunosuppressive drugs in the management of malignant and severe rheumatoid arthritis. *Proc. Roy. Soc. Med.*, 60:130–33, 1967.

Karnofsky, D. A.: Late effects of immunosuppressive anticancer drugs. *Fed. Proc.*, 26:925–33, 1967.

Kaufman, J. J.; Dignam, W.; Goodwin, W. E.; Martin, D. C.; Goldman, R.; and Maxwell, M. H.: Successful normal childbirth after kidney transplantation. *J.A.M.A.*, 200:338–41, 1967.

Kelly, R. M., and Baker, W. H.: Progestational agents in the treatment of carcinoma of the endometrium. *Cancer Res.*, 25:1190–92, 1965.

Kennedy, B. J.: Androgenic hormone therapy in lymphatic leukemia. *J.A.M.A.*, 190:1130–33, 1964.

———: Hormone therapy for advanced breast cancer. *Cancer*, 18:1551–57, 1965.

Kidd, J. G.: Regression of transplanted lymphomas induced *in vivo* by means of normal guinea pig serum. *J. Exp. Med.*, 98:565–81, 1953.

Klein, G.: Plenary Session Papers, XII Congress of International Society of Hematology, 1968, p. 15.

Klein, G.; Klein, E.; and Clifford, P.: Search for host defenses in Burkitt's lymphoma: membrane immunofluorescence tests on biopsies and tissue culture lines. *Cancer Res.*, 27:2510–20, 1967.

Krakoff, I. H., and Murphy, M. L.: Hyperuricemia in neoplastic disease in children: prevention with allopurinol, a xanthine oxidase inhibitor. *Pediatrics*, 41:52–56, 1968.

Lacher, M. J., and Durant, J. R.: Combined vinblastine and chlorambucil therapy of Hodgkin's disease. *Ann. Intern. Med.*, 62:468–76, 1965.

Laird, A. K.: Dynamics of tumor growth. *Brit. J. Cancer*, 18:490–502, 1964.

———: Dynamics of tumor growth: comparison of growth rates and extrapolation of growth curve to one cell. *Brit. J. Cancer*, 19:278–91, 1965.

Lambert, C. J.; Shad, H. H.; Urschel, H. C., Jr.; and Paulson, D. L.: The treatment of malignant pleural effusions by closed trocar tube drainage. *Ann. Thorac. Surg.*, 3:1–5, 1967.

Laster, W. R., Jr.; Mayo, J. G.; Simpson-Herren, L.; Griswald, D. P., Jr.; Lloyd, H. H.; Schabel, F. M., Jr.; and Skipper, H. E.: Success and failure in the treatment of solid tumors. II. Kinetic parameters and "cell cure" of moderately advanced carcinoma 755. *Cancer Chemother. Rep.*, 53:169–88, 1969.

Lawrence, W., Jr.: Current status of regional therapy. *New York Med.*, 63:2359–75, 2518–34, 1963.

Lemon, H. M.: Prednisone therapy of advanced mammary cancer. *Cancer*, 12:93–107, 1959.

Louria, D. B.: Treatment of infections arising in patients with neoplasms. *Mod. Treatment*, 3:1093–98, 1966.

Luce, J. R.; Bodey, G. P.; and Frei, E.: The systemic approach to cancer therapy. *Hosp. Pract.*, 2:42–55, 1967.

Luyendijk, W., and Van Beusekom, G. Th.: Chemotherapy of cerebral gliomas with intra-carotid methotrexate infusion. *Acta Neurochir.*, 15:234–48, 1966.

McCredie, J. A.; Inch, W. R.; Kruuv, J.; and Watson, T. A.: The rate of tumor growth in animals. *Growth*, 29:331–47, 1965.

Martin, D. S.; Hayworth, P.; Fugmann, R. A.; English, R.; and McNeill, H. W.: Combination therapy with cyclophosphamide and zymosan on a spontaneous mammary cancer in mice. *Cancer Res.*, 24:652–54, 1964.

Mathe, G.; Amiel, J. L.; Schwarzenberg, L.; Cattan, A.; and Schneider, M.: Treatment of acute leukemia by allogenic bone marrow graft. *Progr. Clin. Cancer*, 3:309–19, 1967.

Mathe, G.; Amiel, J. L.; Schwarzenberg, L.; Schneider, M.; Cattan, A.; Schlumberger, J. R.; Hayat, M.; and deVassal, F.: Active immunotherapy for acute lymphoblastic leukemia. *Lancet*, 1:697–99, 1969.

Mauer, A. M., and Fisher, V.: Characteristics of cell proliferation in four patients with untreated acute leukemia. *Blood*, 28:428–45, 1966.

Mendelsohn, M. L.: The kinetics of tumor cell proliferation. In *Cellular Radiation Biology*. M.D. Anderson Hospital and Tumor Institute. Williams & Wilkins Co., Baltimore, 1965, pp. 499–513.

Midgley, A. R.: Radioimmunoassay: a method for human chorionic gonadotropin and human luteinizing hormone. *Endocrinology*, 79:10–18, 1966.

Miescher, P. A., and Riethmuller, D.: Diagnosis and treatment of systemic lupus erythematosus. *Seminar Hemat.*, 2:1–28, 1965.

Mitchell, M. S.; Wade, M. E.; DeConti, R. C.; Bertino, J. R.; and Calabresi, P.: Immunosuppressive effects of cytosine arabinoside and methotrexate in man. *Ann. Intern. Med.*, 70:535–47, 1969.

Mitchell, M. S.; Wawro, M. W.; DeContil R. C.; Kaplan, S. R.; Papac, R.; and Bertino, J. R.: Effectiveness of high-dose infusions of methotrexate followed by leucovorin in carcinoma of the head and neck. *Cancer Res.*, 28:1088–94, 1968.

Mittleman, A.; Grinbert, R.; and Dao, Til.: Clinical experience with vincristine in women with breast cancer. *Proc. Amer. Ass. Cancer Res.*, 2:367, 1963.

Moore, E. W.; Thomas, L. B.; Shaw, R. K.; and Freireich, E. J.: The central nervous system in acute leukemia: a postmortem study of 117 consecutive cases, with particular reference to hemorrhage, leukemic infiltrations and the syndrome of meningeal leukemia. *Arch. Intern. Med.* (*Chicago*), 105:451–68, 1960.

Moore, F. D.; Woodrow, S. I.; Aliapoulious, M. A.; and Wilson, R. E.: Carcinoma of the breast. A decade of new results with old concepts. *New Eng. J. Med.*, 277:293–96; 343–50; 411–16; 460–68, 1967.

Oettgen, H. R.; Old, L. J.; Boyse, E. A.; Cambell, H. A.; Phillips, F. S.; Clarkson, B. D.; Tallal, L.; Leeper, R. D.; Schwartz, M. K.; and Kim, J. H.: Inhibition of leukemias in man by L-asparaginase. *Cancer Res.*, 27:2619–31, 1967.

Oettgen, H. R., and Schulten, H. K.: Hemmung maligner neoplasien des menschen durch L-asparaginase. *Klin. Wschr.*, 47:65–71, 1969.

Oliverio, V. T., and Zubrod, O. G.: Clinical pharmacology of the effective antitumor drugs. *Ann. Rev. Pharmacol.*, 5:335–56, 1965.

Osserman, E. F., and Lawlor, D. P.: Serum and urinary lysozyme (muramidase) in monocytic and mono-myelocytic leukemia. *J. Exp. Med.*, 124:921–52, 1966.

Penn, I.; Hammond, W.; Brettschneider, L.; and Starze, T. E.: Malignant lymphomas in transplantation patients. *Transplant Proc.*, 1:106–12, 1969.

Perillie, P. E.; Kaplan, S. S.; Lefkowitz, E.; Rogaway, W.; and Finch, S. C.: Studies of muramidase (lysozyme) in leukemia. *J.A.M.A.*, 203:317–22, 1968.

Rall, D. P., and Homan, E. R.: Possible approaches to selective toxicity: new concepts in cancer chemotherapy. *Cancer Chemother. Rep.*, 51:247–51, 1967.

Rieselbach, R. E.; Morse, E. E.; Rall, D. P.; Frei, E., III; and Freireich, E. J.: Intrathecal aminopterin therapy of meningeal leukemia. *Arch. Intern. Med.* (*Chicago*), 111:620–30, 1963.

Ross, G. T.; Goldstein, D. P.; Hertz, R.; Lipsett, M. B.; and Odell, W. D.: Sequential use of methotrexate and actinomycin D in the treatment of metastatic choriocarcinoma and related trophoblastic diseases in women. *Amer. J. Obstet. Gynec.*, 93:223–29, 1965.

Salmon, S. E., and Smith, B. A.: Immunoglobulin synthesis and total body tumor cell number in IgG multiple myeloma. *J. Clin. Invest.*, 49:1114–21, 1970.

Santos, G. W.: Immunosuppressive drugs. *Fed. Proc.*, 26:907–13, 1967.

————: The pharmacology of immunosuppressive drugs. *Pharmacol. for Physicians*, 2:1–6, 1968.

Santos, G. W.; Sensenbrenner, L. L.; Burke, P. J.; Coloin, O. M.; Owens, A. H., Jr.; Bias, W.; and Slavin, R.: Marrow transplantation in man utilizing cyclophosphamide: Summary of Baltimore experiences. *Exp. Hematol.*, 20:78–81, 1970.

Sartorelli, A. C.: Approaches to the combination chemotherapy of transplantable neoplasms. *Progr. Exp. Tumor Res.*, 6:228–88, 1965.

Sartorelli, A. C., and Creasey, W. A.: Cancer chemotherapy. *Ann. Rev. Pharmacol.*, 9:51–72, 1969.

Schabel, F. M., Jr.: Drug treatment of malignant tumors of man and animals: a rational approach to cancer chemotherapy. *Southern Med. Bull.*, 57:40–46, 1969.

Schwartz, R. S.: Symposium on immunosuppressive drugs. II. Immunosuppressive drugs. *Fed. Proc.*, 26:914–17, 1967.

Senn, J. S.; Till, J. E.; Siminovitch, L.; and McCulloch, E. A.: Colony formation in vitro from single-cell suspensions of human bone marrow. *Exp. Hemat.*, 13:24–26, 1967.

Serpick, A. A.; Lowenbraun, S.; and DeVita, V. T.: Combination chemotherapy of lymphosarcoma and reticulum cell sarcoma. *Proc. Amer. Ass. Cancer Res.*, 10:78, 1969.

Skipper, H. E.: Biochemical, biological, pharmacologic, toxicologic, kinetic and clinical (subhuman and human) relationships. *Cancer*, 21:600–10, 1968.

Skipper, H. E.; Schabel, F. M., Jr.; and Wilcox, W. S.: Experimental evaluation of potential anticancer agents. XIII. On the criteria kinetics associated with "curability" of experimental leukemia. *Cancer Chemother. Rep.*, 35:3–111, 1964.

————: Experimental evaluation of potential anticancer agents. XIV. Further study of certain basic concepts underlying chemotherapy of leukemia. *Cancer Chemother. Rep.*, 45:5–28, 1965.

————: Experimental evaluation of potential anticancer agents. XXI. Scheduling or arabinosylcytosine to take advantage of its S-phase specificity against leukemia cells. *Cancer Chemother. Rep.*, 51:125–65, 1967.

Skurkovich, S. V.; Makhonova, L. A.; Reznichenko, F. M.; and Chervonskiy, G. I.: Treatment of children with acute leukemia by passive cyclic immunization with autoplasma and autoleukocytes operated during the remission period. *Blood*, 33:186–97, 1969.

Southam, C. M.: Evidence for cancer-specific antigens of man. *Progr. Exp. Tumor Res.*, 9:1–39, 1967.

Southwest Cancer Chemotherapy Group: Vincristine (leurocristine) sulfate in the treatment of children with metastatic Wilms' tumor. *Pediatrics*, 32:880–87, 1963.

Steel, G. G.: Cell loss as a factor in the growth rate of human tumors. *Europ. J. Cancer*, 3:381–87, 1967.

Stutman, O.: Absence of carcinogen-induced immune depression in mice resistant to methylcholanthrene oncogenesis. *Proc. Amer. Ass. Cancer Res.*, 10:89, 1969.

Sullivan, R. D.; Miller, E.; and Sikes, M. P.: Antimetabolite-metabolite combination cancer chemotherapy. Effects of intra-arterial methotrexate-intramuscular citrovorum factor therapy in human cancer. *Cancer*, 12:1248–62, 1959.

Sullivan, R. D.; Young, C. W.; Miller, E.; Glatstein, N.; Clarkson, B.; and Burchenal, J. H.: The clinical effects of the continuous administration of fluorinated pyrimidines (5-fluorouracil and 5-fluoro-2′-deoxyuridine). *Cancer Chemother. Rep.*, 8:77–83, 1960.

Swanson, M., and Schwartz, R. S.: Immunosuppressive therapy. *New Eng. J. Med.*, 277:163–70, 1967.

Thomas, E. D.: Bone Marrow Conference. *Exp. Hematol.*, 1970.

Till, J. E., and McCulloch, E. A.: A direct measurement of the radiation sensitivity of normal mouse bone marrow cells. *Radiat. Res.*, 14:213–22, 1961.

Ultmann, J. E.: Diagnosis and treatment of neoplastic effusions. *CA*, 12:42–50, 1962.

Valeriote, F. A., and Bruce, W. R.: Comparison of the sensitivity of hematopoietic colony-forming cells in different proliferative states to vinblastine. *J. Nat. Cancer Inst.*, 38:393–99, 1967.

Valeriote, F. A.; Bruce, W. R.; and Meeker, B. E.: Synergistic action of cyclophosphamide and 1,3-bis-(2-chloroethyl)-1-nitrosourea on a transplanted murine lymphoma. *J. Nat. Cancer Inst.*, 40:935–44, 1968a.

Valeriote, F. A.; Collins, D. C.; and Bruce, W. R.: Hematological recovery in the mouse following single doses of gamma radiation and cyclophosphamide. *Radiat. Res.*, 33:501–11, 1968b.

Venditti, J. M., and Goldin, A.: Drug synergism in antineoplastic chemotherapy. *Advance Chemother.*, 1:397–498, 1964.

Venditti, J. M.; Humphreys, S. R.; Mantel, N. M.; and Goldin, A.: Combined treatment of advanced leukemia in mice with amethopterin and 6-mercaptopurine. *J. Nat. Cancer Inst.*, 17:631–38, 1956.

Videbaek, A.: Chlornaphazin (Erysan®) may induce cancer of the urinary bladder. *Acta Med. Scand.*, 176:45–50, 1964.

Welch, A. D.: The problem of drug resistance in cancer chemotherapy. *Cancer Res.*, 19:359–71, 1959.

Wilcox, W. S.: The last surviving cancer cell: the chances of killing it. *Cancer Chemother. Rep.*, 50:541–42, 1966.

Wilcox, W. S.; Griswold, D. P.; Laster, W. R., Jr.; Schabel, F. M., Jr.; and Skipper, H. E.: Experimental evaluation of potential anticancer agents. XVII. Kinetics of growth and regression after treatment of certain solid tumors. *Cancer Chemother. Rep.*, 47:27–39, 1965.

Wolberg, W. H.: The effect of 5-fluorouracil on DNA-thymidine synthesis in human tumors. *Cancer Res.*, 29:2137–44, 1969.

Young, R. C., and DeVita, V. T.: Cell cycle characteristics of human solid tumors *in vivo*. *Cell Tissue Kinet.*, 3:285–90, 1970.

Young, R. C.; DeVita, V. T.; and Perry, S.: The thymidine-14C and 3H double-labeling technic in the study of the cell cycle of L-1210 leukemia ascites tumor *in vivo*. *Cancer Res.*, 29:1581–84, 1969.

Chapter 13

GENETIC DISORDERS

Hibbard E. Williams

The late appearance of this chapter in a textbook of clinical pharmacology should not lead to implications concerning the importance of this subject. Despite the antiquity of therapeutics, the importance of genetic factors in the use of drugs is one of the newest subdisciplines of pharmacology. In fact, its importance has been appreciated only during the past decade, when an amazing and long-overdue emphasis has been placed on "pharmacogenetics" by the impressive investigations of human geneticists and clinical pharmacologists. Beginning with the teratogenicity of drugs, pharmacogenetics has come to involve several other areas of clinical pharmacology, including the differences in individual responses to drugs, the precipitation of genetic disorders by drugs, the modification of drug effects by genetic diseases, and the effects of drugs on chromosomal structure. Although pharmacogenetic topics have been discussed in each of the preceding chapters, this chapter presents principles important in the role of genetic factors in the rational use of drugs.

The expression of genetic diseases is extremely varied. Mutations that produce lethal cellular alterations in the developing sperm, ovum, or zygote are probably quite common. The mutagens involved in severe defects include various forms of radiation, infectious agents, and, more recently recognized, a number of drugs. Although the exact mechanism by which drugs and chemical agents are mutagenic is largely unknown, the significance of these effects cannot be underestimated. All drugs must be considered potential mutagens until sufficient experience with them eliminates such dangers. This is a feat of no small magnitude, since an effect of drugs on developing germ tissue may not express itself for several generations. Until accurate quantitative means become available for the convenient testing of mutagenicity, any drug must be used with care in any patient within the reproductive age. In all cases of infertility or increased fetal wastage, drugs must be suspected as possible etiologic agents. Because of the difficulties in either objectively convicting or acquitting drugs in the production of lethal mutations, extensive drug testing of new drugs must be supported and the identification and reporting of possible culprits by watchful physicians strongly encouraged.

Another level of genetic expression includes the clinically recognizable congenital anomalies or hereditary metabolic diseases. Drugs play many roles at this level. As with lethal mutations, drugs may be incriminated as etiologic factors in a number of congenital anomalies, the thalidomide example affording the widest evidence of this problem. In a more positive sense, drugs may be useful in the management of certain hereditary metabolic disorders. In the adrenogenital syndrome and in goitrous cretinism, the use of cortisone and thyroid hormone, respectively, is often curative. Use of allopurinol is often helpful in preventing the accumulation of uric acid in hereditary forms of gout (Klinenberg, 1969). Attempts to stimulate new enzyme synthesis in certain enzyme deficiency states, such as some hyperbilirubinemias, or administration of the missing or defective enzyme, have occasionally been successful (Scriver, 1969). Such methods offer promise for better treatment of hereditary metabolic diseases.

On a more subtle level, altered genetic expression may be manifested by abnormalities in drug metabolism. In this form the genetic disorder generally lacks specific phenotypic expression until drug therapy is introduced, often for unrelated, nongenetic disease. A familiar example of this problem is the identification of rapid and slow inactivators of isoniazid (Evans, 1968), a phenomenon that has no known clinical importance in the absence of drug therapy. Another genetic expression is the precipitation of disease by drugs. As an example, the initiation of oxidant drug therapy may lead to the precipitation of hemolytic crises in patients with glucose-6-phosphate dehydrogenase deficiency, although phenotypic expression of the abnormality may be lacking under normal conditions (Kirkman, 1968). Similarly, use of succinylcholine anesthesia in the otherwise normal patient with pseudo-cholinesterase deficiency leads to prolonged apnea (Evans, 1968). *Principle: The role of drugs in the etiology and precipitation of genetic disorders is often overlooked because of their wide variety of clinical expressions. By keeping in mind the various ways in which drugs and genetic disorders may interact, the physician may more frequently and accurately recognize the importance of therapeutic agents in genetic disease.*

CATEGORIES OF DRUGS AND THERAPEUTIC PRINCIPLES

Inherited Differences in Drug Metabolism

This category of pharmacogenetics is a new but rapidly expanding area of investigation, fostered to a large extent by the recognition that hereditarily determined differences in drug metabolism are extraordinarily common. Many advances in this area awaited the elucidation of the complex factors that determine the pharmacokinetics of drugs. Many determinants of pharmacokinetic behavior of drugs are affected by genetic factors, i.e., absorption, transport of drug in blood and across cell membranes, enzymatic metabolism, conjugation, and excretion. A mutation affecting any step in this complex pathway could lead to a recognizable disturbance in drug pharmacokinetics, which undoubtedly occurs much more frequently than is currently recognized. Such recognition is often dependent on the application of correct methods for identification of differences in drug metabolism. Studies of drug concentrations in blood in sample populations may show a bimodal or discontinuous variation that suggests genetic influences on drug metabolism. This approach to the study of isoniazid metabolism has revealed that nearly half the individuals in the United States are "slow inactivators" of isoniazid (Evans *et al.*, 1960). Studies in mono- and dizygotic twins have shown that genetic factors are responsible for individual differences in the metabolism of several drugs (Vesell and Page, 1968a, 1968b, 1968c).

The clinical response to drugs may suggest clues to genetic factors or to genetic-environmental interactions. The unexpected appearance of toxic symptoms to a drug may indicate a genetically determined defect in its metabolism or excretion. An increased requirement for a drug to achieve a desired clinical effect may represent a hereditarily determined resistance to drug action. Recognition of the mechanism for the resistance may allow the rational determination of drug dosage in such individuals. Unfortunately, clinical clues alone cannot be relied upon to identify the many genetic influences on drug metabolism; the large therapeutic index of most drugs tends to hinder recognition of variations in metabolism. More sophisticated and detailed approaches to drug testing in various populations will be necessary to bring out these metabolic aberrations. *Principle: Hereditarily determined factors in drug metabolism and excretion may play a major role in determining drug effectiveness in the individual patient. These factors may be quantitatively more important in determining the response to a drug than are nongenetic differences in intrinsic drug effectiveness. In any untoward drug effect, consider genetic influences.*

Genetic Disorders That Modify Response to Drugs

A number of hereditary disorders can affect an individual's response to a drug. The prototype of this phenomenon is the syndrome of primaquine-sensitive hemolytic anemia, caused by hereditarily determined glucose-6-phosphate dehydrogenase deficiency of erythrocytes (Kirkman, 1968). The symptoms of acute intermittent porphyria may be precipitated by administration of barbiturates (Schmid, 1966). Patients with the Crigler-Najjar syndrome, a deficiency in the glucuronyl transferase system, demonstrate impaired glucuronide conjugation of drugs such as salicylates (Kalow, 1962) (see Chapters 15 and 16). Vasopressin-resistant diabetes insipidus and pseudohypoparathyroidism are examples of defective responsiveness of receptors to hormones (Relkin, 1968; Potts and Deftos, 1969). In the Lesch-Nyhan syndrome (in which excessive purine synthesis occurs), azathioprine administration fails to inhibit *de-novo* synthesis of purines (Kelley *et al.*, 1967).

This group of diverse examples emphasizes the variety of clinical syndromes and therapeutic agents that may interrelate when an underlying genetic disorder exists. As with disorders of drug metabolism, any unusual response to a drug should raise the suspicion of an underlying, previously undiagnosed genetic disorder. A diagnosis of idiopathic hypertrophic subaortic stenosis may be suggested by aggravation of heart failure by digitalis, acute intermittent porphyria considered by the astute physician when the typical symptoms appear after the use of barbiturates, or inherited narrow-angle glaucoma suspected when symptoms of increased intraocular pressure follow atropine administration. *Principle: Consider the presence of a genetic disorder when an unusual clinical response to drug administration is observed.*

Direct Effects of Drugs on the Genotype

The development of techniques for morphologic analysis of human chromosomes has led to speculations concerning the association of certain diseases with altered chromosomal structure. The various sex chromosome anomalies, such as Turner's syndrome and Klinefelter's syndrome, the autosomal trisomic and monosomic states, and the deletion and translocation syndromes indicate the wide variety of clinical problems associated with karyotypic abnormalities. In addition, the high incidence of malignant disease in many conditions known to be associated with coexistent chromosomal abnormalities, e.g., Bloom's syndrome (German *et al.*, 1965), Fanconi's anemia (Swift and Hirschhorn, 1966), and xeroderma pigmentosa (Cleaver, 1968), has focused attention on factors affecting genotype.

Recently, drugs have been incriminated in the production of abnormal genotypes. Although many of these studies have been conducted in highly unphysiologic environments, the reported appearance of abnormal chromosomal forms in patients taking lysergic acid diethylamide (LSD) has raised a number of questions about the clinical importance of such findings and about the frequency of abnormalities following the administration of any exogenous compound (Hirschhorn and Cohen, 1968). Although the role of drugs in the production of significant genotypic abnormalities cannot yet be defined accurately, the experience with thalidomide and the few observations with LSD should raise the danger signal in this fledgling area of pharmacogenetics. Considerable experimental data must be gathered before the significance of these effects can be determined. Until this is done, all drugs must be suspected of having genotypic effects that may require several generations for full expression. The legacy of these important early studies is expanded investigation of the genotypic effects of drugs in future generations.

Treatment of Metabolic Diseases of Genetic Origin

Pharmacogenetics affords one of the most challenging and potentially rewarding aspects of therapeutics for both the geneticist and the clinical pharmacologist. The rational use of therapeutic agents in the treatment of hereditary metabolic disorders is dependent upon a number of factors: accurate early diagnosis, a thorough understanding of pathogenetic mechanisms, knowledge of the mode of transmission and methods for detection of heterozygous carriers, and prognosis of the untreated disease. Although knowledge of these factors is rather primitive for many rare genetic diseases, the recent elucidation of specific pathogenetic defects in several inborn errors of metabolism has led to the development of many unique and successful forms of treatment (Scriver, 1969).

The clinical manifestations of several hereditary metabolic disorders may be similar regardless of variations in their specific enzymatic defect. Consider the following metabolic sequence in which each letter represents a substrate or product, and E_1, E_2, and E_3 represent specific enzymes:

$$A \xrightarrow{E_1} B \xrightarrow{E_2} C \xrightarrow{E_3} D$$
$$C \longrightarrow F$$

As a result of a block in the conversion of C to D owing to a defect in enzyme E_3, four major consequences could result: (1) loss of the product D; (2) accumulation of the substrate C; (3) accumulation of more remote precursors A and B (assuming enzymes E_1 and E_2 are reversible); and (4) production of alternate product F.

A consideration of type 1 glycogen storage disease, secondary to a deficiency of glucose-6-phosphatase, serves as an example (Field, 1966). In this condition the clinical manifestations are related to the four metabolic consequences listed above. In the presence of the specific enzyme defect: (1) loss of the product, glucose, leads to hypoglycemia; (2) accumulation of the substrate, glucose-6-phosphate, may account for many intracellular abnormalities; (3) accumulation of a more remote precursor, glycogen, leads to hepatomegaly; and (4) the production of alternate products, lactate and uric acid, accounts for the acidosis and hyperuricemia seen in this disorder.

The treatment of any hereditary metabolic disorder requires a thorough understanding of its metabolic abnormalities. Therapeutic measures can then be directed toward specific correction or amelioration of each particular abnormality.

Supplying the Missing Product. This approach has been successful in the treatment of several inborn errors of metabolism. Frequent carbohydrate feedings prevent hypoglycemia in patients with the glycogen storage diseases (Field, 1966). Administration of thyroxine to the patient with familial goiter secondary to an enzymatic defect in thyroxine synthesis (Stanbury, 1966), or cortisone administration to the patient with the adrenogenital syndrome (Stempfel and Tomkins, 1966), effectively reverses all the clinical manifestations of these disorders. Oral therapy with uridine in orotic aciduria, a rare disorder of pyrimidine synthesis, has reversed the complicating megaloblastic anemia (Smith et al., 1966).

In enzymatic disorders associated with a structural abnormality in the enzyme that decreases its affinity for substrate, administration of very large amounts of substrate might allow sufficient product synthesis to prevent symptoms related to deficient product supply. This theoretic approach to treatment of an enzymatic defect has not yet found direct application.

Prevention of Substrate Accumulation. This approach to therapy has received wide attention in recent years because of its apparent effectiveness in preventing permanent disability in certain metabolic disorders. A low phenylalanine diet in the treatment of phenylketonuria has prevented severe mental retardation in these patients (Anderson and Swaiman, 1967). Similar methods have been attempted with variable success in the treatment of maple syrup urine disease (Westall, 1963), galactosemia (Komrower, 1967), hereditary fructose intolerance (Froesch et al., 1963), and Refsum's disease (Steinberg et al., 1967).

Prevention of Alternate Product Synthesis. Although the methods for prevention of substrate accumulation may limit alternate product formation, other unique methods have been developed to handle this complication. The use of specific enzyme inhibitors has met with limited but often dramatic success. Allopurinol, a xanthine oxidase inhibitor, reduces serum and urine uric acid levels in patients with hyperuricemia, regardless of the underlying cause of the purine disorder (Klinenberg, 1969) (see Chapter 3). In primary hyperoxaluria, excessive oxalate production may be affected by certain inhibitors of oxalate synthesis (Williams

and Smith, 1968; Smith et al., 1971). These promising results indicate the importance of this type of approach to therapy of genetic metabolic diseases as well as to therapy of certain acquired disorders that may be associated with alterations in metabolic pathways.

Enzyme Induction. This form of therapy attacks the clinical and biochemical problem in a direct fashion by induction of enzyme synthesis. Although attractive in theory, this form of treatment has been largely unsuccessful, perhaps owing in many cases to the complete absence of intracellular mechanisms necessary for specific enzyme synthesis. Barbiturate therapy in one form of the Crigler-Najjar syndrome (hepatic uridyl-transferase deficiency) has lowered the serum concentration of unconjugated bilirubin, presumably by enzyme induction (Yaffe et al., 1966). Presumed induction of glucose-6-phosphatase has been reported in a single complicated case of a combined deficiency of both debranching enzyme and the phosphatase (Moses et al., 1966). Enzyme induction may explain the presumed benefit of large-dose pyridoxine therapy in the several hereditary conditions known to be responsive to this vitamin, such as cystathioninuria (Frimpter, 1965) and xanthurenicaciduria (Tada et al., 1967). Compared with the previously described approaches to treatment, this method must be considered a relative failure, although more accurate knowledge of the mechanisms controlling enzyme induction may lead to greater success in the future.

Enzyme Replacement. As with enzyme induction, replacement is one of the more theoretically attractive treatments of genetic metabolic diseases. For several reasons it has met with limited success (Scriver, 1969). Many enzyme preparations are antigenic and eventually lead to severe allergic reactions. Enzymes usually function intracellularly; transport of the enzyme across cell membranes may be limiting. In addition, the short half-life of administered protein preparations, presumably related to rapid intravascular catabolism, makes long-term use of any enzyme preparation relatively impractical.

The most successful application of this technique has been in the replacement of intravascular enzymes. The administration of purified preparations of factor VIII to patients with classic hemophilia is successful in acute hemorrhagic episodes (Ratnoff, 1966). The administration of a partly purified preparation of pseudocholinesterase to patients with deficiency of this plasma enzyme may lessen apnea produced by drugs (Goedde et al., 1968). In certain hereditary dysgammaglobulinemias, regular treatment with gamma globulin preparations decreases the incidence of bacterial infections (Bearn and Cleve, 1966).

The use of enzymes in intracellular enzyme deficiencies is more disappointing. The study of Hug and Schubert typifies the difficulties encountered in this area (Hug and Schubert, 1967). These investigators administered a fungal preparation of α-1,4-glucosidase to a patient with the lysosomal disorder type II glycogen storage disease. Repeated liver biopsies demonstrated uptake of the enzyme by the hepatic parenchymal cells (perhaps by pinocytosis), and encapsulation within phagosomes and subsequently lysosomes, followed by a reduction in the amount of stored intralysosomal glycogen. Unfortunately, the patient succumbed after several weeks of therapy. The importance of this study lies in the demonstration of hepatic uptake of the enzyme and of partial correction of the metabolic abnormality. With the future development of synthetic protein and enzyme preparations with less likelihood of allergic reactions, this approach to therapy may become one of the most effective forms of therapy for metabolic diseases of genetic origin. *In vitro* studies using cultured human cells have already demonstrated the value of this approach to the treatment of genetic diseases (Porter *et al.*, 1971).

Recent studies of the pathogenesis of a rare inborn error of metabolism termed methylmalonic aciduria have emphasized the use of coenzyme therapy as a mode of treatment in certain genetic diseases (Rosenberg and Scriver, 1969). Methylmalonic aciduria, one of a growing list of vitamin-dependency syndromes, is associated with severe metabolic acidosis, growth retardation, and accumulation of methylmalonic acid in blood and urine. Clinical improvement and reduction in methylmalonic acid excretion follow administration of large doses of vitamin B_{12} (1 mg/day) (Rosenberg *et al.*, 1968a). The underlying defect in this disorder now appears to be a defect in the synthesis of the cobamide coenzyme essential for normal methylmalonyl CoA isomerase activity (Rosenberg *et al.*, 1968b).

Compensatory Therapy. This approach to the treatment of inborn errors attempts to prevent the clinical complications of the disease without directly affecting the metabolic abnormality. The use of phosphate salts in the treatment of primary hyperoxaluria increases the solubility of calcium oxalate, without affecting the synthesis or excretion of oxalate (Williams and Smith, 1968). Cystinuria has successfully been treated with penicillamine, which leads to the excretion of soluble, mixed disulfide products of cysteine and penicillamine,

thereby reducing the likelihood of cystine stone formation (Crawhall and Watts, 1968). Unfortunately, the toxicity of penicillamine limits its practical usefulness in this disease.

Compensatory therapy can effectively prevent some of the clinical manifestations of certain metabolic disorders, such as prevention of uric acid stones in gout or bicarbonate therapy in renal tubular acidosis. Since it represents an indirect approach, it cannot be considered curative, and other complications of the disease not affected by the therapy must be prevented.

Two further points concerning the treatment of genetic diseases require comment. First, not all genetic metabolic diseases require treatment. Pentosuria, essential fructosuria, histidinemia, and Gilbert's disease are inborn errors of metabolism often unassociated with clinical manifestations, and therapy is unnecessary. Since these disorders may occasionally be confused with other more serious conditions, their accurate diagnosis is essential. Second, perhaps the most important form of treatment of genetic disease is prevention. The impact of genetic counseling on an enlightened patient population can reduce the incidence of many serious genetic problems, and in every way can be considered a basic therapeutic maneuver.

Principle: The effectiveness of any therapeutic maneuver can often be directly related to the extent of knowledge concerning pathogenetic mechanisms. Application of this knowledge to the individual patient should lead to rational and successful treatment programs.

SPECIFIC DISEASE STATES

Inherited Differences in Drug Metabolism

Metabolism of Isoniazid. Isoniazid has been extensively investigated since its introduction for the treatment of tuberculosis in the early 1950s. Observations of the rate of drug disappearance from the blood and of the proportion of drug products excreted in the urine suggested that variations in the metabolism of the drug existed in man. The study of Evans and coworkers demonstrated a bimodal distribution of plasma concentrations of isoniazid following oral administration of the drug to 267 subjects (Evans *et al.*, 1960). This finding suggested the presence of two populations, rapid and slow metabolizers. The studies of Bönicke and Lisboa in twins given isoniazid further suggested that these differences in metabolism might be related to genetic factors (Bönicke and Lisboa, 1957). Evans assumed that isoniazid metabolism is controlled at one locus by two autosomal allelic genes, and that slow inactivation is inherited as a recessive trait (Evans *et al.*,

1960). In this manner he was able to predict by genetic analysis the number of children of each phenotype to be expected from matings representing the three possible phenotypic combinations. These studies have also indicated that nearly one-half of the U.S. population metabolizes isoniazid slowly and therefore is homozygous for the recessive gene. Such a high percentage of a recessive gene suggests a selective biologic advantage (as in the case of hemoglobin S, resistant to *falciparum* malaria), but to date none has been associated with slow metabolism of isoniazid.

The hepatic metabolism of isoniazid occurs primarily by transacetylation. This enzyme system, which is noninducible, may act on several substrates in addition to isoniazid, including hydralazine and some sulfonamides (Evans and White, 1964). Attempts to demonstrate significant qualitative differences in the N-acetyltransferase obtained from livers of slow and rapid "acetylators" of isoniazid have largely been unsuccessful, and at the present time no definite enzymologic difference can be shown between slow and rapid "acetylators" (Jenne, 1965; Weber and Cohen, 1968). Because this enzyme system utilizes more than one substrate, interactions between isoniazid and hydralazine can be demonstrated. Competitive inhibition of isoniazid acetylation by hydralazine has been shown in partly purified liver preparations (Jenne, 1965). *In vitro* studies have shown that less acetylation of hydralazine occurs in liver preparations from "slow acetylators" of isoniazid than from "rapid acetylators" (Evans and White, 1964). Similar findings have been reported with sulfamethoxypyridazine, and clinical observations with phenelzine and diphenylhydantoin have suggested increased toxicity of these drugs in patients who acetylate isoniazid slowly (Kutt et al., 1966).

The clinical significance of these interesting observations is varied: (1) Patients who inactivate isoniazid slowly are more likely to develop peripheral neuropathy from the drug; this can be prevented by simultaneous administration of pyridoxine (Kalow, 1962). Despite increased toxicity in such patients, no definite improvement in the clinical effectiveness of isoniazid in the treatment of tuberculosis has been observed. Although tuberculosis cavities may close more rapidly and sputum cultures may revert to normal more quickly in patients who acetylate the drug slowly, no significant difference in clinical response can be identified between patients who acetylate the drug slowly or rapidly, after 6 months of therapy. (2) Side effects of hydralazine therapy (lupus-like syndrome and peripheral neuropathy) appear to be more common in patients who inactivate isoniazid slowly (Perry et al., 1967). (3) The severe side effects of the antidepressant drug phenelzine seem to occur more frequently in patients who acetylate isoniazid slowly (Evans et al., 1965). (4) Similarly, the toxic effects of diphenylhydantoin are more common in "slow acetylators" than in "rapid acetylators" of isoniazid, when tuberculous patients with epilepsy receive both drugs (Kutt et al., 1966). This effect may represent a drug interaction on a molecular enzymatic level (i.e., competition for enzyme-binding sites). *Principle: An understanding of the metabolism of drugs and of the genetic factors controlling metabolism is essential for the rational use of drugs in man.*

Metabolism of Succinylcholine. Shortly after the neuromuscular-blocking drug succinylcholine was introduced as an adjunct to anesthesia, a small number of patients developed prolonged apnea following the administration of a single dose of this drug. A familial occurrence of this increased sensitivity to succinylcholine was disclosed, suggesting the possibility of a genetic defect in the metabolism of the drug.

The metabolism of succinylcholine in man normally occurs by enzymatic hydrolysis of the ester linkage between succinic acid and the two choline molecules. The enzymatic reaction is effected by a normal plasma esterase, pseudocholinesterase. In normal individuals this enzyme rapidly converts succinylcholine to succinylmonocholine, allowing very little of the parent compound to reach its myoneural receptor sites (LaDu, 1969). Studies in patients who have developed prolonged apnea following succinylcholine administration demonstrate a qualitative rather than a quantitative defect in plasma pseudocholinesterase (Kalow and Davies, 1958; Kalow, 1960). The enzyme in these sensitive subjects has a lower affinity for choline ester substrates, including dibucaine, and is therefore less susceptible to inhibition by dibucaine, a known esterase inhibitor (Kalow and Genest, 1957). Using the percentage of inhibition of esterase activity by dibucaine as a measure of the qualitative enzyme abnormality, 20% inhibition is found in subjects known to be sensitive to the drug and about 60% inhibition is noted in the parents and other relatives of these patients (Kalow and Gunn, 1957). These findings suggest that the clinical sensitivity to the drug is inherited as an autosomal recessive trait. The genetic frequency of this abnormality is approximately 1 in 2500 (LaDu, 1969).

At least three other variants of plasma pseudocholinesterase have been described in man. A qualitatively abnormal enzyme, resistant to fluoride inhibition, has been described in some patients sensitive to succinylcholine (Harris and Whittaker, 1961). A few patients have a nearly complete absence of plasma pseudocholinesterase (Kattamis et al., 1967). In a family with several members *resistant* to succinylcholine, a threefold *increase* in the activity of plasma pseudocholinesterase was demonstrated (Neitlich, 1966). In addition, a number of other variants of pseudocholinesterase have been described (Whittaker, 1970). In all these situations a very important observation deserves emphasis. *In the absence of succinylcholine administration, no known clinical abnormalities occur as a result of the mutant enzyme. This finding raises the question of the normal function of this enzyme.*

An interesting approach to the therapy of prolonged apnea in succinylcholine sensitivity has been proposed (Goedde et al., 1968). These investigators found that administration of lyophilized normal human pseudocholinesterase to sensitive individuals shortened the period of apnea. This observation demonstrates one of the few examples of the successful treatment of an inborn error of metabolism by replacement of the defective enzyme. Unfortunately, difficulties in transport of enzymes across cells, rapid destruction of the administered enzyme, and the possibility of allergic reactions have limited the usefulness of this approach in the treatment of intracellular enzymatic defects.

Although a number of drugs appear to be metabolized by hydrolysis of ester linkages (procaine, procainamide, aspirin), the effect of pseudocholinesterase abnormalities on the metabolism of drugs other than succinylcholine has not been shown.

In addition to these two important examples of inherited difference in drug metabolism, genetic factors may play a role in the metabolism and pharmacologic effects of several other drugs (Table 13–1).

Table 13–1. DRUGS FOR WHICH INHERITED DIFFERENCES IN METABOLISM HAVE BEEN SHOWN

Isoniazid
Succinylcholine
Hydralazine
Diphenylhydantoin
Nitrites
Allopurinol
Acetophenetidin
Phenylbutazone
Antipyrine
Coumarin anticoagulants

Metabolism of the Coumarin Anticoagulants. The previous examples represent increased

sensitivity to the actions of a drug. Fewer instances of inherited resistance to the effects of a drug have been demonstrated. The most carefully studied example of this phenomenon is the inherited resistance to the coumarin anticoagulant drugs (O'Reilly et al., 1964). Dominantly inherited resistance to the coumarin anticoagulants was observed in two kindreds. The requirement for the anticoagulant in affected subjects was approximately 20 times the usual dose (O'Reilly et al., 1968). No defect in the metabolism of the drug or in binding to plasma proteins could be detected. In addition to resistance to the anticoagulant drugs, these patients demonstrated unusual sensitivity to the antidotal effects of vitamin K, suggesting modified receptor affinity for both vitamin K and the coumarin anticoagulants (O'Reilly et al., 1968).

A similar resistance to the anticoagulant effects of coumarin drugs was reported in another patient (Lewis et al., 1967). In this study the mechanism of resistance appeared to be related to rapid metabolism of the drug. *Principle: Genetic as well as environmental influences should be suspected in any individual showing an inadequate response to a drug. Although there are few specific examples of hereditarily determined resistance to drugs, the recognition of this phenomenon will undoubtedly lead to further identification of such resistance.*

Genetic Disorders That Modify Response to Drugs

Another major area of pharmacogenetics includes those genetic disorders that predispose to abnormal drug reactions. In addition to its inherent therapeutic implications, this problem involves the diagnostic importance of drugs in patients with genetic disorders. Many genetic disorders associated with an altered drug response are first recognized and diagnosed after drug therapy precipitates symptoms characteristic of the disorder.

Drug-Induced Hemolytic Anemia. Since the recognition that primaquine-induced hemolytic anemia is related to a specific deficiency in erythrocyte glucose-6-phosphate dehydrogenase (G-6-PD), the importance of enzyme deficiencies in the erythrocyte as causes of hemolytic states has been extensively documented. Certain inborn errors of erythrocyte metabolism are among the most prevalent hereditary enzyme defects in man. Several enzymatic defects in the red cell have been described (Table 13–2), mostly involving enzymes in either the pentose phosphate pathway or the glycolytic pathway (Beutler, 1968). Drug-induced hemolysis is most often seen in the pentose phosphate pathway.

Table 13–2. INHERITED DEFECTS IN ERYTH-
ROCYTE ENZYMES ASSOCIATED WITH
HEMOLYSIS

Glucose-6-phosphate dehydrogenase
6-Phosphogluconate dehydrogenase
Pyruvate kinase
Triosephosphate isomerase
2,3-Diphosphoglycerate mutase
Glutathione reductase
Adenosine triphosphatase
Hexokinase
Glyceraldehyde-3-phosphate dehydrogenase

Table 13–3. DRUGS CAPABLE OF INDUCING
HEMOLYSIS IN GLUCOSE-6-PHOSPHATE-
DEFICIENT INDIVIDUALS

Antimalarials	*Sulfonamides*
Primaquine	Sulfanilamide
Pamaquine	Sulfacetamide
Pentaquine	Sulfapyridine
Quinacrine	Sulfisoxazole
Quinine	Salicylazosulfapyridine
Quinocide	Sulfamethoxypyridazine
Analgesics and	
Antipyretics	*Sulfones*
Acetylsalicylic acid	Thiazolsulfone
Acetanilid	Sulfoxone
Acetophenetidin	Diaminodiphenylsulfone
Antipyrine	
Aminopyrine	
Nitrofurans	*Others*
Nitrofurantoin	Naphthalene
Nitrofurazone	Phenylhydrazine
Furazolidone	Dimercaprol
Furaltadone	Probenecid
	Chloramphenicol
	Quinidine
	Trinitrotoluene
	Vitamin K

Although minor clinical differences exist in these various enzyme deficiency states, glucose-6-phosphate dehydrogenase deficiency serves as a prototype of this important phenomenon.

Glucose-6-phosphate dehydrogenase controls the initial step in the pentose phosphate pathway, bringing about the oxidation of glucose-6-phosphate to 6-phosphogluconate, a reaction coupled to the reduction of NADP to NADPH. In the erythrocyte, NADPH is important in maintaining glutathione in its reduced form. Many oxidant drugs increase the rate of oxidation of glutathione, putting demands on the intracellular supply of NADPH for maintenance of glutathione in the reduced form (Kirkman, 1968). In patients with a deficiency of erythrocyte G-6-PD, administration of oxidant drugs leads to an increased demand for NADPH, which cannot be met because of the enzyme deficiency; oxidized glutathione accumulates, and by mechanisms as yet unknown, erythrocyte membrane integrity is disrupted and hemolysis occurs (Carson, 1968). The drugs capable of precipitating hemolysis in the G-6-PD-deficient individual are listed in Table 13–3. Although the rate of hemolysis usually seems unrelated to drug dosage, in three instances it may be dose related: sulfisoxazole, acetylsalicylic acid in Caucasians, and vitamin K in newborns (Kirkman, 1968). In some cases a drug-disease synergism may result in different degrees of hemolysis under different conditions (McCaffrey *et al.*, 1971).

Certain drugs cause hemolysis more readily in Caucasians than in Blacks with G-6-PD deficiency, owing to a biochemical heterogeneity in this disorder (Kirkman, 1968). Leukocytes from G-6-PD-deficient Caucasians are more deficient in the enzyme than leukocytes from Black subjects with the erythrocyte deficiency (Kirkman, 1968). A large number of biochemically distinct variants of G-6-PD have been described, classified to a large extent by differences in electrophoretic mobility of G-6-PD, but variations have also been shown in other

physicochemical properties, including pH optimum, thermostability, and Km values for both glucose-6-phosphate and NADP (Kirkman, 1968). The common G-6-PD variant in American Blacks differs from normal G-6-PD by a single amino acid substitution (Yoshida, 1967).

In addition to biochemical heterogeneity, clinical differences have been demonstrated. In some patients, despite an abnormality in the G-6-PD enzyme, no clinical symptoms are encountered. In other patients, drugs induce hemolysis, but normal reticulocyte counts are present in the absence of drug administration. In still other patients, chronic hemolytic anemia is present even in the absence of drug administration. When enzyme activity is greater than 30% of normal, hemolysis rarely occurs (Kirkman, 1968). Below 30% enzyme activity, hemolysis is common, but its severity is unrelated to the measured enzyme level.

Racial and geographic differences in G-6-PD deficiency also occur (Beutler, 1968). Nearly 15% of American Black males have a deficiency of G-6-PD; a much smaller percentage is found in American Caucasians. Specific variants of the enzyme are common in certain geographic areas, e.g., Indonesia, New Guinea, and Sardinia. In certain areas of Africa, G-6-PD deficiency is prevalent, suggesting that the erythrocytes of deficient individuals may be relatively resistant to malaria (Clarke *et al.*, 1968). The inheritance pattern of all variants of G-6-PD is X linked.

The importance of recognizing drug-induced hemolytic states and identifying the underlying abnormality is emphasized by these studies. In many individuals administration of a drug leads to initial diagnosis. Mature red cells have less G-6-PD activity than young red cells (Marks *et al.*, 1958). For this reason, diagnosis of G-6-PD deficiency may be difficult during acute hemolysis because of the presence of large numbers of young red cells in the circulation. Specific diagnosis may not be possible in these individuals until the hemolysis is reduced and older red cells increase in number.

Several hereditary disorders are thought to represent relative end-organ failure to a specific hormone. These anomalies include nephrogenic diabetes insipidus, vitamin D-resistant rickets, testicular feminization, and pseudohypoparathyroidism. In this type of genetic disorder, altered drug response plays an important role in both diagnosis and treatment.

Nephrogenic Diabetes Insipidus. Nephrogenic or vasopressin-resistant diabetes insipidus is a hereditary disorder characterized by polyuria, polydipsia, and the excretion of persistently hypotonic urine. The administration of vasopressin to affected individuals fails to alter the urinary concentrating ability, although other physiologic effects of the hormone remain intact. The disease is more common in males and appears to be inherited as an X-linked character (Relkin, 1968). The pathogenesis of the disease is unknown, but evidence suggests an insensitivity of the renal tubules to the action of vasopressin. Diagnosis is first based on the demonstration of diabetes insipidus by dehydration tests or on the failure of intravenous hypertonic saline administration to bring about a decrease in urine volume and an increase in urine tonicity (Hickey and Hare, 1944). If a negative result occurs, 0.1 unit of aqueous vasopressin is administered, which should produce maximal antidiuresis within 20 to 30 minutes. In the absence of significant renal disease, failure to respond to vasopressin confirms the diagnosis of nephrogenic diabetes insipidus.

The treatment of this disorder is dependent upon the definition of the underlying pathogenetic mechanisms. In diabetes insipidus secondary to pituitary or hypothalamic disease, vasopressin is indicated. In nephrogenic diabetes insipidus, the failure of the renal tubules to respond to vasopressin precludes its use. In the presence of an intact thirst mechanism, most patients with diabetes insipidus can remain in fluid balance simply by controlling their own fluid intake. If this becomes a significant practical problem drug therapy may be indicated.

An advance in the treatment of nephrogenic diabetes insipidus has been the recognition that administration of chlorothiazide may double urine osmolality and halve urine volume (Kennedy and Crawford, 1959). Although the precise mechanism of this action is unknown, the depletion of total body sodium following chlorothiazide therapy probably results in the reabsorption of greater amounts of sodium in the proximal tubule. This, in turn, leads to the delivery of less fluid to the distal tubule, limiting the volume of water available for excretion (Earley and Orloff, 1962; Skadhauge, 1966). Although chlorpropamide has been useful in ordinary diabetes insipidus, it has not been effective in nephrogenic diabetes insipidus (Arduino *et al.*, 1966; Relkin, 1968). *Principle: A thorough understanding of pathogenetic mechanisms allows an accurate and rational approach to therapy. The recognition of nephrogenic diabetes insipidus as a genetic disease transmitted as an X-linked trait makes genetic counseling and early diagnosis in susceptible infants more successful.*

Numerous additional examples of the modification of drug action by genetic disorders have been documented (Table 13–4). Patients defi-

Table 13–4. MODIFICATION OF DRUG ACTION BY GENETIC DISORDERS

DRUG	GENETIC DISORDER
Sulfonamides, nitrites, acetanilid	Erythrocyte diaphorase deficiency
Sulfonamides, nitrites	Hemoglobin H
Sulfonamides, primaquine	Hemoglobin Zurich
Barbiturates, estrogens, sulfonamides	Acute intermittent porphyria
Corticosteroids	Glaucoma
Anesthetic agents	Sickle-cell anemia
Salicylates, menthol, corticosteroids	Crigler-Najjar syndrome
Aminopyrine, menthol	Pentosuria
Atropine	Mongolism
Norepinephrine	Familial dysautonomia

cient in erythrocyte diaphorase develop methemoglobinemia when given sulfonamides, nitrites, and acetanilid (Cawein *et al.*, 1964). Patients with variants of the hemoglobin molecule, e.g., hemoglobin H (Rigas and Koler, 1961) and hemoglobin Zurich (Frick *et al.*, 1962), may be subject to hemolysis when exposed to sulfonamide drugs. Patients with acute intermittent porphyria may demonstrate a marked precipitation of symptoms following the administration of barbiturates, estrogens, sulfonamides, or diphenylhydantoin (Tschudy, 1968). Certain corticosteroid preparations worsen ocular symptoms in patients with a particular form of inherited glaucoma (Armaly, 1968). Patients with sickle-cell anemia may develop symptoms of infarction secondary to hypoxia following administration of anesthetic agents. In the Crigler-Najjar syndrome, in which hepatic glucuronyl tranferase activity is absent, decreased conjugation of salicylates, menthol, and certain corticosteroids has been observed (Kalow, 1962). A large variety of clinical problems may be encountered with the use of drugs in certain genetic disorders; an understanding of the basic pathogenetic mechanism of the disease may often explain the basis of the drug-disease interaction.

The tendency of patients to respond to some drugs may correlate with their genetic markers. Some patients with certain ABO blood groups are more prone to thrombosis while taking oral contraceptive agents than patients with different blood groups (see Chapter 8). Although such observations may only record correlations and do not imply a chemical or physiologic predisposition to a response to a drug based on the function associated with the genetic marker per se, prospective studies that attempt to correlate known adverse reactions with noticeable and easily documented phenotypic or genotypic characteristics will probably be successful. Such correlations can be useful in making therapeutic decisions, even though the observation of correlation may not explain the pathogenesis of the unusual drug effect.

Direct Effects of Drugs on the Genotype

The mutagenic and teratogenic properties of drugs have been recognized for many years. Many drugs have been incriminated in this phenomenon, including antibiotics, alkylating agents, nitroso compounds, and a miscellaneous group such as thalidomide and lysergic acid diethylamide (LSD). Only in the past 5 years, with the development of proper testing methods, has some insight into this problem been gained. The development of techniques for chromosome analysis and for the culture of human cells *in vitro* has led to some interesting and provocative observations of drug effects on the genotype (Hirschhorn and Cohen, 1968). The recent studies with LSD serve as an example of this problem.

The testing systems used for the study of LSD and other drugs involve analysis of chromosomes obtained from cells (usually lymphocytes) grown in tissue culture, often stimulated by phytohemagglutinin. Chromosomal abnormalities induced in such cells by known mutagenic agents such as irradiation and certain viruses include chromatid breaks (a discontinuity of chromatin material), isochromatid or chromosome breaks, structural rearrangements of chromatin material (translocations, ring chromosomes, or dicentric chromosomes), endoreduplication, and polyploidy (Hirschhorn and Cohen, 1968). Using these procedures, several reports of LSD-induced damage to chromosomes have appeared. Grown in the presence of varying concentrations of LSD, chromosome and chromatid breaks occurred four times more frequently in LSD-treated lymphocytes than in control cells (Cohen et al., 1967a, 1967b; Hirschhorn and Cohen, 1968). In addition to the "break" figures, a number of chromosome exchange and dicentric figures were found in treated but not in control cells.

In vivo studies have yielded similar results (Cohen et al., 1967b). Chromosome break frequencies in normal subjects showed a break frequency of 2.0 to 5.5% (mean 3.8%) compared to a frequency of 5.3 to 25.1% (mean 13.2%) in 18 adults who ingested LSD. Chromatid and chromosome breaks were the most common abnormalities, but exchange figures were also seen with increased frequency in the drug group. No correlation could be established between the chromosomal abnormalities and drug dose or the interval between the last dose and the time of the cell culture. Early studies of chromosome breaks in children of mothers who ingested LSD during pregnancy suggest an increased frequency of chromosomal abnormalities (Hirschhorn and Cohen, 1968). These studies with LSD have been instrumental in initiating an evaluation of the effects of many drugs on the genotype. Increased frequencies of chromosomal breakage have been reported in patients taking chlorpromazine and diphenhydramine (Hirschhorn and Cohen, 1968) and in patients treated with perphenazine (Nielsen et al., 1969). Undoubtedly more reports will be forthcoming, incriminating many other drugs and chemicals in this phenomenon. An unanswered question is the significance of tissue culture findings to phenotypic abnormalities. Although isolated reports have appeared of congenital malformations in children whose parents have taken LSD, the proof of a direct relationship has not been established, despite the likelihood of its existence (Zellweger et al., 1967; Grossbard et al. 1968)., Several genetic disorders emphasize the clinical significance of these studies. The autosomal recessive diseases, Fanconi's anemia, ataxia telangiectasia, and Bloom's syndrome, are associated with chromosomal abnormalities similar to those described above, and the incidence of neoplastic diseases is markedly increased in these disorders.

A further serious concern of these findings is the potential effect of drugs such as LSD on germ cells. Difficulties in obtaining appropriate cells have restricted study in this area. Unfortunately, many chromosomal abnormalities, such as balanced translocations, may be carried for generations before their clinical significance becomes apparent. Such dangers underscore the need for expanded evaluation of the role of drugs in altering the genotype.

These observations are only the first steps in a new field. Their implications are frightening. As new techniques for the evaluation of the genetic influence of drugs on cultured cells become available, drug testing must be expanded. Such studies should help alleviate the uncertainty and anxiety about our current therapy.

REFERENCES

Anderson, J. A., and Swaiman, K. F.: Phenylketonuria and allied metabolic diseases: Proceedings of a conference held at Washington, D.C., April 6–8, 1966. Children's Bureau, Washington, D.C., 1967.

Arduino, F.; Ferraz, F. P. J.; and Rodrigues, J.: Antidiuretic action of chlorpropamide in idiopathic diabetes insipidus. *J. Clin. Endocrinol.*, 26:1325–28, 1966.

Armaly, M. F.: Genetic factors related to glaucoma. *Ann. N.Y. Acad. Sci.*, 151:861–75, 1968.

Bearn, A. G., and Cleve, H.: Genetic variations in the serum proteins. In Stanbury, J. B.; Wyngaarden, J. B.; and Fredrickson, D. S. (eds.): *The Metabolic Basis of Inherited Disease*. McGraw-Hill Book Co., New York, 1966, pp. 1321–42.

Beutler, E.: *Hereditary Disorders of Erythrocyte Metabolism*. Grune & Stratton, New York, 1968.

Bönicke, R., and Lisboa, B. P.: Über die Erbbedingtheit der intraindividuellen Konstanz der Isoniazidausscheidung beim Menschen. *Naturwissenschaften*, 44:314, 1957.

Carson, P. E.: Hemolysis due to inherited erythrocyte enzyme deficiencies. *Ann. N.Y. Acad. Sci.*, 151:765–76, 1968.

Cawein, M.; Behlen, C. H.; Lappat, E. J.; and Cohn, J. E.: Hereditary diaphorase deficiency and methemoglobinemia. *Arch. Intern. Med. (Chicago)*, 113:578–85, 1964.

Clarke, C. A.; Evans, D. A.; Harris, R.; McConnell, R. B.; and Woodrow, J. C.: Genetics in medicine: a review. Pharmacogenetics. *Quart. J. Med.*, 37:183–219, 1968.

Cleaver, J. E.: Defective repair of replication of DNA in xeroderma pigmentosum. *Nature*, 218:652–56, 1968.

Cohen, M. M.; Hirschhorn, K.; and Frosch, W. A.: *In vivo* and *in vitro* chromosomal damage induced by LSD-25. *New Eng. J. Med.*, 277:1043–49, 1967a.

Cohen, M. M.; Marinello, M. J.; and Back, N.: Chromosomal damage in human leukocytes induced by lysergic acid diethylamide. *Science*, 155:1417–19, 1967b.

Crawhall, J. C., and Watts, R. W. E.: Cystinuria. *Amer. J. Med.*, 45:736–55, 1968.

Earley, L. E., and Orloff, J.: The mechanism of antidiuresis associated with the administration of hydro-

chlorothiazide to patients with vasopressin-resistant diabetes insipidus. *J. Clin. Invest.*, 41:1988–97, 1962.

Evans, D. A. P.: Genetic variations in the acetylation of isoniazid and other drugs. *Ann. N.Y. Acad. Sci.*, 151:723–33, 1968.

Evans, D. A. P.; Davison, K.; and Pratt, R. T. C.: The influence of acetylator phenotype on the effects of treating depression with phenelzine. *Clin. Pharmacol. Ther.*, 6:430–35, 1965.

Evans, D. A. P.; Manley, K. A.; and McKusick, V. A.: Genetic control of isoniazid metabolism in man. *Brit. Med. J.*, 2:485–91, 1960.

Evans, D. A. P., and White, T. A.: Human acetylation polymorphism. *J. Lab. Clin. Med.*, 63:394–403, 1964.

Field, R. A.: Glycogen deposition diseases. In Stanbury, J. B.; Wyngaarden, J. B.; and Fredrickson, D. S. (eds.): *The Metabolic Basis of Inherited Disease*. McGraw-Hill Book Co., New York, 1966, pp. 141–77.

Frick, P. G.; Hitzig, W. H.; and Betke, K.: Hemoglobin Zurich: I. A new hemoglobin anomaly associated with acute hemolytic episodes with inclusion bodies after sulfonamide therapy. *Blood*, 20:261–71, 1962.

Frimpter, G. W.: Cystathioninuria: nature of the defect. *Science*, 149:1095–96, 1965.

Froesch, E. R.; Wolf, H. P.; Baitsch, H.; Prader, A.; and Labhart, A.: Hereditary fructose intolerance: an inborn defect of hepatic fructose-1-phosphate splitting aldolase. *Amer. J. Med.*, 34:151–67, 1963.

German, J.; Archibald, R.; and Bloom, D.: Chromosomal breakage in a rare and probably genetically determined syndrome of man. *Science*, 148:506–507, 1965.

Goedde, H. W.; Altland, K.; and Schloot, W.: Therapy of prolonged apnea after suxamethonium with purified pseudocholinesterase: new data on kinetics of the hydrolysis of succinylcholine and succinylmonocholine and further data on N-acetyltransferase polymorphism. *Ann. N.Y. Acad. Sci.*, 151:742–52, 1968.

Grossbard, L.; Rosen, D.; McGilvray, E.; deCapoa, A.; Miller, O.; and Bank, A.: Acute leukemia with PH′-like chromosome in an LSD user. *J.A.M.A.*, 205:791–93, 1968.

Harris, H., and Whittaker, M.: Differential inhibition of human serum cholinesterase with fluoride: recognition of two new phenotypes. *Nature*, 191:496–98, 1961.

Hickey, R. C., and Hare, K.: The renal excretion of chloride and water in diabetes insipidus. *J. Clin. Invest.*, 23:768–75, 1944.

Hirschhorn, K., and Cohen, M. M.: Drug-induced chromosomal aberrations. *Ann. N.Y. Acad. Sci.*, 151:977–87, 1968.

Hug, G., and Schubert, W. K.: Lysosomes in type II glycogenosis: changes during administration of extract from *Aspergillus niger*. *J. Cell Biol.*, 35:C1–C6, 1967.

Jenne, J. W.: Partial purification and properties of the isoniazid transacetylase in human liver: its relationship to the acetylation of *p*-aminosalicylic acid. *J. Clin. Invest.*, 44:1992–2002, 1965.

Kalow, W.: Cholinesterase types. Ciba Foundation Symposium, *Biochemistry of Human Genetics*. Little, Brown and Co., Boston, 1960, pp. 39–56.

———: *Pharmacogenetics: Heredity and the Response to Drugs*. W. N. Saunders Co., Philadelphia, 1962.

Kalow, W., and Davies, R. O.: The activity of various esterase inhibitors towards atypical human serum cholinesterase. *Biochem. Pharmacol.*, 1:183–92, 1958.

Kalow, W., and Genest, K.: A method for the detection of atypical forms of human serum cholinesterase: determination of dibucaine numbers. *Canad. J. Biochem. Physiol.*, 35:339–46, 1957.

Kalow, W., and Gunn, D. R.: The relation between dose of succinylcholine and duration of apnea in man. *J. Pharmacol. Exp. Ther.*, 120:203–14, 1957.

Kattamis, C.; Davies, D.; and Lehmann, H.: The silent serum cholinesterase gene. *Acta. Genet.*, **17**:299–303, 1967.

Kelley, W. N.; Rosenbloom, F. M.; and Seegmiller, J. E.: The effects of azathioprine (Imuran) on purine synthesis in clinical disorders of purine metabolism. *J. Clin. Invest.*, **46**:1518–29, 1967.

Kennedy, G. C., and Crawford, J. D.: Treatment of diabetes insipidus with hydrochlorothiazide. *Lancet*, **1**:866–67, 1959.

Kirkman, H. N.: Glucose-6-phosphate dehydrogenase variants and drug-induced hemolysis. *Ann. N.Y. Acad. Sci.*, **151**:753–64, 1968.

Klinenberg, J. R.: Current concepts of hyperuricemia and gout. *Calif. Med.*, **110**:231–40, 1969.

Komrower, G. M.: Galactosemia. *Proc. Roy. Soc. Med.*, **60**:1155–57, 1967.

Kutt, H.; Winters, W.; and McDowell, F.: Depression of parahydroxylation of diphenylhydantoin by antituberculosis chemotherapy. *Neurology*, **16**:594–602, 1966.

LaDu, B. N.: Pharmacogenetics. *Med. Clin. N. Amer.*, **53**:839–55, 1969.

Lewis, R. J.; Spivack, M.; and Spaet, T. H.: Warfarin resistance. *Amer. J. Med.*, **42**:620–24, 1967.

McCaffrey, R. P.; Wahab, M. F. A.; and Robertson, R. P.: Chloramphenicol-induced hemolysis in Caucasian glucose-6-phosphate dehydrogenase deficiency. *Ann. Intern. Med.*, **74**:722–26, 1971.

Marks, P.; Johnson, A. B.; Hirschberg, E.; and Banks, J.: Studies on the mechanism of aging of human red blood cells. *Ann. N.Y. Acad. Sci.*, **75**:95–105, 1958.

Moses, S. W.; Levin, S.; Chayoth, R.; and Steinitz, K.: Enzyme induction in a case of glycogen storage disease. *Pediatrics*, **38**:111–21, 1966.

Neitlich, H. W.: Increased plasma cholinesterase activity and succinylcholine resistance: a genetic variant. *J. Clin. Invest.*, **45**:380–87, 1966.

Nielsen, J.; Friedrich, U.; and Tsuboli, T.: Chromosome abnormalities in patients treated with chlorpromazine, perphenazine, and lysergide. *Brit. Med. J.*, **3**:634–36, 1969.

O'Reilly, R. A.; Aggeler, P. M.; Hoag, M. S.; Leong, L. S.; and Kropatkin, M. L.: Hereditary transmission of exceptional resistance to coumarin anticoagulant drugs: the first reported kindred. *New Eng. J. Med.*, **271**:809–15, 1964.

O'Reilly, R. A.; Pool, J. G.; and Aggeler, P. M.: Hereditary resistance to coumarin anticoagulant drugs in man and rat. *Ann. N.Y. Acad. Sci.*, **151**:913–31, 1968.

Perry, H. M., Jr.; Sakamoto, A.; and Tan, E. M.: Relationship of acetylating enzyme to hydralazine toxicity. *J. Lab. Clin. Med.*, **70**:1020–21, 1967.

Porter, N. T.; Fluharty, A. L.; and Kihara, H.: Correction of abnormal cerebroside sulfate metabolism in cultured metachromatic leukodystrophy fibroblasts. *Science*, **172**:1263–65, 1971.

Potts, J. T., Jr., and Deftos, L. J.: Parathyroid hormone, thyrocalcitonin, vitamin D, bone and bone mineral metabolism. In Bondy, P. K. (ed.): *Diseases of Metabolism: Endocrinology and Nutrition*, 6th ed. W. B. Saunders Co., Philadelphia, 1969, pp. 904–1082.

Ratnoff, O. D.: Hereditary disorders of hemostasis. In Stanbury, J. B.; Wyngaarden, J. B.; and Fredrickson D. S. (eds.): *The Metabolic Basis of Inherited Disease*. McGraw-Hill Book Co., New York, 1966, pp. 1137–75.

Relkin, R.: Inherited forms of diabetes insipidus and diagnostic drug applications. *Ann. N.Y. Acad. Sci.*, **151**:880–86, 1968.

Rigas, D. A., and Koler, R. D.: Decreased erythrocyte survival in hemoglobin H disease as a result of the abnormal properties of hemoglobin H: the benefit of splenectomy. *Blood*, **18**:1–17, 1961.

Rosenberg, L. E.; Lilljeqvist, A.-Ch.; and Hsia, Y. E.: Methylmalonic aciduria: metabolic block localization and vitamin B_{12} dependency. *Science*, **162**:805–807, 1968a.

———: Methylmalonic aciduria: an inborn error leading to metabolic acidosis, long-chain ketonuria and intermittent hyperglycinemia. *New Eng. J. Med.*, **278**:1319–22, 1968b.

Rosenberg, L. E., and Scriver, C. R.: Disorders of amino acid metabolism. In Bondy, P. K. (ed.): *Diseases of Metabolism: Genetics and Metabolism*, 6th ed. W. B. Saunders Co., Philadelphia, 1969, pp. 366–515.

Schmid, R.: The porphyrias. In Stanbury, J. B.; Wyngaarden, J. B.; and Fredrickson, D. S. (eds.): *The Metabolic Basis of Inherited Disease*. McGraw-Hill Book Co., New York, 1966, pp. 813–70.

Scriver, C. R.: Treatment of inherited disease: realized and potential. *Med. Clin. N. Amer.*, **53**:941–63, 1969.

Skadhauge, E.: Studies of the antidiuresis induced by natrichloriuretic drugs in rats with diabetes insipidus. *Quart. J. Exp. Physiol.*, **51**:297–310, 1966.

Smith, L. H., Jr.; Bauer, R.; and Williams, H. E.: Oxalate and glycolate synthesis by hemic cells. *J. Lab. Clin. Med.*, in press, 1971.

Smith, L. H., Jr.; Huguley, C. M., Jr.; and Bain, J. A.: Hereditary orotic aciduria. In Stanbury, J. B.; Wyngaarden, J. B.; and Fredrickson, D. S. (eds.): *The Metabolic Basis of Inherited Disease*. McGraw-Hill Book Co., New York, 1966, pp. 739–58.

Stanbury, J. B.: Familial goiter. In Stanbury, J. B.; Wyngaarden, J. B.; and Fredrickson, D. S. (eds.): *The Metabolic Basis of Inherited Disease*. McGraw-Hill Book Co., New York, 1966, pp. 215–57.

Steinberg, D.; Mize, C. E.; Avignan, J.; Fales, H. M.; Eldjarn, L.; Try, K.; Stokke, O.; and Refsum, S.: Studies on the metabolic error in Refsum's disease. *J. Clin. Invest.*, **46**:313–22, 1967.

Stempfel, R. S., Jr., and Tomkins, G. M.: Congenital virilizing adrenocortical hyperplasia: the adrenogenital syndrome. In Stanbury, J. B.; Wyngaarden, J. B.; and Fredrickson, D. S. (eds.): *The Metabolic Basis of Inherited Disease*, McGraw-Hill Book Co., New York, 1966, pp. 635–64.

Swift, M. R., and Hirschhorn, K.: Fanconi's anemia: inherited susceptibility to chromosome breakage in various tissues. *Ann. Intern. Med.*, **65**:496–503, 1966.

Tada, K.; Yokoyama, Y.; Nakagawa, H.; Yoshida, T.; and Arakawa, T.: Vitamin B_6 dependent xanthurenic aciduria (the second report). *Tohoku J. Exp. Med.*, **93**:115–24, 1967.

Tschudy, D. P.: Clinical aspects of drug reactions in hereditary hepatic porphyria. *Ann. N.Y. Acad. Sci.*, **151**:850–60, 1968.

Vesell, E. S., and Page, J. G.: Genetic control of dicumarol levels in man. *J. Clin. Invest.*, **47**:2657–63, 1968a.

———: Genetic control of drug levels in man: phenylbutazone. *Science*, **159**:1479–80, 1968b.

———: Genetic control of drug levels in man: antipyrine. *Ibid.*, **161**:72–73, 1968c.

Weber, W. W., and Cohen, S. N.: The mechanism of isoniazid acetylation by human N-acetyltransferase. *Biochim. Biophys. Acta*, **151**:276–78, 1968.

Westall, R. G.: Dietary treatment of a child with maple syrup urine disease: branched-chain keto aciduria. *Arch. Dis. Child.* (*Chicago*), **38**:485–91, 1963.

Whittaker, M.: Genetic aspects of succinylcholine sensitivity. *Anesthesiology*, **32**:143–50, 1970.

Williams, H. E., and Smith, L. H., Jr.: Disorders of oxalate metabolism. *Amer. J. Med.*, **45**:715–35, 1968.

Yaffe, S. J.; Levy, G.; Natsuzawa, T.; and Baliah, T.: Enhancement of glucuronide-conjugating capacity in a hyperbilirubinemic infant due to apparent enzyme induction by phenobarbital. *New Eng. J. Med.*, **275**:1461–65, 1966.

Yoshida, A.: A single amino acid substitution (asparagine to aspartic acid) between normal (B+) and the common Negro variant (A+) of human glucose-6-phosphate dehydrogenase. *Proc. Nat. Acad. Sci.*, **57**:835–40, 1967.

Zellweger, H.; McDonald, J. S.; and Abbo, G.: Is lysergic acid diethylamide a teratogen? *Lancet*, **2**: 1066–68, 1967.

UNIT III

RECOGNITION AND EVALUATION OF EFFECTS OF DRUG ADMINISTRATION

Chapter 14

UNRECOGNIZED THERAPEUTIC MEASURES, INCLUDING PLACEBO

Henry R. Bourne

One guiding principle underlies most of the chapters of this book: The clinician who understands both the pathophysiology of a disease state and the mechanism of action of the drugs he selects will be able to provide specific and effective therapy. However, the practicing physician often deals with clinical situations in which many facts are unexplained. Even on the few occasions when he understands both disease and drug, his patient's condition may change for no known reason. *Principle: In the course of any disease, improvement or deterioration of the individual patient may be totally or partly independent of drug effects.* If we ignore this principle, we do so at risk to our patients. Recognition of phenomena in a patient's course that are independent of drug therapy may lead to more effective care of the sick. In his attempt to understand these unexpected enigmas, the physician should follow the same procedure as any other scientist: (1) he must first ask the right questions; i.e., he must specify precisely what it is he does not understand; (2) he must seek understanding, either from interpretation of data or from actual experiment; and (3) he must act upon the tentative conclusions reached, in effect performing another set of experiments to verify or negate his hypothesis.

A patient with bronchial asthma, for example, often foils every attempt at treatment based exclusively on our understanding of disease and drugs:

A 36-year-old woman has suffered from attacks of asthma for the past 5 years. Each attack is characterized by paroxysms of coughing, wheezing, and breathlessness, associated with variable sputum production. Initially, attacks were relieved by isoproterenol by aerosol or aminophylline suppositories, but over the past 8 months many episodes have required visits to the emergency room for parenteral therapy (epinephrine, intravenous fluids, and rectal or intravenous aminophylline). In the past 4 months she has been admitted twice to the hospital. A brief course of corticosteroid administration helped to terminate the last major attack, 4 weeks ago. For the past 2 weeks she has suffered almost constant wheezing and breathlessness, culminating in her present admission after two doses of parenteral epinephrine produced no improvement. You are called, and asked whether corticosteroid therapy should be instituted, and whether it may be necessary on a chronic basis.

The complete history, physical examination, and laboratory results, omitted in this brief account of a complicated illness, would be at your fingertips. You nonetheless might be at a loss as to what course to follow.

First, you must identify the most important question. Is the issue really "Prednisone, yes or no?" Other questions should be answered first:

Why is this patient's condition worsening? Asked another way: Why has her previous therapy not been effective? The most likely answer might be either that the knowledge of the disease process is incomplete, or that the drugs are not specifically effective in altering the pathologic process. Although such answers are common in many clinical settings, asthma may be notoriously difficult to understand. What makes this particular patient refractory to treatment that has been effective in the majority of patients and previously even in her own illness? Could there be a genetically determined abnormality, as suggested by an atopic family history? Could her emotional state contribute to the worsening of objective disease? Is another illness present, such as sinusitis, bronchiectasis, or diseases characterized by disordered immune responses (periarteritis nodosa)? Does her environment expose her to antigens that trigger allergic responses, or to dry air that might make it difficult for her to eliminate sputum? Is she in fact taking her medicines as prescribed? Are unrecognized emotional stresses increasing her symptoms? Such contributory factors may express themselves predominantly as asthma but require specialized therapy in addition to measures that will reverse bronchospasm.

Many elusive factors may affect the course of any disease and may interfere with or potentiate the effects of any drug. Awareness of these factors and a routine thorough search for them will improve patient care:

1. **Variability Among Patients.** Age, sex, and genetic makeup of the individual may determine the course of disease or the response to treatment. Even more important, though less well understood, is the patient's psychologic makeup.

2. **Variability in the Environment.** Physical or chemical changes in the habitat of patients may affect both disease and therapy.

3. **Variability in Compliance—Whether the Patient Takes His Drugs.** This thought is always applicable, whether the patient improves or whether his condition deteriorates.

4. **Variability of the Disease.** This factor must be considered equally as carefully in individual patients as it is in the design and interpretation of experimental clinical trials.

5. **Variability of Response to Placebo.** The placebo effect can interfere with evaluation of therapy. When recognized and understood, however, the placebo effect assumes a prominent therapeutic role.

Because pharmacotherapy may be so effective and is becoming more firmly based in science, other therapeutic measures, which may seem superficially less rational and scientific, are often neglected or unrecognized. The medical student or clinician may become so enamored of the certainties of biochemistry, physiology, laboratory tests, and precise pharmacologic mechanisms that he may forget that "certainty" is not always possible in science or in medicine. The essence of both clinical problems and science lies in the unanswered question.

Precisely because they are not easy to quantitate or understand, variations among individual patients should be important to the physician. Withering did not discover the usefulness of foxglove for treating dropsy as a result of facts learned in medical school, but because he asked new questions and searched for the answers. Even though our store of facts has grown, the physician still has a similar opportunity every time he sees a patient. An event that appears to lack a physiologic or pharmacologic basis should be explored and explained in order to improve treatment (Figure 14–1). Significant contributions to medical knowledge have been made by physicians who feel compelled to recognize and explain clinical mysteries. Thus pharmacogenetic diseases have been discovered, and new drugs developed based on observation of unwanted side effects (see Chapter 18).

THE PATIENT AS AN INDIVIDUAL

Other than primary diseases, what characteristics differentiate patients from each other and give rise both to difficulties and to opportunities in treatment?

Age and Sex

The patient's age and sex are placed prominently at the beginning of every history. However, these "vital statistics" often are not used as determinants of therapeutic decisions. How nice, but how useless, to know that the gender of a 42-year-old man with coronary disease is a statistical determinant of his problem, or that the age of the octogenarian with gram-negative septicemia may drastically decrease his chance of survival. Many correlations are statistically significant but are also empiric and the mechanism is unknown. When we have clues to a mechanism, however, therapeutic implications may follow.

Physicians have long believed that old people need less digitalis glycoside than do younger people to produce an inotropic effect, and that toxicity is more likely in the elderly taking "usual" doses. One reason for the belief is now apparent: Old people, even those with normal blood creatinine concentrations, generally have decreased renal function (creatinine clearance). Digoxin, which is largely eliminated by the kidney, has a much longer half-life in older

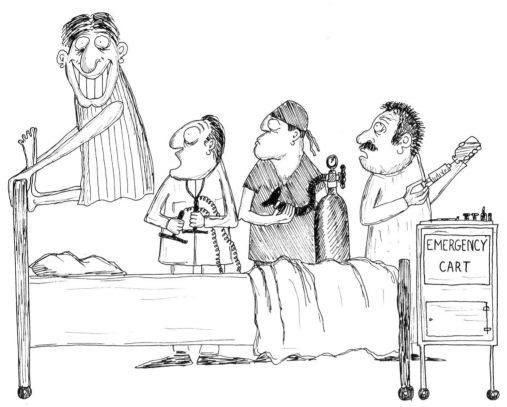

Figure 14–1. "Come back so we can resuscitate you!" (Often in management of patients an event will appear to lack a physiologic or pharmacologic basis.)

patients (Ewy *et al.*, 1969). The same concept may prove applicable in the treatment of the elderly for hypertension with alpha-methyldopa, for diabetes with chlorpropamide, or for arrhythmias with procainamide, all drugs largely excreted in the urine.

What of treatment with oral anticoagulants, metabolized by the liver? We do not know whether older people need smaller doses of these drugs for a given anticoagulant effect, but such a discovery would not be surprising. If true, would changes in metabolism of drug or decreased rates of synthesis of clotting factors by aged hepatic enzyme systems be more critical for the altered response to a standard dose of drug? We know something about liver function in early life, e.g., the "gray baby" syndrome caused by chloramphenicol administered to neonates who are not able to metabolize the drug (Weiss *et al.*, 1960), but we need to know more about the changes in hepatic function related to each of the extremes in age.

What of other organ systems affected by aging? Does diminution of sympathetic circula-tory reflexes in the elderly (Appenzeller and Descarries, 1964) affect the sensitivity of older people to antihypertensive agents like guanethi-dine? Might the vasodilators advocated for treatment of peripheral (or cerebral) arterial insufficiency in old people actually *increase* the risk of cerebral ischemia, both because sym-pathetic reflexes may be less effective and because the cerebral circulation may lose its ability to dilate in response to normal stimuli (e.g., increased arterial pCO_2) (Fazekas *et al.*, 1953)? These questions should be asked even if they have not yet been answered. ***Principle: The age of a patient, young or old, may change either the ability of target organs to respond to drugs or the ability of normal systems to dispose of a drug or to oppose its effects.*** Therapy that takes these changes into account should be more effective and less likely to cause toxicity.

Sex differences in some species (probably not human beings) are associated with great differ-ences in rates of drug metabolism (Quinn *et al.*, 1958; Conney, 1967). Sex differences influence the severity of some diseases, e.g., hypertension (greater end-organ damage in men) or mammary carcinoma (usually swiftly fatal in the rare man with the disease). The patient's sex is important in planning therapy, chiefly because it may partly determine his prognosis, and therefore the urgency and intensity of therapy. In hypertensive patients, vigorous treatment effectively diminishes morbidity and mortality in men with diastolic blood pressures of 115 mm Hg or greater (Veterans Administration Cooperative Study Group, 1967). Since the prognosis for women with the same degree of hypertension is considerably better (Schweitzer *et al.*, 1965), efficacy of drug therapy is more difficult to prove conclusively in females. Until such a study is done, the implication for the clinician faced with a hypertensive woman patient is clear, though difficult to quantify: At any given level of pretreatment blood pressure, the physician may be willing to risk less chance of toxicity; i.e., he will treat less vigorously in a woman than in a man, since his certainty of preventing end-organ changes of hypertension is less. If end-organ changes are present (cardiac, renal, cerebral, or retinal damage), therapy should be as vigorous as necessary (see Chapter 5).

Heredity

The genetic makeup of the patient may critically affect drug therapy. Although pharmacogenetics is a relatively new field, many abnormal responses to drugs can be traced to a genetic basis (see Chapter 13). In a few cases, such as the primaquine sensitivity of patients with glucose-6-phosphate dehydrogenase (G-6-PD) deficiency, our knowledge may have predictive value: By noting one phenotypic characteristic (black skin or Mediterranean origin), we are led to suspect another, G-6-PD deficiency, and to plan our antibiotic and antipyretic therapy accordingly (see Chapter 15).

In most cases, the predictive value of our knowledge is not so great. Nonetheless, many responses to drugs that are initially called "idiosyncratic" are later shown to stem from inherited differences in the patient. For example, at least one patient who required an unusually large dose of digoxin for control of atrial arrhythmias was found to inactivate the drug by a unique pathway (Luchi and Gruber, 1968). A group of patients unusually susceptible to diphenylhydantoin toxicity inactivate the drug more slowly than "normals," probably because of an inherited defect of drug metabolism (Kutt *et al.*, 1964). Patients can inherit decreased sensitivity to certain oral anticoagulants due to abnormal metabolism of the drugs (O'Reilly *et al.*, 1964). Patients given both barbiturates and oral anticoagulants do not always exhibit resistance to the oral anticoagulants as might be expected on the basis of induction of metabolic enzymes. This variability in response may be due in part to genetically determined differences in hepatic enzymes, as suggested by studies in twins (Vessell and Page, 1968).

These examples can teach us that: (1) An unpredictable response to drugs may be the hallmark of an inherited abnormality, rather than an "idiosyncratic" reaction. *Principle: When an event is labeled "idiosyncratic" a potentially important question should be raised about a new physiologic or pharmacologic mechanism.* (2) Recognition of inherited variations depends upon a measurable, accurate, and reproducible index of drug toxicity or effect. This index may be very simple and economical and often is related to careful observation of gross physical or chemical changes. The investigative effort directed at drug interactions involving the oral anticoagulants and inherited abnormalities of their metabolism originated in observations of the changes in the prothrombin time, a test performed in most clinical laboratories. Measurement of drug concentrations in plasma or tissue confirmed the mechanism, but did not lead to the original discovery. *Principle: Drug effects must be quantifiable and reproducible before genetically determined abnormal drug effects can be detected.*

The Psyche: Mind over Matter

The patient's psyche may be one determinant of the course of his disease, e.g., angina pectoris, peptic ulcer, asthma, and some psychiatric disorders. Students of therapeutics should ask how changes in the patient's mental or emotional life may aid or interfere with the treatment of his "physical" disorder. Can we use our knowledge of psychic influence on disease to make therapy more effective?

Some data to answer these questions are respectably "scientific," even physiologic; the real limit to our knowledge is our failure to understand or test the emotional state responsible for the target organ effects we observe. What are the "afferent" pathways leading to fear, for example? How are central nervous processes deranged in the anxiety state or in mental depression? Both psychoanalytic theory and concepts of operant conditioning offer plausible but incomplete answers to these questions (see Chapter 11). Virtually all the target organs of psychosomatic disease (the bronchus, heart, peripheral resistance vessels controlling blood pressure, the mucosa of the upper gastrointestinal tract, the colon, etc.) are richly supplied with autonomic nerves that can be operantly conditioned. In addition, certain emotional states, especially anxiety and fear, are associated with effects on target organs mediated by hormones or autonomic nerves (e.g., increased blood pressure, heart rate, or gastric acid secretion) (Forsham, 1968). These responses can modify or even reverse the effects of potent drugs (Wolf, 1959, 1970).

Even without detailed knowledge of pathogenesis, physicians can often allay anxiety, assuage fear, and help bring meaning into the life of the most despondent invalid. No cookbook recipe can explain how this is done. Perhaps the best therapeutic advice is contained in the quotation: "The secret of the care of the patient is in caring for the patient" (Peabody, 1927). The physician must actually talk with his patients and seek to understand their problems. He must not routinely substitute a pill for his time if he is to provide proper care for problems labeled "psychosomatic." For beginning students, some principles of "psychosomatic therapeutics" can be outlined.

The psychologic "set" of a patient may affect the course of nonpsychosomatic diseases. Pre-existing depressive symptoms can prolong the subjective symptoms of illness in patients with viral influenza (Imboden et al., 1961). Likewise, a patient's attitude toward his myocardial infarction may be one determinant of his prognosis; in general, patients who are frankly anxious and afraid of dying have a greater chance of doing so than those who deny the possibility of dying. It seems likely that the well-known psychologic mechanism of denial may have definite survival value (Hackett et al., 1968). Regardless of cause, there is a temporal relation between increased urinary excretion of catecholamines and untoward events, especially arrhythmias, in patients with acute myocardial infarction (Valori et al., 1967; Januszewicz et al., 1968; Jewitt et al., 1969). Although no definite evidence has been presented that increased catecholamines caused the arrhythmias or that the excess secretion of catecholamines was related primarily to psychologic set, in some cases this appeared quite likely. The therapeutic implications of these studies have not been systematically tested, but it seems likely that if anxiety is effectively allayed through greater confidence in medical support, the possibility of recovery increases. The period of convalescence following discharge from the hospital after a myocardial infarction is notoriously fraught with emotional difficulties which may require a physician's careful intervention (Wishnie et al., 1971). *Principle: A humanistic and therapeutically efficacious goal of a physician is to allay his patient's fear.* In acutely ill patients who may

be almost literally at the mercy of their autonomic nervous system, alleviation of fear may be specifically therapeutic and may make the difference between a successful outcome and death.

At least one excellent study has shown that the supporting role of the physician can make a significant difference in the outcome of the postoperative state. Anesthesiologists in a large hospital divided 97 preoperative patients into two randomly selected groups. One group received the routine preoperative visit and preoperative medications appropriate to the particular surgery involved. The other group had, in addition, more intensive contact with the anesthesiologist, who discussed the nature, causes, and course of normal postoperative pain. Both groups underwent elective intra-abdominal operations of equal risk. The "treated" patients required significantly less analgesic medication (by almost 50%) and their surgeons, who were not aware of the study, sent them home 2.7 days earlier than the control group (Egbert et al., 1964). The study gives an important clue to one of the most vital elements in such support: honest, straightforward communication between physicians and patients. Extrapolation of these results to other clinical situations may be justified, especially to situations where the patient's apprehension and ignorance regarding his illness may affect his ability to follow a plan of treatment. Often, no drug can substitute for planned, effective communication between doctor and patient. This communication may potentiate the effectiveness of drugs or other therapy and may reduce toxicity as well.

Communication between doctor and patient, however honest and straightforward, can, like any therapeutic measure, produce adverse effects. A chance remark or even an inadvertent facial expression may be as dangerous as the forgetful addition of spironolactone to the regimen of a patient already receiving potassium chloride. Much may be lost by the honest statement to a patient in cardiogenic shock that his chances of survival are less than 20%. Probably the only way the clinician can reduce the risks of advice is to have a conscious, well-formulated plan of management of his patient's psychic problems. *Principle: The physician should strive to make every question, every instruction, and every seemingly chance remark therapeutic, or at least not harmful.*

An alternative way of managing psychic problems, especially anxiety, is to use drugs. Narcotics, analgesics, sedatives, "tranquilizing" agents, and antidepressant medications can play indispensable roles in the treatment of many patients (see Chapter 11). Several therapeutic principles apply particularly to the psychotropic drugs:

1. *There must be a clear-cut indication for use of any drug.* The routine use of the nightly sleeping pill often represents little more than a reflex (perhaps protective for the doctor who may be called in the middle of the night because Mrs. Maloney cannot sleep) and may be potentially harmful for the patient (see Chapter 16). Before writing such an order the physician should assure himself that a sleeping medication may genuinely help the individual patient, before subjecting that patient to the risk of drug interactions, allergic reactions, drug fever, or other toxic effects (see Chapters 16 and 17).

2. *Definite goals of treatment, as well as criteria for drug effectiveness, are as necessary in the treatment of any individual patient with emotional problems as in the most sophisticated clinical trial.* Chlordiazepoxide and diazepam, two of the best-selling minor tranquilizers, are undoubtedly effective and useful drugs in certain clinical situations. Many patients now receiving these drugs might receive different treatment if the desired therapeutic effects were measured as carefully as those of agents used, for example, to treat metastatic carcinoma of the breast. Periodic assessment of a patient's emotional state may seem less scientific than looking for regression of metastatic lesions on x-ray, but the usefulness of such an assessment may be nearly as great, in terms of patient comfort and avoidance of unnecessary drug toxicity (see Chapter 11). If target symptoms of psychotropic therapy are so vague that they cannot be assessed, drug treatment is certainly ill advised.

3. *None of the psychoses or neuroses seen in medical patients have been fully explained on a biochemical basis. Furthermore, the mode of action of the psychotropic agents remains largely unknown.* The ability to measure psychotropic effects in a more reproducible way will better define the spectrum of indications for psychotropic drugs. At present, however, the physician should realize that much pharmacotherapy for psychiatric indications is no more "scientific" than was Osler's suggestion of arsenic for pernicious anemia (contrast this with Osler's comments on treatment of neurasthenia, quoted at the end of this chapter). Before ordering Metrazol to "pep up" an old lady in a nursing home (as suggested in drug advertisements), the physician should reflect that his knowledge of human nature, even in old ladies, probably surpasses his (or anybody else's) knowledge of the action of Metrazol. Perhaps in some cases that knowledge of human nature will provide clues to therapy that might be more effective than a drug.

4. *No psychotropic drug yet developed acts only on "the mind," separately from the body.* Although the drugs used to affect the emotional life of patients lack specificity, these drugs produce effects that are more predictable and less changeable than the effects that result from ordinary human relationships. Nonetheless, for some of the psychic ills of men, the relationship between patient and doctor may provide a channel for the only truly specific, consistent, and predictable therapy available, i.e., compassion and understanding.

ENVIRONMENT

The phenotype of each organism is the result of interplay between its genetic material and the influence of environment. The phenotypic disorder of a man with genotypic deficiency of glucose-6-phosphate dehydrogenase would seldom be expressed without the presence of drugs in the individual's environment. Similarly, for a vast array of nongenetic disorders, the disease state is a result of the interplay between the host, the primary agent or cause of the disease, and environmental influences. Such influences can determine whether the disease becomes clinically expressed, its course, and some of its complications. Furthermore, the environment may drastically alter the response of disease to any kind of therapy.

Examples include those physical or chemical factors in the environment known to be the primary cause of disease, or major positive or negative influences, including (1) the air patients breathe, or substances within it (cigarette smoking and carcinoma of the lung, or the pneumoconioses); (2) food (consumption of certain lipids and atherosclerosis; licorice and aldosteronism); (3) water (fluoride ion and prevention of dental caries; "hardness" of water and heart disease [Anderson et al., 1969]); (4) climate (the geographic distribution of malaria); and (5) more exotic substances (ingestion of clay or starch producing iron-deficiency anemia, paint chips producing lead poisoning, or the plethora of over-the-counter drugs, tonics, and remedies, each capable of producing its own disorder).

Relatively protected from many of the ravages of nature, people may suffer from side effects of technology itself. The physician must realize that as technology becomes increasingly complex and far reaching, patients may become subject to environmental influences that are more subtle, but no less important. The physician will not become aware of these influences unless he looks for them. Two examples:

1. How many physicians consider the potential ability of substances "incidentally" present

in the patient's environment to alter the patient's metabolism of drugs administered with therapeutic intent? The ability of many insecticides, including DDT, to induce hepatic microsomal enzyme systems, thereby speeding metabolism of other drugs, has been demonstrated in animals (Hart and Fouts, 1963, 1965), and recently in man (Kolmodin *et al.*, 1969). Workers in a Swedish factory who were repeatedly exposed to a number of chlorinated insecticides metabolized the anti-inflammatory drug antipyrine significantly faster than control subjects. Exposure to DDT is unavoidable for almost everyone in the United States; some foodstuffs contain at least 5 ppm of the compound, a concentration sufficient to change metabolism of many drugs in animals. Admittedly, no one knows whether such effects are of clinical importance. Nor do we know, for example, what effect smoking cigarettes may have on metabolism of drugs, though the activity of at least one "detoxifying" enzyme, benzpyrene reductase, has been elevated in placentas delivered from cigarette-smoking mothers (Welch *et al.*, 1968).

2. Over the last few years, radiologists found that the normal range of values for the uptake of radioactive iodine by the thyroid gland was slowly decreasing. At least one explanation has been offered (Pittman *et al.*, 1969): A technical change in the process of baking bread has led to the incorporation of considerably more iodine into the American diet; as a consequence, iodine trapping by the thyroid appears to be relatively less avid in the average normal subject. Thus, radioactive iodine uptake tests in many normal people give values considered diagnostic of hypothyroidism 10 years ago. Also, a patient with genuinely low thyroid function whose baker still baked bread in the old way might run the risk of having his disease missed by a test whose normal range was based on a different population. *Principle: Unrecognized environmental influences may seriously impair the effectiveness of drug therapy, either directly, by affecting drug metabolism or effect, or indirectly, by making interpretation of diagnostic tests difficult.*

Environmental factors may unmask disease, as well as hide it: coma in hypothyroid patients can be precipitated with the onset of winter; addisonian crisis is more likely during hot summer days, when salt and water depletion are frequent. We do not know why peptic ulcer is so common in the spring. The environmental changes most often caused by physicians themselves are those associated with hospitalization. Such a seemingly simple procedure as putting a patient into a hospital may carry with it a drastically high risk. Older patients may become disoriented after only a few days of bed rest and separation from their normal surroundings. Bed rest may precipitate coma, formation of urinary calculi, or renal failure due to the hypercalcemia that may first appear in hospitalized patients with breast cancer with bone metastases, multiple myeloma, hyperparathyroidism, etc. After a myocardial infarction or hip fracture, postural hypotension may be exacerbated, especially in the aged patient at bed rest (Fareeduddin and Abelmann, 1969). A patient with impaired defense mechanisms may become infected by drug-resistant "hospital" strains of microorganisms such as *Staph. aureus*. Changes in the patient's environment may unmask occult disease, e.g., atropine given to a patient with unsuspected glaucoma, or may cause deterioration of a patient with already diagnosed disease. *Principle: The potential beneficial effects of hospitalization, like those of any drug, must be weighed against potential toxicity.*

COMPLIANCE WITH THE THERAPEUTIC REGIMEN

At some point in the course of every difficult problem in medical management the thoughtful physician asks himself: "Is my patient actually taking the drug I have prescribed?" Perhaps such a question should be routine. For example:

A 66-year-old widow was admitted to a hospital for treatment of acute myocardial infarction in May. Her illness was complicated by the development of mild congestive heart failure, for which she was placed on digoxin, 0.25 mg per day. During the 3 weeks following discharge she complained of increasing dyspnea on climbing two flights of stairs and deepening depression related to her lonely, disease-limited life. She felt she simply must get out of her third-story apartment in a "dangerous" section of the city. Mild cardiomegaly was noted on physical examination. The intern following her in clinic gave emotional support, raised her digoxin to two pills per day, and referred her to the social service department. By early August her condition improved: she had moved into a first-floor apartment with a niece and was much happier. In addition, her exertional dyspnea and cardiomegaly had disappeared, and she was eager to take on a part-time job as a babysitter.

Secretly congratulating himself for a job well done, the intern told his patient that she was doing so well that he might soon be able to allow her to discontinue her digoxin. "I'm sorry, doctor," said the patient, "you've been so good to me that I really have to tell you something. After I got out of the hospital I never took any of those heart pills. I am a Christian Scientist."

This story's happy ending, for the patient at least, should not obscure the important lessons it contains: A physician hardly ever knows all the facts; he is likely to interpret the facts that are available in terms of response of patho-physiologic processes to drug therapy, especially if the outcome is favorable; and the real sequence of cause and effect may be quite different, since even objective changes in the patient's condition may stem from "nonspecific" changes in the environment (a first-floor apartment), or from the natural course of the disease in question (recovery of normal cardiac reserve following healing of a myocardial infarction). These generalizations may apply equally well to situations in which the patient is actually "going downhill," or even when no change in his condition can be detected.

Noncompliance: Documentation and Consequences

Patients often fail to comply with a medical regimen. Careful study of 40 outpatients receiving a total of 143 different medications in a university medical clinic revealed that only 10% were taking their medications exactly as prescribed (Malahy, 1966). Of the total number of errors, omission of one or more doses accounted for 19.7%, incorrect dosage for 14.5%, incorrect timing or sequence of medications for 33.7%, and discontinuation of medication for 7.7%. Studies of chemotherapy for tuberculosis have shown that from 50 to 90% of patients fail to take their medicines as prescribed, and many do not take them at all (Dixon et al., 1957; Breite, 1959; Berry et al., 1962; Preston and Miller, 1964; Maddock, 1967; Moulding et al., 1970). The rumor that grass outside the windows of tuberculosis sanitariums dies of PAS toxicity may be well founded. Similarly, in one study only 50% of children given oral prophylaxis for rheumatic fever actually took their drugs as prescribed (Feinstein et al., 1959). Compliance with instructions to take penicillin for documented streptococcal infections in children is not much better; in one study, 82% of patients had discontinued medication by the ninth day (Bergman and Werner, 1963). Two studies demonstrated that one-third of pregnant women fail to take their oral iron as prescribed (Benstead and Theobald, 1952; Bonnar et al., 1969). Other studies have shown noncompliance with antacid therapy for duodenal ulcer (Roth and Berger, 1960; Caron and Roth, 1968), chemoprophylaxis against malaria (Gilroy, 1952), tranquilizer or antidepressant medication for psychiatric disorders (Willcox et al., 1965), insulin or diet for diabetes (Watkins et al., 1967), and diet instructions for treatment of obesity (Glennon, 1966).

The degree of a patient's compliance with his regimen is almost impossible to judge without objective evidence; direct-interview techniques have repeatedly failed to detect noncompliance detected by other means (Feinstein et al., 1959; Gordis et al., 1969), and the physician's judgment as to the compliance of a particular patient is more often wrong than right (Preston and Miller, 1964; Caron and Roth, 1968).

Failure to take medications may be even more difficult to predict than to detect (Davis, 1967), chiefly because potential causes are numerous and poorly understood. Many investigators have studied the influence of such factors as patient attitudes, education, and socioeconomic status, duration of disease, age, and sex, with inconsistent results (Davis and Eichhorn, 1963; MacDonald et al., 1963). Two clues appeared in the careful study of 40 outpatients noted above, only 4 of whom were taking their drugs exactly as prescribed (Malahy, 1966): (1) although age and education did not correlate with medication errors, the total number of medications correlated very well; (2) when questioned at home, patients failed to understand the purpose of 71 of the total of 143 drugs prescribed, despite careful instruction by doctors and nurses. Many instances of failure to comply with a medical regimen may simply result from failure to understand complicated instructions.

A patient's presence in a hospital is no guarantee that drugs will be administered as ordered. Careful observation of nine nurses in a university hospital revealed that for every six drug doses ordered, an error was made in one (Barker and McConnell, 1962). Of all errors, 37% were simple omissions of an ordered dose, and 18% were administration of a drug not ordered. The remainder, numerically less frequent but potentially as dangerous, included wrong time for the dose, under- and overdose, extra dose, and wrong dose form. Another study showed that medication errors by nurses increased logarithmically with the number of different drugs prescribed (Vere, 1965). The therapeutic implications of such a finding should be obvious.

What are the consequences of incorrect drug administration, either because of poor compliance with doctor's orders by a patient at home, or because of medication errors in a hospital? Failure to take medicine correctly can severely influence the effectiveness of therapy; recurrence of streptococcal pharyngitis is definitely more frequent in patients who fail to complete the prescribed course of treatment (Mohler et al., 1956), and recurrent attacks of rheumatic fever are more common in patients who fail to continue their antibiotic prophylaxis (Feinstein et al., 1959). In some cases, noncompliance with a regimen may make little or no difference in results, as in chronic antacid treatment of peptic ulcer (Roth and Berger, 1960). If failure to take a medicine makes no difference in therapy, it seems likely that the medicine is ineffective. Failure to comply with a drug regimen might even be therapeutic if the regimen is inappropriate. Similarly, the absence of a single untoward event related to medication error in the hospital study cited (Barker and McConnell, 1962) suggests that many of the medicines prescribed for those inpatients may not have been absolutely necessary. At least, the specific dose and frequency of many of the drugs ordered were relatively less important than the prescribing physician may have thought. *Principle: The physician should decide which drugs are of marginal importance and which ones are crucial. Of the former, some may actually be discarded; with the latter, he should take measures necessary to assure their correct administration.*

Remedies for Noncompliance

How can medication errors or "noncompliance" be prevented? Medication errors or incorrect self-administration of drugs must first be suspected. When therapy is not optimally effective, the physician should suspect that his patient is not taking his drug (or is receiving another drug not prescribed). Noncompliance should be suspected at all times, even when things are going well, for only in this way can the effects of treatment versus the natural course of the disease be properly judged.

Medication errors or noncompliance must then be detected. For certain drugs, this can be exceedingly simple; a straightforward test for stool iron gives unequivocal evidence as to whether a patient is taking ferrous sulfate. Other methods, ranging from pill counting (unreliable in some cases) to assay for drug or drug metabolites in urine, have been tried (Roth et al., 1970). Often, nonleading questions as to "side effects" may be revealing, e.g., dry mouth for anticholinergics, tachycardia for sympathomimetic amines given for asthma, or the sensation of "fullness in the head" after nitroglycerin. Absence of such effects may be a clue to failure of compliance by the patient or to inadequate dosage. Pharmacologically inactive material may be added to the tablet or capsule and sought in urine or blood. Riboflavin, which can be detected by its fluorescence in the urine, has been used in a few clinical trials, such as the Veterans Administration study of drug treatment for hypertension, where greater than 50% of patients were found to be noncompliers (Veterans Administration Cooperative Study Group, 1967). Riboflavin could be used by practicing physicians as well, when documentation of drug administration is crucial to decisions about further therapy, e.g., during hormone replacement in hypothyroid patients.

The patient or some reliable member of the family must thoroughly understand the medical regimen, including the underlying rationale as well as details of dosage and timing. The physician should take time to explain, and often to write in detail, the regimen to be followed. Each drug should be referred to by name (color alone will not suffice). It may even be useful to tape sample pills to a piece of cardboard, with accompanying instructions for administration of each. Most important, each return visit of an outpatient should be devoted in part to a review of the drug regimen, complete with a count of the actual pills in labeled bottles. It may be useful periodically to have a patient bring all contents of a home medicine chest to the clinic. As suggested in one study (Malahy, 1966), surprises may be in store, such as the discovery that one patient was taking two different digitalis preparations without knowing the name or purpose of either.

To be effective, every medical regimen should be as simple as possible. The fewer the pills, and the fewer the separate times for their administration, the more likely the patient will be to take them correctly. Nurses are also less likely to make medication errors when they have fewer pills to distribute. Thus, knowledge of the kinetics of a drug should suggest appropriate intervals between doses (see Chapter 2). The long half-life and slow onset of action of drugs like guanethidine, thyroid hormone, and digitoxin should allow their administration once daily. One possible justification of fixed-dose drug combinations may be that the patient need take fewer pills. The hypothesis that prepared combinations of drugs are taken more faithfully than drugs in separate preparations has not been tested. There are compelling reasons *not* to use most of these preparations (see Chapter 15).

If noncompliance with a regimen is strongly suspected or documented, direct steps should be taken to correct the situation.

Principle: Failure to comply with a medical regimen can be dangerous, but can usually be prevented by appropriate measures. Noncompliance will not be detected unless it is either tested for in a routine manner or suspected and specifically investigated.

VARIABILITY OF DISEASE

Awareness of possible variations in the natural history of any disease process may affect decisions in therapeutics. Examples include the transient "cure" of diabetes that may follow the first correction of ketoacidosis in a juvenile diabetic; the "cure" of hypertension that may follow an acute myocardial infarction; the gratifying disappearance (in some cases) of signs of progression of "malignant" hypertension when blood pressure is brought under control; and the bewildering fluctuations in activity of diseases such as regional enteritis, pheochromocytoma, and carcinoid tumors, which make frequent reassessment of therapy mandatory, even (or especially) when the patient is doing well.

PLACEBO EFFECT

This chapter has reviewed several critical variables that the physician often fails to appreciate. The placebo effect, closely intertwined with all these variables, is often the last to be appreciated, but it may be recognized, analyzed, and even measured. Most important, rational use of the placebo effect may result in effective therapy (Bourne, 1971).

Definition, History, and Classification of the Placebo Effect

In Latin the verb *placebo* means, "I shall please." The certainty of such a prediction is qualified in the definition of a placebo by Shapiro: "Any therapeutic procedure (or that component of any therapeutic procedure) which is objectively without specific activity for the condition being treated" (Shapiro, 1964). The placebo itself must be distinguished from the placebo effect, which may or may not occur in any given situation. Shapiro defines the placebo effect as "the psychological, physiological, or psychophysiological effect of any medication or procedure given with therapeutic intent, which is independent of or minimally related to the pharmacologic effects of the medication or to the specific effects of the procedure, and which operates through a psychological mechanism" (Shapiro, 1959).

Such definitions sound cumbersome and vague because they state what the placebo and placebo effect are *not*, rather than what they *are*. The modern concept of a placebo did not and could not develop until it could be contrasted with truly specific treatment (Shapiro, 1960). If we remember that there were very few truly effective remedies available only 7 or 8 decades ago, we can agree with Shapiro that "the history of medical treatment for the most part until relatively recently is the history of the placebo effect, since almost all medications until recently were placebos" (Shapiro, 1959). It may be a mistake, however, to look on the placebo as a relic of bygone days, or useful only as a control versus more specific therapy in therapeutic trials. A great deal of the practicing

physician's therapy is truly "placebo" in the primary sense of "I shall please." More important, such placebo therapy can be quite effective.

The placebo is most effective when (1) the doctor knows he is giving it; (2) he knows why he is giving it, and what results he may reasonably expect, good or bad; and (3) he attempts to judge whether or not it is effective and changes his therapy when necessary. *Principle: The placebo effect should be suspected whenever principles of pathophysiology and pharmacology fail to explain a change in the patient's course (for better or worse). The placebo effect is likely to be most important in those therapeutic situations in which pathophysiology is most poorly understood, and when drugs or other specific treatments are least successful.*

Vehicle of Administration. Placebos are most commonly thought of as pills or injections that simulate administration of an active drug. More dramatic interventions, such as surgery, can produce definite positive (or negative) placebo effects, e.g., the many varieties of cardiac surgery for angina (Dimond *et al.*, 1960). Many gastroenterologists suspect they are observing the placebo effect when dietary restriction helps a patient with gastrointestinal symptoms (see Chapter 4). In peptic ulcer, for example, no good evidence exists that rigid dietary restriction helps the patient, and some think it may do more harm than good (Hendrix, 1968). The vast variety of therapeutic and diagnostic procedures performed by physicians and their assistants undoubtedly exert considerable placebo effect, from simple blood drawing to barium enema or cardiac catheterization. Although it has not been systematically tested, no one doubts the "I shall please" effect resulting from the simple act of taking a medical history and performing a physical examination. Certainly no physician is ever likely to alleviate chronic tension headache without these latter two procedures, and perhaps in some patients no further treatment, placebo or otherwise, may be necessary. The last and most important vehicle for administration of a placebo is the physician himself, whose appearance, attitudes, prestige, emotional responsiveness, and understanding form the groundwork for effectiveness of any form of placebo or active drug.

"Pure" versus "Impure" Placebo. The pure placebo is a substance administered as a drug, or a procedure performed, that could have no conceivable physiologic or pharmacologic effect on the patient. An impure placebo is a substance or procedure with potential pharmacologic or physiologic effects, although not necessarily on the particular disease process in question (e.g., vitamin B_{12} for weakness and fatigue in the absence of pernicious anemia). It is important to recognize that no truly "pure" placebo really exists. Even fructose or lactose can produce definite (and very unpleasant) physiologic effects in patients who are "intolerant" to those substances.

Positive versus Negative Placebo Effects. A placebo effect need not always be beneficial and may be frankly toxic; dermatitis medicamentosa and angioneurotic edema have resulted from placebo therapy (Wolf and Pinsky, 1954). More subtle but equally important negative placebo effects must occur when the physician himself, by virtue of a moment of inattention, a raised eyebrow, or a transient look of disgust, loses the trust of his patient.

Planned versus Unconscious or Inadvertent Placebo. In drug trials or clinical investigation, the physician's awareness of the presence of a placebo can drastically affect the outcome of a study, hence the importance of the double-blind technique (see Chapter 1). In clinical practice the physician's awareness of placebo effects will almost always be an advantage in therapy. Unplanned or inadvertent placebo medication

may be directed more at "pleasing" the physician than at helping the patient.

Such a "classification" is necessarily arbitrary and the four categories are not exclusive or all inclusive. Still, if we know the "vehicle" of administration for the placebo, its "purity," whether the effect was positive or negative, and whether the physician was or was not aware of the potential placebo nature of the therapy in question, we can approach a better understanding of a wide spectrum of therapeutic interventions.

Evidence for the Widespread Significance of the Placebo Effect

Because of its usefulness in therapeutic trials, the placebo has been studied extensively in a wide variety of conditions (Figure 14–2). As a result, we know that placebo therapy can produce effects in almost any disease state. A study that shows no response to placebo medication might almost be suspected of lack of objectivity on that ground. More than a decade ago, Beecher was able to collect data on placebo therapy in 1082 patients with conditions that included postoperative wound pain, cough,

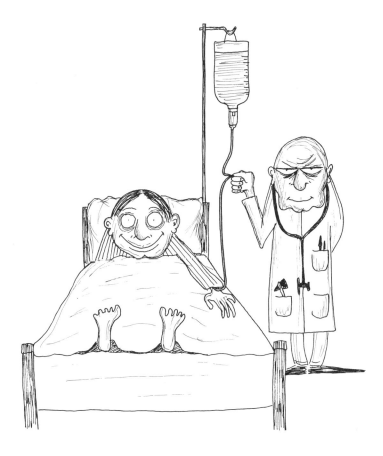

Figure 14–2. The placebo has not been displaced by the wonders of twentieth-century science. It plays an important role in the daily practice of most physicians.

mood changes, angina pectoris, headache, sea-sickness, anxiety and tension, and the common cold (Beecher, 1955). Satisfactory relief by a placebo was achieved in 35% of these patients. A similar review today adds many other conditions to this list, including status asthmaticus (Wayne, 1956), hypertension (Shapiro, 1956), mental depression (Overall et al., 1962; Hollister et al., 1967), and many other diseases. The percentage of relief might not be so high in these diseases, but in virtually every study a considerable number of patients have been helped by placebo medication.

The placebo has not been displaced by the wonders of twentieth-century science. Paradoxically, discovery of the "wonder drugs" such as penicillin may actually have made the placebo more effective today than it was in the nineteenth century, because of the generally increased "faith" of both patients and doctors in the efficacy of drugs. For example: (1) A study of treatment for the common cold (National Disease and Therapeutic Index, 1958–1968) revealed that 31% of patients received a prescription for a "broad-spectrum" or "medium-spectrum" antibiotic, 22% received penicillin, and 6% sulfonamides, none of which could possibly have had any beneficial specific pharmacologic effect on the viral infection per se. (2) Thousands of doses of vitamin B_{12} are administered yearly at considerable expense to patients without pernicious anemia. (3) A similar drug with even less scientific justification is a combination of vitamin B_{12} and intrinsic factor, administered orally, which in 1966 was prescribed 434,000 times to patients 65 years old or older, at a total retail price of greater than two million dollars. (4) Often, when more than one drug is included in a pill, at least one of the drugs is in fact placebo (perhaps as much for the doctor as for the patient), e.g., the antifungal component of several formerly popular pills also containing tetracycline has been pronounced unnecessary by the National Research Council. The combinations have been withdrawn from the market (683,000 prescriptions of one of these combinations were given to patients 65 years old and older in 1966, at a total retail price of 3.7 million dollars) (Task Force on Prescription Drugs, 1968; National Research Council, 1969).

Similar examples could be listed ad nauseam; instead, the reader should attempt to classify each of these instances according to the scheme given above. He will find that most are "impure" placebos, that the potential negative or toxic effects may often seem to outweigh putative beneficial effects, and that many of these placebos probably are of the "inadvertent" or "unconscious" variety.

Mechanism of the Placebo Effect

Despite widespread use of placebo medication, the way in which it produces its undeniably powerful effects is not well understood. The need for greater understanding is imperative. As Pickering has put it: "To rely on data, the nature of which one does not understand, is the first step in losing intellectual honesty. The doctor is particularly vulnerable to a loss of this kind, since so much of therapeutics is based on suggestion. And the loss naturally leaves him and his patients the poorer" (Pickering, (1955).

Whatever the mechanism involved, two requirements for any placebo effect are absolutely necessary: (1) The disease process itself, or the symptoms it produces, must be capable of variable intensity, both over time and in different patients. In some cases the resilience of the host, and powerful defense mechanisms developed through evolution, can protect against and even cure disease. Severe acidosis and cardiac arrest are unlikely to be susceptible to placebo therapy, precisely because they represent failure of defense mechanisms. The importance of this resilience is underlined by the long history of "success" of medicine and of physicians through centuries in which virtually no specific therapy was available. In other cases, it may simply be that subjective symptoms vary, and their cause (e.g., gastric hyperacidity) or assessment by the central nervous system may be influenced by psychologic factors. For example, consider the effects of placebo therapy in reducing the pain of headache (Beecher, 1955) or the erstwhile popularity of Krebiozen as an anticancer drug. (2) There must be a doctor-patient relationship, actual or implied. Patients may obtain relief from over-the-counter medications (e.g., the frequent relief of tension headache immediately after ingestion of aspirin, long before the drug can be absorbed) without the intervention of a physician, but the prestige of physicians as "healers" with a multitude of wonder drugs may lend magic to aspirin, cathartics, antihistamines, and other drugs available with or without a prescription. In general, however, it is the actual dynamic relationship between physician and patient that makes the placebo most effective.

Closer examination of the doctor-patient relationship affords important clues to understanding the placebo effect. One common denominator in virtually all patients is *fear*. Another, common to patients and physicians, is *hope*. Another way of describing the same phenomena is to use the central psychoanalytic concept of *transference*; a patient may transfer emotions originally directed at certain objects in his past environment (parents, teachers, other physicians, food, physical comfort, etc.) onto new objects (physician, nurse, medical student, or pills, injections, and even machines, such as ECG monitors in a coronary-care unit or a cobalt radiotherapy unit). Implicit in the concept of transference is the idea that any sort of emotion, positive or negative, may be transferred, e.g., trust or distrust, love or hate, hope or disappointment. In psychotherapy, for example, good results are definitely related to the patient's previous positive expectations as to results of treatment (Frank *et al.*, 1963). Another implication is that the physician is also capable of transferring his own feelings from past emotional foci to his patients or his drugs.

The concept of transference may not be literally "true" and certainly is difficult to test objectively. Operant conditioning experiments in animals and man are more easily quantified, but confirm the same conclusions. Past experience of the organism may profoundly affect responses to new environmental stimuli. More specifically, behavior in a new situation can often be determined by the "reward" or "punishment" that occurred in association with certain types of behavior in the past (Brady, 1960; DiCara, 1970) (see Chapter 15). Translated into the therapeutic situation, the good or bad results of contact with drugs and physicians in the past might partly determine the results of anything perceived as "treatment" in the present. In addition to overt behavior, autonomic responses may be altered by purely "psychologic" stimuli in the past; e.g., gastric acid secretion or heart rate may be affected by stimuli of which the subject may not be aware on a conscious level (Katkin and Murray, 1968).

In the context of either "transference" or "operant conditioning," the placebo response comes into sharper focus. Placebo responses occur much more frequently when the end point of therapy is overt behavior (e.g., in psychiatry [Lesse, 1962]), subjective sensation (e.g., nausea and vomiting [Wolf *et al.*, 1957], or postoperative pain [Lasagna *et al.*, 1954]), which can be modified by previously formed attitudes of patients, or a variable that is under hormonal or autonomic control (e.g., gastric acidity [Wolf, 1950], bronchoconstriction in asthma [Wayne, 1956], blood pressure [Ayman, 1930]). Conversely, placebo responses are unlikely when the therapeutic end point is not susceptible to such control (e.g., regression of metastatic tumor nodules in the lung or radiologic joint changes in rheumatoid arthritis). Placebo responses are less common in protracted disease states with an unremitting downhill course (Lesse, 1962), perhaps partly because the patient's past experience

may have favored negative transference. In psychotherapy, placebo response is much more likely in patients whose symptoms are predominantly somatic (Campbell and Rosenbaum, 1967), possibly because these patients have well-developed "reflexes" controlling their awareness of subjective physical sensations. In general, increased anxiety and increased "stressfulness" of the situation make placebo effects more likely (Beecher, 1955; Lesse, 1962; Campbell and Rosenbaum, 1967), though not always (Rickels and Downing, 1967). Accordingly, normal control subjects are probably less likely to obtain positive or negative effects from a placebo than are truly sick patients. One reason may be that in stress situations the patient is "set" for transference, or that he falls back on conditioned responses when rational predictions about his future course seem impossible.

Much attention has been paid to the problem of defining a "placebo reactor." An extremely well-designed study (Lasagna *et al.*, 1954) showed that certain patients differed markedly from others in their response to placebo (saline) injections for severe postoperative pain. Of 162 postoperative patients, 14% experienced consistent analgesia from placebo, comparable to that from the active drug morphine. Another group, the "nonreactors" (31%), consistently failed to obtain analgesia from placebo, and the responses of the remaining 55% were inconsistent. These workers emphasized several points: It was impossible for an observer to determine by conversation or examination, even in retrospect, whether any individual patient might be a placebo reactor or nonreactor. Nonetheless, when the two extreme groups were taken as a whole, certain general characteristics of both groups could be outlined. By psychologic testing, the reactor group was found to be more outgoing, more dependent on outside stimulation from the environment for emotional satisfaction, more favorably disposed to hospitalization, more concerned with "visceral" or pelvic complaints (constipation, etc.), somewhat more anxious, and perhaps less mature than the nonreactor group. Most significantly, the nonreactor group appeared to respond less well to genuine analgesic medication than the reactors and required more doses of morphine for a longer time postoperatively.

Such a study illustrates how difficult it is to predict whether an individual patient will respond to placebo medication. The chief difference between the two groups in Lasagna's study simply may be that the nonreactors suffered more severe pain (despite the fact that "severity" of their operations was the same in both groups) (Trouton, 1957). Other studies have not been able to define such groups easily (Knowles and Lucas, 1960; Campbell and Rosenbaum, 1967). Occasionally a consistent placebo reactor on one day may be a nonreactor on another day (Wolf et al., 1957).

However, certain generalizations prominent in medical folklore related to the placebo are not true. Contrary to what one might guess, the "hypersuggestible" typical hysterical personality does not predispose to positive or negative placebo reactions (Lesse, 1962). Similarly, women are not more likely than men to receive relief from a placebo (Trouton, 1957). A positive reaction to placebo does not mean that the pain, discomfort, or disease state is "only psychologic" and not "real." Conversely, a negative reaction to placebo does not mean that the disease state *is* "real."

If a true personality type typical of the placebo reactor exists, it is expressed to some degree in almost every patient, since the mechanisms responsible for the placebo effect are probably operative in everyone. (Analogy: Try to define a type of patient whose congestive heart failure will consistently respond to digitalis.) *Principle: The physician who wishes to make best use of placebo therapy should concentrate not on the personality "type" of his patient so much as on the disease process he is treating and the environmental and emotional stresses active in his patient.*

Rational Use of the Placebo in Drug Trials and Clinical Practice

Use of a placebo medication or procedure in therapeutic trials has become almost standard. The placebo is useful in scientific drug trials because its effect can be seen in almost any therapeutic setting. In its simplest form, the placebo is valuable as a necessary "control," in the same way that comparison of corticosteroids plus acetylsalicylic acid (ASA) versus ASA alone in rheumatoid arthritis would require ASA in the control group. Real-life situations are not so simple, and use of the placebo may require more thought.

In some cases no "placebo group" may be necessary at all. If one mode of therapy has definitely been shown to have genuine benefit, that therapy, not placebo, should be the "control." For example, in testing new drugs for symptomatic relief in rheumatoid arthritis, a demonstrated superiority to placebo medication is worse than useless, since (1) the placebo group has been deprived of active medication (aspirin) and (2) the real question, "Is new drug X superior to conventional therapy?" has not been answered. The story of indomethacin,

superior to placebo (Wanka et al., 1964) but not to aspirin (Pinals and Frank, 1967), and carrying considerable serious toxicity (Lövgren and Allander, 1964; Robindon, 1965), is a case in point.

In some cases, the best use of a "pure" placebo may simply be to separate from a study a group of patients who respond to any pill. The remaining patients then can be used to demonstrate more clearly a difference between two or more active drugs (Friend, 1969). The superiority of aspirin to codeine and morphine (all by oral route) in moderate postoperative pain was much more clear-cut if "placebo reactors" were removed from all treatment groups (Beecher et al., 1953).

Use of the "pure" or "true" placebo carries with it a serious drawback in some drug trials (Jick, 1969). Because many "active" drugs produce symptoms or signs that become detectable by either the patient or the physician, a "pure" placebo may make a double-blind experiment invalid, since the doctor or patient may accurately guess which patients are receiving which medication.

In judging any published drug trial, a most important item will be the investigators' definition of the end point of therapy. An end point must be determined before the study begins, because of the potential bias that might be introduced by stopping the study prematurely, when the results "look good," and in order to set up appropriate means of measuring the desired therapeutic effect. The end point must be definite, measurable, and reproducible from test to test, whether it be a certain concentration of blood sugar or subjective relief of pain, discomfort, or anxiety. Similarly, all potential toxicities must be defined before the study begins and acceptable limits fixed for each; appropriate indices of these toxic effects must be followed.

Investigators who do not fulfill these requirements for a drug trial are open to criticism on moral as well as scientific grounds. They may endanger patients who are deprived for longer than necessary of a drug that does work, or who are exposed to a toxic or ineffective drug. The same criteria of drug effect and toxicity should be applied to the placebo medication in the drug trial. We should not fail, however, to make precisely these same demands of our use of placebo (or active) medication in daily clinical practice. A doctor who prescribes "green pills" for anxiety or "yellow pills" for premenstrual tension may or may not look on these pills as placebos. He always is obligated to follow the results of his therapy as carefully as he would with digitalis, chlorambucil, or amphotericin B.

Because it is often given for indefinite complaints, and because its mechanism is poorly understood, decision on the use of the placebo may be cavalier. In addition, the twentieth-century physician may have a faintly shamefaced attitude toward using placebo and is often reluctant to admit he is using it (Hofling, 1955). Quite possibly, the physician's honest recognition that he is contemplating using a placebo could improve his effective use of it, by making him think carefully about why he has chosen that particular drug. *Principle: In the emotionally "charged" atmosphere of many doctor-patient relationships, the physician must always be maximally aware of his own and his patient's feelings, in order to make placebo therapy specific.*

Rational Use of the Placebo: Indications

Clear-cut indications are required before a placebo is used. There should be a rational expectation that the placebo may prove effective in a well-defined therapeutic situation. Many such indications will arise. Two general classes of indications for placebo are common enough to be mentioned. We can extract from them principles applicable in other management problems.

If carefully controlled trials have shown placebo to be effective in ameliorating a disease state, physicians should seriously consider using it. For example, a large study (Overall *et al.*, 1962) on the treatment of mild mental depression showed that a group of patients responded quite well to placebo in 3 weeks, just as well as other groups treated with an inhibitor of monoamine oxidase or with dextroamphetamine-amobarbital, and almost as well as a parallel group treated with imipramine. At the end of 12 weeks, results in the four groups were identical. A later study by the same group (Hollister *et al.*, 1967) attempted to eliminate possible placebo reactors by administering placebo tablets to 133 depressed patients before they were placed on active drugs. Thirty-two patients (25%) responded so well to the placebo that they could not be included in the drug trial (see Chapter 11). Both studies demonstrate the same point: Many depressed patients recover when given almost any sort of pill (or spontaneously). Recovery frequently may occur after as short a period as a week, but is in fact *usual* after 3 months.

Thus many depressed patients may profit from a short course of placebo therapy. Severely depressed or suicidal patients would certainly not be candidates for placebo. A large fraction of the remaining group with less severe depression might respond very well to placebos and

would not be subject to the toxicities of the tricyclic antidepressants (Coull *et al.*, 1970). In addition, a suicide attempt with placebo tablets will surely fail.

Another type of indication for the use of a placebo arises in the extremely common situation in which no drug is indicated, but the patient cannot be convinced and requires or demands something tangible that he can define as "treatment." Often a pill, a diet, a strict prohibition of certain additives, or even repeated blood tests are desired by a patient because of his past experience with other doctors, with another disease, or even with another patient, e.g., the exhaustive evaluation for malignancy demanded by a patient whose father died of cancer. Possibly the demand may be iatrogenic, but by a more roundabout path; many patients (and probably many doctors) are victims of the "magic bullet" theory of therapeutics and refuse to be "cured" without an active intervention.

In such cases the rational physician may be forced to choose between giving medicine he is sure will have no beneficial pharmacologic effects versus giving no therapy and allowing his patient to go to another doctor who may be more of an "activist" than he. If these are the only true alternatives, a placebo is superior to any active drug with dubious indications (thyroid extract for weakness without true myxedema, nikethamide as a "pepper-up" in the mornings, vitamins for "tired blood," antibiotics for viral coryza, etc.).

Preservation of the doctor-patient relationship cannot be justified in order to continue pecuniary or emotional gains for the physician, although Molière was neither the first nor the last to note that such motives often constitute an indication for placebo in the real world. Similarly, one other common justification for the placebo—to "get that patient off my back"—cannot be condoned. Rational use of the placebo absolutely requires that the physician follow his patient for evidence of therapeutic effect. He cannot do so in the absence of a strong and continuing relationship with his patient. *Principle: A patient's demand for drug treatment may justify the use of a placebo if pathology requiring active treatment has been ruled out, and if a truly useful purpose can be served by offering an intervention that the patient can interpret as "treatment."*

The need for placebo medication can and should be limited. The physician may offer a placebo with the statement that it should first ameliorate, then abolish, the symptoms. If the symptoms do disappear, he can stop the placebo. If they do not, the physician must stop the placebo, since it is ineffective. *Principle: It is almost as important to know when to stop a drug as when to start it. This is equally true of placebo.*

Rational Use of the Placebo: Toxicity

The potential toxicity of any impure placebo should be obvious, simply as a result of the known toxic properties of the active drug involved. Other possible toxic effects of any placebo medication are more subtle, but no less real.

The foremost potential toxicity of a placebo is that of overlooking a condition for which more specific treatment might be indicated. No physician would ever knowingly withhold active therapy for any disease serious enough to warrant treatment. In practical terms the issue is often crucial, however, since the placebo may provide an appealing substitute for the sometimes arduous task of diagnosis.

A 48-year-old Negro woman had been complaining for 6 months of increasing weakness and lassitude, with loss of appetite and occasional "dizzy spells," all occurring in a setting of intense marital difficulties. Although her hemoglobin was said to be normal, she was given weekly injections of vitamin B_{12} 5 weeks prior to admission. In mid-January she was brought to the emergency room nearly comatose and suffered a cardiac arrest shortly after arrival. With intubation, external cardiac massage, epinephrine, alkali, and cardioversion from ventricular fibrillation to normal sinus rhythm she recovered. At this point prearrest serum electrolytes were reported, revealing Na^+ 124, K^+ 7.8. Further questioning revealed that her skin and mucous membranes had been turning blacker over the past 6 to 8 months. Her idiopathic Addison's disease was confirmed by laboratory tests and responded well to replacement with adrenal corticosteroids.

It seems likely that in this case the vitamin B_{12} was a more effective placebo for the doctor than for the patient. *Principle: The physician who wishes to use a placebo must secure his diagnosis, just as before use of any drug.*

The life-crippling habituation potential of many chronically administered drugs is familiar to the clinician, and the placebo is no exception. Every physician has seen patients with peptic ulcer whose lives are severely limited by a compulsively designed diet, which is probably without definite effects on their gastric acid production or duodenal mucosa, and unfortunate patients on a demanding gluten-free diet who never have had sprue.

Use of a placebo may foster the mistaken conception that symptoms are due to physical causes, when in fact they are not. If placebo administration is unconscious on the part of the doctor, he may fall victim to the same misconception.

Purely ethical considerations, such as the physician's laudable hesitation about outright lying, may occasionally be outweighed by the physician's duty to alleviate suffering. Discovery by a patient that he has been "tricked," even if he was tricked into feeling better, may cause more suffering than was present in the first place and may destroy the ability of doctor and patient to work together. Like any drug toxicity, this one may be best avoided if it is anticipated before therapy is begun. In some patients such a possibility might constitute a strong contraindication to placebo therapy; in others it might dictate shorter duration of therapy. Alternatively, such toxicity may be avoided in some cases by careful explanation that the pill (actually placebo) is being given as a trial, that its mechanism of action is not well understood, but that it is unlikely to prove toxic. It may even be stated that a placebo effect is possible, but that if the pill works this is unimportant. In the setting of a strong relation between doctor and patient, such an explanation will place the placebo in a proper light, even if its true nature is discovered by the patient. In the absence of such a relationship between doctor and patient the placebo should not be administered.

The placebo may be used as a therapeutic trial, to "see if it will work" (other modes of therapy being unavailable or inappropriate), but the clinician is often wrong if he attempts to judge from the effects of a placebo whether the symptoms treated were primarily psychologic in nature. Relief of pain by sterile saline injection does not mean the pain had no physical cause; similarly, the failure of saline to alleviate pain often has little bearing on whether the pain was physical or psychologic in origin.

Principles: (1) Know what you are treating, and why. (2) Attempt to define the placebo nature of your treatment, and its mechanism. Ask whether that mechanism can apply in the clinical situation at hand. (3) Formulate a therapeutic plan in advance, including realistic goals to be achieved over a definite period. (4) Measure the results of placebo treatment carefully. (5) If the therapeutic goals are achieved, placebo medication can be stopped or gradually tapered. If the goals have not been reached, or if there are signs of impending toxicity, the placebo should be discontinued.

To summarize the placebo effect, we can do no better than to quote Osler's prescription for treatment of neurasthenia, a condition for which he eschewed the use of drugs (Osler, 1918):

> The use of religious ideas and practices may be most helpful, and this has come into vogue in various forms, as Christian Science, Emmanuelism, Mental Healing, *etc.* It is an old story. In all

ages, and in all lands, the prayer of faith, to use the words of St. James, has healed the sick; and we must remember that amid the Aesculapian cult, the most elaborate and beautiful system of faith healing the world has seen, scientific medicine took its rise. As a profession, consciously or unconsciously, more often the latter, faith has been one of our most valuable assets, and Galen expressed a great truth when he said: "He cures most successfully in whom the people have the greatest confidence." It is in these cases of neurasthenia and psychasthenia, the weak brothers and the weak sisters, that the personal character of the physician comes into play, and once let him gain the confidence of the patient, he can work just the same sort of miracle as Our Lady of Lourdes or Ste. Anne de Beaupre. Three elements are necessary: first, a strong personality in whom the individual has faith—Christ, Buddha, Aesculapius (in the days of Greece), one of the saints, or, what has served the turn of common humanity very well, a physician. Secondly, certain accessories— a shrine, a sanctuary, the services of a temple, or for us a hospital or its equivalent, with a skillful nurse. Thirdly, a suggestion, either of the "only believe," "feel it," "will it" attitude of mind, which is the essence of every cult and creed, or of the active belief in the assurance of the physician that the precious boon of health is within reach.

REFERENCES

Anderson, T. W.; LeRiche, W. H.; and MacKay, J. S.: Sudden death and ischemic heart disease. Correlation with hardness of local water supply. *New Eng. J. Med.,* **280**:805–807, 1969.

Appenzeller, O., and Descarries, L.: Circulatory reflexes in patients with cerebrovascular disease. *New Eng. J. Med.,* **271**:820–23, 1964.

Ayman, D.: An evaluation of therapeutic results in essential hypertension. *J.A.M.A.,* **95**:246–49, 1930.

Barker, K. N., and McConnell, W. E.: How to detect medication errors. *Mod. Hosp.,* **99**:95–106, 1962.

Beecher, H. K.: The powerful placebo. *J.A.M.A.,* **159**:1602–1606, 1955.

Beecher, H. K.; Keats, A. S.; Mosteller, F.; and Lasagna, L.: The effectiveness of oral analgesics (morphine, codeine, acetylsalicylic acid) and the problem of placebo "reactors" and "non-reactors." *J. Pharmacol. Exp. Ther.,* **109**:393–400, 1953.

Benstead, N., and Theobald, G. W.: Iron and "physiological" anemia of pregnancy. *Brit. Med. J.,* **1**:407–10, 1952.

Bergman, A. B., and Werner R. J.: Failure of children to receive penicillin by mouth. *New Eng. J. Med.,* **268**:1334–38, 1963.

Berry, D.; Ross, A.; Huempfner, H.; and Deuschle, K.: Self-medication behavior as measured by urine chemical tests in domiciliary tuberculous patients. *Amer. Rev. Resp. Dis.,* **86**:1–7, 1962.

Bonnar, J.; Goldberg, A.; and Smith, J. A.: Do pregnant women take their iron? *Lancet,* **1**:457–58, 1969.

Bourne, H.: The placebo—a frequently unappreciated opportunity in therapeutics. *Rat. Drug Ther.,* in press, 1971.

Brady, J. V.: Emotional behavior. In Field, J. (ed.): *Handbook of Physiology.* American Physiological Society, Washington, D.C., 1960, pp. 1529–52.

Breite, M. J.: Urine test for the detection of PAS in ambulatory tuberculous patients. *Amer. Rev. Tuberc.,* **79**:672, 1959.

Campbell, J. H., and Rosenbaum, P.: Placebo effect and symptom relief in psychotherapy. *Arch. Gen. Psychiat. (Chicago),* **16**:364–68, 1967.

Caron, H. S., and Roth, H. P.: Patients' cooperation with a medical regimen. Difficulties in identifying the noncooperator. *J.A.M.A.,* **203**:922–26, 1968.

Conney, A. H.: Pharmacological implications of microsomal enzyme induction. *Pharmacol. Rev.,* **19**:317–66, 1967.

Coull, D. C.; Crooks, J.; Dingwall-Fordyce, I.; Scott, A. M.; and Weir, R. D.: Amitriptyline and cardiac disease. Risks of sudden death identified by monitoring system. *Lancet,* **2**:590–91, 1970.

Davis, M. S.: Predicting non-compliant behavior. *J. Health Soc. Behav.,* **8**:265–71, 1967.

Davis, M. S., and Eichhorn, R. L.: Compliance with medical regimens: a panel study. *J. Health Hum. Behav.,* **4**:240–49, 1963.

DiCara, L. V.: Learning in the autonomic nervous system. *Sci. Amer.,* **222**:31–39, 1970.

Dimond, E. G.; Kittle, C. F.; and Crockett, J. E.: Comparison of internal mammary artery ligation and sham operation for angina pectoris. *Amer. J. Cardiol.,* **5**:483–86, 1960.

Dixon, W. M.; Shadling, P.; and Wootton, I. D.: Out-patient PAS therapy. *Lancet,* **2**:871–72, 1957.

Egbert, L. D.; Battit, G. E.; Welch, C. E.; and Bartlett, M. K.: Reduction of postoperative pain by encouragement and instruction of patients. A study of doctor-patient rapport. *New Eng. J. Med.,* **270**:825–27, 1964.

Ewy, G. A.; Kapadia, G. G.; Yao, L.; Lullin, M.; and Marcus, F. I.: Digoxin metabolism in the elderly. *Circulation,* **39**:449–53, 1969.

Fareeduddin, K., and Abelmann, W. H.: Impaired orthostatic tolerance after bed rest in patients with myocardial infarction. *New Eng. J. Med.,* **280**:345–50, 1969.

Fazekas, J. F.; Bessman, A. N.; Cotsonas, N. J., Jr.; and Alman, R. W.: Cerebral hemodynamics in cerebral arteriosclerosis. *J. Gerontol.,* **8**:137–45, 1953.

Feinstein, A. R.; Wood, H. F.; Epstein, J. A.; Tarante, A.; Simpson, R.; and Tursky, E.: A controlled study of three methods of prophylaxis against streptococcal infection in a population of rheumatic children. II. Results of the first three years of the study, including methods for evaluating the maintenance of oral prophylaxis. *New Eng. J. Med.,* **260**:697–702, 1959.

Forsham, P. H.: The adrenal cortex. In Williams, R. H. (ed.): *Textbook of Endocrinology.* W. B. Saunders Co., Philadelphia, 1968, pp. 287–379.

Frank, J. D.; Nash, E. H.; Stone, A. R.; and Imber, S. D.: Immediate and long-term symptomatic course of psychiatric outpatients. *Amer. J. Psychiat.,* **120**:429–39, 1963.

Friend, D. G.: The ubiquitous placebo. *Med. Counterpoint,* Nov., 1969, pp. 18–20.

Gilroy, A. B.: Investigation of prognanil prophylaxis and co-existing parasitemia. *Ann. Trop. Med. Parasit.,* **46**:72–84, 1952.

Glennon, J. A.: Weight reduction: an enigma. *Arch. Intern. Med. (Chicago),* **118**:1–2, 1966.

Gordis, L.; Markowitz, M.; and Lilienfeld, A. M.: The inaccuracy in using interviews to estimate patient reliability in taking medications at home. *Med. Care,* **7**:49–54, 1969.

Hackett, T. P.; Cassem, N. H.; and Wishnie, H. A.: The coronary care unit. An appraisal of its psychologic hazards. *New Eng. J. Med.,* **279**:1365–70, 1968.

Hart, L. G., and Fouts, J. R.: Effects of acute and

chronic DDT administration on hepatic microsomal drug metabolism in the rat. *Proc. Soc. Exp. Biol. Med.*, 114:388–92, 1963.

———: Further studies on the stimulation of hepatic microsomal drug metabolizing enzymes by DDT and its analogs. *Arch. Exp. Path. Pharmacol.*, 249:486–500, 1965.

Hendrix, T. R.: Abdominal pain. In Harvey, A. M.; Cluff, L. E.; Johns, R. J.; Owens, A. H.; Rabinowitz, D.; and Ross, R. S. (eds.); *The Principles and Practice of Medicine.* Appleton-Century-Crofts, New York, 1968, pp. 916–40.

Hofling, C. K.: The place of placebos in medical practice. *Gen. Pract.*, 11:103–107, 1955.

Hollister, L. E.; Overall, J. E.; Shelton, J.; Pennington, V.; Kimball, I.; and Johnson, M.: Drug therapy of depression. Amitriptyline, perphenazine, and their combination in different syndromes. *Arch. Gen. Psychiat. (Chicago)*, 17:486–93, 1967.

Imboden, J. B.; Canter, A.; and Cluff, L. E.: Convalescence from influenza. A study of the psychological and clinical determinants. *Arch. Intern. Med. (Chicago)*, 108:393–99, 1961.

Januszewicz, W.; Sznajderman, M.; Wocial, B.; and Preibisz, J.: Urinary excretion of free norepinephrine and free epinephrine in patients with acute myocardial infarction in relation to its clinical course. *Amer. Heart J.*, 76:345–52, 1968.

Jewitt, D. E.; Reid, D.; Thomas, M.; Mercer, C. J.; Valori, C.; and Shillingford, J. P.: Free noradrenaline and adrenaline excretion in relation to the development of cardiac arrhythmias and heart-failure in patients with acute myocardial infarction. *Lancet*, 1:635–41, 1969.

Jick, H.: Experimental models for the clinical evaluation of drugs. *Med. Counterpoint*, Nov., 1969, pp. 41–44.

Katkin, E. S., and Murray, E. W.: Instrumental conditioning of autonomically mediated behavior: theoretical and methodological issues. *Psychol. Bull.*, 70:52–68, 1968.

Knowles, J. B., and Lucas, C. J.: Experimental studies of the placebo response. *J. Ment. Sci.*, 106:231–40, 1960.

Kolmodin, B.; Azarnoff, D. L.; and Sjöqvist, F.: Effect of environmental factors on drug metabolism: decreased plasma half-life of antipyrine in workers exposed to chlorinated hydrocarbon insecticides. *Clin. Pharmacol. Ther.*, 10:638–42, 1969.

Kutt, H.; Wolk, M.; Scherman, R.; and McDowell, F.: Insufficient parahydroxylation as a cause of diphenylhydantoin toxicity. *Neurology*, 14:542–48, 1964.

Lasagna, L.; Mosteller, F.; vonFelsinger, J. M.; and Beecher, H. K.: A study of the placebo response. *Amer. J. Med.*, 16:770–79, 1954.

Lesse, S.: Placebo reactions in psychotherapy. *Dis. Nerv. Syst.*, 23:313–19, 1962.

Lövgren, O., and Allander, E.: Side effects of indomethacin. *Brit. Med. J.*, 1:118, 1964.

Luchi, R. J., and Gruber, J. W.: Unusually large digitalis requirements. A study of altered digoxin metabolism. *Amer. J. Med.*, 45:322–28, 1968.

MacDonald, M. E.; Hagberg, K. L.; and Grossman, B. J.: Social factors in relation to participation in followup care of rheumatic fever. *J. Pediat.*, 62:503–13, 1963.

Maddock, R. K.: Patient cooperation in taking medicines. A study involving isoniazid and aminosalicylic acid. *J.A.M.A.*, 199:169–72, 1967.

Malahy, B.: The effect of instruction and labeling on the number of medication errors made by patients at home. *Amer. J. Hosp. Pharm.*, 23:283–92, 1966.

Mohler, D. N.; Wallin, D. G.; Dreyfus, E. G.; and Bakst, H. J.: Studies in the home treatment of streptococcal disease. II. A comparison of the efficacy of oral administration of penicillin and intramuscular injection of benzathine penicillin in the treatment of streptococcal pharyngitis. *New Eng. J. Med.*, 254:45–50, 1956.

Moulding, T.; Omstad, G. D.; and Sbarbaro, J. A.: Supervision of outpatient drug therapy with the medication monitor. *Ann. Intern. Med.*, 73:559–64, 1970.

National Disease and Therapeutic Index: Reference File. Diagnosis: Common Cold, 1958–1968. Lea Associates, Inc., Ambler, Pa., 1969.

National Research Council (Division of Medical Sciences): White paper on fixed combinations of antimicrobial agents. In *Drug Efficacy Study*, National Academy of Sciences, Washington, D.C., 1969, pp. 123–39.

O'Reilly, R. A.; Aggeler, P. M.; Hoag, M. S.; Leong, L. S.; and Kropatkin, M. L.: Hereditary transmission of exceptional resistance to coumarin anticoagulant drugs. *New Eng. J. Med.*, 271:809–15, 1964.

Osler, W.: *The Principles and Practice of Medicine.* D. Appleton and Co., New York, 1918.

Overall, J. E.; Hollister, L. E.; Pokorny, A. D.; Casey, J. F.; and Katz, G.: Drug therapy in depressions. Controlled evaluation of imipramine, isocarboxazide, dextroamphetamine-amobarbital, and placebo. *Clin. Pharmacol. Ther.*, 3:16–22, 1962.

Peabody, F. W.: The care of the patient. *J.A.M.A.*, 88:877–82, 1927.

Pickering, G. W.: Disorders of contemporary society and their impact on medicine. *Ann. Intern. Med.*, 43:919–29, 1955.

Pinals, R. S., and Frank, S.: Relative efficacy of indomethacin and acetylsalicylic acid in rheumatoid arthritis. *New Eng. J. Med.*, 276:512–14, 1967.

Pittman, J. A., Jr.; Dailey, G. E., III; and Beschi, R. J.: Changing normal values for thyroidal radioiodine uptake. *New Eng. J. Med.*, 280:1431–34, 1969.

Preston, D. F., and Miller, F. L.: The tuberculosis outpatient's defection from therapy. *Amer. J. Med. Sci.*, 247:21–25, 1964.

Quinn, G. P.; Axelrod, J.; and Brodie, B. B.: Species, strain, and sex differences in metabolism of hexobarbitone, amidopyrine, antipyrine, and aniline. *Biochem. Pharmacol.*, 1:152–59, 1958.

Rickels, K., and Downing, R. W.: Drug- and placebo-treated neurotic outpatients. Pretreatment levels of manifest anxiety, clinical improvement, and side reactions. *Arch. Gen. Psychiat. (Chicago)*, 16:369–72, 1967.

Robindon, R.: Indomethacin in rheumatic disease. A clinical assessment. *Med. J. Aust.*, 1:266–69, 1965.

Roth, H. P., and Berger, D. G.: Studies on patient cooperation in ulcer treatment. I. Observation of actual as compared to prescribed antacid intake on hospital ward. *Gastroenterology*, 38:630–33, 1960.

Roth, H. P.; Caron, H. S.; and Hsi, B. P.: Measuring intake of a prescribed medication. A bottle count and a tracer technique compared. *Clin. Pharmacol. Ther.*, 11:228–37, 1970.

Schweitzer, M. D.; Gearing, F. R.; and Perera, G. A.: The epidemiology of primary hypertension. Present status. *J. Chron. Dis.*, 18:847–57, 1965.

Shapiro, A. K.: The placebo effect in the history of medical treatment: implications for psychiatry. *Amer. J. Psychiat.*, 116:298–304, 1959.

———: A contribution to the history of the placebo effect. *Behav. Sci.*, 5:109–35, 1960.

———: Factors contributing to the placebo effect. Their implications for psychotherapy. *Amer. J. Psychother.*, 18 (Suppl. 1):73–88, 1964.

Shapiro, A. P.: Consideration of multiple variables in evaluation of hypotensive drugs. *J.A.M.A.*, 160:30–39, 1956.

Task Force on Prescription Drugs: Background Papers: The drug users. U.S. Dept. of Health, Education and Welfare, Washington, D.C., 1968.

Trouton, D. S.: Placebos and their psychological effects. *J. Ment. Sci.*, **103**:344–54, 1957.

Valori, C.; Thomas, M.; and Shillingford, J.: Free noradrenaline and adrenaline excretion in relation to clinical syndromes following myocardial infarction. *Amer. J. Cardiol.*, **20**:605–17, 1967.

Vere, D. W.: Errors of complex prescribing. *Lancet*, **1**:370–73, 1965.

Vessell, E. S., and Page, J. G.: Genetic control of dicumarol levels in man. *J. Clin. Invest.*, **47**:2657–63, 1968.

Veterans Administration Cooperative Study Group on Antihypertensive Agents: Effects of treatment on morbidity in hypertension. Results in patients with diastolic blood pressures averaging 115 through 129 mm Hg. *J.A.M.A.*, **202**:1028–34, 1967.

Wanka, J.; Jones, L. I.; Wood, P. H. N.; and Dixon, A. St. J.: Indomethacin in rheumatic diseases. Controlled clinical trial. *Ann. Rheum. Dis.*, **23**:218–25, 1964.

Watkins, J. D.; Williams, T. F.; Martin, D. A.; Hogan, M. D.; and Anderson, E.: A study of diabetic patients at home. *Amer. J. Public Health*, **57**:452–59, 1967.

Wayne, E. J.: Placebos. *Brit. Med. J.*, **2**:157, 1956.

Weiss, C. F.; Glazko, A. J.; and Weston, J. K.: Chlor-amphenicol in the new born infant. A physiological explanation of its toxicity when given in excessive doses. *New Eng. J. Med.*, **262**:787–94, 1960.

Welch, R. M.; Harrison, Y. E.; Conney, A. H.; Poppers, P. J.; and Finster, M.: Cigarette smoking. Stimulatory effect on metabolism of 3,4-benzpyrene by enzymes in human placenta. *Science*, **160**:541–42, 1968.

Willcox, D. R.; Gillan, R.; and Hare, E. H.: Do psychiatric outpatients take their drugs? *Brit. Med. J.*, **2**:790–92, 1965.

Wishnie, H. A.; Hackett, T. P.; and Cassem, N. H.: Psychological hazards of convalescence following myocardial infarction. *J.A.M.A.*, **215**:1292–96, 1971.

Wolf, S.: Effects of suggestion and conditioning on the action of chemical agents in human subjects. The pharmacology of placebos. *J. Clin. Invest.*, **29**:100–109, 1950.

————: The pharmacology of placebos. *Pharmacol. Rev.*, **11**:689–704, 1959.

————: Emotions and the autonomic nervous system. *Arch. Intern. Med. (Chicago)*, **126**:1024–30, 1970.

Wolf, S.; Doering, C. R.; Clark, M. L.; and Hagans, J. A.: Chance distribution and the placebo "reactor." *J. Lab. Clin. Med.*, **49**:837–41, 1957.

Wolf, S., and Pinsky, R. H.: Effects of placebo administration and occurrence of toxic reactions. *J.A.M.A.*, **155**:339–41, 1954.

Chapter 15

DRUG REACTIONS

Kenneth L. Melmon and *Howard F. Morrelli*

We are a pill-taking society. During Osler's era most pills were innocuous (Keynes, 1968) (see Chapter 1). Now the dangers of taking drugs are considerably greater; a recent review presented the disturbing facts that (1) reactions increase as pill taking increases; (2) pill taking is more common now than in the past two to three decades; and (3) reactions are more severe than they were 5 years ago, although about 80% of reactions could be prevented without reducing the therapeutic effects of the drugs. Physicians have not recognized the reactions they have caused; they can learn to do so and to treat or even prevent them.

This chapter reviews the inappropriate prescription habits of doctors; it documents the consequences of indiscriminate use of drugs and describes an approach to prevent reactions.

Why do we take or prescribe pills so freely? Perhaps the habit can be explained by applying the principles of operant conditioning (Schuster and Thompson, 1969). Operant conditioning attributes taking an action to the favorable consequences of prior similar actions. Because the placebo effect is great, the consequence of the first pill-taking event was undoubtedly satisfying. In other words, regardless of why man took the first pill, he took the second pill because he liked the effect of the first one (Lewin, 1964). Figure 15–1 illustrates the final result of reinforced conditioning: the well-intentioned clinician, gratified by his experience with successive administration of drugs, ultimately believes that pills should be given for each complaint and that pills will cure almost irrespective of the disease or the drug's pharmacologic effect (Maronde *et al.*, 1969; Stolley and Lasagna, 1969).

Drugs have been developed that change biochemical and physiologic processes and, if properly used, alter the course of disease favorably. In a sense, the operant conditioning described above has been fortunate as it has stimulated academic and commercial interests to investigate and produce effective drugs. However, progress is a two-edged sword; the advances that have made drugs effective have increased both their availability and potential toxicity. If a considerable number of drugs are given or taken primarily because of "reflex" or conditioning (a doctor writes prescriptions for about 75% of his patients), many of the drugs will be inappropriate and toxicity will occur frequently (Palmer, 1969; Stolley and Lasagna, 1969; Lennard *et al.*, 1970; Melmon, 1971).

What can be done about this problem? Public education should decrease the public's demand for pills (Bean, 1950) and reduce the incidence of drug reactions. Education in clinical pharmacology must be strengthened to fill such gaps in physicians' training as pharmacokinetics (McIntyre, 1968; Lasagna, 1969; Melmon and Morrelli, 1969; Wagner, 1969). Postgraduate education stressing evaluation of a physician's

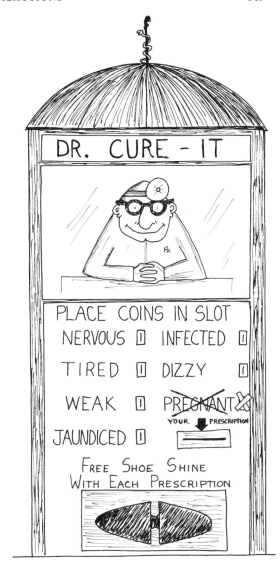

Figure 15–1. Consequences of reinforced conditioning.

approach to treatment must be made more attractive to practitioners (Overall and Tupin, 1969). Physicians must no longer be satisfied with the *Physicians' Desk Reference* and drug advertising as sole sources of drug information (Smith, 1968). We must help educate industrial "detail men" or provide convincing evidence of their shortcomings (Palmer, 1969). Perhaps equally important is the need to strengthen (both scientifically and economically) the governmental regulatory agencies responsible for the control of drugs (Modell, 1967; Editorial, 1969).

Prescriptions are given well out of proportion to their most generously estimated need. In the United States, chloromycetin is given in more doses than are required to cure all infections responsive to the drug. Osler was correct, but

somewhat optimistic, when he said, "One of the duties of the physician is to educate the masses not to take medicine" (Bean, 1950). The physician's primary duty is to educate himself to withhold drugs when they are unnecessary and to educate patients to avoid drugs in some ailments. Formerly, a major consequence of prescribing for symptoms was a delay in the diagnosis of disease. Inappropriate prescribing may now result in (1) lack of use of effective therapy for a life-threatening but curable disease; (2) the production of severe toxicity; (3) prolongation of a disease state; or (4) the development of a disorder to which a patient would otherwise not be subject. For example, patients may suffer teratogenicity (Cohlan, 1969) from thalidomide, ulceration of the bowel from potassium chloride, intramural intestinal hemorrhage from anticoagulants, retinal disorders from phenothiazines, cardiac failure from propranolol, changes in carbohydrate tolerance from diuretics, liver damage from many drugs, renal tubular acidosis from antibiotics (McCurdy et al., 1968), neuropathies from anticancer agents (Sandler et al., 1969), and aseptic necrosis of bone from corticosteroids (Meyler and Peck, 1968). *Principle: Drug administration can create diseases.*

Are these hazards of therapeutics as rare as they are commonly assumed to be? Only recently have data appeared on the personal, public, and economic consequences of the misuse of drugs. These are true drug reactions, and their consequences are great.

DEFINITION OF A DRUG REACTION

A drug reaction includes all unwanted consequences of drug administration, even administration of the wrong drug (or drugs) to the wrong patient in the wrong dosage (form, amount, route, or interval), at the wrong time, or for the wrong disease. Any single "wrong" may result in unwanted effects and therefore may cause a reaction. Ideally, the right drug, in the right dosage, in the right patient, at the right time for the right disease would produce no reactions. Regardless of his wisdom and conscientious approach, the therapist occasionally makes therapeutic decisions that entail a risk of drug reactions. He is forced to accept and indeed to make provision for side effects; when he gives antitumor agents, for example, he knowingly takes the risk of causing pancytopenia.

THE CLASSIC DRUG REACTION

Considerable attention has been focused on the standard or classic manifestations of drug reactions, their pathogenesis, and the means for detecting and treating them. Excellent and complete reviews on this subject are widely available in current literature (Goodman and Gilman, 1970). Classic drug reactions include those symptoms related to the individual's immunologic response to standard doses of drug (hypersensitivity or meta reactions), his inordinate response to usual or less-than-usual doses (idiosyncrasy or hyperreactivity), or his predictable responses to an overdose of the drug or a drug combination.

Hypersensitivity

Hypersensitivity to a drug is dependent on many factors. The drug or its metabolites must be antigenic or capable of acting as a haptene to stimulate antibody production. Exposure to the drug allows antibody production and antigen-antibody interaction. Despite the exposure of many people to drugs of many varieties, hypersensitivity reactions account for only 6 to 10% of all drug reactions (Borda et al., 1968), and few drugs cause hypersensitivity.

A detailed analysis of penicillin allergy is useful as a model of hypersensitivity reactions. The penicillin preparation (Stewart, 1967; Kovotzer and Haddad, 1970; Stewart and McGovern, 1970) and its route and rate of administration (Westerman et al., 1966) may determine the type of antibody produced and, therefore, the type of reaction. Exposure to drug may not be obvious (e.g., a patient taking a vaccine containing penicillin or drinking milk from cows treated for mastitis with penicillin). Although physicians may carefully seek evidence of previous exposure or reaction, the information may not be available from the patient or his records (Smith et al., 1966). For example, the indiscriminate and inappropriate use of penicillin, sometimes without the knowledge of the patient, often makes an accurate account of previous drug exposure impossible (Stolley and Lasagna, 1969). However, reactions to penicillin are likely to occur in patients who have previously reacted to penicillin or other drugs, and in patients who are atopic (Smith et al., 1966).

The skin-sensitizing (IgE) antibodies in penicillin allergy are most commonly developed to the penicilloyl metabolite of penicillin ("major" determinant). IgE is thought to be responsible for anaphylactic reactions and may also be produced in response to the unaltered drug or to another metabolite (e.g., penaldate, penicilloate, or penicillamine) (Levine, 1966; Turk and Baker, 1968). IgM and IgG antibodies may be produced after exposure of patients to penicillin and are usually specific for the penicilloyl metabolite ("major" determinant).

The "minor" determinants (unaltered drug or other drug metabolites) may be responsible for disastrous allergic reactions, and the nomenclature (major and minor determinants) is misleading. Better terms might be "frequent" and "infrequent" determinants. There are many possible determinants of antigenicity after administration of penicillin (Table 15–1).

Although IgE antibodies may cause immediate anaphylactic reactions, the significance of IgM and IgG antibodies is less clear. IgG antibodies may act as blocking antibodies to prevent or modify the course of reactions in patients who are skin-test sensitive to antigen but who develop skin rashes rather than anaphylaxis on exposure to the allergen. In some patients, the concentration of IgG falls during the acute allergic reaction and rises during the recovery period.

Table 15–1. DETERMINANTS OF ANTIGENICITY AFTER ADMINSTRATION OF PENICILLIN

TYPE OF ANTIBODY	IgM	IgG	IgE (REAGIN, OR SKIN-SENSITIZING ANTIBODY)
Svedberg sedimentation	19S	7S	
Agglutination of penicillin-incubated erythrocytes			
Saline	+++	+	
Serum	+++	+++	
Antigenic determinants	Major ?Minor	Major ?Minor	Major and minor
Role	?Exanthems	Blocking hemolysis	Immediate anaphylaxis Early urticarial

Hemagglutinating antibodies (IgG) are usually specific for the penicilloyl determinant, but these antibodies may be found in 60 to 100% of populations, if sensitive methods for their detection are used. Although patients with a history of allergy have higher concentrations of IgG than normals, it is not known if these antibodies are responsible for most reactions. In addition, lymphocytes from patients allergic to penicillin are more rapidly transformed by penicillin *in vitro* than are those taken from normals. This observation suggests that some lymphocytes have been "sensitized" to components of the penicillins. These lymphocytes, on contact with the antigen, release a substance that causes blood monocytes to migrate across endothelial linings of vessels, become converted to macrophages, and destroy tissues by release of lysosomal enzymes. This hypothesis may explain those allergic reactions to penicillin that simulate serum sickness.

Skin-testing procedures are necessary to evaluate the propensity of a given individual to react to penicillin, since serologic tests have no predictive value (Adkinson *et al.*, 1971). Research procedures, such as basophil degranulation tests or the passive transfer of IgE to monkeys, are impracticable for clinical use. Skin testing with unmodified penicillin is associated with an unacceptable incidence of severe reactions. Since penicilloyl is known to be the frequent (major) antigenic determinant, it is combined with polymerized polylysine to create a test substance less allergenic than either unmodified drug or penicilloyl combined with a complex protein.

Skin testing for IgE may reveal positive tests for penicilloyl polylysine (PPL), penicillin, or both. Seventeen studies of 2332 patients with a history of allergy who were skin tested with PPL antigen showed positive responses to PPL in 17 to 91%, most groups reporting 40 to 60%. These investigations tested 22,462 individuals with no history of penicillin allergy and found positive reactions in 0 to 10% (Table 15–2).

In seven studies (410 patients), comparing skin tests with PPL and penicillin in patients with a positive history of reaction, a higher percentage of positive reactions was obtained with PPL than with penicillin (50% vs. 25%).

Although the initial experience with PPL antigen versus "minor" or infrequent antigen indicated that anaphylactic reactions were much more common when the patient had a positive skin test to the minor determinant antigens, some patients have positive skin tests to PPL alone and develop anaphylactic reactions when penicillin is given (Rosenblum, 1968). When the skin test is positive, penicillin should not be used, since appropriate alternate antibiotics are usually available. If penicillin must be used, desensitization (producing, in essence, multiple but small and controllable reactions) should precede full-scale therapy.

The following recommendations for use of penicillin (slightly modified) have been proposed by a committee of experts of the World Health Organization:

1. Always have an emergency kit available for treatment of allergic reactions.

2. Always obtain an exact history of the patient's previous contact with penicillin, previous penicillin reactions, and allergic diathesis. In infants less than 3 months old, ask about penicillin allergy in the mother.

3. Do not give penicillin to patients with a previous history of reactions; indications for administration of penicillin are severely restricted in patients with an allergic diathesis (EDITORS NOTE: a disputable point in certain infections, such as subacute bacterial endocarditis).

4. If possible, refer patients with suspected penicillin allergy to a center capable of performing both skin tests and immunologic tests to provide the patient with objective diagnosis and permanent records.

5. Always tell the patient that he is going to receive penicillin.

6. Do not use penicillins topically.

7. Avoid the use of penicillinase-resistant penicillins unless there is a known infection with penicillinase-producing staphylococci. Owing to the cross-sensitivity of the semisynthetic penicillins (all have the 6-aminopenicillanic acid nucleus) there is no security in changing to one of these drugs. Although less frequent, cross-reactions may also occur with cephalosporins.

Table 15–2. ANTIBODY TITERS IN BLOOD AFTER PENICILLIN ADMINISTRATION: NONREACTORS VS. REACTORS*

ANTIBODY PRODUCED	PERCENTAGE OF PATIENTS WITH ANTIBODY PRODUCED		
A. *Nonreactors*	*No Recent Treatment* (112 *patients*)	*Treatment with Moderate Doses* (103 *patients*)	*Treatment with High Doses* (12 *patients*)
None	3	0	0
IgM	77	61	92
IgG plus IgM	17	30	8
IgE plus IgG and IgM	3	8	0
Major and minor determinants plus IgG and IgM	0	1	0

	PERCENTAGE OF PATIENTS WITH ANTIBODY TITERS WHO DEVELOPED:				
B. *Reactors* (7 *to* 14 *days after initiaton of treatment*)	*Immediate Reactions* (12 *patients*)	*Accelerated Reactions* (10 *patients*)	*Late Urticaria* (11 *patients*)	*Urticaria Plus Arthralgia* (16 *patients*)	*Skin Rash* (15 *patients*)
IgM	0	0	0	0	58
IgM (high titers)	0	0	0	0	32
IgE plus IgG and IgM	0	60	91	0	5
Minor determinant plus IgM	42	0	0	56	0
Minor determinant plus IgG and IgM	16	0	0	25	0
Minor determinant plus IgE, IgG and IgM	42	40	9	19	5

* Data for this table were compiled from Parker *et al.*, 1962; Brown *et al.*, 1964; Levine, 1966; Voss *et al.*, 1966; and Idsoe *et al.*, 1968. Available data do not permit calculation of the frequency of reactions, which is reported to vary from 0.7% to 10% in various studies. Among the reactions, anaphylaxis may occur in about 0.0015% to 0.004%, with a fatality rate of 0.00015% to 0.0002%.

8. To avoid contamination, use disposable equipment for penicillins when possible.

9. Observe all patients receiving penicillin for at least one-half hour after injection.

Summary Principles: (1) When seeking possible reactors, a history may be helpful, but a negative history should not exclude further testing with agents incapable of stimulating production of causative antibody. Penicillin scratch or conjunctival tests can be dangerous, as they can cause severe reactions and stimulate antibody production. *(2) When hypersensitivity is present but the drug must be used, small doses given at frequent intervals may minimize the effects of hypersensitivity. However, if the drug is again indicated after a drugless interval, the "desensitizing" procedure must be repeated. (3) Because we are unwittingly exposed to many drugs, as in foods* (Harber and Levine, 1969), *the incidence of hypersensitivity may increase. (4) A therapist must always be ready to treat the most severe forms of hypersensitivity, and antidotes must always be considered before administering dangerous drugs.*

The pathogenesis of hypersensitivity is similar for a number of drugs that stimulate antibody production and result in tissue-damaging antigen-antibody reactions. The sequence of events is identical to that seen in an acute inflammatory response elicited by other antigen-antibody interactions, with or without complement, and is dependent on local tissue response or response of the formed elements in blood (see Chapter 9). The morphologic changes in the microvasculature are characteristic of the acute inflammatory lesion, and similar therapeutic maneuvers aimed at preventing or reversing the acute disease are effective in many varieties of hypersensitivity (Miller and Melmon, 1970) (see Chapter 9). These observations oversimplify the events in hypersensitivity responses associated with drugs; minor but important variations occur (see Chapter 18). These variations are important when therapy of a specific event is considered. For example, if the complement system is unimportant in the development of a reaction to penicillin, there is no purpose in trying to prevent its activation by using anticomplementary drugs. However, once a host of reactions has been initiated by different drugs, a number of therapeutic agents with broad anti-inflammatory, bronchodilating, or antihistaminic actions might be useful.

The manifestations of hypersensitivity depend on the drug's dose and distribution and on host factors (La Du, 1971), including the distribution, quantity, and quality of the antibody (see Chapters 13 and 18). After penicillin administration, urticaria, maculopapular rashes, local reactions, angioedema, anaphylaxis, and fever can occur, simultaneously or in some sequence.

Unusual syndromes have been described that are probably due to the distribution of the drug and the manifestations of hypersensitivity. The Stevens-Johnson syndrome is characterized by lesions in various mucous membranes and is classically caused by phenolphthalein and a variety of other drugs such as sulfonamides. There is no difference between the pathogenesis of this syndrome and that caused by other drugs that induce hypersensitivity. Some antigen-antibody dependent reactions (e.g., photo-allergic phenomena) require more than the drug for manifestations of sensitivity (Harber and Levine, 1969). Likewise, some hypersensitivity reactions do not depend on antigen-antibody reactions, but apparently produce similar chemical and morphologic changes directly in tissues. Some drugs, such as demethylchlortetracycline, produce photosensitivity reactions in skin exposed to ultraviolet radiation. These reactions are classified as phototoxic; they depend on the presence of drug in skin and on the drug's ability to emit tissue-damaging energy when exposed to a source of ultraviolet radiation. Another type of sensitivity to a drug is caused by the direct and severe irritant effects of the drug on the tissues it reaches in high concentration. Dermatologists and internists frequently encounter such reactions that should not be classified as "hypersensitivity" because they are dose dependent, often predictable and preventable, and would occur in the majority of the population exposed to the toxic dose of the drug. The most effective treatment of these lesions is prevention. *Principle: Common factors in the pathogenesis of disease states should be sought in order to select treatment that can alter the course or manifestations of the disease state.*

The decision to treat a reaction is influenced by its severity, the likelihood of its duration, and the toxicity of the methods used to treat it. The type of treatment depends on how the causative agent was administered (if a deposit of long-acting penicillin is used, it cannot be conveniently removed; orally administered drug can be discontinued) or the severity of the reaction. Simple withdrawal of the drug, with or without use of antihistamines, may be sufficient to manage mild urticaria, but this would be inadequate for serum sickness or anaphylaxis. Likewise, isoproterenol, antihistamines, and assisted ventilation would be ineffective in reversing the leukopenia or thrombocytopenia caused by antigen-antibody interaction affecting the granulocyte or platelet. *Principles: (1) No simple formula for the treatment of a "drug reaction" can be derived. Application of this principle makes the therapy of reactions precise and avoids further drug reactions. (2) A therapist should distinguish between drugs that prevent a reaction and those that nonspecifically reverse the sequelae of the reaction. (3) When considering treatment of reactions, the severity of the manifestations must be considered before the therapeutic plan is set.*

Idiosyncratic Reactions to Drugs

Idiosyncratic reactions occur in only a small number of patients and include both predictable pharmacologic effects after inordinately small doses of drug and unusual effects of drugs. When the response could be expected on the basis of the known pharmacology of the drug but occurs at unusually low doses, the patients are classified as hyperresponders. However, most idiosyncratic reactions are not related to the known pharmacology of the drug, and their pathogenesis is as poorly understood as the pathogenesis of "primary," "essential," or "idiopathic" disease. Idiosyncrasy excludes those reactions based on known genetic abnormalities and the allergic or meta reactions. Though all the effects of a drug cannot be predicted in all men, the physician must be able to recognize and treat unusual manifestations of a drug's effect. The existence of idiosyncrasy implies that a risk always accompanies the administration of a drug, that if a drug reaction occurs the manifestations will not be predictable, and that the therapy of such reactions must be individualized. The number of idiosyncratic reactions in most series is less than 5% (Borda et al., 1968). As more knowledge of the pharmacology of drugs becomes available, many of these reactions are likely to be removed from the idiosyncratic category. Thalidomide provides one example of the benefits of knowledge in this area. Although the teratogenic effects were once considered idiosyncratic, understanding of the metabolism of the drug, and of the fact that a metabolite is an alkylating agent, has led to the reclassification of this "reaction."

Predictable and Preventable Drug Reactions

The unusual and unpredictable responses to drug administration, i.e., classic reactions (allergic and idiosyncratic), make up less than 20 to 30% of drug reactions. Because they are unpredictable and often unavoidable, they constitute the assumed risk associated with drug therapy. However, if 20 to 30% of drug reactions are unpredictable, the remaining 70 to 80% of reactions must be predictable and potentially avoidable.

The most frequent examples of drug toxicity (drug reactions) are direct extensions of the intended pharmacologic action of the drug (e.g., hypoglycemia due to excess of insulin), or from unwanted but inseparable secondary pharmacologic effects of a drug (e.g., hypoglycemic reactions due to blockade of epinephrine's effects by propranolol). These drug reactions may be preventable and their prevention may not alter the therapeutic benefit of the drug or alternative drugs. The prevention of this type of drug reaction is illustrated by the use of digitalis. Digitalis is unquestionably indicated for the treatment of congestive heart failure. The beneficial effects of the drug are primarily related to its ability to increase myocardial contractility and cardiac output (see Chapter 5). As the dose is increased, the myocardial contractile force rapidly increases, and potassium is lost from the cells. However, nearly maximum contractile force is developed before potassium loss is sufficient to cause major changes in chronotropic activity or, presumably, other conduction effects. Therefore "digitalization" usually precedes electrocardiographic evidence of increased ventricular irritability.

It is likely that lethal doses of digitalis in animals are roughly comparable to those for man; in animals, the lethal dose is five to ten times the minimal effective dose responsible for increasing contractile forces, and when arrhythmias occur, approximately 60% of the lethal dose has been given. Why, then, do some therapists feel that it is necessary to produce toxicity (ventricular premature contractions) before digitalis administration is adequate? The major reason may be that a clinical dictum has not been updated by available facts and that the old objectives have not been replaced by measurements of changes in hemodynamics or in renal function produced by digitalis. These changes represent the therapeutic objectives and should be measured directly. Digitalis has a relatively wide therapeutic index (ratio of beneficial to adverse effects), but if facts are ignored the margin of safety narrows.

Ten per cent of patients taking digitalis alone show evidence of toxicity, and toxicity appears in 17 to 35% of patients taking digitalis and diuretics (Hurwitz and Wade, 1969); digitalis accounts for 21% of all drug reactions in hospitals and in at least one study such reactions were lethal in 30% of the cases (Ogilvie and Ruedy, 1967). Once the patient on digitalis therapy evidences conduction abnormalities, he is taking close to the LD_{50} dose. Therapeutic,

not toxic, effects should be followed to prevent digitalis toxicity. *Principle: Application of valid pharmacologic data to clinical settings allows optimal therapy. Disregard for the high therapeutic index of a drug is hazardous.*

CONSEQUENCES OF DRUG REACTIONS

1. Eighteen to thirty percent of patients in hospitals have a drug reaction (Seidl *et al.*, 1966; Hoddinott *et al.*, 1967).

2. Drug reactions account for 3 to 5% of hospital admissions (Seidl *et al.*, 1966; Hurwitz, 1969a).

3. Thirty percent of patients admitted for a drug reaction have a reaction to the same or another drug during the same hospitalization.

4. Patients with reactions have a considerably longer stay in the hospital (11.4 days without reaction and 28.7 days with reaction [Seidl *et al.*, 1966]; 12.0 days without reaction and 20.8 days with reaction [Schimmel, 1964]; 11.6 ± 7.8 [S.D.] days without reaction and 20.5 ± 12.3 days with reaction [Ogilvie and Ruedy, 1967]).

5. The economic consequences of drug reactions in hospitals are staggering. When the average patient stay of 12 days is raised to 14 days because of drug reactions, then 1/7 of hospital days are devoted to the care of drug reactions. The estimated dollar cost of such hospitalization alone is close to $3 billion a year (Task Force on Prescription Drugs, 1969). To this must be added immeasurable human suffering, as well as economic consequences to the patient and to society.

6. In approximately 29% of patients, the reactions are severe (Ogilvie and Ruedy, 1967). The most discouraging finding is that most of these reactions are avoidable (Ogilvie and Ruedy, 1967; Borda *et al.*, 1968).

Principles: (1) The availability of potent new drugs and the use of drug combinations will decrease even further the ratio of classic to preventable reactions. (2) The physician can often avoid causing drug reactions, but if they occur he should recognize and treat them promptly. (3) If therapists fail in their responsibility, higher rates of drug reactions and even further increases in the hazards of reactions may result (MacDonald and MacKay, 1964). Unless the medical profession responds, the physician may remain unable to recognize when he is using new or dangerous drugs (Melmon *et al.*, 1970), the disturbing and publicly recognized course of inappropriate drug prescribing may continue, and the government may attempt to control therapeutics in ineffective and repugnant ways (Cooper, 1968a, 1968b, 1968c, 1968d, 1968e; Comment, 1969a, 1969b, 1969c). We must improve our therapeutic skills and convince patients that they do not need drugs. The diseases of medical progress are largely predictable and preventable drug effects.

RECOGNITION OF DRUG REACTIONS

Lasagna proposed the following dicta: (1) No clinically useful drug is devoid of toxicity. (2) No human should be exposed to needless risk. (3) The harm to present and future generations caused by lack of adequate remedies for many diseases makes it imperative that new drugs, despite their attendant hazards, continue to be introduced into research and practice. If the therapist accepts these dicta, he accepts a commitment to understand the effects of drugs in disease, the predisposing factors to drug reactions, and the effects of disease on drugs before he uses them.

Most data on drug reactions have become available only recently. Drug reactions have increased in number and severity because of (1) the increased availability of potent prescription drugs; (2) public exposure to drugs used or produced industrially that enter the environment; (3) the availability of potent drugs without prescription; and (4) the availability of illicit preparations (Sheps and Shapiro, 1962; Boyd, 1968; Risebrough et al., 1968; Schachter, 1968; Scott, 1968; Wyckoff et al., 1968; Abelson, 1969; Jelliffe et al., 1969; Smith, 1969a, 1969b). More information is needed about the reasons people take drugs and the increasing number of people who depend on them (Freedman, 1966; Smith, 1969a; Wheeler and Edmonds, 1969), the potential toxicity of such drugs (Auerbach and Rugowski, 1967; Bewley, 1967; Geber, 1967; Sparkes et al., 1968; Hirschhorn, 1969), and some of the economic waste and personal tragedy associated with problems such as drug addiction (meperidine addiction in physicians removes about 300 of them from practice each year) (Garb, 1969; Farnsworth, 1970). There is increasing awareness of the problems created by polypharmacy (Monroe and Cluff, 1968), the effect of drugs in complicating therapy or invalidating laboratory tests (Batsakis et al., 1968; Bogusz, 1968), the effects of drugs on genes (Motulsky, 1969), the ways to separate drug reactors from nonreactors (Reidenberg and Lowenthal, 1968), and the factors that predispose patients to drug reactions (Hurwitz, 1969a, 1969b; Johnson, 1969; Peters and Marcoux, 1969; La Du, 1971).

There are multiple reasons for our current lack of adequate data on drug reactions. Drug reactions often cannot be viewed as clear-cut cause-and-effect events. Lasagna has described the absence of the "light-switch" phenomenon in some drug reactions, i.e., lack of apparent proximate cause (Lasagna, 1969). For instance, the long-term effects of certain drugs may not be seen for generations after they have been administered. After administration of an alkylating agent for the treatment of a neoplastic disease, its effects on germ tissue may not be seen until the following generation, or until subtle genetic abnormalities appear late in life or after administration of other drugs (see Chapter 13).

Drugs that concentrate in certain tissues, e.g., phenothiazines in the retina or antimalarial agents in the lens, can cause damage long after the drug has been discontinued. The maximum concentration of the drug in these tissues may not be reached until after administration has ceased, and the concentration may remain high for prolonged periods (Leopold, 1968) (see Chapter 2). Thus a reaction may appear long after drug administration has commenced and may continue well after administration has ceased.

Another difficulty in relating cause and effect is presented by the "drug reaction" consisting of one agent diminishing the effect of a second agent. In fact whenever a compound fails to produce expected results, alteration in its absorption, metabolism, or elimination should be considered; the lack of therapeutic effectiveness must be considered an adverse effect of drug administration. *Principle: If objectives of efficacy have not been predetermined, lack of efficacy is difficult to recognize, and such "reactions" are difficult to identify.*

Yet another obstacle increases the difficulty in proving a cause-and-effect relationship in drug toxicity. Data on errors in drug administration in hospitals are surprising (Crooks et al., 1965). The error rate in drug administration is quite high and increases as the number and doses of drugs increase (Leading Article, 1965; Barker, 1969; Arnhold et al., 1970). If substantial error rates are apparent even with the professional supervision provided in hospitals, the unreliability of drug administration in less supervised circumstances is probably equally high. One must know whether the patient suspected of a drug reaction has or has not taken the drug in question (Gordis et al., 1969).

Another obstacle to recognition of drug toxicity is the physician's low index of suspicion. A physician is naturally reluctant to think that his treatment contributes to a patient's disability. It is easier to attribute new symptoms in a patient to an extension of his underlying disease, rather than to obvious or occult drug toxicity. In one study, house officers responsible for treating inpatients were asked whether drug reactions had occurred. A substantial proportion of the patients considered by the house officers to be free of drug reactions had actually experienced drug toxicity or reaction as determined by objective notes in the patient's chart or by routine laboratory data obtained during the course of hospitalization. All too frequently, laboratory data or new symptoms that do not "fit" into the anticipated course of a disease are ignored. Although it may be recognized that a patient with glucose-6-phosphate dehydrogenase deficiency will almost certainly develop hemolysis when given pamaquine, some therapists do not recognize and therefore do not anticipate that other anilines used as diuretics or uricosuric agents can also cause hemolysis. Life-threatening clinical situations often lead to irrational use of drugs, and the drama, urgency, and hopelessness of the situation mask the effects of drug reactions. When a patient develops ventricular premature beats and is given lidocaine, it is the rare physician who recognizes that lidocaine may intensify the arrhythmia, and who questions continuing the drug even after multifocal premature ventricular contractions become obvious, persist, and seem to occur close to the time of drug administration. When the patient develops intractable ventricular tachycardia, it is attributed to disappointing and hopeless deterioration of the patient's clinical condition rather than to possible lidocaine toxicity. Not until central nervous system manifestations occur is the drug toxicity recognized and a "drug reaction"

reported or at least considered by the physician (see Chapter 5).

The problems encountered in recognizing drug toxicity are illustrated by a patient with tuberculosis taking a large dose of para-aminosalicylic acid who developed fever, skin rash, hyperventilation, and a bleeding tendency attributed to hematogenous spread of the tuberculosis. As his temperature continued to rise, acetylsalicylic acid was administered as an antipyretic. To the amazement of the clinicians, clear evidence of salicylism became apparent even though they thought relatively small doses of salicylates were being given. Considerable time passed before the physicians recognized that the symptoms were related to their prescriptions and not to infection! Figure 15–2 illustrates the attitude that sometimes prevents physicians from "seeing the forest for the trees" during an adverse drug reaction.

Another obstacle to recognition of reactions is that drugs are used excessively either singly or in combination (it is rare to find an individual or even a clinical study that simply tests the effect of one agent). Polypharmacy has become a way of life for the American public. Physicians frequently prescribe multiple therapeutic agents simultaneously, but even when a single drug is prescribed, the ingestion pattern of a patient may vary. Over-the-counter preparations contain agents capable of influencing the metabolism, absorption, and elimination of many drugs. For instance, the antihistamines can

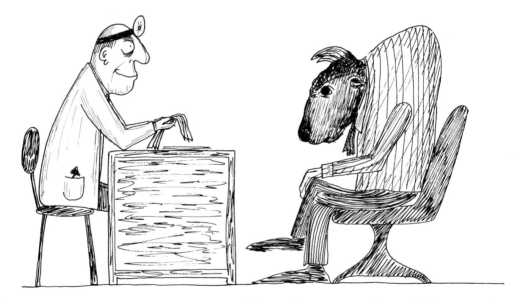

"Cut back to 20 pills a day, George. That rash on your thumb bothers me."

Figure 15–2. *Et tu*, doctor?

influence the metabolism of a variety of therapeutic agents (see Chapter 16) and may themselves become less or more effective depending on the other compounds used for the disease state. In a clinical situation involving polypharmacy, a "suspected reaction" may be easy to recognize but difficult to relate to a single drug (Figure 15–2).

Poor reporting of drug reactions has minimized the apparent incidence of drug toxicity in the United States. Reporting in the past has relied on the volition of the physician or hospital staff; the quality of the data that have been gathered is deplorable. Millions of dollars were spent by the American Medical Association and the Food and Drug Administration on drug reaction programs that have been relatively ineffective (Long, 1967).

Things are not, however, entirely bleak. We can learn how to recognize reactions (Koch-Weser et al., 1969); we can learn why patients do or do not comply with their doctor's prescriptions (Feinstein et al., 1959; Schwartz et al., 1962; Paul et al., 1965; Willcox et al., 1965; Davis, 1966; Malahy, 1966; Davis, 1968; Bonnar et al., 1969). We can decrease errors in drug administration and at least be able to trust that the patient actually takes what is prescribed for him (Crooks et al., 1965; Vere, 1965; Hynniman et al., 1970; Moulding et al., 1970) (see Chapter 14).

Reporting systems can be improved so that they furnish precise information (Wintrobe, 1965; Sidel et al., 1967; Borda et al., 1968). An effective study must include a consistent and complete patient population representative of a community's medical experience and must include information on all drugs given to the patients and careful observations for the presence of drug reactions. Until this has been done, the true incidence and severity of toxicity for any given compound will remain unknown. Centers can be developed to handle and conduct research on problems of drug abuse (Meyers and Smith, 1968). Drug information and referral centers can help in patient and physician education (Ma and Edmonds, 1969), and voluntary programs can improve prescription practices. Physicians can exploit the talents of paramedical personnel who have already proved able to predict, detect, and report drug reactions in hospitals (Visconti and Smith, 1967). These "paramedics" also have established methods for obtaining information from the past experience of drug administration (Borda et al., 1968; Kunin and Dierks, 1969; Visconti, 1969) and are actively assisting physicians in making decisions related to clinical drug interactions and in running data retrieval systems. Paramedical personnel can prepare and administer prescribed drugs, take drug histories from patients, and search for chemical-chemical interactions to explain changes in laboratory tests that may either herald or be misinterpreted as drug reactions. Lack of objectivity in discovering drug reactions may be overcome by the judicious use of laboratory tests to determine the concentration of suspected drugs and their metabolites in plasma or tissues. In addition, suspected allergic phenomena can be documented by the appearance of antibody to the drug in question or by the disappearance of complement if the reaction is dependent on complement activation or consumption.

Many new concepts must be assimilated by the therapist before drug misuse can be corrected. Some of these are detailed in the next section of this chapter. Recognition that a lack of knowledge alone may significantly increase the suffering of patients should be sufficient stimulus to the therapist to equip himself with thorough and critical knowledge of the drugs he uses. *Principle: Sound knowledge is requisite to safe therapeutics.*

At the same time, the therapist should understand that his personal experience may contribute to a total body of knowledge but cannot substitute for the larger experience (see Chapter 1). *Principle: Personal experience can never substitute for judgment based on a composite of methodically obtained facts.*

APPROACH TO THE PREVENTION OF DRUG REACTIONS

As mentioned previously, the practice of polypharmacy has recently increased; the average patient in a hospital receives from six to ten drugs simultaneously. At this level of multiple-drug administration, the adverse reaction rate is 7 to 10%. Many patients receive more than 20 drugs simultaneously. Under such circumstances the patient has at least a 40% chance of developing adverse reactions to one or more of the drugs (see Chapter 16). *Principle: Only when specific objectives have been established should drugs be added to an existing regimen. The benefit-to-risk ratio for each drug decreases when many are given.*

When additional drugs are added to a regimen, evaluation should be made both of the effects of the new drug and of the continuing effect of the previous drug(s). With such an approach, toxicity and drug interactions might be detected and perhaps the chances of severe toxicity diminished. The careless administration of multiple drugs simultaneously not only leads to unpredictable side effects, but also makes it almost impossible to attribute a therapeutic effect or an adverse reaction to any specific agent (see Chapter 16). The termination of all therapy may then become mandatory.

The use of fixed-dosage forms of drugs is generally unwise. The major drawbacks to fixed-dosage combinations are: (1) a maximum effect of a single agent may not be detected or determined, and therefore the need for the second drug cannot be established; (2) the effects of the second drug cannot be maximized without increasing the dose of the first drug; (3) the use of two drugs predisposes to drug reactions; and (4) many drug combinations have fixed doses such that both toxicity and efficacy will be unlikely.

Pharmacologic Principles That May Help to Prevent Drug Reactions

Most responses to drugs are dose dependent. Although the dose-response curve of a single drug effect is predictable, most drugs have a number of effects, each of which may have a different dose-response curve. An adverse effect of a drug may be anticipated by knowing its likelihood of occurrence in comparison with the more desirable effects of the drug. The chemical nature of the drug may often be helpful in prediction of possible undue increases or decreases in the concentration of the drug in plasma. Certain diseases alter absorption, metabolism, or excretion of drugs, and since the adverse effects of many drugs are directly related to their tissue or blood concentration, a relationship exists between pharmacokinetics and drug reactions (Thomson et al., 1969; Wagner, 1969).

It is useful to know the polarity (degree of water solubility) of drugs. Highly polar drugs, readily dissolved in water, are relatively slowly absorbed and almost invariably depend on renal excretion for their elimination. Polar compounds such as thiazides, mecamylamine, and mercurial diuretics are likely to accumulate in individuals with decreased renal function. Ability to recognize the chemical characteristics that determine polarity and pK_a (Perrin, 1965) facilitates the prediction of drug accumulation in disease states. Nonpolar compounds are usually well absorbed by virtue of their solubility in lipid-rich cell membranes, are usually extensively bound to plasma proteins, and often require metabolism by the liver (see Chapter 2). Thus in an individual who is given phenothiazines, bishydroxycoumarin, quinidine, phenylbutazone, or antimalarials (all nonpolar compounds), hepatic function and serum protein concentration should be studied lest standard doses given at standard intervals cause

undesirable effects. *Principle: The chemical nature of a drug may be used to predict its absorption, distribution, metabolism, and excretion, and therefore its likelihood of causing toxicity in certain disorders.*

There are additional benefits in recognizing chemical similarities between agents. If a drug produces an adverse effect, drugs of similar chemical composition should be administered with caution. An individual with glucose-6-phosphate dehydrogenase deficiency should not be given aniline derivatives; if he requires analgesics, phenacetin should be omitted; if antibiotics are needed, sulfanilamide and nitrofurantoin should be avoided; if he develops diabetes mellitus, tolbutamide should not be given; and if a uricosuric agent is necessary, probenecid should be avoided. Figure 15-3 demonstrates the chemical similarities between agents used for widely different therapeutic purposes; reaction to one agent may forecast reaction to the others. When alternative drugs are used for the same therapeutic purpose, a drug reaction or toxic event may be avoided. In clinical settings when drugs of similar chemical composition are given with different therapeutic intent, adverse reactions may result. Compounds such as nicotinic acid, nicotinamide, and iproniazid are metabolized rapidly in a patient who is a "rapid acetylator" of isoniazid. If rapid acetylation of the chemically related compounds is expected, it is no surprise if their therapeutic effects are absent at standard doses (see Chapter 13).

Certain chemical groupings predictably produce drug toxicity. If an individual is sensitive to a hydrazine-containing compound (e.g., he develops liver damage), other hydrazines may cause the same effect. A variety of amino-containing and nitro-containing compounds may produce methemoglobinemia (Kalow, 1962). A person sensitive to industrial organic compounds such as nitrobenzene or nitroaniline may develop methemoglobinemia when taking sulfanilamides, sulfathiazoles, phenacetin, or acetanilid. Inorganic compounds, such as potassium nitrate, are capable of producing the same biochemical abnormality.

Adverse effects can occur if the undesirable effect of one drug is similar to and perhaps additive to that of another compound. Phenothiazines have atropine-like qualities; if they are added to antihistaminics with similar properties, atropinism may ensue. The less obvious pharmacologic effects of drugs must be considered in order to avoid combinations that create clinically important reactions (see Chaper 16).

Competitive inhibitors of the pharmacologic effects of endogenous amines can produce drug

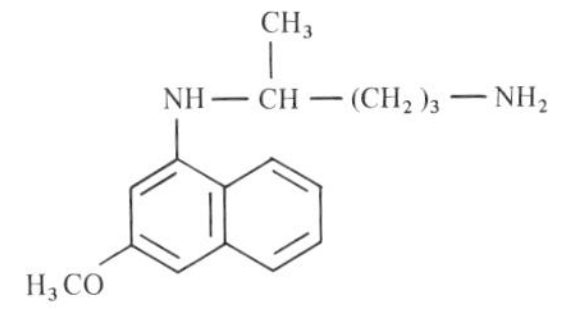

Primaquine (antimalarial)

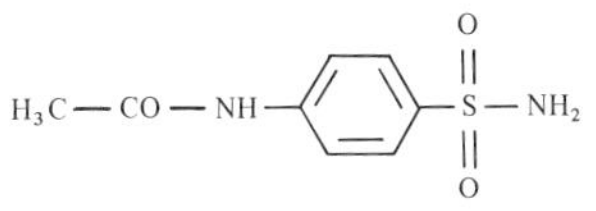

N^4-Acetylsulfanilamide (antibiotic)

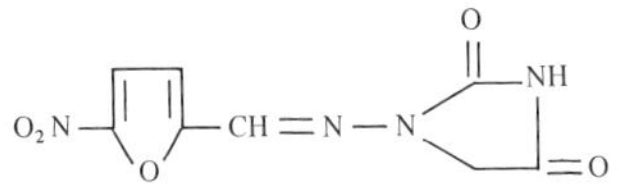

Nitrofurantoin (antibiotic)

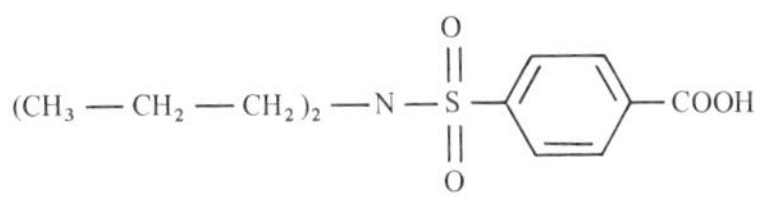

Probenecid (uricosuric)

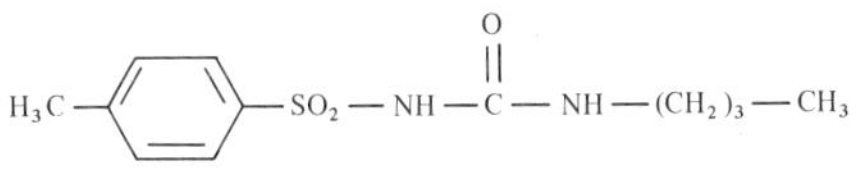

Tolbutamide – a sulfonylurea (hypoglycemic)

Figure 15–3.   Analogs of aniline or oxidants that may cause hemolytic anemia in patients with glucose-6-phosphate dehydrogenase deficiency. One advantage of knowing chemical similarities between drugs is that their therapeutic or "side" effects often can be anticipated or predicted. Each of these drugs can cause oxidation of hemoglobins. A number of other drugs are closely related chemically, and some sulfonylurea compounds may be capable of the same oxidation. Therefore, if a patient develops hemolysis while taking one of these drugs, great caution is necessary in using probenecid as a uricosuric agent, or tolbutamide as an orally active hypoglycemic agent. The relationship between hydrazine groups and monoamine oxidase inhibition predisposes to this effect after use of nitrofurantoin.

reactions by acting as partial agonists. By virtue of their close chemical similarities to the endogenous catecholamines, some of the adrenergic blocking drugs transiently elicit sympathomimetic effects (Goodman and Gilman, 1970). Antihistaminics may initially mimic the effects of histamine, either by acting directly as histaminic agents or by releasing histamine from endogenous tissue sites. Antagonists of a given effect of an endogenous substance may not antagonize *all* the pharmacologic effects of the agonist at all receptor sites. Incomplete antagonism may account for the retroperitoneal fibrosis associated with methysergide administration (see Chapter 18). Knowing the chemical composition of available antagonists may allow choices that prevent the possible synergistic effects of the "antagonists" with selected pharmacologic effects of the "agonist." Chlorpromazine may be an alternative choice to a number of other antagonists because it is a multipotent competitive agent that has relatively little chemical relationship to histamine, catecholamines, acetylcholine, or kinins, but is capable of competitively interfering with the peripheral effects of each.

Physiologic Variables That May Predispose to Unusual Drug Effects

A number of physiological variables can alter the pharmacokinetics or pharmacology of drugs, and therefore their effects. Among the important determinants of the effects of a drug are the physiologic state of the patient and the pathophysiology of his disease. Physicians "know" that pediatric doses differ from those for adults and that genetic differences influence response to some agents (Nagao and Mauer, 1969; La Du, 1971), but rarely consider differences between the young adult and the geriatric population. The neonate and the older individual have different responses to drugs (Jick et al., 1968). Age seems to be a major variable influencing the likelihood of adverse drug reactions (Ewy et al., 1969). The pediatric and geriatric populations are on the extremes of a spectrum of responses, in which developmental pharmacology and degeneration of organ function play major roles in the accumulation of drugs. The incidence of adverse drug reactions is highest in the very young and very old. In patients 60 to 70 years old, the risk of a drug reaction is almost double that in adults 30 to 40 years old. In the neonate, drug-conjugating enzymes in the liver may be immature, the absorption of drugs from the gut may be different than in adults, and the responsiveness of tissues to any given concentration of drug may vary from that expected in adults. An example of dissimilarities in drug effect in the child versus adult is the enhanced response of the newborn to catecholamines. The relative inability of the neonate's liver to conjugate bilirubin may be directly related to its inability to conjugate a large number of drugs and to the accumulation of these drugs when they are given in standard doses. Therefore chloramphenicol, codeine, morphine, phenolphthalein, salicylamide, and a host of other nonpolar compounds requiring hepatic conjugation should be given in lower-than-standard doses to the very young.

Data on the differing responses to drugs of the neonate and young child compared to the adult are incomplete. However, *the known differences in pharmacokinetics and pharmacology in infants and children must be considered if toxic effects are to be avoided.*

Body weight and fitness may modify a drug's effect. As previously observed, a nonpolar compound is more likely to distribute in adipose tissue than is a water-soluble agent. An obese person may demonstrate relatively little effect of the drug for a rather prolonged time if the expected effects involve nonfat-containing tissues. Once effects are seen, they may persist even after administration is terminated, as the drug migrates from fat stores to receptors. Conversely, a thin individual may demonstrate a pronounced effect rather quickly after a low total dose of a drug with high lipid solubility (e.g., pentobarbital), and the duration of the effect after discontinuation may be considerably shorter than in the obese patient.

Although considerable emphasis has been given to differences in drug effect in animals of different sex, there is little evidence of major differences in effect of most drugs between men and women.

Minor changes in acid-base balance that are considered to be within the normal range may greatly influence the requirements for drugs under different conditions. For this reason, it is useful to divide drugs into acids and bases (see Chapters 2 and 16). For example, the renal clearance of some drugs is remarkably affected by changes in the pH of urine. In acidic urine, weakly acidic drugs such as sulfonamide, salicylic acid, or phenobarbital are found in relatively low concentration, as opposed to weak bases such as antihistaminics or amphetamine. The opposite is true if the urine is alkaline. Application of this information not only aids in the use of a drug but may also provide methods to accelerate elimination of a drug overdose (see Chapters 16 and 17).

The importance of other physiologic variables that can modify drug effects is less clear. Some foods affect the gastrointestinal absorption rate and hence the concentration of different drugs in blood (see Chapters 2, 4, and 16). Absorption of drugs can be altered by unusual eating habits or by disease states that affect the function of the small bowel or its contents. Amino acid accumulation during the course of uremia or fluid accumulation within the lumen of the bowel during ileus can change the way that drugs are transported, particularly if the drugs are either amino acids or highly polar weak acids. Although precise absorption data related to a drug may not be available, the chemistry of the drug should be considered in terms of the rate of intestinal absorption.

Disease States That Predispose to Drug Reactions

Certain diseases seem to predispose to a drug reaction. These are probably best divided into two categories. The first comprises those diseases in which multiple therapy is often unavoidable (infectious diseases, psychiatric disorders, and diseases of the cardiovascular system). Digitalis, quinidine, antimicrobials, insulin, and antihypertensives produced 60% of reactions in one study (Seidl *et al.*, 1966).

The second group of diseases that predispose to drug reactions are those that primarily affect the organs of absorption, metabolism, or excretion. In diseases of the liver and in acquired renal failure or congenital renal disease (such as renal tubular acidosis), metabolism of drugs and excretion of drugs and drug products can be altered.

Although considerable information has been acquired related to the principles of pharmacokinetics, relatively little laboratory or clinical research has been conducted in the alteration of a drug's kinetics by disease states (see Chapters 2 and 5). Experimentation is required to determine whether a priori thoughts related to the kinetics of drugs in diseases can be clinically useful. Alterations in drug absorption from the gastrointestinal tract may occur during external compression of the bowel with obstruction and alteration of bowel flora, pernicious anemia, and regional enteritis, but complete data are not available. However suggestive the incomplete data may be, the physician must rely on demonstration of drug effects in the individual patient to determine whether therapy is successful.

The role of protein binding of drugs is discussed in Chapter 2. Whether dysproteinemic states can substantially change the availability of drugs to receptor sites has not yet been studied, but patients with hypoalbuminemia should be approached with this possibility in mind. In treating such patients with digitalis, a lower initial dose of digitoxin (which is ordinarily bound to albumin) might be used, since an enhanced effect may theoretically be obtained. The reverse might be true of drugs that bind to globulins in hyperglobulinemic states, but study is required to determine the clinical importance of these speculations.

A multitude of diseases can alter the pharmacology of drugs. Unfortunately, whether disease states alter pharmacology via pharmacokinetics (see Chapter 2) or by changing receptor sensitivity has not been well investigated. The majority of investigations related to disease-induced changes in pharmacology are discussed in Chapters 3, 4, and 5. Most genetic abnormalities that become phenotypically evident after drug administration or those that alter drug responses can be mimicked by acquired disease (see Chapter 13). For instance, the conjugating ability of the liver is decreased in the Crigler-Najjar syndrome, and the half-life of substances that are excreted by conjugation is prolonged. Acquired liver disease may produce the same type of abnormality. A case in point is the difference between the half-life of cortisol in normal individuals, those with Crigler-Najjar syndrome, and those with acquired liver disease. In normal subjects the half-life is approximately 28 minutes; it can be as long as 35 minutes in patients with acquired liver disease and 70 minutes or more in patients with Crigler-Najjar syndrome (Kalow, 1962). Thyroid disorders also influence the clearance of cortisol. A number of genetic abnormalities can probably be discovered by carefully observing drug effects in a large number of patients. Unusual effects of drugs due to genetic abnormalities in animals have later been detected in humans. Animal data predict that esterolytic enzyme deficiencies will be found in man, in addition to the presently postulated cholinesterase deficiencies. Search should be made in man for the atropinase abnormalities found in rabbits. Drug-induced congenital malformations (mutations) after cortisone administration in animals conceivably may be witnessed in man. The species differences among animals in metabolism of barbiturates and antipyrine, in the effects of anesthetics and hormones, in the response to histamine, in hepatic toxicity of hydrazine-containing compounds, and in reserpine-induced lactation are prototypes of genetic variations found in animals and may portend the same for man. The search for possible unexpected or untoward effects of drugs may lead the physician to discover genetic abnormalities (see Chapter 13). The alert practicing physician is in a much better position to detect these subtle abnormalities than is the man who spends most of his time in the laboratory, divorced from clinical therapeutics.

Other Factors Predisposing to Drug Reactions

A number of drug reactions are probably created by overly hopeful expectations of drug therapy; e.g., digitalis toxicity often occurs in clinical situations in which digitalis has least efficacy (congestive heart failure secondary to mitral insufficiency, extremely severe aortic stenosis, or a very large arteriovenous shunt). Benefits of digitalis in such situations are minimal, despite a major increase in myocardial contractility. Therefore, the physician is tempted to increase doses until toxic levels are reached. Even when toxic effects are finally apparent, little therapeutic benefit has been obtained but the life of the patient is endangered. Although digitalis toxicity may be a blatant example of how heroics can lead to toxicity, analogous circumstances are associated with the administration of sedatives, antibiotics, analgesics, diuretics, anti-inflammatory agents, corticosteroids, oral hypoglycemic agents, and a host of other potent chemicals. *Principle: The use of a drug for a disorder unresponsive to it can lead to drug overdose.*

This does not preclude, however, the possible requirements of inordinately large doses of a drug before the desired effect is obtained. The simple commitment to treat requires that the drug be given in doses sufficient to produce an effect. If well-laid plans for observation of drug effect are made before its administration, failure to find effects after appropriately increasing the dose or shortening the interval between doses may indicate the need for even further increases in drug dosage. If no effect is obtained after increasing doses and if appropriate assays for the compound are unavailable, an alternate route of administration is advisable. This approach, for example, might avoid the relatively useless continued administration of intramuscular diphenylhydantoin (see Chapter 2).

Data are unavailable on the effects of prolonged administration of most drugs. Indeed, the toxicity of a number of drugs on the market was undetected until uncommon toxicities were revealed by many patient-years of exposure. If careful observations had not been made by the physicians administering the drugs, the cataracts associated with MER-29, the teratogenicity of thalidomide, the ototoxicity of streptomycin, the nephrotoxicity of outdated tetracyclines, the potential toxicity of saline (Shapiro *et al.*, 1971), and even the gastrointestinal bleeding produced by aspirin or ethacrynic acid (Slone *et al.*, 1969) would not have become common knowledge. *Principle: Continuing vigil must be maintained for unusual or changing effects produced by a drug even though the drug has been given safely for long periods.*

To summarize: The most direct and meaningful first step that can and must be taken by therapists is the use of already available information on preventing and detecting drug reactions. Knowledge of the pharmacology of drugs allows prediction of toxicity even under extraordinary circumstances. Failure to apply available knowledge is perhaps the major factor in the increasing incidence of drug reactions. The increase in drug reaction rates can be attributed to the more frequent use of potent pharmacologic agents without a corresponding increase in the knowledge of the chemistry and pharmacology of the drug and of the disease process for which it is used. *Principle: Diminution of drug reaction rates requires the same knowledge that permits optimal therapeutic effects of drugs.*

Adverse reactions occur in every physician's practice. His recognition of the reaction depends on his knowledge of the pharmacology of the drugs he uses and on his ability to recognize that he may cause reactions despite his good intentions. Unless all the pharmacologic effects of a drug are appreciated, new symptoms may be falsely ascribed to extension or complications of the disease rather than to drug toxicity or reaction. Our success in preventing adverse reactions is critically dependent on our capacity for acquiring and using valid information. *Principle: Drug effects must be continually assessed to lessen the likelihood of producing toxicity.*

Finally, as Dr. R. H. Moser has stated, "Progress is often painful" (Moser, 1969). At times the broadening expanse of medical knowledge seems overwhelming; to keep abreast of trends in diagnosis and therapy appears to be an impossible undertaking. Yet this continuing intellectual challenge generates the vitality that is the very essence of the practice of medicine.

REFERENCES

Abelson, P. H.: Persistent pesticides. *Science,* **164**:633, 1969.

Adkinson, N. F., Jr.; Thompson, W. L.; Maddrey, W. C.; and Lichtenstein, L. M.: Routine use of penicillin skin testing on an inpatient service. *New Eng. J. Med.,* **285**:22–24, 1971.

Arnhold, R. G.; Adebonojo, F. O.; Callas, E. R.; Callas, J.; Carte, E.; and Stein, R. C.: Patients and prescriptions. Comprehension and compliance with medical instructions in a suburban pediatric practice. *Clin. Pediat.* (*Phila.*), **9**:648–51, 1970.

Auerbach, R., and Rugowski, J. A.: Lysergic acid diethylamide: effect of embryos. *Science,* **157**:1325–26, 1967.

Barker, K. N.: The effects of an experimental medication system on medication errors and costs. Part one: introduction and errors study. Part two: the cost study. *Amer. J. Hosp. Pharm.,* **26**:324–33, 388–97, 1969.

Batsakis, J. G.; Preston, J. A.; Briere, R. O.; and Giesen, P. C.: Iatrogenic aberrations of serum enzyme activity. *Clin. Biochem.,* **2**:125–33, 1968.

Bean, W. B. (ed.): *Sir William Osler: Aphorisms from His Bedside Teachings and Writings.* Henry Schuman, Inc., New York, 1950.

Bewley, T. H.: Adverse reactions from the illicit use of lysergide. *Brit. Med. J.,* **3**:28–30, 1967.

Bogusz, M.: Influence of insecticides on the activity of some enzymes contained in human serum. *Clin. Chim. Acta,* **19**:367–69, 1968.

Bonnar, J.; Goldberg, A.; and Smith, J. A.: Do pregnant women take their iron? *Lancet,* **1**:457–58, 1969.

Borda, I. T.; Slone, D.; and Jick, H.: Assessment of adverse reactions within a drug surveillance program. *J.A.M.A.,* **205**:645–47, 1968.

Boyd, E. M.: Analgesic abuse: maximal tolerated daily doses of acetylsalicylic acid. *Canad. Med. Ass. J.,* **99**:790–98, 1968.

Brown, B. B.; Price, E. V.; and Moore, M. B.: Penicilloyl-polylysine as an intradermal test of penicillin sensitivity. *J.A.M.A.,* **189**:599–604, 1964.

Cohlan, S. Q.: The teratogenicity of drugs in man. *Pharmacol. for Physicians,* **3**:Aug., 1969.

Comment: Adverse effects of drugs frequently used as diagnostic aids. *Med. Let. Drugs Ther.,* **11**:49–52, 1969a.

————: Senator Nelson versus the prescribing physician. *Med. World News*:15–18, Jan. 31, 1969b.

————: Towards more legislation on drugs. *Nature,* **221**:408–409, 1969c.

Cooper, J. D.: U.S. seen as "consultant" to M.D.'s on prescribing. *Med. Tribune,* April 22, 1968a.

————: Information anomaly posed by patterns of prescribing. *Med. Tribune,* April 25, 1968b.

————: All-purpose guide can burden M.D.'s without adding a benefit. *Med. Tribune,* April 29, 1968c.

————: Form of prescribing control by government called issue. *Med. Tribune,* May 2, 1968d.

————: Ideas are offered for new start. *Med. Tribune,* May 6, 1968e.

Crooks, J.; Clark, C. G.; Caie, H. B.; and Mawson, W. B.: Prescribing and administration of drugs in hospital. *Lancet,* **1**:373–78, 1965.

Davis, M. S.: Variations in patients' compliance with doctors' orders: analysis of congruence between survey responses and results of empirical investigations. *J. Med. Educ.,* **41**:1037–48, 1966.

————: Physiologic, psychological, and demographic factors in patient compliance with doctor's orders. *Med. Care,* **6**:115–22, 1968.

Editorial: The drug efficacy study. *New Eng. J. Med.,* **280**:1177–79, 1969.

Ewy, G. A.; Kapadia, G. G.; Yao, L.; Lullin, M.; and Marcus, F. I.: Digoxin metabolism in the elderly. *Circulation,* **39**:449–53, 1969.

Farnsworth, D. L.: Drug dependence among physicians. *New Eng. J. Med.,* **282**:392–93, 1970.

Feinstein, A. R.; Wood, H. F.; Epstein, J. A.; Taranta, A.; Simpson, R.; and Tursky, E.: A controlled study of three methods of prophylaxis against streptococcal infection in a population of rheumatic children. II. Results of the first three years of the study, including methods for evaluating the maintenance of oral prophylaxis. *New Eng. J. Med.,* **260**:697–702, 1959.

Freedman, A. M.: Drug addiction: an eclectic view. *J.A.M.A.,* **197**:878–82, 1966.

Garb, S.: Drug addiction in physicians. *Anesth. Analg.* (*Cleve*), **48**:129–33, 1969.

Geber, W. F.: Congenital malformations induced by mescaline, lysergic acid diethylamide, and bromolysergic acid in the hamster. *Science,* **158**:265–67, 1967.

Goodman, L. S., and Gilman, A. (eds.): *The Pharmacologic Basis of Therapeutics,* 4th ed. The Macmillan Co., New York, 1970.

Gordis, L.; Markowitz, M.; and Lilienfeld, A. N.: The inaccuracy in using interviews to estimate patient reliability in taking medications at home. *Med. Care,* **7**:49–54, 1969.

Harber, L. C., and Levine, G. M.: Photosensitivity

dermatitis from household products. *G.P.*, **39**:95–101, 1969.

Hirschhorn, K.: LSD and chromosomal damage. *Hosp. Pract.*, pp. 98–103, Feb. 1969.

Hoddinott, B. C.; Gowdey, C. W.; Coulter, W. K.; and Parker, J. M.: Drug reactions and errors in administration on a medical ward. *Canad. Med. Ass. J.*, **97**:1001–6, 1967.

Hurwitz, N.: Predisposing factors in adverse reactions to drugs. *Brit. Med. J.*, **1**:536–39, 1969a.

————: Admissions to hospital due to drugs. *Brit. Med. J.*, **1**:539–40, 1969b.

Hurwitz, N., and Wade, O. L.: Intensive hospital monitoring of adverse reactions to drugs. *Brit. Med. J.*, **1**:531–36, 1969.

Hynniman, C. E.; Conrad, W. F.; Urgh, W. A.; Rudnick, B. R.; and Parker, P. F.: A comparison of medication errors under the University of Kentucky unit dose system and traditional drug distribution systems in four hospitals. *Amer. J. Hosp. Pharm.*, **27**:802–14, 1970.

Idsoe, O.; Guthe, T.; Willcox, R. R.; *et al.*: Nature and extent of penicillin side-reactions, with particular reference to fatalities from anaphylactic shock. *Bull. W.H.O.*, **38**:159–88, 1968.

Jelliffe, R. W.; Hill, D.; Tatter, D.; and Lewis, E. L., Jr.: Death from weight-control pills: a case report with objective postmortem confirmation. *J.A.M.A.*, **208**:1843–47, 1969.

Jick, H.; Slone, D.; Borda, I. T.; and Shapiro, S.: Efficacy and toxicity of heparin in relation to age and sex. *New Eng. J. Med.*, **279**:284–86, 1968.

Johnson, J. E., III: The detection of drug allergy. *Pharmacol. for Physicians*, **3**:June, 1969.

Kalow, W.: *Pharmacogenetics: Heredity and the Response to Drugs.* W. B. Saunders Co., Philadelphia, 1962.

Keynes, G.: The Oslerian tradition. *Brit. Med. J.*, **2**:599–604, 1968.

Koch-Weser, J.; Sidel, V. W.; Sweet, R. H.; Kanarek, P.; and Eaton, A. E.: Factors determining physician reporting of adverse drug reactions. Comparison of 2000 spontaneous reports with surveillance studies at the Massachusetts General Hospital. *New Eng. J. Med.*, **280**:20–26, 1969.

Kovotzer, J., and Haddad, Z.: *In vitro* detection of human IgE mediated immediate hypersensitivity reaction to pollens and penicillin by a modified rat mast cell degranulation technique. *J. Allergy*, **45**:126, 1970.

Kunin, C. M., and Dierks, J. W.: A physician-pharmacist voluntary program to improve prescription practices. *New Eng. J. Med.*, **280**:1442–46, 1969.

La Du, B. N., Jr.: The genetics of drug reactions. *Hosp. Pract.*, **6**:97–107, 1971.

Lasagna, L.: In *Drug Research Report* ("The Blue Sheet"), May 14, 1969, pp. 17–21.

Leading Article: Drugs in hospital. *Lancet*, **1**:361–62, 1965.

Lennard, H. L.; Epstein, L. J.; Bernstein, A.; and Ransom, D. C.: Hazards implicit in prescribing psychoactive drugs. *Science*, **169**:438–41, 1970.

Leopold, I. H.: Ocular complications of drugs: visual changes. *J.A.M.A.*, **205**:631–33, 1968.

Levine, B. B.: Immunologic mechanisms of penicillin allergy. *New Eng. J. Med.*, **275**:115–25, 1966.

Lewin, L.: *Phantastica, Narcotic and Stimulating Drugs.* Dutton, New York, 1964.

Long, J. W.: F.D.A.'s adverse drug reaction information system. *Drug Inf. Bull.*, 114–19, July–Sept., 1967.

Ma, H., and Edmonds, C.: Drug referral centre. *Med. J. Aust.*, **2**:289–91, 1969.

McCurdy, D. K.; Frederic, M.; and Elkinton, J. R.: Renal tubular acidosis due to amphotericin B. *New Eng. J. Med.*, **278**:124–31, 1968.

MacDonald, M. G., and MacKay, B. R.: Adverse drug reactions. Experience of Mary Fletcher Hospital during 1962. *J.A.M.A.*, **190**:1071–74, 1964.

McIntyre, A. R.: Flexner, pharmacology, and the future. *J. Clin. Pharmacol.*, **8**:278–80, 1968.

Malahy, B.: The effect of instruction and labeling on the number of medication errors made by patients at home. *Amer. J. Hosp. Pharm.*, **23**:283–92, 1966.

Maronde, R. F.; Burks, D.; Lee, P. V.; Light, P.; McCarron, M. M.; McCary, M.; and Seibert, S.: Physician prescribing practices. A computer based study. *Amer. J. Hosp. Pharm.*, **26**:566–73, 1969.

Melmon, K. L.: Preventable drug reactions—causes and cures. *New Eng. J. Med.*, **284**:1361–68, 1971.

Melmon, K. L.; Grossman, M.; and Morris, R. C., Jr.: Emerging assets and liabilities of a committee on human welfare and experimentation. *New Eng. J. Med.*, 1970, in press.

Melmon, K. L., and Morrelli, H. F.: The need to test the efficacy of the instructional aspects of clinical pharmacology. *Clin. Pharmacol. Ther.*, **10**:431–35, 1969.

Meyers, F. M., and Smith, D. E.: Drug abuse: recommendations for California treatment and research facilities. *Calif. Med.*, **109**:191–97, 1968.

Meyler, L., and Peck, H. M. (eds.): *Drug-Induced Diseases.* Excerpta Medica Foundation, Amsterdam, 1968.

Miller, R. L., and Melmon, K. L.: The related roles of histamine, serotonin and bradykinin in the pathogenesis of inflammation. *Series Haematol.*, 1970, in press.

Modell, W.: FDA censorship. *Clin. Pharmacol. Ther.*, **8**:359–61, 1967.

Monroe, J. F., and Cluff, L. E.: Problems with multiple drugs. *Int. Anesth. Clin.*, **6**:19–31, 1968.

Moser, R. H. (ed.): *Diseases of Medical Progress*, 3rd ed. Charles C Thomas, Springfield, Ill., 1969.

Motulsky, A. G.: Drugs and genes. *Ann. Intern. Med.*, **70**:1269–72, 1969.

Moulding, T.; Onstad, G. D.; and Sbarbaro, J. A.: Supervision of outpatient drug therapy with the medication monitor. *Ann. Intern. Med.*, **73**:559–64, 1970.

Nagao, R., and Mauer, A. M.: Concordance for drug-induced aplastic anemia in identical twins. *New Eng. J. Med.*, **281**:7–11, 1969.

Ogilvie, R. I., and Ruedy, J.: Adverse drug reactions during hospitalization. *Canad. Med. Ass. J.*, **97**:1450–57, 1967.

Overall, J. E., and Tupin, J. P.: Investigation of clinical outcome in a doctor's choice treatment setting. *Dis. Nerv. Syst.*, **30**:305–13, 1969.

Palmer, R. F.: Drug misuse and physician education. *Clin. Pharmacol. Ther.*, **10**:1–4, 1969.

Parker, C. W.; deWeck, A. L.; Kern, M.; and Eisen, H. N.: The preparation and some properties of penicillenic acid derivatives relevant to penicillin hypersensitivity. *J. Exp. Med.*, **115**:803, 1962.

Paul, I. H.; Langs, R. J.; and Barr, H. L.: Individual differences in the recall of a drug experience. *J. Nerv. Ment. Dis.*, **140**:132–45, 1965.

Perrin, D. D.: *Dissociation Constants of Organic Bases in Aqueous Solution.* Butterworths, London, 1965.

Peters, G. A., and Marcoux, J. P.: Some adverse drug reactions common in the postoperative period. *Surg. Clin. N. Amer.*, **49**:1123–35, 1969.

Reidenberg, M. M., and Lowenthal, D. T.: Adverse nondrug reactions. *New Eng. J. Med.*, **279**:678–79, 1968.

Risebrough, R. W.; Huggett, R. J.; Griffin, J. J.; and Goldberg, E. D.: Pesticides: transatlantic movements in the Northeast Trades. *Science*, **159**:1233–36, 1968.

Rosenblum, A. H.: Penicillin allergy. *J. Allergy*, **42**:309–18, 1968.

Sandler, S. G.; Tobin, W.; and Henderson, E. S.: Vincristine-induced neuropathy: a clinical study of fifty leukemic patients. *Neurology*, **19**:367–74, 1969.

Schachter, S.: Obesity and eating. *Science*, **161**:751–56, 1968.

Schimmel, E. M.: The hazards of hospitalization. *Ann. Intern. Med.*, **60**:100–10, 1964.

Schuster, C. R., and Thompson, T.: Self administration of and behavioral dependence on drugs. *Ann. Rev. Pharmacol.*, **9**:483–502, 1969.

Schwartz, D.; Wang, M.; Zeitz, L.; and Goss, M. E. W.: Medication errors made by elderly, chronically ill patients. *Amer. J. Public Health*, **52**:2018–29, 1962.

Scott, R. B.: A survey of deaths and critical illnesses in association with the use of intrauterine devices. *Int. J. Fertil.*, **13**:297–300, 1968.

Seidl, L. G.; Thornton, G. F.; Smith, J. W.; and Cluff, L. E.: Studies on the epidemiology of adverse drug reactions. III. Reactions in patients on a general medical service. *Johns Hopkins Hosp. Bull.*, **119**:299–315, 1966.

Shapiro, S.; Slone, D.; Lewis, D. P.; and Jick, H.: Fatal drug reactions among medical inpatients. *J.A.M.A.*, **216**:467–72, 1971.

Sheps, M. C., and Shapiro, A. P.: Physician's responsibility in age of therapeutic plenty. *Circulation*, **25**:399–407, 1932.

Sidel, V. W.; Koch-Weser, J.; Barnett, G. O.; and Eaton, A.: Drug utilization and adverse reactions in a general hospital. *Hospitals*, **41**:80–88, 1967.

Slone, D.; Jick, H.; Lewis, G. P.; Shapiro, S.; and Miettinen, O. S.: Intravenously given ethacrynic acid and gastrointestinal bleeding. *J.A.M.A.*, **209**:1668–71, 1969.

Smith, D. E.: Changing drug patterns in the Haight-Ashbury. *Calif. Med.*, **110**:151–57, 1969a.

———: Use of LSD in the Haight-Ashbury: observations at a neighborhood clinic. *Calif. Med.*, **110**:472–76, 1969b.

Smith, J. W.; Johnson, J. E., III; and Cluff, L. E.: Studies on the epidemiology of adverse drug reactions. II. An evaluation of penicillin allergy. *New Eng. J. Med.*, **274**:998–1002, 1966.

Smith, M. C.: Drug advertising as a source of therapeutic information. *Amer. J. Hosp. Pharm.*, **25**:305–309, 1968.

Sparkes, R. S.; Melnyk, J.; and Bozzetti, L. P.: Chromosomal effect *in vivo* of exposure to lysergic acid diethylamide. *Science*, **160**:1343–45, 1968.

Stewart, G. T.: Macromolecular residues contributing to the allergenicity of penicillins and cephalosporins. *Antimicrob. Agents Chemother.*, pp. 543–49, 1967.

Stewart, G. T., and McGovern, J. P.: *Penicillin Allergy —Clinical and Immunological Aspects.* Charles C Thomas, Springfield, Ill., 1970.

Stolley, P. D.: Prescribing patterns of physicians. *J. Chronic Dis.*, **22**:395–405, 1969.

Stolley, P. D., and Lasagna, L.: Prescribing patterns of physicians. *J. Chron. Dis.*, **22**:395–405, 1969.

Task Force on Prescription Drugs: Final report. U.S. Dept. of Health, Education and Welfare, Washington, D.C., 1969.

Thomson, P.; Rowland, M.; Cohn, K.; Steinbrunn, W.; and Melmon, K. L.: Critical differences in the pharmacokinetics of lidocaine between normal (N) and congestive heart failure (HF) patients. *Clin. Res.*, **17**:140, 1969.

Turk, J. L., and Baker, H.: Drug reactions III. Immunoglobulin class E–anaphylactic antibodies. *Brit. J. Dermatol.*, **80**:622–24, 1968.

Vere, D. W.: Errors of complex prescribing. *Lancet*, **1**:370–73, 1965.

Visconti, A. J.: Use of drug interaction information in patient medication records. *Amer. J. Hosp. Pharm.*, **26**:378–87, 1969.

Visconti, A. J., and Smith, M. C.: The role of hospital personnel in reporting adverse drug reactions. *Amer. J. Hosp. Pharm.*, **24**:273–75, 1967.

Voss, H. E.; Redmond, A. P.; and Levine, B. B.: Clinical detection of the potential allergic reactor to penicillin by immunologic tests. *J.A.M.A.*, **196**:679–83, 1966.

Wagner, J. G.: Aspects of pharmacokinetics and biopharmaceutics in relation to drug activity. *Amer. J. Pharm.*, **141**:5–20, 1969.

Westerman, G.; Corman, A.; Stelos, P.; and Nodine, J. H.: Adverse reactions to penicillin: a review of treatment. *J.A.M.A.*, **198**:173–74, 1966.

Wheeler, L., and Edmonds, C.: A profile of drug takers. *Med. J. Aust.*, **2**:291–94, 1969.

Willcox, D. R. C.; Gillan, R.; and Hare, E. H.: Do psychiatric out-patients take their drugs? *Brit. Med. J.*, **2**:790–92, 1965.

Wintrobe, M. M.: Reporting of adverse reactions to drugs. *Ann. Intern. Med.*, **62**:170–74, 1965.

Wyckoff, D. W.; Davies, J. E.; Barquet, A.; and Davis, J. H.: Diagnostic and therapeutic problems of parathion poisonings. *Ann. Intern. Med.*, **68**:875–82, 1968.

Chapter 16

DRUG INTERACTIONS

Howard F. Morrelli and *Kenneth L. Melmon*

Drug interactions are the sequelae attending the simultaneous use of two or more drugs. The interaction may result in enhanced or diminished drug effect and may be useful or harmful. Useful drug interactions are represented by combinations of agents used to lower the blood pressure, in which one drug lowers the cardiac output and another the peripheral vascular resistance. Regrettably, numerous drug interactions are harmful and may be recognized only when severe toxicity occurs.

Knowledge of drug interactions enables a physician to prevent drug toxicity. He may be able to recognize drug-induced symptoms readily and to provide accurate and specific therapy for the patient. Even if the drug-induced toxicity is severe or life threatening, it may be amenable to correct diagnosis and treatment.

Drug interactions may involve physicochemical combinations of the drugs or direct competition for protein-binding sites, receptor sites, or clearance mechanisms. They also may be more complex, the pharmacologic effects of one drug altering the patient's response to another drug. This chapter discusses drug-drug and drug-patient-drug interactions. The topics of drug-induced diseases and drug-induced abnormalities in laboratory tests are discussed more fully in Chapters 15 and 18. For example, at least 35 drugs either can truly increase serum concentrations of glutamic oxaloacetic transaminase (SGOT) or can interfere with the

chemical assay. A recent review described modification of 80 common laboratory test values by an average of at least ten drugs (Elking and Karat, 1968).

When a new symptom appears in a disease state treated with a drug, and either the disease or the drug may cause the symptom, the physician is in a diagnostic dilemma. If the patient takes several drugs, and if two or more drugs may cause the new symptom as may the underlying disease, or if two drugs in concert elicit symptoms that would not otherwise appear, the physician is in a diagnostic quandary. Consider the plight of the consultant invited to help manage a ventricular arrhythmia in a patient with acute myocardial infarction and congestive heart failure, who has been given digitalis, propranolol, quinidine, and a thiazide diuretic. Should he stop all drugs, or add another (lidocaine, potassium chloride, diphenylhydantoin, or isoproterenol)? Should he add another drug to "pour oil on troubled waters" or would he be "adding coals to the fire"? The decision would hinge on the sequence in which the symptoms had developed, the manner in which drugs had been given, other symptoms or signs, and laboratory data such as serum electrolytes and blood quinidine concentration. Knowledge of drug interactions is crucial in solving such complex problems, but the interactions are presented here in simpler contexts.

CLINICAL IMPORTANCE OF DRUG INTERACTIONS

Drug interactions are most obviously important if they result in hemorrhage, hypoglycemic coma, seizures, or a hypertensive crisis (Wishinsky *et al.*, 1962; Horwitz *et al.*, 1964; Sjoqvist, 1965; Aggeler *et al.*, 1967; Hussar, 1970; Editorial, 1971). A variety of more subtle interactions may alter drug effects in ways subliminal to conventional clinical analysis (Prescott, 1969). If a potent antihypertensive agent does not "work," the physician may overlook the actions of another drug and may ascribe the resistance to the patient's disease (Leishman *et al.*, 1963).

The precise incidence of adverse reactions to single drugs is unknown. The reports are incomplete and not necessarily accurate, and present methods of reporting drug reactions do not take into consideration the total amount of drug in use (Lasagna, 1965). It is even more difficult to identify the population affected by drug interactions. Clinical pharmacologists may recognize drug interactions as the basis for an adverse effect more regularly than do internists, who tend to report such effects as reactions to single drugs (Ogilvie and Ruedy, 1967; Borda *et al.*, 1968). The ability of internists to recognize drug interactions may be encumbered by (1) lack of information on drug interactions; (2) the tendency of physicians to attribute new symptoms during treatment to the underlying disease; (3) the tendency to ascribe a severe drug reaction to the patient's idiosyncratic response to a single drug, rather than to a drug interaction; (4) relative lack of training in pharmacokinetics, resulting in the use of therapeutic agents as "tonics" rather than as chemicals with known or predictable absorption, distribution, and excretion (see Chapter 2); and (5) the large number (more than 100) of drugs involved in drug interactions, which tends to preclude their memorization and ready recall. In addition, even when the physician knows the drugs and dosage prescribed, multiple-drug therapy leads to mistakes in drug administration (Vere, 1965) (see Chapter 15). Even in hospitals, the errors include administration of wrong drugs (Simmons *et al.*, 1968) (see Chapter 15).

As clinical awareness of the possibility of drug interactions has increased, numerous case reports and more comprehensive studies of drug interactions in man have appeared. Epidemiologic studies demonstrate that the rate of adverse reactions to drugs increases from 4.2% when five or fewer drugs are given, to 45% when 20 or more drugs are prescribed (Smith *et al.*, 1966). Although other factors might account for this extraordinary incidence of reactions, the exponential increase may imply a synergistic rather than a simple additive effect of multiple-drug therapy.

Although this chapter emphasizes the hazards of polypharmacy, it should not be construed as a plea to return to the practice of therapeutic nihilism. Medical research and the pharmaceutical industry have produced a host of potent, relatively specific, and effective therapeutic agents. These drugs cannot be withheld from a patient whose disease may be ameliorated by their use. Regrettably, the blessings attending enhanced potency and efficacy of drugs have been accompanied by increased toxicity. *Principle: The more potent the agent, the higher the risk of toxicity, either by exaggeration of the intended effect, or as an inevitable ancillary action seen concomitantly with the intended effect.* This liability applies even more strongly to multiple-drug therapy.

RECOGNITION AND PREVENTION OF DRUG INTERACTIONS

The rationale for drug choice and the therapeutic goals and guidelines for therapeutic or toxic effects must be firmly established on both clinical and pharmacologic grounds before the use of multiple drugs can be justified. When polypharmacy is unavoidable, knowledge of the frequency and mechanisms of drug interaction is essential. A properly informed physician can detect drug interactions early and avoid serious toxicity, or he may intentionally allow a drug interaction to occur. For example, he may give a sedative drug to a patient on chronic anticoagulant therapy and readjust the dose of anticoagulant to the new "steady state" of enhanced hepatic metabolism of anticoagulant; discontinuation of the sedative requires readjustment of the anticoagulant dose according to the patient's prothrombin time. *Principle: The physician must know the risks and set clearly defined therapeutic goals and guidelines to therapeutic or toxic effects. Drug interactions per se are no threat to a patient; a physician's ignorance of an interaction is dangerous.* Even the usually disastrous hypertensive reactions occurring in patients taking monoamine-oxidase-inhibiting drugs who ingest tyramine-containing foods or sympathomimetic drugs may have therapeutic application, as has been suggested in the treatment of the severe hypotension seen in profound degrees of autonomic insufficiency (Seller, 1969). *Principle: Knowledge of drug interactions not only may prevent toxicity, but also may lead to therapeutic innovations* (see Chapter 18).

The number of drugs presently known to be

involved in drug interactions is too great to permit their memorization by trade or generic names. Classification of interactions by pharmacologic type, chemical nature of drugs likely to be involved, and pharmacokinetic mechanism of interaction is feasible and provides a logical framework that fosters the transference of information to clinical settings (Solomon *et al.*, 1971). The classification of interactions presented in this chapter should facilitate the evaluation of drugs, as it utilizes reasoning rather than recall. It should also enable the physician to recognize previously unreported drug interactions, based on similarities to other drugs known to cause interactions.

The pharmacologic effect of a drug or of its active metabolite is related to the free concentration of the active substance at its receptor site. The receptor site may be intracellular, as with phenobarbital, or extracellular, as with mecamylamine (Inversine). The free concentration of drug or active drug metabolite may increase or decrease as a result of (1) direct physical or chemical combination of two drugs; (2) altered gastrointestinal absorption or competition for protein-binding sites or receptor sites; (3) altered drug metabolism by induction or inhibition of drug-metabolizing enzymes; (4) changes in acid-base equilibrium that influence the distribution and renal clearance of some drugs; and (5) alterations of hemodynamic or renal tubular function that influence rates of renal excretion. In addition, pharmacologically induced changes in a patient may render him sensitive or resistant to the effects of another agent. Examples of commonly used drugs are discussed for each of these mechanisms; more detailed listings of drugs are given in the tables.

Direct Chemical or Physical Interactions

Our appreciation of drugs as therapeutic agents may diminish our awareness of their important chemical or physical properties. These properties account for interactions that may be therapeutically useful or harmful. For example, the anticoagulant effect of heparin, an acid, may be reversed by protamine, a base. Other basic drugs, such as antihistamines, phenothiazines, and certain antibiotics, if given in stoichiometrically appropriate quantities, may also counter heparin's effects, as shown *in vitro*, and *in vivo* in dogs (Nelson *et al.*, 1959). Although we recognize the chelating properties of ethylenediaminetetraacetate in treating selected cases of hypercalcemia or lead poisoning, we are less likely to assign this chemical property to the tetracycline antibiotics. Tetracyclines are chelating agents, and gastrointestinal absorption of

these drugs is inhibited when they are given simultaneously with antacids containing multivalent cations (Ca^{++}, Mg^{++}, or Al^{+++}) or with iron (Dearborn *et al.*, 1957; Kunin and Finland, 1961).

Cholestyramine, a drug used to bind bile salts within the gastrointestinal lumen in patients with pruritus associated with biliary cirrhosis, may also bind a number of drugs, preventing their absorption (Wagner, 1961; Council on Drugs, 1966). A therapeutic trial of corticosteroids might be invalidated by the simultaneous ingestion of cholestyramine. Cholestyramine also prevents the gastrointestinal absorption of thyroxine (Northcutt *et al.*, 1969). Other complex polymers that bind bile salts within the gastrointestinal lumen may bind other drugs, and the dosage schedule must be adjusted to allow their absorption. Kaolin, a hydrated aluminum silicate, is a commonly used adsorbent for the treatment of diarrhea; it adsorbs drugs and limits the gastrointestinal absorption of lincomycin (Wagner, 1961).

Many drugs are chemically or physically incompatible in solution and cannot safely be admixed for intravenous use (Simberkoff *et al.*, 1970). One study identified 104 such drugs, some of which were incompatible with as many as 20 other drugs or vehicles (Pelissier and Burgee, 1968). A few antibiotics commonly given intravenously and some of their incompatibilities are listed in Table 16–1. If the physical or chemical incompatibility results in precipitation of the agents and a "great white cloud" forms in the solution intended for intravenous use, the nurse or patient usually takes action to prevent its administration. If the incompatibility results in the formation of complexes of drugs that do not precipitate, inactive drug or a toxic complex may unwittingly be given. *Principle: Considerable sophistication in pharmaceutical chemistry is required to predict the results of addition of drugs to fluids for intravenous use. Drugs should not be added to intravenous fluids without prior review by a pharmaceutical chemist or a knowledgeable pharmacist.*

Pills and tablets are not simply containers for active drug. They vary widely in composition and in the manner and degree to which they are physically compressed. These variations can result in differences in drug absorption rate and in pharmacologic availability. Until the pharmaceutical manufacturers agree, or the Food and Drug Administration requires, that drugs must have therapeutic as well as generic equivalence, a change in brands may result in a change in the effective dose of a drug (Caminetsky, 1963; Carter, 1963; Gwilt *et al.*, 1963; Braverman and Ingbar, 1964; Levy, 1964; Leonards and Levy,

Table 16–1. CHEMICAL OR PHYSICAL IN-COMPATIBILITIES OF SOME ANTIBIOTICS COMMONLY GIVEN BY INTRAVENOUS INFUSION*

DRUG	INCOMPATIBLE WITH
Amphotericin B (Fungizone)	Diphenhydramine Penicillin G Solutions of pH less than 6 or more than 7 Tetracyclines Water for injection with preservative
Cephalothin sodium (Keflin)	Aminophylline Barbiturates Calcium chloride Calcium gluconate Chloramphenicol Diphenylhydantoin Erythromycin Heparin Kanamycin Metaraminol Norepinephrine Phenothiazines Polymyxin B Protein hydrolysates Sulfadiazine Sulfisoxazole Tetracyclines Vancomycin
Chloramphenicol	Aminophylline Barbiturates Cephalothin Dimenhydrinate Diphenhydramine Diphenylhydantoin Erythromycin Hydrocortisone Hydroxyzine Polymyxin B Prochlorperazine Protein hydrolysates Sulfadiazine Sulfisoxazole Tetracyclines Vancomycin Vitamin B complex
Colistimethate (Coly-Mycin)	Cephalothin Chlortetracycline Erythromycin Hydrocortisone Hydroxyzine
Erythromycin gluceptate	Aminophylline Barbiturates Cephalothin Chloramphenicol Colistimethate Diphenylhydantoin Heparin Prochlorperazine Protein hydrolysates

DRUG	INCOMPATIBLE WITH
	Riboflavin Tetracyclines Vitamin B with C
Kanamycin sulfate (Kantrex)	Barbiturates Calcium gluconate Cephalothin Diphenylhydantoin Heparin Hydrocortisone Methicillin Prochlorperazine Sodium bicarbonate Sulfisoxazole Vitamin B with C
Lincomycin (Lincocin)	Diphenylhydantoin Penicillin G Protein hydrolysates
Penicillin G	Amphotericin B Ascorbic acid Chlorpheniramine Chlorpromazine Dexamethasone Diphenylhydantoin Ephedrine Heparin Hydroxyzine Lincomycin Metaraminol Phenobarbital Phenylephrine Prochlorperazine

* Abstracted and modified from *Drug Information Service Newsletter*, Alta Bates Community Hospital, 1:No. 7–8, Aug.-Sept., 1969, with the permission of the author, Kay Yamagata, Pharm.D.

1965; Lu *et al.*, 1965; McKendry *et al.*, 1965; O'Reilly *et al.*, 1966; Schamberg, 1969).

Drug Interactions in Gastrointestinal Absorption

Many factors influence drug absorption from the gastrointestinal tract. In addition to the dissolution rate of the ingested drug, gastric emptying time, gut motility, and blood flow may be important determinants of absorption (Prescott, 1969). Drugs appear to be absorbed in their nonionized form (Hogben *et al.*, 1959). Many drugs are weak acids or weak bases, and the proportion of ionized to nonionized drug is dependent on the pK_a of the drug and on the pH of the drug's milieu. Some drugs in nonionized form are nonpolar or highly soluble in lipids and quickly cross lipid-rich cell membranes. In ionized form they are polar or water soluble, and their transfer across cell membranes is relatively slow. The observation of relatively rapid absorption of weak acids in the alkaline small bowel has led to the hypothesis that the pH of the fluid in immediate contact with the cell surface is lower than that of the fluid in the gastrointestinal lumen (Hogben *et al.*, 1959). Perhaps the large surface area of the small bowel or the high rate of intestinal blood flow counters the pH effects that would theoretically limit the rate of gastrointestinal absorption of weak acids. The pH gradient effect may lead to accumulation in the stomach of ionized drugs that are weak bases, and gastric analysis for alkaline drugs may be positive long after ingestion. Gastric washing to remove such drugs is not as efficacious as one might predict on the basis of pH gradient effect alone, since gastric blood flow is small.

In animal studies, drugs that reduce gut motility appear to slow gastrointestinal absorption of several drugs (Frey and Kampmann, 1966; Consolo, 1968). The clinical relevance of these studies is unknown, nor have the effects of repeated gastric suction been studied to determine whether significant amounts of basic drugs are removed.

In addition to chemical or physical binding within the gastrointestinal lumen, some drugs may alter the rate at which other drugs are transported across the mucosal membrane or may alter the ability of the gastrointestinal mucosa to metabolize drugs to inactive substances. Barbiturates reduce the gastrointestinal absorption of intact griseofulvin (Busfield *et al.*, 1963) and of bishydroxycoumarin (Aggeler and O'Reilly, 1966, 1969).

Some drugs, such as iron, are best absorbed when the gastric content is highly acidic; other drugs, such as the penicillins, vary in their resistance to gastric acidity and degree of absorption, depending upon whether or not the drug is taken with meals. Information regarding optimal administration of drug relative to food intake should be obtained when using unfamiliar drugs.

Promazine absorption is impaired in humans given an antidiarrhea mixture containing attapulgite and citrus pectin (Sorby and Liu, 1966). Animal studies have indicated increased or decreased drug absorption after intake of a variety of substances, including caffeine (Goto *et al.*, 1968), surface-active agents (Aoki *et al.*, 1969), and ethylenediaminetetraacetate (Kakemi *et al.*, 1968). The clinical significance of these findings has not been established. Drugs that resemble natural foodstuffs, such as amino acids, purines, and pyrimidines (alpha-methyldopa and purine and pyrimidine analogs for cancer chemotherapy), should be investigated to determine whether they, like foods, require active mucosal transport and whether competition for absorption occurs. Transport mechanisms in renal tubules are similar to those in the gut. Competition for renal tubular reabsorption of amino acids occurs during the use of alpha-methyldopa, and an aminoaciduria is induced (Weiner, 1967). Relatively specific defects in absorption may be seen; e.g., diphenylhydantoin and other anticonvulsants impair the absorption of folic acid (see Chapter 11).

Drug Interactions in Protein Binding

Many drugs are reversibly bound to plasma or tissue proteins (Table 16–2) and when bound they are pharmacologically inert. Displacement of a drug from its binding protein allows the drug to act, but also facilitates its metabolism or excretion. One drug may displace another from protein-binding sites, depending on the relative amounts and affinity constants of each drug for mutual binding sites and on the degree to which the binding sites are saturated by the first drug. Sulfonylurea oral hypoglycemic agents are avidly bound to protein (Wishinsky *et al.*, 1962) and may be displaced from their binding protein to cause hypoglycemia when sulfaphenazole is added. Other sulfonamides with similar affinity for protein binding do not duplicate this response; thus this explanation for the interaction is speculative. The prolonged tolbutamide effect may be caused by diminished hepatic or renal clearance of the drug, but it is possible that the tolbutamide is displaced to a tissue protein that releases it more slowly. Phenylbutazone and salicylates are also thought to enhance tolbutamide's effect by this mechanism (Brodie, 1965).

Phenylbutazone can displace warfarin from its binding protein and induce acute bleeding. When phenylbutazone is chronically administered, it induces enhanced hepatic metabolism of warfarin; a biphasic effect is seen during its administration (Aggeler *et al.*, 1967). Additional drugs believed to enhance warfarin's prothrombinopenic effects by displacing it from plasma proteins include clofibrate (Atromid-S), diphenylhydantoin (Dilantin), mefenamic acid (Ponstel), oxyphenbutazone (Tandearil), and salicylates (Eisen, 1964; Fox, 1964; Aggeler *et al.*, 1967; Comment, 1967; Schrogie and Solomon, 1967; Coldwell and Zawidzka, 1968; Hunninghake and Azarnoff, 1968). Acetaminophen and phenyramidol (Analexin) potentiate the effects of several anticoagulant drugs; although this has been ascribed to changes in anticoagulant metabolism, changes in protein

Table 16–2. INTERACTIONS IN TRANSPORT*

	PERCENT BINDING DRUG A	PERCENT BINDING DRUG B
Plasma	1 free	0.1 free
	9 bound	0.9 bound
Cells	1 free	0.1 free
	89 bound	98.9 bound

A-TYPE DRUGS	B-TYPE DRUGS
Pamaquine, quinine	Quinacrine
Tolbutamide	Sulfaphenazole, phenylbutazone, salicylates
Warfarin and other oral anticoagulant drugs, acetaminophen	Phenylbutazone, salicylates, clofibrate, diphenylhydantoin
Warfarin	Oxyphenbutazone, sulfinpyrazone, mefenamic acid
Bilirubin	Salicylates, sulfonamides
Methotrexate	Salicylates, sulfonamides
Quinine	Pyrimethamine
Sulfaethylthiadiazole	Phenylbutazone
Sulfonamide antibiotics	Phenylbutazone, oxyphenbutazone, sulfinpyrazone, warfarin, salicylates, probenecid, tolbutamide

* Many drugs, particularly acids, are reversibly bound to plasma and tissue proteins. Only a free drug exerts pharmacologic effect. If a very highly bound B-type drug is given with a moderately bound A-type drug, the bound form of the latter is displaced, enhancing A's effects. See text for qualifications.

binding have not been excluded (Carter, 1965; Antlitz et al., 1968; Antlitz and Awalt, 1969).

Amethopterin (methotrexate), a drug useful in treating leukemia and used in selected cases of severe psoriasis, may be displaced by highly acidic and protein-bound drugs such as salicylates and sulfonamides, causing pancytopenia (Dixon et al., 1965). A similar interaction appears critical in antimalarial therapy. Quinacrine (Mepacrine, Atabrine) is very highly protein bound. If pamaquine (Aminoquin, Plasmochin) is given simultaneously or shortly after quinacrine, the gastrointestinal and hematologic toxicities of pamaquine may be seen (Zubrod et al., 1948; Blount, 1967). Quinine is not so avidly bound to proteins as pyrimethamine, and if the two drugs are given simultaneously in conventional doses, severe quinine toxicity including cinchonism and bone marrow depression may be produced (Blount, 1967). High initial blood levels of quinine were reported after a single dose of pyrimethamine and sulphorthodimethoxine and continuing doses of quinine

(Brooks et al., 1969). Pyrimethamine and sulphorthodimethoxine disappear slowly after single-dose administration, as they are released slowly from tissue-binding proteins. It seems reasonable to attribute the initially high quinine levels to displacement from protein-binding sites that continued until the concentrations of sulphorthodimethoxine and pyrimethamine were reduced.

Endogenous substances can be released from protein-binding sites when highly protein-bound drugs are administered. Bilirubin is normally bound to plasma proteins (O'Dell, 1959). Bilirubin may be displaced from proteins and may contribute to the occurrence of kernicterus in neonates if salicylates or sulfonamides are given during the neonatal period (Silverman et al., 1956).

Drug interactions based on competition for protein-binding sites are not always adverse. The antibacterial activity of sulfonamides, particularly the long-acting agents that are more highly protein bound (inactive), can be enhanced by several acidic, highly protein-bound drugs (Anton, 1960, 1968; Garrod et al., 1969). This displacement probably shortens the duration of the antibiotic effect by promoting clearance of free drug (Anton, 1961). However, the relatively high incidence of severe allergic reactions to long-acting sulfonamides precludes their use under most circumstances.

For drugs that are very highly protein bound (i.e., more than 90% of the drug is present in the blood), even a minor percentage change in protein binding (2 to 5%) results in a doubling or trebling of the concentration of the free drug. All the drugs mentioned in this section are highly protein bound and, except for the antimalarials, are acidic. *Principle: When it is mandatory to use combinations of drugs that are highly protein bound, adjustments in dosage may be required. Unexpected drug toxicity during multiple therapy should lead the physician to look for an interaction during transport and to seek information regarding the protein-binding characteristics of the drugs prescribed for the patient* (Meyer and Guttman, 1968). Many clinical reports on drug toxicity attribute interactions to diminished metabolism of one drug by the action of another; interactions in transport should not be prematurely excluded as an underlying or contributing factor.

Drug Interactions at the Receptor Site

Drug effects ultimately occur as a result of binding to specialized areas on or within cells, known as receptor sites (Ehrenpreis et al., 1969). The amount of drug in association with receptor sites depends upon the amount of drug in the body, its accessibility to the receptor site, and the affinity constant of the drug for the receptor (the ratio of association to dissociation constants of the drug for the receptor). The association of a drug with the receptor may result in a detectable effect, such as vasoconstriction when norepinephrine acts upon vascular alpha-adrenergic receptors. Other drugs may have a high affinity for receptor sites or may be present in such large quantities that they may associate with the receptor, eliciting no detectable effect of their own, but preventing access of pharmacologically active agents to the receptor. Atropine elicits no pharmacologic effect itself; it has a high affinity constant for some of the receptor sites responsive to acetylcholine and competitively prevents acetylcholine from reaching receptor sites where it is active. Atropine's blockade of the receptor can be reversed by drugs that allow acetylcholine to accumulate and compete for receptor sites. These agents include the cholinesterase inhibitors (neostigmine, physostigmine, and edrophonium).

Antihistamines, phenothiazines, tricyclic antidepressants (imipramine group), and antiparkinsonian agents share with atropine the ability to block access of acetylcholine to its receptors (see Chapters 11 and 18). After substantial intake of these drugs singly or, at lower doses, after the simultaneous intake of several drugs, impressive degrees of "atropinization" may occur; symptoms include visual disturbances, fever, dry mouth, sinus tachycardia and other arrhythmias, gastrointestinal ileus, and bladder atony. Central nervous system symptoms compatible with central cholinergic blockade may appear, including confusion, hallucinations, and coma (see Chapter 11).

Drugs that block acetylcholine receptor sites are relatively specific for a given category of receptors. Atropine and the drugs mentioned above act chiefly on the peripheral parasympathetic receptors, and perhaps centrally. Other competitive antagonists of acetylcholine are selective for another cholinergic receptor, the motor end plates of muscle. D-Tubocurarine and gallamine act in this way to induce hyperpolarization (Koelle, 1965). The curariform effect is mimicked by certain antibiotics (neomycin, kanamycin, streptomycin, and colistimethate), and muscle paralysis, manifested as apnea, may be induced by excessive doses of these drugs or by conventional doses in patients with renal failure (Pridgen, 1956; Brazil and Corrado, 1957; Fisk, 1961; Bush, 1962; Wolinsky and Hines, 1962; Ream, 1963; Parisi and Kaplan, 1965; Anthony and Louis, 1966; Barlow and Groesbeek, 1966; Gold and Richardson, 1966; Pohlmann, 1966; Zauder

et al., 1966; Lindesmith et al., 1968). This reaction is reversible with drugs such as neostigmine that increase concentrations of acetylcholine at the receptor.

Some antiadrenergic agents compete for receptor sites. Phentolamine (Regitine) competitively blocks the effects of the alpha-stimulating drug norepinephrine; phenoxybenzamine (Dibenzyline) induces a competitive block at low doses and a noncompetitive block at high doses, by binding very tightly to the receptor. Beta stimulation by isoproterenol (Isuprel) is specifically and competitively blocked by appropriate doses of propranolol (Inderal). Newer drugs that block beta receptors may be specific for receptors in single organs, such as the heart or blood vessels (Wilkenfeld and Levy, 1968; Areskog and Adolfsson, 1969). Propranolol has generalized beta-blocking properties, including the ability to block the beta-mediated metabolic effects of epinephrine (Brown et al., 1968). This latter effect may be unwelcome, as it may lead to hypoglycemic reactions in patients taking oral hypoglycemic agents or insulin (Abramson et al., 1966; Kotler et al., 1966; Cowell and Hetenyi, 1969; Erill, 1969). The tachycardia and wide pulse pressure characteristic of ordinary hypoglycemic reactions are not seen during propranolol therapy, but sweating and pallor reportedly are present (Kotler et al., 1966). Adrenergic blocking agents may induce other metabolic changes in response to infusions of insulin, arginine, thyroid-stimulating hormone, and nicotinic acid, but the clinical significance of these effects is not clear (Lincova et al., 1968; Blackard and Heidingsfelder, 1969; Ghouri and Haley, 1969; Levey et al., 1969; Strauch et al., 1969; Vance et al., 1969). Phenothiazines and imipramines (tricyclic antidepressants) have alpha-adrenergic blocking ability, and caution is required in the selection of pressor agents and doses of drug necessary to reverse hypotension (see Chapter 18).

The adrenergic neuron and its granules are receptors for the storage of norepinephrine. Norepinephrine has high affinity but no apparent activity at this site. Guanethidine (Ismelin) must be taken up by adrenergic neurons before it can deplete granular stores of norepinephrine and prevent physiologic release of neuronal norepinephrine stores (Nies and Melmon, 1967). A variety of substances interfere with adrenergic neuronal uptake of guanethidine or cause its release from the neuron, thereby interfering with its antihypertensive effect. Of clinical importance are imipramine, amphetamine, ephedrine, and possibly reserpine (Day and Rand, 1963; Brodie et al., 1965; Mitchell

Table 16-3. INTERACTIONS AT THE RECEPTOR SITE*

Drug A + receptor $\xrightarrow{k}$ Drug A–receptor complex ⟶ Response

Drug B + receptor $\xrightarrow{K}$ Drug B–receptor complex ⟶ No response

RECEPTOR	A-TYPE DRUGS	B-TYPE DRUGS
Vessel alpha receptor	Norepinephrine	Phentolamine, imipramines, phenothiazines, phenoxybenzamine
Vessel beta receptor	Isoproterenol	Propranolol
Cardiac sinoatrial node	Acetylcholine	Atropine, antihistamines, phenothiazines, imipramines, antiparkinsonian agents
Neuromuscular junction	Acetylcholine	d-Tubocurarine
Neuromuscular junction	Succinylcholine	Gallamine, kanamycin, colistimethate, neomycin, streptomycin
Adrenergic neuron	Norepinephrine	Metaraminol
Adrenergic neuron	Norepinephrine	Guanethidine
Liver cell	Vitamin K	Coumadin, salicylates, propylthiouracil, aminosalicylic acid, anabolic steroids, chloramphenicol, d-thyroxine

* Some drugs, like A, combine with receptors to form a complex that elicits a response. The concentration of A and its affinity (k) for the receptor are determinants of the response. Other drugs, like B, have affinity (K) for the receptor, but the complex elicits no response. If the concentration of B or its affinity constant (K) is higher than A's, no response will be detected. See text for description of interactions.

et al., 1967; Abrams, 1969; Hanahoe *et al.*, 1969).

Hypertension following an excessive dose of guanethidine or after amphetamine administration in a patient taking guanethidine can be effectively treated with an alpha-blocking drug. Although the muscle-end-plate-polarizing effects of antibiotics with curariform action may be reversed by cholinesterase inhibitors, this therapy is contraindicated during decamethonium (depolarizing) paralysis (Goodman and Gilman, 1970). Some interactions of this type are listed in Table 16-3. *Principle: Knowledge of the mechanisms of action of drugs and of their interactions is the key to proper drug administration, limits adverse effects, and allows the proper choice of effective countermeasures if an adverse reaction occurs.*

Drug Interactions Due to Accelerated Drug Metabolism

Many drugs and other foreign compounds are metabolized by hepatic and possibly other microsomal enzymes. Enzymatic activity changes a nonpolar drug to a polar metabolite, usually renders drugs pharmacologically inert, and provides a mechanism for renal clearance of the metabolite. Occasionally the metabolite of the original drug retains pharmacologic activity, as is the case with most oral hypoglycemic agents, phenoxybenzamine, and cyclophosphamide (Cytoxan). Drugs and a variety of agents present in the environment (particularly insecticides and plant poisons) are capable of enhancing the activity of these enzymes (Conney, 1967;

Welch *et al.*, 1967; Wattenberg *et al.*, 1968). Not only is the inducing agent metabolized more quickly, but a variety of other drugs and endogenous compounds, such as cortisol, bilirubin, and the sex steroids, may also be affected (Conney *et al.*, 1965). Table 16-4 lists some of the more than 200 agents known to induce their own metabolism or the metabolism of other drugs. Most of these listings have been abstracted from recent reviews of the literature (Conney, 1967; Kuntzman, 1969; Prescott, 1969). Many of the data on enzyme induction have been obtained from animal studies and may not be fully applicable to man. *Principle: Any drug that is lipid soluble at physiologic pH should be considered a candidate for enzyme-inducing capability, and this effect should be looked for in patients on combination drug therapy.* This chapter does not attempt to reiterate the detailed information available elsewhere regarding differences in types of enzyme induction or influences of other manipulations on the induction process.

Barbiturates, which are often considered relatively innocuous drugs, are potent microsomal enzyme stimulators and can affect the metabolism of several drugs, as indicated in Table 16-4. Warfarin and bishydroxycoumarin, for example, are metabolized more rapidly after the administration of barbiturates. While a patient is receiving a barbiturate, larger doses of anticoagulants are required to maintain the therapeutic range of prothrombin time. If the sedative drug is discontinued, the required dose of anticoagulant decreases. Unless the anti-

Table 16–4. DRUGS THAT INDUCE THEIR OWN METABOLISM OR THE METABOLISM OF OTHER DRUGS

Drugs That Enhance Their Own Metabolism

Aminopyrine	Meprobamate
Chlorcyclizine	Pentobarbital
Chlordiazepoxide	Phenobarbital
Chlorpromazine	Phenylbutazone
DDT	Probenecid
Glutethimide	Tolbutamide
Hexobarbital	

Drugs That Enhance the Metabolism of Other Drugs or Substances

INDUCING AGENT	DRUG(S) OR SUBSTANCE(S) AFFECTED
Phenobarbital	Barbiturates
	Phenylbutazone
	Warfarin
	Bishydroxycoumarin
	Diphenylhydantoin
	Testosterone
	Progesterone
	Cortisol
	Griseofulvin
	Digitoxin
	Estradiol
	Androsterone
	Chloramphenicol
	Bilirubin
	Thyroxine
Diphenylhydantoin	Corticosteroids and sex steroid hormones
Chlorcyclizine	Corticosteroids and sex steroid hormones
Norchlorcyclizine	Corticosteroids and sex steroid hormones
Orphenadrine	Corticosteroids and sex steroid hormones
Phenylbutazone	Corticosteroids and sex steroid hormones
Chlordane	Corticosteroids and sex steroid hormones
DDT	Corticosteroids and sex steroid hormones
	Thyroxine
n-Phenylbarbital	Corticosteroids and sex steroid hormones
Amobarbital	Warfarin
Secobarbital	Warfarin
Meprobamate	Warfarin
Griseofulvin	Warfarin
Ethchlorvinol	Warfarin
Haloperidol	Warfarin
Chloral hydrate	Bishydroxycoumarin
	Warfarin
Heptabarbital	Bishydroxycoumarin
Barbiturates	Ethylbiscoumacetate
Glutethimide	Ethylbiscoumacetate
	Warfarin

INDUCING AGENT	DRUG(S) OR SUBSTANCE(S) AFFECTED
Alcohol	Tolbutamide
Barbital	Bilirubin
	Acenocoumarin
Phenothiazines	Benzpyrene

coagulant dose is diminished, bleeding may ensue. Other drugs have similar effects (see Table 16–4) (Fox, 1964; Burns and Conney, 1965; Cucinell *et al.*, 1965; Elias, 1965; Cucinell *et al.*, 1966; van Dam *et al.*, 1966; Weiner, 1966; Cullen and Catalano, 1967; Hoffbrand and Kininmonth, 1967; Formiller and Cohon, 1969). *Principle: The fact that an interaction occurs does not preclude the use of two drugs simultaneously. Appropriate manipulation of the dose of an anticoagulant, based on prothrombin times and on administration or discontinuation of an enzyme-inducing drug, is acceptable and safe.*

Drug interactions based on induction of drug-metabolizing microsomal enzymes should be suspected if a patient requires an increased dose of a drug after a new drug is added to his therapeutic regimen. If a patient develops an unexpected sensitivity to a drug, his record should be reviewed to determine whether a drug was recently discontinued from his therapeutic program. Clinicians are in an excellent position to detect clinically important drug interactions; the mechanism of the interaction can later be defined by more refined techniques (Sotaniemi *et al.*, 1970; Kutt and Fouts, 1971).

Drug Interactions Apparently Due to Inhibited Drug Metabolism

A number of drug interactions are apparently based on inhibition of metabolism of one drug by another. This effect could be produced by irreversible inhibition of an enzyme responsible for the metabolism of the first drug, or by competition as a substrate for the same drug-metabolizing enzyme (Levy and Yamada, 1971). Allopurinol, a xanthine oxidase inhibitor, prolongs the half-life and intensifies the effects of a given dose of substituted purines, such as 6-mercaptopurine, since the latter drugs are metabolized by xanthine oxidase. Profound bone marrow toxicity occurs unless the dose of 6-mercaptopurine is decreased during allopurinol therapy (Elion *et al.*, 1963; DeConti and Calabrisi, 1966).

Table 16–5 lists examples of reactions thought to be caused by inhibition of metabolism of one drug by another. The hypoglycemic effects of tolbutamide (Orinase) and the toxic effects of

Table 16–5. DRUG INTERACTIONS APPARENTLY DUE TO INHIBITED DRUG METABOLISM

DRUG METABOLIZED SLOWLY	DRUG INHIBITING DRUG'S METABOLISM	
Diphenylhydantoin	Bishydroxycoumarin Disulfiram Isonicotinic acid p-Aminosalicylic acid Cycloserine Phenylbutazone	Phenyramidol Sulfaphenazole Sulthiame Methylphenidate Chloramphenicol
Bishydroxycoumarin	Chloramphenicol Phenyramidol	Phenylbutazone Oxyphenbutazone
Tolbutamide	Monoamine oxidase inhibitors Phenylbutazone Probenecid Sulfaphenazole	Salicylates Phenyramidol Alcohol Chloramphenicol
Hexabarbital	Progesterone Norethynodrel	Aminosalicylic acid Metyrapone

6-Substituted purines:
  6-Mercaptopurine
  6-Methylthiopurine
  6-Propylthiopurine
  6-Chloropurine
	Allopurinol	

Oxyphenbutazone Pethidine, promazine Nortriptyline	Methandrostanolone Oral contraceptives Hydrocortisone	

Substances Eliciting Toxic Reactions During Monoamine Oxidase Inhibition:

Catecholamines	Hypoglycemic agents
Catecholamine-releasing agents	Narcotics Chloral hydrate
Tyramine, including food sources	Antiparkinsonian agents Cocaine
Phenothiazines	Diuretics
Tricyclic antidepressants	Antihypertensive agents
Amphetamines	Sedatives
Barbiturates	

diphenylhydantoin (Dilantin) have been attributed to inhibition of the metabolism of these drugs by bishydroxycoumarin (Dicumarol) (Hansen *et al.*, 1966; Kristensen and Hansen, 1967).

Several drugs have caused hypoglycemic reactions in patients previously stable during therapy with tolbutamide; possibly the metabolism of tolbutamide is inhibited by such agents as phenylbutazone (Butazolidin), probenecid (Benemid), sulfaphenazole (Orisul), salicylates, phenyramidol (Analexin), and perhaps alcohol in some alcoholic patients (Stowers *et al.*, 1959; Field *et al.*, 1967; Solomon and Schrogie, 1967; Arky *et al.*, 1968; Brook *et al.*, 1968; Peaston and Finnegan, 1968).

Diphenylhydantoin has produced toxicity at a previously nontoxic dose when the therapeutic program was changed to include any one of a large number of drugs, including bishydroxycoumarin, disulfiram (Antabuse), antituber-

culous drugs, phenylbutazone (Butazolidin), phenyramidol (Analexin), sulfaphenazole (Sulfabid, Orisul), and sulthiame (Murray, 1962; Hansen *et al.*, 1966; Kiorboe, 1966; Kutt *et al.*, 1966; Olesen, 1966; Comment, 1967; Olesen, 1967; Solomon and Schrogie, 1967; Hansen *et al.*, 1968; Kutt *et al.*, 1968; Landy, 1968; Lucas, 1968; Brennan *et al.*, 1970). More recently, methylphenidate (Ritalin) has been reported to interact with both the anticonvulsants and ethylbiscoumacetate (Tromexan), and chloramphenicol has slowed the clearance of tolbutamide, diphenylhydantoin, and bishydroxycoumarin (Christensen and Skovsted, 1969; Garrettson *et al.*, 1969).

Oral contraceptive agents reduce the rate of drug metabolism in animals. Pregnant women and women taking oral contraceptives metabolize pethidine (Demerol, Tubex) and promazine (Sparine) more slowly than do controls (Crawford and Rudofsky, 1966). In animals, prednisolone decreases metabolism of cyclophosphamide to its active form (Hayakawa *et al.*, 1969), and hydrocortisone and testosterone inhibit metabolism of nortriptyline (Aventyl) (Bahr *et al.*, 1970). Although corticosteroids are commonly thought to be relatively safe, caution is required in the routine use of even short-term massive doses of these drugs. Other steroid drugs such as spironolactone have been shown to impair the metabolism of bishydroxycoumarin (Solymoss *et al.*, 1970; Vesell *et al.*, 1970).

The monoamine-oxidase-inhibiting drugs pargyline (Eutonyl) and tranylcypromine (Parnate) interact with many drugs. During monoamine oxidase inhibition, catecholamines and catecholamine-releasing agents (including tyramine in certain foods) may produce fatal hypertensive reactions (Horwitz *et al.*, 1964; Sjoqvist, 1965). Enzyme systems other than monoamine oxidase may be nonspecifically inhibited during therapy with these drugs, accounting entirely or in part for the enhanced effects of sedatives, narcotics, anesthetics, antiparkinsonian agents, antihypertensive agents, the tricyclic (imipramine) antidepressants, phenothiazines, and hypoglycemic agents (Sjoqvist, 1965). These reactions may result in death or in serious morbidity (Luby and Domino, 1961; Mason, 1962; Sjoqvist, 1965). Other hydrazine derivatives may have monoamine-oxidase-inhibiting properties in addition to the primary pharmacologic effect for which the drugs are usually intended, e.g., procarbazine (Matulane), a cancer chemotherapeutic agent (Mann and Hutchison, 1967). It may be unwise to ascribe all the adverse effects of monoamine oxidase inhibition to that action alone; some evidence suggests that the hypoglycemia seen during monoamine oxidase inhibition may be related to the presence of the hydrazine group common to many monoamine-oxidase-inhibiting drugs and other agents, and not to inhibition of the enzyme itself, as hypoglycemia is not elicited by the nonhydrazine-containing drug pargyline (Potter *et al.*, 1969). *Principle: The monoamine oxidase inhibitors exemplify the relative lack of specificity of most drugs, even those "scientifically tailored" for a specific purpose. A drug may elicit unexpected actions either because intake of the agent was not anticipated (e.g., tyramine) or because its chemical structure (e.g., the hydrazine group) exerts effects independent of the effect for which the drug was designed. Even when the physician thinks he understands the mechanism of action of a drug, he should be on the alert for unexpected effects.*

There are distressingly few guidelines to permit prospective identification of drugs that may inhibit the metabolism of other agents.

Monoamine oxidase inhibitors, anticoagulants, hypoglycemic agents, and diphenylhydantoin merit particular attention because of known interactions. These effects may have been detected early because they are severe; more subtle interactions may be more difficult to recognize. *Principle: Assessment of a patient's therapeutic response and guidelines for drug effect and toxicity should always be established before initiation of therapy. This principle holds particularly for drugs added to a previously stable regimen, to allow early detection and reduction in severity of reactions due to inhibition of drug metabolism.*

Influence of Acid-Base Balance on Drug Distribution and Clearance

Physicians may alter the acidity of body fluids with therapeutic intent, or as an unwanted but pharmacologically inherent effect of drugs used for other purposes. Systemic alkalosis, with or without paradoxical aciduria, may occur during therapy with thiazide diuretics. Conversely, systemic acidosis with an alkaline urine results from the use of carbonic acid anhydrase inhibitors in glaucoma. These effects may produce major changes in drug distribution or in renal clearance of drugs, thereby altering the concentration of free drug at its receptor site (Beckett *et al.*, 1970).

Table 16–6 illustrates the effects on drug distribution of pH gradients between fluids in different body compartments. The diffusion of lipid-soluble weak acids and bases depends in part on their state of ionization in a given milieu. Ionized drugs diffuse slowly across lipid-rich cell membranes. Intracellular fluid is normally more acidic than plasma; hence the rapidly diffusing form of the drug, its nonionized form, tends to exit from cells and to be converted to its ionized form in the relatively alkaline milieu of plasma. An alkaline drug subject to pH partitioning accumulates within cells.

Changes in plasma pH alter the ratio of extracellular to intracellular concentration of drugs subject to pH gradient partitioning. The pharmacologic effect depends upon whether the receptor for the drug is intracellular or extracellular. Plasma concentrations of phenobarbital diminish during acute respiratory acidosis, and coma deepens as the drug enters cells, where it is active. Mechanical ventilation or alkalinization of extracellular fluids with bicarbonate results in extracellular accumulation of phenobarbital, lessening its effects (Waddell and Butler, 1957). Alkalinizing not only the extracellular fluid but also the renal tubular urine to an even greater degree than plasma

Table 16-6. INFLUENCE OF pH ON DRUG ABSORPTION, DISTRI-
BUTION, AND EXCRETION*

PROCESS	DRUG A (WEAK ACID)	DRUG B (WEAK BASE)
Gastric absorption	Relatively rapid	Relatively slow
Small-bowel absorption	Relatively slow	Relatively rapid
Plasma/cell ratio	High	Low
Renal clearance in:		
Acid urine	Low	High
Alkaline urine	High	Low
	Sulfonamides	Antihistamines
	Salicylic acid	Mecamylamine
	Phenobarbital	Amphetamine
		Quinidine

* The diffusion of lipid-soluble weak acids and bases depends in part upon their
state of ionization in a given milieu. Ionized drugs diffuse across lipid-rich cell
membranes poorly. Intracellular sites are more acidic than plasma; hence
alkaline drugs accumulate in cells. Other factors such as extensive protein
binding, degree of lipid solubility, and partition coefficient may alter the
predicted effect based upon pK_a of the drug alone.

creates a pH gradient cascade from within cells
to urine that can greatly facilitate renal clearance of phenobarbital in intoxicated patients
(see Chapter 18). Other chemical features of
drugs, such as their affinity for plasma and tissue
proteins and their partition coefficient at
physiologic pH, may not permit distribution
along pH gradients as predicted by the pK_a of
the drug and the pH of body fluids. Highly
protein-bound and very nonpolar drugs do not
behave in the manner described above (see
Chapter 2).

Mecamylamine is a weak base with an extracellular site of action. Imposition of an acute
extracellular acidosis favors its extracellular
accumulation, enhances its free concentration at
receptor sites, and causes hypotension (Payne
and Rowe, 1957). *Principle: Enhanced renal
clearance of a weak base requires induction of an
acid diuresis.* This procedure is efficacious for
the removal of some drugs, such as amphetamine (Beckett and Rowland, 1965) or quinidine
(Gerhardt et al., 1969).

Table 16-6 lists the influence of pH gradients
on absorption, distribution, and renal clearance
of drugs subject to pH gradient partitioning. A
change in therapeutic effect of a drug or the
appearance of toxicity under circumstances in
which the pH of body fluids has been altered
should suggest the possibility of this influence
(Milne, 1965). High affinity for plasma and tissue
proteins and nonpolarity of ionized drugs may
render the effects of pH partitioning less
important (see Chapters 2 and 17).

Drug Interactions Due to Altered Renal Clearance

Alterations in glomerular filtration, renal
tubular reabsorption, or secretion rate may
influence drug clearance. Although acute reduction in the glomerular filtration rate during
drug therapy is relatively uncommon, several
drugs can directly alter tubular reabsorption or
secretion of drugs. Hypoglycemia has occurred
when acetohexamide was given concurrently
with phenylbutazone, a drug that appears to
slow the renal clearance of the active metabolite
of acetohexamide (hydroxyhexamide) (Field
et al., 1967). Probenecid retards renal tubular
secretion of penicillin, and salicylates diminish
the uricosuric action of probenecid.

Changes in urinary pH induced by disease, or
as a result of therapy with ammonium chloride,
sodium bicarbonate, thiazides, or acetazolamide,
may profoundly influence the renal excretion of
many drugs that are weak acids or bases. Weak

acids are absorbed poorly from alkaline urine in the renal tubular lumina, and weak bases are reabsorbed poorly from acid urine. Accordingly, weak acids like phenobarbital or salicylic acid have high renal clearance in alkaline urine, and basic drugs such as amphetamine or mecamylamine have high renal clearance when the urine is acid (Milne, 1965).

Some drugs are specifically intended to alter renal tubular function (Weiner et al., 1960). Spironolactone interferes with the effects of aldosterone on the renal tubule, and triamterene exerts a direct tubular effect, enhancing sodium clearance and reducing potassium clearance. The potassium content of the diet and use of salt substitutes must be considered, in addition to the usual avoidance of potassium chloride supplements, during therapy with these agents.

Interactions with the Psychotherapeutic Drugs

The phenothiazines are useful in psychotic disorders requiring tranquilization. When used alone, they impose side effects such as orthostatic hypotension, cholinergic blockade, and signs of parkinsonism that are acceptable in treatment of psychotic behavior. These adverse effects are not necessarily justifiable in patients with mild degrees of anxiety or agitation (see Chapter 11). Phenothiazines potentiate the central nervous system effects of barbiturates, alcohol, and narcotics. Severe extrapyramidal reactions and hypertensive crises may be seen if phenothiazines are used with monoamine oxidase inhibitors. Complex changes in cardiovascular function are observed during phenothiazine administration (Jarvik, 1965). Central and peripheral effects may lead to postural hypotension. Care must be taken in the selection of a pressor agent with relatively pure alpha-stimulating activity (Barsa and Saunders, 1964; Inglis and Barrow, 1965).

Phenothiazines lower the seizure threshold in animals, and when equally effective drugs are available for treatment of agitation in patients who may have an underlying tendency to seizures, such as epilepsy or delirium tremens, phenothiazines should be avoided. This contraindication is particularly applicable in patients who take other agents that lower the seizure threshold, such as the tricyclic antidepressants.

Ventricular tachycardia has been reported during phenothiazine therapy and poisoning (Desautels et al., 1964; Hollister and Kosek, 1965; Schoonmaker et al., 1966). The electrophysiologic effects and the changes in cardiac electrolyte composition induced by phenothiazines resemble those produced by quinidine (Kelly et al., 1963; Madan and Pendse, 1963;

Ban and St. Jean, 1964; Burton et al., 1967). The arrhythmia tends to be paroxysmal, resembling the arrhythmias induced by quinidine (Selzer and Wray, 1964). In the periods of normal sinus rhythm intervening between runs of ventricular tachycardia, a prolonged Q–T interval may be seen. Although a definitive statement about management of such arrhythmias cannot be made on the basis of controlled clinical trials, such an arrhythmia would theoretically be treated in a manner analogous to therapy for quinidine toxicity; procainamide and quinidine would be less desirable than diphenylhydantoin, isoproterenol, induction of an alkalosis to lower serum potassium, or electrical defibrillation with pacing. Diphenylhydantoin and isoproterenol can counter the effects of quinidine that depress intraventricular conductivity; these drugs should be useful in phenothiazine-induced ventricular tachycardia, but this has not been well documented. *Principle: In any form of therapy, the therapeutic goal should be predetermined (e.g., control of the arrhythmia, return of Q–T interval to normal) and the possibility of drug toxicity considered (e.g., appearance of diphenylhydantoin's central nervous system toxicity, unacceptable degrees of sinus tachycardia, or paradoxical hypotension from isoproterenol); alternative methods should be utilized if initial interventions fail.*

The tricyclic antidepressants have largely supplanted the monoamine oxidase inhibitors for treatment of depression. Although safer than the monoamine oxidase inhibitors, they have impressive toxicity in their own right (see Chapter 18), and they interact with many drugs. Their atropine-like activity is at least additive with that of the phenothiazines, antihistamines, and antiparkinsonian agents. Their cardiac effects resemble those of quinidine and the phenothiazines, but in intoxicated patients the occurrence of sudden death due to arrhythmias and congestive heart failure has been particularly frequent (Freeman et al., 1969).

Use of the tricyclic antidepressants along with or shortly after discontinuation of monoamine oxidase inhibitors has resulted in hyperexcitation, hyperpyrexia, and seizures, as well as in severe atropinism (Brachfeld et al., 1963; Jarecki, 1963; Goldberg, 1964; Lockett and Milner, 1965). These drugs are antagonistic to the antihypertensive action of guanethidine (Stone et al., 1964; Mitchell et al., 1967). Some preliminary reports suggesting a similar antagonism of the antihypertensive effects of reserpine and alpha-methyldopa (Aldomet) have appeared (White, 1965), but the clinical significance of these effects is not established.

The benzodiazepine antianxiety agents (Librium, Valium, Serax) have enjoyed a relatively benign reputation when used alone, but respiratory depression has been reported when chlordiazepoxide was given to patients intoxicated with other sedatives (Bell, 1969). These drugs also seem to potentiate the anticholinergic effects of the tricyclic antidepressants (Kane and Taylor, 1963; Abdou, 1966). As with other centrally acting agents, alcohol is best avoided during therapy with antidepressants (Landauer et al., 1969).

The tricyclic antidepressants have both direct and indirect effects on cardiovascular physiology. They impair adrenergic neuronal uptake of norepinephrine, rendering the patient potentially sensitive to the effects of norepinephrine; they are also peripheral blockers of alpha-adrenergic-stimulating agents, may cause postural hypotension, and appear to have direct depressant effects on myocardial contractility in addition to the anticholinergic effects that may lead to tachycardia (see Chapter 18).

Large doses of hydrocortisone (Bahr et al., 1970) and methylphenidate (Medical News, 1969) impair hepatic clearance of tricyclic antidepressants. Barbiturates, by stimulating hepatic microsomal enzyme activity, might decrease the effects of the tricyclic antidepressants, but there is considerable individual variation in plasma concentration of drug in patients taking a constant dose, suggesting the possibility of genetic differences in clearance or in antecedent enzyme induction.

Drug Interactions Due to Effects Elicited by a Previously Administered Drug

Drug toxicity may appear as the result of subtle changes induced in the patient by another drug. Thiazide diuretics, by causing potassium loss, may predispose patients to digitalis toxicity. Reserpine depletes myocardial stores of norepinephrine, and bradycardia may be seen when digitalis is given (Roberts et al., 1963). Catecholamine-depleting drugs, such as reserpine or guanethidine, may produce a state of denervation supersensitivity or may interfere with adrenergic neuronal uptake of norepinephrine, making such patients supersensitive to the effects of infused norepinephrine (Dollery, 1965). Propranolol inhibits beta-mediated sympathetic responses and may blunt the cardiovascular response to the hypoglycemia caused by insulin or sulfonylureas (Abramson et al., 1966).

During hormonal replacement in patients with myxedema, the dose of barbiturates and digitalis must be increased to maintain the same therapeutic effect (Doherty and Perkins, 1966). Thyroid replacement therapy promotes catabolism of preformed clotting factors and decreases the dose requirement of anticoagulant drugs that interfere with synthesis of clotting factors (Lowenthal and Fisher, 1957). Antibiotic therapy alters bowel flora that normally synthesize vitamin K and therefore reduces the dose of warfarin needed to induce a given degree of prothrombinopenia. Certain antibiotic combinations, especially those combining a bacteriostatic with a bactericidal agent, may be antagonistic in their antibacterial effect; in most clinical settings, these combinations may be avoided (Wallace et al., 1967; Jawetz, 1968). The onset and termination of action of spironolactone as an aldosterone antagonist are relatively slow, allowing for the induction of hyperkalemia during and for a few days after its use, if large amounts of potassium salts are given. A similar electrolyte abnormality may be seen when heparin is chronically administered, as it also acts as an aldosterone antagonist. Salt substitutes may be rich in potassium ion and may cause hyperkalemia. The potent natriuretic combination of spironolactone and triamterene may frequently elicit hyperkalemia. By altering the metabolism of dexamethasone and metyrapone, diphenylhydantoin may influence the results of tests of adrenal function (Werk et al., 1969; Jubiz et al., 1970).

Drug therapy may alter a patient's responsiveness to other drugs in numerous ways. *Principle: The best operational approach for the physician is to abandon attempts to memorize lists of known incompatibilities in favor of approaching the patient with these questions: (1) How does the patient's disease potentially modify his responsiveness to a drug? (2) Has any therapy influenced the pathophysiologic abnormalities originally present so that the patient's responsiveness to a drug is altered? (3) What are the effects of treatment that are known to alter the patient's physiologic and/or biochemical homeostatic mechanisms? Consideration of these questions can prevent drug interactions.*

This chapter has emphasized the importance of drug interactions that can occur during administration of commonly used drugs. Mechanisms of the interactions and means for detecting and preventing adverse drug interactions have been outlined. Other reviews of drug interactions offer different emphases (Birkenhead, 1965; Gillette, 1967; McIver, 1967; Schrogie, 1968; Stuart, 1968; Block and Lamy, 1969; Dunphy, 1969; Editorial, 1969; Hussar, 1969; Prescott, 1969; Visconti, 1969; Zupko, 1969; Azarnoff and Hurwitz, 1970).

The magnitude and complexity of the problem of drug interactions are illustrated by the recognized interactions involving the oral anticoagulants (Table 16–7) (Kleinman and Griner,

Table 16–7. ORAL ANTICOAGULANT INTER-ACTIONS

Diminished anticoagulant effects

Cholestyramine
Vitamin K
Barbiturates
Ethchlorvynol
Glutethimide
Griseofulvin
Meprobamate
Diphenylhydantoin
Chloral hydrate
Phenylbutazone (late)
Chlorpromazine
Haloperidol
?Antihistamines
?Chlordane, DDT

Enhanced anticoagulant effects

Aspirin, *p*-aminosalicylic acid
Propylthiouracil, methylthiouracil
Quinidine
Acetaminophen
Phenylbutazone (early)
Antibiotics
Oxyphenbutazone, sulfinpyrazone
Phenyramidol
Dextrothyroxine
Levothyroxine
Clofibrate
Androsterone
Chloramphenicol

1970; Robinson and Sylwester, 1970; Sigell and Flessa, 1970; Griner *et al.*, 1971). This long list will undoubtedly lengthen. The physician must keep current, but it is difficult to read all the numerous articles on drug interactions. Review articles are helpful (Morrelli and Melmon, 1968; Robinson and Sylwester, 1970), as are publications such as the *Medical Letter*, *Clinical Alert*, and the Food and Drug Administration *Clinical Experience Abstracts*.

The physician can avoid or detect drug interactions through continual awareness of the possibility of their occurrence, avoidance of multiple-drug therapy whenever possible, and careful monitoring of drug effects when new agents are introduced into a previously stable drug program. If evidence of enhanced or diminished drug activity is seen when another drug is added to or subtracted from a therapeutic regimen, an interaction should be suspected. *Principle: Maintenance of detailed medical records, with a statement about all drugs taken by the patient, including prescriptions by other physicians and proprietary medications, is a necessary step in preventive medicine.*

The number of drugs involved in interactions and their complex interplay with disease states may eventually lend itself to computer methodology. Storage of information on known interactions and the prediction of likely interactions based on the chemical and pharmacologic nature of the drugs in given disease states should be no formidable task for a computer programmer. Given access to such a program, physicians might receive early warning about the potential hazards to be encountered in a wide variety of clinical circumstances. Despite such an innovation, the physician's role remains the same, i.e., his prerogatives in prescribing medications, his ultimate responsibility for his patient's safety, and his efforts in careful clinical observation that lead to the detection of previously unrecognized drug interactions.

REFERENCES

Abdou, F. A.: Elavil-Librium combination. *Amer. J. Psychiat.*, **120**:1204, 1966.
Abrams, W. B.: The mechanisms of action of antihypertensive drugs. *Dis. Chest*, **55**:148–59, 1969.
Abramson, E. A.; Arky, R. A.; and Woeber, K. A.: Effects of propranolol on the hormonal and metabolic responses to insulin-induced hypoglycaemia. *Lancet*, **2**:1386–89, 1966.
Aggeler, P. M., and O'Reilly, R. A.: The pharmacological basis of oral anticoagulant therapy. *Thromb. Diath. Haemorr. Suppl.*, **21**:227–56, 1966.
———: Effect of heptabarbital on the response to bishydroxycoumarin in man. *J. Lab. Clin. Med.*, **74**: 229–38, 1969.
Aggeler, P. M.; O'Reilly, R. A.; Leong, L.; and Kowitz, P. E.: Potentiation of anticoagulant effect of warfarin by phenylbutazone. *New Eng. J. Med.*, **276**:496–501, 1967.
Anthony, M. A., and Louis, D. L.: Apnea due to intramuscular colistin therapy. Report of a case. *Ohio Med. J.*, **62**:336–38, 1966.
Antlitz, A. M., and Awalt, L. F.: A double blind study of acetaminophen used in conjunction with oral anticoagulant therapy. *Curr. Ther. Res.*, **11**:360–61, 1969.
Antlitz, A. M.; Mead, J. A.; and Tolentino, M. A.: Potentiation of oral anticoagulant therapy by acetaminophen. *Curr. Ther. Res.*, **10**:501–507, 1968.
Anton, A. H.: The relation between the binding of sulfonamides of albumin and their antibacterial efficacy. *J. Pharmacol. Exp. Ther.*, **129**:282–90, 1960.
———: A drug induced change in the distribution and renal excretion of sulfonamides. *J. Pharmacol. Exp. Ther.*, **134**:291–303, 1961.
———: The effect of disease, drugs, and dilution on the binding of sulfonamides in human plasma. *Clin. Pharmacol. Ther.*, **9**:561–67, 1968.
Aoki, M.; Kamada, A.; Yata, N.; Kisimoto, K.; Mugino, C.; Sakaguchi, H.; Tanabe, K.; and Mimura, I.: Studies on absorption of drugs. IV. Effects of surface active agents on intestinal absorption of drugs. *Chem. Pharm. Bull.*, **17**:1109–14, 1969.
Areskog, N. H., and Adolfsson, L.: Effects of a cardioselective beta-adrenergic blocker (I.C.I. 50172) at exercise in angina pectoris. *Brit. Med. J.*, **2**:601–603, 1969.
Arky, R. A.; Veverbrants, E.; and Abramson, E. A.: Irreversible hypoglycemia: a complication of alcohol and insulin. *J.A.M.A.*, **206**:575–78, 1968.

Azarnoff, D. L., and Hurwitz, A.: Drug interactions. *Pharmacol. for Physicians*, **4**:1–7, Feb., 1970.

Bahr, C.; Sjoqvist, F.; and Orrhenius, S.: The inhibitory effect of hydrocortisone and testosterone on the plasma disappearance of nortriptyline in the dog and the perfused rat liver. *Europ. J. Pharmacol.*, **9**:106–10, 1970.

Ban, T. A., and St. Jean, A.: The effect of phenothiazines on the electrocardiogram. *Canad. Med. Ass. J.*, **91**:537–40, 1964.

Barlow, M. B., and Groesbeek, A.: Apparent potentiation of neuromuscular block by antibiotics. *S. Afr. Med. J.*, **40**:135–36, 1966.

Barsa, J., and Saunders, J. C.: A comparative study of tranylcypromine and pargyline. *Psychopharmacologia*, **6**:295–98, 1964.

Beckett, A. H.; Kourounakis, P.; Vaughan, D. P.; and Mitchard, M.: The absorption, blood concentrations and excretion of pentazocine after oral, intramuscular, or rectal administration to man. *J. Pharm. Pharmacol.*, **22**:169S–74S, 1970.

Beckett, A. H., and Rowland, M.: Determination and identification of amphetamine in urine. *J. Pharm. Pharmacol.*, **17**:59–60, 1965.

Bell, D. S.: Dangers of treatment of status epilepticus with diazepam. *Brit. Med. J.*, **1**:159–61, 1969.

Birkenhead, Lord C.: Symposium #7: Clinical effects of interactions between drugs. *Proc. Roy. Soc. Med.*, **58**:943–99, 1965.

Blackard, W. G., and Heidingsfelder, S. A.: Effect of adrenergic receptor blockade on nicotinic acid-induced plasma FFA rebound. *Metabolism*, **18**:226–33, 1969.

Block, L. H., and Lamy, P. P.: Drug interactions with emphasis on o-t-c drugs. *J. Amer. Pharm. Ass.*, **NS9**:202–206, 1969.

Blount, R. E.: Management of chloroquine-resistant falciparum malaria. *Arch. Intern. Med. (Chicago)*, **199**:557–60, 1967.

Borda, I. T.; Slone, D.; and Jick, H.: Assessment of adverse reactions within a drug surveillance program. *J.A.M.A.*, **205**:645–47, 1968.

Brachfeld, J.; Wirtshafter, A.; and Wolfe, S.: Imipramine-tranylcypromine incompatibility: near fatal toxic reaction. *J.A.M.A.*, **186**:1172–73, 1963.

Braverman, L. E., and Ingbar, S. H.: Anomalous effects of certain preparations of desiccated thyroid on serum protein-bound iodine. *New Eng. J. Med.*, **270**:439–42, 1964.

Brazil, O. V., and Corrado, A. P.: The curariform action of streptomycin. *J. Pharmacol. Exp. Ther.*, **120**:452–59, 1957.

Brennan, R., *et al.*: Diphenylhydantoin intoxication attendant to slow-inactivation of isoniazid. *Neurology*, **20**:687–93, 1970.

Brodie, B. B.: Displacement of one drug by another from carrier or receptor sites. *Proc. Roy. Soc. Med.*, **58**:946–55, 1965.

Brodie, B. B.; Chang, C. C.; and Costa, E.: On the mechanism of action of guanethidine and bretylium. *Brit. J. Pharmacol.*, **25**:171–78, 1965.

Brook, R.; Schrogie, J. J.; and Solomon, H. M.: Failure of probenecid to inhibit the rate of metabolism of tolbutamide in man. *Clin. Pharmacol. Ther.*, **9**:314–17, 1968.

Brooks, M. H.; Malloy, J. P.; Bartelloni, P. J.; Sheehy, T. W.; and Barry, K. G.: Quinine, pyrimethamine, and sulphorthodimethoxine: clinical response, plasma levels, and urinary excretion during the initial attack of naturally acquired falciparum malaria. *Clin. Pharmacol. Ther.*, **10**:85–91, 1969.

Brown, J. H.; Riggilo, D. A.; and Dungan, K. W.: Oral effectiveness of beta adrenergic antagonists in preventing epinephrine-induced metabolic response. *J. Pharmacol. Exp. Ther.*, **163**:25–35, 1968.

Burns, J. J., and Conney, A. H.: Enzyme stimulation and inhibition in the metabolism of drugs. *Proc. Roy. Soc. Med.*, **58**:955–60, 1965.

Burns, J. J.; Welch, R. M.; and Conney, A. H.: Drug effects on enzymes. *Clin. Pharmacol.*, **2**:67–75, 1967.

Burton, R.; Beli, G. E.; and Huston, J. R.: Water and electrolyte content of the rat heart after thioridazine administration. *J. Clin. Pharmacol.*, **7**:271–74, 1967.

Busfield, D.; Child, K. J.; Atkinson, R. M.; and Tomich, E. G.: An effect of phenobarbitone on blood levels of griseofulvin in man. *Lancet*, **2**:1042–43, 1963.

Bush, G. H.: Antibiotic paralysis. *Brit. Med. J.*, **2**:1062–63, 1962.

Caminetsky, S.: Substitution for brand-name drugs. *Canad. Med. Ass. J.*, **88**:950, 1963.

Carter, A. K.: Substitution for brand-named drugs. *Canad. Med. Ass. J.*, **88**:98, 1963.

Carter, S. A.: Potentiation of the effect of orally administered anticoagulants by phenyramidol hydrochloride. *New Eng. J. Med.*, **273**:423–26, 1965.

Christensen, L. K., and Skovsted, L.: Inhibition of drug metabolism by chloramphenicol. *Lancet*, **2**:1397–99, 1969.

Coldwell, B. B., and Zawidzka, A.: Effect of acute administration of acetylsalicylic acid on the prothrombin activity of bishydroxycoumarin-treated rats. *Blood*, **32**:945–49, 1968.

Comment: Anticoagulants—multiple drug therapy. *Clin. Alert*, No. 165, Aug. 5, 1967.

Conney, A. H.: Pharmacological implications of microsomal enzyme induction. *Pharmacol. Rev.*, **19**:317–66, 1967.

Conney, A. H.; Jacobson, M.; and Schneidman, K.: Induction of liver microsomal cortisol 6β-hydroxylase by diphenylhydantoin or phenobarbital: an explanation for the increased excretion of 6-hydroxycortisol in humans treated with these drugs. *Life Sci.*, **4**:1091–98, 1965.

Consolo, S. F.: An interaction between desipramine and phenylbutazone. *J. Pharm. Pharmacol.*, **20**:574–75, 1968.

Council on Drugs: An antipruritic agent for primary biliary cirrhosis and cholestatic jaundice: cholestyramine resin (Cuemid). *J.A.M.A.*, **197**:261–62, 1966.

Cowell, J. W. F., and Hetenyi, G.: The effect of phenoxybenzamine and propranolol and their combination on the restoration of glucose homeostasis after insulin induced hypoglycemia. *Arch. Int. Pharmacodyn.*, **178**:412–22, 1969.

Crawford, J. S., and Rudofsky, S.: Some alterations in the pattern of drug metabolism associated with pregnancy, oral contraceptives and the newly-born. *Brit. J. Anaesth.*, **38**:446–54, 1966.

Cucinell, S. A.; Conney, A. H.; Sansur, M. S.; and Burns, J. J.: Drug interactions in man. I. Lowering effect of phenobarbital on plasma levels of bishydroxycoumarin (DicumarolR) and diphenylhydantoin (DilantinR). *Clin. Pharmacol. Ther.*, **6**:420–29, 1965.

Cucinell, S. A.; Odessky, L.; Weiss, M.; and Dayton, P. G.: The effect of chloral hydrate on bishydroxycoumarin metabolism: a fatal outcome. *J.A.M.A.*, **197**:366–68, 1966.

Cullen, S. I., and Catalano, P. M.: Griseofulvin-warfarin antagonism. *J.A.M.A.*, **199**:582–83, 1967.

Day, M. D., and Rand, M. J.: Evidence for a competitive antagonism of guanethidine by dexamphetamine. *Brit. J. Pharmacol.*, **20**:17–28, 1963.

Dearborn, E. H.; Litchfield, J. T., Jr.; Eisner, H. J.; Corbett, J. J.; and Dunnett, C. W.: The effect of various substances on the absorption of tetracycline in rats. *Antibiot. Med.*, **4**:627–41, 1957.

DeConti, R. C., and Calabrisi, P.: Use of allopurinol for prevention and control of hyperuricemia in patients with neoplastic disease. *New Eng. J. Med.*, **274**:481–86, 1966.

Desautels, S.; Filteau, C.; and St. Jean, A.: Ventricular tachycardia associated with administration of thioridazine hydrochloride (Mellaril): report of a case with a favourable outcome. *Canad. Med. Ass. J.*, **90**:1030–31, 1964.

Dixon, R. L.; Henderson, E. S.; and Rall, D. P.: Plasma protein binding of methotrexate and its displacement by various drugs. *Fed. Proc.*, **24**:454, 1965.

Doherty, J. E., and Perkins, W. H.: Digoxin metabolism in hypo- and hyperthyroidism. Studies with tritiated digoxin in thyroid disease. *Ann. Intern. Med.*, **64**:489–507, 1966.

Dollery, C. T.: Physiological and pharmacological interactions of antihypertensive drugs. *Proc. Roy. Soc. Med.*, **58**:983–87, 1965.

Dunphy, T. W.: Drug interactions. *Amer. J. Hosp. Pharm.*, **26**:367–77, 1969.

Editorial: Drug interactions. *Amer. J. Pharm.*, **141**:107–108, 1969.

Editorial: Drug interactions—a problem. *J.A.M.A.*, **216**:2005, 1971.

Ehrenpreis, S.; Fleisch, J. H.; and Mittag, T. W.: Approaches to the molecular nature of pharmacological receptors. *Pharmacol. Rev.*, **21**:131–81, 1969.

Eisen, M. J.: Combined effect of sodium warfarin and phenylbutazone. *J.A.M.A.*, **189**:64–65, 1964.

Elias, R. A.: Effect of various drugs on anticoagulant dosage. In Nichol, E. S. (ed.): *Anticoagulant Therapy in Ischemic Heart Disease.* Grune & Stratton, New York, 1965, p. 443.

Elion, G. B.; Callahan, S.; Nathan, H.; Bieber, S.; Rundles, R. W.; and Hitchings, G. H.: Potentiation by inhibition of drug degradation: 6-substituted purines and xanthine oxidase. *Biochem. Pharmacol.*, **12**:85–93, 1963.

Elking, M. P., and Karat, H. F.: Drug induced modifications of laboratory test values. *Amer. J. Hosp. Pharm.*, **25**:484–519, 1968.

Erill, S.: Persistence of the hypoglycemic effect of tolbutamide after block of beta-adrenergic receptors. *Arch. Int. Pharmacodyn.*, **177**:286–89, 1969.

Field, J. B.; Ohta, M.; Boyle, C.; and Remer, A.: Potentiation of acetohexamide hypoglycemia by phenylbutazone. *New Eng. J. Med.*, **277**:889–94, 1967.

Fisk, G. C.: Respiratory paralysis after a large dose of streptomycin: report of a case. *Brit. Med. J.*, **1**:556–57, 1961.

Formiller, M., and Cohon, M. S.: Coumarin and indandione anticoagulants: potentiators and antagonists. *Amer. J. Hosp. Pharm.*, **26**:574–82, 1969.

Fox, S. L.: Potentiation of anticoagulants caused by pyrazole compounds. *J.A.M.A.*, **188**:320–21, 1964.

Freeman, J. W.; Mundy, G. R.; Beattie, R. R.; and Ryan, C.: Cardiac abnormalities in poisoning with tricyclic antidepressants. *Brit. Med. J.*, **2**:610–11, 1969.

Frey, H. H., and Kampmann, E.: Interaction of amphetamine with anticonvulsant drugs. II. Effect of amphetamine on the absorption of anticonvulsant drugs. *Acta Pharmacol. Toxicol.*, **24**:310–16, 1966.

Garrettson, L. K.; Perel, J. M.; and Dayton, P. G.: Methylphenidate interaction with both anticonvulsants and ethyl biscoumacetate. *J.A.M.A.*, **207**:2053–56, 1969.

Garrod, L. P.; James, D. G.; and Lewis, A. A. G.: The synergy of trimethoprim and sulphonamides. *Postgrad. Med. J.*, **45**:Suppl., Nov. 1969.

Gerhardt, R. E.; Knouss, R. F.; Thyrum, P. T.; Luchi, R. J.; and Morris, J. J., Jr.: Quinidine excretion in aciduria and alkaluria. *Ann. Intern. Med.*, **71**:927–33, 1969.

Ghouri, M. S. K., and Haley, T. J.: Structure-activity relationships in the adrenergic-blocking agents. *J. Pharmaceut. Sci.*, **58**:511–38, 1969.

Gillette, J. R.: Theoretical aspects of drug interactions. In Siegler, P. E., and Moyer, J. H., III (eds.): *Animal and Clinical Pharmacological Techniques in Drug Evaluation.* Year Book Medical Publishers, Chicago, 1967, pp. 48–66.

Gold, G. N., and Richardson, A. P., Jr.: An unusual case of neuromuscular blockade seen with therapeutic blood levels of colistin methanesulfonate (Coly-Mycin). *Amer. J. Med.*, **41**:316–21, 1966.

Goldberg, L. I.: Monoamine oxidase inhibitors: adverse reactions and possible mechanisms. *J.A.M.A.*, **190**:456–62, 1964.

Goodman, L. S., and Gilman, A. (eds.): *The Pharmacological Basis of Therapeutics*, 4th ed. The Macmillan Co., New York, 1970.

Goto, S.; Takamatsu, R.; Shibao, M.; and Iguchi, S.: Effect of combination of pharmaceuticals on gastrointestinal absorption. Combination of caffeine with a few absorbable drugs. *Chem. Pharm. Bull.*, **16**:332–37, 1968.

Griner, P. F.; Raisz, L. G.; Rickles, F. R.; Wiesner, P. J.; and Odoroff, C. L.: Chloral hydrate and warfarin interaction: clinical significance? *Ann. Intern. Med.*, **74**:540–43, 1971.

Gwilt, J. R.; Robertson, A.; Goldman, L.; and Blanchard, A. W.: The absorption characteristics of paracetamol tablets in man. *J. Pharm. Pharmacol.*, **15**:445–53, 1963.

Hanahoe, T. H. P.; Ireson, J. D.; and Large, B. J.: Interactions between guanethidine and inhibitors of noradrenaline uptake. *Arch. Int. Pharmacodyn. Ther.*, **82**:349–53, 1969.

Hansen, J. M.; Kristensen, M.; and Skovsted, L.: Sulthiame (Ospolot R) as inhibitor of diphenylhydantoin metabolism. *Epilepsia*, **9**:17–22, 1968.

Hansen, J. M.; Kristensen, M.; Skovsted, L.; and Christensen, L. K.: Dicoumarol-induced diphenylhydantoin intoxication. *Lancet*, **2**:265–66, 1966.

Hayakawa, T.; Kanai, N.; Yamada, R.; Kuroda, R.; Higashi, H.; Mogami, H.; and Jinnai, D.: Effect of steroid hormone on activation of Endoxan (cyclophosphamide). *Biochem. Pharmacol.*, **18**:129–35, 1969.

Hoffbrand, B. I., and Kininmonth, D. A.: Potentiation of anticoagulants. *Brit. Med. J.*, **2**:838–39, 1967.

Hogben, C. A. M.; Tocco, D. J.; Brodie, B. B.; and Schanker, L. S.: On the mechanism of intestinal absorption of drugs. *J. Pharmacol. Exp. Ther.*, **125**:275–82, 1959.

Hollister, L. E., and Kosek, J. C.: Sudden death during treatment with phenothiazine derivatives. *J.A.M.A.*, **192**:1035–38, 1965.

Horwitz, D.; Lovenberg, W.; Engelman, K.; and Sjoerdsma, A.: Monoamine oxidase inhibitors, tyramine, and cheese. *J.A.M.A.*, **188**:1108–10, 1964.

Hunninghake, D. B., and Azarnoff, D. L.: Drug interactions with warfarin. *Arch. Intern. Med. (Chicago)*, **121**:349–52, 1968.

Hussar, D. A.: Tabular compilation of drug interactions. *Amer. J. Pharm.*, **141**:109–56, 1969.

———: The hypoglycemic agents—their interactions. *J. Amer. Pharm. Ass.*, **NS10**:619–24, 1970.

Inglis, J. M., and Barrow, M. E. H.: Premedication, a reassessment. *Proc. Roy. Soc. Med.*, **58**:29–32, 1965.

Jarecki, H. G.: Combined amitriptyline and phenelzine poisoning. *Amer. J. Psychiat.*, **120**:189, 1963.

Jarvik, M. E.: Drugs used in the treatment of psychiatric disorders. In Goodman, L. S., and Gilman, A. (eds.): *The Pharmacologic Basis of Therapeutics*, 3rd ed. The Macmillan Co., New York, 1965, pp. 159–214.

Jawetz, E.: The use of combinations of antimicrobial drugs. *Ann. Rev. Pharmacol.*, **8**:151–70, 1968.

Jubiz, W.; Levinson, R. A.; Meikle, A. W.; West, C. D.; and Tyler, F. H.: Absorption and conjugation of metyrapone during diphenylhydantoin therapy: mechanism of the abnormal response to oral metyrapone. *Endocrinology*, **86**:328–31, 1970.

Kakemi, K.; Sezaki, H.; Hayashi, M.; and Nadai, T.: Absorption and excretion of drugs. XXXVII. Effect of Ca^{++} on the absorption of tetracycline from the small intestine. *Chem. Pharm. Bull.*, **16**:2206–12, 1968.

Kane, F. J., and Taylor, T. W.: A toxic reaction to combined Elavil-Librium therapy. *Amer. J. Psychiat.*, **119**:1179–80, 1963.

Kelly, H. G.; Fay, J. E.; and Laverty, S. G.: Thioridazine hydrochloride (Mellaril): its effect on the electrocardiogram and a report of two fatalities with electrocardiographic abnormalities. *Canad. Med. Ass. J.*, **89**:546–54, 1963.

Kiorboe, E.: Phenytoin intoxication during treatment with AntabuseR (disulfiram). *Epilepsia*, **7**:246–49, 1966.

Kleinman, P. D., and Griner, P. F.: Studies of the epidemiology of anticoagulant-drug interactions. *Arch. Intern. Med. (Chicago)*, **126**:522–23, 1970.

Koelle, G. B.: Neuromuscular blocking agents. In Goodman, L. S., and Gilman, A. (eds.): *The Pharmacologic Basis of Therapeutics*, 3rd ed. The Macmillan Co., New York, 1965, pp. 596–613.

Kotler, M. N.; Berman, L.; and Rubenstein, A. H.: Hypoglycaemia precipitated by propranolol. *Lancet*, **2**:1389–90, 1966.

Kristensen, M., and Hansen, J. M.: Potentiation of the tolbutamide effect by dicoumarol. *Diabetes*, **16**:211–14, 1967.

Kunin, C. M., and Finland, M.: Clinical pharmacology of the tetracycline antibiotics. *Clin. Pharmacol. Ther.*, **2**:51–69, 1961.

Kuntzman, R.: Drugs and enzyme induction. *Ann. Rev. Pharmacol.*, **9**:21–36, 1969.

Kutt, H., and Fouts, J. R.: Diphenylhydantoin metabolism by rat liver microsomes and some of the effects of drug or chemical pretreatment on diphenylhydantoin metabolism by rat liver microsomal preparations. *J. Pharmacol. Exp. Ther.*, **176**:11–26, 1971.

Kutt, H.; Verebely, K.; and McDowell, F.: Inhibition of diphenylhydantoin metabolism in rats and rat liver microsomes by antitubercular drugs. *Neurology*, **18**:706–10, 1968.

Kutt, H.; Winters, W.; and McDowell, F. H.: Depression of parahydroxylation of diphenylhydantoin by antituberculosis chemotherapy. *Neurology*, **16**:594–602, 1966.

Landauer, A. A.; Milner, G.; and Patman, J.: Alcohol and amitriptyline effects on skills related to driving behavior. *Science*, **163**:1467–68, 1969.

Landy, P. G.: "Dilantin" overdosage. *Med. J. Aust.*, **2**:639, 1968.

Lasagna, L.: Drug toxicity in man: the problem and the challenge. *Ann. N.Y. Acad. Sci.*, **123**:312–15, 1965.

Leishman, A. W. D.; Matthews, H. L.; and Smith, A. J.: Antagonism of guanethidine by imipramine. *Lancet*, **1**:112, 1963.

Leonards, J. R., and Levy, G.: Absorption and metabolism of aspirin administered in enteric-coated tablets. *J.A.M.A.*, **193**:99–104, 1965.

Levey, G. S.; Roth, J.; and Pastan, I.: Effect of propranolol and phentolamine on canine and bovine responses to TSH. *Endocrinology*, **84**:1009–15, 1969.

Levy, G.: Effect of dosage from properties on therapeutic efficacy of tolbutamide tablets. *Canad. Med. Ass. J.*, **90**:978–79, 1964.

Levy, G., and Yamada, H.: Drug biotransformation interactions in man. III: Acetaminophen and salicylamide. *J. Pharm. Sci.*, **60**:215–21, 1971.

Lincova, D.; Cernohorsky, M.; Cepelik, J.; and Wenke, M.: Effects of ring-methylated beta-adrenergic blocking agents on isoproterenol-induced free fatty acid mobilization. *Biochem. Pharmacol.*, **17**:2375–80, 1968.

Lindesmith, L. A.; Baines, R. D.; Bigelow, D. B.; and Petty, T. L.: Reversible respiratory paralysis associated with polymyxin therapy. *Ann. Intern. Med.*, **68**:318–27, 1968.

Lockett, M. F., and Milner, G.: Combining the antidepressant drugs. *Brit. Med. J.*, **1**:921, 1965.

Lowenthal, I., and Fisher, L. M.: The effect of thyroid function in the prothrombin time response to warfarin in rats. *Experientia*, **13**:253–54, 1957.

Lu, F. C.; Rice, W. B.; and Mainville, C. W.: A comparative study of some brands of tolbutamide available in Canada. II. Pharmaceutical aspects. *Canad. Med. Ass. J.*, **92**:1166–69, 1965.

Luby, E. D., and Domino, E. F.: Toxicity from large doses of imipramine and an MAO inhibitor in suicidal intent. *J.A.M.A.*, **177**:68–69, 1961.

Lucas, B. G.: Dilantin overdosage. *Med. J. Aust.*, **2**:639–40, 1968.

McIver, A. K.: Drug interactions. *Pharm. J.*, **199**:205–10, 1967.

McKendry, J. B. R.; Lu, F. C.; Bickerton, D.; and Hancharyk, G.: A comparative study of some brands of tolbutamide available in Canada. I. Clinical aspects. *Canad. Med. Ass. J.*, **92**:1106–9, 1965.

Madan, B. R., and Pendse, V. K.: Antiarrhythmic activity of thioridazine hydrochloride (Mellaril). *Amer. J. Cardiol.*, **11**:78–81, 1963.

Mann, A. M., and Hutchison, J. L.: Manic reaction associated with procarbazine hydrochloride therapy of Hodgkin's disease. *Canad. Med. Ass. J.*, **97**:1350–53, 1967.

Mason, A.: Fatal reaction associated with tranylcypromine and methylamphetamine. *Lancet*, **1**:1073, 1962.

Medical News: Stimulant augments antidepressant. *J.A.M.A.*, **208**:1616, 1969.

Meyer, M. C., and Guttman, D. E.: The binding of drugs by plasma proteins. *J. Pharmaceut. Sci.*, **57**:895–918, 1968.

Milne, M. D.: Influence of acid-base balance on efficacy and toxicity of drugs. *Proc. Roy. Soc. Med.*, **58**:961–63, 1965.

Mitchell, J. R.; Arias, L.; and Oates, J. A.: Antagonism of the antihypertensive action of guanethidine sulfate by desipramine hydrochloride. *J.A.M.A.*, **202**:973–76, 1967.

Morrelli, H. F., and Melmon, K. L.: The clinician's approach to drug interactions. *Calif. Med.*, **109**:380–89, 1968.

Murray, F. J.: Outbreak of unexpected reactions among epileptics taking isoniazid. *Amer. Rev. Resp. Dis.*, **86**:729–32, 1962.

Nelson, R. M.; Frank, C. G.; and Mason, J. O.: The antiheparin properties of the antihistamines, tranquilizers, and certain antibiotics. *Surg. Forum*, **9**:146–50, 1959.

Nies, A. S., and Melmon, K. L.: Recent concepts in the clinical pharmacology of antihypertensive drugs. *Calif. Med.*, **106**:388–99, 1967.

Northcutt, R. C.; Stiel, J. N.; Hollifield, J. W.; and Stant, E. G.: The influence of cholestyramine on thyroxine absorption. *J.A.M.A.*, **208**:1857–61, 1969.

O'Dell, G. B.: Studies in kernicterus. I. The protein binding of bilirubin. *J. Clin. Invest.*, **38**:823–33, 1959.

Ogilvie, R. I., and Ruedy, J.: Adverse drug reactions during hospitalization. *Canad. Med. Ass. J.*, **97**:1445–50, 1450–57, 1967.

Olesen, O. V.: Disulfiram (AntabuseR) as inhibitor of phenytoin metabolism. *Acta Pharmacol. Toxicol.*, **24**:317–22, 1966.

————: The influence of disulfiram and calcium carbimide on the serum diphenylhydantoin. *Arch. Neurol. (Chicago)*, 16:642–44, 1967.

O'Reilly, R. A.; Nelson, E.; and Levy, G.: Physicochemical and physiologic factors affecting the absorption of warfarin in man. *J. Pharmaceut. Sci.*, 55:435–37, 1966.

Parisi, A. F., and Kaplan, M. H.: Apnea during treatment with sodium colistimethate. *J.A.M.A.*, 194:298–99, 1965.

Payne, J. P., and Rowe, G. G.: The effects of mecamylamine in the cat as modified by the administration of carbon dioxide. *Brit. J. Pharmacol.*, 12:457–60, 1957.

Peaston, M. J. T., and Finnegan, P.: A case of combined poisoning with chlorpropamide, acetylsalicylic acid and paracetamol. *Brit. J. Clin. Pract.*, 22:30–31, 1968.

Pelissier, N. A., and Burgee, S. L., Jr.: Guide to incompatibilities. *Hosp. Pharm.*, 3:15–32, 1968.

Pohlmann, G.: Respiratory arrest associated with intravenous administration of polymyxin B sulfate. *J.A.M.A.*, 196:181–83, 1966.

Potter, W. Z.; Zaharko, D. S.; and Beck, L. V.: Possible role of hydrazine group in hypoglycemia associated with the use of certain monoamine-oxidase inhibitors (MAOI's). *Diabetes*, 18:538–41, 1969.

Prescott, L. F.: Pharmacokinetic drug interactions. *Lancet*, 2:1239–43, 1969.

Pridgen, J. E.: Respiratory arrest thought to be due to intraperitoneal neomycin. *Surgery*, 40:571–74, 1956.

Ream, C. R.: Respiratory and cardiac arrest after intravenous administration of kanamycin with reversal of toxic effects by neostigmine. *Ann. Intern. Med.*, 59:384–87, 1963.

Roberts, J.; Ito, R.; Reilly, J.; and Carioli, V. J.: Influence of reserpine and beta TM 10 on digitalis induced ventricular arrhythmia. *Circ. Res.*, 13:149–58, 1963.

Robinson, D. S., and Sylwester, D.: Interaction of commonly prescribed drugs and warfarin. *Ann. Intern. Med.*, 72:853–56, 1970.

Schamberg, I. L.: Therapeutic equivalence of prescription drugs. *J. Clin. Pharmacol.*, 9:205–16, 1969.

Schoonmaker, F. W.; Osteen, R. T.; and Greenfield, J. C., Jr.: Thioridazine (Mellaril^R)-induced ventricular tachycardia controlled with an artificial pacemaker. *Ann. Intern. Med.*, 65:1076–78, 1966.

Schrogie, J. J.: Drug interactions. FDA Papers, U.S. Department of Health, Education, and Welfare, Washington, Nov., 1968.

Schrogie, J. J., and Solomon, H. M.: The anticoagulant response to bishydroxycoumarin. II. The effect of D-thyroxin, clofibrate and norethandrolone. *Clin. Pharmacol. Ther.*, 8:70–77, 1967.

Seller, R. H.: Idiopathic orthostatic hypertension. Report of successful treatment with a new form of therapy. *Amer. J. Cardiol.*, 23:838–44, 1969.

Selzer, A., and Wray, H.: Paroxysmal ventricular fibrillation occurring during treatment of chronic atrial arrhythmias: quinidine syncope. *Circulation*, 35:17–26, 1964.

Sigell, L. T., and Flessa, H. C.: Drug interactions with anticoagulants. *J.A.M.A.*, 214:2035–38, 1970.

Silverman, W. A.; Andersen, D. H.; Blane, W. A.; and Crozier, D. N.: A difference in mortality rate and incidence of kernicterus among premature infants allotted to two prophylatic antibacterial regimens. *Pediatrics*, 18:614–25, 1956.

Simberkoff, M. S.; Thomas, L.; McGregor, D.; Shenkein, I.; and Levine, B. B.: Inactivation of penicillins by carbohydrate solutions at alkaline pH. *New Eng. J. Med.*, 283:116–19, 1970.

Simmons, M.; Parker, J. M.; Gowdy, C. W.; and Coulter, W. K.: Adverse drug reactions during hospitalization. *Canad. Med. Ass. J.*, 98:175, 1968.

Sjoqvist, F.: Psychotropic drugs. II. Interaction between monoamine oxidase (MAO) inhibitors and other substances. *Proc. Roy. Soc. Med.*, 58:967–78, 1965.

Smith, J. W.; Seidl, L. G.; and Cluff, L. E.: Studies on the epidemiology of adverse drug reactions. V. Clinical factors influencing susceptibility. *Ann. Intern. Med.*, 65:629–40, 1966.

Solomon, H. M.; Barakat, M. J.; and Ashley, C. J.: Mechanisms of drug interaction. *J.A.M.A.*, 216:1997–99, 1971.

Solomon, H. M., and Schrogie, J. J.: The effect of phenyramidol on the metabolism of diphenylhydantoin. *Clin. Pharmacol. Ther.*, 8:554–56, 1967.

Solymoss, B.; Varga, S.; Krajny, M.; and Werringloer, J.: Influence of spironolactone and other steroids on the enzymatic decay and anticoagulant activity of bishydroxycoumarin. *Thromb. Diath. Haemorrh.*, 23:562–68, 1970.

Sorby, D. L., and Liu, G.: Effects of adsorbents on drug absorption. II. Effect of an antidiarrhea mixture on promazine absorption. *J. Pharm. Sci.*, 55:504–10, 1966.

Sotaniemi, E.; Arvela, P.; Hakkarainen, H.; and Huhti, E.: The clinical significance of microsomal enzyme induction in the therapy of epileptic patients. *Ann. Clin. Res.*, 2:223–27, 1970.

Stone, C. A.; Porter, C. C.; Stavorski, J. M.; Ludden, C. T.; and Totaro, J. A.: Antagonism of certain effects of catecholamine-depleting agents by antidepressant and related drugs. *J. Pharmacol. Exp. Ther.*, 144:196–204, 1964.

Stowers, J. M.; Constable, L. W.; and Hunter, R. B.: A clinical and pharmacological comparison of chlorpropamide and other sulfonylureas. *Ann. N.Y. Acad. Sci.*, 74:689–95, 1959.

Strauch, G.; Modigliani, E.; and Bricaire, H.: Growth hormone response to arginine in normal and hyperthyroid females under propranolol. *J. Clin. Endocr.*, 29:606–608, 1969.

Stuart, D. M.: Drug metabolism. I. Basic fundamentals. II. Drug interactions. *Pharmindex*, Sept. and Oct., 1968.

Vance, J. E.; Buchanan, K. D.; O'Hara, D.; Williams, R. H.; and Porte, D.: Insulin and glucagon responses in subjects with pheochromocytoma: effects of alpha adrenergic blockade. *J. Clin. Endocr.*, 29:911–16, 1969.

van Dam, E. E.; Overkamp, M.; and Haanen, C.: The interaction of drugs. *Lancet*, 2:1027, 1966.

Vere, D. W.: Errors of complex prescribing. *Lancet*, 1:370–73, 1965.

Vesell, E. S.; Passananti, G. T.; and Greene, F. E.: Impairment of drug metabolism in man by allopurinol and nortriptyline. *New Eng. J. Med.*, 283:1484–88, 1970.

Visconti, J. A.: Use of drug interaction information in patient medication records. *Amer. J. Hosp. Pharm.*, 26:378–87, 1969.

Waddell, W. J., and Butler, T. C.: The distribution and excretion of phenobarbital. *J. Clin. Invest.*, 36:1217–26, 1957.

Wagner, J. G.: Biopharmaceutics: absorption aspects. *J. Pharm. Sci.*, 50:539–87, 1961.

Wallace, J. F.; Smith, R. H.; Garcia, M.; and Petersdorf, R. G.: Studies on the pathogenesis of meningitis. VI. Antagonism between penicillin and chloramphenicol in experimental pneumococcal meningitis. *J. Lab. Clin. Med.*, 70:408–18, 1967.

Wattenberg, L. W.; Leong, J. L.; and Galbraith, A. R.: Induction of increased benzapyrene hydroxylase activity in pulmonary tissue *in vitro*. *Proc. Soc. Exp. Biol. Med.*, 127:467–69, 1968.

Weiner, I. M.: Mechanisms of drug absorption and excretion. The renal excretion of drugs and related compounds. *Ann. Rev. Pharmacol.*, **7**:39–56, 1967.

Weiner, I. M.; Washington, J. A., III; and Mudge, G. H.: On the mechanism of action of probenecid on renal tubular secretion. *Bull. Johns Hopkins Hosp.*, **106**:33–46, 1960.

Weiner, M.: Effect of centrally active drugs on the action of coumarin anticoagulants. *Nature*, **212**:1599–1600, 1966.

Welch, R. M.; Harrison, Y. E.; and Burns, J. J.: Implications of enzyme induction in drug toxicity studies. *Toxicol. Appl. Pharmacol.*, **10**:340–51, 1967.

Werk, E. E., Jr.; Choi, Y.; Sholiton, L.; Olinger, C.; and Haque, N.: Interference in the effect of dexamethasone by diphenylhydantoin. *New Eng. J. Med.*, **281**:3234, 1969.

White, A. G.: Methyldopa and amitriptyline. *Lancet*, **2**:441, 1965.

Wilkenfeld, B. E., and Levy, B.: Adrenergic blocking properties of MJ 1999 and butoxamine on cardiac vascular beta-receptors. *Arch. Int. Pharmacodyn.*, **176**:218–32, 1968.

Wishinsky, H.; Glasser, E. J.; and Perkal, S.: Protein interactions of sulfonylurea compounds. *Diabetes*, **2** (Suppl):18–25, 1962.

Wolinsky, E., and Hines, J. D.: Neurotoxic and nephrotoxic effects of colistin in patients with renal disease. *New Eng. J. Med.*, **266**:759–62, 1962.

Zauder, H. L.; Barton, N.; Bennett, E. J.; and Lore, J.: Colistimethate as a cause of postoperative apnoea. *Canad. Anaesth. Soc. J.*, **13**:607–10, 1966.

Zubrod, C. G.; Kennedy, T. J.; and Shannon, J. A.: Studies on the chemotherapy of human malarias. VIII. The physiological disposition of pamaquine. *J. Clin. Invest.*, **27**:114–20, 1948.

Zupko, A. G.: A new professional responsibility—drug interactions, I. *Pharmacy Times*, Sept.-Oct., 1969.

Chapter 17

RATIONAL THERAPY OF DRUG OVERDOSAGE

Howard F. Morrelli

Prompt, accurate diagnosis and precise management of patients intoxicated by therapeutic agents afford the clinician a relatively uncommon opportunity in medicine, i.e., to completely reverse a moribund state. Even if the overdose is intentionally taken, appropriate therapy and psychiatric treatment may have gratifying results (Fahy *et al.*, 1970; Ianzito, 1970).

This chapter describes the unique manifestations of poisoning with selected drugs and demonstrates the process used to evaluate clinical literature and to make therapeutic decisions. It attempts to explain intoxicated states in pathophysiologic, pharmacologic, and pharmacokinetic terms. Emphasis on the general principles of diagnosis and treatment of intoxication in relation to selected agents may provide an approach that is more broadly applicable to other drugs and toxic substances. This approach illustrates how rational therapeutic maneuvers are developed and applied to treat the patient as a whole, to manage specific toxic symptoms, and to enhance clearance of the drug, if the latter is possible and necessary. It is more important to learn the process or method of approach to the problem than to memorize details. Facts such as the pK_a or polarity of a drug can be found

quickly in reference material. The use of examples in this chapter is solely to demonstrate the applicability of general principles. *Learn the principles or reasons for the conclusions drawn as demonstrated by the use of data. Certain types of data are keys to proper therapeutic decisions. If the reasons for using the data are clear and the derived principles useful, the physician will obtain the data when necessary.*

GENERAL MEASURES TO SUSTAIN LIFE

Successful therapy of poisoned patients largely depends on the physician's ability to provide expert supportive care. Most of this chapter dwells on specifics of individual drugs, to demonstrate how to acquire and utilize information in therapy, but general measures to keep the patient alive are equally crucial determinants of the outcome of therapeutic interventions. Given the theoretical alternatives of access to good patient monitoring systems versus precise information about the type and dose of central nervous system depressants ingested, experienced clinicians would pick the former. If the patient lives, he eventually metabolizes and/or excretes the drug. The best results in patients poisoned with barbiturates have been obtained by supportive care alone (Henderson and Merrill, 1966).

Poisoning with drugs commonly causes coma, seizures, respiratory depression, and/or shock. Coma should not cause great alarm; anesthesiologists induce it regularly. The principles of management learned in the operating suite are eminently applicable to drug-induced coma. An adequate airway must be ensured, with ventilation supported artificially as dictated by arterial pCO_2 and pO_2 measurements. To prevent aspiration pneumonia and atelectasis, endotracheal intubation, pulmonary toilet, and intermittent full inflation of the lungs are required. The eyes should be protected from trauma, and artificial tear fluid should be used if tearing is suppressed. Compression injuries of peripheral nerves must be avoided, and the patient must be frequently "turned" to prevent decubitus ulcers (Mandy and Ackerman, 1970). If coma is prolonged, physical therapy should be employed to prevent joint deformities. Careful attention to leg wrapping may reduce the incidence of venous stasis, phlebothrombosis, and pulmonary embolism. Fluid and electrolyte therapy must be tailored to the needs of the individual patient and followed by daily measurement of weight, volume of urine, and serum electrolytes. Simultaneous determinations of serum and urinary osmolality may be indicated if inappropriate secretion of antidiuretic hormone is suspected (Bartter and Schwartz, 1967). Stimulant drugs to lessen coma are generally best avoided, as their efficacy is slight and the hazard of inducing seizures is substantial (Myschetzky, 1961). After ingestion of most depressant drugs, coma lasts a day or two; intensive supportive care should prevent the sequelae of coma in most patients (Nilsson and Eyrich, 1950; Clemmesen, 1954; Thorstrand, 1965).

If seizures occur, etiologies other than direct drug effect (e.g., inadequacy of cerebral perfusion, hypoxemia, respiratory alkalosis, or hypoglycemia) should be considered. The literature contains relatively little information on treatment of drug-induced seizures. In theory, barbiturates that add to central nervous system depression should be avoided. Even diazepam may synergize with other depressants, producing respiratory arrest or hypotension (Bell, 1969). If diphenylhydantoin is used, large loading doses given in small intravenous increments should be utilized, analogous to therapy for cardiac arrhythmias (Bigger et al., 1968) (see Chapter 5).

Hypotension in poisoning may have complex etiologies. The patient's blood volume and state of hydration should be evaluated early and measured frequently. If fullness of neck veins is difficult to evaluate, the central venous pressure may be monitored as a guide to adequacy of volume replacement. If the drug has direct depressant effects on the myocardium, rises in the pulmonary artery pressure may be a more sensitive indicator of early left-sided heart failure than the central venous pressure. If the blood pressure is difficult to measure by auscultation, an arterial catheter manometer may be helpful. Optimally, measurements of cardiac output and peripheral vascular resistance should guide therapy.

If volume and hydration are adequate, the decision to increase blood pressure depends on whether tissue perfusion is adequate. In comatose patients, symptoms of cerebrovascular insufficiency or angina are absent, but decreases in the patient's hourly urine output and increasing differences between the arterial and mixed central venous pO_2 remain as signs of poor perfusion (see Chapter 5). Poor tissue perfusion leads to acidosis with decreasing concentrations of serum CO_2-combining power (usually referred to as $HCO_3{}^-$), and if the respiratory center, carotid or aortic bodies, and respiratory muscle function are intact, hyperventilation with decreasing pCO_2 may result. During acidosis or hypotension, the pCO_2 serves as a guide to adequacy of therapy. Lactic acidosis may appear in this setting and has a high mortality rate unless treated early (Tranquada, 1964). Treatment of metabolic acidosis in shock is discussed in Chapter 3.

Additional clues to the severity of the hypotension include signs of sympathetic nervous system overactivity: pallor, cold extremities, cyanosis of digits due to stasis, pupillary dilation, tachycardia, decrease in bowel sounds, and sweating. Because drug intoxication may mimic or mask some of these findings, critical signs may sometimes be lacking.

The blood pressure is determined by the cardiac output and the peripheral vascular resistance. When the cardiac output declines, signs of overactivity of the sympathetic nervous system may appear. Warm extremities and a bounding cardiac apical impulse may indicate that the hypotension is mostly due to a decrease in the peripheral vascular resistance. It would be advantageous and it is sometimes mandatory to have readily available means for measuring cardiac output and peripheral vascular resistance. Assuming normality of the blood volume, beta-adrenergic stimulators to increase cardiac output or alpha-adrenergic stimulators to increase peripheral vascular resistance may be necessary, depending on the physiologic defect present (see Chapter 5 for a more complete discussion of the treatment of shock).

Acute renal failure, as manifested by oliguria, may occur despite response of shock to therapy. Urine abnormalities and a progressive rise in serum concentrations of creatinine and blood urea nitrogen should be detected early to alert the physician to the possibility of volume overload and the potential need for dialysis (Bluemle et al., 1959; Franklin and Merrill, 1960; Maher and Schreiner, 1961; Schreiner, 1970; Simon and Krumlovsky, 1971).

Principle: The physician's natural fascination with the intricacies of the pharmacology of a toxic drug and the possible ways of removing it should not diminish his attention to the all-important details of caring for the intoxicated patient. Fortunately, the body can eliminate most drugs in a predictable length of time. Any intervention aimed at shortening this time carries with it predictable risks. Only by weighing the risks of intervention against those of coma can rational decisions be made. After treatment or prevention of the immediately life-threatening symptoms of respiratory arrest, shock, and renal failure, a sequence of questions should be posed and answered as fully as possible:

1. What has been ingested (one or more drugs, dose, dose form, etc.)?

2. How serious is the intoxication?

  a. Clinical status of the patient (depth of coma, respiratory depression, etc.).

  b. Alleged dose intake, blood concentration of drug.

  c. Intrinsic "lethality" of the drug (mortality among intoxicated patients).

3. What are the characteristic toxic and unique effects of the agent, and the therapy of such effects (tendency for the drug to cause specific derangements such as respiratory alkalosis or arrhythmias)?

4. Can and/or should the drug be removed from the patient (gastric lavage, diuresis, dialysis)?

5. Are there any features of the patient that may modify the course of the intoxication or its therapy (hepatic, renal or cardiac disease, etc.)?

SALICYLATE INTOXICATION

What Has Been Ingested?

Voluntary reports to the *National Clearinghouse for Poison Control Centers* described 107,000 ingestions of salicylate in 1967. The true incidence of ingestions is undoubtedly greater. In children less than 5 years of age (86% of the cases voluntarily reported), accidental intake was blamed, whereas in teen-agers and adults more than half the ingestions were allegedly volitional (Crotty, 1968).

Salicylate intoxication is most commonly due to ingestion of acetylsalicylic acid (aspirin). Intoxications with salicylic acid, sodium salicylate, phenylsalicylate, or methylsalicylate (oil of wintergreen) are relatively rare. Oil-of-wintergreen ingestion is particularly feared by pediatricians, probably because a large dose of salicylate is usually taken in this form of intoxication (Done, 1965).

The dosage form of ingested salicylate is a determinant of its rate of gastrointestinal absorption. Liquid effervescent mixtures and buffered tablets are absorbed more quickly than are plain tablets (Leonards, 1963). After intake of therapeutic doses of aspirin, peak levels in plasma are seen in 30 to 60 minutes. Enteric-coated tablets of aspirin vary widely in the rate and completeness of absorption. Occasionally, a lag phase as long as 20 hours is seen before absorption is complete (Levy and Hollister, 1964). Some aspirin tablets are relatively insoluble, forming an aspirin mass that serves as a continuing source for aspirin absorption (Done, 1965; Matthew *et al.*, 1966). These last two situations are suggested when serum salicylate concentrations do not fall (or even rise) long after ingestion; this finding would obviously influence therapeutic interventions. *Principle: The dose form of a drug is a determinant of the clinical condition of the patient* (see Chapter 2).

Although acetylsalicylic acid and sodium salicylate have somewhat different pharmacologic effects (Samter, 1969), sodium salicylate is too irritating for oral use. During gastrointestinal absorption and as a result of plasma esterase activity, acetylsalicylic acid is deacetylated to salicylate within an hour. Accordingly, by the time most patients who have taken acetylsalicylic acid are seen medically, their toxic manifestations are due to salicylate. In rare circumstances, slow absorption might conceivably permit a continuing level of acetylsalicylate.

How Serious Is the Intoxication?

Clinical Status of the Patient. Salicylate intoxication during the course of therapeutic administration of aspirin may differ from that seen after single toxic doses. The therapeutic dose of aspirin is near its toxic dose. Since the elimination of this drug is dose dependent, i.e., the half-life of the drug is progressively longer at higher tissue and blood concentrations of the drug, toxic doses may accumulate on a fixed-dosage regimen. In adults, this process would likely be recognized by the onset of hyperpnea and tinnitus, and severe toxicity would be avoided. In infants and young children, these symptoms could be elusive, allowing development of more severe metabolic and electrolyte abnormalities. In acute poisonings, even in children less than 4 years of age, metabolic acidosis usually appears about 12 hours after respiratory alkalosis (Done, 1965). These considerations and findings lend credence to the empiric observations of clinicians that young children chronically poisoned are even sicker than children acutely intoxicated. *Principle: The course and severity of poisoning are influenced not* *only by dose, but also by chemical form and concentration of the drug, formulation for administration, and the acute or chronic circumstances of its development.*

Alleged Dose Intake. Initial attempts to correlate blood concentrations of salicylate obtained on admission with the degree of severity of intoxication and the eventual outcome of the patient were unsatisfactory. A more reliable correlation was found between outcome and estimates of the probable concentration of drug shortly after ingestion (Done, 1960). At conventional therapeutic doses of aspirin, the half-life of salicylate is approximately 2 to 5 hours. After toxic doses of the drug (10 to 20 g), the half-life of salicylate is nearly 20 hours. Utilizing the half-life appropriate for poisoning, one can calculate the approximate concentration of drug in blood shortly after ingestion with the formula:

$$\log S_0 = \log S_1 + 0.015\,T$$

where S_0 is the early concentration of salicylate; S_1, the first observed salicylate concentration; T, the time interval in hours since ingestion of the drug; and 0.015, a factor to correct for the loss of salicylate in the time between ingestion and hospitalization.

Utilizing this correction factor, the following correlations between S_0 and clinical severity have been derived (Done, 1960):

S_0	SEVERITY
50 mg/100 ml	Not intoxicated
50 to 80 mg/100 ml	Mildly intoxicated
80 to 110 mg/100 ml	Moderately intoxicated
110 to 160 mg/100 ml	Severely intoxicated
160 mg/100 ml	Usually lethal

This calculation does not take into account changes in clearance (half-life) imposed by renal disease, continuing gastrointestinal absorption of residual drug, or the effects of interventions to promote salicylate clearance (e.g., induction of an alkaline diuresis). In addition to the influence on rate of clearance of very high concentrations in blood, young children clear similar doses of the drug more slowly than do adults (Done, 1962, 1965). In infants 4 to 8 months old, a salicylate half-life of 30 hours has been found (Done, 1965). Some authors have suggested the possibility that very high salicylate levels diminish the clearance capacity for salicylates on the basis of enzyme inhibition (Sturman *et al.*, 1968). *Principle: Predictions of clinical course and anticipated changes in laboratory data must be made on the basis of available tools, but*

deviations from the "rules" occur and require exploration and explanation, lest important diagnostic considerations or therapeutic steps be omitted.

Intrinsic "Lethality" of the Drug. Although aspirin overdose may be lethal, most patients need either no hospitalization, or hospitalization for only a day or two (Crotty, 1968). Prolonged treatment is usually not required only because relatively small doses are ingested, since there is good correlation between estimated initial blood levels and mortality. Operationally, the clinician should assume the worst and should attend his patient closely until the course of events permits him to act otherwise.

What Are the Characteristic Toxic and Unique Effects of the Drug, and the Therapy of Such Effects?

Respiratory Alkalosis; Metabolic Acidosis. The acid-base status to be expected in patients with salicylate intoxication is not clearly defined in the literature, presumably because (1) physicians tended to report on patients of different ages, i.e., children vs. adults; (2) timing of observations varied in relation to the patient's course and severity of intoxication, with failure to compare similar patients at similar times; (3) tools in the past have been relatively inadequate to evaluate acid-base balance; (4) the distinctions were not made between acute and chronic toxicity; and (5) other disease processes were not considered.

Observation of the patient is more critical to therapy than are clinical rules of thumb, such as "infants and young children are almost always acidotic; older children and adults are almost always alkalotic." The clinical rule is generally true: In adults, the effect of salicylate on the respiratory center (induction of a profound respiratory alkalosis) almost always outweighs the metabolic effects of the drug (increased acid formation). In infants and young children, at least later in the course of salicylate intoxication, the metabolic generation of acid exceeds the capacity of the lungs, kidneys, and buffer systems, resulting in acidosis (Done, 1965). Acidosis may be seen in older children and adults (Proudfoot and Brown, 1969), but it is sufficiently uncommon that its presence should alert clinicians to the possibility of complicating renal disease or chronic toxicity. The acid-base status of the individual patient must be defined by measurement of arterial pH and pCO_2. An adult with serum electrolytes of sodium, 143 mEq per liter; potassium, 3.5 mEq per liter; bicarbonate, 15 mEq per liter; and chloride, 98 mEq per liter; and a urinary pH of 5.0 could have respiratory alkalosis with paradoxical aciduria (discussed below) or lactic acidosis! Arterial blood pH and pCO_2 measurements quickly distinguish between these states.

Arterial pH is a much better test than concentrations of serum electrolytes to discriminate between metabolic acidosis and respiratory alkalosis. Since the therapy of these disorders is so different, the distinction must be made precisely. *Principle: Diagnosis of a suspected abnormality must be confirmed by the most sensitive techniques available.*

Attempts to control respiratory alkalosis by increasing the pCO_2 of inspired air or by using anesthetics or barbiturates to decrease respiratory center sensitivity are not well tolerated or recommended (Smith and Smith, 1966). Animals intoxicated with salicylates are sensitive to the depressant effects of barbiturates (Rapaport and Guest, 1945; Coldwell and Solomonraj, 1968), suggesting danger in the use of these drugs. Correction of metabolic acidosis is discussed in the section on salicylate clearance.

Water Balance. Patients with salicylate intoxication may have profound degrees of dehydration due to water loss via vomiting, sweating, fever, and hyperpnea. The extent of the water deficit may be masked by concomitant sodium loss, with a relatively normal serum electrolyte "panel" resulting from combined depletion. Clinical signs of dehydration, e.g., poor tissue turgor, dry mucous membranes (other than oral, because of the hyperpnea), flat neck veins, high urinary specific gravity, and an elevated hematocrit, may provide clues to the degree of dehydration. As an alkaline diuresis may be desirable in therapy of salicylate intoxication, water losses must be fully corrected. When clinical signs are equivocal, the central venous pressure can be monitored as a guide to volume replacement.

Sodium Balance. Sodium losses in salicylate intoxication appear as a consequence of vomiting, sweating, or a therapeutic diuresis. The degree of loss and guides for adequacy of replacement are similar to those for water balance.

Potassium Balance. In addition to loss of potassium via vomiting and sweating, renal potassium losses may be great as a consequence of respiratory alkalosis, sodium depletion, and/or dehydration (Mudge et al., 1950; Robin et al., 1959; Beveridge et al., 1964). Total-body potassium stores cannot be estimated on the basis of the serum potassium alone, as there is no necessary correlation between the two values. Alkalosis is usually associated with hypokalemia as potassium enters cells; the converse applies during acidosis. Measurements of total-body potassium (radioactive potassium space)

in states of potassium depletion have shown a range of potassium depletion of 1 to 10 mEq potassium/kg body weight. An acidotic patient with hypokalemia would probably be at the upper end of this spectrum, for purposes of gross estimation of deficits (Moore et al., 1953; Maffly and Edelman, 1961). The electrocardiogram may be utilized both to approximate the severity of potassium deficits and to serve as a monitor of replacement rates. At the high intravenous rates of potassium replacement that may be required in salicylate intoxication, the electrocardiogram must be monitored frequently or continually.

Urinary pH. Insufficient stress has been placed on the influence of salicylate intoxication on urinary pH. The finding of paradoxical aciduria is common in salicylate intoxication (Robin et al., 1959; Done, 1965). The inappropriate secretion of an acid urine is probably a combined result of respiratory alkalosis, sodium depletion, and potassium depletion (Schwartz and Relman, 1967). Correction of the aciduria by bicarbonate administration alone may be hazardous and difficult (Done, 1968). Continuing sodium and potassium deficiencies favor the renal secretion of acid, and correction of these deficiencies helps to attain an alkaline diuresis. In sodium and/or potassium depletion states, the unavailability of these ions in the distal tubules of the kidney may necessitate renal losses of hydrogen to accompany poorly reabsorbed anions (phosphates, sulfates, etc.). Repletion of sodium and potassium ions may be the key to achieving an alkaline diuresis. Alkalinization of the urine, even in patients with moderately severe respiratory alkalosis, has been accomplished with bicarbonate, without aggravation of the alkalosis (Cumming et al., 1964). Frequent determinations of arterial pH are required during this form of therapy. The role of urine pH in salicylate clearance is discussed below.

Other Disorders in Salicylate Intoxication. In addition to the major problems in acid-base and fluid-electrolyte balance, a variety of other disorders may appear in salicylate intoxication, including (1) hyperthermia as a function of increased metabolic rate, and (2) appearance of an "anion gap" in acidotic patients (particularly children); i.e., the remainder between the sum of sodium and potassium and the sum of bicarbonate and chloride ($[Na^+ + K^+] - [HCO_3^- + Cl^-]$) is greater than the usual value of 15 mEq and is probably due to accumulation of organic acids, as high concentrations of salicylates may inhibit enzymatic activity of the Krebs cycle (Winters, 1963).

In very high doses, salicylates may cause bleeding by direct effects on vessels and blood platelets, or by inhibiting synthesis of blood-clotting factors (Smith and Smith, 1966). Bleeding is uncommon in salicylate poisoning, but in testing the patient's prothrombin time the physician must remember that the clotting factor with the shortest "half-life" is factor VII (4 to 6 hours). Depression of prothrombin time may not appear for 24 to 36 hours, even if synthesis of clotting factors is completely inhibited, and depression is reversible with vitamin K_1. Chronic intoxication may be a more likely setting for prothrombinopenia.

Evidence of mild renal damage, with small amounts of urinary protein and increased numbers of renal tubular cells, is relatively non-specific. Acute renal failure may be due to decreased renal perfusion and is not necessarily evidence of direct salicylate nephrotoxicity (Smith and Smith, 1966).

Pulmonary edema has been reported in salicylate intoxications, particularly in patients with rheumatic fever carditis or other underlying heart disease. This could be related to the sodium-retaining properties of the drug seen with chronic intake or to excessive sodium replacement in therapy of acute poisoning (Smith and Smith, 1966). Severe acidosis shifts blood from the peripheral to the central circulation and might favor the appearance of pulmonary edema.

Can the Drug Be Removed from the Patient?

Induction of Emesis and Gastric Lavage. It is surprising that the efficacy of these manipulations has not been established in humans. Emesis or lavage fluid has not been analyzed sufficiently often for salicylate content, particularly in relation to ingested dose, to establish the efficiency of the procedures (Done, 1968; Levy and Yaffe, 1968; Done, 1969). Studies in animals have shown superiority of induced emesis to gastric lavage, but the clinical relevance of these experimental studies (and similar studies done with a variety of drugs) is obscured by the contrast between the early induction of emesis by drugs and the relatively long time required for gastric lavage (Arnold et al., 1959; Abdallah and Tye, 1967; Corby et al., 1967). The experimental induction of emesis shortly after ingestion is not comparable to the usual clinical setting of a lag time between ingestion and therapy.

Apomorphine appears to be a more potent emetic than ipecac in puppies and seems to act more rapidly in humans, but may have central nervous system depressant effects that make its use less desirable (Robertson, 1962; Berry and Lambdin, 1963; Sturkey, 1966; Corby et al.,

1967; Done, 1968). Mechanically induced emesis is less effective than drug-induced vomiting (Dabbous et al., 1965). The "course record" for salicylate removal by any method appears to be 20,340 mg of aspirin, by lavage, 9 hours after ingestion (Matthew et al., 1966). In normal volunteers, a greater reduction in serum salicylate was obtained by oral-activated charcoal and apomorphine than with either therapy given alone, but the therapy was given 30 minutes after intake of aspirin (Decker et al., 1969).

Aspirin delays gastric emptying time, and occasionally considerable aspirin may be removed, either by induction of emesis or by gastric lavage, while protecting the comatose patient from aspiration of emesis fluid. *Principle: Gastric lavage or drug-induced emesis seems advisable, if the patient can be protected from aspiration pneumonia. The basis for this procedure rests more on the rare-to-occasional recovery of large quantities of drug than on verification of its routine efficacy by studies in man.*

Measures to Enhance the Renal Clearance of Salicylate. After gastrointestinal absorption of acetylsalicylic acid and its conversion to salicylate, the drug is cleared by conjugation with glycine or with phenolic and glucuronic acids or is excreted unchanged in the urine. After an aspirin dose of 0.3 g, only 2 to 5% appears unchanged in the urine.

When the amount of salicylate in the body is more than 0.3 g, the capacity to form salicyluric acid is exceeded. The half-life for elimination gradually increases with dose; at very high doses it approaches 20 hours and elimination occurs almost exclusively by urinary excretion of unaltered salicylate (Levy and Matsuzawa, 1967).

The measured excretion of unchanged salicylate is the net effect of glomerular filtration of plasma water, active secretion of drug into proximal tubular fluid, and passive reabsorption in the distal convoluted tubules. When passive reabsorption exceeds the first two processes, no salicylate appears in the urine.

Important determinants of the tubular reabsorption of salicylate are the urinary pH and the urine flow rate. The driving force for reabsorption of salicylate is the difference between the concentration of nonionized drug in the luminal fluid and that in the peritubular blood vessels, since nonionized drugs cross cell membranes quickly and ionized drugs slowly (see Chapter 2). The pK_a of salicylate is 3.0. As urinary pH increases from 5.0 to 8.0, the fraction of ionized salicylate increases, decreasing tubular reabsorption and increasing urinary excretion of salicylate. At urine pH less than 6.0, salicylate is almost completely reabsorbed; increasing the urine pH from 7.0 to 8.0 increases the excretion rate fivefold (MacPherson *et al.*, 1955). Superficially, one might not predict that a small change in urine pH would have such a profound effect on salicylate clearance, since the percentage of ionized salicylate (pK_a 3.0) changes little in the pH shift from 7.0 to 8.0. Although the change in percentage is small, the amount of salicylate filtered and secreted into tubular urine is so great that the quantity subject to excretion is large (see Chapter 2).

Since the proportion of salicylate bound to plasma albumin decreases with high concentrations of the drug, the amount available for glomerular filtration increases. Alkalinization of the tubular urine "traps" ionized salicylate in tubular urine and promotes its clearance. At urine pH 8.0, the renal clearance of salicylate is greater than inulin clearance (Gutman *et al.*, 1955), a finding that confirms the importance of glomerular filtration, renal tubular secretion of salicylate into tubular urine, and the ionic "trapping" effect (see Chapter 2).

The clinical efficacy of alkaline diuresis as a maneuver to enhance salicylate clearance has been shown (Cumming *et al.*, 1964). Concerns about the potential hazards of aggravating a pre-existent respiratory alkalosis by bicarbonate therapy are reasonable, and appropriate serial monitoring of arterial blood pH is an important prerequisite to this form of therapy. *Principle: Detailed knowledge about the pharmacokinetics of a drug may allow rational therapeutic interventions.*

The central nervous system symptoms arising from metabolic acidosis could transiently worsen during parenteral alkalinizing therapy. The pCO_2, pH, and bicarbonate concentrations of arterial blood increase simultaneously during alkalinization therapy. Since CO_2 is diffusible into cerebrospinal fluid much more quickly than bicarbonate, cerebrospinal fluid pH may *diminish* after parenteral administration of bicarbonate (Posner and Plum, 1967). The lag phase between arterial blood and cerebrospinal fluid equilibria of bicarbonate and pH also accounts in part for the tendency of acidotic patients to continue to hyperventilate after arterial pH is restored to normal. If a patient's acidosis is corrected fully and quickly by parenteral bicarbonate therapy, an alkalosis may ensue.

Carbonic-anhydrase-inhibiting drugs (e.g., acetazolamide) alkalinize the urine successfully (Schwartz *et al.*, 1959; Feuerstein *et al.*, 1960), but have the theoretic disadvantages of increasing urinary sodium losses, causing neurologic disturbances, and, in effect, imposing a drug-induced disease (renal tubular acidosis) in the patient being treated for intoxication. *Principle: When a disorder can be recognized, and its pathophysiologic changes identified with fair certainty, as in the case of salicylate intoxication (the recognition of sodium, water, and potassium deficiency with an acid-base abnormality), a direct therapeutic approach is more attractive than the imposition of another pharmacologic change in the patient.*

Similarly, although one osmotically active drug, tromethamine (THAM), has been reported to increase the renal clearance of salicylate (Strauss, 1968), osmotic diuretics may cause pulmonary edema or renal damage; the buffering effect of tromethamine is poor compared to that of bicarbonate therapy (Bleich and Schwartz, 1966). The use of osmotic diuretics alone, without simultaneous attempts to alkalinize the urine, fails to enhance salicylate clearance, as salicylate clearance remains almost constant at different flow rates of persistently acid urine (Done, 1968).

One cannot take the position that proper fluid and electrolyte therapy is unequivocally superior to alkalinization of the urine with acetazolamide or tromethamine, since a controlled clinical trial has not compared the efficacy and toxicity of these methods. In fact, controlled series have not verified the assumption that enhancing clearance of the drug reduces morbidity or mortality. Since the undesirable metabolic effects of salicylates appear late in the course of intoxication, their appearance could possibly be prevented or reduced by removing the drug. Pending controlled trials that disprove the efficacy of maneuvers to enhance salicylate clearance, one may justifiably induce an alkaline diuresis in patients with moderate to severe intoxication unless complications or other disease states necessitate dialysis.

Other Means of Salicylate Clearance. Exchange blood transfusion, peritoneal dialysis with and without additives to "trap" salicylate in the dialysis fluid, and extracorporeal hemodialysis have been advocated for therapy of salicylate intoxication (as well as for intoxication with other drugs) (Adams *et al.*, 1957; Radebaugh and Emery, 1957; Spritz *et al.*, 1959; Elliot and Crichton, 1960; Ettledorf *et al.*, 1961; James *et al.*, 1962; Summitt and Ettledorf, 1964; Smith and Smith, 1966; Done, 1968; Mattocks, 1969).

These maneuvers may be necessary in patients with poor renal function, refractory shock, or congestive heart failure, or in situations when electrolyte balance otherwise is difficult to obtain. The usual response to alkaline diuresis probably warrants reservation of these dramatic and potentially harmful procedures for special circumstances. Some of the studies cited above were done in animals; in the laboratory setting, complicated dialysis techniques may be initiated shortly after intoxication. The clinical availability of methods to initiate an alkaline diuresis is generally much greater than the ability to begin hemodialysis or peritoneal dialysis with special additives. *Principle: Methods of detoxification must be critically analyzed for their relevance to clinical circumstances.*

Other Considerations of the Patient with Salicylate Intoxication That May Influence Therapy

Renal Disease, Shock, and Congestive Heart Failure. Patients have been mentioned as candidates for dialytic therapy because of impaired renal clearance mechanisms and/or difficulties in achieving the desired changes in acid-base and fluid-electrolyte balance. Hemodialysis is a formidable technical problem in infants; hence peritoneal dialysis is preferred (Done, 1968).

Diabetes. Salicylate intoxication may induce hypoglycemia, most commonly in infancy (Done, 1968). Diabetic patients taking oral hypoglycemic agents can develop hypoglycemia even while taking therapeutic doses of salicylates (Cherner *et al.*, 1963).

Bleeding Disorders. The bleeding defect of von Willebrand's disease is aggravated by salicylates (Quick, 1969; Samter, 1969). Hemophiliacs or patients taking anticoagulants may bleed after taking aspirin (Kaneshiro *et al.*, 1969; Packham and Mustard, 1969).

Aspirin poisoning is common and may be lethal. The severity of the intoxication may be estimated by calculating the blood concentration of salicylate present shortly after ingestion, based on the time lag between ingestion and initial observation of the patient. Laboratory tests should determine the degree of the known pathophysiologic and biochemical abnormalities induced by salicylates, and these disorders should be corrected directly. Based on the pharmacokinetic data provided, induction of an alkaline diuresis or a dialysis procedure should be considered in all but mildly intoxicated patients. Similar considerations should be applied to almost all intoxications.

BARBITURATE INTOXICATION

What Has Been Ingested?

Important differences in prognosis and therapeutic interventions are found among intoxica-

tions with the barbiturates. Emergency management of coma with respiratory depression and/or shock is standard for the group, but interventions to enhance clearance of the drug from the patient are quite variable in their efficacy. Patients who suicidally ingest barbiturates often combine the drug with other depressants, particularly alcohol (Henderson and Merrill, 1966). The toxic effect of barbiturates plus alcohol may be more than simply additive (McKown *et al.*, 1963). Blood alcohol determinations are usually available and should be included in toxicologic screening procedures. *Principle: Identification of a single intoxicant does not exclude effects of other drugs.*

The increasing availability of psychoactive agents makes it likely that intoxications with multiple agents will increase. Shock, hypothermia, pulmonary edema, and bradycardia may suggest meprobamate intoxication (Davis *et al.*, 1968). Parkinsonian neurologic features, orthostatic hypotension, signs of cholinergic blockade, and electrocardiographic changes with a prolonged Q-T interval suggest the presence of a phenothiazine drug (Hollister, 1966; Brophy, 1967). Mydriasis, dry mouth, intestinal ileus, bladder atony, and tachycardia are compatible with the cholinergic blockade characteristic of severe glutethimide intoxication (Sharpless, 1965). A period of agitation, delirium, and/or seizures antecedent to the comatose phase, cholinergic blockade, and cardiac arrhythmias may suggest the presence of a tricyclic antidepressant (Davis *et al.*, 1968). Striking increases in motor activity, hallucinations, diaphoresis, and hyperpyrexia, particularly if associated with hypertension, should suggest intoxication with monoamine oxidase inhibitors or amphetamine (Matthew *et al.*, 1966). The admixture of clinical signs due to several drugs may make the precise recognition of these drugs difficult. Physicians should know common combinations of drugs that are used for intentional overdose or are used in clinical settings that can lead to or are commonly associated with intoxication. When these patterns are known, the therapist can anticipate the alteration in the course, the appearance of unusual complications, and the need to modify therapeutic measures created by additional drugs.

How Serious Is the Intoxication?

Clinical Signs. A classification (page 613) of intoxication (slightly modified) has been suggested as a guide to therapeutic interventions and prognosis (Henderson and Merrill, 1966).

Emergency therapy of hypoxia and hypercapnea, or restoration of the blood pressure to

SEVERITY OF INTOXICATION	CHARACTERISTICS
0	Asleep, but can be aroused and can answer questions
I	Semicomatose, withdraws from painful stimuli, reflexes intact
II	Comatose, does not withdraw from painful stimuli, no respiratory or circulatory depression, most reflexes intact
III	Comatose, most or all reflexes absent, but without depression of respiration or circulation
IV	Comatose, reflexes absent. Respiratory depression with cyanosis or circulatory failure and shock, or both

normal by replacement of volume, may result in prompt improvement in the patient in the same way as in the patient with salicylate poisoning. Acute respiratory acidosis increases the quantity of the ionized form of barbiturate in blood and allows the intracellular accumulation of the drug, where it exerts its effects. Correction of the respiratory acidosis favors extracellular movement of the drug and lightens coma. Conversely, continuing gastrointestinal absorption of the drug, particularly after intestinal ileus is corrected, may deepen coma later in the course of the intoxication. Serial observations of the patient are required to detect this process. *Principle: There are several potential determinants of depth of coma in barbiturate intoxications. Profound coma may be a stimulus to utilize aggressive measures to promote drug clearance.*

Alleged Dose Intake and Serum Concentration of the Drug. Fatal doses for some barbiturates have been given as phenobarbital, 5.0 g; barbital, 10.0 g; pentobarbital and secobarbital, 3.0 g (Berman *et al.*, 1956). Frequently, the ingested dose is unknown, and when combinations of drugs have been taken, one cannot be reassured by a "small" dose of barbiturate. There is a very poor correlation between blood concentrations of barbiturates on admission to the hospital and length of coma (Henderson and Merrill, 1966). However, extrapolation of the observed blood concentration of drug on admission to the concentration predicted shortly after ingestion can be attempted for phenobarbital, based on a plasma disappearance rate of 0.7% per hour (Fazekas *et al.*, 1956). Extrapolation is not as successful as with salicylates, as the pK_a of phenobarbital is 7.24, allowing for major variation in the ionized/nonionized ratio of drug within the range of pH values seen

clinically. Changes in pH may significantly alter brain concentration of barbiturate, the crucial determinant of depth and duration of coma (Waddell and Butler, 1957). Further, chronic administration of barbiturates may alter the central nervous system responsiveness to barbiturates and results in the induction of hepatic microsomal enzymes that accelerate barbiturate's metabolism to its inactive metabolites (Burns and Conney, 1965). In the case of short-acting barbiturates, the extrapolation of observed blood level to time "zero" blood level would probably be even less worthwhile. The pK_a of pentobarbital is 7.96, making the fraction of nonionized drug much less susceptible to major changes within the range of arterial pH compatible with life. The short-acting barbiturates have much higher protein-binding affinity and lipid solubility, which favors their entry into cells regardless of pH partitioning effects. Furthermore, a commonly used laboratory assay procedure for the short-acting barbiturates fails to distinguish between active drug and inactive metabolite (Bloomer, 1965). *Principle: Knowledge of a drug's chemical nature and its pharmacokinetic behavior is essential to an understanding of the clinical significance of concentrations of a toxic substance in blood.*

Despite the limitations in prognostic value of barbiturate concentrations in blood, serial determinations of blood barbiturate may be helpful in identifying those patients who have ingested other depressant drugs (very deep coma, but low blood barbiturate level) or those who have continuing gastrointestinal absorption (unchanging or increasing concentrations) or may provide clues to the presence of otherwise obscure hepatic, renal, or thyroid disease.

Intrinsic "Lethality" of the Drug. How does one evaluate prognosis and the need for special forms of intervention? The mortality of comatose patients with barbiturate intoxication has been reported from 1.0 to 12.7% (Plum and Swanson, 1957; Ferguson and Grace, 1961; Maher *et al.*, 1962). It is difficult to assign "lethality" to a drug, particularly when coma is prolonged, since the complications in comatose patients (e.g., infection) may be the determinants of eventual outcome. The most conservative programs employed in treatment are associated with greater survival (Hadden *et al.*, 1969). Strong inferences from these results cannot be made, as too many other variables, such as ancillary therapy and availability of intensive-care units, would render an uncontrolled comparison invalid. In relative terms, the lethality of glutethimide intoxication appears to be greater than that of barbiturates (Maher *et al.*,

1962), whereas relatively few deaths ensue in phenothiazine intoxication (Davis *et al.*, 1968).

What Are the Characteristic Toxic and Unique Effects of the Agent, and the Therapy of Such Effects?

Central Nervous System. Depression may be profound, accounting for hypothermia, coma, and respiratory depression. The depression is dose dependent and, for the longer-acting agents such as phenobarbital, is related in part to pH gradient-determined partitioning of drug into cells. Redistribution of phenobarbital may be accomplished by alkalinization of extracellular fluids. Attempts to reverse the central nervous system depression with stimulant drugs have been abandoned on the basis of excessive induction of seizures, with postictal depression (Myschetzky, 1961). Unless shock is present, cerebral blood flow and oxygen consumption are normal in barbiturate intoxication (Malmlund, 1968). EEG monitoring should be employed when available to follow patients (Haider *et al.*, 1971).

Cardiovascular System. The cardiovascular response to barbiturate intoxication is complex and probably involves central and autonomic nervous system effects, as well as possible direct depressant effects on peripheral vessels and myocardial contractility. Very high concentrations of barbiturates in blood are necessary to demonstrate the latter effect in animals (Price, 1960). In addition, hypotension associated with barbiturate administration may be related to vasodilation rather than to myocardial depression (MacCannell, 1969). In man, blood volume replacement is usually sufficient to restore the blood pressure. The merits and liabilities of alpha- and beta-stimulating and blocking drugs in the management of shock are discussed in Chapter 5. Pulmonary and cerebral edema may appear in the course of severe barbiturate intoxication, but little is known about their pathophysiologic bases; therefore, treatment is supportive.

Renal Response to Barbiturate Intoxication. Barbiturates directly inhibit renal tubular reabsorption of sodium. However, they also release antidiuretic hormone, and the hypotensive effects of the drug tend to diminish renal perfusion and may elicit acute tubular necrosis. These competing effects of the drug make it necessary to assess the patient's blood volume and serum electrolyte concentrations in order to properly treat the hypotension and oliguria.

Can and/or Should the Drug Be Removed from the Patient?

Phenobarbital. Extracorporeal dialysis, peritoneal dialysis, or alkaline diuresis with or without osmotic agents enhances the clearance of pharmacologically active drug. Clearance rates have been given as 33 to 43 ml per minute and 48 to 72 ml per minute for extracorporeal dialysis, 12.6 ml per minute for peritoneal dialysis, and 17 ml per minute for alkaline osmotic diuresis (Kyle *et al.*, 1953; Sunshine and Leonards, 1954; Berman *et al.*, 1956; Dobos *et al.*, 1961; Ohlsson and Fristedt, 1962; Myschetzky and Lassen, 1963; Berman and Vogelsang, 1964; Knochel *et al.*, 1964). Theoretically, removal of active drug should shorten the length of coma and improve survival. However, the lowest mortality rates reported in barbiturate intoxication are by those investigators who used conservative measures alone (Nilsson and Eyrich, 1950; Clemmesen, 1954). The discrepancy between various reports could be due to hazards imposed by the dialysis procedures themselves (Maher and Schreiner, 1965) and could reflect less satisfactory conservative maneuvers during dialysis, or a combination of the tendencies of both treatment and drug to cause a common complication (e.g., both barbiturate intoxication and peritoneal dialysis predispose to pulmonary atelectasis). Furthermore, the patients treated by these different interventions may not be comparable. Theoretically, the safest method (probably alkaline diuresis) should logically be preferred to the more dramatic interventions of peritoneal or extracorporeal dialysis. These constraints have no pertinence in severe renal failure, shock, massive intoxication, cardiac failure, and perhaps severe liver disease, in which other considerations (including compromised barbiturate clearance) affect the therapeutic decision. The clearance of phenobarbital follows first-order pharmacokinetics; i.e., the amount cleared in a unit of time is proportional to tissue and blood concentrations of drug and, barring complications, considerable drug is cleared early. When dialysis is tested in animals, the procedure is begun immediately or shortly after drug administration and is highly efficient in removing a large percentage of drug. These data may not be fairly extrapolated to the clinical setting, where considerable time ordinarily elapses between drug intake and hemodialysis. In many clinical settings it may be far easier and quicker to initiate an alkaline diuresis than to await hemodialysis.

Clearly, the decision to utilize any procedure to rid the patient of phenobarbital is open to question. In very severely intoxicated patients, one might argue that shortening of coma's duration or prevention of the severe cardiovascular sequelae of very high concentrations of phenobarbital in blood justifies the risks of the available methods, but studies in comparable patients are required to prove the contention. *Principle: Even the most attractive theoretic considerations and data obtained from animal studies must be verified for efficacy and lack of toxicity in man prior to their acceptance.*

Pentobarbital and Amobarbital. Clearance rates for extracorporeal and peritoneal dialysis of these drugs are reportedly similar to those for phenobarbital (Kyle *et al.*, 1953; Sunshine and Leonards, 1954; Berman *et al.*, 1956; Berman and Vogelsang, 1964; Knochel and Barry, 1965). This finding is inconsistent with the known differences in the chemical nature of these drugs. The short-acting barbiturates are less polar and have higher affinity constants for protein, and their pK_as do not favor pH partitioning. In fact, the studies reporting favorable clearance rates for pentobarbital and amobarbital contained a systematic error. The methodology for measurement of drug did not distinguish between active drug and inactive drug metabolite. The clearance of inactive drug metabolite is enhanced by the interventions, but not clearance of the drug itself (Bloomer, 1965). In retrospect, the efficacy ascribed to dialytic therapy for intoxication with short-acting barbiturates may have been based on methodologic error and observer bias. Current clinical reports of the therapeutic efficacy of dialytic procedures for other psychoactive agents must be scrutinized in the light of this experience. *Principle: Therapeutic interventions must be confirmed in the appropriate clinical context by controlled studies.*

Some form of dialysis may be in order for some patients intoxicated with short-acting barbiturates, but a means for identifying these patients is needed. When gas-liquid chromatographic or thin-layer chromatographic analyses become more available to clinicians, perhaps patients can be found who have sufficiently high blood concentrations of unaltered drug to merit the institution of dialysis. Lacking these procedures, the therapist must weigh the available evidence carefully. Even the most aggressive may do well to recall the words of Thomas Hardy:

And ill it therefore suits
The mood of one of my high temperature
To pause inactive while await me means
Of desperate cure for these so desperate ills!
The Dynasts, Part 1, Act IV, scene iii

The conservative position in regard to dialysis should not preclude the use of this intervention in massively intoxicated patients (Linton *et al.*, 1964; Maher and Schreiner, 1968). Even in this setting, however, one should attempt to assay dialysis fluid for unaltered drug by the most specific methods available, to verify the efficacy of the procedure (Teehan *et al.*, 1970; Mandelbaum and Simon, 1971).

Features of the Patient That May Modify the Course of the Intoxication or Its Therapy

Most patient features that may modify the intoxication or its therapy have been cited in the preceding discussion (e.g., the use of dialytic therapy in patients with either poor renal function, congestive heart failure, or possibly severe liver disease). Hypothyroid patients metabolize some drugs more slowly than do normal patients. Hypothermia slows the rate of drug metabolism (Kalser *et al.*, 1969). Chronic drug intake allows the development of central nervous system tolerance to the depressant effects of barbiturates and induces hepatic microsomal enzyme systems that normally metabolize barbiturates. The chronic intake of barbiturates or glutethimide may result in a state of drug dependency, and withdrawal manifestations may be seen as the patient recovers from the intoxication if the drug is abruptly discontinued.

OTHER COMMON INGESTANTS: PSYCHOACTIVE AGENTS

Certain data are useful in making therapeutic decisions in the management of other common intoxications. Psychoactive agents are chosen for review because they are commonly used, not because they present unique problems in management. When treating intoxication, the physician should first obtain the answers to the questions listed in the outline previously discussed. He should then consider the principles of the approach common to all intoxications, seek helpful information, avoid the pitfalls of therapeutic decision based on irrelevant data, and measure whether his maneuvers are actually helpful in accomplishing his objective.

Glutethimide

In 1966, 2,882,000 prescriptions for glutethimide (Doriden) were written for patients 65 years of age or older (Task Force on Prescription Drugs, 1968). The drug is no more efficacious than barbiturates or other sedatives, it has dependency liability, and the mortality rate of patients taking 20 tablets or more has been 45% (Maher *et al.*, 1962). Glutethimide was introduced as a drug with less toxicity and addiction liability than the barbiturates. Although these initial claims were refuted, glutethimide still sells well. The data on its adverse effects have apparently eluded or failed to impress practitioners. Perhaps the availability of some of the newer sedatives that thus far have been free of dependency liability and impressive lethality will erode the glutethimide market, even if only by the promotional efforts for the new drugs.

Hypotension seems to be particularly important in glutethimide intoxication. The central nervous system depression fluctuates. This effect could result from late gastrointestinal absorption of the drug owing to its limited solubility, from reversal of ileus seen as a consequence of the atropinic effects of the drug, or even from the drug's substantial enterohepatic circulation.

Glutethimide is nonpolar and enters cells quickly, accounting both for its rapid onset of action and for the difficulty in its removal by water dialysis (Kier et al., 1958; Schreiner et al., 1958; Chandler et al., 1959; Barbour, 1960; Goldbaum et al., 1962; Maher et al., 1962; Maher and Schreiner, 1961; McDonald et al., 1963). The lipid solubility of the drug has led to attempts to enhance its clearance by use of oily dialysis fluids (Shinaberger et al., 1965; Ginn et al., 1968). An interesting approach has been to hemoperfuse through a charcoal column to remove the drug (De Myttenaere et al., 1967).

In reviewing the literature bearing on dialysis treatment of glutethimide intoxication, one should recall the early results with dialysis of the short-acting barbiturates. Do the methods used for drug assay discriminate between active drug and its metabolite? Would oil dialysis across a *cellophane* membrane be more efficient than water dialysis?

Although there are favorable reports on the efficacy of water and oil dialysis procedures, these interventions have utilized either spectrophotometric determination or thin-layer chromatographic assay for the drug (Shinaberger et al., 1965; Graeme, 1968; Rejent and Klendshoj, 1968). Gas-liquid chromatography is more sensitive and specific than the methods utilized thus far in clinical studies (Gary et al., 1968). Pending even more rigorous demonstration that dialysis procedures remove unaltered drug, the questions in the preceding paragraph must remain open (Chazan and Cohen, 1969).

The fraction of glutethimide excreted into the bile as the glucuronide conjugate may possibly return to the patient as *free* glutethimide, if gastrointestinal flora can deconjugate the drug-glucuronide complex. This possibility should be quantitated because if it is substantial, catharsis and/or antibiotic suppression of gastrointestinal flora may be an efficacious means of enhancing drug clearance (Keberle et al., 1962; Charyton, 1970; Maher, 1970). This speculation is not intended to stimulate the therapist to embark on such a treatment program. However, the information can be employed to devise experimental models for therapy based on an interesting aspect of the pharmacokinetics of the drug and can later be applied in the clinical setting if preliminary work warrants.

Glutethimide poisoning differs in important ways from barbiturate intoxication; glutethimide causes cholinergic blockade and has different pharmacokinetic behavior. These factors account for the unusual clinical manifestations of poisoning and its course and determine the feasibility of possible maneuvers to rid the patient of excess drug. *Principle: Agents given for identical therapeutic goals may have different toxic potential; this factor must be considered in selection of drugs.*

Meprobamate

In 1966, for patients 65 years of age or older, 770,000 prescriptions for meprobamate were written; simultaneously, 2,035,000 prescriptions for the somewhat more expensive Equanil, and 885,000 prescriptions for the most expensive equivalent, Miltown, were written (Task Force on Prescription Drugs, 1968).

Nearly 700 cases of meprobamate intoxication have been reported (Davis et al., 1968). The average dose taken in severe intoxications was listed as 12.7 g, or about 30 of the larger tablets. Patients with meprobamate overdose may have hypotension, bradycardia, hypothermia, shock, and pulmonary edema (Davis et al., 1968).

Meprobamate is dialysable, and dialysis may be considered in patients with very severe intoxication and serious hepatic or renal disease (Dyment et al., 1965; Maddock and Bloomer, 1967; Mouton et al., 1967). The spontaneous clearance is approximately 8.5 mg/100 ml per hour, a much faster rate than that of barbiturates or glutethimide (Maddock and Bloomer, 1967); this fact should be kept in mind when considering dialysis.

Benzodiazepines

Toxicologic experience with these drugs, chlordiazepoxide (Librium), diazepam (Valium), and oxazepam (Serax), has been relatively limited and relatively benign. These agents have been available for a shorter time than the drugs described above, but they are sold in large quantities (Task Force on Prescription Drugs, 1968). Chlordiazepoxide has an unusually long half-life, with high concentrations remaining in blood 24 hours after administration of a large oral dose (Randall, 1961). Although intoxication with chlordiazepoxide has been benign compared to that with other psychoactive agents (Zbinden et al., 1961; Hollister, 1965; Brophy,

1967), the drug may synergize with other central nervous system depressants to cause respiratory arrest or hypotension (Bell, 1969).

Some authors have suggested that in view of the long half-life of the drug in plasma, dialysis should be used to shorten the duration of coma in patients with chlordiazepoxide intoxication (Hollister, 1965). One patient who had ingested several depressant drugs underwent hemodialysis with a reduction in blood chlordiazepoxide level from about 2.5 mg/100 ml to 1.0 mg/100 ml in 10 hours (Cruz et al., 1967). The latter authors were unable to lower blood concentrations of chlordiazepoxide in dogs by hemodialysis, and the dialysis fluid in the patient reported revealed no chlordiazepoxide (the assay used was sensitive to 0.1 mg/ml). Assuming the concentration of chlordiazepoxide in the dialysis fluid was just below this figure, one may calculate the volume of dialysis fluid necessary to remove 100 mg of drug: 1000 liters! Chlordiazepoxide can cross a cellophane membrane (Haig et al., 1967), but the relevance of this in vitro finding to clinical settings remains unestablished. In uncomplicated cases, the symptoms are mild and duration of coma is relatively short. Conservative therapy is recommended until definitive studies of the efficacy of dialysis are available.

Phenothiazines

Since therapy of coma induced by the phenothiazines differs little from that of other drugs, and since the mortality of phenothiazine intoxication may be more importantly related to complications of coma and to the cardiovascular effects of these agents, the student is referred to other sources for general descriptions of phenothiazine intoxication (Hollister, 1965; Davis et al., 1968). In brief, patients intoxicated with phenothiazines may have a period of agitation, hyperactivity, or seizures prior to the depressed state, particularly if they have ingested one of the less sedative phenothiazines such as fluphenazine (Prolixin), perphenazine (Trilafon), or trifluoperazine (Stelazine) (Barker and Kerr, 1960; Cilliers, 1960; Campbell, 1961; Chicoine, 1961; Beighton and Wilkinson, 1967). Mortality in phenothiazine intoxication has been relatively low and occasionally is caused by an unanticipated late "respiratory arrest" (possibly due to unrecognized cardiac arrest).

Parkinsonian symptoms or more severe extrapyramidal reactions may occur even after relatively small doses of phenothiazines. The more severe reactions may cause great discomfort, resembling tetanus. These symptoms ordinarily respond to conventional antiparkinsonian agents such as benztropine (Cogentin) or

trihexyphenidyl (Artane) (Gunn and Goldman, 1967; Simpson and Angus, 1970). Acute, severe reactions may dramatically respond to parenteral diphenhydramine (Benadryl). If diphenhydramine is given intravenously, this must be done slowly, with electrocardiographic monitoring, as the drug may induce arrhythmias. The antiparkinsonian agents and antihistaminic drugs have atropine-like effects that may add to those of the phenothiazines.

Even at therapeutic doses, phenothiazines may cause orthostatic hypotension (Curry et al., 1970a). Hypotension and tachycardia may be seen after intravenous administration. These effects are thought to be related to central effects of the drug, direct depressant effects on the myocardium and vasculature, and alphaadrenergic blockade (Jarvik, 1965). If hypotension complicates the course of a patient intoxicated with a phenothiazine, and if the patient does not respond to volume replacement and the recumbent position, pressor therapy may be required. Selection of the pressor agent requires some thought. Alpha-mimetic (vasoconstrictor) effects are desired; accordingly norepinephrine or methoxamine (Vasoxyl) is appropriate. If one were to give an agent with both alpha-mimetic- and beta-mimetic-stimulating properties during alpha-adrenergic blockade, only the beta (vasodilatory) effects might be manifested and hypotension might result. Drugs such as epinephrine or metaraminol (Aramine) should be avoided.

Sudden death has occurred during therapy with phenothiazine drugs and has been attributed to "respiratory arrest." Ventricular tachycardia similar to that induced by quinidine has been seen in patients intoxicated with phenothiazines (Kelly et al., 1963; Madan and Pendse, 1963; Ban and St. Jean, 1964; Desautels et al., 1964; Selzer and Wray, 1964; Hollister, 1965; Schoonmaker et al., 1966; Burton et al., 1967; Feder, 1967). The electrocardiogram should be examined for increases in the Q-T and QRS intervals. If ventricular tachycardia develops, it should be treated in a manner analogous to quinidine-induced ventricular tachycardia (see Chapter 5). *Principle: Search for signs of all the known pharmacologic effects of a drug in intoxicated states.*

Phenothiazines are rapidly absorbed from the gastrointestinal tract and are highly bound to plasma proteins (Curry et al., 1970b). The liver produces a number of metabolites whose pharmacologic activity is unknown. The metabolites are excreted principally via the biliary system, where they may enter an enterohepatic cycle. Relatively little drug appears in the urine. These characteristics suggest that hemodialysis and peritoneal dialysis would be ineffective in removing the drug. If enhanced renal clearance is sought, assuming that a renal tubular secretion mechanism is available for phenothiazines analogous to that proved for the organic base chlorprothixene (Taractan), an *acid* diuresis might be worthy of trial. Phenothiazines are weak bases, and acidification of tubular urine might "trap" poorly reabsorbed ionized drug in the urine. Regrettably, the only report on diuretic therapy for phenothiazine toxicity found only 16 mg of drug in 7.5 liters of urine obtained during a 17-hour period (Beighton and Wilkinson, 1967). This study, however, utilized a means of diuresis that resulted in *alkalinization* of the urine (Lee and Ames, 1965). The utility of induction of an acid diuresis, or of enhancement of gastrointestinal losses of the drug, remains to be evaluated and should be compared to simple supportive care. *Principle: "Negative" results in a therapeutic trial must be scrutinized as closely as "positive" results to verify the conclusions drawn.*

Dibenzazepines (Tricyclic Antidepressants)

This category of drugs includes imipramine (Tofranil), amitriptyline (Elavil), nortriptyline (Aventyl), desipramine (Norpramin), and protriptyline (Vivactil). Severe to fatal intoxications with imipramine and amitriptyline have been caused by intake of 1 to 3 g of drug (Davis *et al.*, 1968).

These compounds are highly nonpolar and have pK_a values of approximately 8 to 9 (Bickel and Weder, 1969). The drugs are metabolized by hepatic microsomal enzymes, and only a small percentage of unaltered drug appears in the urine. There is as much as a tenfold variation in the plasma concentration of drug among individuals taking the same dose. The individual variation in drug clearance may be due to genetic differences in hepatic microsomal enzyme activity (Hammer *et al.*, 1969). It may be difficult to estimate the severity of intoxication in an individual patient on the basis of ingested quantity of drug alone. In addition, some patients may become comatose shortly after ingestion, or as long as 6 hours later (Ayd, 1969). Accordingly, it may be impossible to predict the ultimate severity of the intoxication on the basis of early findings. Agitation, delirium, and seizures may precede the onset of coma, and seizures may continue during the comatose phase. Agitation or delirium may also be seen during recovery from coma.

Impressive degrees of cholinergic blockade are described in this intoxication, including ileus, bladder atony, mydriasis, and thirst (Ayd, 1969; Davis and Termini, 1969).

Arrhythmias, including sinus tachycardia, atrial fibrillation, atrial flutter, atrioventricular block, ventricular tachycardia, and ventricular flutter, have been reported (Ramsay, 1967; Barnes *et al.*, 1968; Alexander and Niño, 1969; Freyschuss *et al.*, 1970; Sueblinvong and Wilson, 1969; Coull *et al.*, 1970; Williams and Sherter, 1971). A "characteristic" electrocardiographic finding of prolonged intraventricular conduction (wide QRS complex) with striking ST segment depression has been reported (Barnes *et al.*, 1968). The arrhythmias have been attributed to cholinergic blockade and are responsive to physostigmine, isoproterenol, or electrical pacing. Inspection of the electrocardiograms reproduced in the literature reveals striking prolongation of the Q-T interval in many instances (Harthorne *et al.*, 1963; Barnes *et al.*, 1968; Sueblinvong and Wilson, 1969). The high incidence of these arrhythmias and electrocardiographic changes in dibenzazepine intoxication, contrasted with those following atropine administration (Gravenstein *et al.*, 1969), implies that the drugs have a direct myocardial effect in addition to the sequelae of cholinergic blockade. Studies of the tricyclic antidepressants have been conducted in rabbit atria. These studies show a quinidine-like effect to be present that is reversed by isoproterenol (Matsuo, 1967) (see Chapter 5).

Although desipramine and amitriptyline potentiate the pressor effects of norepinephrine *in vitro*, possibly by inhibiting adrenergic neuronal uptake of norepinephrine (Besendorf *et al.*, 1962; Kaumann *et al.*, 1965), they also block alpha-adrenergic receptors (Scriabine, 1969). Hypotension may be severe in patients intoxicated with these drugs, and if these patients are unresponsive to volume replacement, pressor therapy is indicated. As in phenothiazine intoxication, "paradoxical" hypotension has been reported after metaraminol administration in imipramine intoxication; however, the patient responded to norepinephrine (Harthorne *et al.*, 1963). Imipramine may depress myocardial contractility, but the depression is reversible by ouabain (Laddu and Somani, 1969).

Some patients, particularly in the presence of underlying cardiovascular disease, have developed congestive heart failure during the course of poisoning with dibenzazepines (Cairncross and Gershon, 1962). Digitalization would seem advisable if cardiac failure develops.

Disturbances of body temperature may occur, with hyperthermia being a major problem in some patients. A hypothermic blanket may be required.

Some of the central nervous system manifestations of cholinergic blockade, such as delirium and agitation, may be countered with physostigmine, which can cross the blood-brain barrier.

Attempts to enhance clearance of these agents by diuresis or dialytic therapy have failed (Harthorne *et al.*, 1963; Halle and Collipp, 1969). Failure of these interventions could have been predicted on the basis of the drug's chemical nature. An early report on diuretic therapy claimed success, but the patient was comatose for 48 hours (a common duration) and a nonspecific method of assay for the drug was employed (Prout *et al.*, 1965). In rats, attempts to enhance renal clearance by acid diuresis failed (Bickel and Weder, 1969). Neither this approach, gastric lavage (possibly effective by virtue of pH gradient partitioning), nor hemoperfusion through adsorbents has been reported in man. Supportive measures may be sufficient in most intoxications, even if a new method to remove the drug becomes available.

These drugs should not be prescribed promiscuously for minor depression or in place of non-drug therapy of depression (see Chapters 11 and 14). Depressed patients may be covertly suicidal; if suicidal intent is even remotely suspected, the physician may diminish the availability of drug by dispensing small numbers of pills at more frequent intervals or by giving the prescription to a responsible family member for administration.

Summary Principles: (1) Treat the patient, then his poison. Conservative therapy to control symptoms common to many drugs may be enough to permit survival. Do not let the patient die of respiratory arrest or shock while you are on the telephone to a poison control center. ***(2) If possible, find out what has been ingested.*** This provides a guide to the severity of poisoning and to any unique features of the intoxication that may warrant specific monitoring or therapy. ***(3) Attempt to establish the severity of the intoxication and, after consideration of factors such as concurrent diseases of the liver or kidney, decide whether or not the drug can and/or should be removed. (4) Read the clinical literature on poisoning with the suspected drug or drugs with great care, to acquire and analyze all data needed to make therapeutic decisions.*** Follow the guidelines for evaluation of clinical studies given in Chapter 1.

REFERENCES

Abdallah, A. H., and Tye, A.: A comparison of the efficacy of emetic drugs and stomach lavage. *Amer. J. Dis. Child.*, 113:571–75, 1967.

Adams, J. T.; Bigler, J. A.; and Green, O. C.: A case of methyl salicylate intoxication treated by exchange transfusion. *J.A.M.A.*, 165:1563–65, 1957.

Alexander, C. S., and Niño, A.: Cardiovascular complications in young patients taking psychotropic drugs. *Amer. Heart J.*, 78:757–69, 1969.

Arnold, F. J.,; Hodges, J. B., Jr.; Barla, R. A., Jr.; Spector, S.; Sunshine, I.; and Wedgwood, R. J.: Evaluation of the efficacy of lavage and induced emesis in the treatment of salicylate poisoning. *Pediatrics*, 23:286–301, 1959.

Ayd, F. J.: Desipramine: a reappraisal after seven years. *Med. Counterpoint*, pp. 41–46, 1969.

Ban, T. A., and St. Jean, A.: The effect of phenothiazines on the electrocardiogram. *Canad. Med. Ass. J.*, 91:537–40, 1964.

Barbour, B. H.: Peritoneal dialysis in the management of dialysable poisons. *Clin. Res.*, 8:114, 1960.

Barker, J. C., and Kerr, E. M.: Overdose of trifluoperazine. *Lancet*, 2:1304, 1960.

Barnes, R. J.; Kong, S. M.; and Wu, R. W.: Electrocardiographic changes in amitriptyline poisoning. *Brit. Med. J.*, 3:222–23, 1968.

Bartter, F. C., and Schwartz, W. B.: The syndrome of inappropriate secretion of antidiuretic hormone. *Amer. J. Med.*, 42:790–806, 1967.

Beighton, P. H., and Wilkinson, D. J.: Trifluoperazine overdosage. *Practitioner*, 199:73–74, 1967.

Bell, D. S.: Dangers of treatment of status epilepticus with diazepam. *Brit. Med. J.*, 1:159–61, 1969.

Berman, L. B.; Jeghers, H.; Schreiner, G. E.; and Pallotta, A. J.: Hemodialysis, an effective therapy for acute barbiturate poisoning. *J.A.M.A.*, 161:820–27, 1956.

Berman, L. B., and Vogelsang, P.: Removal rates for barbiturates using two types of peritoneal dialysis. *New Eng. J. Med.*, 270:77–80, 1964.

Berry, F. A., and Lambdin, M. A.: Apomorphine and levallorphan tartrate in acute poisonings. *Amer. J. Dis. Child.*, 105:160–63, 1963.

Besendorf, H.; Steiner, F. A.; and Hurlimann, A.: (Laroxyl) ein neues Antidepressivum mit sedierender Wirdung. *Schweiz. Med. Wschr.*, 92:4244–46, 1962.

Beveridge, G. W.; Forshall, W.; Munro, J. F.; Owen, J. A.; and Weston, D. A. G.: Acute salicylate poisoning in adults. *Lancet*, 1:1406–12, 1964.

Bickel, M. H., and Weder, H. J.: Buccal absorption and other properties of pharmacokinetic importance of imipramine and its metabolites. *J. Pharm. Pharmacol.*, 21:160–68, 1969.

Bigger, J. T., Jr.; Schmidt, D. H.; and Kutt, K.: Relationship between the plasma level of diphenylhydantoin sodium and its cardiac antiarrhythmic effects. *Circulation*, 38:363–74, 1968.

Bleich, H. L., and Schwartz, W. B.: Tris buffer (THAM): an appraisal of its physiologic effects and clinical usefulness. *New Eng. J. Med.*, 274:782–87, 1966.

Bloomer, H. A.: Limited usefulness of alkaline diuresis and peritoneal dialysis in pentobarbital intoxication. *New Eng. J. Med.*, 272:1309–13, 1965.

Bluemle, L. W., Jr.; Webster, G. D., Jr.; and Elkinton, J. R.: Acute tubular necrosis. Analysis of one hundred cases with respect to mortality, complications, and treatment with and without dialysis. *Arch. Intern. Med. (Chicago)*, 104:180–97, 1959.

Brophy, J. J.: Suicide attempts with psychotherapeutic drugs. *Arch. Gen. Psychiat. (Chicago)*, 17:652–57, 1967.

Burns, J. J., and Conney, A. H.: Enzyme stimulation and inhibition in the metabolism of drugs. *Proc. Roy. Soc. Med.*, 59:955–60, 1965.

Burton, R.; Bell, G. E.; and Huston, J. R.: Water and electrolyte content of the rat heart after thioridazine administration. *J. Clin. Pharmcol.*, 7:271–74, 1967.

Cairncross, K. D., and Gershon, S.: A pharmacological basis for the cardiovascular complications of imipramine medication. *Med. J. Aust.*, **11**:372–75, 1962.

Campbell, F. A.: Suicidal attempts by overdose of perphenazine (Sentazin trilafon). *J. Irish Med. Ass.*, **48**:116, 1961.

Chandler, B. F.; Meroney, W. H.; Czarnecki, S. W.; Herman, R. H.; Cheitlin, M. D., Goldbaum, L. E.; and Herndon, E. G.: Artificial hemodialysis in management of glutethimide intoxication. *J.A.M.A.*, **170**:914–17, 1959.

Charytan, C.: The enterohepatic circulation in glutethimide intoxication. *Clin. Pharmacol. Ther.*, **11**:816–20, 1970.

Chazan, J. A., and Cohen, J. J.: Clinical spectrum of glutethimide intoxication. *J.A.M.A.*, **208**:837–39, 1969.

Cherner, R.; Groppe, C. W., Jr.; and Rupp, J. J.: Prolonged tolbutamide-induced hypoglycemia. *J.A.M.A.*, **185**:883–84, 1963.

Chicoine, L.: Intoxication caused by derivatives of phenothiazine. Review and report on 25 cases. *Un. Med. Canada*, **90**:469–74, 1961.

Cilliers, A. J.: Perphenazine poisoning: a case report. *Med. Proc. (S. Afr.)*, **6**:93–95, 1960.

Clemmesen, C.: New line of treatment in barbiturate poisoning. *Acta Med. Scand.*, **148**:83–89, 1954.

Coldwell, B. B., and Solomonraj, G.: The effect of barbiturates on salicylate metabolism in the rat. *Clin. Toxicol.*, **1**:431–44, 1968.

Corby, D. G.; Lisciandro, R. C.; Lehman, R. H.; and Decker, W. J.: The efficiency of methods used to evacuate the stomach after acute ingestions. *Pediatrics*, **40**:871–80, 1967.

Coull, D. C.; Crooks, J.; Dingwall-Fordyce, I.; Scott, A. M.; and Weir, R. D.: Amitriptyline and cardiac disease. Risk of sudden death identified by monitoring system. *Lancet*, **2**:590–91, 1970.

Crotty, J. J.: The epidemiology of salicylate poisoning. *Clin. Toxicol.*, **1**:381–86, 1968.

Cruz, I. A.; Cramer, N. C.; and Parrish, A. E.: Hemodialysis in chlordiazepoxide toxicity. *J.A.M.A.*, **202**:438–40, 1967.

Cumming, G.; Dukes, D. C.; and Widdowson, G.: Alkaline diuresis in treatment of aspirin poisoning. *Brit. Med. J.*, **2**:1033–36, 1964.

Curry, S. H.; Davis, J. M.; Janowsky, D. S.; and Marshall, J. H. L.: Factors affecting chlorpromazine plasma levels in psychiatric patients. *Arch. Gen. Psychiatry*, **22**:209–15, 1970a.

Curry, S. H.; Marshall, J. H. L.; Davis, J. M.; and Janowsky, D. S.: Chlorpromazine plasma levels and effects. *Arch. Gen. Psychiatry*, **22**:289–96, 1970b.

Dabbous, I. A.; Bergman, A. B.; and Robertson, W. O.: The ineffectiveness of mechanically induced vomiting. *J. Pediat.*, **66**:952–54, 1965.

Davis, J. M.; Bartlett, E.; and Termini, B. A.: Overdosage of psychotropic drugs: a review. *Dis. Nerv. Syst.*, **29**:157–64, 246–56, 1968.

Davis, J. M., and Termini, B. A.: Attempted suicide with psychotropic drugs: diagnosis and treatment. *Med. Counterpoint*, pp. 59–64, 1969.

Decker, W. J.; Shpall, R. A.; Corby, D. G.; Combs, H. F.; and Payne, C. E.: Inhibition of aspirin absorption by activated charcoal and apomorphine. *Clin. Pharm. Ther.*, **10**:710–13, 1969.

De Myttenaere, M. H.; Maher, J. F.; and Schreiner, G. E.: Hemoperfusion through a charcoal column for glutethimide poisoning. *Trans. Amer. Soc. Artif. Intern. Organs*, **13**:190–98, 1967.

Desautels, S.; Filteau, C.; and St. Joan, A.: Ventricular tachycardia associated with administration of thioridazine hydrochloride (Mellaril): report of a case with a favourable outcome. *Canad. Med. Ass. J.*, **90**:1030–31, 1964.

Dobos, J. K.; Phillips, J.; and Covo, G. A.: Acute barbiturate intoxication. *J.A.M.A.*, **176**:268–72, 1961.

Done, A. K.: Salicylate intoxication. Significance of measurements of salicylate in blood in cases of acute ingestion. *Pediatrics*, **26**:800–807, 1960.

——: Proceedings, 41st Ross Pediatric Research Conference (C. D. May, ed.). Ross Laboratories, Columbus, 1962, p. 83.

——: Salicylate poisoning. *J.A.M.A.*, **192**:770–72, 1965.

——: Treatment of salicylate poisoning: review of personal and published experiences. *Clin. Toxicol.*, **1**:451–67, 1968.

——: Pharmacologic principles in the treatment of poisoning. *Pharmacol. Physicians*, **3**:1–10, July, 1969.

Dyment, P. G.; Curtis, D. D.; and Gourrich, G. E.: Meprobamate poisoning treated by peritoneal dialysis. *J. Pediat.*, **67**:124–26, 1965.

Elliot, G. B., and Crichton, J. U.: Peritoneal dialysis in salicylate intoxication. *Lancet*, **2**:840–42, 1960.

Ettledorf, J. N.; Dobbins, W. T.; Summett, R. L.; Rainwater, W. T.; and Fischer, R. L.: Intermittent peritoneal dialysis using 5 per cent albumin in the treatment of salicylate intoxication in children. *J. Pediat.*, **58**:226–36, 1961.

Fahy, T. J.; Brocklebank, J. T.; and Ashby, D. W.: Syndromes of self poisoning. *Irish J. Med. Sci.*, **3**:497–503, 1970.

Fazekas, J. F.; Goldbaum, L. R.; Kappanyi, T.; and Shea, J. G.: Study on the effect of overdose of pentylenetetrazol and barbiturate combinations in human volunteers. *Amer. J. Med. Sci.*, **231**:531–41, 1956.

Feder, S. L.: The use of psychotherapeutic drugs. *Med. Clin. N. Amer.*, **51**:1453–66, 1967.

Ferguson, M. J., and Grace, W. J.: The conservative management of barbiturate intoxication: experience with 95 unconscious patients. *Ann. Intern. Med.*, **54**:726–33, 1961.

Feuerstein, R. C.; Fineberg, L.; and Fleishman, E.: The use of acetozoleamide in the therapy of salicylate poisoning. *Pediatrics*, **25**:215–27, 1960.

Franklin, S. S., and Merrill, J. P.: Acute renal failure. *New Eng. J. Med.*, **262**:711–18, 761–67, 1960.

Freyschuss, U.; Sjoqvist, F.; Tuck, D.; and Asberg, M.: Circulatory effects in man of nortriptyline, a tricyclic antidepressant drug. *Pharmacol. Clinica*, **2**:68–71, 1970.

Gary, N. E.; Dotzler, P.; Maher, J. F.; and Schreiner, G. E.: Determinations of glutethimide in serum: an evaluation of thin-layer chromatography method compared to spectrophotometric analysis. *Clin. Toxicol.*, **1**:273–79, 1968.

Ginn, H. E.; Anderson, K. E.; Mercier, R. K.; Stevens, T. W.; and Matter, B. J.: Camphor intoxication treated by lipid dialysis. *J.A.M.A.*, **203**:230–31, 1968.

Goldbaum, L. R.; Williams, M. A.; and Maher, J. F.: Determination of glutethimide (Doriden) in tissues and its distribution in the body. *Fed. Proc.*, **21**:180, 1962.

Graeme, J. L.: Acute overdosage of hypnotic-sedative-tranquilizer drugs with special reference to glutethimide. *Clin. Toxicol.*, **1**:135–42, 1968.

Gravenstein, J. S.; Ariet, M.; and Thornby, J. I.: Atropine on the electrocardiogram. *Clin. Pharmacol. Ther.*, **10**:660–66, 1969.

Gunn, D. R., and Goldman, D.: Extrapyramidal and other effects induced by neuroleptic agents. *Int. J. Neuropsychiat.*, **3**:131–40, 1967.

Gutman, A. B.; Yu, T. F.; and Sirata, J. H.: A study, by simultaneous clearance techniques, of salicylate excretion in man. Effect of alkalination of the urine by bicarbonate administration; effect of probenecid. *J. Clin. Invest.*, **34**:711–21, 1955.

Hadden, J.; Johnson, K.; Smith, S.; Price, L.; and Giardina, E.: Acute barbiturate intoxication. *J.A.M.A.*, **209**:893–900, 1969.

Haider, I.; Matthew, H.; and Oswald, I.: Electroencephalographic changes in acute drug poisoning. *Electroencephalogr. Clin. Neurophysiol.*, **30**:23–31, 1971.

Haig, O. G.; Easterling, R. E.; and Weller, J. M.: Removal of chlordiazepoxide by dialysis. *Clin. Res.*, **15**:359, 1967.

Halle, M. A., and Collipp, P. J.: Amitriptyline hydrochloride poisoning, unsuccessful treatment by peritoneal dialysis. *N. Y. State J. Med.*, **69**:1434–36, 1969.

Hammer, W.; Martens, S.; and Sjoqvist, F.: A comparative study of the metabolism of desmethylimipramine, nortriptyline, oxyphenylbutazone in man. *Clin. Pharmacol. Ther.*, **10**:44–49, 1969.

Harthorne, J. W.; Marcus, A. M.; and Kaye, M.: Management of massive imipramine overdosage with mannitol and artificial dialysis. *New Eng. J. Med.*, **268**:33–36, 1963.

Henderson, L. W., and Merrill, J. P.: Treatment of barbiturate intoxication. *Ann. Intern. Med.*, **64**:876–90, 1966.

Hollister, L.: Toxicity of psychotherapeutic drugs. *Practitioner*, **194**:72–84, 1965.

———: Overdoses of psychotherapeutic drugs. *Clin. Pharmacol. Ther.*, **7**:142–46, 1966.

Hollister, L. E., and Kosek, J. C.: Sudden death during treatment with phenothiazine derivatives. *J.A.M.A.*, **192**:1035–38, 1965.

Ianzito, B. M.: Attempted suicide by drug ingestion. *Dis. Nerv. Syst.*, **31**:453–58, 1970.

James, J. A.; Kimbell, L.; and Read, W. T.: Experimental salicylate intoxication. I. Comparison of exchange transfusion, intermittent peritoneal lavage and hemodialysis as a means for removing salicylate. *Pediatrics*, **29**:442–47, 1962.

Jarvik, M. E.: Drugs used in the treatment of psychiatric disorders. In Goodman, L. S., and Gilman, A. (eds.): *The Pharmacologic Basis of Therapuetics*, 3rd ed. The Macmillan Co., New York, 1965.

Kalser, S. C.; Kelly, M. P.; Forbes, E. B.; and Randolph, M. M.: Drug metabolism in hypothermia. Uptake, metabolism, and biliary excretion of pentobarbital-2-C^{14} by the isolated, perfused fat liver in hypothermia and euthermia. *J. Pharmacol. Exp. Ther.*, **170**:145–53, 1969.

Kaneshiro, M. M.; Mielke, C. H., Jr.; Kasper, C. K.; and Rapaport, S. I.: Bleeding time after aspirin in disorders of intrinsic clotting. *New Eng. J. Med.*, **281**:1039–42, 1969.

Kaumann, A.; Basso, N.; and Aramendia, J.: The cardiovascular effects of N-(γ-methylaminopropyl-imino-dibenzyl) HCl (desmethylimipramine) and guanethidine. *J. Pharmacol. Exp. Ther.*, **147**:54–64, 1965.

Keberle, H.; Hoffmann, K.; and Bernhard, K.: The metabolism of glutethimide (Doriden®). *Experientia*, **18**:105–11, 1962.

Kelly, H. G.; Fay, J. E.; and Laverty, S. F.: Thioridazine hydrochloride (Mellaril): its effect on the electrocardiogram and a report of two fatalities with electrocardiographic abnormalities. *Canad. Med. Ass. J.*, **89**:546–54, 1963.

Kier, L. C.; Whitehead, R. W.; and White, W. C.: Blood and urine levels in glutethimide (Doriden) intoxication. *J.A.M.A.*, **166**:1861–62, 1958.

Knochel, J. P., and Barry, K. G.: THAM dialysis: an experimental method to study diffusion of certain weak acids *in vivo*. II. Secobarbital. *J. Lab. Clin. Med.*, **65**:361–69, 1965.

Knochel, J. P.; Clayton, L. E.; and Smith, W. L.: Intraperitoneal THAM: an effective method to enhance phenobarbital removal during peritoneal dialysis. *J. Lab. Clin. Med.*, **64**:257–68, 1964.

Kyle, L. H.; Jeghers, H.; Walsh, W. P.; Doolan, T. D.; Wishinsky, H.; and Pallotta, A.: The application of hemodialysis to the treatment of barbiturate poisoning. *J. Clin. Invest.*, **32**:364–71, 1953.

Laddu, A. R., and Somani, P.: Desipramine toxicity and its treatment. *Toxicol. Appl. Pharmacol.*, **15**:287–94, 1969.

Lee, H. A., and Ames, A. C.: Hemodialysis in severe barbiturate poisoning. *Brit. Med. J.*, **1**:1217–19, 1965.

Leonards, J. R.: The influence of solubility on the rate of gastrointestinal absorption of aspirin. *Clin. Pharmacol. Ther.*, **4**:476–79, 1963.

Levy, G., and Hollister, L. E.: Failure of U.S.P. disintegration test to assess physiological availability of enteric coated tablets. *N. Y. J. Med.*, **64**:3002–3005, 1964.

Levy, G., and Matsuzawa, T.: Pharmacokinetics of salicylate elimination in man. *J. Pharmacol. Exp. Ther.*, **156**:285–93, 1967.

Levy, G., and Yaffe, S. J.: The study of salicylate pharmacokinetics in intoxicated infants and children. *Clin. Toxicol.*, **1**:409–24, 1968.

Linton, A. L.; Luke, R. G.; Speirs, I.; and Kennedy, A. C.: Forced diuresis and hemodialysis in severe barbiturate intoxication. *Lancet*, **1**:1008–10, 1964.

MacCannell, K. L.: The effect of barbiturates on regional blood flow. *Canad. Anaesth. Soc. J.*, **16**:1–6, 1969.

McDonald, D. F.; Greene, W. M.; Kretchmar, L.; and O'Brien, G.: Experiences in acute glutethimide (Doriden) intoxication. Superiority of extracorporeal dialysis over peritoneal dialysis. *Invest. Urol.*, **1**:127–33, 1963.

McKown, C. H.; Verhulst, H. L.; and Crotty, J. J.: Overdosage effects and danger from tranquilizing drugs. *J.A.M.A.*, **185**:425–30, 1963.

MacPherson, C. R.; Milne, M. D.; and Evans, B. M.: The excretion of salicylate. *Brit. J. Pharmacol.*, **10**:484–89, 1955.

Madan, D. R., and Pendse, V. K.: Antiarrhythmic activity of thioridazine hydrochloride (Mellaril). *Amer. J. Cardiol.*, **11**:78–81, 1963.

Maddock, R. K., Jr., and Bloomer, H. A.: Meprobamate overdosage. *J.A.M.A.*, **201**:999–1003, 1967.

Maffly, R. H., and Edelman, I. S.: The role of sodium, potassium and water in the hypo-osmotic states of heart failure. *Progr. Cardiov. Dis.*, **4**:88–104, 1961.

Maher, J. F.: Determinants of serum half-life of glutethimide in intoxicated patients. *J. Pharmacol. Exp. Ther.*, **174**:450–55, 1970.

Maher, J. F., and Schreiner, G. E.: Acute glutethimide intoxication: experience with hemodialysis. *Trans. Amer. Soc. Artif. Intern. Organs*, **7**:100–109, 1961.

———: Cause of death in acute renal failure. *Arch. Intern. (Chicago)*, **110**:493–504, 1962.

———: Hazards and complications of dialysis. *New Eng. J. Med.*, **273**:370–77, 1965.

———: The dialysis of poisons and drugs. *Trans. Amer. Soc. Artif. Intern. Organs*, **14**:440–53, 1968.

Maher, J. F.; Schreiner, G. E.; and Vestervelt, F. B., Jr.: Acute glutethimide intoxication. I. Clinical experience (22 patients) compared to acute barbiturate intoxication (63 patients). *Amer. J. Med.*, **33**:70–82, 1962.

Malmlund, H.: Cerebral blood flow and oxygen consumption in barbiturate poisoning. *Acta Med. Scand.*, **184**:373–77, 1968.

Mandelbaum, J. M., and Simon, N. M.: Severe methyprylon intoxication treated by hemodialysis. *J.A.M.A.*, **216**:139–40, 1971.

Mandy, S., and Ackerman, A. B.: Characteristic traumatic skin lesions in drug-induced coma. *J.A.M.A.*, **213**:253–56, 1970.

Matsuo, S.: Comparative effects of imipramine and propranolol on the transmembrane potentials of the isolated rabbit atria. *Jap. J. Pharmacol.*, **17**:279–86, 1967.

Matthew, H.; Mackintosh, T. F.; Tompsett, S. L.; and Cameron, J. C.: Gastric aspiration and lavage in acute poisoning. *Brit. Med. J.*, **1**:1333–37, 1966.

Mattocks, A. M.: Accelerated removal of salicylate by additives in peritoneal dialysis fluid. *J. Pharm. Sci.*, **58**:595–98, 1969.

Moore, F. D.; Edelman, I. S.; Olney, J. M.; James, A. H.; Brooks, L.; and Wilson, G.: Body sodium and potassium. III. Inter-related trends in alimentary, renal and cardiovascular disease; lack of correlation between body stores and plasma concentration. *Metabolism*, **3**:334–50, 1953.

Mouton, D. E.; Cohen, R. J.; and Barrett, O., Jr.: Meprobamate poisoning: successful treatment with peritoneal dialysis. *Amer. J. Med. Sci.*, **253**:706–709, 1967.

Mudge, G. H.; Foulks, J.; and Gilman, A.: Renal secretion of potassium in the dog during cellular dehydration. *Amer. J. Physiol.*, **161**:159–66, 1950.

Myschetzky, A.: The significance of megimide in the treatment of barbiturate poisoning. *Danish Med. Bull.*, **8**:33–36, 1961.

Myschetzky, A., and Lassen, N. A.: Urea-induced osmotic diuresis and alkalinization of urine in acute barbiturate intoxication. *J.A.M.A.*, **185**:936–42, 1963.

Nilsson, E., and Eyrich, B.: On treatment of barbiturate poisoning. *Acta Med. Scand.*, **137**:381–89, 1950.

Ohlsson, W. T. L., and Fristedt, B. I.: Blood lavage in acute barbiturate poisoning. Ten years' experience. *Lancet*, **2**:12–17, 1962.

Packham, M. A., and Mustard, T. F.: The effect of pyrazole compounds on thrombin-induced platelet aggregation. *Proc. Soc. Exp. Biol. Med.*, **130**:72–75, 1969.

Plum, F., and Swanson, A. G.: Barbiturate poisoning treated by physiological methods. *J.A.M.A.*, **163**:827–35, 1957.

Posner, J. B., and Plum, F.: Spinal fluid pH and neurologic symptoms in systemic acidosis. *New Eng. J. Med.*, **277**:605–13, 1967.

Price, H. L.: General anesthesia and circulatory homeostasis. *Physiol. Rev.*, **40**:187–218, 1960.

Proudfoot, A. T., and Brown, S. S.: Acidaemia and salicylate poisoning in adults. *Brit. Med. J.*, **1**:547–50, 1969.

Prout, B. J.; Young, J.; and Goddard, P.: Imipramine poisoning in childhood and suggested treatment. *Brit. Med. J.*, **1**:972, 1965.

Quick, A. J.: Aspirin, alcohol, and gastric haemorrhage. *Lancet*, **1**:623, 1969.

Radebaugh, J. F., and Emery, F. C.: Salicylate poisoning. Treatment with replacement transfusion. *J. Maine Med. Ass.*, **48**:437–40, 1957.

Ramsay, I. D.: Survival after imipramine poisoning. *Lancet*, **2**:1308–9, 1967.

Randall, L. C.: Pharmacology of chlordiazepoxide (Librium). *Dis. Nerv. Syst., Suppl.*, **22**:7–15, 1961.

Rapaport, S., and Guest, G. M.: The effect of salicylates on the electrolyte structure of blood plasma. I. Respiratory alkalosis in monkeys and dogs after sodium and methyl salicylate: the influence of hypnotic drugs and of sodium bicarbonate on salicylate poisoning. *J. Clin. Invest.*, **24**:759–69, 1945.

Rejent, T. A., and Klendshoj, N. C.: Rapid determination of glutethimide in biological fluids. A comparison of the thin-layer chromatographic method with gas-chromatographic methods. *Clin. Toxicol.*, **1**:143–48, 1968.

Robertson, W. O.: Syrup of ipecac—a slow or fast emetic. *Amer. J. Dis. Child.*, **103**:58–61, 1962.

Robin, E. O.; Davis, M. D.; and Rees, S. B.: Salicylate intoxication with special reference to the development of hypokalemia. *Amer. J. Med.*, **26**:869–82, 1959.

Samter, M.: The acetyl- in aspirin. *Ann. Intern. Med.*, **71**:208–209, 1969.

Schoonmaker, F. W.; Osteen, R. T.; and Greenfield, J. C., Jr.: Thioridazine (Mellaril[R])-induced ventricular tachycardia controlled with an artificial pacemaker. *Ann. Intern. Med.*, **65**:1076–78, 1966.

Schreiner, G. E.: Dialysis of poisons and drugs—annual review. *Trans. Amer. Soc. Artif. Intern. Organs*, **16**:544–68, 1970.

Schreiner, G. E.; Berman, L. B.; Kovach, R.; and Bloomer, H. A.: Acute glutethimide (Doriden) poisoning. The use of bemegride (Megimide) and hemodialysis. *Arch. Intern. Med. (Chicago)*, **101**:899–911, 1958.

Schwartz, R.; Fellers, F. K.; Knapp, J.; and Yaffe, C.: The renal response to administration of acetozoleamide during salicylate intoxication. *Pediatrics*, **23**:1103–14, 1959.

Schwartz, W. B., and Relman, A. S.: Effects of electrolyte disorders on renal structure and function. *New Eng. J. Med.*, **267**:383–89, 452–58, 1967.

Scriabine, A.: Some observations on the adrenergic blocking of activity of desipramine and amitriptyline on aortic strips of rabbits. *Experientia*, **25**:164–65, 1969.

Selzer, A., and Wray, J.: Quinidine syncope. Paroxysmal ventricular fibrillation occurring during treatment of chronic atrial arrhythmias. *Circulation*, **40**:17–26, 1964.

Sharpless, S. K.: Hypnotics and sedatives. In Goodman, L. S., and Gilman, A. (eds.): *The Pharmacological Basis of Therapeutics*, 3rd ed. The Macmillan Co., New York, 1965.

Shinaberger, J. H.; Shear, L.; Clayton, L. E.; *et al.*: Dialysis for intoxication with lipid soluble drugs: enhancement of glutethimide extraction with lipid dialysate. *Trans. Amer. Soc. Artif. Intern. Organs*, **11**:76–82, 1965.

Simon, N. M., and Krumlovsky, F. A.: The role of dialysis in the treatment of poisoning. *Rational Drug Ther.*, **5**:1–7, March, 1971.

Simpson, G. M., and Angus, J. W. S.: Drug induced extrapyramidal disorders. *Acta Psychiatr. Scand.*, **212**:1–58, 1970.

Smith, M. J. H., and Smith, P. K.: *The Salicylates. A Critical Bibliographic Review.* John Wiley & Sons, Interscience Publishers, New York, 1966.

Spritz, N. S.; Fahey, T. J.; Thompson, D. D.; and Rubin, A. L.: The use of extracorporeal hemodialysis in the treatment of salicylate intoxication in a 2-year-old child. *Pediatrics*, **24**:540–43, 1959.

Strauss, J.: Tris-(hydroxymethyl)-amino-methane (THAM): a pediatric evaluation. *Pediatrics*, **41**:667–89, 1968.

Sturkey, H. C.: Ipecac syrup. Its use as an emetic in poison control. *J. Pediat.*, **69**:139–41, 1966.

Sturman, J. A.; Dawkins, P. D.; McArthur, N.; and Smith, M. J. H.: The distribution of salicylate in mouse tissues after intraperitoneal injection. *J. Pharm. Pharmacol.*, **20**:58–63, 1968.

Sueblinvong, V., and Wilson, J. F.: Myocardial damage due to imipramine intoxication. *J. Pediat.*, **74**:375–78, 1969.

Summitt, R. L., and Ettledorf, J. N.: Salicylate intoxication in children: experience with peritoneal dialysis and alkalinization of the urine. *J. Pediat.*, **64**:803–14, 1964.

Sunshine, I., and Leonards, J. R.: Use of artificial

kidney for removal of barbiturates in dogs. *Proc. Soc. Exp. Biol. Med.*, **86**:638–41, 1954.

Task Force on Prescription Drugs. The Drug Users. U.S. Department of Health, Education and Welfare, U.S. Govt. Printing Office, Washington, D.C., 1968, p. 50.

Teehan, B. P.; Maher, J. F.; Carey, J. J. H.; Flynn, P. D.; and Schreiner, G. E.: Acute ethchlorvynol (Placidyl®) intoxication. *Ann. Intern. Med.*, **72**:875–82, 1970.

Thorstrand, C.: A ten year study of the mortality rate due to hypnotic and sedative intoxications. *Opuscula Med. (Stockh.)*, **10**:270, 1965.

Tranquada, R. E.: Lactic acidosis. *Calif. Med.*, **101**:450–61, 1964.

Waddell, W. T., and Butler, T. C.: The distribution and excretion of phenobarbital. *J. Clin. Invest.*, **36**:1217–26, 1957.

Williams, R. B., Jr., and Sherter, C.: Cardiac complications of tricyclic antidepressant therapy. *Ann. Intern. Med.*, **74**:395–98, 1971.

Winters, R. W.: Acid-base disturbances, and the treatment of salicylate intoxication. In Dixon, A. St. J.; Martin, B. K.; Smith, M. J. H.; and Wood, P. H. N. (eds.): *Salicylates: An International Symposium.* Little, Brown & Co., Boston, 1963, pp. 270–80.

Zbinden, G.; Bagdon, R. E.; Keith, E. F.; Phillips, R. D.; and Randall, L. O.: Experimental and clinical toxicology of chlordiazepoxide (Librium R). *Toxicol. Appl. Pharmacol.*, **3**:619–37, 1961.

Chapter 18

DRUG MODELS OF DISEASE: SWEET USES OF ADVERSITY

Leo E. Hollister

Sweet are the uses of adversity, which like the toad, ugly and venomous, wears
yet a precious jewel in its head.

As You Like It, Act 2, scene 1

The purpose of this chapter is to demonstrate that although unexpected reactions to drugs are generally unwanted, some may provide new therapeutic applications of drugs or useful models of naturally occurring diseases. The classification of various mechanisms and specific types of drug reactions is mentioned in Chapters 15–17 of this book and elsewhere (Whipple *et al.*, 1965; Meyler and Peck, 1968). Observant and astute clinicians must recognize unwanted or unexpected reactions to a drug so that the reaction may be turned to good use.

THERAPEUTIC APPLICATIONS OF SIDE EFFECTS

The saying that "today's side effect may be tomorrow's therapeutic effect" is an exaggeration, but there are examples of its truth. Unexpected or unwanted effects of a drug eventually may be exploited and the drug used for purposes other than the original intent (Table 18–1). In some instances, the same drug is used for the new purpose; in others, derivatives of the original drug are synthesized to exploit the

Table 18–1. EXAMPLES OF SIDE EFFECTS OF DRUGS TURNED TO THERAPEUTIC USE

PROTOTYPE DRUG	PROPOSED USE	SIDE EFFECT	DERIVED USE OR CLASS OF DRUGS
Novasurol	Antitreponemal	Diuresis	Mercurial diuretics
Sulfanilamide	Antibacterial	Hypoglycemia	Sulfonylureas
		Diuresis	Carbonic anhydrase inhibitors
			Thiazides
		Thyroid inhibition	Thiouracils
Amphetamine	Stimulant	Appetite suppression	Anorexiants
Iproniazid	Antituberculosis	Euphoria	Antidepressant
Chlorpromazine	Antihistaminic	Sedation	Phenothiazine antipsychotics
Reserpine	Antihypertensive	Sedation	Antipsychotic
Meprobamate	Muscle relaxant	Sedation	Antianxiety
Imipramine	Antipsychotic	Antidepression	Tricyclic antidepressants
Diazoxide	Antihypertensive	Hyperglycemia	Hyperglycemic
Nalorphine	Narcotic antagonist	Analgesia	Agonist-antagonist analgesics

therapeutic actions more effectively. Serendipity may lead to most instances of establishing new uses for old drugs, but usually, as Pasteur said, "Chance favors the prepared mind."

No drug has a single pharmacologic effect. Consequently, many of the unwanted effects of drugs in one specific clinical condition become desirable in others. Almost all examples of employment of unwanted effects depend on an intrinsic pharmacologic action of a drug rather than on an idiosyncratic response of a patient. *Principle: Clinical evaluations of new and old drugs must include all signs of pharmacologic effect, not just those presumed to be important for the intended therapeutic result. Sometimes unexpected reactions can be turned to rewarding uses.*

SIDE EFFECTS OF DRUGS AS MODELS FOR DISEASE

Study of models of spontaneously occurring diseases of unknown pathogenesis may lead to definition of their cause and permit rational treatment of the illness. Several animal models of disease have been found, but they are often restricted to a single species or are due to some rare genetic variant (Frenkel *et al.*, 1969). These models are therefore of limited value for application to diseases in man. However, unwanted effects of therapeutic agents have provided very close models of some diseases in man. Four examples have been chosen from the incomplete list shown in Table 18–2. These examples illustrate the contributions models may make toward the understanding and treatment of human disorders.

The Catecholamine Hypothesis of Depression

Soon after reserpine (Serpasil) was used clinically as an antipsychotic and antihypertensive agent, it was noted that some patients became depressed. The depressive reactions to the drug often were indistinguishable from spontaneously occurring depressions. Many reactions persisted after the drug was withdrawn, necessitating electroconvulsive therapy. Some drug-induced depressions led to suicide. These reactions suggested that the drug-induced depression could provide a model for naturally occurring depressions. The discovery that reserpine depleted stores of serotonin and norepinephrine in the central nervous system led to the proposal that naturally occurring depressions might be associated with decreased availability of norepinephrine at central adrenergic synapses. This observation also focused attention on the possible physiologic function of these amines in the nervous system and provided a hypothesis to explain the actions of centrally

acting drugs (Pletscher *et al.*, 1956). Presumably, if depletion of amines is associated with sedation, an increase in brain amines should be associated with stimulation or euphoria. *Principle: A description of the pharmacologic effects of a drug should always distinguish between reliable fact and working hypothesis. The former can lead to predictable effects and to rational innovation in drug use. The latter may do the same, but use of the drug could as easily lead to a new hypothesis.*

Iproniazid (Marsilid) produced central nervous system stimulation and euphoria in patients with tuberculosis. In addition to its antituberculosis activity, it was found to be a potent inhibitor of monoamine oxidase, an enzyme largely responsible for the intraneuronal oxidation of amines in the nervous system. When evidence indicated that treatment with iproniazid increased the concentration of amines in the brain, the drug was proposed as an antidepressant. Early clinical experience was favorable, and a number of monoamine oxidase inhibitors (MAOI) were introduced for the clinical treatment of depression (Zeller and Barsky, 1952).

The mechanism of action of amphetamines, which were known to be effective central nervous system stimulants, was reinvestigated to determine their effect on brain amines (Burn, 1960). Pretreatment of animals with reserpine, by depleting the neuronal content of norepinephrine, abolished the stimulating effects of amphetamine (Benzedrine). The major mechanism of amphetamine stimulation was ascribed to that previously found for tyramine. Tyramine is a potent sympathomimetic agent that acts indirectly by increasing the release of norepinephrine (see Chapter 5). Alternatively, amphetamines may act as weak transmitters or may impede the neuron's reuptake of released norepinephrine.

Imipramine (Tofranil), with a chemical structure and many pharmacologic actions similar to those of chlorpromazine, initially seemed to provide an exception to the rule. Its clinical antidepressant action was surprising, for it had been synthesized as a modified phenothiazine antipsychotic (see Chapter 11). The crucial difference in action between imipramine and chlorpromazine (Thorazine) was that the former potentiated sympathetic responses whereas the latter blocked them (Gyermek, 1966). The reasons for this difference are not entirely clear. Imipramine and other related tricyclic compounds augment sympathetic responses by blocking the uptake of norepinephrine after its release from neurons.

The present model of the central adrenergic

Table 18–2. EXAMPLES OF DRUG-INDUCED MODELS OF HUMAN DISEASE

DISEASE	DRUGS
Skin	
Hyperpigmentation	Busulfan, chlorpromazine
Hirsutism	Diazoxide
Ichthyosis	Triparanol, butyrophenones
Stevens-Johnson syndrome	Sulfonamides, antibiotics, others
Respiratory	
Interstitial pulmonary fibrosis	Nitrofurantoin, busulfan
Hemic	
Ineffective erythropoiesis	Chloramphenicol, cycloserine, pyrazinamide
Thrombocytopenic purpura	Quinidine, digitalis, others
Megaloblastic anemia	Anticonvulsants, pyrimethamine
Hemolytic anemia	Immunologic: penicillin, methyldopa, stibophen
	Metabolic: antimalarials, analgesics, others
Lymphoma	Hydantoin anticonvulsants
Gastrointestinal	
Cholestatic jaundice of pregnancy	Oral contraceptives
Xanthomatous biliary cirrhosis	Chlorpromazine
Hemorrhagic pancreatitis	Steroids, diuretics, indomethacin, phenindione, immunosuppressants
Duodenal ulcer	Reserpine, ?corticosteroids
Urinary system	
Nephrotic syndrome	Penicillamine, trimethadione, gold salts, others
Renal tubular acidosis	Carbonic anhydrase inhibitors, outdated tetracycline, amphotericin B
Endocrine	
Diabetes mellitus	Diuretics, oral contraceptives
Hypoglycemia	Alcohol, propoxyphene, salicylates, sulfonylureas
Hypercalcemia	Thiazides, vitamin D
Metabolic—nutritional	
Xanthinuria	Allopurinol
Porphyrias	Barbiturates
Gout	Diuretics
Malabsorption syndrome	Neomycin
Elevated serum lipids	Oral contraceptives
Nervous system	
Parkinson syndrome	Antipsychotics
Seizures	Phenothiazines
Neuromuscular syndrome (myasthenia-like)	Chloroquine, steroids, alcohol, colistimethate, others
Special senses	
Retinitis pigmentosa	Thioridazine, chloroquine
Cataract	Steroids
Psychiatric disorders	
Depression	Reserpine
Schizophrenia	Amphetamine-like drugs (abuse range of doses)
Anxiety states	Sympathomimetics (therapeutic range of doses)
Others	
Retroperitoneal fibrosis	Methysergide
Systemic lupus erythematosus	Hydralazine, procainamide, anticonvulsants, antituberculous drugs
Infectious mononucleosis	Antituberculous drugs
Cardiomyopathies	Sympathomimetics, digitalis, antiarrhythmics, antipsychotics

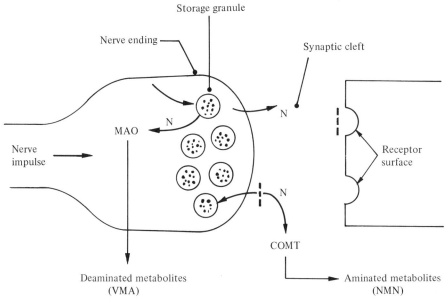

Figure 18–1. Model of central noradrenergic synapse. Transmitter (norepinephrine) is synthesized, stored in storage granules, and oxidized intraneuronally by monoamine oxidase (*MAO*), producing deaminated metabolites, such as vanilmandelic acid (*VMA*). Nerve impulse releases norepinephrine (*N*) into synaptic cleft for access to receptor. Drugs such as chlorpromazine are believed to block access to receptor (solid bar). Some released transmitter is O-methylated by catechol-O-methyltransferase (*COMT*), producing aminated metabolites such as normetanephrine (*NMN*). Some returns to the nerve ending for further storage; drugs such as tricyclic antidepressants are believed to impair this reuptake (cross-hatched bar).

synapse and the sites of action of these drugs are shown in Figure 18–1. When a nerve impulse or drug activates the sympathetic fiber, norepinephrine is released from storage granules located at the ends of the fiber near the synaptic cleft. After synaptic transmission, most of the norepinephrine is taken back into the neuron for further storage. The norepinephrine that is not reabsorbed is catabolized by the enzyme catechol-O-methyltransferase to produce normetanephrine. Both these actions are rapid, setting a time limit on the process of synaptic transmission. Within the neuron, synthesis and degradation of norepinephrine are in a state of dynamic equilibrium, some norepinephrine constantly being catabolized by monoamine oxidase. The end products of this intraneuronal pathway are deaminated metabolites, primarily 3-methoxy-4-hydroxymandelic acid (vanilmandelic acid, VMA). Thus VMA is derived mainly from the endogenous turnover of catecholamines. On the other hand, only release of norepinephrine at the synapse results in the production of normetanephrine, the excretion of which is used as an index for turnover of released and physiologically active norepinephrine.

The norepinephrine hypothesis proposes that depressive reactions are associated with a diminished amount of physiologically available norepinephrine at the central adrenergic synapses (Bunney and Davis, 1965; Schildkraut et al., 1967). Antidepressants may rectify this deficiency through several possible mechanisms (see Table 18–3). On the other hand, drugs that provoke depression or control mania seem to reduce the amount of norepinephrine available at the synapse. *Principle: An elegant hypothesis, which attempts to explain both the biochemical basis for a disorder and the mechanisms of action of drugs used to treat it, is very seductive. However, hypotheses must be tested to determine whether they can be accepted.*

The norepinephrine hypothesis of depression may be criticized on a number of counts. First, the data are indirect and relate to pharmacologic studies done in animals; in man, study is limited to urinary excretion of catecholamines and their metabolites, which may not accurately reflect events in the central nervous system. Second, some investigators believe too much emphasis has been placed on norepinephrine, to the exclusion of other amines. Possibly the dynamic balance between aminergic systems is

Table 18-3. DRUG EFFECTS ON NORADRENERGIC SYNAPSES*

DRUG	CLINICAL EFFECT	EFFECT AT SYNAPSE	POTENTIAL MECHANISM
Reserpine	Antipsychotic	Depletion	Decreases intraneuronal storage
Amphetamine	Stimulant	Increase	Releases norepinephrine from neurons; ?inhibits neuronal reuptake
MAO inhibitors	Antidepressant	Increase	Inhibits intraneuronal deamination
Tricyclics	Antidepressant	Increase	Inhibits neuronal reuptake

* Modified from Schildkraut, J. J.; Schanberg, S. M.; Breese, G. R.; and Kopin, I. J.: Norepinephrine metabolism and drugs used in the affective disorders: a possible mechanism of action. *Amer. J. Psychiat.*, **124**: 54–62, 1967.

of greater importance than the state of one. Third, some clinical exceptions to the rule have occurred; neither alpha-methylparatyrosine nor parachlorphenylalanine has produced depression in man (Gershon *et al.*, 1967). The former, a specific inhibitor of tyrosine hydroxylase, should decrease the content of both norepinephrine and dopamine in the central nervous system. The latter inhibits the synthesis of 5-hydroxytryptamine (serotonin). Finally, the capricious effects of antidepressants in clinical situations contrast with their predictable behavior in the laboratory. Not all drugs that fit the theory are equally useful clinically, and the most useful of all (the tricyclics) seem increasingly limited to a very small segment of depressive syndromes (see Chapter 11). *Principle: A continuing dialogue between clinical and animal pharmacologists is required if drug-induced models of disease are to be exploited fully. Hypotheses must always be clinically relevant.*

Drug-Induced Retroperitoneal Fibrosis

The association between retroperitoneal fibrosis and chronic administration of methysergide maleate (Sansert) has suggested clues to the etiology of this rare disorder. The disease evoked by methysergide resembles the naturally occurring disease, but on discontinuation of methysergide, the disorder is usually reversed. More subtle forms of the disorder may be recognized as patients treated with methysergide are surveyed routinely.

A case of retroperitoneal fibrosis was first described in 1948; over 300 cases have been reported since. All cases were considered to be idiopathic until 1961, when the syndrome was first associated with use of methysergide. Since then, reports of drug-related retroperitoneal fibrosis have surpassed the number of cases regarded as "idiopathic" (Graham *et al.*, 1966).

Both the idiopathic and drug-induced forms of the disorder have similar clinical presentations. Initial complaints are vague, but generally include aches or pains in the lower back or lower extremities. Other patients may first be seen for unexplained hypertension. The characteristic sign of the disease is obstruction of the ureter that may be unilateral and minimal or bilateral and severe, resulting in irreversible renal damage. Signs of obstructive vascular disease may be manifested by intermittent claudication, the Leriche syndrome, or decreased sexual potency. Some instances of a generalized fibrotic disorder have occurred, with heart murmurs, pleuropulmonary fibrosis, Riedel's struma of the thyroid, or other sites of fibrosis.

The anatomic distribution of fibrosis is periaortic, beginning near the aortic bifurcation, and may spread laterally. The fibrotic process tends to draw the ureters medially, the left being most affected because it is closer to the aorta at the point of bifurcation. The perivascular distribution may extend upward toward the thoracic aorta or downward along the iliac vessels. Early stages of the pathologic process are characterized by infiltration with lymphocytes and plasma cells with diminution in fat cells and fibrosis. Later mature dense connective tissue with extensive collagen deposition is found (Mitchinson, 1969).

The localization of fibrosis around the aorta strongly suggests a vascular origin of the disease. Methysergide, possibly by causing spasm in the aorta, its peripheral branches, or its vasa vasorum, might permit a leakage of materials through the aortic wall that stimulates the growth of fibrous tissue. Such materials might be plasma proteins or lipoproteins. Arterial and arteriolar constriction is a pharmacologic effect of many ergot derivatives. Thus retroperitoneal fibrosis has been described in patients who have used ergotamine tartrate and is seen in diseases such as the carcinoid syndrome characterized in part by excessive serotonin production.

Several other possible explanations for this association may be considered. The serotonin content of tissues may be increased even by an agent that may antagonize some of its effects. Analogous simultaneous antagonism and additive pharmacologic effects are seen with some antiadrenergic and antihistaminic drugs. The serotonin content of the brain is increased following administration of lysergic acid diethylamide, a compound chemically related to methysergide that also has powerful antiserotonin effects. If methysergide acts similarly, prolonged exposure to high levels of free serotonin in tissues could lead to other pharmacologic effects. Serotonin does promote fibrosis in pulmonary tissue, heart valves, the endocardium, and the retroperitoneal space of animals and man. Some indication that methysergide may act similarly to lysergic acid diethylamide is provided by a report of two cases of retroperitoneal fibrosis elicited by the latter drug (Aptekar and Mitchinson, 1970).

As only 1% of patients exposed to chronic treatment with methysergide develop retroperitoneal fibrosis, the effect may be analogous to the uncovering of latent systemic lupus erythematosus by a variety of drugs, including hydralazine and procainamide. In such a concept of the disease, susceptibility of the patient is the critical factor. A recent report of retroperitoneal fibrosis associated with hydralazine therapy suggests this mechanism. The nature of the inflammatory reaction has also suggested an autoimmune reaction, presumably elicited by the drug. *Principle: Although many "reasons" for the action of a drug may be conjectural, the conjectures may have useful unifying and practical implications.*

The development of retroperitoneal fibrosis during treatment with methysergide has provided many clues to its pathogenesis, despite the fact that it has not provided an answer to the etiology of the spontaneous disease. Perhaps this disease ultimately may be considered solely a sequel of drug or environmental agent exposure. The description of "spontaneous" retroperitoneal fibrosis dates from 1948, when antihistamines became freely available. Since then, a great variety of other drugs that might affect neurohumors, vascular tone, or connective tissue have been introduced, such as atropine-like agents, reserpine, autonomic blocking drugs, corticosteroids, and other anti-inflammatory drugs. Little evidence presently incriminates these drugs, but once a new complication has been described for one drug, it is often found to be associated with other agents. Further investigation is required to determine whether methysergide only provides a model for a disease or whether it may be one of numerous pharmacologic agents that might cause the disease. However, such clinically useful investigation might never have been initiated had clinicians been casual about their use of the drug and failed to establish its relationship to an unexpected side effect.

Drug-Induced Hemolytic Anemias

Hemolytic anemia associated with 8-aminoquinoline antimalarial drugs was first noted with administration of pamaquine naphthoate in 1926 (Prankerd, 1962). Subsequently, congeners (pentaquine phosphate, isopentaquine, and primaquine), as well as members of other drug classes (sulfonamides, acetanilid, and phenacetin), were found to produce this disorder. Although these drugs are different pharmacologically, they are all potent oxidants, the common property they share in provoking hemolytic anemia. *Principle: In searching for a common mechanism of action among a diverse group of drugs, consider biochemical as well as pharmacologic properties* (see Chapter 15).

In this disorder, the primary defect lies in the erythrocyte. Cells labeled with ^{51}Cr from a sensitive individual are destroyed when transfused to an insensitive individual subsequently given primaquine; conversely, cells from nonsensitive individuals are spared when transfused to a sensitive subject subsequently exposed to the drug. Biochemical studies indicate that susceptible cells have abnormally low concentrations of reduced glutathione and increased amounts of oxidized glutathione. Failure to maintain adequate amounts of reduced glutathione is due to a severe deficiency of an enzyme involved in the metabolic pathway, glucose-6-phosphate dehydrogenase (G-6-PD). Systematic studies of the concentration of this enzyme in large groups of people indicate that the abnormality is a genetic trait carried on the X chromosome with variable expression in heterozygous female carriers. The elucidation of the factors predisposing to drug-induced anemias provided one of the first examples of the interaction of genetic factors with drugs (Motulsky and Stamatoyannopoulos, 1966) (see Chapter 13).

People deficient in G-6-PD are the largest group of patients with red-cell biochemical abnormalities that predispose to hemolysis on exposure to drugs. A few cases of nonspherocytic hemolytic anemia have also been traced to this disorder, but in these cases the presence of oxidant drugs was required. Additional biochemical abnormalities in erythrocytes sensitive to the hemolytic action of drugs include deficiencies of glutathione reductase and phosphogluconic dehydrogenase (enzymes also involved in the reduction of glutathione), as well as deficiency of glutathione itself. When an oxidant drug increases the amount of hydrogen peroxide in the cell, oxidized glutathione, a disulfide, accumulates. This agent may interact with hemoglobin to alter metabolic activities of the cell, rendering it more susceptible to destruction. The increased peroxides also may damage the cell (Beutler, 1969).

Unstable hemoglobins account for another group of drug-induced hemolytic anemias. More than 12 abnormal hemoglobins have been described. Each abnormal hemoglobin has some alteration of amino acid residues at or near the distal or proximal histidyl residues of the alpha or beta chains. Not all abnormal hemoglobins "sensitize" the cell to the same drugs involved in G-6-PD deficiency. At times, stress no greater than infection or fever may cause hemolysis of such cells. Unstable hemoglobins are readily denatured to insoluble aggregates or may have a weak heme-globin bond. Although the exact mechanism by which they produce hemolysis is not known, it very likely differs only slightly among the abnormal hemoglobins.

Abnormal plasma factors may also play a role in the drug-induced hemolytic anemias (Carstairs, 1968). An immunologic mechanism for such anemias was discovered in 1956 when stibophen (Fuadin) administration resulted in hemolysis. Subsequently, two different types of immune mechanisms were found to play a role in hemolytic anemias associated with penicillin and methyldopa (Aldomet). Based on observations of the effects of these drugs, three different mechanisms of drug-dependent immune hemolytic anemia have been discovered.

The stibophen type of immune hemolytic anemia is associated with an antibody that agglutinates or lyses cells solely in the presence of the drug. The antigen may be a complex of drug either with a component of the erythrocyte or with a plasma protein. The antigen is adsorbed onto the cells. The penicillin type differs in that very large amounts of drug must be present, bound to erythrocytes. Although most patients receiving penicillin develop antipenicillin antibodies, only those who also have IgG antibodies develop hemolysis. Methyldopa need not be present for the occurrence of hemolytic reactions associated with its use. Possibly the drug binds to erythrocytes and cross-links proteins to them, altering their antigenicity. Another possibility is that the drug may alter the body's response to its own cells.

The elucidation of the mechanism of action of drug-induced hemolytic anemias has broadened our concept of hemolytic disorders and has explained some instances of "idiopathic nonspherocytic anemia" or even unusual drug reactions. The full spectrum of mechanisms must be defined so that the role of exogenous agents and endogenous defects or of their interaction becomes clear. Then the therapist is better able to predict the likelihood of a drug-induced disease, to avoid creating the circumstances that may cause it, and to remedy the problem if it appears. *Principle: The same end result from several drugs does not imply a common mechanism.*

Antipsychotic Drugs and Parkinson's Disease

The antipsychotic drugs reserpine and chlorpromazine evoke an extrapyramidal syndrome that closely mimics Parkinson's disease. This drug-induced syndrome is amenable to conventional pharmacotherapy of Parkinson's disease. To many psychopharmacologists, this novel adverse effect constitutes a valuable model for the study of a puzzling illness.

As the mechanism of action of the antipsychotic drugs was being studied, a series of unrelated discoveries led to the hypothesis that the manifestations of Parkinson's disease were associated with a deficiency of dopamine in the nuclei and tracts of the extrapyramidal system and that alleviation of this deficiency might ameliorate the disorder. These discoveries can be summarized in four major sections:

1. Reserpine decreased the capacity of storage granules at nerve endings to bind a variety of biogenic amines, including serotonin, norepinephrine, and dopamine (Bein, 1956). Chlorpromazine did not alter the storage, release, or turnover of these amines, but impaired access of the amines to receptors by impairing their transport across the membrane of the nerve ending (Berti and Shore, 1967). Thus both types of antipsychotic drugs were found to interfere with the action of neurotransmitters. The relative importance of each specific biogenic amine in producing antipsychotic effects is unclear; the focus of attention has moved from serotonin and norepinephrine to the current favorite, dopamine.

2. Biochemical mapping of the brain disclosed that distribution of these amines was uneven. The greatest concentration of norepinephrine was in the hypothalamus, whereas that of dopamine was in the corpus striatum, which contained little norepinephrine (Carlsson, 1959). As early as 1957, dopamine had been thought to be a neurotransmitter per se rather than simply a precursor to norepinephrine. The uneven distribution of the two amines tended to support this concept.

3. Beginning in 1960, chemical examination of the brains of 40 patients with either drug-induced Parkinson's disease or the post-encephalitic Parkinson syndrome revealed a marked decrease in dopamine content in the corpus striatum, as well as in the caudate nucleus, substantia nigra, and globus pallidus (Hornykiewicz, 1966). This critical discovery set the stage for development of the dopamine hypothesis, which could explain both the biochemical pathology of naturally occurring disease and the biochemical mechanism of an unusual neurologic side effect of drug therapy.

4. A tract between the substantia nigra and corpus striatum is dependent on dopamine as a neurotransmitter (Anden et al., 1966; Poirier et al., 1966). Dopamine also inhibits nerve-cell activity. Fluorescent microscopic techniques have refined the gross biochemical outline of this system and have proved that drugs that evoke extrapyramidal syndromes deplete this system of dopamine.

Over the next several years, attempts were made to treat patients with Parkinson's disease with dihydroxyphenylalanine (dopa) (Birkmayer and Hornykiewicz, 1962). The blood-brain barrier was impervious to dopamine itself, but allowed its precursor, levodopa, to pass. As the brain possesses the enzymes necessary to convert dopa to dopamine, administration of levodopa was a logical step to increase dopamine content in the brain. Despite reports of transitory alleviation of symptoms by either oral or intravenous administration of levodopa to patients with Parkinson's disease, the effect was minimal or too brief, discouraging most workers. One group of workers finally achieved success with extraordinarily high oral doses of levodopa (Cotzias et al., 1967). *Principle: No drug should be considered a failure until it has been used in doses that produce either the desired effect or intolerable adverse effects.*

This new pharmacologic approach to treatment has been evaluated in a substantial number of patients. Results with levodopa are far superior to those from previously available drug therapy. The evidence from uncontrolled, separate studies is so convincing that an expert review committee refused a proposal for a large-scale double-blind comparison of the drug with placebo or conventional therapy on the grounds that prior experiences provided historic controls adequate to prove efficacy. The first group to use levodopa successfully reported on 28 patients treated chronically, with dramatic improvement in 10, marked improvement in 10 others, and moderate or modest improvement in the rest (Cotzias et al., 1969). Results of long-term treatment in the hands of others has been comparable (Campbell, 1970). Although choreiform movements and adverse mental effects have been bothersome and puzzling complications of treatment (the latter could be relevant to the role of dopamine in schizophrenia), they have not yet limited the clinical use of this most promising treatment.

Summary Principles: (1) Unwanted or unexpected effects of drugs are not always bad. Past experience shows that some reactions may provide clues to new uses for old drugs or may stimulate the development of new classes of drugs to exploit the newly found effect. Effects of drugs may also provide useful models of human disease, adding new dimensions to our understanding of their pathogenesis and, at least in one recent and dramatic example, leading to a completely novel therapeutic approach to a chronic, disabling illness. (2) Physicians are loath to recognize and report drug reactions in their patients (see Chapter 15). Failure to do so may deprive us of valuable insights.

REFERENCES

Anden, N. E.; Fuxe, K. H.; and Hamburger, B.: A quantitative study on the nigroneostriatal dopamine neurone system in the rat. *Acta Physiol. Scand.*, **67**:306–12, 1966.

Aptekar, R. G., and Mitchinson, M. J.: Retroperitoneal fibrosis in two patients previously exposed to LSD. *Calif. Med.*, **113**:77–79, 1970.

Bein, J. H.: Pharmacology of rauwolfia. *Pharmacol. Rev.*, **8**:435–83, 1956.

Berti, F., and Shore, P. A.: A kinetic analysis of drugs that inhibit the adrenergic neuronal membrane amine pump. *Biochem. Pharmacol.*, **16**:2091–94, 1967.

Beutler, E.: Drug-induced hemolytic anemia. *Pharmacol. Rev.*, **21**:73–103, 1969.

Birkmayer, W., and Hornykiewicz, O.: The L-DOPA effect in Parkinson's syndrome in man: on the pathogenesis and treatment of Parkinson akinesis. *Arch. Psychiat. Nervenkr.*, **203**:560–74, 1962.

Bunney, W. E., and Davis, J. M.: Norepinephrine in depressive reactions: a review. *Arch. Gen. Psychiat. (Chicago)*, **13**:483–94, 1965.

Burn, J. H.: Tyramine and other amines as noradrenaline-releasing substances. In Vane, J. R.: Wolstenholme, G. E. W.; and O'Conner, M. (eds.): *Adrenergic Mechanisms.* J. & A. Churchill, Ltd., London, 1960, pp. 326–36.

Campbell, J. G.: Long-term treatment of Parkinson's disease with levodopa. *Neurology (Minneap.)*, **20** (No. 12, Part 2), 18–19, 1970.

Carlsson, A.: The occurrence, distribution and physiological role of catecholamines in the nervous system. *Pharmacol. Rev.*, **11**:449–93, 1959.

Carstairs, K.: Drug-induced immune haemolysis. *Proc. Roy. Soc. Med.*, **61**:1309, 1968.

Cotzias, G. C.; Papavasiliou, P. S.; and Gellene, R.: Modification of parkinsonism. Chronic treatment with l-dopa. *New Eng. J. Med.*, **280**:337–44, 1969.

Cotzias, G. C.; Van Woert, M. H.; and Schifferm, L. M.: Aromatic amino acids and modification of parkinsonism. *New Eng. J. Med.*, **276**:374–79, 1967.

Frenkel, J. F., Moderator et al.: Symposium: choice of animal models for the study of disease processes in man. *Fed. Proc.*, **28**:160–215, 1969.

Gershon, S.; Hekemian, L. J.; Floyd, A., Jr.; and Hollister, L. E.: A-methyl-p-tyrosine (AMT) in schizophrenia. *Psychopharmacologia*, **11**:189–94, 1967.

Graham, J. R.; Suby, H. I.; LeCompte, P. R.; and Sadowsky, N. L.: Fibrotic disorders associated with methysergide therapy for headache. *New Eng. J. Med.*, **274**:359–68, 1966.

Gyermek, L.: The pharmacology of imipramine and related antidepressants. *Int. Rev. Neurobiol.*, **9**:95–143, 1966.

Hornykiewicz, O.: Dopamine (3-hydroxytriptamine) and brain function. *Pharmacol. Rev.*, **18**:925–64, 1966.

Meyler, L., and Peck, H. M.: *Drug-Induced Diseases*, Vol. III. Excerpta Medica Foundation, Amsterdam, 1968.

Mitchinson, M. J.: Systematic idiopathic fibrosis. Dissertation for the degree of M.D. (Cantab.), 1969.

Motulsky, A. G., and Stamatoyannopoulos, G.: Clinical implications of glucose-6-phosphate dehydrogenase deficiency. *Ann. Intern. Med.*, **65**:1329–34, 1966.

Pletscher, A.; Shore, P. A.; and Brodie, B. B.: Serotonin as mediator of reserpine action in brain. *J. Pharmacol. Exp. Ther.*, **116**:84–89, 1956.

Poirier, L. J.; Sourkes, T. L.; Bouvier, G.; Boucher, R.; and Carabin, S.: Striatal amines, experimental tremor and the effect of harmaline in the monkey. *Brain*, **89**:37–52, 1966.

Prankerd, T. A. J.: Hemolytic effects of drugs and chemical agents. *Clin. Pharmacol. Ther.*, **4**:334–50, 1962.

Schildkraut, J. J.; Schanberg, S. M.; Breese, G. R.; and Kopin, I. J.: Norepinephrine metabolism and drugs used in the affective disorders: a possible mechanism of action. *Amer. J. Psychiat.*, **124**:54–62, 1967.

Whipple, H. E.; Spitzer, M. I.; and Burns, J. J.: Evaluation and mechanisms of drug toxicity. *Ann. N.Y. Acad. Sci.*, **123**:1–366, 1965.

Zeller, A. A., and Barsky, J.: *In vivo* inhibition of liver and brain monoamine oxidase by 1-isonicotinyl-2-isopropylhydrazine. *Proc. Soc. Exp. Biol. Med.*, **81**:459, 1952.

UNIT IV
CLINICAL EXAMPLES OF THE USE OF DRUGS

PROGRAMMED CASES IN THERAPEUTICS

Howard F. Morrelli

This unit is intended to demonstrate the application of the principles presented in earlier sections of the book to actual cases. The programmed format cannot substitute for supervised clinical experience as a teaching method, but it can simulate the process utilized by clinicians in solving problems, i.e., sorting data, formulating hypotheses, making therapeutic decisions, and evaluating the patient's response to therapy.

Programmers of instructional material vary in their opinions about the value of different formats. Some contend that the student should always be led to select the correct answer, so that he does not learn incorrect information. Other types of instructional goals, particularly those stressing recall of information, are better served by presenting the subject material and requesting its recall later in the program. The subject material contained here is too complex to permit use of a highly structured program. The answers to the questions posed include as many plausible answers as possible, even if they are incorrect, to attract the student to the answer section to learn why a "reasonable-sounding" answer is not optimal for the case under discussion. More difficult questions are included in some of the answers in an attempt to challenge the better-informed student.

These programs have been "field tested" in a student group ranging from third-year medical school to third-year medical residents in house-staff training. It is recommended that no more than one program be completed at a sitting, and that the student write down the answers he selects prior to proceeding to the answers, to reinforce for himself what he does and does not understand.

CASE #1

W. L. is a 36-year-old married black man admitted from the emergency room with a chief complaint of severe headaches. He had enjoyed good health through high school and had served in the Army for two years without abnormalities being described at induction or discharge physical examination. At an employment physical examination 6 years prior to admission he was told he had high blood pressure, but he did not seek medical assistance until 4 years prior to admission, when he developed morning headaches, which cleared before noon. Complete physical findings at that time were not available to the present physician, but blood pressure was reportedly 180/120. He was treated with oral reserpine and thiazide diuretics, but took these inconsistently because the pills made him feel "washed out" and "weak." Although his initial response to reserpine and thiazide was good, he developed resistance, and alpha-methyldopa was added to his regimen. This program also failed to control his blood pressure, and therapy was switched to guanethidine, 25 mg p.o. daily, and thiazide diuretics twice daily. His response was initially adequate, but he developed resistance to guanethidine when an antidepressant drug was added to his medication. In an attempt to compensate for this, furosemide, 40 mg t.i.d., was given instead of his thiazide diuretic. Two weeks prior to admission he felt "weak" and decided to stop his drugs. Three days prior to admission he developed headaches, and when he was examined in the emergency room, his blood pressure was 260/160, pulse 86; ocular fundi showed fresh hemorrhages, exudates, arteriolar spasm, and papilledema. Neck veins were flat. Lungs were clear. Cardiac impulse was in the fifth left intercostal space 2 cm lateral to the midclavicular line, forceful and sustained. A_2 was loud, a loud S_4 was audible at the apex, and no murmurs were heard. Peripheral pulses were of appropriate amplitude and synchrone; no bruits were heard. Abdominal examination and neurologic examination were within normal limits.

Laboratory data included hemoglobin, 11.0; hematocrit, 32; white-blood-cell count, 11,000; differential cell count, normal. Urinalysis: specific gravity, 1.012; protein, 4+; glucose, acetone neg.; pH, 6.0. Sediment 1 to 2 white blood cells, 5 to 10 red blood cells per high-power field. No casts. Na^+, 130; K^+, 3.0; Cl^-, 89; HCO_3^-, 33 mEq per liter;

creatinine, 7.0 mg/100 ml; albumin/globulin ratio, 3.5/3.6; blood urea nitrogen, 120; cholesterol, 180; uric acid, 9.0 mg/100 ml; calcium, 8.0 mEq per liter; phosphorus, 6.2 mg/100 ml. Two-hour postprandial glucose, 200 mg/100 ml; arterial pH, 7.45; pCO_2, 32; pO_2, 100. Stool guaiac negative.

Chest film showed left ventricular configuration of the heart, with clear lung fields. Electrocardiogram revealed increased voltage in leads representing the left ventricle, S-T segments were depressed, T waves were flat, and U waves were prominent.

Therapy was initiated with small doses of intravenous and oral alpha-methyldopa plus oral thiazides. By the next morning his blood pressure was 180/110 supine and 90/60 standing (he didn't stand long!). Pulse rate supine was 80; standing it was 84.

Q-1. The abrupt onset of severe hypertension and headaches in this patient, where blood pressure control has recently been reasonably good, is probably due to:

    A. Recent discontinuation of his medications.   See A-I*

    B. Relentless progress of a renal disease.   See A-II

    C. Moderate hypertension causing subarachnoid bleeding or an intra-cerebral hematoma with profound sympathetic discharge.   See A-III

    D. A dissecting aortic aneurysm.   See A-IV

Q-2. The patient failed to take his medicines early in his treatment course because of "weakness." Which of the following are probably responsible?

    A. Reserpine was causing depression.   See A-V

    B. Diuretics were causing sodium depletion; weakness was a symptom of volume depletion.   See A-VI

    C. Diuretics were causing potassium depletion, a known cause of muscle weakness.   See A-VII

    D. The patient developed impotence on reserpine but was shy about volunteering this information and claimed "weakness" instead.   See A-VIII

Q-3. The addition of alpha-methyldopa to his initial treatment with reserpine and thiazide diuretic was:

    A. A reasonable attempt to use two antihypertensive drugs of moderate potency to get additive effects, to control the blood pressure without imposing the unwanted effects of a single more potent antihypertensive drug.   See A-IX

    B. Theoretically sound because alpha-methyldopa has sufficiently potent direct depressant effects on the peripheral vascular resistance to synergize with reserpine.   See A-X

    C. Theoretically unsound because the pressor response to tyramine is restored in patients given alpha-methyldopa during chronic reserpinization.   See A-XI

    D. Unsuccessful owing to the rapidly progressive nature of his disease.   See A-XII

Q-4. The patient had a good initial response to guanethidine, but temporally associated with prescription of an antidepressant drug, the patient's blood pressure rose. Which of the following are reasonable explanations for this sequence of events?

    A. Antidepressant drugs make hypertension much more severe.   See A-XIII

    B. Most psychoactive agents are alkaloids or amines, and physiochemical considerations would make it likely that they would combine directly with guanethidine.   See A-XIV

    C. Antidepressant drugs have access to the CNS, whereas guanethidine does not, acting only on peripheral adrenergic neurons; hence it is unlikely that the events are causally related.   See A-XV

    D. None of the above.   See A-XVI

Q-5. On entry to the hospital, a number of findings were present that influence

* Answers relating to Case #1 appear on pages 638–42.

the rate at which it is desirable to lower the blood pressure. Rank these signs in order of clinical importance from 1 to 7 and state why rank order was given for each.

See A-XVII

A. Level of the blood pressure.
B. Recent stopping of all antihypertensive drugs.
C. Ocular fundi abnormalities.
D. Presence of headaches.
E. Degree of proteinuria.
F. Signs of left ventricular hypertrophy.
G. Rate of rise of blood pressure.

Q-6. At the time of admission, which of the following laboratory tests are likelier due to his diuretic treatment and which to his disease?

See A-XVIII

LABORATORY TEST	TREATMENT	DISEASE

Na^+, 130
K^+, 3.0
CO_2, 33
Cl^-, 89
2-hour p.c. glucose, 200 mg/100 ml
Uric acid, 9.0 mg/100 ml
Creatinine, 7.0 mg/100 ml; BUN, 120 mg/100 ml
Ca^{++}, 8.0 mEq per liter; PO_4^{3-}, 6.4 mg/100 ml

Q-7. What potential complications or concomitants of severe hypertension could account for the patient's laboratory findings of:

A. Hyponatremia.   See A-XIX
B. Hypokalemic, hypochloremic alkalosis.   See A-XX
C. Glucose intolerance, hyperuricemia.   See A-XXI
D. Discordant elevation of BUN relative to creatinine (usual ratio in uncomplicated uremia is 10:1).   See A-XXII

Q-8. The presence of uremia in this patient (pick one or more):

A. Contraindicates the use of potent antihypertensive drugs, for fear of reducing renal perfusion and increasing uremia.   See A-XXIII
B. Indicates that control of hypertension may be partly or completely effective in restoring renal function to normal.   See A-XXIV
C. Does not greatly influence the decision about lowering the blood pressure.   See A-XXV
D. May influence the specific drug chosen based on its major mechanism of action.   See A-XXVI

Q-9. The patient's blood pressure responded dramatically to a small amount of alpha-methyldopa in the supine position, but he had undue orthostatic hypotension without compensatory tachycardia on standing. This probably:

A. Represents a drug effect magnified by the disease or its complications.   See A-XXVII
B. Represents an idiosyncratic sensitivity that will permit management at low doses of the drug.   See A-XXVIII
C. Represents undue pharmacologic effect of a drug that is ordinarily cleared by the kidneys.   See A-XXIX
D. Is compatible with an otherwise latent myocardial infarction.   See A-XXX

Q-10. Which of the following are important determinants of the blood pressure (check one or more)?

A. Blood volume.   See A-XXXI
B. Cardiac contractility.
C. Autonomic nervous system function.

D. Peripheral vascular resistance.

E. Venous tone.

F. Absence of obstructive valvular or vascular disease, or pericardial disease.

G. Intact adrenocortical function.

Q-11. Based upon the patient's history, physical findings, and laboratory data, which of the following are likely additives to the antihypertensive effects of the alpha-methyldopa? Comment in space provided, evidence pro or con from the case protocol.

A. Blood volume._____ See A-XXXII

B. Cardiac contractility. _____ See A-XXXIII

C. Autonomic nervous system function. _____

_____ See A-XXXIV

D. Peripheral vascular resistance. _____ See A-XXXV

E. Venous tone. _____ See A-XXXVI

F. Obstructive or pericardial lesion._____

_____ See A-XXXVII

G. Adrenocortical function. _____ See A-XXXVIII

Q-12. The patient has been found to have severe orthostatic hypotension probably as a result of drug effect, plus the effects of hypovolemia and sodium and potassium depletion. Appropriate steps to take are:

A. Transfuse 1 to 2 units of whole blood, monitoring the blood pressure. See A-XXXIX

B. Stop all antihypertensive therapy until his blood pressure is stable. See A-XL

C. Put the patient in the reverse Trendelenburg position. See A-XLI

D. Continue present program, capitalizing on the synergistic features to lower the pressure at low-dose requirements of alpha-methyldopa. See A-XLII

Q-13. The reverse Trendelenburg position lowers the blood pressure in patients taking adrenergic-depleting or ganglionic blocking drugs because:

A. They are "gravity-assisting" drugs that cause venous pooling. See A-XLIII

B. The hydrostatic pressure in the arterial tree is directly lowered in the cranial vessels by this maneuver. See A-XLIV

C. Normal reflexes for maintaining erect blood pressure are compromised by these drugs. See A-XLV

D. Myocardial stores of norepinephrine are depleted by these drugs. See A-XLVI

A-I

Very good. This is a fact you have to "know" and hence is representative of the need for a baseline fund of information in some clinical situations, as the mechanism for "rebound accelerated or malignant hypertension" is not established. The clinical rule of thumb is that patients with documented diastolic BPs greater than 120 prior to antihypertensive Rx are likely to "rebound" if antihypertensive drugs are stopped abruptly.

A-II

One cannot totally exclude chronic renal disease such as glomerulonephritis, but the recent rate of deterioration would require the additional diagnosis of acute exacerbation of acute nephritis, since chronic renal disease is *chronic*. A later question deals further with the differential diagnosis of hypertension versus renal

disease of other etiologies and whether this critically influences early antihypertensive therapy.

A-III

This happens rarely, but is not likely in this patient since there are no profound CNS symptoms such as coma or localizing neurologic signs to permit the diagnosis of intracerebral hematoma, nor is stiff neck, a hallmark of subarachnoid bleeding, mentioned in the case protocol. At least you picked a logically correct answer; try another response.

A-IV

This patient is a reasonable candidate for dissecting aortic aneurysm with his long-standing antecedent hypertension, and aneurysms may occur without classical features, but in absence of *any* clue to the presence of aortic aneurysm, choosing this diagnosis "first" is guessmanship. Try another answer.

A-V

O.K. It happens and may be described in nonspecific terms. You really need more historic information to permit this diagnosis alone.

A-VI

Not bad, but you would have to postulate additional conditions like constant severe restriction of sodium intake by diet or a renal lesion to use this explanation, since the decrease in total-body sodium as a result of thiazide administration is transient in patients on a normal sodium intake. A later question returns to this issue.

A-VII

Probably a little better choice than the alternatives, since renal conservation mechanisms for potassium are less potent than those for Na^+, and there is later evidence for K^+ depletion. A more detailed history of what he meant by "weakness" would have been helpful.

A-VIII

This answer is more pharmacologically correct than medically. One assumes the veracity of a patient's statements unless there is substantial evidence to the contrary. Had the question included a direction to ask the patient about impotence as part of his "weakness" it would be acceptable, but still relatively unlikely, as impotence is a more regular complaint with the more potent adrenergic-depleting (guanethidine) or ganglionic blocking (mecamylamine) drugs, than with reserpine.

A-IX

Balderdash! Quit thinking about therapeutic agents as tonics, and focus on their physiologic mechanism of action or known biochemical effects. If important and potent agents are to be given, the literature must be reviewed prior to their individual or combined use. Failure to do this results in fatal reactions, e.g., combination use of monoamine oxidase inhibitors plus catechol-releasing agents. If you selected this choice, reread Chapter 5.

A-X

If you knew that alpha-methyldopa has direct action on the peripheral vascular resistance, this is a reasonable choice. Regrettably, the potency of alpha-methyldopa in this regard is only mild, as are most agents available for antihypertensive therapy, including thiazides and hydralazine. If one speculated that reserpine and alpha-methyldopa might interact adversely, or if that were known, use of another drug to decrease peripheral resistance during sympathetic blockade or depletion might be a better choice.

A-XI

This is probably the best choice among the alternatives provided. At least the statements are true. In addition to the restoration of tyramine sensitivity, catechol fluorescence reappears in adrenergic neurons when alpha-methyldopa is given to reserpine-depleted animals. These lines of evidence suggest that reserpine fails to deplete adrenergic neurons of alpha-methylnorepinephrine. Theoretically, this could result in either enhanced or diminished antihypertensive action: If alpha-methylnorepinephrine is not released well by physiologic stimuli, and if norepinephrine is depleted in a major way, enhanced antihypertensive action might be expected. If alpha-methylnorepinephrine is released at reasonable rates, fewer antihypertensive effects would be predicted. At conventional clinical doses, little additive antihypertensive effect is seen, but one should be prepared for an unusual antihypertensive effect at higher dose levels. Go on to the next question.

A-XII

Lazy answer not uncommonly given by physicians when their patients fail to respond as predicted to their random application of drug therapy. Try another answer.

A-XIII

Not unless the patient has a pheochromocytoma or has been treated with monoamine oxidase inhibitors like pargyline, then takes amphetamine or a tricyclic antidepressant like imipramine.

A-XIV

Guanethidine is a base. Try another answer.

A-XV

You've been had! The statement is true, but does not exclude the possibility that the drugs interact peripherally. (See A-XVI.)

A-XVI

Yes. If the adrenergic neuron is considered as a "receptor" for norepinephrine, guanethidine may be thought of as a competitor for norepinephrine's receptor sites in granules for storage of norepinephrine. Guanethidine then reduces adrenergic neuronal stores of norepinephrine and limits the capacity of the neuron to "take up" circulating norepinephrine. The tricyclic antidepressants and amphetamines appear to compete even more successfully than guanethidine for the mutual storage sites, liberating norepinephrine with abolition or reversal of guanethidine's antihypertensive effects.

A-XVII

1. *Ocular fundi.* Acute severe changes, demonstrating vascular damage.
2. *Rate of rise of BP.* An ominous sign clinically.
3. *Degree of proteinuria.* Maybe, but not as certain as 1 and 2, as it could be due to *other* renal disease, and the "4+" report is only semiquantitative.
4. *Level of the blood pressure.* A pretty good indication of severity, but some patients have this level of blood pressure elevation without the more important signs of acute vascular damage.
5. *Recent stopping of all antihypertensive drugs.* As an isolated feature this is unimportant. It becomes very important in association with findings of accelerated or malignant hypertension, and in this context would warrant a rank order of 3.
6. *Presence of headaches.* May correlate with signs of CNS damage or may be a relatively nonspecific symptom. If convinced of relation to BP, rank high.
7. *Left ventricular hypertrophy.* Probably a sign of more long-standing disease.

(This question emphasizes the principle that acute vascular damage is an important determinant of the need to treat. Look for disease, not numbers.)

A-XVIII

Diuretic therapy could cause all the laboratory test abnormalities listed in the question:

Hyponatremia and hypokalemia by virtue of total-body cation depletion. Hypovolemia could cause the abnormal BUN/creatinine ratio. Alkalosis and hypochloremia, particularly in view of moderate uremia, suggest the possibility of potassium depletion alkalosis with paradoxical aciduria.

Thiazides and furosemide may cause glucose intolerance, but K^+ depletion and uremia can also cause glucose intolerance. Thiazides and furosemide may cause hyperuricemia, but the level of hyperuricemia in this patient is not disproportionate to his uremia. Diuretics, particularly the more potent ones, can cause increases in urinary calcium, but only rarely do they cause frank hypocalcemia. His hypocalcemia and increased serum phosphate are more suggestive of chronic azotemia.

The diuretics may have added to other mechanisms accounting for the laboratory

test abnormalities, but since they have been omitted for the past 2 weeks, alternative explanations for these findings would be advantageous as a prelude to therapy. Proceed to Question 7.

A-XIX

1. Profound sodium diuresis seen during severe hypertensive crises.
2. Renal disease with loss of ability to conserve sodium at normal rates: relative sodium wasting.

A-XX

Secondary hyperaldosteronism due to (1) low blood volume, or (2) release of renin during acute renal hypertensive damage, eliciting aldosterone secretion in response to angiotensin release.

A-XXI

Uremic state.

A-XXII

A prerenal cause like congestive heart failure, severely impaired cardiac output; a catabolic state; infection; gastrointestinal bleeding; or a postrenal cause like obstructive uropathy. Based on the clinical findings given, one would probably suspect blood volume depletion.

A-XXIII

Treatment of the hypertension is required, as the mortality of untreated accelerated or malignant hypertension is 85% in one year. At least half of these patients show significant improvement in renal function if the blood pressure is lowered. Some patients show a transient deterioration in renal function that clears with continued antihypertensive therapy.

A-XXIV

It is more commonly *partly* effective than *completely* effective in restoring renal function, since two vascular lesions are present in hypertensive renal disease: a reversible acute vasculitis affecting small vessels, and a more chronic, irreversible atherosclerosis of large vessels.

A-XXV

Right. See A-XXIII, and select another alternative if you picked this alone.

A-XXVI

Probably true. If the patient responds to agents that act chiefly (hydralazine) or in part (alpha-methyldopa) by decreasing the peripheral vascular resistance, as opposed to drugs that decrease cardiac output by pooling blood in veins (ganglionic blockers, potent antiadrenergics), renal perfusion may be maintained as much as possible. Select another answer if you picked this one alone.

A-XXVII

O.K. You didn't get fooled. Proceed to Question 10.

A-XXVIII

"Pollyanna" answer of a type not rare in unskilled therapeutics. You should exhaust reasonable positive alternatives before accepting a negative one. Try another answer.

A-XXIX

Not the *worst* available choice, but fails to deal with other known pharmacologic actions of alpha-methyldopa when it is initiated, for instance, lethargy. If this were uncomplicated excessive drug action, why is the patient alert?

A-XXX

Good try, since it relates the pathophysiology of the patient to an unexpected drug effect. Other complications in this patient are more likely than silent myocardial infarction to account for the sensitivity to alpha-methyldopa.

A-XXXI

All should be checked.

A-XXXII

Blood volume. Good. The mild anemia shown by slightly low hematocrit may be misleading if there is concurrent plasma volume depletion. Hypovolemia is suggested by flat neck veins, abnormal ratio of BUN/creatinine. This was the case, as shown by ^{51}Cr blood volume reduction of 30% in both RBC mass and plasma volume. Reduction of blood volume would be expected to synergize with the effect of a drug that decreases adrenergic action and decreases the peripheral vascular resistance. Another mechanism was also likely involved. Select an additional answer.

A-XXXIII

No good clinical signs of impaired contractility are given in the protocol, e.g., S_3 gallop, signs of heart failure, low pulse pressure. Hence this is not very likely.

A-XXXIV

Underlying impairment of autonomic nervous system function, if it affected the adrenergic component, could add to the adrenergic-depleting action of alpha-methyldopa. This patient is chronically potassium depleted, a

condition in which baroreceptor function is poor. Part of his excessive response to alpha-methyldopa is likely due to this mechanism. (In retrospect, it would have been helpful to examine his blood pressure and pulse rate supine and erect and with Valsalva's maneuver prior to treatment.)

A-XXXV

No clinical description, such as flushed, warm skin or bruit over an AV anastomosis, was given to implicate diminished peripheral resistance. Try another answer.

A-XXXVI

O.K. answer if you related it to low blood volume or autonomic nervous system function, q.v.

A-XXXVII

No physical signs of these diseases were described. Try another answer.

A-XXXVIII

It is true that adrenal steroids are thought to exert a "permissive role" in norepinephrine effects on vessels, i.e., that a vasoconstrictor response to norepinephrine is suboptimal in the absence of cortisol; but one would have to postulate Addison's disease in this patient to utilize this mechanism and this would be unlikely given a hypertensive patient with no hyperkalemia.

A-XXXIX

Blood transfusion is a dangerous intervention. It is used when there is clear need. This patient's orthostatic hypotension can be managed in other ways. Transfusion of blood may increase the blood pressure, and there is no evidence that patients in uremia fare better at "normal" hematocrits than at levels of 25 to 30. Try another answer.

A-XL

This error is not uncommonly made and would predictably result in a second episode of "rebound malignant hypertension."

A-XLI

Quite right. This is discussed in more detail in the next question.

A-XLII

The continuing effects of hypovolemia and electrolyte depletion will make the patient more responsive to the antihypertensive effects of nearly any antihypertensive drug, but his response is not to be considered "desirable" and a basis for continuing treatment, since the hypovolemia will reduce his renal function, and chronic potassium depletion may result in arrhythmias, renal dysfunction, pyelonephritis, and "weakness." The electrolyte abnormalities should be treated independently of the drug therapy required for his hypertension. Sodium deprivation is no longer felt to be a good method of reducing the blood pressure, as it may cause deterioration in renal function.

A-XLIII

Yes. The principal mechanism of action of most of the potent antihypertensive drugs is a reduction in cardiac output by this mechanism. Another answer is O.K., but not as good as this one.

A-XLIV

If this occurs, it is trivial compared to other important mechanisms. Choose another answer.

A-XLV

True, but not as good as one of the other answers because it is so obviously true and does not give a mechanism for the action.

A-XLVI

True for some of the drugs, but not all in these categories; ganglionic blocking drugs do not deplete myocardial norepinephrine. The depletion of cardiac norepinephrine probably does not account for much of the antihypertensive action of the adrenergic-depleting drugs, but it may be responsible for congestive heart failure at toxic levels.

Follow-up: After correction of blood volume and electrolyte abnormalities, the patient was readily controlled on alpha-methyldopa and thiazide diuretics.

CASE #2

A 29-year-old white woman was first noted to be hypertensive at the conclusion of her second full-term pregnancy. She noted some feelings of being flushed at that time. She was not known to be hypertensive again until 3 years later, during the third trimester of her third pregnancy, which was complicated by placenta praevia requiring cesarean section. She had no other findings such as edema or proteinuria suggestive of pre-eclampsia. She was well for about 1 year until 6 weeks prior to her hospital admission, when she was found to have hypertension, and laboratory studies showed mild diabetes. She was treated with an oral contraceptive agent. In the weeks before admission to the hospital she complained of spells, consisting of hot sweats with flushing and a clammy sensation. On occasion, she felt cardiac palpitations and a sensation of pressure in her head. In the few days prior to admission she felt dizzy and weak on getting up rapidly from sitting or lying. There was no family history of cardiovascular disease. Physical examination on admission revealed blood pressure of 150/85 lying, with a pulse rate of 98, and 115/80 standing, with a pulse rate rising to 120. Funduscopic examination showed minimal arteriolar narrowing. Cardiac examination was unremarkable except for occasional premature ventricular contractions. Urinary studies demonstrated catechol excretion rates of 600 to 900 mg per day, metanephrines of 16 to 21 mg per day, and vanilmandelic acid of 20 to 25 mg per day.

Q-1. Please list a complete differential diagnosis for this patient. See A-I*

Q-2. Which of the diagnostic possibilities listed in Question 1 would you consider to be the most likely based on all the data provided, assuming no important positive findings have been omitted from the protocol? Diagnostic choice:
A. Essential hypertension. See A-II
B. Renovascular hypertension. See A-III
C. Toxemia of pregnancy. See A-IV
D. Aldosteronism. See A-V
E. Coarctation of aorta. See A-VI
F. Cushing's disease. See A-VII
G. Primary renal disease. See A-VIII
H. Pheochromocytoma. See A-IX

* Answers relating to Case #2 appear on pages 645–52.

Q-3. Which of the following substances are subject to falsely high apparent urinary excretion rates in patients suspected of having a pheochromocytoma?
A. Catecholamines.
B. Metanephrines.
C. Vanilmandelic acid.
D. All the above.   See A-X

Q-4. What are the substances and the mechanism of spurious induction of high excretion rates for:
A. Catecholamines.   See A-XI
B. Metanephrines.   See A-XII
C. Vanilmandelic acid.   See A-XIII

Q-5. Administration of pharmacologic agents to patients suspected of having a pheochromocytoma is sometimes useful in supporting the diagnosis. List the agents.   See A-XIV

Q-6. How often are pharmacologic tests for the presence of a pheochromocytoma positive in patients with the disease?   See XV
A. 100%
B. 90%
C. 75%
D. 50%

Q-7. Which of the tests in the earlier question would be indicated for the patient under discussion?   See A-XVI

Q-8. The diagnosis of a pheochromocytoma is secure, and large quantities of catechols and their metabolites are being excreted; therefore:
A. It is somewhat urgent that the tumor be removed to prevent a fatal or crippling hypertensive stroke in a young mother. Surgery should be scheduled within a few days.   See A-XVII
B. The large quantities of catechols being excreted suggest a malignant process. Even if the tumor is presently benign, it may become malignant. Surgery is indicated within a few weeks.   See A-XVIII
C. The data presented localize the tumor to the abdomen; no further delays need be incurred by diagnostic studies, and the patient may be explored forthwith.   See A-XIX
D. I cannot recommend surgery now.   See A-XX

Q-9. It is clear that the patient has a large pheochromocytoma, and that it probably secretes predominantly norepinephrine (most pheochromocytomas do). In view of this, why doesn't the patient have hypertension at the time of the examination?
A. The tumor secretes intermittently, accounting for the normal blood pressure at the time of the examination. Serial blood pressure determinations are required.   See A-XXI
B. The tumor is secreting large amounts of epinephrine. Epinephrine has both alpha (constricting) and beta (dilating) effects on the vessels determining the peripheral vascular resistance. The beta effects would be expected to dilate sufficient vessels in the peripheral vascular resistance to prevent diastolic hypertension.   See A-XXII
C. Despite the continuing effects of excessive catecholamines on cardiac and vessel function, the patient is a good candidate for hypovolemia, and/or ganglionic blockage, and/or heart disease to account for the absence of hypertension.   See A-XXIII

Q-10. Beside the following list of antihypertensive agents, write (I) if you think the drug is indicated now, (D) if the drug would be of dubious value, or (C) if you have reason to believe the drug is contraindicated.

See A-XXIV

Hydralazine
Mecamylamine
Trimethaphan
Thiazide diuretics
Nitroprusside
Phentolamine

Reserpine
Alpha-methyldopa
Guanethidine
Phenoxybenzamine
Propranolol
Pargyline

Q-11. In the previous question, reserpine, guanethidine, and alpha-methyldopa were considered to be contraindicated in this patient because:
A. They might obscure further tests of catecholamine secretion or excretion necessary for diagnosis.
B. They might cause hypertension.
C. They are excessively potent as antihypertensive agents and might induce shock.

See A-XXV

Q-12. In the earlier question, hydralazine, mecamylamine, trimethaphan, thiazides, nitroprusside, and pargyline were considered to be of doubtful value or contraindicated in this patient because:
A. They might obscure further tests of catecholamine secretion or excretion necessary for diagnosis.
B. They are not clearly indicated at present.
C. They might cause shock or hypertension.
D. The hypertension of pheochromocytoma requires specific adrenergic blocking therapy.

See A-XXVI
See A-XXVII
See A-XXVIII

See A-XXIX

Q-13. In the previous question, propranolol was considered to be of doubtful value or possibly indicated in this patient because (pick one or more):
A. Presence of premature ventricular contractions constitutes an indication for its use.
B. Although the tumor secretes relatively little epinephrine compared to norepinephrine, the beta-stimulating effects of both of these may cause serious arrhythmias.
C. The cardiac depressant actions of propranolol should be avoided in a patient with possible myocardial damage; hence its use is not unequivocally indicated.

See A-XXX

See A-XXXI

See A-XXXII

Q-14. In considering the treatment of pheochromocytoma generally, it has been decided that phentolamine and phenoxybenzamine are each useful since they are alpha-adrenergic blocking agents. In selecting a drug for this patient, which of the following would you feel is most applicable?
A. The two drugs are equivalent, either may be employed.
B. Phentolamine has a quicker onset of action and is preferable.
C. Phenoxybenzamine has a later onset of action, since it is metabolized to an active agent that induces noncompetitive blockade, and is therefore preferable.

See A-XXXIII
See A-XXXIV

See A-XXXV

Q-15. Assuming that phentolamine or phenoxybenzamine is a correct choice for therapy of the patient described, what was the principal object of the treatment?
A. Treatment of the pheochromocytoma.
B. Control of the patient's hypertension.
C. Control of the patient's arrhythmia.
D. Control of the patient's postural hypotension.

See A-XXXVI
See A-XXXVII
See A-XXXVIII
See A-XXXIX

Q-16. How large should the initial doses of the alpha-adrenergic blocking drug be? Justify your choice of the following:
    A. Small.   See A-XL
    B. Medium.   See A-XLI
    C. Large.   See A-XLII

Q-17. If the tumor is localized to the abdomen, how soon should surgery be done after initial control of the patient's symptoms, i.e., a few days?
    A. At once.   See A-XLIII
    B. After 2 to 3 weeks.   See A-XLIV
    C. Six months later.   See A-XLV

Q-18. Which symptoms, physical findings, or laboratory tests would persist (mark + alongside choice) or be absent (mark − alongside choice) during adequate pharmacologic control of the patient with phentolamine or phenoxybenzamine? These findings will permit assessment of the adequacy of the treatment and determine when the patient is properly prepared for surgery.   See A-XLVI
    A. Hypovolemia.
    B. Sweating.
    C. High excretion rates of catecholamines and their metabolites.
    D. Hypertension.
    E. Postural hypotension.
    F. Palpitations.
    G. Elevated 2-hr postprandial blood sugar.
    H. T-wave inversion in the electrocardiogram.
    I. Elevated plasma free fatty acids.

Q-19. If the prolonged administration of phenoxybenzamine had resulted in complete irreversible alpha receptor blockade, what drug could be given to increase the peripheral vascular resistance, if hypotension occurred at the time of surgery and the hypotension was refractory to volume replacement?   See A-LI

A-I

Essential hypertension.
Renovascular hypertension.
Toxemia of pregnancy.
Aldosteronism.
Coarctation of the aorta.
Cushing's disease.
Primary renal disease with secondary hypertension.
Pheochromocytoma.
(Proceed to Question 2.)

A-II

Essential hypertension: wrong answer. Certainly the most likely on the basis of statistical probability, since essential hypertension accounts for at least 80% of all cases of hypertension, but this diagnosis would be inappropriate in a patient who describes paroxysmal symptoms, has a striking degree of postural hypotension not readily assignable to essential hypertension, and whose laboratory findings strongly suggest an alternative diagnosis. Try another.

A-III

Renovascular hypertension: nice try but no cigar! The consideration of renovascular hypertension in a young female with recent onset of hypertension is a good thought, but this diagnosis is not particularly likely in view of her normal blood pressure recorded at the time of examination. The degree of postural change is unusual, unless one were to postulate secondary hyperaldosteronism (loss of baroreceptor function is a feature of primary and secondary hyperaldosteronism). This latter possibility is excluded by the fact that her pressure is presently normal, and secondary aldosteronism is a feature of very severe hypertension. To make the diagnosis of renovascular hypertension one would have been assisted by the presence of an epigastric bruit or an IVP showing a small kidney on one side. In addition, a timed-sequence IVP would most likely show delayed filling of the ischemic kidney with hyperconcentration of dye on later films on the same side (due to increased reabsorption of water from the ischemic kidney), leading to confirmatory tests such as aortography and/or differential renal function tests.

A-IV

Toxemia of pregnancy: wrong. This might have been considered at the time of her last pregnancy when mild hypertension was noted, i.e., possible pre-eclampsia, but there is no current suggestion of pregnancy given in the protocol, and since she has been on birth control pills, this diagnosis is unlikely. On the other hand, you should have considered the possibility of birth-control-pill–induced hypertension. This clinical entity has been reported frequently in the literature, and although its ultimate mechanism remains obscure, it may be associated with high aldosterone secretion rates, electrolyte abnormalities, and postural hypotension. One may be reasonably certain that this is not the sole explanation for her disease, as she was known to be hypertensive prior to administration of the birth control pill.

A-V

Aldosteronism: a very good thought in a young female with mild hypertension, essentially normal fundi, and loss of baroreceptor reflexes. The diagnosis of hypertension secondary to an aldosterone-secreting tumor would be very unlikely in the absence of hypokalemia, which was not described in the protocol. Hypokalemia may be absent in aldosteronism if the patient has been on a low-sodium diet or has been taking sodium-depleting agents like thiazides, since there will be no sodium available for distal tubular exchange with potassium. Further, this diagnosis is not particularly likely in a patient with a good history of flushing and paroxysmal symptoms. If you considered seriously the diagnosis of an aldosterone-secreting tumor and if this was further suggested by hypokalemia, but aldosterone secretion rates were normal or low, excessive ingestion of licorice would have been an alternative possibility. Some cases of aldosteronism are characterized by normal, but continuously high, levels of aldosterone secretion that are not suppressible by DOCA. An unusually rare cause of hypertension with many features suggesting aldosteronism is the lack of 17-beta hydroxylase in the adrenal cortex, resulting in high excretion rates of DOCA, which are reversible by treatment with cortisol.

A-VI

Coarctation of the aorta: a very poor first choice in the absence of cardiac murmurs, cardiac enlargement, sustained hypertension, and discrepancies in amplitude or timing of the peripheral pulses.

A-VII

Cushing's disease: hypertension is a feature of Cushing's disease, but when present is accompanied by other gross features of the syndrome such as truncal obesity, muscle weakness, bruising, and thin skin. This diagnosis ignores the paroxysmal nature of the patient's symptoms and critical pieces of laboratory data provided in the protocol. Try another diagnosis.

A-VIII

Primary renal disease: with an extraordinary exception, neither acute nor chronic renal disease would be expected to cause hypertension in the absence of abnormalities of the urinary sediment or of abnormal renal function tests. You should review your basic concepts regarding the diagnosis of significant renal disease. Try another diagnosis.

A-IX

Pheochromocytoma: an unusual cause of hypertension, but clearly the diagnosis of first choice in this patient because of the history of flushing and paroxysmal symptoms, and possibly because of the premature ventricular contractions noted on the physical examination, the postural hypotension, and the abnormally high urinary excretion rates of catecholamines and their metabolites (in the absence of interfering substances). You have demonstrated insight into the preliminaries of the diagnosis of pheochromocytoma. Proceed to the more difficult questions.

A-X

D. All the above. Proceed to next question for discussion of mechanisms of spurious elevation.

A-XI

A. Catecholamines: catechols such as epinephrine or isoproterenol given for bronchospasm can increase the urinary excretion rate of catecholamines since they are catechols. Most assay procedures for catechols depend on fluorescent techniques; accordingly, drugs with high fluorescence, such as alpha-methyldopa, tetracyclines, ephedrine, or phenothiazines, may cause confusion. Administration of large amounts of catechol-depleting antihypertensive drugs such as reserpine or guanethidine might conceivably increase urinary catecholamines temporarily (this has not been studied), but their chronic administration is known *not* to interfere.

A-XII

B. Metanephrines: monamine oxidase inhibitors given for hypertension or depression (pargyline or tranylcypromine) would increase the urinary excretion of metanephrines and decrease the urinary excretion of vanilmandelic acid, since monoamine oxidase converts the former to the latter in the normal metabolic sequence of catecholamines. Certain other drugs given for infection (INH) or cancer (procarbazine) may have monamine-oxidase-blocking properties and may cause confusion.

A-XIII

C. Vanilmandelic acid: this substance may be assayed by fluorescent methods that may also detect other phenolic acids whose presence in the urine is determined by ingestion of foods with a high content of phenolic compounds, such as coffee, vanilla, nuts, and certain fruits and vegetables.

A-XIV

Pharmacologic tests that may be useful in supporting the diagnosis of pheochromocytoma:
Phentolamine (alpha-adrenergic-blocking agent).
Tyramine (catechol-releasing agent).
Histamine (catechol-releasing agent).
Glucagon (mechanism uncertain).

A-XV

C. 75%.

A-XVI

None. It may be tempting to suggest a stimulation test, i.e., tyramine, histamine, glucagon, or tilt table to increase the blood pressure, since the patient is normotensive at the time of examination. On the other hand, these stimulation procedures may elicit a profound hypertensive response and must only be done with phentolamine immediately available to reverse the reaction. The major reason for not proceeding with stimulation procedures in this patient is the fact that the available urinary studies are diagnostic. Catechol test is 90% accurate, VMA 95% accurate, metanephrine probably near 100% accurate. There is no need to embark upon a potentially dangerous test in this patient. Pharmacologic tests are useful as screening devices of fair validity when one strongly suspects a pheochromocytoma in a patient with equivocal urinary excretion rates of catechols or their metabolites, or when one needs to know at once whether a patient has a pheochromocytoma in urgent circumstances such as malignant hypertensive crisis when one is contemplating the use of catechol-releasing

agents (e.g., guanethidine) as part of the acute management.

A-XVII

A. One is anxious to prevent further damage to the patient by the tumor; however, to operate at once without locating the tumor, without adequate pharmacologic control of the symptoms being caused by the tumor products, and without consideration of means to minimize the effects of massive catecholamine release during induction of anesthesia or manipulation of the tumor would show bad judgment. Is the tumor in the chest or the abdominal cavity?

A-XVIII

B. Wrong answer. The large quantities of tumor products suggest either a sizable tumor or multiple smaller tumors, but they have no meaning in terms of malignancy. There is no evidence that benign pheochromocytomas become malignant. The histology of pheochromocytomas is confusing, as they may show cellular pleomorphism and encroachment upon veins. The diagnosis of malignancy depends upon evidence of metastatic involvement of other organs, although urinary excretion of primitive catechols such as dopamine or its metabolite (homovanillic acid) may be highly suggestive.

A-XIX

C. The data (especially the large quantities of catechol metabolites) suggest a large pheochromocytoma, but are inadequate to localize the tumor. Preliminary data suggest strongly that if the tumor secretes large amounts of ephinephrine (15% of the total catecholamines) it is located in one or both adrenals or in the organ of Zuckerkandl. These organs contain the enzyme phenylethanolamine N-methyl transferase, which is necessary for the conversion of norepinephrine to epinephrine. No other tissue and few tumors located elsewhere have thus far been reported to contain this enzyme. Additional steps to localize the tumor include skull films, chest x-rays, intravenous pyelography with tomograms, and sampling of venous blood along the caval systems for catecholamine levels.

A-XX

D. Right on! Please review responses to the alternative choices given in A-XVII, A-XVIII, and A-XIX. In addition to the objections listed, there are some unexplained clinical findings in the patient that require explanation before either surgical or medical treatment can be initiated. Proceed to the next question.

A-XXI

A. A good thought, but the very large quantities of urinary catechols and their metabolites make this suggestion relatively unlikely. Intermittent secretors tend to have smaller daily quantities of tumor product, and it may be necessary to collect the first available urine specimen after a brief hypertensive crisis to demonstrate the abnormal secretion and excretion rate of catecholamines (uncommonly). Subsequent blood pressure determinations around the clock failed to demonstrate hypertension. Postural hypotension with tachycardia persisted. Try one of the other answers.

A-XXII

B. A fair speculation, but this response ignores the well-known pharmacologic effects of large amounts of parenteral epinephrine: striking systolic and usually diastolic hypertension due to the combined effects of alpha and beta stimulation of both the heart (dramatic increase in cardiac output) and the peripheral vascular resistance. If you tried answers A and B before answer C, try thinking about the physiologic determinants of the blood pressure, and how these individually or in combination might be altered by a pheochromocytoma to account for lack of hypertension despite catechol excess. Then see A-XXIII.

A-XXIII

C. Excellent. Long-standing excesses of catecholamines might be expected to (1) reduce the blood volume (see Chapter 5), thereby limiting venous return, cardiac output, and blood pressure response; (2) induce ganglionic blockage, by analogy to the ganglionic blocking action of catechols demonstrated in the experimental model of the superior cervical ganglion in the cat; (3) induce a lesion of the heart that would inhibit cardiac output in response to catechol excess, limiting the hypertensive response. Catechol-induced myocardial lesions would include myocardiopathy and myocardial infarction. The patient developed tachycardia on standing. This is more compatible with hypovolemia than ganglionic blockade. The patient's blood volume was found to be reduced by 25%. No evidence for ganglionic blockade was found. In addition, the patient developed T-wave inversion in ECG leads I, aVL, V3-6 over the course of a few days, suggesting an acute myocardial process. Proceed to the next question.

A-XXIV

Hydralazine (D or C)   Reserpine (C)
Mecamylamine (D or C) Methyldopa (C)

Trimethaphan (D or C) Guanethidine (C)
Thiazides (D or C)   Phenoxybenzamine (I)
Nitroprusside (D or C) Propranolol (D or I)
Phentolamine (I)   Pargyline (D or C)

A-XXV

C. Although these drugs might influence the tests for pheochromocytoma, and parenteral or large doses of them may induce hypotension in essential hypertension, the major concern about their use in pheochromocytoma is their suspected potential for release of catecholamines from the tumor and "saturated" adrenergic neurons, precipitating a hypertensive crisis. Unless you are confident about the mechanism of action of all the drugs listed in this question sequence, reread Chapter 5 before proceeding.

A-XXVI

A. Wrong answer. Only pargyline among this group would be expected to interfere with excretion tests. The hypotensive action of the monoamine-oxidase-inhibiting drug depends on the synthesis of octopamine, a false neurotransmitter that is either released instead of norepinephrine or limits the production of norepinephrine by feedback inhibition of synthetic enzymes. There is no assurance that this sequence would ensue in a patient with a pheochromocytoma; hence pargyline is of dubious value. An interesting approach to the management of *malignant* pheochromocytoma has been the use of alpha-methyltyrosine, which inhibits the enzyme tyrosine hydroxylase, rate limiting in the synthesis of catecholamines.

A-XXVII

B. Quite right! This patient is normotensive, and the drugs listed would not be particularly indicated even if the patient was hypertensive, as more specific means are available for treatment.

Choice of any of these drugs for this patient is inappropriate since she is *normotensive*. Selection of this category of drugs by a physician would indicate that his approach to therapeutics was by "recipe"; i.e., a disease (pheochromocytoma or hypertension) elicits a reflex response to administer an antihypertensive agent without due reflection on the pathophysiology of the patient's symptoms.

A-XXVIII

C. Possibly, but not the best answer among the alternatives provided. Hypotension might result from the more potent drugs of this list, and reflexly, large amounts of catechols might be released. Hypertension would not be expected as a result of the direct effects of these drugs.

A-XXIX

D. A true statement, but selection of this answer is not as correct as one of the alternatives, since the statement does not apply to this patient who is *normotensive*. Try another answer.

A-XXX

A. Correct, at least some of the time! If one were reasonably sure that an arrhythmia appearing in a patient with a pheochromocytoma were due to the effects of catecholamines alone, and especially if it persisted when the hypertension had been controlled with alpha-adrenergic blocking drugs, or if the arrhythmia were serious, unassociated with congestive heart failure, and refractory to more conventional antiarrhythmic drugs like lidocaine, propranolol would certainly be in order.

Some physicians have recommended the use of propranolol routinely as a part of the preoperative management of patients with pheochromocytoma to "prevent" arrhythmias. The utility of this practice has not been compared to use of alpha blocking therapy alone, which commonly improves cardiac rhythm by reducing hypertension or by partly blocking cardiac alpha and beta receptors (overlapping effect of alpha blockers).

One or more of the alternative answers are also correct; pick one.

A-XXXI

B. True, but it may be possible to control the arrhythmia by means of alpha blocking agents to control the hypertension, since hypertension increases left ventricular tension, a cause of arrhythmias. Further, the blocking effect of alpha blocking agents is not restricted to alpha receptors (at least it appears so in the heart), as their use in pheochromocytoma appears to alleviate certain of the cardiac events one would ordinarily assign to beta stimulation. See A-XXX for additional discussion. How about answer C?

A-XXXII

C. Correct. This patient has a cardiac lesion as indicated by her electrocardiogram, and possibly her arrhythmia is related to heart disease as opposed to catechol effects. Propranolol may cause congestive heart failure; patients with acute myocardial infarction fare less well than controls in studies of its use in acute myocardial infarction. One or both of the alternative answers is also correct; return to them.

A-XXXIII

A. Try thinking about other qualities that drugs have in addition to their principal desired

pharmacologic action, i.e., kinetics and how this influences duration of action, reversible versus irreversible blockade, and degree of blockade expected, before selecting one of the alternative answers.

A-XXXIV

B. Phentolamine. It is true that the quick onset of action is useful in certain circumstances in pheochromocytoma, such as a hypertensive crisis appearing prior to therapy, or during surgery despite good preoperative control. The short half-life of this drug, however, requires that it be given every 4 to 6 hours by mouth to maintain complete control. Patients find this inconvenient, and even those with the best of intentions may "forget" a dose, with hypertension ensuing. If large doses are given by mouth, gastrointestinal irritation with nausea, vomiting, and diarrhea may occur. Try answer C.

A-XXXV

C. Phenoxybenzamine. This is probably the best choice for this patient, but not for the reason cited in the question. There is no theoretic advantage to the drug's requirement for metabolism prior to pharmacologic activity; nor is the fact that a noncompetitive or non-equilibrium alpha-adrenergic blockade is imposed of necessary therapeutic benefit. The latter quality confers a long duration of action; this is useful since drugs taken once or twice daily are less likely to be "forgotten" than are drugs taken many times daily. "Breakthrough" of hypertension is less likely, even though phenoxybenzamine can be given every 12 hours, contrasted with the need to give phentolamine every 4 to 6 hours. The problem of equilibrium versus nonequilibrium blockade is considered in a later question.

A-XXXVI

A. "Treatment of the pheochromocytoma" is the worst possible choice among the possibilities listed, as it implies that the name of a disease alone suffices to elicit a therapeutic response. Treatment should be directed toward the pathophysiologic manifestations of the disease detectable by history, physical examination, and laboratory data or special tests. Review the case history and try another response!

A-XXXVII

B. "Control of the patient's hypertension" is the second *worst* answer to this question among the alternatives listed. The patient is not hypertensive at the time of the examination, and you were given the additional information that frequent observations of the blood pressure never disclosed hypertension. If you selected this answer with the intent of preventing potential episodes of hypertension in the future, due to massive release of catechols, you're excused, but another answer can be defended with greater ease for the patient *at present*.

A-XXXVIII
C. "Control of the patient's arrhythmia"; not bad, but not as good as another choice. Try again.

A-XXXIX
D. "Control of the patient's postural hypotension." Excellent. This seemingly paradoxical choice depends upon a good understanding of the pathophysiology of the disease to be treated. The alpha blocking agent was chosen to overcome the long-standing effects of excessive alpha-adrenergic stimulation of the peripheral vascular resistance and heart that had led to hypovolemia with a reduced cardiac reserve and output, hence to postural hypotension. If the hypovolemia had been more severe, causing even a greater degree of postural hypotension, it could have been treated directly by saline infusions (but at the risk of causing hypertension).

A-XL
A. Small. Excellent choice. There is a tendency for physicians to be more impressed by numbers reported by the laboratory than by their own examination and reflection upon physical findings. In this patient the attending physicians were impressed by the large quantities of catecholamines present in the urine and began treatment with a large dose of phenoxybenzamine. This caused a striking increase in the postural hypotension and several syncopal episodes. Small doses were tolerated well, however, and as the patient recovered from the excessive effects of catechols, particularly with respect to hypovolemia, she tolerated, and in fact required, more substantial doses of the drug. Had due consideration been given to the patient's normal blood pressure at rest with postural hypotension, this potentially dangerous sequence could have been avoided.

A-XLI
B. Medium. Perhaps justifiable as an answer, but be brave, try one of the others.

A-XLII
C. Large. Incorrect choice for this patient. Review your thinking about the pathophysiol-

ogy of the patient's symptoms and select one of the remaining alternatives.

A-XLIII
A. *At once*: wrong answer. Don't panic; weigh the advantages and potential disadvantages of early versus late surgery, and try one of the other alternative answers.

A-XLIV
B. Controversial answer. There is some anxiety about removing the tumor to prevent hypertensive catastrophes, but good medical control is possible; a relatively long time interval is desirable to permit recovery of homeostatic mechanisms of blood pressure control on rational grounds and is successful on empiric grounds (as determined by morbidity and mortality of surgery done immediately versus after a "cooling-off" period of medical management). In addition, since one could not be certain of the patient's cardiac lesion (i.e., silent myocardial infarction versus catechol myocardiopathy), and since the mortality of *any* surgery shortly after acute myocardial infarction is high, it was deemed advisable to treat the patient for 6 weeks to 3 months before surgical intervention, assuming good patient cooperation and follow-up, and a good response to medical therapy.

A-XLV
C. Controversial question. There is some anxiety about removing the tumor to prevent a hypertensive stroke in a young mother. On the other hand, good medical control is possible, and a relatively long time interval to permit recovery of homeostatic mechanisms of BP control is desirable on rational grounds, and successful on empiric grounds. Since we cannot be certain of her cardiac lesion (i.e., silent myocardial infarction versus catechol myocardiopathy), and since the mortality of *any* surgery shortly after acute myocardial infarction is very high, it was deemed advisable to treat the patient for 6 weeks to 3 months before surgical intervention, assuming good patient cooperation, follow-up, and excellent control of symptoms and findings by medical therapy.

A-XLVI
Hypovolemia $(-)0$
Sweating $(-)0$
High excretion rates of catecholamines and their metabolites $(+)\#$
Hypertension $(-)0$
Postural hypotension $(-)0$
Palpitations $(-)0$
Elevated 2-hr postprandial blood sugar $(+)*$

T-wave inversion in the electrocardiogram (−)**

Elevated plasma free fatty acids (+)*

If you erred in an answer marked 0 see A-XLVII; if marked # see A-XLVIII; if marked * see A-XLIX; if marked ** see A-L.

A-XLVII

Items marked 0 are findings usually assignable to the alpha mimetic effects of catecholamines, and should be absent during adequate pharmacologic therapy. A potential exception is the symptom of palpitation, or the presence of premature beats on examination of the patient; these may be due to beta effects of catecholamines, and although they are usually controlled by alpha-adrenergic blocking drugs, they may require additional therapy as indicated earlier in this question series.

A-XLVIII

The *blocking* drugs would not be expected to influence the tumor's secretion or the patient's excretion of catecholamines or their metabolites.

A-XLIX

These findings are due to excessive catecholamine activity, but are metabolic effects of *beta* mimetic overactivity and might persist during *alpha* blocking therapy.

A-L

Ideally, one would hope for a cardiac lesion that was reversible by therapy as reflected by return of the electrocardiogram to normal. If the patient had a subendocardial infarction and 6 months elapsed between the time of infarction and surgery, T-wave changes from inversion to or at least toward normal would be expected.

A-LI

Angiotensin. This peptide is a direct vasoconstrictor that acts independently from catecholamine receptors.

ADDENDUM

This case demonstrates particularly well the need for precise analysis of all the patient's findings in terms of their pathophysiologic significance before drug therapy is begun. Although it is clear that the patient has a pheochromocytoma with striking increase in both catecholamine and catecholamine metabolite excretion, the choice of therapy with an alpha-blocking agent cannot be made routinely. The facts that the patient has no striking hypertension at present and has orthostatic hypotension and postural tachycardia warrant scrutiny prior to therapy. These findings are present despite large circulating quantities of catecholamines, which must increase peripheral vascular resistance strikingly. A tentative explanation might be that the patient's tumor was secreting solely epinephrine, and that the beta effects accounted for the tachycardia and diastolic blood pressures of 80. On the other hand, it is known that patients with pheochromocytoma rarely secrete epinephrine alone. Most tumors secrete only 15 to 20% of the total catecholamines as epinephrine, and it is further known that large quantities of epinephrine itself cause systolic and diastolic hypertension. Accordingly, the explanation for the patient's current cardiovascular findings must lie elsewhere. Other determinants of the blood pressure are the blood volume and cardiac output. Some patients who have a pheochromocytoma develop hypovolemia, possibly on the basis of prolonged catechol excess. At least in experimental circumstances, high concentrations of catecholamines may induce ganglionic blockade, but this does not seem to pertain to this patient in view of her striking tachycardia in response to postural hypotension. Last, the cardiac output may have been influenced directly by effects of the pheochromocytoma that caused an acute myocardial infarction or induced a catechol myocardiopathy. An ECG taken on admission was compared to tracings made 1 month previously; comparison showed the appearance of T-wave inversion in the anterolateral leads. Although serum enzyme concentrations did not confirm the presence of an acute myocardial infarction, the rapid appearance of the T-wave changes is perhaps more suggestive of an acute subendocardial infarction than of a catechol myocardiopathy. In summary, in this patient who has had a massive increase in catecholamine secretion, the absence of hypertension is assignable to the dual effects of hypovolemia and an acute myocardial process. A long-acting agent, such as phenoxybenzamine, would be somewhat preferable to the shorter-acting phentolamine for the patient's convenience and for longer duration of action. One would predict that the initial doses of the drugs should be small, with increments being given as a patient recovers from the hypovolemic state and the acute myocardial process. The patient's follow-up is of interest: On the basis of the very large catechol excretion, a sizable dose of phenoxybenzamine, 50 mg, was given as the initial dose. The patient's postural hypotension was greatly increased and she had two syncopal episodes on standing. Subsequently, the patient was given 10 mg of phenoxybenzamine twice daily. The patient was kept at bedrest until blood measurements returned to normal, and at the end of 1 week she could stand without hypotension or tachycardia. When she was seen in a follow-up examination 6 weeks later, it was necessary to increase her phenoxybenzamine dosage to prevent symptoms of catechol excess that were appearing before her second daily dose. An electrocardiogram showed that T waves were returning toward normal. One would anticipate that her phenoxybenzamine dose will further increase with continued recovery. Surgery was scheduled 6 months after the acute myocardial insult, after she was closely followed in the hospital to be sure that complete pharmacologic control of catechol excess had been achieved to reaffirm the normality of her blood volume; a large pheochromocytoma was removed without difficulty.

CASE #3

D. R. F. is a 37-year-old white married woman with known diabetes mellitus who entered an emergency room in coma. She had a 24-hour history of flu-like symptoms prior to entry that included vomiting, diarrhea, malaise, productive cough, and possibly fever. On the evening of admission the patient was found unresponsive on the bathroom floor. Her insulin and dietary intake on the day of admission were unknown, but her insulin was usually given in a single daily injection of 20 units PZI insulin with 40 units of NPH, with little dietary restriction. Since the original diagnosis of diabetes 6 years ago, her control had been "poor" owing to irregular insulin intake in part, and she had been hospitalized on two prior occasions for diabetic ketosis without coma.

On admission she was completely unresponsive to pain, hypotensive (70/50), hyperpneic (28), and appeared severely dehydrated. Oral temperature was 37.2° C. Examination of the chest showed bibasilar râles, but save for sinus tachycardia, the cardiac examination was within normal limits. Admitting weight was 50 kg.

Laboratory studies showed hematocrit, 51; white blood count, 42,000 with a "left shift"; urinalysis showed 4+ glucose and ketones. Serum sodium, 120 mEq per liter; potassium, 7.2 mEq per liter; bicarbonate, 6.0 mEq per liter; chloride, 89 mEq per liter; creatinine, 5.6 mg/100 ml; glucose, 1496 mg/100 ml; ketones, "large" at 1:8 dilution. Arterial blood gases showed pH, 6.91; pCO_2, 17; pO_2, 98. ECG showed sinus tachycardia with peaking of the T waves on a narrow base. Chest x-ray showed bilateral basal infiltrates.

Therapy over the next 10 hours consisted of 300 units of regular insulin given intravenously and a like quantity given subcutaneously, with 8 liters of fluids containing 1170 mEq sodium, 200 mEq potassium, 370 mEq bicarbonate, and 1000 mEq chloride. At the end of this therapy the patient had a blood pressure of 130/80; urine output had increased to 400 ml per hour. Serum sodium was 152 mEq per liter; potassium, 3.6 mEq per liter; bicarbonate, 26 mEq per liter; chloride, 117 mEq per liter; glucose, 251 mg/100 ml. Arterial gases showed pH, 7.41; pCO_2, 21; pO_2, 80. The patient was now alert and responsive to questions, but disoriented and apprehensive.

Q-1. Which of the following statements is probably true regarding the patient's insulin therapy? Select one or more.
A. PZI and NPH insulins should not be given in the same syringe. See A-I*
B. Subcutaneous insulin should have been avoided when the patient was initially seen in coma. See A-II
C. The best indicator for the timing and size of subsequent doses of insulin is the blood sugar level. See A-III
D. Patients like this require much more than their daily maintenance insulin dose to bring them out of coma because they are acidotic. See A-IV

Q-2. A better way to have given this patient insulin would have been to:
A. Look up the average first 24-hour insulin dose requirements for patients in diabetic coma in a text or review article on diabetic coma

* Answers to questions relating to Case #3 appear on pages 654–58.

and give that amount in equal fourths every 6 hours intravenously.   See A-V

B. Take the dose arrived upon by the process listed above and infuse it uniformly over the 24 hours.   See A-VI

C. Take the dose arrived upon by the process listed in A and plan on giving it in intravenous boli at intervals of 1 or 2 hours, with the early doses being bigger than the later doses.   See A-VII

D. Follow the plan listed in C, but double the insulin dose every hour or 2 if there is no reduction in the ketones and blood sugar, anticipating a potential insulin requirement of 20,000 to 30,000 units of insulin in the first 24 hours.   See A-VIII

Q-3.   At times the ketosis of diabetic coma, as measured by serial dilution of serum applied to commercially available Acetest tablets, fails to diminish or even increases during treatment with insulin. This could be due to (pick one or more):

A. Intake of aspirin.   See A-IX
B. Insufficient insulin.   See A-X
C. Starvation ketosis.   See A-XI
D. Therapeutic effect of insulin.   See A-XII

Q-4.   On the basis of the admitting history, physical examination, and laboratory tests, which of the following derangements in total body composition is likely, and if more than one of the statements are true, rank them in order of probable quantitative deficit or excess?

A. Total body sodium is decreased.   See A-XIII
B. Total body sodium is increased.   See A-XIV
C. Total body water is decreased.   See A-XV
D. Total body water is increased.   See A-XVI
E. Total body potassium is increased.   See A-XVII
F. Total body potassium is decreased.   See A-XVIII

Q-5.   The patient's electrolytes on admission and the degree of acidosis reflected in the arterial gas studies (pick one or more):

A. Very strongly suggest the possibility of lactic acidosis since there is an "anion gap" of 32 mEq per liter.   See A-XXII

B. Are compatible with either lactic acidosis or this patient's disease.   See A-XXIII

C. Call for sufficient sodium bicarbonate therapy to bring the venous bicarbonate quickly to at least 24 mEq per liter.   See A-XXIV

D. Reflect an acidosis severe enough to account for the coma. Treatment with intravenous bicarbonate should lessen the patient's coma.   See A-XXV

Q-6.   How does one monitor patients for response following treatment with the following agents in diabetic ketoacidosis?

A. Sodium.   See A-XXIX
B. Water.   See A-XXX
C. Insulin.   See A-XXXI
D. Potassium.   See A-XXXII

Q-7.   At what time during the treatment of ketoacidosis and at what rate should potassium chloride replacement be given (pick one or more)?

A. Shortly after institution of insulin and bicarbonate therapy, as these treatments cause potassium to enter cells.   See A-XXXIII

B. When the electrocardiogram becomes normal or shows signs of hypokalemia.   See A-XXXIV

C. No faster than 15 mEq potassium per hour for fear of causing local venous pain, thrombophlebitis, or hyperkalemia.   See A-XXXV

D. As fast as necessary.   See A-XXXVI

Q-8. The likeliest etiology of the patient's episode of ketoacidosis is:

    A. Bacterial pneumonia.   See A-XXXVII

    B. Influenza.   See A-XXXVIII

    C. Insufficient daily insulin.   See A-XXXIX

    D. Congestive heart failure.   See A-XL

Q-9. How should the pneumonia be managed?

    A. Do sputum and blood cultures; withhold antibiotic therapy until bacteriologic confirmation of the diagnosis is available to guide antibiotic selection.   See A-XLI

    B. Start penicillin intravenously, 60 million units daily.   See A-XLII

    C. Start cephalosporin and kanamycin.   See A-XLIII

    D. Start a synthetic penicillin resistant to penicillinase, kanamycin, and polymyxin B.   See A-XLIV

    E. None of the above is an attractive choice.   See A-XLV

A-I

True. PZI insulin contains an excess of protamine that combines with the insulin in NPH insulin and converts the mixture essentially to PZI insulin. The earlier hypoglycemic effects of NPH insulin will not be observed, and the long duration of action of PZI insulin or of the PZI-NPH mixture is considered to be undesirable as it may lead to early-morning hypoglycemic reactions and/or Somogyi effects. Another answer in this series is also correct.

A-II

Concur entirely. There is no guarantee that the patient's subcutaneous blood flow will be sufficiently normal in her dehydrated and hypotensive state to permit its absorption; it might in fact fail to be absorbed until her cardiovascular status is returned to normal and may be responsible for a late hypoglycemic reaction. Patients in ketoacidosis should receive their insulin intravenously. Another of the answers to Question Q-1 is correct; select one or more.

A-III

No. It is true that following the blood sugars in treatment of diabetic coma is necessary to ensure therapeutic effect and to prevent hypoglycemic reactions, but selecting this answer ignores another important pathophysiologic event in diabetic coma that importantly alters response to insulin. Try another answer.

A-IV

No. Patients with acidosis of similar severity, but different etiologies, like uremia or lactic acidosis, are not so extremely resistant to the effects of insulin. Correcting the acidosis of diabetic coma does not result in a great reduction in the insulin requirement. Patients with nonketotic, hyperosmolar diabetic coma with similar degrees of elevation in blood sugar and mild acidosis respond to comparatively small doses of insulin and would predictably become seriously hypoglycemic if given the quantity of insulin customarily used in ketoacidosis. There is an excellent correlation between the diminution of serum ketones and the return of patient's sensitivity to insulin's effects. This implies that the ketones in some way interfere with insulin's action, possibly by competing for receptor sites. Further, it provides the physician with an important bedside diagnostic tool in following the patient's response to treatment. Try another answer.

A-V

No. This is probably the worst choice among the possible alternatives listed, as it indicates that there has been no consideration of the duration of action or "half-life" of regular insulin given intravenously, and of the tendency of diabetic ketosis to be insulin resistant when the ketosis is maximal. Try another answer.

A-VI

No. This is probably the second worst choice among the alternatives listed. It is better than A-V since it attempts to utilize the short half-life of insulin, or at least compensates for it by constant infusion, but the theoretic advantages of this administration tend to be outweighed by the technical difficulty of constant intravenous infusion therapy in clinical practice unless special apparatus like an infusion syringe pump is available. This answer also fails to take into account the effect of ketosis on insulin resistance early in treatment. Try another answer.

A-VII

This is the second best answer, since it takes into consideration the duration of action of regular insulin given intravenously and the antagonism of insulin's effects by ketosis early in the treatment program. (See A-VIII.)

A-VIII

This is probably the best answer among the alternatives listed since it takes into account the duration of action of insulin given intravenously and the effect of ketosis on producing insulin resistance early in the treatment period; it further considers the possibility that the patient may have developed "insulin resistance" for another reason and may in fact require tens of thousands of units of insulin in the first 24 hours. It also indicates that the reader has learned the principle that the proper dose of a drug is that which elicits the desired pharmacologic effect or toxicity, and that dosage constraints gleaned from even large series of patients cannot be applied to all individuals with the disease.

A-IX

Yes. Salicylates give a false-positive Acetest reaction for ketones. In the urine test, boiling of the urine volatilizes ketones but not salicylates, permitting their differentiation. Try another answer.

A-X

Yes. Try another answer.

A-XI

Yes. Relative carbohydrate lack would favor lipolysis and generate ketosis analogous to that seen in starvation. It has been shown that patients receiving glucose in addition to or in place of electrolyte solutions recover from ketosis faster than patients treated solely by insulin and electrolyte solutions. Try another answer.

A-XII

Yes. Acetest tablets measure ketone bodies, but do not detect beta-hydroxybutyrate. Beta-hydroxybutyrate is converted to ketones more rapidly as ketoacidosis is corrected. An initial rise in ketones could be interpreted as a sign of therapeutic response, although it is not the principal therapeutic effect intended.

A-XIII

Yes. Rank the order of severity 2. Estimate depletion in milliequivalents. (See A-XIX.)

A-XIV

No. In certain states, like congestive heart failure, cirrhosis, or the nephrotic syndrome, total body sodium may be increased despite hyponatremia, but when this is the case the patients have obvious ascites or peripheral edema. This patient was described as being dehydrated.

A-XV

Yes. Give *two* possible explanations for the patient's hyponatremia *other* than the greater depletion of total body sodium than of total body water. Rank order of severity 1. (See A-XX.)

A-XVI

No. This choice would account for hyponatremia but is incompatible with all other available evidence in the patient's history and physical findings.

A-XVII

No. There are no recognized clinical situations in which an excess of total body potassium is known to occur. The hyperkalemia seen is more directly related to her severe acidosis and may occur even when total body potassium stores are depleted. If you picked this answer you need to review principles of fluid and electrolyte balance.

A-XVIII

Yes. Rank order 3. Calculate her potassium deficit in milliequivalents. (See A-XXI.)

A-XIX

Calculation of sodium deficits in diabetic ketoacidosis is somewhat more complicated than estimation of sodium deficits in simple sodium depletion encountered in sweating, with water losses compensated for by drinking. In this example, for instance, one may not simply subtract the observed serum sodium from the desired serum sodium and multiply the remainder times the sodium space (total body water or about 50% of total body weight in kilograms). It is necessary to estimate the effect of the hyperglycemia on reduction of the serum sodium (by moving water from intracellular compartment to extracellular compartment) and the degree of total body water loss before one can appropriately interpret the observed serum sodium. The osmolar effect of the glucose can be roughly approximated by dividing the blood glucose by 20. (This is not so accurate as dividing by the molecular weight of glucose, 180.16, and changing milligrams/100 ml to grams per liter, but is easy, fast, and close enough to the more accurate method that it is useful, and hence used more often.) In this patient, one could ascribe about 75 milliosmoles of activity to the glucose present in blood. Since sodium chloride has twice the osmolar activity of glucose (two ions versus one) a change in serum sodium by a factor of about 37.5 mEq per liter would generate a similar osmolar change. If we add this figure to the patient's observed serum sodium of 120 mEq per liter, we arrive at a "corrected" serum sodium of 157 mEq per liter. Estimating her "corrected" serum sodium permits one to state that the patient is relatively more deficient in water than in sodium (excluding the other mechanism of hyponatremia listed in A-XX). Estimating that her dehydration is severe, or 10% of her weight in kilograms, or 5 liters, one could calculate that the addition of 5 liters of water to her total body water, simultaneous with the reduction in her blood sugar, would reduce her "corrected" serum sodium from 157 mEq per liter to 123 mEq per liter. To achieve a serum sodium of 136 mEq per liter the patient would need $136 - 123 = 13$ mEq per liter in 30 liters (new total body water), or about 390 mEq Na^+. Calculations of this sort were not done in ordering the patient's fluids in the first 10 hours, and she developed hypernatremia.

A-XX

As discussed in Answer A-XIX, hyperglycemia lowers the serum sodium by shifting water from within cells to the extracellular compartment. Hyperlipidemic states may artificially "lower" the apparent serum sodium by occupying space in the pipette ordinarily occupied by plasma water. Sodium ions do not enter the lipid phase of plasma; if the lipid phase is substantial it will reduce the plasma water in any given volume, and though the sodium concentration is normal in the water phase of plasma or serum, the sodium content of 1 ml of a lipid serum will be less than that of normal serum.

A-XXI

Some authors relate intracellular cation depletion (chiefly potassium) to extracellular cation depletion (chiefly sodium) and infer an approximate depletion of potassium from the estimated sodium depletion. Empiric measurement of total body potassium with radioactive potassium has shown a range of mild potassium depletion (1 mEq/kg body weight) to severe potassium depletion (10 mEq/kg body weight). Since this patient is hyperkalemic, one could guess that she is probably moderately depleted, approximately 250 mEq. Had she been hypokalemic with her acidosis, it would have been appropriate to consider her severely depleted, in the range of 500 mEq.

A-XXII

Maybe, but there are at least two other reasons for this patient to have an abnormal "anion gap." What are they? Try another answer.

A-XXIII

Good idea to think of lactic acidosis as a complication of diabetic ketoacidosis, particularly since the patient is hypotensive and may not be perfusing tissues well. On the other hand, the anion gap could be due to high blood levels of acetoacetate and beta-hydroxybutyrate, in addition to renal retention of sulfate, phosphate, and urate (the patient's creatinine was elevated; ketones reduce the renal clearance of urate). If the patient failed to respond to insulin and perhaps to modest doses of sodium bicarbonate in terms of venous bicarbonate and arterial pH, lactic acidosis would seem more likely, and intensive therapy with bicarbonate might be needed. (Reconsider C and D; unless certain, see A-XXIV and A-XXV.)

A-XXIV

How much bicarbonate would be required to do this? (See A-XXVI.) There are data in the patient's record that indicate giving this much bicarbonate might induce an alkalosis. What are the data, and what are the reasons for this? (See A-XXVII.)

A-XXV

The acidosis is severe enough to account for the coma, but treatment with bicarbonate might increase the depth of coma by *decreasing* brain pH. How? Is there a clue in the protocol that there is a discrepancy between brain pH and arterial pH? (See A-XXVIII and Chapter 17.)

A-XXVI

In the normal patient, bicarbonate space is approximately 0.4 times body weight in kilograms. To attain a venous CO_2 content of 24 would require $24 - 7 = 17$ times $20 = 340$ mEq bicarbonate.

A-XXVII

Following treatment with 370 mEq bicarbonate the venous CO_2 content rose to 26 mEq per liter and the arterial pH rose to 7.41. The pCO_2, however, remained low at 21. The patient continued to hyperventilate. The patient will probably become alkalotic for respiratory and metabolic reasons. Why? (See A-XXVIII.)

A-XXVIII

Cerebrospinal fluid pH may drop after bicarbonate therapy in diabetic ketoacidosis. Bicarbonate therapy increases peripheral bicarbonate and pCO_2 levels. CO_2 is rapidly diffusible into the central nervous system, but bicarbonate diffuses into the brain slowly; increasing cerebrospinal fluid pCO_2 without a corresponding increase in bicarbonate would lower brain pH. At a time when the peripheral pH was normal, the patient continued to be disoriented and apprehensive, possibly signs of only partly corrected or even diminished cerebrospinal fluid pH. Additional evidence of continuing brain acidosis is the low pCO_2. In addition to the continuing respiratory component favoring alkalosis, insulin therapy will result in the metabolism of ketones and beta-hydroxybutyrate to bicarbonate, which could account for a metabolic contribution to alkalosis. The kidney may excrete inappropriate amounts of ammonia and acid after correction of acidosis. These considerations lead one to conclude that if bicarbonate is used in diabetic acidosis, the acidosis should be only partly corrected toward normal.

A-XXIX
Clinical evaluation of dehydration or inspection of cervical venous pressure, or, if greater precision is required, measurement of overhydration, weights, blood pressure, pulse rate, central venous pressure, urine volumes per hour, and serum electrolytes.

A-XXX
Same as A-XXIX.

A-XXXI
Blood glucose and serum ketones.

A-XXXII
Electrocardiogram: hyperkalemia causes tall, peaked T waves with a narrow T-wave base; more severe changes include broadening of the QRS complex, atrial arrest, and ventricular arrhythmias. Classic changes of hypokalemia include loss of amplitude of the T wave, appearance of U waves, S-T segment, intraventricular conduction defects, and ventricular arrhythmias. The correlation between ECG and serum K^+ is imperfect. Physical examination: muscle weakness, loss of deep tendon reflexes; respiratory arrest may occur in hypokalemia; agitation may be seen in hyperkalemia.
Serum electrolytes: the ECG and physical examination are necessary owing to the lag phase between drawing of blood, measurement, and reporting of serum levels by the laboratory. Serum potassium may change very quickly during treatment of diabetic ketoacidosis.

A-XXXIII
Not a good choice. The statement is true, but does not specify a means for following the adequacy of treatment. Try another answer.

A-XXXIV
Yes. The electrocardiogram is a fairly reliable way of monitoring the patient for adequacy of treatment and avoidance of hyperkalemia. At rapid rates of potassium replacement it must be monitored constantly, as serum potassium may change abruptly. Serial serum potassium concentrations should be obtained to correlate retrospectively with the ECG findings. Another answer is also correct.

A-XXXV
Clinical "rules" of this type, including the variety that says "no more than 30 or 60 mEq per liter potassium in intravenous feedings," are useful when they alert physicians to the dangers of high rates of potassium administration, including those listed in the question; but if one has convincing evidence that the patient is not responding to this rate of replacement, higher rates are required. There should be compelling evidence in favor of continuing hypokalemia when very high rates of potassium replacement are initiated, and the physician must be in constant attendance to prevent hyperkalemia. Try another answer.

A-XXXVI
Yes. Higher rates of infusion may be necessary, but require constant monitoring of the electrocardiogram by a physician to preclude induction of hyperkalemia. See Answer A-XXXIV for additional discussion. Another answer in this series is also correct.

A-XXXVII
Yes. See A-XXXVIII, A-XXXIX, and A-XL if you were uncertain about this choice.

A-XXXVIII
Would be unlikely to cause the physical finding of bibasilar râles and infiltrates described on chest film, although influenza may have been complicated by pneumonia. Try another answer.

A-XXXIX
Possible, but less likely than an infection. Try another answer.

A-XL
Congestive heart failure could present with bibasilar râles and a chest x-ray showing basilar "infiltrates," but there was no mention of antecedent cardiac disease, no cardiomegaly was described, and there was peripheral dehydration. Another answer is more likely.

A-XLI
In some situations it is possible to await bacteriologic information before proceeding with treatment, especially in chronic infections. In

this patient the probabilities are great that she would die of the infection if it were not treated promptly. Logically, this would be a correct answer, but operationally the hazards of delaying treatment outweigh the benefits to be accrued by waiting for cultures. Antibiotic selection may be guided by gram-stain examination of the sputum, especially a specimen obtained by transtracheal aspiration, if the specimen shows a preponderance of one organism. Try another answer.

A-XLII

Some would support this course of action since the patient has not been hospitalized recently, or known to be exposed to sources of resistant staphylococci. Others would counter that since the patient is a diabetic and unable to cope normally with infections, she should be given antibiotics effective against most gram-positive cocci and most gram-negative rods, if preliminary screening procedures like sputum gram stain fail to reveal a preponderant organism type. Cultures should, of course, be taken prior to initiation of any antibiotic therapy. Which of the patient's electrolyte abnormalities might be aggravated by this treatment? (See A-XLVI.) Try another answer.

A-XLIII

This selection can be defended, but does not "cover" the patient for the possibility of *Pseudomonas* infection. Which of these antibiotics, if selected after cultures are obtained, must be given in reduced dosage to this patient? (See A-XLVII.) Try another answer.

A-XLIV

This selection can also be defended after cultures are obtained, but exposes the patient to the side effects of three drugs. What important side effects would be expected if conventional doses of these drugs were given to this patient? (See A-XLVIII.) Try another answer.

A-XLV

Agreed, particularly if one is unable to personally evaluate the patient for degree of "toxicity" or severity of the infection. This type of judgment comes from seeing many cases and is not readily verbalized, but includes patient's listlessness, diminution in skin perfusion, sometimes apprehension or the appearance of great fatigue; signs of excessive sympathetic nervous system activity may also be present.

A-XLVI

Potassium balance. Penicillin G is ordinarily marketed as a potassium salt with about 1.6 mEq per million units penicillin. At this dose level the patient would receive almost 100 mEq potassium in addition to her intended supplements.

A-XLVII

Kanamycin. The patient had azotemia on admission; kanamycin is cleared by the kidney and causes toxicity if given in full doses during renal failure.

A-XLVIII

Renal damage, deafness, and neuromuscular blockade. The renal clearance of both kanamycin and polymyxin is reduced in uremia.

CASE #4

A 48-year-old divorced white woman presented herself to a physician with a 3-month history of frequent substernal chest pains. She was vague about the details and character of the chest pain, but it was clear that it had bothered her frequently and for long periods over this time. On examining her, the physician noted that she was mildly intoxicated and had an odor of alcohol on her breath. He also noted an irregular pulse. An ECG taken in his office showed an anterior wall myocardial infarction of indeterminate age and frequent premature ventricular contractions. She was advised to enter the hospital, but she refused and went home. The following morning she decided to be hospitalized, presented herself for admission, and was placed in the coronary-care unit with continuous monitoring of her electrocardiogram. Laboratory data revealed a normal hematocrit and white blood count. Urinalysis showed a specific gravity of 1.010, with a pH of 5.0. She was begun on quinidine, 400 mg p.o. every 4 hours, and had received three doses by 9:00 P.M. the day of admission. At 11:00 P.M. on the same day she had a sudden onset of seizures and cardiovascular collapse; the electrocardiographic monitor showed a rapid, somewhat irregular ventricular rate of approximately 130 beats per minute with wide QRS complexes and no apparent P waves (see representative segment of her ECG given below). The assumption was made that the patient had ventricular tachycardia, and direct current defibrillation was immediately applied; normal sinus rhythm was restored, but 30 seconds later the arrhythmia recurred. Fifty milligrams of lidocaine were administered intravenously, and cardioversion was again effective in restoring sinus rhythm. The patient regained consciousness and for several minutes appeared stable, which, for the first time, provided an opportunity to appraise her overall situation.

Electrocardiogram during arrhythmia
Lead II

Electrocardiogram after cardioversion
Lead II

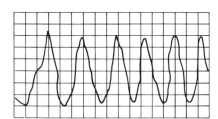

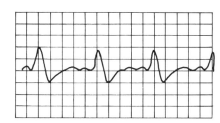

Q-1. Given the above information, one should:

A. Digitalize the patient.   See A-I*

B. Start ventricular pacing.   See A-II

C. Begin an infusion of lidocaine at 1 to 4 mg per minute.   See A-III

D. Notify the hospital chaplain that the patient is critically ill.   See A-IV

E. Try propranolol.   See A-V

Q-2. Was it rational to use lidocaine to treat the arrhythmia?   See A-VI

Q-3. What arrhythmias could cause the ECG appearance given in the protocol?   See A-VII

Q-4. The fact that the rhythm was slightly irregular favors the possibility that the pacemaker is ventricular. Why is it critical to characterize the arrhythmia more definitely, if possible?   See A-VIII

Q-5. The patient had a recurrence of her arrhythmia, again successfully terminated by cardioversion; exploratory ECG leads during the episodes identified P waves at a rate of 80 per minute unrelated to the QRS complexes; hence the patient had ventricular tachycardia. What are the possible causes of her arrhythmia in diagnostic categories? Formulate a differential diagnosis.   See A-X

In an attempt to define what factors might be contributing to this patient's recurrent life-threatening arrhythmia, a history was obtained that was not very helpful because of her obtundation and confusion. It was apparent that she had been drinking, but it was impossible to ascertain how extensive her drinking had been. She denied intake of any medications. She had had diarrhea, three to ten loose stools per day, for several weeks. She denied vomiting. She denied symptoms of dyspnea on exertion, orthopnea, paroxysmal nocturnal dyspnea, and edema. She stated that she had been eating normal amounts of food, although a subsequent history obtained from her son stated that she had been eating very little. On physical examination, she was small (weight, 88 lb; height, 4 ft, 10 in.). Her blood pressure was 90/60, pulse was 120 per minute and regular. She was somnolent and mildly confused when awake. There was no jaundice or spider angiomata. Examination of the head and neck was unremarkable, Chvostek's sign was negative. Her neck veins were not distended. Her lungs were clear to auscultation. Her heart was not enlarged, the first cardiac tone was soft, a third heart sound was heard, but there were no cardiac murmurs. The abdomen was soft, no organomegaly or masses were felt, bowel tones were absent. Peripheral pulses were normal, no bruits were heard. There was no peripheral edema, but moiedema was present. Reflexes were symmetric but hypoactive. She was weak.

* Answers to questions relating to Case #4 appear on pages 661–65.

Before anything further could be done the patient had another bout of ventricular tachycardia, again responding to cardioversion.

Q-6.   Given the additional information about the patient's status, which diag-
         nostic etiologies seem most likely, and what is the evidence for the various
         possibilities?   See A-XII

Q-7.   What are the principal mechanisms whereby arrhythmias like this are
         generated?   See A-XIII

Q-8.   What drugs resemble quinidine in their effect on the electrocardiogram as
         shown in A-XIV?   See A-XVI

Q-9.   What drugs will reverse all or some of the electrocardiographic effects of
         quinidine?   See A-XVII

Q-10.   The patient's physician felt there were sufficient clinical signs of potassium
         depletion to permit initiation of intravenous potassium chloride as long as
         he remained at the bedside, monitoring the electrocardiogram. Despite
         this, and later laboratory confirmation of serum sodium, 134 mEq per
         liter; potassium, 2.3 mEq per liter; bicarbonate, 33 mEq per liter; and
         chloride, 103 mEq per liter, the patient continued to have repeated epi-
         sodes of ventricular tachycardia, and the physician decided to counter the
         effects of quinidine with one of the following. Which would you have
         selected, and why?
         A. Digitalis.   See A-XVIII
         B. Diphenylhydantoin.   See A-XIX
         C. Calcium ion.   See A-XX
         D. Lidocaine.   See A-XXI
         E. Isoproterenol.   See A-XXII

Q-11.   Quinidine concentration in serum drawn at 11:30 P.M. the evening of the
         arrhythmia was eventually reported to be 10 mg per liter; a follow-up
         determination the following morning showed a quinidine level of 15 mg
         per liter, presumably reflecting:
         A. A laboratory error.   See A-XXIV
         B. Improved gastrointestinal absorption of quinidine during the night. See A-XXV
         C. Correction of metabolic alkalosis shifted quinidine from within cells
            to extracellular loci.   See A-XXVI
         D. A genetic defect in quinidine metabolism.   See A-XXVII

Q-12.   The patient was given serial intravenous injections of 100 mg of diphenyl-
         hydantoin to a total dosage of 700 mg. Temporally associated with this
         she continued to have PVCs but had no further bouts of ventricular tachy-
         cardia, and her ECG reverted to a pattern of normal-duration QRS com-
         plexes and Q-T interval by 6:00 A.M. the following morning. At noon that
         day she was given diphenylhydantoin, 100 mg intramuscularly every 6
         hours, and intravenous infusion of lidocaine, 3 to 4 mg per minute. She
         continued to have PVCs, but had no further runs of ventricular tachy-
         cardia. This sequence suggests:
         A. Continuing efficacy of diphenylhydantoin.   See A-XVIII
         B. Spontaneous recovery from quinidine intoxication.   See A-XXIX
         C. Efficacy of lidocaine in combating quinidine toxicity.   See A-XXX
         D. Another etiology for the premature ventricular contractions.   See A-XXXI

Q-13.   Lidocaine was continued at a rate of 3 to 4 mg per minute and the pre-
         mature ventricular contractions continued. On the second day of this
         therapy the patient became agitated and had hallucinations. Lidocaine
         toxicity was suspected, the drug was discontinued, and 12 hours later the

patient cleared of these symptoms, but she remained lethargic and somnolent. Premature ventricular contractions continued. The patient should have (pick one or more):

A. A blood glucose determination.   See A-XXXII
B. A serum electrolyte determination.   See A-XXXIII
C. No more lidocaine.   See A-XXXIV
D. Treatment for delirium tremens.   See A-XXXV

A-I

No. The data provided are insufficient to permit this action. If you chose this answer, it may be that you have learned to treat electrocardiograms rather than patients, and that when arrhythmias appeared that did not respond to "cardiac depressants," a cardiac "stimulant" should be tried. This approach is no longer tenable. Try another answer.

A-II

Not a bad choice if you specifically intended to use pacing as an interim measure prophylactically to prevent a recurrence of the arrhythmia and to "buy time" to get additional information and analyze the patient's problem more fully. It is a bad choice if you intended to treat the patient solely by this intervention, as the protocol indicates that at this moment she appears fairly stable and we have not yet ascertained what the arrhythmia *is*, what its likely pathophysiologic basis may be, and what pharmacologic effect of antiarrhythmic agents might be useful based on these considerations. Try another answer.

A-III

No. The data provided are insufficient to permit this action. You are not yet certain of the type of arrhythmia the patient has had, have not considered the potential pathophysiologic mechanisms of the arrhythmia, and have not thought enough about diseases the patient may have to permit rational choice of an antiarrhythmic agent based on its pharmacologic effects. Try another answer.

A-IV

This is the best answer among the alternatives listed, assuming you additionally intend to get more information about the patient, and to think about what disease may have caused the arrhythmia and by what disturbances in cardiac function these arrhythmias are produced so that an antiarrhythmic agent can be selected rationally.

A-V

No. The data provided are insufficient to permit this action. There is thus far no evidence of excessive catecholamine activity. If you chose this answer you may have fallen into the trap of trying "that new drug" when older drugs appeared to fail. Try another answer.

A-VI

No. Rational therapy consists of drug selection based on pharmacologic action to specifically counter a pathophysiologic process. The use of lidocaine is, however, justifiable on the basis of games theory. Actions based on games theory come into play when clinical circumstances prevent full analysis of a patient's problem, (i.e., a precise diagnosis) and when the patient's illness is so severe that the physician must guess at what is most probably going on and act on that guess. In this case the physician felt that the arrhythmia was most likely ventricular tachycardia due to acute myocardial infarction, and since lidocaine has been demonstrated to be efficacious for this arrhythmia empirically, he was entitled to give it. Now that the patient is stable, he is obliged to abandon therapy based on games theory, to proceed to a differential diagnosis of her disease, including consideration of the pathophysiologic mechanisms that might cause her arrhythmia, and then to treat rationally.

A-VII

A. Atrial fibrillation with complete heart block and independent ventricular tachycardia.
B. Paroxysmal atrial tachycardia with aberrant intraventricular conduction.
C. Nodal tachycardia with aberrant intraventricular conduction.
D. Atrial flutter with atrioventricular block and aberrant intraventricular conduction.
E. Sinus tachycardia with aberrant intraventricular conduction.
F. Ventricular tachycardia.

A-VIII

If the patient has third-degree AV block, one could not give quinidine or procainamide for fear of suppressing ventricular activity entirely, unless a cardiac pacemaker wire were secured in the ventricle. Alternatively, if the patient has a supraventricular arrhythmia, treatment will likely be different from that for a ventricular focus. How does one characterize the arrhythmia further? (See A-IX.)

A-IX

If the arrhythmia recurs, do multiple exploratory chest leads, esophageal, and even right atrial leads to find activity of P waves and their relation to the QRS complexes. Verifying the arrhythmia permits one to treat with a much greater degree of confidence than otherwise.

A-X

A. Acute myocardial infarction.
B. Quinidine intoxication.
C. Delirium tremens, with respiratory arrest and hypoxia.
D. Electrolyte abnormalities.
E. Congestive heart failure secondary to atherosclerotic heart disease.
F. Alcoholic myocardiopathy.

What steps should be taken to evaluate each of the above possibilities? (See A-XI.)

A-XI

A. Acute myocardial infarction: history, physical examination, serial electrocardiograms, serial serum enzyme determinations (SGOT, LDH, CPK).
B. Quinidine intoxication: ECG (prolonged QRS, Q-T interval), serum quinidine levels.
C. Physical examination: stigmata of excessive alcohol intake, tremor, agitation, hallucinations, confusion, recurrent seizures associated with respiratory arrest.
D. Electrolyte abnormalities: given the history of alcohol intake, one might suspect potassium depletion, associated with muscle weakness and perhaps loss of deep tendon reflexes. ECG changes could demonstrate loss of T waves, appearance of U waves, S-T segment depression, and premature ventricular contractions. In view of the alcoholic history, magnesium depletion should also be considered, but is less likely than potassium depletion.
    Hypercalcemia can present with mental confusion, and ECG changes could include shortening of the Q-T interval, S-T segment depression, and premature ventricular contractions.
E. Congestive heart failure: history of dyspnea on exertion, nocturia, paroxysmal nocturnal dyspnea, etc. Physical findings of cardiomegaly, gallop, edema, pulmonary congestion, and cardiomegaly on chest film.
F. Alcoholic myocardiopathy: physical findings of cardiomegaly and congestive heart failure. ECG might show conduction defects.

A-XII

Acute myocardial infarction: recent history of chest pain, acute or indeterminate-age anterior wall infarction pattern on ECG, arrhythmia.

Potassium depletion: history of drinking with poor nutritional intake, chronic diarrhea, absent bowel sounds, muscle weakness, hyporeflexia, ECG conduction delay, long apparent Q-T (possibly Q-U) interval. Urine specific gravity of 1.010 could represent isosthenuria of kaliopenic nephropathy, and urine pH of 5.0 could be due to the "paradoxical aciduria" seen during the alkalosis of potassium depletion.

Quinidine intoxication: sizable dose ordered for a patient of small body size. ECG changes of conduction defect, apparent long Q-T interval.

In order to optimally select drug therapy for the patient, it is necessary to be familiar with the potential pathophysiologic mechanisms causing the patient's arrhythmia and the pharmacologic means of modifying these.

A-XIII

Changes in automaticity related to rates of spontaneous diastolic depolarization, changes in threshold or maximum diastolic potential. Diagram these (A-XIV).

Changes in conductivity in the Purkinje tissue that may lead to premature ventricular contractions or ventricular tachycardia. Diagram these (A-XV).

A-XIV

A normal depolarization and repolarization sequence, characteristic of pacing and conducting cardiac tissues. Ventricular muscle has no phase 4.

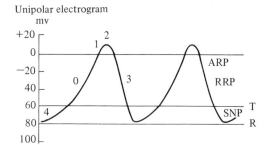

Unipolar electrogram

Corresponding surface electrocardiogram

0 = Action potential   T = Threshold
1 = Positive overshoot   R = Resting potential
2 = Slow repolarization
3 = Rapid repolarization

ARP = Absolute refractory period
RRP = Relative refractory period
SNP = Supernormal excitability potential

A depolarization sequence with rapid "phase 4" or spontaneous diastolic depolarization leading to a more rapid pacemaker rate that could "take over" from a slower supraventricular focus. Rapid spontaneous diastolic depolarization occurs in Purkinje tissue adjacent to an area of myocardial infarction.

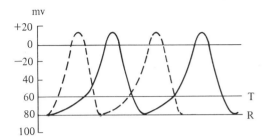

A depolarization sequence modified by changes in the threshold potential that initiates rapid depolarization. Hypercalcemia increases the threshold, hypocalcemia decreases it.

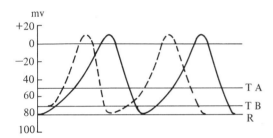

Effect of changing maximum diastolic potential on rate of pacemaker activity. During hypokalemia the maximum diastolic potential is greater (more negative) and the late phase of rapid repolarization is prolonged.

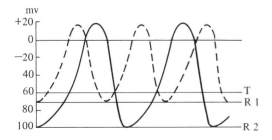

Effect of quinidine on the electrocardiogram: phase 4 slows, amplitude and rate of rise of the action potential are less, repolarization (hence refractory period) is lengthened.

Electrogram

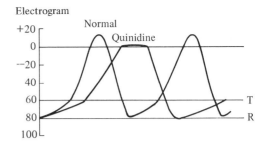

Electrocardiogram after quinidine

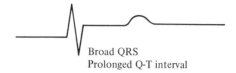

Broad QRS
Prolonged Q-T interval

A-XV
Impaired conductivity and ventricular arrhythmias:

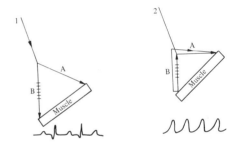

In 1 above is shown a division of Purkinje bundle marked B where conduction is slower than in its A fiber. If conduction is sufficiently delayed, time will elapse for muscle repolarization, so that it is able to respond to the delayed impulse traversing the B fiber.

In 2 above is diagrammed a branch of Purkinje tissue whose anterograde conduction is totally blocked in the B fiber. The B fiber is able to conduct an impulse in a retrograde manner; following depolarization initiated by the A fiber, the B fiber sets up a circular conduction pathway that causes ventricular tachycardia.

A-XVI
Procainamide.
Phenothiazines, possibly imipramine.

A-XVII
Diphenylhydantoin.
Lidocaine.
Isoproterenol.
Digitalis.
Calcium ion.

A-XVIII

Digitalis is probably not an ideal choice in the complex situation described since it is so long acting, and its effects on impairing conduction might summate with those of quinidine to worsen the arrhythmia.

A-XIX

A good choice. It has been learned that one can give intravenous diphenylhydantoin in small doses repeatedly, monitoring the patient for correction of the arrhythmia and signs of CNS toxicity (vertigo, nystagmus, incoordination). Patients who have responded to diphenyl-hydantoin have done so at doses smaller than those needed to induce CNS toxicity. Action of dilantin: slows phase 4, but restores prolonged phase 0 and 2 in depressed conducting tissue, improving conductivity.

A-XX

Pharmacologically correct, but difficult to monitor clinically because of the long time lag between drawing blood for serum calcium measurement and the report by the laboratory.

A-XXI

A good choice if you knew it could reverse the electrocardiogram effects of quinidine. If it can reverse quinidine's effects, why didn't it prevent recurrent ventricular tachycardia on its first use? (See A-XXIII.)

A-XXII

A good answer if you selected this drug to try to improve cardiac conductivity, but some might be reluctant to start this agent in a potentially hypovolemic patient. Another answer is probably better.

A-XXIII

One cannot say whether or not lidocaine would have prevented recurrences, as only one bolus was given, and the pharmacologic effects of a bolus of lidocaine persist for only 20 to 30 minutes.

A-XXIV

Probably not. Assay procedure is reliable.

A-XXV

Probably the best among the alternatives provided. Correction of hypokalemia-induced ileus could permit further absorption of quinidine.

A-XXVI

No. Provision of additional hydrogen ions to the extracellular compartment would render more ionized quinidine in that compartment, but the degree of shift should not be this great considering the pK_a of the drug, the likely degree of shift in the patient's pH, and the high tissue affinity of quinidine.

A-XXVII

Possible, but has not yet been described, and toxicity would have been expected earlier.

A-XXVIII

No. Intramuscular dilantin is so poorly absorbed that blood levels are too low to exert antiarrhythmic action. Try another answer.

A-XXIX

Possible. Assuming maximal absorption of drug by 6:00 A.M., she might have substantially cleared the drug over the next 6 hours. Try another answer.

A-XXX

Possible, but it is about time for the patient to begin spontaneous recovery if the arrhythmia was induced by quinidine alone. Try another answer.

A-XXXI

Probably the best choice among the alternatives listed, as it is always good to reconsider additional diagnostic possibilities if the patient continues to have difficulties despite correction of known or initially suspected problems.

A-XXXII

Yes. Hypoglycemia is not uncommon in alcoholics early in their hospitalization. This patient's blood sugar was normal. Try another answer.

A-XXXIII

Yes. Hypomagnesemia could account for the CNS and cardiac findings. On measurement it was 1.1 mg/100 ml, and following replacement therapy with magnesium the patient's mental status became normal and the premature ventricular contractions disappeared.

A-XXXIV

This answer is acceptable if it was selected primarily on the basis of its lack of efficacy in controlling the arrhythmia at relatively high dosage rates, but not if this answer was selected on the basis of attribution of the CNS signs to lidocaine toxicity, as they cleared long after lidocaine was discontinued. Try another answer.

A-XXXV

Acceptable answer, but another answer is also acceptable, and probably better. The patient had an uneventful subsequent hospital course. She was discharged on the twenty-first hospital day feeling well, with normal serum electrolytes, evolving T-wave abnormalities of a recent myocardial infarction, and in normal sinus rhythm on no medications.

CASE #5

R. B., a 63-year-old white married man, was admitted to the hospital with a 2-month history of increasing breathlessness and edema. Nine years earlier, he had had an aortic valve replaced by a prosthesis because of aortic stenosis. His postoperative course was complicated by wound infection and mediastinitis. His chest wound closed by secondary intention. Three years after this procedure, symptoms of heart failure reappeared, and at cardiac catheterization a 50-mm-Hg gradient across the aortic valve was found. He was treated with digitalis and diuretics and responded well. Three years later, his symptoms of heart failure became worse despite continued digitalis and chlorothiazide. His symptoms became worse very gradually during the next 2 years, and he was hospitalized for treatment of congestive heart failure; an electrocardiogram showed an old myocardial infarction. At that hospitalization he was additionally found to have hepatosplenomegaly, ascites, esophageal varices, and an anemia refractory to iron therapy. He responded to bed rest; sodium restriction; digoxin, 0.25 mg daily; and an increase in chlorothiazide from 0.5 g once daily to the same dose twice daily. During the year before admission the patient once again had a gradual return of progressively severe congestive heart failure. In the 2 months before admission his digoxin was increased from 0.25 mg daily to 0.25 mg twice daily; his chlorothiazide was discontinued and replaced by furosemide, 40 mg twice daily, but the patient had increasing fluid retention.

Physical examination found an elderly thin white man in no acute distress lying recumbent. Blood pressure was 100/60; pulse, 100 and irregular; respiratory rate, 24. His face was slightly flushed. His neck veins were distended to the angle of the mandible with the patient sitting upright; prominent V waves were noted in the cervical venous pulse. Chest excursion was restricted. On auscultation of the chest, bibasilar rales were audible halfway to the scapulae. The heart was enlarged to the anterior axillary line in the sixth intercostal space. The prosthetic heart sounds were loud, followed by a grade III/VI systolic murmur of loudest intensity at the right base. The abdomen was tensely distended; a fluid wave was demonstrated. The liver edge was not felt, but the spleen was palpable 8 cm below the costal margin. There was abundant sacral and leg edema. Neurologic examination was described as normal.

Admitting laboratory data included: white blood count, 3500, with 82% polymorphonuclears and 18% lymphocytes; platelet count, 90,000; packed-cell volume, 25%; erythrocyte sedimentation rate, 25 mm per hour. Urinalysis showed specific gravity of 1.010; pH of 5.0; no proteinuria, glucosuria, or ketonuria. Microscopic examination found 1 to 3 WBCs per low-power field. Serum electrolytes were: sodium, 136 mEq per liter; potassium, 3.9 mEq per liter; bicarbonate, 24 mEq per liter; chloride, 102 mEq per liter; creatinine, 2.3 mg/100 ml; blood urea nitrogen, 47 mg/100 ml. Haptoglobins were absent, serum iron was 44 with total serum iron-binding capacity of 452 mg/100 ml. Magnesium was 3.1 mEq per liter; calcium, 8.6 mEq per liter. A 24-hour urine collection contained 2 mEq sodium and 60 mEq potassium.

In an attempt to achieve a diuresis, furosemide, 40 mg daily, plus hydrochlorothiazide was administered in addition to his digoxin, 0.25 mg twice daily. After 3 days of therapy his weight remained constant, but he complained of lethargy, and was confused; on passive dorsiflexion of the wrist a "flapping" tremor developed (asterixis).

Q-1. On this admission, the patient may be considered representative of "refractory" congestive heart failure. In formulating plans for his therapy, which of the following diseases should be considered in the differential diagnosis of refractory heart failure (pick one or more)?
A. Inadequate drug therapy. See A-I*
B. Excessive sodium intake despite adequate drug therapy. See A-II
C. Apathetic thyrotoxicosis. See A-III
D. Subacute bacterial endocarditis. See A-IV

* Answers to questions relating to Case #5 appear on pages 668–73.

E. Multiple small pulmonary emboli.   See A-V
F. Occult myocardial infarction.   See A-VI
G. Congestive heart failure due to anemia.   See A-VII
H. Faulty aortic valve prosthesis.   See A-VIII
I. Digitalis toxicity.   See A-IX
J. Another answer   See A-X

Q-2. The serum creatinine of 2.3 mg/100 ml and the blood urea nitrogen of 47 mg/100 ml suggest (pick one or more):
A. Serious intrinsic renal disease.   See A-XII
B. Bleeding esophageal varices.   See A-XIII
C. A hepatorenal syndrome.   See A-XIV
D. Congestive heart failure.   See A-XV
E. Obstructive uropathy.   See A-XVI

Q-3. The initial 24-hour urine collection contained 2 mEq sodium and 60 mEq potassium. These values indicate (pick one or more):
A. Rigid dietary sodium restriction.   See A-XVII
B. Excessive dietary potassium.   See A-XVIII
C. Congestive heart failure.   See A-XIX
D. A renal lesion impairing sodium excretion.   See A-XX
E. Primary aldosteronism.   See A-XXI
F. Secondary aldosteronism.   See A-XXII

Q-4. What is the site of action and presumed mechanism of action of the following diuretics?
A. Acetazolamide.   See A-XXIV
B. Thiazides.   See A-XXV
C. Organic mercurials.   See A-XXVI
D. Furosemide.   See A-XXVII
E. Ethacrynic acid.   See A-XXVIII
F. Spironolactone.   See A-XXIX
G. Triamterene.   See A-XXX
H. Aminophylline.   See A-XXXI

Q-5. Following 3 days of the new diuretic program, the patient developed somnolence, confusion, and asterixis. Based on the information given in the case protocol, these symptoms are likeliest due to:
A. Cerebrovascular thrombosis incidental to dehydration.   See A-XXXII
B. Hyponatremic central nervous system signs.   See A-XXXIII
C. Hypokalemia.   See A-XXXIV
D. Hepatic coma.   See A-XXXV
E. Azotemia.   See A-XXXVI

Q-6. After 3 days of the combination therapy with furosemide and hydrochlorothiazide, the patient had a serum sodium of 126 mEq per liter; potassium, 5.1 mEq per liter; chloride, 98 mEq per liter; bicarbonate, 23 mEq per liter; creatinine, 2.3 mg/100 ml; 24-hour urine sample contained 4 mEq sodium and 256 mEq potassium. The next step should be (pick one or more):
A. Suspect total body potassium depletion despite the normal serum potassium. Start potassium gluconate by mouth.   See A-XXXVII
B. Increase the dose of furosemide to as much as 400 mg daily.   See A-XXXVIII
C. Stop the diuretics being given.   See A-XXXIX
D. The oral dose range of hydrochlorothiazide is 25 to 100 mg; that of methyclothiazide is 5 to 10 mg. Hence the latter drug is more potent and should be substituted for the former.   See XL

E. Start ethacrynic acid. See XLI
F. Give hypertonic saline to return the serum sodium to normal. See XLII
G. Start spironolactone, monitoring serum electrolytes as a guide to effective dose range. See XLIII
H. Do measurements of serum ammonia and aldosterone secretion rate before proceeding further. See XLIV

Q-7. The patient was begun on spironolactone, 25 mg by mouth three times daily. Urine sodium excretion increased to 20 mEq per day, but urine potassium excretion remained at 180 mEq per day and there was little weight loss. Increasing the spironolactone to 200 mg daily increased urine sodium loss rates to 60 mEq daily, but urine potassium continued at 180 mEq daily. At this juncture the serum sodium was 133 mEq per liter; potassium, 5.3 mEq per liter; chloride, 105 mEq per liter; and bicarbonate, 22 mEq per liter. To enhance sodium excretion one should (pick one or more):
A. Start chlorothiazide. See A-XLVI
B. Increase the dose of spironolactone. See A-XLVII
C. Start triamterene. See A-XLVIII
D. Restrict oral fluids. See A-XLIX

Q-8. The patient was given triamterene, 100 mg by mouth twice daily, in addition to the spironolactone therapy. On this combination his urine sodium rose to nearly 200 mEq daily and urine potassium diminished to 60 mEq daily. The patient began to lose weight at a rate of 1 kg daily and blood urea nitrogen fell from its initial value of 47 to 29 mg/100 ml.
A. Why did the blood urea nitrogen fall? See A-L
B. What side effects of this treatment program may appear? See A-LI

Q-9. On the fourth day of the combination therapy serum sodium was 130 mEq per liter, potassium was 6.0 mEq per liter, chloride was 103 mEq per liter, and bicarbonate, 22 mEq per liter. One should immediately (pick one or more):
A. Stop all drugs. See A-LII
B. Do an electrocardiogram See A-LIII
C. Give insulin and glucose intravenously. See A-LIV
D. Restrict dietary potassium. See A-LV
E. Examine the patient and repeat the electrolyte determinations. See A-LVI
F. Start a sodium-potassium exchange ion by mouth. See A-LVII

Q-10. The patient's hyperkalemia was never life threatening, but did not diminish despite dietary restriction in potassium intake, and when his serum potassium rose to 6.7 mEq per liter a sodium-potassium ion-exchange resin was given for a few days. Triamterene was discontinued and replaced by chlorothiazide, 500 mg by mouth twice daily. On this combination the patient continued to diurese even though he had lost 13 kg in weight in the preceding 2 weeks. On the day of discharge from the hospital his serum sodium was 126 mEq per liter; potassium, 5.1 mEq per liter; chloride, 102 mEq per liter; and bicarbonate, 23 mEq per liter. Serum creatinine was 1.0 mg/100 ml and blood urea nitrogen was 60 mg/100 ml. The patient was discharged on digoxin 0.25 mg twice daily, spironolactone 200 mg daily, and chlorothiazide 1 g daily. A week later he visited a private physician in another city, complaining of weakness and fatigability on exertion. The physician interpreted his complaints and physical findings as those of congestive heart failure and gave ethacrynic acid intravenously. An immediate and brisk diuresis ensued but was complicated by the onset of severe muscle cramps and faintness on rising from the recumbent position. On examination he had moderate ascites, trace ankle edema, full but not distended neck veins, and orthostatic hypotension, and he weighed 4 kg less than at his recent hospital discharge.

What accounts for the new symptoms?   See A-LIX

What clue was present at the time of hospital discharge that this might occur?   See A-LX

How should this episode be treated?   See A-LXI

How can one prevent a recurrence of this in the future?   See A-LXII

A-I
True, but if you chose this first or only, you're probably cued by the nature of this textbook, as all the other possibilities listed should be considered and excluded before accepting the diagnosis of refractory heart failure or inadequate drug therapy and embarking upon therapy with potent drugs in high doses, for fear of inducing drug toxicity unnecessarily.

A-II
Yes. A complete dietary history should be obtained. Other answers are also correct; try more.

A-III
Yes. Re-examine the patient with this diagnosis in mind; order thyroid function studies if in doubt. Other answers are correct; try more.

A-IV
Yes. Re-examine the patient with this in mind; it is probably worthwhile to do blood cultures. Rheumatoid factor and possibly ear lobe blood histiocytes may be increased nonspecifically in endocarditis; consider doing these tests in patients on antibiotics for other conditions when the diagnosis of endocarditis is considered. Other answers are also correct; try more.

A-V
Yes. Review history for episodes of transient dyspnea with or without signs of pulmonary infarction (hemoptysis, pleurisy). Do lung scan if in doubt. Other answers are correct; try more.

A-VI
Yes. Do serial electrocardiograms, serum enzymes to exclude this possibility. Other answers are also correct; try more.

A-VII
Yes. Anemia can increase the severity of congestive heart failure. An isotopic determination of the patient's red-cell mass and plasma volume will distinguish whether he has a deficit of red blood cells or an excessive increase in plasma volume to direct therapy. Other answers are also correct; try more.

A-VIII
Yes. If physical findings had included atypical prosthetic heart sounds or if the patient eventually failed to respond to therapy, cardiac catheterization would be in order. Other answers are correct; try more.

A-IX
Yes. Digitalis toxicity may present solely as increasing severity of congestive heart failure, but this is relatively uncommon. Should be more strongly considered if the patient fails to respond to additional therapy. Other answers are correct; try more.

A-X
Yes. There are even fewer common causes of refractory heart failure or the appearance of it, such as primary lung disease, arteriovenous anastamoses, constrictive pericarditis, and Laennec's cirrhosis, but these and others seem to cause less difficulty than the suggestions listed in A-I through A-IX. What evidence is presented in the protocol that suggests the diagnosis of hepatic cirrhosis on a basis of congestive heart failure? (See A-XI.)

A-XI
Long-standing severe heart failure, high venous pressure, esophageal varices, severe ascites, and splenomegaly.

A-XII
Not a very good choice. Serious intrinsic renal disease would have a greater elevation in the serum creatinine. The blood urea nitrogen/creatinine ratio is usually 10:1. In this patient the blood urea nitrogen/creatinine ratio is nearly 20:1, suggesting an extrarenal reason for the discrepant elevation of the blood urea nitrogen. Try another answer.

A-XIII
Good thought. Gastrointestinal bleeding does increase the blood urea nitrogen. Do serial hematocrits and stools for occult blood. Consider gastric aspiration for blood. Other answers in the alternatives are also correct; try another.

A-XIV

Not a very good choice, since the hepatic disease associated with the hepatorenal syndrome is very severe and includes intense jaundice, not described in this patient. Try another answer.

A-XV

Yes. Prerenal causes of azotemia such as hypotension, hypovolemia, and congestive heart failure characteristically have higher elevations in blood urea nitrogen than in serum creatinine. Other alternatives in this series are also correct; try another.

A-XVI

Yes. Postrenal causes of azotemia are associated with increases in blood urea nitrogen disproportionate to increases in serum creatinine. Review the patient's history for potential causes of obstructive uropathy; if no clues are found, another etiology is more likely. Try another answer.

A-XVII

Probably not. A rigid restriction in dietary sodium is a 0.5-g-sodium diet, which contains 6 to 7 mEq of sodium. Try another answer.

A-XVIII

No. Conventional diets contain 50 to 150 mEq of potassium. Try another answer.

A-XIX

Yes. Characteristically in congestive heart failure the urine sodium is low and the potassium high. This could be due to increased proximal tubular reabsorption of sodium such that any residual sodium reaching the distal tubules undergoes exchange with potassium under the influence of excessive aldosterone excretion. An explanation for the same finding in patients with congestive heart failure but normal aldosterone secretion rates invokes the possibility that there is a change in intrarenal blood flow to favor glomerular filtration into long rather than short tubules. If this is true, the time in which the tubular urine has contact with tubular epithelium will be relatively long, permitting even normal amounts of aldosterone to effect a relatively enhanced potassium-sodium exchange.

A-XX

No. The renal lesions likely to be associated with very low urine sodium excretion rates are the nephrotic syndrome and terminal renal failure; no evidence for either of these is given in the protocol. During early and moderate renal failure urine sodium losses may be substantial and fixed.

A-XXI

Not a good idea to add an additional disease unless the findings are otherwise inexplicable. Try another answer. If you picked this answer, how did you account for the normal serum potassium and modest urinary potassium? (See A-XXIII.)

A-XXII

Maybe. See A-XIX for an alternative explanation. If you picked this answer, how did you account for the normal serum potassium and modest urinary potassium? (See A-XXIII.)

A-XXIII

There is so little sodium ion reaching the distal tubular exchange site on the basis of proximal sodium reabsorption that relatively little exchange can take place. This may occur in primary aldosteronism after sodium-restricted diets and use of diuretics, but is not very likely in this patient.

A-XXIV

Acetazolamide and dichlorphenamide are noncompetitive inhibitors of carbonic anhydrase in the kidney and other tissues. Its renal effects appear to be those of limiting hydrogen ion generation and availability such that renal tubular reabsorption of bicarbonate is limited. Accordingly, during carbonic anhydrase inhibition, urinary bicarbonate levels rise and are accompanied by elevated excretion of sodium and potassium ions. During a bicarbonate diuresis, the kidney is unable to excrete normal amounts of titratable acid and ammonia. Chronic therapy produces a systemic acidosis with alkaline urine, which eventually blunts the diuretic response to the drug. It is thought that the effect on carbonic anhydrase involves the entire length of the renal tubule (see Chapter 3).

A-XXV

Thiazide diuretics are organic acids that appear to impair active reabsorption of sodium in the distal convoluted tubule. In vitro studies have shown that these drugs inhibit oxygen consumption and adenosine triphosphate generation, presumptive evidence that these drugs reduce energy required for active sodium reabsorption. Since more sodium is presented to the distal tubule, sodium potassium exchange is enhanced, particularly if the edematous state is complicated by secondary hyperaldosteronism, and hypokalemia with or without hypochloremic alkalosis may be produced. Water losses may not be as great as sodium, potassium, and chloride losses, so that hyponatremia may be seen (see Chapter 3).

A-XXVI

Organic mercurials appear to act at the ascending limb of the loop of Henle or more distally, inhibiting the active reabsorption of sodium ion. Free-water clearance is not increased to the same degree as is seen with agents that act on the proximal tubule, such as mannitol. Depending upon the amount of sodium presented to the distal tubule, urine flow rates, and the influence of aldosterone, varying amounts of potassium are excreted. Organic mercurials may induce a hypochloremic alkalosis, which interferes with the diuretic action of the drugs. Diuresis may be augmented by inducing a hyperchloremic acidosis (see Chapter 3).

A-XXVII

Furosemide acts at the loop of Henle and distally. It is potent, having a maximal level of activity 1 hour after administration, compared to thiazides, whose maximal activity occurs during the third or fourth hour. The duration of action of furosemide is 6 to 7 hours. Urine electrolyte composition after furosemide is subject to the same variables as those described for the thiazides. There is dispute in the literature as to whether or not an enhanced diuresis is seen when thiazides are given simultaneously with furosemide; there is agreement that no increased diuresis ensues when ethacrynic acid is given with furosemide.

A-XXVIII

Ethacrynic acid appears to impair sodium reabsorption at the loop of Henle. Its potency and very prompt onset of action cause problems in volume depletion and electrolyte imbalance, but it may be efficacious when other diuretics fail, e.g., during alkalosis, acidosis, or renal insufficiency. Distal tubular exchange mechanisms of potassium and hydrogen ion for sodium are intact during ethacrynic acid diuresis, so that final urinary electrolyte composition is variable depending on aldosterone secretion, etc.

A-XXIX

Aldosterone may act upon the nucleus of renal tubular cells as a derepressor of DNA-controlled synthesis of RNA, which controls the synthesis of new proteins, including potentially a carrier protein for the sodium-potassium exchange. Spironolactone acts as a competitive inhibitor of aldosterone. It acts at the distal tubule to promote the clearance of sodium and to diminish the clearance of potassium. The dose required to produce this effect depends upon the amount of aldosterone present, but may be much greater than the amount to be found in commercially prepared fixed combinations of spironolactone plus a thiazide diuretic.

A-XXX

Triamterene acts directly on the renal tubule to increase sodium excretion and to decrease potassium excretion. It is not an aldosterone antagonist. The effects on sodium and potassium excretion are synergistic with those of spironolactone, the combination of drugs producing much greater changes in electrolyte excretion than either drug alone. This potent combination may be complicated by volume depletion, prerenal azotemia, and/or hyperkalemia.

A-XXXI

Aminophylline and theophylline are modest diuretics taken alone, but may importantly potentiate other diuretics by increasing cardiac output and glomerular filtration in addition to reducing renal tubular reabsorption of sodium.

A-XXXII

A terrible choice. The protocol specifies that the patient had no weight loss, nor was a massive diuresis described. Try again.

A-XXXIII

Possible, as diuretics tend to cause a greater loss of electrolytes than of water. In addition, some patients with congestive heart failure secrete excessive amounts of antidiuretic hormone, or their kidneys behave as though there were an excessive secretion of antidiuretic hormone by reabsorbing an undue amount of water from the glomerular filtrate. This patient also is a likely candidate for cardiac cirrhosis, and patients with cirrhosis commonly become hyponatremic after diuretic therapy. The degree of hyponatremia seen in congestive heart failure and cirrhosis is relatively mild, and usually develops relatively gradually, so that it is relatively unlikely that the mental symptoms shown by the patient are caused by this. It would be appropriate to request an electrolyte panel. Try another answer.

A-XXXIV

Hypokalemia is a common occurrence in either congestive heart failure or cirrhosis treated by diuretics, but hypokalemia alone would not be expected to produce this mental picture unless weakness of respiratory muscles had induced carbon dioxide narcosis. Try another answer.

A-XXXV

Yes. Hepatic coma is not uncommon after diuretic therapy. The precise mechanism is not entirely clear, but there is a good correlation between systemic alkalosis induced by diuretics and hepatic coma, possibly because the alkalosis causes increased renal retention of ammonia and favors the cerebrospinal fluid concentration of ammonia.

A-XXXVI

A bad choice. Although azotemia, particularly of the prerenal variety, is a common complication of cirrhosis treated with diuretics probably on the basis of hypovolemia, it rarely becomes severe unless the patient spontaneously progresses to the hepatorenal syndrome. No mention of oliguria was made. Further, the patient has physical findings of an expanded blood volume. Try again.

A-XXXVII

It is appropriate to consider the possibility of total-body-potassium depletion. A reduction in the intracellular potassium concentration, which is the chief determinant of intracellular osmolarity, might well be associated with a secondary reduction in extracellular osmolarity, which in turn is principally determined by the serum sodium concentration. Both the hyponatremia and high urine loss rates of potassium point to this possibility. Serum potassium does not correlate well with total body potassium. This answer is incorrect, however, as one would not expect potassium gluconate to reverse the deficiency. The patient has had a substantial drop in serum chloride. During chloride depletion states, less sodium ion is reabsorbed by the proximal renal tubule, permitting a greater degree of sodium–hydrogen ion and potassium ion exchange by the distal tubule. This process will continue unless chloride ion is replaced as well as potassium ion.

A-XXXVIII

Doubtful choice. The very low urinary sodium and very high urinary potassium suggest secondary hyperaldosteronism or intrarenal redistribution of blood flow to long tubules, permitting maximal sodium-potassium exchange. This would continue if a greater blockade of proximal reabsorption of sodium were induced. Try another answer.

A-XXXIX

Good choice, as the signs of early hepatic coma are ominous. How do you intend to elicit a diuresis? (See A-XLV.)

A-XL

No. Diuretics of the thiazide category have been advertised as being "more potent" on the basis that a few milligrams of one drug are equivalent in diuretic efficacy to several hundred milligrams of another, but this has no practical relevance, as increasing the dosage of the "low-milligram" drug does not increase saluresis; in other words, it is marketed at or near its maximal dose-response level of efficacy. Be aware of this intellectual canard in promotional drug literature.

A-XLI

Doubtful choice. The very low urinary sodium and very high urinary potassium suggest secondary hyperaldosteronism or intrarenal redistribution of blood flow to glomeruli with long renal tubules favoring maximal sodium-potassium exchange. This would continue even if a greater degree of proximal tubular blockade of sodium ion were induced. Try another answer.

A-XLII

Terrible choice. The serum sodium is not so low as to be alarming (unless you thought it dropped from its initial value to the new state within hours, which is unlikely). The patient has had no major diuresis in which sodium was lost, and since ascites and edema were described and must still be present in the absence of a major diuresis, his total body sodium is greatly increased. Try another answer.

A-XLIII

Spironolactone, yes; serum electrolytes alone, no. What would be an important monitor of spironolactone's effect? (See A-XLV.)

A-XLIV

Logically correct but operationally inappropriate. The presence of early hepatic coma requires action earlier than the time ordinarily required to obtain these tests, and on the basis of the clinical material one can reasonably proceed with a treatment program. Try another answer.

A-XLV

Since the data provided indicate that the patient is probably undergoing extensive distal tubular sodium-potassium exchange, it would be reasonable to attempt to interfere with this process with spironolactone with or without triamterene (with which it is synergistic), then to add agents that interfere with more proximal reabsorption of sodium ion, starting with agents of modest potency such as the thiazides and progressing as needed to more potent agents such as furosemide or ethacrynic acid, monitoring daily urine sodium and potassium excretion rates as a guide to therapy. Serial serum electrolyte determinations, creatinine, and blood urea nitrogen determinations would also be appropriate. Proceed to Question 7.

A-XLVI
Probably not the best alternative since there is still evidence for active sodium-potassium exchange not blocked fully by spironolactone. Try another answer.

A-XLVII
Acceptable choice. Of the remaining alternatives, which would you select if a greater dose of spironolactone did not increase sodium and decrease potassium excretion?

A-XLVIII
Probably the best choice among the alternatives listed. Triamterene acts directly on the renal tubule and is independent of the presence or absence of aldosterone. It is synergistic with spironolactone.

A-XLIX
Probably the worst choice among the alternatives listed. This maneuver might increase the serum sodium, but would not be expected to increase urine sodium losses. Try another answer.

A-L
Improvement in the congestive heart failure diminished the degree of his prerenal azotemia.

A-LI
Hyperkalemia.
Hypovolemia.

A-LII
The degree of hyperkalemia should cause concern, but not alarm. The therapy is very important to the patient and should not be discontinued unless the side effect is severe and is not controlled by other measures. Certainly this should not be done without examination of the patient, repeat electrolyte determination, and review of his electrocardiogram. Try other answers.

A-LIII
Yes. If there are striking changes of hyperkalemia present, particularly involving arrhythmias, more vigorous and speedy methods to lower the serum potassium will be required. In

this case, there were no ECG changes of hyperkalemia. Other answers are also correct.

A-LIV
If the ECG findings had shown marked changes of hyperkalemia, especially including arrhythmias, this step would be appropriate. It would not be good therapy for chronic hyperkalemia, as its effects are transient. Try another answer.

A-LV
Yes, if there is no evidence of functional impairment based on examination of the patient, his electrocardiogram, and a repeat serum electrolyte panel.

A-LVI
Yes. Other answers are also correct.

A-LVII
This is a reasonable consideration in this patient, even though one is ordinarily reluctant to give a sodium-potassium exchange resin to edematous patients as it increases their body sodium. In this patient the unusually favorable sodium/potassium excretion ratio might permit its use chronically. Other answers are correct. Can you think of a drug that might increase urinary potassium? (See A-LVIII.)

A-LVIII
Giving a thiazide diuretic, furosemide, or ethacrynic acid might block more proximal tubular reabsorption of sodium, increasing the amount of sodium available for potassium exchange by the distal tubule. To prevent a massive diuresis one would begin with the weakest agent and progress in dose and potency upward as needed.

A-LIX
The patient has been overtreated with regard to diuretics, even though he has residual ascites and trace peripheral edema. Some patients with chronic heart failure have a decrease in their cardiac output if they are treated with diuretics to "dry weight." Their cardiac output and exercise tolerance are better when they are slightly congested. Hypokalemia should also have been a consideration in view of the weakness and orthostatic hypotension, but it was not present. The muscle cramps might have led one to consider renal losses of calcium or magnesium from the chronic and acute diuretic therapy, but his serum values were normal.

A-LX
The rise in blood urea nitrogen might have provided a clue that the patient's cardiac output,

hence renal perfusion, was decreasing. He also should have been examined for bladder distention, since a postrenal cause would increase the blood urea nitrogen selectively.

A-LXI

Stop the diuretics; liberalize sodium intake until weakness and orthostatic hypotension have cleared.

A-LXII

Find the weight and degree of edema and ascites at which the patient has minimal symptoms and optimal exercise tolerance. Try to correlate these with the lowest blood urea nitrogen that can be obtained; use diuretics intermittently to achieve this degree of compensation.

CASE #6

A 22-year-old unmarried white woman was admitted following ingestion of sodium acetylsalicylate and a proprietary sleeping compound containing an antihistamine and scopolamine. The patient had enjoyed good physical health in the past, but was hospitalized a year earlier for an acute schizophrenic reaction. She had been under psychiatric care, taking thioridazine and trifluoperazine.

Early in the afternoon of the day of admission she had taken 36 tablets of the sleeping compound and 100 sodium acetylsalicylate tablets. At 4:00 P.M. she attempted to throw herself under an autombile and was brought to another hospital. Gastric lavage was performed, the lavage containing 150 mg/100 ml sodium acetylsalicylate; the corresponding serum level was 12.5 mg/100 ml.* She was then transferred to the university hospital.

Past medical history and review of systems were noncontributory to the present illness.

Blood pressure was 160/90, respirations were 48 per minute, pulse rate was 160 beats per minute, the rectal temperature was 40° C. The patient was semicomatose, flushed, and flaccid, but responded to painful stimuli. Pupils were fixed and dilated. Examination of the chest showed a few basilar râles on the right; respirations were deep and rapid. Examination of the heart was unremarkable; the abdomen revealed absent bowel sounds but was soft. The extremities demonstrated no abnormalities; deep tendon reflexes were exaggerated. There were bilateral extensor plantar reponses.

Admitting laboratory data included: hematocrit of 50%; hemoglobin, 16.6; white blood count, 31,000 with a left shift. Urinalysis showed specific gravity of 1.013; pH, 6.0; no glucose, acetone, or bilirubin; sediment negative. Blood glucose was 102 mg/100 ml; serum sodium was 129 mEq per liter; potassium, 3.6 mEq per liter; chloride, 94 mEq per liter; bicarbonate, 12.3 mEq per liter.

Chest x-ray was unremarkable. Electrocardiogram showed sinus tachycardia with intermittent right-bundle-branch block.

Q-1. In view of the low serum salicylate concentration, the patient's symptoms are best explained by:
1. Synergistic effects of thioridazine, trifluoperazine, antihistamine, and scopolamine, producing severe atropine-like intoxication.   See A-I†
2. Salicylate intoxication.   See A-II
3. Lactic acidosis.   See A-III
4. Atropine-like intoxication plus salicylate intoxication.   See A-IV

Q-2. Based on the hyperpnea, serum electrolytes, and urine pH one can state that:
1. The patient is almost certainly acidotic.   See A-VII
2. The patient is almost certainly alkalotic.   See A-VIII
3. It is equally likely that the patient is either alkalotic or acidotic.   See A-IX
4. The salicylate intoxication is more severe than the serum level of 12.5 mg/100 ml would suggest.   See A-X

* Done at an emergency room shortly after 4:00 P.M. en route to the hospital.
† Answers to questions relating to Case #6 appear on pages 675–79.

Q-3.   Which of the following disorders may be seen during salicylate intoxication? For the disorders selected, give a pathophysiologic basis if it is known and suggest therapy.

1. Acid-base imbalance.   See A-XI
2. Electrolyte imbalance.   See A-XII
3. Hyperthermia.   See A-XIII
4. Pulmonary edema.   See A-XIV
5. Renal damage.   See A-XV
6. Hemorrhage.   See A-XVI

Q-4.   Which of the following might be expected as a result of the combined intake of thioridazine, trifluoperazine, antihistamine, and scopolamine (pick one or more)?

1. Seizures.   See A-XVIII
2. Hyperthermia.   See A-XIX
3. Hypothermia.   See A-XX
4. Hypotension.   See A-XXI
5. Cardiac arrhythmias.   See A-XXII
6. Coma.   See A-XXIII
7. Ileus.   See A-XXIV

Q-5.   Orally ingested salicylates are absorbed rapidly from the stomach and small intestine. Salicylates are rapidly distributed throughout body tissues. In plasma, acetylsalicylate is rapidly hydrolyzed to salicylate. At conventional dose levels, most of the salicylate is metabolized by the hepatic microsomal enzymes. The chief metabolic products are glycine or glucuronide conjugates, and a small fraction is metabolized to gentisic acid. Only a small percentage of ingested salicylate appears in the urine at conventional doses. After massive salicylate intake, the metabolic pathways for salicylate clearance become saturated, and considerable unaltered salicylate appears in the urine. Accordingly, the following (pick one or more) are reasonable methods for facilitating salicylate clearance from the body:

1. Gastric lavage.   See A-XXVI
2. Alkaline diuresis.   See A-XXVII
3. Osmotic diuresis.   See A-XXVIII
4. Acidification of the urine.   See A-XXIX
5. Exchange transfusion.   See A-XXX
6. Peritoneal dialysis.   See A-XXXI
7. Hemodialysis.   See A-XXXII
8. Administration of phenobarbital to induce greater activity of hepatic microsomal enzymes.   See A-XXXIII

Q-6.   How would increasing plasma pH affect the plasma level of salicylate?   See A-XXXVIII

Q-7.   Which of the following therapeutic interventions would be appropriate for the patient described in the protocol? Why or why not?

1. Acetazolamide.   See A-XXXIX
2. Sodium and potassium chloride intravenously.   See A-XL
3. A thiazide.   See A-XLI
4. Sodium bicarbonate intravenously.   See A-XLII

Q-8.   How will the clearance of phenothiazines, antihistamines, and scopolamine be influenced by the steps taken to increase renal clearance of salicylates?   See A-XLIII

Q-9.   An alkaline diuresis will greatly augment the renal clearance of phenobarbital. Although the pK_a of thiopental is quite similar to that of phenobarbital, alkaline diuresis has essentially no effect on its renal clearance. Why not?   See A-XLIV

Q-10. A single serum salicylate determination does not correlate particularly well with the ultimate outcome of the patient intoxicated with salicylates. What are the reasons for this?   See A-XLV

A-I

A synergistic response to these drugs may elicit a profound atropine-like reaction including fever, mental symptoms, dry mouth, fixed dilated pupils, absence of bowel sounds, dry skin, and tachycardia. If this is solely present, why is the patient so hyperpneic? Try another answer.

A-II

Salicylate intoxication could account for almost all the findings, but there is a discordance in the neurologic findings that precludes this diagnosis alone. What is it? (See A-V.)

A-III

Lactic acidosis should always be suspected in seriously ill patients with an anion gap. Would an elevated blood lactate clinch this diagnosis? (See A-VI.)

A-IV

Yes. Important signs of intoxication with both drug types are present. Proceed to next question.

A-V

If the central nervous system signs were due to aspirin ingestion alone, and if her pupils were fixed and dilated, it is unlikely that her ability to respond to external stimuli would have been maintained. The ocular findings are probably due to an atropine-like intoxication.

A-VI

No. Part of the anion gap could be due to salicylate. Blood lactate levels are high during hyperventilation. It has not yet been established that the patient is acidotic (see Chapter 17).

A-VII

Many students are misled into selecting this alternative, mostly on the basis of an acid urine. Acidosis is relatively rare in adults intoxicated with salicylates, unless there has been hypotension with acute renal failure or hypoxia with lactic acidosis. In profound sodium and potassium depletion states, a paradoxical aciduria may be seen even with systemic alkalosis. Arterial blood gases and pH are necessary to make the distinction. Try another answer.

A-VIII

This would be a reasonable choice if you recalled that metabolic acidosis is relatively rare in adults intoxicated by salicylates. The degree of reduction in venous bicarbonate is rather extreme, and if you calculated the pCO_2 reduction necessary to achieve this level, you would find it to be so low as to strain your credulity. Hence you probably were not entitled to the "certainly" part of the statement. Try another answer. Do not fail to get arterial blood gases and pH whenever the distinction is important.

A-IX

It is not equally likely that the patient is acidotic or alkalotic. Alkalosis is much more common in adults intoxicated with salicylates than acidosis. In children acidosis is more common; at least this is true in infants. Arterial gases and pH are needed to confirm the suspicion of severe respiratory alkalosis. Try another answer.

A-X

Yes. The drugs that the patient has taken with atropine-like effects in intoxicated states would not produce this degree of acidosis unless acute renal failure on the basis of hypotension, or lactic acidosis on the basis of hypoxemia, had been present. Neither was described. Aspirin intoxication may produce a severe respiratory alkalosis in adults. This patient's arterial gases showed pH, 7.60; pCO_2, 13.2; pO_2, 80. One of the points emphasized by this set of questions is the need for this determination whenever there is any doubt about the differential diagnosis of acidosis vs. alkalosis. Knowing that the respiratory alkalosis is severe permits one to infer that the salicylate intoxication is severe. The initial value reported as 12.5 mg/100 ml was in error by a factor of tenfold. A repeat salicylate level was 160 mg/100 ml!

A-XI

Yes. In adults, the most common finding is respiratory alkalosis, due to direct stimulation of the brain respiratory center. It is important to obtain serial blood gas studies during either intervention to ensure proper attainment of pCO_2, pO_2 and pH. In infants and very young children one is more likely to find a metabolic acidosis. Salicylates appear to uncouple oxidative phosphorylation, increasing the rate of carbon dioxide formation. Additionally they may interfere with metabolic processes that lead to an accumulation of organic acids in the blood. Treatment for this would consist of sodium bicarbonate therapy, monitoring blood pH, pCO_2, and pO_2. Other answers in this series are correct; try more.

A-XII

Yes. Electrolyte disturbances in salicylate intoxication may be complex and severe. They will be discussed under the headings of water, sodium, and potassium losses.

Water

Water losses in salicylate intoxication may be severe due to vomiting, sweating, hyperpnea, and hyperthermia. The degree of dehydration must be estimated on clinical findings such as cervical venous pressure, weight loss, tissue turgor, and hypotension, as sodium losses occur simultaneously and the serum electrolytes may show a normal or low serum sodium despite major water losses. Water should be replaced as 5% glucose in water or by saline solutions depending upon estimated electrolyte losses.

Sodium

Sodium is lost during salicylate intoxication via vomiting, sweating, and renal losses. The serum sodium may or may not reflect total body sodium accurately, owing to changes in total body water described above. An estimate of degree of dehydration should be made and related to the observed serum sodium to permit more accurate estimation of sodium deficit.

Potassium

Potassium losses occur through vomiting, sweating, and renal losses. The renal losses are augmented by respiratory alkalosis, by dehydration, and, if hypovolemia is present, by secondary hyperaldosteronism. Treatment consists of intravenous potassium chloride at a rate sufficient to correct electrocardiographic abnormalities without inducing those of hyperkalemia. Serum and urinary electrolytes are additional useful guides to the rate and adequacy of replacement. Hypokalemia in salicylate intoxication may require vigorous replacement therapy. If the sodium and potassium chloride replacement is not adequate, a metabolic alkalosis with paradoxical aciduria will continue; as will be discussed later, this may reduce renal clearance of salicylate.

A-XIII

Hyperthermia usually occurs only in infants and young children and is probably due to the metabolic effects of the drug. It would be treated by sponge baths or a hypothermia blanket as needed.

A-XIV

Sodium retention occurs during chronic high-dose therapy with salicylates. In patients without heart disease, this may be seen simply as a reduction in the hematocrit due to expansion of the plasma volume. In patients with heart disease, pulmonary edema may be produced. The mechanism for the sodium retention is not known. Pulmonary edema has been reported in salicylate intoxication, but it is rare. Replacement of excessive quantities of sodium could be responsible for pulmonary edema, and the central venous pressure should be monitored if large quantities of sodium are given. Other answers are correct.

A-XV

Renal damage of two types has been described in salicylate intoxication. Slight degrees of proteinuria and an increase in the cellular elements of the urine may be found, which clear on withdrawal of the drug. Acute renal failure may occur if dehydration leads to shock. Occurrence of the latter would probably constitute an indication for a dialysis procedure to clear the patient of azotemia and salicylates. Other answers are correct.

A-XVI

Hemorrhage occurs in salicylate intoxication for several reasons. Salicylate is a vitamin K antagonist in the liver; hence prothrombin time decreases. It may have direct effects on vessels and lead to petechial bleeding, or it may interfere with platelet adhesiveness to account for petechiae. Would a normal prothrombin time on the day of admission exclude an important effect of salicylates on the patient's level of clotting factors? Why or why not? (See A-XVII.)

A-XVII

Vitamin K promotes the synthesis of clotting factors; the other determinant of their blood level is their catabolic rate. If synthesis of clotting factors is arrested by high levels of salicylate (or warfarin), the clotting factors will diminish in blood in accordance with their varying catabolic rates. The clotting factor with the shortest "half-life" is factor VII, with a half-life of 2 to 6 hours. Relatively large reduction in clotting factors is needed to slow clotting or prothrombin time. The effect of salicylates on the prothrombin time may not be seen for one or two days. Repeated determinations of the prothrombin time would be needed to ascertain whether or not therapy with vitamin K was needed.

A-XVIII

Yes. Phenothiazines and antihistamines lower the seizure threshold.

A-XIX

Yes. The atropine-like side effects of phenothiazines and antihistamines plus the effect of scopolamine would very likely induce fever. Other answers in this series are correct.

A-XX

The central effects of phenothiazines could induce hypothermia or poikilothermia. Other answers are also correct.

A-XXI

Phenothiazines exert central and peripheral effects that lead to hypotension. Both phenothiazines and antihistamines have quinidine-like effects and might depress cardiac output. The peripheral effects of phenothiazines on the circulation resemble those of alpha-blocking or beta-stimulating agents. How does this affect the type of sympathomimetic agent used to treat hypotension during phenothiazine therapy? (See A-XXV.) Other answers are correct.

A-XXII

Yes. The atropine-like effects of these drugs could result in a sinus tachycardia, or their quinidine-like effects could lead to conduction defects and paroxysmal ventricular tachycardia. Other answers are also correct.

A-XXIII

Yes. Other answers are also correct.

A-XXIV

Yes. This and other signs of cholinergic blockage should be sought in patients intoxicated with these drugs. Other answers are also correct.

A-XXV

Since phenothiazines are alpha-receptor blocking agents (or beta-receptor "facilitating" agents), one would select a pressor that acts directly on receptors and has no beta-stimulating activity. If an agent with mixed alpha- and beta-stimulating properties were given during alpha receptor blockage, one might see beta-mediated vasodilation with paradoxical hypotension. Methoxamine would be a good choice, or one could avoid the alpha-beta receptor mech-

anisms and induce vasoconstriction with angiotensin. Proceed to Question 5.

A-XXVI

Gastric lavage is indicated in salicylate intoxication even several hours after the ingestion, as gastric emptying may be delayed and considerable unabsorbed drug may be present in the stomach. After complete gastrointestinal absorption of salicylates, gastric lavage would remove relatively little drug by diffusion across the gastric mucosa compared to a drug like amphetamine. Why? (See A-XXXIV.) Try another answer.

A-XXVII

Yes. The pK_a of salicylates is acid, and at high rates of urine flow it is possible to increase the renal clearance eight- to tenfold by alkalinizing the urine. Why? (See A-XXXVII.) Other answers are also correct.

A-XXVIII

Osmotic diuretics would increase urine flow rates and hence the renal clearance of salicylates, but they are less efficient than alkalinizing the urine at high rates of urine flow. Some osmotic diuretics tend to cause renal damage directly, or may cause volume depletion, shock, and acute tubular necrosis. They would be given with considerable circumspection, if at all, in salicylate intoxication. Try another answer.

A-XXIX

Certainly not. Try another answer.

A-XXX

Useful procedure in infants and young children, but not ordinarily applicable to adults. Try another answer.

A-XXXI

Peritoneal dialysis could be used to remove salicylates, but it is a relatively slow method. What type of dialysate would remove the greatest quantity of salicylate in a given time interval? (See A-XXXV.) Try other answers.

A-XXXII

Hemodialysis would remove considerable salicylate, especially if it were introduced early in the course of the intoxication when blood salicylate levels were at their peak. Regrettably, there is often delay of several hours in setting up the equipment; hence alkaline urinary diuresis may be more practicable. Hemodialysis would certainly be appropriate if renal failure were present. Investigations in dogs treated by hemodialysis showed this to be more efficient than other means of treatment, but the study is not necessarily applicable to poisoned humans, as the hemodialysis was initiated immediately after administration of the salicylate, when their blood levels were very high. Try another answer.

A-XXXIII

No. Phenobarbital does induce hepatic microsomal enzymes, but the effect takes at least several days. Neither would this procedure increase the amount of glycine necessary for conjugation with salicylates. Try another answer.

A-XXXIV

Gastric contents are quite acid relative to blood. Since salicylates are acid, they would be predominantly in nonionized form in the lumen of the stomach. Nonionized drugs cross cell membranes, which are lipid rich, much more quickly than ionized drugs, which are polar or water soluble. Ion trapping, the accumulation of higher concentrations of ionized drug across a cell barrier, would favor a high plasma concentration of salicylate. Conversely, drugs that are weak bases accumulate in acid gastric contents, the gastric concentration being many times greater than blood concentration. Even for these drugs, gastric lavage is a relatively slow means of removing the drug. Why? (See A-XXXVI.)

A-XXXV

An alkaline dialysate containing high concentrations of albumin would theoretically be ideal, to utilize "ion-trapping" effect of ionizing more salicylate in the peritoneal cavity than in the blood and to take advantage of the affinity of salicylate for albumin binding. Regrettably, the patient would become alkalotic if alkaline dialysate were used, and the expense of adding albumin to the dialysate is very great compared to the slight increase in efficiency of the dialysis procedure so obtained.

A-XXXVI

Gastric blood flow is such a small fraction of the cardiac output that, even were the gastric blood completely cleared of its drug content, relatively little drug would be removed from the patient as a whole.

A-XXXVII

The pK_a of salicylates is acid. In alkaline urine the salicylate is almost entirely ionized, hence water soluble, with only a small fraction present in nonionized or lipid-soluble form. Water-soluble ions cross lipid-rich cell membranes poorly; an "ion-trapping" gradient can be set up between plasma and tubular urine favoring tubular retention and excretion of salicylate.

A-XXXVIII

The initial effect would be to increase plasma levels. Intracellular sites are normally more acidic than plasma, and the "ion-trapping" effect described in A-XXXVII would favor a higher extracellular than intracellular concentration of salicylate. This would be enhanced by increasing plasma pH and would in turn promote renal clearance. Proceed to Question 7.

A-XXXIX

Possibly. This drug would alkalinize the urine and might increase urine flow rates, but since there is fair evidence for sodium and potassium depletion, these ions should be replaced if acetazolamide were to be given. The induction of a systemic acidosis by acetazolamide is not desirable, but this could be compensated for by giving sodium bicarbonate. Try other answers.

A-XL

Yes. There is good evidence for sodium and potassium depletion given in the protocol. Depletion of these ions probably accounts for the paradoxical aciduria described; unless it is treated, it will be difficult to alkalinize the urine and thereby promote the renal clearance of salicylates. Try additional answers.

A-XLI

Bad guess. This drug would probably aggravate the sodium and potassium depletion, and although some thiazide diuretics are modest inhibitors of carbonic anhydrase, the effect is in all probability too modest to alkalinize the patient's urine. Try another answer; almost any is better than this choice.

A-XLII

Good choice. It would require constant supervision to embark upon sodium bicarbonate therapy in a patient with respiratory alkalosis of this degree of severity, but it has been done successfully, monitoring arterial blood pH, urine pH, serum electrolytes, and electrocardiogram to prevent the appearance of hypokalemia. Sodium and potassium chloride should be given in addition, based on the clinical evidence for depletion of these electrolytes. If this was your only choice in the series, try other answers.

A-XLIII

Phenothiazines, antihistamines, and scopolamine are very basic (high-pK_a) drugs; their renal clearance will be diminished by alkalinization of the urine. Since the patient's serum salicylate was so extremely elevated, and since the atropine-like side effects of these drugs seemed serious but not as life threatening as the salicylate intoxication, it was decided to promote the renal clearance of salicylates by alkalinizing the urine. Proceed to Question 9.

A-XLIV

Thiopental is so intrinsically lipid soluble, and is bound to plasma and brain proteins to such a greater degree than phenobarbital, that relatively little free thiopental is presented to the kidney for "ion trapping" to occur. Information about lipid solubility and protein-binding characteristics of a drug is needed in addition to its pK_a to predict what results will be seen on alkalinizing or acidifying the urine.

A-XLV

A single serum determination may have been drawn before gastrointestinal absorption of the drug was complete. Serial determinations of salicylate levels will ascertain whether absorption is continuing, and whether or not hepatic metabolism and renal clearance mechanisms are adequate. Salicylates are cleared by first-order kinetics at toxic levels. The higher the blood level, the more drug is cleared in a given unit of time. A log concentration of blood concentration plotted against time in hours gives a straight line. In untreated patients the half-life of salicylates is 20 hours. Given this information, one can take the salicylate level obtained when the patient is first seen and relate that level to the interval between ingestion of the drug and the time the observation was made, to estimate what the highest salicylate level must have been prior to the time of observation. This value correlates better with ultimate course than does a randomly obtained blood salicylate level.

Comment: The patient survived this episode of intoxication. Her serum salicylates remained elevated for longer than one would have predicted, either because of continuing gastrointestinal absorption or because she was treated solely with large amounts of saline and potassium chloride. Her urine pH did not become alkaline until 36 to 48 hours had elapsed. In restrospect, she probably should have been treated with sodium bicarbonate or acetazolamide to hasten renal clearance of the salicylates. Her leukocytosis was due to an aspiration pneumonia, which responded uneventfully to antibiotic therapy. After her medical management she was transferred to a psychiatric hospital for additional therapy.

CASE #7

A 29-year-old married woman was admitted with complaints of weight loss, tachycardia, fever, and joint pains. She was in good health until 6 months before admission, when she developed thyrotoxicosis. She was begun on therapy with iodothiouracil, 100 mg p.o. three times daily. In the next 4 to 6 weeks she gradually improved symptomatically and had a diminution in thyroid size and in the concentration of serum-protein-bound iodine. Two months prior to admission the iodothiouracil therapy was discontinued. One month later she noted a gradual return of her initial symptoms of hyperthyroidism; the iodothiouracil therapy was reinitiated at the above dose.

One week prior to admission she developed arthritis with joint effusions, severe diffuse abdominal pain, and high spiking fever. She was suspected to have a serum sickness reaction to the iodothiouracil and was placed upon a single daily dose of 60 mg of hydrocortisone. The height and spiking quality of the patient's fever led to the addition of parenteral ampicillin therapy.

Despite these interventions, she became sicker, developing bouts of paroxysmal atrial tachycardia with rapid ventricular response rates and persistently high fever. She was thought to be in thyroid storm and was transferred to a university hospital for further management.

Family history revealed her mother had had thyrotoxicosis. There was no past history of allergic reactions in the patient or her family.

Physical examination on admission disclosed a rectal temperature of 40° C, blood pressure of 110/80, and pulse rate of 144 per minute and irregular. The patient was in acute distress, confused, lethargic, and dehydrated. Ocular findings revealed nystagmus to upward and lateral gaze, lid lag, and impaired convergence. Her thyroid gland was three to four times normal size, and a loud systolic and diastolic bruit was audible over it. The patient's lungs were clear; no cardiomegaly was detected; neck veins were flat when the patient was recumbent. Abdominal examination showed slight tenderness in the right lower quadrant. Bowel sounds were present. On pelvic examination, one observer detected a tender right adnexal mass. Knee joints showed effusions and tenderness. There was a fine tremor of the outstretched hands and generalized muscle weakness, but save for the nystagmus and mental confusion her neurologic examination was within normal limits.

Laboratory studies included a hematocrit of 35%, white-blood-cell count of 20,000 with a predominance of polymorphonuclear leukocytes. Urinalysis was normal. Cultures of blood, urine, spinal fluid, sputum, and stool were reported as "no growth." Lumbar puncture revealed an opening pressure that was normal, but the spinal fluid contained 30 leukocytes/ml. Spinal fluid smears and cultures for tuberculosis, fungi, and bacteria were negative. Radiographic studies of her skull, chest, and abdomen were interpreted as normal. Electrocardiogram was interpreted as atrial tachycardia or flutter with varying degrees of atrioventricular block. Serum thyroxine concentration was 15 μg/100 ml; the thyroidal radioactive iodine uptake was 80% at 2 hours.

On the basis of this information, the patient was thought to have "thyroid storm" and possibly an occult bacterial infection. Therapy was initiated with 25 mg methimazole by mouth four times daily, 20 mg propranolol p.o. four times daily, 10 mg prednisone by mouth every 8 hours, 15 mg phenobarbital by mouth every 6 hours, 500 mg kanamycin intramuscularly every 12 hours, and 2.5 g cephalosporin intravenously every 6 hours. She was also given 1 g of sodium iodide intravenously on the first hospital day.

Q-1.   The patient's initial response to therapy with iodothiouracil 6 months before the present admission was gratifying. Her clinical relapse when therapy was discontinued was (pick one or more):

A. A clue to the possibility that the patient was under emotional stress.   See A-I*

B. Predictable and avoidable.   See A-II

C. A calculated risk of treatment of thyrotoxicosis with oral therapy, occurring in 10 to 20% of patients.   See A-III

D. Extremely unfortunate, but unavoidable since the disease undergoes spontaneous exacerbations and remissions.   See A-IV

Q-2.   As an outpatient, the patient did not respond to the 60 mg of hydrocortisone given for the suspected serum sickness reaction to iodothiouracil. Her failure to respond is probably due to the following (pick one or more:

A. Diagnosis of serum sickness reaction is incorrect.   See A-VI

B. Dose of hydrocortisone is inappropriate in thyrotoxicosis.   See A-VII

C. Dose of hydrocortisone is inappropriate for serum sickness.   See A-VIII

D. Inappropriate selection of type of steroid. The patient should have been given daily doses of a much more potent anti-inflammatory steroid preparation such as dexamethasone.   See A-IX

Q-3.   The use of iodothiouracil as the initial antithyroid drug therapy is open to some question since (pick one or more):

A. It may cause bone marrow depression, predisposing to sepsis.   See A-XII

B. Since it is used infrequently in the United States, its obscure toxic effects may not be readily recognized.   See A-XIII

C. Its iodine content may cause hypersensitivity reactions.   See A-XIV

D. Its iodine content may cause difficulty in maintaining control of thyrotoxicosis.   See A-XV

Q-4.   Which of the following statements can be made about the therapy with antibiotics given to the patient (pick one or more)?

A. The treatment of the patient with ampicillin was warranted on the basis of the severity of her clinical features, the striking leukocytosis, and the high spiking fever.   See A-XVII

* Answers to questions relating to Case #7 appear on pages 682–86.

   B. Switching the patient from ampicillin to kanamycin and cephalosporin was necessary, as she had failed to respond to an antibiotic
with a narrower antibacterial spectrum   See A-XVIII

   C. The therapy should be modified to a single drug if cultures demonstrate a single organism or be discontinued if all cultures are negative,
to prevent the appearance of a resistant organism.   See A-XIX

   D. The therapy might conceivably introduce confusion in interpreting a
positive edrophonium test for myasthenia, which may be associated
with thyrotoxicosis.   See A-XX

Q-5.* In view of the patient's failure to respond to the therapy as listed, a review
of the initial diagnosis is in order. How would you evaluate the patient
for each of the following possibilities?

   A. Inadequately treated serum sickness reaction.   See A-XXII

   B. Bacterial sepsis.   See A-XXIII

   C. Right-lower-quadrant peritonitis.   See A-XXIV

   D. Gonococcal pelvic inflammatory disease with gonococcal arthritis.   See A-XXV

   E. Inadequately treated thyrotoxicosis.   See A-XXVI

   F. Disseminated intravascular coagulation.   See A-XXVII

Q-6. In severe thyrotoxicosis, the heart behaves as though it were "sensitive"
to the beta effects of catecholamines, and attempts to deplete catecholamines with reserpine or guanethidine have been alleged to influence
cardiac symptomatology in a favorable manner. More recently, it has
been shown that propranolol can decrease the pulse rate and cardiac
output in patients with thyrotoxicosis. Propranolol is also known to
decrease ventricular response rates in atrial fibrillation by decreasing
atrioventricular conduction. How would you respond to the following
statements made about anti-adrenergic therapy for the cardiovascular
manifestations of thyrotoxicosis?

   A. In the reserpine and guanethidine studies, effective antithyroid
therapy was given simultaneously with the adrenergic-depleting drugs.
The cardiovascular improvement was not apparent for several days
to 1 week, but it takes this long for the full effects of reserpine or
guanethidine to be seen, when given in conventional manner. Which
therapy caused the improvement?   See A-XXVIII

   B. It is not surprising that propranolol decreases pulse rate and cardiac
output in thyrotoxicosis. Although the studies thus far available are
not controlled and not compared to conventional therapy, the demonstrated effects of propranolol are welcome enough to warrant its
use in nearly all patients with thyrotoxicosis.   See A-XXIX

Q-7. It has long been asserted that the heart in patients with thyrotoxicosis is
unduly "sensitive" to the effects of digitalis, i.e., that such patients
develop ventricular irritability more regularly than euthyroid
patients. This is somewhat surprising in view of the known enhanced
clearance of digoxin in thyrotoxicosis. How would you respond to the
following statements?

   A. Perhaps it is true that the heart is unduly responsive to the effects of
catecholamines during thyrotoxicosis. If so, the effects of digitalis on
cardiac automaticity might summate with those of catecholamines to
cause ventricular irritability.   See A-XXX

   B. Atrial fibrillation is a very common arrhythmia in serious thyrotoxicosis. Perhaps physicians have attempted to control the ventricular response rate to the usual level of 60 to 90 beats per minute, and
this degree of reduction of ventricular response rate is inappropriate
for patients with an elevated metabolic rate and some "need" for a
tachycardia, even at rest. Attempts to "force" so slow a ventricular

 * Read the paragraph following A-XX before proceeding with this question.

response rate might require such large amounts of digitalis for its
effects on atrioventricular conduction as to induce ventricular
irritability.   See A-XXXI

C. The statements in A and B above seem rather speculative, but alert
to me the possibility of avoiding digitalis toxicity, and might even
lead me to consider the use of propranolol in cases where control of
ventricular rate is difficult with digitalis alone.   See A-XXXII

Q-8.* The patient is "going downhill" rapidly. Which of the following steps
would you take at this time?

A. Emergency thyroidectomy.   See A-XXXIII
B. Radioactive iodine therapy in an "ablative" dose.   See A-XXXIV
C. Exchange blood transfusion to remove her extrathyroidal thyroid
hormone pool size.   See A-XXXV
D. Antibiotic sensitivity tests of her *Pseudomonas*.   See A-XXXVI
E. Give heparin for disseminated intravascular coagulation, a known
sequel of *Pseudomonas* sp. sepsis.   See A-XXXVII

A-I
Maybe. Emotional stress is often an antecedent to the onset of thyrotoxicosis and should have been referred to in the history. Another answer is better.

A-II
A relapse was predictable in a sense, in that most patients treated for such a short period of time would go into relapse, but the prediction is not absolute, since some patients would not have relapsed. Given the limitations imposed in applying probability data from a series of similar patients to an individual patient, this answer is probably the best among the alternatives listed. How did you propose to "avoid" the relapse? (See A-V.)

A-III
The calculated-risk portion of this answer is true, but the figures given for relapse rate are far too low. Even after a year's treatment with antithyroid drugs, about 50% of the patients will eventually have a relapse. Try another answer.

A-IV
It is true that the disease undergoes spontaneous exacerbations and remissions, but this does not mean that relapses of this sort are unavoidable. Longer duration of antithyroid therapy by drugs would have a higher probability of inducing a sustained remission. Most patients treated in this way should receive therapy for at least 1 year. Other modes of treatment are available. Try another answer.

A-V
Several possible alternatives are available: Surgical intervention or radioactive iodine

therapy could have been given after initial control of the thyrotoxicosis. If antithyroid drug therapy alone were selected, it would be desirable to have a means of estimating when antithyroid drug therapy could be discontinued. A potential way to evaluate the activity of the disease state after prolonged drug therapy would be to measure the patient's radioactive iodine thyroidal uptake, then repeat the iodine uptake after suppressive doses of triiodothyronine therapy. Failure of the triiodothyronine to suppress thyroidal uptake of iodine would indicate a continuing stimulus to thyroid hyperfunction and would lead to continued antithyroid drug therapy. If the iodine uptake was suppressed, the antithyroid therapy could be discontinued, with careful follow-up being required for possibility of eventual relapse. Proceed to Question 2.

A-VI
It is always a good idea to reevaluate the patient for alternative diagnoses when therapy fails to improve the patient, but there is no special reason to abandon this diagnosis yet. Are there any special laboratory tests that might be ordered to further evaluate the possibility of a serum-sickness drug reaction? (See A-X.) Try another answer.

A-VII
Yes. The turnover rate of adrenal steroids is more rapid than normal in thyrotoxicosis. In the euthyroid state, maintenance doses of hydrocortisone must be given every 6 hours, as the half-life of the of the drug is 90 minutes. In thyrotoxicosis, if high anti-inflammatory levels of the steroid were desired on a continuous basis to suppress very active inflammation, it would be necessary to give the drug every few hours. The

---

* Read the paragraph following A-XXXII before answering Q-8.

dose of phenobarbital was also rather low. Another answer is also correct.

A-VIII
Yes. Single daily or even alternate daily doses of large amounts of hydrocortisone (usually given as one of the synthetic preparations with less sodium-retaining properties) will control allergic or inflammatory conditions of lesser intensity such as the indolent phase of lupus erythematosus, but acute severe inflammatory reactions probably require more sustained levels of steroids for control. How does the daily dosage given to this patient prior to her hospitalization compare with (1) the usual daily adrenal secretion rate of cortisol, (2) the maximal daily secretion rate of cortisol, (3) a usual dose of hydrocortisone or its synthetic equivalent given for intense inflammatory reactions, and (4) so-called "pharmacologic" doses of steroids, where some action other than glucocorticoid or anti-inflammatory action is sought? (See A-XI.) Another answer is also correct.

A-IX
This is a great choice or a poor choice depending upon the reasons it was selected. If you decided the patient needed a more potent anti-inflammatory steroid effect at more frequent intervals, but hesitated to use hydrocortisone for fear of inducing sodium retention, all is well. If you selected this answer believing there was any other important merit in administering a few milligrams of a synthetic preparation as opposed to several hundred milligrams of hydrocortisone, you've been misled, probably by the drug advertising literature. Nor is there a substantial difference among the various preparations in their glucocorticoid effects and their anti-inflammatory effects. Thus far, no synthetic steroid has been developed that dissociates these properties. Glucocorticoid effect is measured to determine milligram potency effect and equivalence to other steroid preparations. For example, ascribing an arbitrary number of 20 to hydrocortisone, equivalent milligram potencies of synthetic steroids become: cortisone, 25; prednisone and prednisolone, 5; methylprednisolone and triamcinolone, 4; paramethasone, 2; betamethasone, 0.75; dexamethasone, 0.75.

A-X
Serum-sickness-type reactions are thought to be mediated by circulating antigen-antibody complexes that fix to tissues, bind complement, and cause cell damage. In this process serum complement levels may be lowered and renal damage may result in the appearance of urinary "light chains" (kappa or lambda chains of globulin).

Regrettably, these tests are not specific for drug reactions. At times, false-positive lupus-erythematosus-cell preparations are found in serum sickness (to be distinguished from drug-induced lupus).

A-XI
Usual daily secretion rates of cortisol are about 30 mg. Maximal daily secretion rate is about 300 mg. Conventional anti-inflammatory doses are usually in the range of 200 to 300 mg daily in divided doses for acute severe inflammatory reactions. Smaller doses given daily or even every other day are successful in controlling more indolent inflammatory processes. Massive doses of adrenal steroids (in excess of 1,000 g hydrocortisone or equivalent) are given for cerebral edema and some leukemias and are advocated by some in the therapy of gram-negative shock, but in these circumstances pharmacologic actions other than anti-inflammatory effects are sought.

A-XII
True, but so do the other thiouracil derivatives. Can this unwanted effect be prevented by doing weekly or twice-weekly complete blood counts? Why or why not? (See A-XVI.) Try another answer.

A-XIII
The infrequent use of a drug does not in itself preclude its use, but it is mandatory for physicians to be fully versed in all the known effects of drugs they intend to prescribe. Try another answer.

A-XIV
True, but another answer in the series may be even better than this choice, as the incidence of allergic reactions to iodide is low.

A-XV
Thiouracils are potent inhibitors of thyroid hormone synthesis, but in the therapy of thyrotoxicosis, the gland must be depleted of preformed thyroid hormone before the thyrotoxicosis subsides. Iodides are helpful in the management of acute thyrotoxicosis with severe symptoms, as they inhibit thyroidal release of thyroid hormone. When the two drugs are given simultaneously, thyroid hormone depletion is slower than when a thiouracil is used alone. If thyroid synthesis is not fully blocked (inadequate or interrupted therapy), the iodine may serve as a substrate for thyroid hormone synthesis, resulting in uncontrolled thyrotoxicosis. When it can be established that thyroid hormone synthesis is blocked, as in the therapy of

thyrotoxicosis with a thiouracil with satisfactory control, iodides may be added after the initial response to reduce the vascularity of the thyroid gland prior to surgery.

A-XVI

Serial white-blood-cell counts are not helpful in this situation. Thyrotoxicosis itself may cause a relative lymphocytosis and introduce confusion with neutrophil suppression. The onset of neutropenia induced by thiouracils is so sudden that weekly or biweekly blood counts have failed to prospectively identify marrow depression. Patients are advised of the possibility of this event, instructed as to warning signs of infection such as pharyngitis and stomatitis, and advised to report these to their physician immediately. The patient's leukocytosis excludes this diagnosis.

A-XVII

Probably not. The suspected diagnosis of serum sickness and thyrotoxicosis is sufficient to account for the leukocytosis and high spiking

fever. The abdominal findings provoke concern, but if cultures are persistently negative, antibiotics may serve to promote the appearance of resistant organisms. Try another answer.

A-XVIII

Probably not. The failure to "respond" to ampicillin may indicate that the patient's major symptoms are unrelated to a bacterial infection. Continued therapy with antibiotics in the absence of positive cultures or clinical response predisposes patients to the appearance of resistant organisms. Try another answer.

A-XIX

Yes. Another answer in this series is also correct.

A-XX

Yes. Kanamycin has curare-like neuromuscular blocking properties that might be countered by edrophonium. This reaction would be much more likely if full doses of kanamycin were given to a uremic patient, as it is cleared entirely by the kidneys.

Despite the therapy described above, the patient's joints became more tender, the white-blood-cell count increased, and the patient continued to appear "toxic." Despite the negative blood cultures, sodium colistimethate was begun. The patient's pulse rate decreased to 90 beats per minute, but after intensive fluid replacement she developed a cardiac middiastolic gallop, râles at the lung bases, and mild cervical venous distention. The propranolol therapy was discontinued. Prednisone was increased to 20 mg by mouth every 4 hours, with a decrease in joint tenderness ensuing. Although the patient was never hypokalemic, she complained of severe muscle weakness and ptosis. A transient improvement in muscle strength was seen when edrophonium was given, but this response was difficult to interpret since the patient was taking ——————? See A-XXI.

A-XXI

Kanamycin and sodium colistimethate. Each of these has curariform effects at the neuromuscular junction.

A-XXII

Look for continuing clinical signs of inflammation, fever, elevation in erythrocyte sedimentation rate, eosinophilia, or status of joint inflammation. In some cases there may be a decreased serum "complement" or the appearance of gamma globulin "light chains" in the urine. It was of great interest, and probably a sign of therapeutic effect, that her joint symptoms improved strikingly when the steroid therapy was increased in dosage and the time interval between doses was diminished.

A-XXIII

Blood cultures. Increase in white-blood-cell count (sometimes a decrease in white-blood-cell count is seen during severe infections). Blood platelets may decrease. Shock may appear,

particularly in gram-negative infections. Repeatedly examine the patient for localizing signs of infection.

A-XXIV

Abdominal paracentesis or transvaginal culdocentesis.

A-XXV

Blood cultures. Arthrocentesis with gram stain and culture of joint fluid. Other bacterial arthritides may be diagnosed in the same way. The patient's prior therapy with ampicillin made gonoccocal infection unlikely.

A-XXVI

Failure of thyroid gland to diminish in size, lack of improvement in blood tests of thyroid function, clinical evidence of continuing hypermetabolism.

A-XXVII

Appearance of bleeding. Diminution in blood platelets, decrease in fibrinogen. Appearance of fragmented and distorted red blood cells on blood smear. Elevation in levels of fibrin split products in blood.

A-XXVIII
Effective antithyroid therapy would be expected to result in a clinical response at about the same time as the antiadrenergic drugs exert their most important effects. The salubrious effects on cardiovascular performance reported by these studies could have been due to the antithyroid therapy alone. Unless the efficacy of norepinephrine depletion can be more convincingly demonstrated, the use of these drugs in thyrotoxicosis cannot be unequivocally recommended.

A-XXIX
Although the effects of propranolol seem most attractive, controlled studies comparing its effects to standard therapy are necessary since the enhanced cardiac output may be a necessary concomitant of the greatly increased metabolic rate in some patients, and decreasing the cardiac output might diminish tissue perfusion unduly. If the therapy were undertaken, monitors for arteriovenous oxygen difference or

blood lactates and lactate/pyruvate ratios should be considered to ensure that the therapy was not harmful. Additionally, a controlled study is necessary to demonstrate superiority to conventional therapy, since propranolol has unwanted effects and, in the patient described here, appeared to cause congestive heart failure.

A-XXX
Maybe. Both catecholamines and digitalis accelerate the slow spontaneous phase of diastolic depolarization of cardiac conducting and pacemaking tissue. Try another answer.

A-XXXI
Conceivably, but clinical data are lacking to prove this speculation. Try another answer.

A-XXXII
Yes, but keep in mind that this use of propranolol has not been thoroughly established on the basis of controlled clinical trials comparing it to standard therapy, and that when more specific blocking agents become available, they may be preferable to propranolol. Proceed to next question.

At this juncture in the patient's course, a culdocentesis was done, and feculent material was obtained. The patient's clinical status was judged to be so precarious that surgery was not elected, because the surgeon was not convinced of the physical findings and asserted that the source of the feculent material could have been puncture of the bowel. Shortly thereafter the patient developed subungual splinter hemorrhages, Roth spots in the ocular fundi, increasing leukocytosis, and jaundice. The patient was taken to surgery, where she was found to have gangrenous perforation of her distal ileum. The involved bowel was removed, and drains were placed. Blood cultures became positive for *Pseudomonas* sp. The pathologic specimen demonstrated diffuse vasculitis. The patient was unable to take oral medications; hence all medications were given parenterally, including methimazole, 25 mg intravenously four times daily. During this time her thyroid diminished in size and her serum thyroxine returned to normal. Despite this intervention and continuing therapy with sodium colistimethate, the patient developed hypotension, a fall in blood platelet count, and an increased prothrombin time, but plasma fibrinogen and red-blood-cell morphology were normal.

A-XXXIII
No. The thyrotoxicosis seems to be under control. Another disease is more likely responsible for her symptoms. Try another answer.

A-XXXIV
No. Thyrotoxicosis seems to be under control. Try another answer.

A-XXXV
Not appropriate for consideration at this juncture, although it is an interesting thought in the phase of thyroid storm. The procedure has not yet been compared to standard therapy to permit critical evaluation of this method of therapy. Try another answer.

A-XXXVI
Yes. One could consider doing this and antibiotic serum bacterial levels, i.e., determining at what dilution her serum is bactericidal for her organism, and adjust antibiotic dosage accordingly, as she is so critically ill and possibly still infected with *Pseudomonas* sp.

A-XXXVII
One would seriously consider the diagnosis of disseminated intravascular coagulation in this patient and determine fibrin split products in her plasma. In the absence of positive laboratory tests for this complication, one could not proceed with heparin therapy. Try another answer.

The patient died the day after surgery, developing widespread petechiae preterminally. Postmortem examination showed massive *Pseudomonas* sepsis involving all organs. Localized abscesses were found in the abdomen and myocardium. Acute necrotizing vasculitis was found in the kidney, bowel, and heart, but this process had spared the central nervous system. The thyroid gland showed evidence of successful therapy. The adrenal glands showed bilateral hemorrhagic necrosis, and there was acute tubular necrosis of her kidneys.

Apparently the infection was not controlled, because of either her steroid therapy, inadequate dose or type of antibiotic therapy, local tissue factors in the abscesses that prevented access of antibiotic to the organisms, inadequate surgical drainage, or all of these in concert. In a highly retrospective analysis of the case, the extensive vasculitis at postmortem leads one to question the therapy with iodides on admission to the university hospital, since it was a likely cause of her initial complaints of serum sickness.

INDEX

A-beta-lipoproteinemia. *See* Vitamin A
Absorption and disposition kinetics, dose-dependent, 49–50
  first-order, 47–48
  intravenous bolus, 39–45
  intravenous infusion, 45–46
  kinetic systems, 48–49
  pharmacologic effect vs. time, 50–51
  prolonged-release dosage forms, 46–47
  volume of distribution, 42–44
Acetaminophen (Tylenol), 495–99
Acetanilid, as analgesic, 495–99
  hemolysis, 541
  induction of methemoglobinemia, 362
Acetazolamide (Diamox), 502–503
Acetohexamide, diabetes mellitus, 302–305
  drug interactions, 596–97
Acetophenazine, as antipsychotic, 463–67
  senile psychoses, 470
Acetophenetidin (phenacetin), as analgesic, 495–99
  hemolysis, 541
  metabolism, 540
Acetylcholine. *See also* Antiarrhythmic agents
  autonomic nervous system, 142–43
  cardiac automaticity, 195–96, 202–203
  drug interactions, 591–92
  effects on His-Purkinje system, 205
  parasympathetic nervous system, 147
  Parkinson's syndrome, 477–79
N-Acetyl-L-cysteine (Mucomyst), 274
DL-Acetylmethadol, 472
Acetylsalicylic acid. *See* Salicylates
N-Acetyltransferase, 539
Acid-base balance. *See also* Fluid and electrolyte replacement; Gastrointestinal disorders; Passage of drugs across membranes; Renal disorders; Respiratory disorders
  acid, production, 67–69
  acidosis, 69–71
  alkalosis, 71–72, 189
  buffers, endogenous, 67
  cardiac automaticity, 195–96, 202–203
  drug interactions, 595–97
  drug reactions, 580
  Henderson-Hasselbalch equation, 66–67
  pK_a, meaning, 66–67
  regulation, 66–72
  respiratory failure, 285–86
  urinary pH, 66–69, 72
Acidophilic adenoma. *See* Pituitary
Acidosis, bronchial asthma, 279
  digitalis toxicity, 191
  insulin action, 297–98
  treatment in shock, 176
Acromegaly. *See also* Endocrine disorders; Pituitary

Acromegaly—(*Cont.*)
  osteoporosis, 337
  pathogenesis, 292–93
  treatment, 322
ACTH. *See* Adrenocorticotropin
Actinomycin D. *See* Dactinomycin
Action potential. *See* Cardiac electrophysiology
Acute tubular necrosis. *See* Diuretics; Renal disorders
Addiction to drugs. *See* Drug abuse
Addison's disease. *See* Adrenals
Adenosine triphosphatase, 541
Adenyl cyclase system, 384–85
ADH. *See* Vasopressin
Adjustment of drug administration. *See* Dosage regimens
Adjustment of therapy. *See* Dosage regimens
Adolescent behavior disorders. *See* Psychiatric disorders
Adrenal steroids. *See also* Corticosteroids; individual agents
  biochemical and physiologic actions, 326–28
  corticosteroid-binding globulin (CBG), 326
  half-life, 326–28
  hematopoietic disorders, 367–68
  mineralocorticoids, 328
  secretion, 326
  structure-activity relationships, 327–28
Adrenalectomy. *See* Cushing's syndrome
Adrenals. *See also* Corticosteroids; Cushing's syndrome
  corticosteroids in nonadrenal disorders, 330–32
  Cushing's syndrome, 329–30
  hyperplasia, congenital, 161–63
  insufficiency, anemia, 361
    produced by corticosteroids, 411
    treatment, 328–29
  oral contraceptives, 342
  physiologic function, 324–28
Adrenergic blocking agents. *See also* Alpha-adrenergic blocking agents; Arrhythmias; Beta-adrenergic blocking agents; Cardiovascular disorders; individual agents
  alpha, 157–58
  angina pectoris, 224–25
  beta, 158–59
  diagnostic use, 164–65
  drug interactions, 591–92
  drug reactions, 578–79
  hyperthyroidism, 316
  indications for use, 157–59
  mechanism of action, 157–59
  receptors, 157–58
Adrenocorticotropin (ACTH). *See also* Corticosteroids; Pituitary
  pituitary physiology, 320

Lysin-8-vasopressin. *See* Vasopressin
Lysosomes, effect of salicylates, 393, 396
   histamine release, 385

Macroglobulinemia, 362
Macrolide antibiotics, 429
Magnesium. *See also* Fluid and electrolyte replacement
   absorption, 113
   antiarrhythmic effects, 207
   deficiency, 113
   digitalis toxicity, 192–93
   replacement, 113
Malabsorption, 113–16. *See also* Gastrointestinal disorders
Malaria, 539
Malignancy. *See* Cancer; individual syndromes
Manic disorders, 467–68
Mannitol, absorption, 28
   hemolytic anemia, 370
   osmotic diuretic properties, 77
   postsurgical obstructive jaundice, 100
Mannose, 295–97
Maple syrup urine disease, 537
Marsilid. *See* Iproniazid
Mast cells, 385, 388–89
Matulane. *See* Procarbazine
Mebutamate (Capla), 455–59
Mecamylamine. *See also* Hypertension
   drug interactions, 595–96
   hypertension, 168–69
   pK_a, 66–67
Mechlorethamine. *See* Nitrogen mustard
Medulloblastoma, 525
Mefenamic acid (Ponstel), 495–99
Megakaryocytes, 365
Melanocyte-stimulating hormone (MSH), Parkinson's syndrome, 479
   pituitary physiology, 320
Melanoma, 525
Melphalan (Alkeran, L-sarcolysin), cancer chemotherapy, 516–26
   polycythemia, 374
Membrane transport of drugs. *See* Passage of drugs across membranes
Menadione (K$_3$). *See* Vitamin K
Menadione sodium bisulfite (Hykinone), 376
Menadione sodium diphosphate (Synkavite), 376
Meningitis, tuberculous, 402–403
Menopausal gonadotropin (HMG), 341
Mental deficiency, 455, 470
Meperidine (Demerol), analgesic properties, 491–95
   drug interactions, 475–76
Mephenytoin (Mesantoin), 501–506
Mephyton (K$_1$). *See* Vitamin K
Meprobamate. *See also* Psychotherapeutic agents
   abuse, 470–71
   anxiety states, 455–59
   drug interactions, 475–76
   intoxication, 612, 616
   metabolism, 472–73
Mepyramine, 390–91
MER-29. *See* Triparanol
6-Mercaptopurine (Purinethol), cancer chemotherapy, 513–26
   drug interactions, 592–95

6-Mercaptopurine (Purinethol)—(*Cont.*)
   hepatic disorders, 102–103
   immunosuppressive properties, 399, 526–29
   rheumatoid arthritis, 408–409
Mercurial diuretics. *See* Diuretics
Mesantoin. *See* Mephenytoin
Mesoridazine (Serentil), 463–67
Metabolic disease, genetic. *See* Genetic disorders
Metaraminol. *See also* Antihypertensive agents
   drug interactions, 591–92
   mechanism of action, 155
   synthesis, 155
Methacycline, 429–30
Methadone (Dolophine), analgesic properties, 491–95
   drug addiction, 471–72
Methalone, 345
Methamphetamine, 472. *See also* Amphetamines
Methaqualone (Quaalude). *See also* Psychotherapeutic agents
   abuse, 470–71
   anxiety states, 458–59
Methemalbumin, 361
Methemoglobin, 361–62
Methenamine, 434–35
Methenolone, 345
Methicillin, antibacterial spectrum, 427–28
   pharmacokinetics, 436–38
Methimazole, 313–15
Methorphan, 491–95
Methotrexate (amethopterin), cancer chemotherapy, 512–26
   dose-dependent kinetics, 49–50
   drug interactions, 411–12, 589–90
   hepatic toxicity, 411–12
   immunosuppressive properties, 399–400, 526–29
   psoriasis, 411–12
   rheumatoid arthritis, 408–409
Methotrimeprazine (Levoprome), 498
Methoxamine, 174
Methsuximide (Celontin), 502–506
Methyldopa. *See* Alpha-methyldopa
Methylparafynol, 485
Methylphenidate (Ritalin). *See also* Psychotherapeutic agents
   abuse, 472
   antidepressant properties, 459–63
   drug interactions, 592–98
   effect on sleep, 489
   hyperkinetic child, 469
Methylprednisolone, 328, 399
Methyltestosterone, 345, 372
Methysergide, drug reactions, 579
   dumping syndrome, 119–20
   inflammation, 390–91
   retroperitoneal fibrosis, 628–29
Metrazole. *See* Pentylenetetrazole
Metyrapone, 329–30
Migraine, 343
Milk. *See* Cow's milk
Milk-alkali syndrome, 117
Milontin. *See* Phensuximide
Mineralocorticoids, 328
Mithramycin, 517
Mitral stenosis. *See* Cardiovascular disorders
Molybdenum, 368